Epileptic Syndromes
In Infancy, Childhood and Adolescence

All the video sequences are available online at:
https://epileptic-syndromes.jle.com/

WITH VIDEO
SUPPLEMENTS

Epileptic Syndromes
In Infancy, Childhood and Adolescence

6th edition with video sequences

Edited by:
Michelle Bureau, Pierre Genton,
Charlotte Dravet, Antonio V. Delgado-Escueta,
Renzo Guerrini, Carlo Alberto Tassinari, Pierre Thomas & Peter Wolf

Video editor
Pierre Thomas

Videos available at: https://epileptic-syndromes.jle.com/

John Libbey EUROTEXT

All the video sequences are available online at:
https://epileptic-syndromes.jle.com/

WITH VIDEO SUPPLEMENTS

ISBN: 978-2-7420-1572-6

Published by
Éditions John Libbey Eurotext
127, avenue de la République, 92120 Montrouge, France
Tél. : +33 (0)1 46 73 06 60
Fax : +33 (0)1 40 84 09 99
e-mail : contact@jle.com
www.jle.com

John Libbey Eurotext
34 Anyard Road, Cobham
Surrey KT11 2LA
United Kingdom

FOREWORD

The first edition of *Epileptic Syndromes in Infancy, Childhood and Adolescence* appeared in 1984 as the proceedings of a workshop of the Commission on Classification and Terminology of the International League against Epilepsy. The workshop took place at the Centre Saint-Paul in Marseille, France, and was initiated and organized by late Joseph Roger, on behalf of the Commission. He, commission chairman Peter Wolf and previous commission chairman Fritz E. Dreifuss had agreed that the coming International Classification of Epileptic Syndromes and Epilepsies (ICESE), like the preceding seizure classification, needed to be based not just on expert opinions but on solid scientific data. For all proposed syndromes, the available data were presented and discussed in detail at the workshop, and the syndromes that passed this critical review were defined and included in the ICESE of 1989. The book which documented this process could be published thanks to the efforts of André Perret, a physician working in the pharmaceutical industry, who provided the necessary sponsorship.

The term "Blue Guide" ("Guide Bleu" in French) was coined by our late friend Pierre Loiseau and bears witness to the widespread use of this volume in clinical practice. Its worldwide distribution was facilitated by the simultaneous publishing of an English and French version.

There were four further editions: in 1992, a major update on the syndromes justified a 2nd edition; in 2002, besides the well-known syndromes, new concepts derived from the major advances in genetics and neuroimaging for aetiology were included in a 3rd edition; in 2005, for the Paris International Epilepsy congress, the 4th edition included a video support illustrating the various seizures and syndromes. The 4th edition was translated into Japanese and into Mandarin Chinese, which furthered its global impact.

Epileptology kept changing, and a 5th edition (in English and French) came out in 2012, and was again translated into Japanese, and, for the first time, into Spanish and a special edition was made for India.

Seven years later, in 2019, this new edition, in English only, includes the most recent advances in our understanding of the epilepsies. The syndromic approach is still its backbone, but has to be adapted in the light of the new (2017) Classification scheme of the International League against Epilepsy. Chapters have been updated, partly rearranged, and still with the video companion. The diversity of editors and authors underlines the objectivity of the modern syndromic approach, which is no longer simply "electroclinical". A large space is dedicated to the rapid advances in genetics and neuroimaging which play a fundamental role in most syndromes.

We hope that the "Blue Guide" will retain its position as a reference textbook for our epileptologist colleagues, for neurologists, neuropediatricians, their pupils and all those with an interest in clinical epileptology or research.

The John Libbey Eurotext staff demonstrated their trademark competence, dedication – and patience.

The Editors

Disclaimer

The editors thank patients and families, who gave their consent for the use of their video recordings associated with this 6th edition. Video sequences should be seen only by the following persons: physicians and other medical staff working in the field of epileptology and scientists involved in clinical or basic epileptological sciences. Video sequences should be played only on personal or institutional computers, as complements and illustrations to the chapters of the hard copy. These sequences are not meant to be copied for public presentations.

CONTENTS

CONTRIBUTORS

Frederick Andermann
Montreal Neurological Hospital and Institute, McGill University, Montreal, Quebec, Canada
Chapter 18. Rasmussen encephalitis

Jérôme Aupy
Bordeaux University Hospital, Department of Clinical Neurosciences, Bordeaux, France
Chapter 20. The syndromes of mesio-temporal lobe epilepsy with hippocampal scleroses and temporal plus epilepsies

Stéphane Auvin
Pediatric Neurology Department, Robert-Debré Children Hospital, University of Paris, France
Chapter 11. Myoclonic epilepsies in infancy and early childhood

Nadia Bahi-Buisson
Pediatric Neurology, Hôpital Necker Enfants-Malades, Paris, France
Chapter 29. Epilepsies and chromosomal disorders

Julia N. Bailey
Epilepsy Genetics and Genomics Labs, Neurology and Research Services, Veterans Affairs Greater Los Angeles Healthcare System, West Los Angeles, USA; Department of Epidemiology, Fielding School of Public Health, University of California, Los Angeles (J.N.B.), USA
Chapter 2. Genetic basis and testing of epileptic syndromes

Thomas Bast
Department of children and adolescents, Epilepsy Centre Kork, Kehl, Germany
Chapter 24. Epilepsy and inborn errors of metabolism

Elinor Ben-Menachem
Institute for Clinical Neurosciences, Sahlgrenska Academy, Goteborg, Sweden
Chapter 20. The syndromes of mesio-temporal lobe epilepsy with hippocampal scleroses and temporal plus epilepsies

Michelle Bureau
Centre Saint-Paul, Henri-Gastaut Hospital, Marseille, France
Chapter 6. Benign neonatal and infantile seizures and epilepsies
Chapter 10. Dravet syndrome (previously severe myoclonic epilepsy in infancy)
Chapter 13. Self-limited focal epilepsies in childhood
Chapter 14. Encephalopathy related to status epilepticus during slow sleep (ESES) including Landau-Kleffner syndrome
Chapter 15. Absence epilepsies
Chapter 30. Progressive myoclonus epilepsies

Carol S. Camfield
Department of Pediatrics, IWK Health Centre and Dalhousie University, Halifax, Nova Scotia, Canada
Chapter 9. Febrile seizures and genetic epilepsy with febrile seizures plus (GEFS+)

Peter R. Camfield
Department of Pediatrics, IWK Health Centre and Dalhousie University, Halifax, Nova Scotia, Canada
Chapter 9. Febrile seizures and genetic epilepsy with febrile seizures plus (GEFS+)

Gaetano Cantalupo
Child Neuropsychiatry Unit, University of Parma, Parma, Italy; Child Neuropsychiatry Unit, University of Verona, Verona, Italy
Chapter 14. Encephalopathy related to status epilepticus during slow sleep (ESES) including Landau-Kleffner syndrome

Roberto H. Caraballo
Department of Neurology, Hospital Nacional de Pediatria "Prof. Dr. Juan P. Garrahan", Buenos Aires, Argentina
Chapter 16. Isolated focal (formerly partial) seizures in adolescence

Chiara Cirelli
Center for Sleep and Consciousness, University of Wisconsin – Madison School of Medicine, Department of Psychiatry, Madison, USA
Chapter 14. Encephalopathy related to status epilepticus during slow sleep (ESES) including Landau-Kleffner syndrome

Patrick Chauvel
Cleveland Clinic and Aix-Marseille University, Marseille, France
Chapter 20. The syndromes of mesio-temporal lobe epilepsy with hippocampal scleroses and temporal plus epilepsies

Catherine Chiron
Inserm U663; University Paris Descartes; Necker Hospital, Paris, France
Chapter 8. Infantile spasms

Harry T. Chugani
Departments of Pediatrics and Neurology, Nemours A.I. du Pont Hospital for Children, Wilmington, DE and Thomas Jefferson University, Philadelphia, USA
Chapter 8. Infantile spasms

Özlem Çokar
Department of Neurology, Haseki Research and Training Hospital, Health Sciences University, Istanbul, Turkey
Chapter 10. Dravet syndrome (previously severe myoclonic epilepsy in infancy)
Chapter 13. Self-limited focal epilepsies in childhood

Valerio Conti
Pediatric Neurology, Neurogenetics and Neurobiology Unit and Laboratories, Neuroscience Department, A. Meyer Children's Hospital, Florence, Italy
Chapter 3. Animal models of epileptic syndromes

Massimo Cossu
Department of Neurosciences, Center for Epilepsy Surgery "C. Munari", Hospital Niguarda, Milan, Italy
Chapter 21. Frontal lobe epilepsy syndromes

Arielle Crespel
Epilepsy Unit, Montpellier, France
Chapter 12. Lennox-Gastaut syndrome
Chapter 19. Epilepsy with generalized tonic-clonic seizures alone

Bernardo Dalla Bernardina
Child Neuropsychiatry Unit, University of Verona, Verona, Italy
Chapter 14. Encephalopathy related to status epilepticus during slow sleep (ESES) including Landau-Kleffner syndrome

Francesca Darra
Child Neuropsychiatry Unit, University of Verona, Verona, Italy
Chapter 14. Encephalopathy related to status epilepticus during slow sleep (ESES) including Landau-Kleffner syndrome

Paola De Liso
Department of Neurosciences, Bambino Gesù Children's Hospital, IRCCS, Rome, Italy
Chapter 6. Benign neonatal and infantile seizures and epilepsies

Maria Del Socorro Gonzalez Sanchez
Saint-Paul Center, Henri Gastaut Hospital, Marseille, France
Chapter 19. Epilepsy with generalized tonic-clonic seizures alone

Antonio V. Delgado-Escueta
Department of Neurology, David Geffen School of Medicine, University of California, Los Angeles, USA; Epilepsy Genetics and Genomics Labs, Neurology and Research Services, Veterans Affairs Greater Los Angeles Healthcare System, West Los Angeles, USA
Chapter 2. Genetic basis and testing of epileptic syndromes
Chapter 20. The syndromes of mesio-temporal lobe epilepsy with hippocampal scleroses and temporal plus epilepsies
Chapter 21. Frontal lobe epilepsy syndromes
Chapter 27. Brain parasitic infections
Chapter 30. Progressive myoclonus epilepsies

Veysi Demirbilek
Department of Neurology, Cerrahpasa Faculty of Medicine, Istanbul University-Cerrahpasa, Istanbul, Turkey
Chapter 13. Self-limited focal epilepsies in childhood

Charlotte Dravet
Centre Saint-Paul, Henri-Gastaut Hospital, Marseille, France; Infantile Neuropsychiatric Unit, Fondazionze Policlinico Universitario A. Gemelli, IRCCS, Catholic University Sacro Cuore, Rome, Italy
Chapter 10. Dravet syndrome (previously severe myoclonic epilepsy in infancy)
Chapter 11. Myoclonic epilepsies in infancy and early childhood

Reyna M. Duron
Epilepsy Genetics and Genomics Labs, Neurology and Research Services, Veterans Affairs Greater Los Angeles Healthcare System, West Los Angeles, USA; Facultad de Ciencias de la Salud, Universidad Tecnológica Centroamericana UNITEC, Tegucigalpa, Honduras
Chapter 2. Genetic basis and testing of epileptic syndromes

Maurizio Elia
IRCCS Oasi Maria SS, Troina (EN), Italy
Chapter 29. Epilepsies and chromosomal disorders

Natalio Fejerman†
Hospital de Pediatrica "Juan P. Garrahan", Buenos Aires, Argentina
Chapter 5. Syndromes and antiepilepsy drugs

Edoardo Ferlazzo
Regional Epilepsy Centre, Bianchi-Melacrino-Morelli Hospital, Reggio Calabria, Italy.
Chapter 12. Lennox-Gastaut syndrome

Stefano Francione
Department of Neurosciences, Center for Epilepsy Surgery "C. Munari", Hospital Niguarda, Milan, Italy
Chapter 21. Frontal lobe epilepsy syndromes

Lucia Fusco
Department of Neuroscience and Neurorehabilitation, Bambino Gesù Children's Hospital, Rome, Italy
Chapter 8. Infantile spasms

Aristea S. Galanopoulou
Saul R. Korey Department of Neurology, Dominick P. Purpura Department of Neuroscience, Laboratory of Development Epilepsy, Montefiore/Einstein Epilepsy Management Center, Albert Einstein College of Medicine and Montefiore Medical Center, Bronx, New York, USA
Chapter 3. Animal models of epileptic syndromes

Hector H. Garcia
Center for Global Health – Tumbes and Department of Microbiology, Universidad Peruana Cayetano Heredia, Lima, Peru; Cysticercosis Unit, Instituto Nacional de Ciencias Neurologicas, Jirón Ancash 1271, Lima, Peru
Chapter 27. Brain parasitic infections

Elena Gardella
Danish Epilepsy Center, Epilepsihospitalet, Dianalund, Filadelfia, Denmark; Syddansk Universitet, Odense, Denmark
Chapter 4. EEG traits and epileptic syndromes

Philippe Gélisse
Epilepsy Unit, Montpellier, France
Chapter 5. Syndromes and antiepilepsy drugs
Chapter 12. Lennox-Gastaut syndrome
Chapter 17. Juvenile myoclonic epilepsies
Chapter 19. Epilepsy with generalized tonic-clonic seizures alone

Pierre Genton
Centre Saint-Paul, Henri-Gastaut Hospital, Marseille, France
Chapter 5. Syndromes and antiepilepsy drugs
Chapter 12. Lennox-Gastaut syndrome
Chapter 15. Absence epilepsies
Chapter 17. Juvenile myoclonic epilepsies
Chapter 19. Epilepsy with generalized tonic-clonic seizures alone
Chapter 30. Progressive myoclonus epilepsies

Giuseppe Gobbi
Child Neurology and Psychiatry Unit, Maggiore "C.A. Pizzardi" Hospital, Bologna, Italy
Chapter 29. Epilepsies and chromosomal disorders

Isidro Gonzales
Cysticercosis Unit, National Institute of Neurological Sciences, Jirón Ancash 1271, Lima, Peru
Chapter 27. Brain parasitic infections

Tiziana Granata
Department of Pediatric Neuroscience, Neurological Institute Foundation "Besta", Milan, Italy
Chapter 18. Rasmussen encephalitis

Renzo Guerrini
Pediatric Neurology Unit and Laboratories, Children's Hospital A. Meyer-University of Florence, Italy
Chapter 10. Dravet syndrome (previously severe myoclonic epilepsy in infancy)
Chapter 11. Myoclonic epilepsies in infancy and early childhood
Chapter 31. Epilepsy and malformations of the cerebral cortex

Édouard Hirsch
Strasbourg University Hospital, Strasbourg, France
Chapter 15. Absence epilepsies

Yushi Inoue
National Epilepsy Centre, Shizuoka Institute of Epilepsy and Neurological Disorders, Shizuoka, Japan
Chapter 28. Complex reflex epilepsies

Pierre Jallon
Thézan des Corbières, France
Chapter 16. Isolated focal (formerly partial) seizures in adolescence

Anna Kaminska
Pediatric Neurology, Hôpital Necker Enfants-Malades, Paris, France
Chapter 29. Epilepsies and chromosomal disorders

Dorothée Kasteleijn-Nolst Trenité
Department of Functional Neurosurgery and Epilepsy, University Medical Center Utrecht, the Netherlands; Faculty of Medicine and Psychology Sapienza, Rome, Italy
Chapter 22. Photosensitivity and syndromes

Christian Korff
Pediatric Neurology, University Hospitals, Geneva, Switzerland
Chapter 24. Epilepsy and inborn errors of metabolism

Greta Macorig
Epilepsy Unit, Montpellier, France
Chapter 12. Lennox-Gastaut syndrome
Chapter 19. Epilepsy with generalized tonic-clonic seizures alone

Roberto Mai
Department of Neurosciences, Center for Epilepsy Surgery "C. Munari", Hospital Niguarda, Milan, Italy
Chapter 21. Frontal lobe epilepsy syndromes

Francesco Mari
Pediatric Neurology Unit and Laboratories, Children's Hospital A. Meyer-University of Florence, Italy
Chapter 11. Myoclonic epilepsies in infancy and early childhood

Carla Marini
Child Neurology Unit, Children's Hospital A. Meyer, Florence, Italy
Chapter 9. Febrile seizures and genetic epilepsy with febrile seizures plus (GEFS+)
Chapter 29. Epilepsies and chromosomal disorders

Nancy A. McNamara
Department of Pediatrics, University of Michigan, Ann Arbor, Michigan, USA
Chapter 9. Febrile seizures and genetic epilepsy with febrile seizures plus (GEFS+)

Marco T. Medina
School of Medical Sciences, University of Honduras, Tegucigalpa, Honduras
Chapter 15. Absence epilepsies
Chapter 17. Juvenile myoclonic epilepsies
Chapter 27. Brain parasitic infections

Stefano Meletti
Department of Biomedical, Metabolic and Neural Science, University of Modena and Reggio Emilia, Italy; Neurology Unit, Azienda Ospedaliera-Universitaria Modena, Italy
Chapter 22. Photosensitivity and syndromes

Roberto Michelucci
IRCCS-Institute of Neurological Sciences of Bologna, Unit of Neurology, Bologna, Italy
Chapter 30. Progressive myoclonus epilepsies

Mathieu Milh
Inserm U910, Faculté de Médecine de la Timone, Department of Paediatric Neurology, Hôpital Timone-Enfants, Marseille, France
Chapter 7. Early severe neonatal and infantile epilepsies

Eli M. Mizrahi
Peter Kellaway Section of Neurophysiology, Department of Neurology, Section of Pediatric Neurology, Department of Pediatrics, Baylor College of Medicine, Houston, USA
Chapter 7. Early severe neonatal and infantile epilepsies

Solomon L. Moshé
Saul R. Korey Department of Neurology, Dominick P. Purpura Department of Neuroscience, Montefiore/Einstein Epilepsy Management Center, Albert Einstein College of Medicine and Montefiore Medical Center, Bronx, New York, USA; Department of Pediatrics, Albert Einstein College of Medicine and Montefiore Medical Center, Bronx, New York, USA
Chapter 3. Animal models of epileptic syndromes

Astrid Nehlig
Inserm U1129, Pediatric Neurology, Necker-Enfants Malades Hospital, Paris-Descartes University, Paris, France
Chapter 3. Animal models of epileptic syndromes

Bernd A. Neubauer
Department of Neuropediatrics, University Hospital Giessen and Marburg (UKGM), Giessen, Germany
Chapter 6. Benign neonatal and infantile seizures and epilepsies

Viet-Huong Nguyen
Epilepsy Genetics and Genomics Labs, Neurology and Research Services, Veterans Affairs Greater Los Angeles Healthcare System, West Los Angeles, USA; Chapman University School of Pharmacy, Orange County, USA
Chapter 2. Genetic basis and testing of epileptic syndromes

Marina Nikanorova
Children Department, Danish Epilepsy Centre, Dianalund, Denmark
Chapter 12. Lennox-Gastaut syndrome

Lino Nobili
Child Neuropsychiatry Unit, IRCCS G. Gaslini Institute, DINOGMI-Department of Neurosciences, Rehabilitation, Ophthalmology, Genetics, Maternal and Child Health, University of Genoa, Genova, Italy
Chapter 21. Frontal lobe epilepsy syndromes

Douglas R. Nordli Jr
Pediatric Epilepsy, Children's Memorial Hospital, Feinberg School of Medicine, Northwestern University, Chicago, USA
Chapter 24. Epilepsy and inborn errors of metabolism

Hirokasu Oguni
Tokyo Women's Medical University, Department of Pediatrics, Tokyo, Japan
Chapter 10. Dravet syndrome (previously severe myoclonic epilepsy in infancy)

Chrysostomos P. Panayiotopoulos
Clinical Neurophysiology Dpt, St Thomas'NHS Foundation Trust, London, United Kingdom
Chapter 13. Self-limited focal epilepsies in childhood

Elena Parrini
Pediatric Neurology Unit and Laboratories, Children's Hospital A. Meyer, University of Florence, Firenze, Italy
Chapter 31. Epilepsy and malformations of the cerebral cortex

Fabienne Picard
Department of Neurology, University Hospital and Medical School of Geneva, Geneva, Switzerland
Chapter 25. Genetically determined focal epilepsies

Perrine Plouin
Clinical Neurophysiology Unit, Necker Enfants Malades Hospital, Paris, France
Chapter 6. Benign neonatal and infantile seizures and epilepsies

Patrizia Riguzzi
IRCCS-Institute of Neurological Sciences of Bologna, Unit of Neurology, Bologna, Italy
Chapter 30. Progressive myoclonus epilepsies

Guido Rubboli
Danish Epilepsy Center, Epilepsihospitalet, Dianalund, Filadelfia, Denmark; University of Copenhagen, Copenhagen, Denmark
Chapter 4. EEG traits and epileptic syndromes
Chapter 14. Encephalopathy related to status epilepticus during slow sleep (ESES) including Landau-Kleffner syndrome
Chapter 22. Photosensitivity and syndromes

Javier Salas-Puig
Epilepsy Unit, Neurology Department, Hospital Universitari Vall d'Hebron, Autonoma University, Barcelona, Spain
Chapter 23. Epileptic syndromes in the elderly

Sofia S. Sanchez
Universidad Pueruana Cayetano Heredia, Lima, Peru; Cysticercosis Unit, Instituto Nacional de Ciencias Neurologicas, Jiron Ancash 1271, Lima, Peru
Chapter 27. Brain parasitic infections

Ingrid E. Scheffer
Epilepsy Research Centre, Department of Medicine, the University of Melbourne, Austin Health, Department of Paediatrics, the University of Melbourne, Royal Children's Hospital, Florey and Murdoch Children's Research Institutes, Melbourne, Australia
Chapter 9. Febrile seizures and genetic epilepsy with febrile seizures plus (GEFS+)
Chapter 25. Genetically determined focal epilepsies

Anna Serafini
Department of Neurology and Neurorehabilitation, University of Illinois, Chicago, USA
Chapter 17. Juvenile myoclonic epilepsies

Jose Maria Serratosa
Neurology Service, University Hospital Jiménez Diaz Foundation, Autonomous University of Madrid and Ciberer, Madrid, Spain
Chapter 2. Genetic basis and testing of epileptic syndromes
Chapter 30. Progressive myoclonus epilepsies

Renee A. Shellhaas
Department of Pediatrics, University of Michigan, Ann Arbor, Michigan, USA
Chapter 9. Febrile seizures and genetic epilepsy with febrile seizures plus (GEFS+)

Barbara Swartz
Hoag Memorial Hospital Presbyterian, Newport Beach, California, and Children's Hospital of Orange County, Orange, USA
Chapter 21. Frontal lobe epilepsy syndromes

Laura Tassi
Department of Neurosciences, Center for Epilepsy Surgery "C. Munari", Hospital Niguarda, Milan, Italy
Chapter 21. Frontal lobe epilepsy syndromes

Carlo Alberto Tassinari
University of Bologna, Bologna, Italy; Neurosciences Department, University of Parma, Parma, Italy
Chapter 4. EEG traits and epileptic syndromes
Chapter 14. Encephalopathy related to status epilepticus during slow sleep (ESES) including Landau-Kleffner syndrome
Chapter 21. Frontal lobe epilepsy syndromes
Chapter 30. Progressive myoclonus epilepsies

Pierre Thomas
Department of Neurology, Pasteur Hospital, Nice, France
Chapter 17. Juvenile myoclonic epilepsies
Chapter 19. Epilepsy with generalized tonic-clonic seizures alone

Giulio Tononi
Center for Sleep and Consciousness, University of Wisconsin – Madison School of Medicine, Department of Psychiatry, Madison, USA
Chapter 14. Encephalopathy related to status epilepticus during slow sleep (ESES) including Landau-Kleffner syndrome

Marina Trivisano
Department of Neurosciences and Neurorehabilitation, Bambino Gesù Children's Hospital, IRCCS, Rome, Italy
Chapter 6. Benign neonatal and infantile seizures and epilepsies
Chapter 8. Infantile spasms

Federico Vigevano
Department of Neurosciences and Neurorehabilitation, Bambino Gesù Children's Hospital, IRCCS, Rome, Italy
Chapter 6. Benign neonatal and infantile seizures and epilepsies
Chapter 8. Infantile spasms

Flavio Villani
Epilespy Monitoring Unit "Paolo Zorzi", Divison of Clinical and Experimental Epileptology, Neurological Institute Foundation "Besta", Milan, Italy
Chapter 18. Rasmussen encephalitis

Angela Vincent
Weatherhall Institute of Molecular Medicine and Nuffield Department of Clinical Neurosciences, John Radcliffe University Hospital, Oxford, United Kingdom
Chapter 26. Autoimmune epilepsies and encephalopathies

Stephan Waltz
Child Neurology, Children's Hospital of Cologne, Cologne, Germany
Chapter 22. Photosensitivity and syndromes

Peter Wolf
Danish Epilepsy Centre Filadelfia, Dianalund, Denmark; Florianópolis, Brazil
Chapter 15. Absence epilepsies
Chapter 28. Complex reflex epilepsies

Sukhvir Wright
School of Life and Health Sciences, Aston University, Birmingham, United Kingdom; Department of Paediatric Neurology, Birmingham Children's Hospital, Birmingham, United Kingdom
Chapter 26. Autoimmune epilepsies and encephalopathies

Elza Márcia Yacubian
São Paulo Federal University, São Paulo, Brazil
Chapter 17. Juvenile myoclonic epilepsies

Sameer Zuberi
Royal Hospital for Children and School Medicine, University of Glasgow, Glasgow, United Kingdom
Chapter 1. Classification, epidemiology, prognosis

CHAPTER 1
CLASSIFICATION, EPIDEMIOLOGY, PROGNOSIS

Sameer Zuberi

Royal Hospital for Children and School Medecine, University of Glasgow, Glasgow, United Kingdom

Classification

Historically, classifications in medicine have served two independent objectives which are to have i) a taxonomic system to organize our views and knowledge; and ii) a diagnostic manual to help categorize the epilepsies in ways that facilitate communication and research (Wolf, 2003). These objectives are not mutually exclusive and are both essential for developing scientific classifications within clinical medicine where the ultimate goal is to improve care for the person with disease. Medical knowledge and the resources from which we draw that knowledge are no longer the sole preserve of the physician and as such medical classifications must have additional objectives. They should facilitate communication with people with epilepsy and their carers as well as informing clinical management. In the xxth century books and journals held in medical libraries were accessible only to doctors and their students, with classification systems evolving to reflect this. We developed a language which aided communication between physicians but excluded those without specialist training and more importantly people with epilepsy and their carers, thus maintaining the unhelpful mystique around the practice of medicine.

Distinct from other areas of scientific practice, in medicine, patients and carers are uniquely invested in understanding the nature and management of disease. The parent or carer is the most passionate advocate for the child and in the xxist century they have easy access to previously unimagined volumes of information and evidence through electronic media. Classifications should aid physicians in making sense of this information for patients and carers and allow people with epilepsy and their families to better communicate with each other. The 2017 ILAE Classification of Seizures and the Epilepsies was developed to reflect advances in knowledge, particularly in relation to how aetiology influences management, and to encourage the use of more straightforward and accessible language. There are many other classification systems which should continue to develop for more specialized purposes within epileptology; for example, anatomical network, pathological or genetic classifications. Rodent model, zebrafish and brain slice researchers should develop classifications for the electrographic events they study but we cannot expect to have an epilepsy classification that fits all events studied by epileptologists. Indeed, if we tried to there may be a danger of placing too much emphasis on the relevance of "seizure" types or aetiologies in these models to what we see in the human.

A clinical classification should be flexible enough to be used in high resource and low resource health care systems. Low resource is in-fact "normal resource" as the majority of people with epilepsy will not have access to specialists in epilepsy, EEG, MRI, metabolic tests and genetic investigations. A classification must work for the clinician who just has a history and a video on a smartphone as well as it does for those who have access to 3T brain MRI, inpatient video-telemetry and whole genome sequencing.

The Framework for Classification of the Epilepsies *(Figure 1)* describes a multi-level and flexible classification which is developed primarily for clinical practice and to inform precision medicine (Scheffer *et al.*, 2017). The link between aetiology, precision medicine and therapeutics is discussed further in the aetiology section below.

Epileptic seizures are a symptom of many different diseases of the brain and a unifying biological classification is not practical or possible with our current levels of knowledge. The framework provides a comprehensive overview of an individual's epilepsy including clinical elements such as seizure types and co-morbidities, epilepsy types inferred from seizure types and EEG, epilepsy syndromes and a

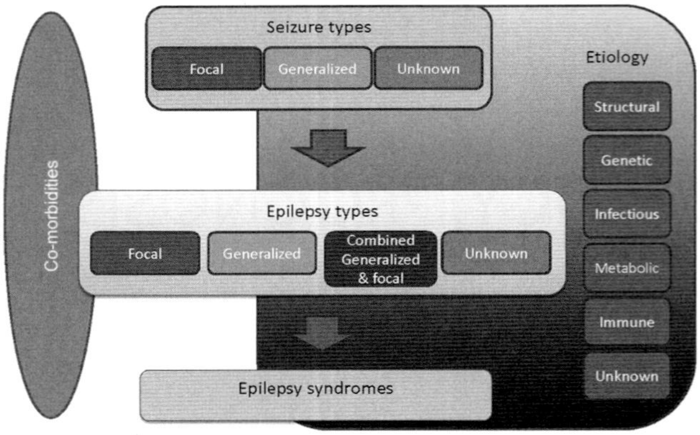

Figure 1 **The 2017 ILAE framework for classification of the epilepsies.**

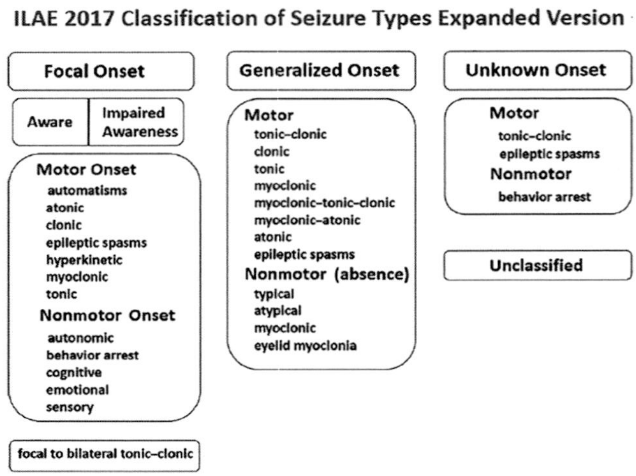

Figure 2 **The 2017 ILAE classification of seizure types.**

consideration of aetiology. In addition to aiding classification the framework leads the physician through the elements required to make a diagnosis and as such takes guidance from previous diagnostic schemes (Engel, 2001).

Seizure types

A seizure is defined as the transient occurrence of signs and or symptoms due to abnormal excessive or synchronous neuronal activity in the brain with a seizure type simply a useful grouping of seizure characteristics for purposes of clinical care, teaching and research (Fisher *et al.*, 2017a). The term seizure in the classification only relates to epileptic seizures and not any non-epileptic events which may be colloquially described as seizures. Almost any human behaviour can be re-capitulated during an epileptic seizure therefore there is always a decision to be made in a classification as to how many seizure types are defined. The ILAE 2017 Classification includes a list of seizure types, defining each type and separating them into those of focal onset, generalised onset and of unknown onset *(Figure 2)*. Additional descriptors, how to map new to old terms and an updated glossary of terms is presented in an instruction manual (Fisher *et al.*, 2017b).

There was a suggestion that the distinction between the focal and generalised seizures be abandoned in the 2010 ILAE Classification Commission proposal however the decision was made to retain these concepts of seizure onset and propagation in the 2017 ILAE Position papers (Berg *et al.*, 2010).

Focal seizures are conceptualized as originating within networks limited to one hemisphere. These may be discretely localized or more widely distributed.

When the seizure evolves to indicate involvement of bilateral networks the terminology *focal to bilateral* is recommended with the seizure types described after the terms focal and bilateral. Two such examples would be *a focal clonic seizure (evolving) to bilateral tonic seizure* or a *focal tonic seizure (evolving) to bilateral clonic seizure*. This provides a more detailed description than the old focal to secondary generalised.

Generalised seizures are conceptualised as originating at some point within, and rapidly engaging, bilaterally distributed networks. These networks may include cortical and sub-cortical structures and no assumption is made on the underlying physiology of network propagation. This is best understood in the cortico-thalamic networks associated with absence seizures however the term generalised does not imply involvement of a specific network (Blumenfeld, 2005).

Generalised seizures in which bilateral networks are rapidly engaged are rarely seen clinically or on EEG in the neonate and it is likely that the distinction between focal and generalised will not be maintained in the proposed ILAE adaptation of the classification for seizures in this age group (see Classification of Seizures in the Neonate).

The 1997–2001 Classification Task Force recommended adopting focal as the exclusive term replacing partial and this is supported in the

2017 ILAE position papers (Engel, 2001). The term partial was seen to imply that a seizure which was only *part* of a seizure and not an event which may be just as clinically significant as a generalised seizure.

Assessment of consciousness, responsiveness and awareness may be extremely challenging or not possible to determine in children, particularly in neonates and young infants. The ILAE chose retained or impaired awareness as a surrogate for all such impairments in focal seizures. Unless it is part of a detailed pre-surgical hypothesis, differentiating between all the different types of impairment of responsiveness, consciousness and awareness is unlikely to influence clinical management. In daily life there may be compromise to an individual's well-being from a failure of responsiveness even if awareness is maintained, whether that compromise is within the learning environment, interacting with others, working with machinery or driving a car.

Some seizure types, which have been well established in clinical practice but not previously listed in ILAE Classifications, are recognised in the 2017 Classification. These include focal spasms, focal myoclonic, focal tonic and the generalised seizure types; myoclonic absence, myoclonic-tonic-clonic, myoclonic-atonic and eyelid myoclonia. Eyelid myoclonia is placed in the non-motor (absence) grouping but could just as reasonably have been placed within the motor category as the myoclonia are more prominent than the absence.

Epilepsy types

In many healthcare settings, indeed for most people with epilepsy worldwide, it may not be possible to classify an epilepsy beyond the seizure types. The classification of an Epilepsy type assumes that the individual has a diagnosis of epilepsy as per the 2014 definition (Fisher *et al.*, 2014). An important feature of the new definition is that individuals may be diagnosed with epilepsy after their first seizure if they are likely to have more seizures. This is exemplified in the first seizure of a genetic epilepsy syndrome which is inherited in an autosomal dominant manner when there is a known family history but is also relevant in the first seizure of a syndrome such as childhood epilepsy with centrotemporal spikes where seizure semiology and EEG support the syndromic diagnosis. The classification of a focal epilepsy type may be straightforward if there is a known pathology such as a right hemiplegia secondary to an antenatal stroke and the seizure type is a focal clonic seizure affecting the right side of the body. When a particular combination of seizures is noted for example generalised tonic clonic seizures, myoclonic seizures and absences it may be possible to say confidently the individual has a generalised epilepsy type. In many circumstances it can be difficult to say whether an individual has a focal or a generalised epilepsy. In the author's view this distinction is the least important in epilepsy classification but has been maintained primarily for historical reasons and for ease of placing disparate, individually rare epilepsies into larger groups for pharmaceutical trials. Seizure types are valuable in guiding the physician to aetiology, treatment approaches and to a syndromic diagnosis. From a nosological perspective the seizure type, the aetiology and the epilepsy syndrome are much more clinically relevant than the epilepsy type. Many epilepsy syndromes discussed in this book are characterised by both focal and generalised seizure types and in many the seizure type and epilepsy type remain unknown. As concepts of epilepsy syndromes evolve and broaden the number of people whose highest level of classification is at this level may diminish.

Epilepsy syndromes

Several definitions have been proposed for what comprises an epilepsy syndrome since the pioneering work in the last century by groups in France, Italy and Germany. The ILAE have not as yet produced an official classification of epilepsy syndromes or position papers on the boundaries of specific epilepsy syndromes though this is planned by the ILAE Nosology and Classification Task Force 2017–2021. Concepts and boundaries of syndromes have changed over the last 50 years as clinicians have defined new syndromes and studied the complex relationship between aetiology, particularly genetic, and syndrome. The various editions of the Guide Bleu have helped clinicians navigate this challenging terrain. The ILAE curated website www.epilepsydiagnosis.org also provides information and videos on syndromes. In the development of the 2017 Classification of Seizures and Epilepsies the most hotly debated issue was whether the syndromes of childhood absence epilepsy, juvenile absence epilepsy, generalised tonic clonic seizures alone and juvenile myoclonic epilepsy should be collectively termed genetic generalised epilepsies (GGE) rather than idiopathic generalised epilepsies (IGE). Idiopathic in the 1989 classification was defined as *an epilepsy of primarily genetic origin in which there is no gross neuroanatomical or neuropathological abnormality* (Commission on Classification and Terminology of the ILAE, 1989). It should be acknowledged that many physicians have used the term incorrectly in epilepsy practice to mean *unknown* rather than primarily genetic. Monogenic twin studies in these syndromes have shown concordance rates of 65–80% (Berkovic *et al.*, 1998). The debate was around several issues including that the vast majority of people with these syndromes do not have a first degree relative with a similar syndrome, that applying the term "genetic" may minimise the impact of other factors including environmental on the expression of disease and the perceived stigma and societal implications on employment and marriage in large parts of the world of the term genetic. A compromise was reached in the position paper with the ILAE recommendation that IGE could still be used as a collective term for the four syndromes but that GGE could be used when the physician was happy to invoke a primarily genetic aetiology (Scheffer *et al.*, 2017).

The 2017 definition of an epilepsy syndrome is a cluster of features incorporating seizure types, EEG, imaging, diurnal features, comorbidities and age dependency (in terms of onset and remission) that tend to occur together (Scheffer *et al.*, 2017). The syndrome may have aetiological, prognostic and treatment implications. This is similar to that proposed by the ILAE in 1989 (Commission on Classification and Terminology of the ILAE, 1989). Traditionally syndromes have been defined by electroclinical features however in the last decade most novel but consistent epilepsy phenotypes have emerged from gene discovery. Cohorts of cases with a shared genetic aetiology have been studied and consistent electroclinical phenotypes emerged (Bahi-Buisson *et al.*, 2008). In this context broad definitions of what constitutes an epilepsy syndrome have a greater clinical utility and could allow us to bring electroclinical entities which share consistent prognosis and management under the umbrella of the epilepsy syndrome.

An epilepsy syndrome is a condition characterised by epileptic seizures in which a consistent cluster of clinical, EEG and investigative features has specific aetiological, management and prognostic implications. An epilepsy syndrome may have one or more aetiologies. When a single aetiology is associated with a consistent epilepsy phenotype, the aetiology, for example a genetic or structural lesion, may best define the syndrome rather than a single clinical feature or an eponym.

This definition would allow childhood absence epilepsy, hippocampal sclerosis with focal seizures, hypothalamic hamartoma with gelastic seizures, and *CDKL5* developmental and epileptic encephalopathy (DEE) to all be classed as epilepsy syndromes. Being inclusive may promote clinical trials in both the well-established electroclinical syndromes and those defined primarily by aetiology (Devinsky *et al.*, 2017, Mullen *et al.*, 2018). The definition is broader and will bring some conceptual challenges which are inevitable in a disease which is defined by a symptom. For example; it is possible that not only will children evolve from one syndrome to another for example Ohtahara syndrome to Infantile Spasms syndrome to Lennox-Gastaut syndrome but they may also have more than one syndrome at one time. For example; Infantile Spasms in a child with *CDKL5* DEE or an individual with childhood epilepsy with centrotemporal spikes may develop encephalopathy with status epilepticus during sleep (ESES). It is still to be determined whether the ILAE adopts a more inclusive approach to syndrome definition.

Aetiology and comorbidities

The desire for personalised or precision medicine has driven the aetiological perspective of the 2017 ILAE Classification (Zuberi & Brunklaus, 2018). Precision medicine can be defined as prevention and therapy which takes individual variability into account. The 2017 ILAE Classification encourages the physician to stratify patients by aetiology at all stages of the diagnostic process. This is not a new concept in epilepsy classification however the focus at all stages of the diagnostic process and the defining of aetiological sub-groups has not been emphasised to this degree previously. An individual's epilepsy should be classified by the most detailed electroclinical description possible in terms of seizure type, epilepsy type and syndrome and this should always be linked to aetiology. If the aetiology is unknown then this should be emphasised thus encouraging the clinician to reconsider aetiology at subsequent consultations.

It is possible to classify by more than one aetiological group. An example would be focal onset infantile spasms associated with a focal cortical dysplasia. If the infant also has a diagnostic variant in the *DEPDC5* gene as a cause of the dysplasia, then the child has both a structural and genetic aetiology. The structural aetiology may lead to epilepsy surgery the genetic aetiology should lead to genetic counselling for the family. An aetiological approach to diagnosis can encourage early epilepsy surgery and potentially improved outcomes (Braun & Cross, 2018). Requesting genetic testing early in a clinical evaluation in infancy may make a diagnosis early, suggest particular therapeutic approaches or avoiding others, prevent invasive investigations, aid in psychological adjustment and counselling for the family and save money for the health service (Brunklaus *et al.*, 2013, de Lange *et al.*, 2018, Howell *et al.*, 2018).

Many of the epilepsies are associated with significant co-morbidities and these should be considered within epilepsy classification. Placing them within the classification framework emphasises their importance and that the epilepsy specialist should acknowledge that addressing them is their responsibility. These comorbidities may be another consequence of the aetiology underlying the epilepsy for example a hemiplegia in a child with an antenatal stroke who has focal seizures or they may be a consequence of the epilepsy, the psychological impact of the epilepsy or side effects of the treatment for the epilepsy. Comorbidities vary from mild specific learning difficulties to profound global intellectual impairment, motor disorders, autism and psychiatric disease. In the severe early onset genetic and developmental epileptic encephalopathies the underlying aetiology is the most important determinant of intellectual outcome and not the epileptic encephalopathy. Assessment and treatment of the co-morbidities independent of management of seizures should not be neglected in people with epilepsy (Brunklaus *et al.*, 2011). In certain epilepsies there is the potential for amelioration of the epileptic encephalopathy through rapid and effective treatment. This is well recognised in infantile spasms with recent evidence indicating that lead time to treat may influence developmental outcome (O'Callaghan *et al.*, 2018).

Classification of seizures and epilepsies in the neonate

Epileptic seizures have the highest age specific incidence in the first few days of life and are the commonest neurological emergency in the neonatal period (Ronen *et al.*, 1999). Seizures in this age group are most frequently symptoms of an acute aetiology and for several reasons the electrographic seizure may have minimal or no clinical correlate. This may be because the immaturity of the neonatal brain allows uncoupling of the electrographic discharge from the clinical features particularly in the critically ill, cooled or encephalopathic patient (Nash *et al.*, 2011). Anti-seizure medications can also result in uncoupling of the clinical and electrographic event (Scher *et al.*, 2003). A sick newborn; intubated, ventilated, sedated and paralysed may have a high seizure burden which may go unrecognised without continuous cerebral function monitor (CFAM) or EEG recording (Murray *et al.*, 2008). These special considerations led the Neonatal Seizure Task Force of the ILAE Commission for Classification and Terminology to propose a modification of the 2017 Classification which is likely to develop into an ILAE position paper by 2019 (Pressler *et al.*, 2018).

Awareness and responsiveness cannot be determined confidently in the neonate and the clinical utility of this descriptor for a focal seizure is limited therefore it is eliminated from the neonatal classification proposal. A clear and clinically relevant distinction between generalised and focal seizures has not been established in seizures in the neonate therefore all seizures are regarded as focal. The classification emphasises the importance of video recording and continuous ampilitude-integrated EEG (aEEG) or EEG monitoring in neonates both to identify the many paroxysmal events which are non-epileptic in nature and to identify electrographic-only seizures or those with limited clinical signs. The framework developed for the neonate could readily be adapted for use in older children and adults with suspected seizures in the intensive care setting.

Epidemiology and prognosis

The epidemiology and prognosis of individual epilepsy syndromes will be covered in the relevant chapters. Prospective population-based studies take time and require precision and consistency in diagnostic evaluation across large cohorts (Thurman *et al.*, 2011). A systematic review and meta-analysis of 222 international studies on epilepsy incidence and prevalence reported a point prevalence of epilepsy of 6.38 per 1,000 persons (95% CI 5.57–7.30), a pooled lifetime prevalence of 7.6 per 1,000 and an incidence rate of 61.44 per 100,000 patient years (95% CI 50.75–74.38) (Fiest *et al.*, 2017). This review identified considerable heterogeneity between studies in relation to sampling methods, case ascertainment and diagnostic methods. Few studies are stratified by epilepsy type or aetiology let alone by epilepsy syndrome. With electronic records and the increasing availability of imaging, genetic and metabolic investigations it is hoped that more robust data will emerge on the incidence of specific early childhood onset syndromes, though the vast majority of studies to date remain retrospective in nature. A prospective study of new onset epilepsy in Iceland attempted to classify all new onset cases of epilepsy at all ages in a period of just over 3 years using the 1989 ILAE Classification (Olafsson *et al.*, 2005). The authors reported a low percentage of specific epilepsy syndromes with the exception being Benign Rolandic Epilepsy in 25 cases comprising 20% of epilepsies with onset in childhood and 5% of the total. Childhood Absence Epilepsy was identified in 7 patients with an incidence of 0.8 per 100,000 patient years with a similar incidence for West syndrome. The authors commented that the 1989 syndromic classification had some flaws in relation to adult onset epilepsy though their study confirmed its usefulness in childhood in the epilepsies. In a prospective cohort in Connecticut 613 children diagnosed with epilepsy from 1993 to 1997 were assessed for syndromic diagnosis at 2 years following diagnosis (Berg *et al.*, 2010). It is notable that 84 children had a change in epilepsy syndrome than that assigned soon after diagnosis. In 24 because the syndrome had evolved but in 60 because of a rectification of the initially assigned syndrome thus emphasising the time needed to make a confident syndromic diagnosis. Half of the syndrome evolutions were to Lennox-Gastaut syndrome. In this paper large non-specific groupings classes such as symptomatic localisation related epilepsies were regarded as syndromes.

It has been argued that as epilepsy course and remission cannot be easily predicted therefore syndrome classification cannot help predict course and remission of epilepsy however long-term syndrome specific outcome data are now emerging (Beghi, 2009). In a Swedish county of 60,192 children aged 1 month to 16 years 205 cases of active epilepsy were identified. 24% had onset in the first year and 50% before 4 years of age (Larsson & Eeg-Olofsson, 2006). A named syndrome could be diagnosed in 49.4% of cases. The percentage with Rolandic epilepsy (17%) and childhood absence epilepsy (5.9%) were similar to the Icelandic data. In a study of new-onset epilepsy and epilepsy syndromes in childhood a specific syndrome was assigned to 28% (99/359) of cases at presentation and in this group the syndromic diagnosis percentage only increased to 29% (105/359) at final follow up (Wirrel, 2011). Only six children developed a definite syndrome over time and only 3 evolved from one syndrome to another. In a retrospective study of children presenting with epilepsy less than one year of age from 1997 through 2006 to the Helsinki Hospital 158 cases were identified, of which 92% were followed to 24 months or death (Gaily *et al.*, 2016). An epilepsy syndrome was identified in 58%

of patients with West syndrome (41/100,000) and benign familial and non-familial infantile epilepsy (22/100,00) the most common syndromes. Genetic aetiologies were identified in 17% of cases however not all children had genetic testing. Many of the well-established clinical epilepsy syndromes of childhood have associated genetic aetiologies. Through early population-based prospective genetic testing linked to deep phenotyping at the onset of epilepsy and thereafter more accurate incidence figures for many of the epilepsy syndromes of infancy, childhood and adolescence will emerge.

REFERENCES ▶

Bahi-Buisson N, Kaminska A, Boddaert N, *et al.* (2008): The three stages of epilepsy in patients with CDKL5 mutations. *Epilepsia* 49: 1027–1037.

Beghi E (2009): The concept of the epilepsy syndrome. How useful is it in clinical practice? *Epilepsia* 50 (Suppl 5): 4–10.

Berg AT, Berkovic SF, Brodie MJ, *et al.* (2010): Revised terminology and concepts for organization of seizures and epilepsies: report of the ILAE Commission on Classification & Terminology, 2005–2009. *Epilepsia* 51: 676–685.

Berkovic SF, Howell RA, Hay DA, *et al.* (1998): Epilepsies in twins: genetics of the major epilepsy syndromes. *Ann Neurol* 43: 435–445.

Blumenfeld H (2005): Cellular and network mechanisms of spike-wave seizures. *Epilepsia* 46 (Suppl 9): 21–33.

Braun KPJ & Cross JH (2018): Paediatric epilepsy surgery: the earlier the better. *Expert Rev Neurother* 18: 261–263.

Brunklaus A, Dorris L, Zuberi SM (2011): Comorbidities and predictors of health-related quality of life in Dravet syndrome. *Epilepsia* 52: 1476–1482.

Brunklaus A, Dorris L, Ellis R, *et al.* (2013): The clinical utility of an SCN1A genetic diagnosis in infantile-onset epilepsy. *Dev Med Child Neurol* 55: 154–161.

Commission of Classification and Terminology of the ILAE (1989): Proposal for revised classification of epilepsies and epileptic syndromes. *Epilepsia* 30: 389–399.

de Lange IM, Gunning B, Sonsma ACM, *et al.* (2018): Influence of contraindicated medication use on cognitive outcome in Dravet syndrome and age at first afebrile seizure as a clinical predictor in SCN1A-related seizure phenotypes. *Epilepsia* 59: 1154–1165.

Devinsky O, Cross JH, Laux L, *et al.* (2017): Trial of cannabidiol for drug-resistant seizures in the Dravet syndrome. *New Engl J Med* 376: 2011–2020.

Engel J (2001): A proposed diagnostic scheme for people with epileptic seizures and with epilepsy: Report of the ILAE task force on classification and terminology. *Epilepsia* 42: 796–803.

Fiest KM, Sauro KM, Wiebe S, *et al.* (2017). Prevalence and incidence of epilepsy. A systematic review and meta-analysis of international studies. *Neurology* 88: 296–303.

Fisher RS, Cross JH, French JA, *et al.* (2017a): Operational classification of seizure types by the International League Against Epilepsy. *Epilepsia* 58: 522–530.

Fisher RS, Cross JH, D'Souza C, *et al.* (2017b): Instruction manual for the ILAE 2017 Operational Classification of Seizure Types. *Epilepsia* 58: 531–542.

Fisher RS, Acevedo C, Arzimanoglou A, *et al.* (2014): ILAE official report: a practical definition of epilepsy. *Epilepsia* 55: 475–482.

Gaily E, Lommi M, Lapatto R. (2016): Incidence and outcome of epilepsy syndromes with onset in the first year of life: A retrospective population-based study. *Epilepsia* 57: 1594–1601.

Howell KB, Eggers S, Dalziel K, *et al.* (2018): A population-based cost-effectiveness study of early genetic testing in severe epilepsies of infancy. *Epilepsia* 59: 1177–1187.

Larsson K, Eeg-Olofsson O (2006): A population based study of epilepsy in children from a Swedish county. *Eur J Paediatr Neurol* 10: 107–113.

Mullen SA, Carney PW, Roten A, *et al.* (2018): Precision therapy for epilepsy due to *KCNT1* mutations: A randomized trial of oral quinidine. *Neurology* 90: e67-e72.

Murray DM, Boylan GB, Ali I, *et al.* (2008): Defining the gap between electrographic seizure burden, clinical expression and staff recognition of neonatal seizures. *Fetal & Neonatal an addition of Arch Dis Child* 93: F187-F191.

Nash KB, Bonifacio SL, Glass HC, *et al.* (2011): Video-EEG monitoring in newborns with hypoxic-ischemic encephalopathy treated with hypothermia. *Neurology* 76: 556–562.

O'Callaghan FJK, Edwards SW, Dietrich F, *et al.* (2018): Vigabatrin with hormonal treatment *versus* hormonal treatment alone (ICISS) for infantile spasms: 18-month outcomes of an open-label randomised controlled trial. *Lancet Child Adolesc Health* 2: 715–725.

Olafsson E, Ludvigsson P, Gudmundsson G, *et al.* (2005): Incidence of unprovoked seizures and epilepsies in Iceland and assessment of the epilepsy syndrome classification: a prospective study. *Lancet Neurol* 4: 627–634.

Pressler RM, Cilio MR, Mizrahi EM, *et al.* (2018): The ILAE Classification of Seizures & the Epilepsies: Modification for Seizures in the Neonate. Proposal from the ILAE Task Force on Neonatal Seizures. https://www.ilae.org/files/dmfile/NeonatalSeizureClassification-ProofForWeb.pdf

Ronen G, Penney S, Andrew W (1999): The epidemiology of clinical neonatal seizures in Newfoundland: A population-based study. *J Pediatr* 134: 71–75.

Scheffer IE, Berkovic S, Capovilla, *et al.* (2017): ILAE classification of the epilepsies. Position paper of the ILAE Commission for Classification and Terminology. *Epilepsia* 58: 512–521.

Scher MS, Alvin J, Gaus L, *et al.* (2003): Uncoupling of EEG-clinical neonatal seizures after antiepileptic drug abuse. *Pediatr Neurol* 28: 277–280.

Thurman DJ, Beghi E, Begley CE, *et al.* (2011): Standards for epidemiological studies and surveillance of epilepsy. *Epilepsia* 52: 2–26.

Wirrell EC, Grossardt BR, Wong-Kisiel LC, *et al.* (2011): Incidence and classification of new-onset epilepsy and epilepsy syndromes in children in Olmsted County, Minnesota from 1980 to 2004: a population-based study. *Epilepsy Res* 95: 110–118.

Wolf P (2003): Of cabbages and kings: some considerations on classifications, diagnostic schemes, semiology, and concepts. *Epilepsia* 44: 1–4.

Zuberi SM & Brunklaus A (2018): Epilepsy in 2017: Precision medicine drives epilepsy classification and therapy. *Nat Rev Neurol* 4: 67–68.

CHAPTER 2

GENETIC BASIS AND TESTING OF EPILEPTIC SYNDROMES

Antonio V. Delgado-Escueta[1,2], Viet-Huong Nguyen[2,3], Reyna M. Duron[2,4], Julia N. Bailey[2,5] and Jose Maria Serratosa[6]

[1] Department of Neurology, David Geffen School of Medicine, University of California, Los Angeles, USA
[2] Epilepsy Genetics and Genomics Labs, Neurology and Research Services, Veterans Affairs Greater Los Angeles Healthcare System, West Los Angeles, USA
[3] Chapman University School of Pharmacy, Orange County, USA
[4] Facultad de Ciencias de la Salud, Universidad Tecnológica Centroamericana UNITEC, Tegucigalpa, Honduras
[5] Department of Epidemiology, Fielding School of Public Health, University of California, Los Angeles (J.N.B.), USA
[6] Neurology Service, University Hospital Jiménez Diaz Foundation, Autonomous University of Madrid and Ciberer, Madrid, Spain

Introduction

"How will genetic testing for epilepsy syndromes change my clinical practice of epilepsy? I am still doing the same thing I was taught as a house physician!"
A frequent question/comment during American Epilepsy Society meetings

The 6th edition of *Epileptic Syndromes in Infancy, Childhood and Adolescence* will be remembered as the editions when genetic testing of the epilepsy syndromes became part of the everyday clinical practice of the epilepsies. Several events that transpired during these editions prompted this development. First was the sequencing of the human genome and, in 2010, the reduction to less than $1,000 per person for the cost of parallel next generation whole exome/genome sequencing (WGS/WES) and, with this, the rise of commercial clinical genome centers. Second was the $215 million NIH investment in the Precision Medicine Initiative and new treatments tailored to the individual's genetic makeup, transforming how treatment is selected for genotyped epilepsies. The third events, which we are still witnessing, are the fruits of these initiatives and the beginning of the end of some fatal diseases. First, cystic fibrosis (Burgener & Moss, 2018), then Werdnig Hoffman spinal muscular atrophy 1 (Mendell JR *et al.*, 2017), and more recently a fatal epilepsy of late infancy and early childhood, Batten disease ceroid-lipofucsinosis 2 (Schulz *et al.*, 2018). One by one, disease mechanisms of fatal epilepsies of infancy, childhood and adolescence, are being targeted by the genius of basic researchers and pharma. By the time this 6th edition comes around in 2019, several of these fatal epilepsies will be undergoing curative treatment trials. Nevertheless, what has been equally important in placing genetic testing of epileptic syndromes into the heart and soul of the clinical practice of epilepsy was maybe the acceptance in 2012 by the American Board of Psychiatry and Neurology (ABPN) for the specialty practice of epileptology, and the start of diplomate examinations. The confluence of all these events – more inexpensive WGS/WES, the rise of commercial clinical genome centers, the Precision Medicine Initiative and the beginning quest to cure fatal epilepsies – are changing the everyday clinical practice of epileptology. And, today, one will not pass the ABPN Epilepsy Board exams if one does not know how to interpret genetic testing of epileptic syndromes.

Thus this chapter aims to i) present the genetic bases of 19 age-dependent genetically based epileptic syndromes and a cartography/chromosomal map of some epilepsy genes *(Table I, Figure 1)*; ii) discuss clinical genetic testing for these epileptic syndromes and their disease causing genetic variants, focusing on genotyping that is of practical use to the clinician/practitioner; iii) guide the epilepsy practitioner on how to decide if genetic variants of these epilepsy genes are pathogenic based on the evidentiary criteria recommended by the American College of Medical Genetics and Genomics and the Association for Molecular Pathology (ACMG-AMP) and summarized in ClinVar (there are now 84 genes considered to cause epilepsy as their primary symptome, 73 genes that cause both neurodevelopmental disability and epilepsy, some 536 genes associated with epilepsy and other systemic abnormalities [Wang *et al.*, 2017]); and iv) focus on how clinical genetic testing is changing how we treat the epileptic syndromes.

Curating the epilepsy genome towards an atlas of the human epilepsy genome

In 1969, Gastaut originally proposed to classify epilepsies into generalized and partial while subdividing generalized epilepsies into primary and secondary (Gastaut, 1969). In 1989, the ILAE Commission on Classification and Terminology developed the ILAE syndrome classification (Commission, 1989) after evaluating all the epilepsy syndromes that, until the early 1980s, had been described mainly by the "Gastaut Marseille" group and the "Janz German" school. This initiative was documented in the first edition of this book (Roger *et al.*, 1985).

Historically, age-dependent genetic epileptic syndromes with normal neurologic status, without prior neurologic insult and without structural lesions on brain imaging acted as probes that cut into heterogeneous groups of specific epilepsies. This introduced new concepts in epileptology over the last four decades as ongoing research in brain imaging and video-EEG recordings of actual seizures further improved and refined our concepts on diagnosis and classification of epilepsy syndromes. Initially, the complexity and variability of phenotypes and overlapping clinical features limited the resolution of phenotype-based classification and confounded epilepsy nosology.

Then, came discovery of epilepsy genes in 1995 and proof of epilepsy causing variants/mutations changed our concepts of epilepsy syndromes into epilepsy diseases (see *Table I* and *Figure 1* for epilepsy gene map/cartography). These are exemplified by germ line disease causing variants/mutations. Variants in the alpha-4 subunit of nACH receptor (CHRNA4) (Steinlein *et al.*, 1995) was the first, then other nACH receptors such as CHRNA2 and CHRNB2 were associated with autosomal dominant nocturnal frontal lobe epilepsy, *KCNQ2*, and *KCNQ3* with benign familial neonatal convulsions (Singh *et al.*, 1998; Charlier *et al.*, 1998; Biervert & Steilein, 1999; Biervert *et al.*, 1998) alpha-2 subunit of GABA-A receptor with "febrile seizures plus syndrome" with absence seizures (Baulac *et al.*, 2001; Wallace *et al.*, 2001), the beta-3 subunit of GABA-A receptor with remitting childhood absence epilepsy (Tanaka *et al.*, 2007), the leucine-rich glioma-inactivated 1 (LGI1) with familial temporal lobe epilepsy with auditory features (Ottman *et al.*, 2010) and *EFHC1* and *ICK* variants with juvenile myoclonic epilepsy (Bailey *et al.*, 2017, 2018).

Interestingly, what sharpened the diagnostic view of the medical community to genetic testing of epilepsy syndromes was the 2001 discovery of somatic recurrent *de novo mutations in a sporadic epilepsy syndrome described by Dravet, e.g.* the alpha1 subunit of the sodium channel *(SCN1A)* arising mainly from paternally derived chromosomes, the beta-1 subunit of sodium channel *(SCN1B)* (Wallace *et al.*, 1998; Escayg *et al.*, 2000, 2001), protocadherin 19 (PCDH19) in X-linked females with Dravet. This recognition of *de novo* mutations in sporadic epilepsies led to whole exome sequencing of developmental disabilities mixed with infantile epileptic encephalopathies such as infantile spasms in West syndrome and Lennox-Dravet syndrome which revealed in 2013, *de novo* variants in *GABRb3, CACNA1A* (calcium channel, voltage–dependent, P/Q type, alpha-1A subunit), *CHD2* (chromodomain helicase-DNA binding protein 2), *FLNA* (FilaminA), *GABRa1, GRIN1* (glutamate receptor, ionotropic, N-methyl-D-aspartate, subunit 1), *GRIN2B* (glutamate receptor, ionotropic, N-methyl-D-aspartate, subunit 2B), *HNRNPU* (heterogenous nuclear ribonucleoprotein U), *IQSEC2* (Intelligence quotient motif and SEC domain containing protein 2 in xp11.22), *MTOR* and *NEDD4L* (neural precursor cell-expressed developmentally down-regulated gene 4-like) (Allen *et al.*, 2013) and, in 2017, *de novo* variants in *NTRK2* (neurotrophic receptor tyrosine kinase 2), *GABRB2, CLTC* (clathrin heavy chain involved in spindle formation), *DHDDS* (dehydrodolichyl diphosphate synthase), *NUS1, RAB11A* (specifies recycling endosomes in formation of autophagosomes during autophagy), *GABBR2* and *SNAP25* (synaptosome associated protein 25, a core component of the N-ethylmaleimide-sensitive factor attachment complex involved in exocytosis) (Hamdan *et al.*, 2017).

With association of disease causing variants with specific epileptic syndromes also came realization of specific antiepileptic drugs as "keys that fit the lock" of disease mechanisms of epileptic syndromes. The concept of "antiepileptic drugs that act as sodium channel blockers worsen genetic epilepsies" has to be modified. *De novo SCN1A* variants Dravet syndrome or epileptic encephalopathy is worse with sodium channel blockers but *de novo SCN8A or SCN2A* variants Dravet syndrome can respond favorably with sodium channel blockers. Some *KCNT1* deficient malignant migrating partial epilepsies in infancy respond to quinidine (Abdelnour *et al.*, 2018) but some to carbamazepine. Sodium channel blockers can also be effective in variant KCNQ2 while ketogenic diet has diverse efficacy in variant *SCN1A, CDKL5, KCNQ2, STXBP1 and SCN2A* (Ko *et al.*, 2018).

When gene-panel sequencing platforms are used by commercial genome centers to screen for potentially pathogenic variants, they are targeting in combination these 84 genes whose mutations are primarily expressed as epilepsies, the 73 epileptic encephalopathies genes *(Table I)* and about 40 genetic diseases whose phenotype significantly include epilepsy *(Table II)*.

Familial and sporadic 15q13.3 microdeletions in idiopathic generalized epilepsies are now explained as precedents for seizures with complex inheritance (Dibbens *et al.*, 2009; Helbig *et al.*, 2009).

Table I **Some epilepsy genes and their phenotypes**

Chromosome	Gene	Phenotype
1p35-31.1	*SLC2A1/Glut1*, glucose transporter type I	Early onset absence epilepsy; also in epilepsy with paroxysmal exercise-induced dyskinesia
1p36	*GABRD* GABA receptor variants E177A and R220H andArg220His	Generalized epilepsy with febrile seizures plus (GEFS+) with absence seizures
1q21-23	*ATP1A2*, sodium potassium ATPase alpha-2 subunit	Familial hemiplegic migraine with epilepsy
1q21	*CHRNB2*, beta 2 subunit of nicotinic acetylecholine receptor	Autosomal dominant nocturnal frontal lobe epilepsy 3
2q22-23	*CACNB4* with *R482X* mutation, calcium channel beta-4 subunit	Idiopathic generalized epilepsy, juvenile myoclonic epilepsy
2q24	*SCN9A* sodium channel alpha-9 subunit	Dravet SMEI syndrome or simple febrile seizures, intractable epilepsy, complex partial seizures with hippocampal scleroses, pain syndromes
2q24	*SCN1A* sodium channel alpha-1 subunit	Intractable childhood epilepsy with generalized tonic clonic seizures (ICEGTC); generalized epilepsies with febrile seizures plus (GEFS+); severe myoclonic epilepsy of infancy of Dravet; febrile seizures 3 (FEB3)
2q24	*SCN3A*, sodium channel alpha-3 subunit	Partial epilepsy
2q23-24.3	*SCN2A*, sodium channel alpha-2 subunit	Benign familial neonatal infantile seizures; febrile and afebrile seizures
4q13-31	*SCARB2/LIMP2*	Progressive myoclonus epilepsy, Unverricht-Lundborg type, also inaction myoclonus-renal failure syndrome
5p13	*EAAT1*; glial glutamate transporter	Episodic ataxia with seizures, migraine, alternating hemiplegia
5q34	*GABRA1*, GABA A receptor alpha-1 subunit	Juvenile myoclonic epilepsy
5q34	*GABRG2*, GABA A receptor gamma-2 subunit	Generalized epilepsy with febrile seizures plus (GEFS+3) and childhood absence; febrile seizures only, Dravet syndrome
6p12-p11	Myoclonin1/*EFHC1* gene	Juvenile myoclonic epilepsy (EJM1)
6p-21.3	*BRD2*, mitogen-activated kinase gene	Juvenile myoclonic epilepsy (EJM2)
6p-22	*EPM2B*, malin ubiquitin ligase	Lafora progressive myoclonus epilepsy
6q24	*EPM2A*, laforin/dual specificity protein phosphatase	Lafora progressive myoclonus epilepsy
7q36	*CNTNAP2*	Focal epilepsy; developmental delay, cortical migration defects
8q24	*KCNQ3*, EBN potassium channel	Benign familial neonatal convulsions
9q33.3-q34.11	*STXBP1/Munc18-1*, syntaxin binding protein1 Sporadi	Sporadic Ohtahara syndrome of early infantile epileptic encephalopathy with EEG suppression bursts
9q33.3-q34.11	*SPTAN1*, alpha-2 spectrin deletion, duplication	Early onset epileptic encephalopathy (early onset West syndrome) with severe hypomyelination
10q22	*KCNMA1*, BK potassium channel alpha subunit	Generalized epilepsy and paroxysmal dyskinesia; nonconvulsive absence seizures

10q24	*LGI1*/Epitempin	Autosomal dominant partial epilepsy with auditory features
11p13	*ELP4* elongator complex gene	Rolandic epilepsy with centrotemporal spikes
11p15.5	*SLC25A22/GC1* encodes mitochondrial glutamate/H +symporters	Neonatal seizures with EEG suppression-burst and hypotonia
11q14-q23	*TSC1* (hamartin) gene	Tuberous sclerosis
12p13	*KCNA1* voltage gated potassium channel	Partial epilepsy, partial epilepsy in episodic ataxia 1
12p13.31	Atrophin binds to a TATA-binding protein which is a cofactor for (CREB) cAMP-responsive element binding protein-dependent transcriptional activation; CREB is inhibited; dominant	Dentato-rubro-pallido-luysian atrophy; CAG repeat; "Haw River" syndrome
12q22-q24.1	*TSC2* (tuberin) gene	Tuberous sclerosis
16p13	*TBC1D24* gene (binds ARF6 which is involved in neurite branching and extension)	Autosomal recessive familial infantile myoclonic epilepsy (FIME)
15q21	*ME2* malic enzyme involved in GABA synthesis	Idiopathic generalized epilepsy
15q11-15	*GABRB3* GABA receptor beta 3 subunit	Remitting childhood absence epilepsy
19p13	*CACNA1-A*, voltage-gated P/Q calcium channel alpha subunit	Absence epilepsy, familial hemiplegic migraine, dominant episodic ataxia2, acetazolamide responsive, spinocerebellar degeneration type 6
19q13	SCN1β, sodium channel beta-1 subunit	Generalized epilepsies with febrile seizures plus
19q13.2	*NACHR* nicotinic acetylcholine receptor alpha-4 subunit	Autosomal dominant nocturnal frontal lobe epilepsy 1
20q	*KCNQ2* potassium channel subunit	Benign familial neonatal convulsions (EBN1)
21q22.3	*CSTB*, cystatin B	Unverricht-Lundborg disease; progressive myoclonus epilepsy Baltic myoclonus (EPM1)
Xp22	*TREX1*,3'-5' DNAexonuclease	Aicardi's syndrome with early infantile epileptic encephalopathy and EEG burst suppression
Xp22	*ARX*, Aristaless related homeobox gene	X linked infantile spasms of West syndrome, spasticity, mental retardation, Partington syndrome (ataxia, mental retardation and dystonia), Ohtahara syndrome, X-linked myoclonic epilepsy
Xp22	*CDKL5*, cyclin dependent kinase like 5 gene	Infantile spasms, hypsarrhythmia, overlapping phenotypes of Angelman syndrome and atypical Rett syndrome
Xq22.1	*PCDH19*, protocadherin 19 gene	Dravet syndrome, epilepsy and mental retardation in females (EFMR)
Xq22	*SPRX2*, secreted sushi-repeat containing protein	Rolandic epilepsy with oral and speech dyspraxia; bilateral perisylvian polymicrogyria
Xq22.3-q23	*DCX*, doublecortin gene	X-linked lissencephaly and subcortical band heterotopia, double cortex syndrome

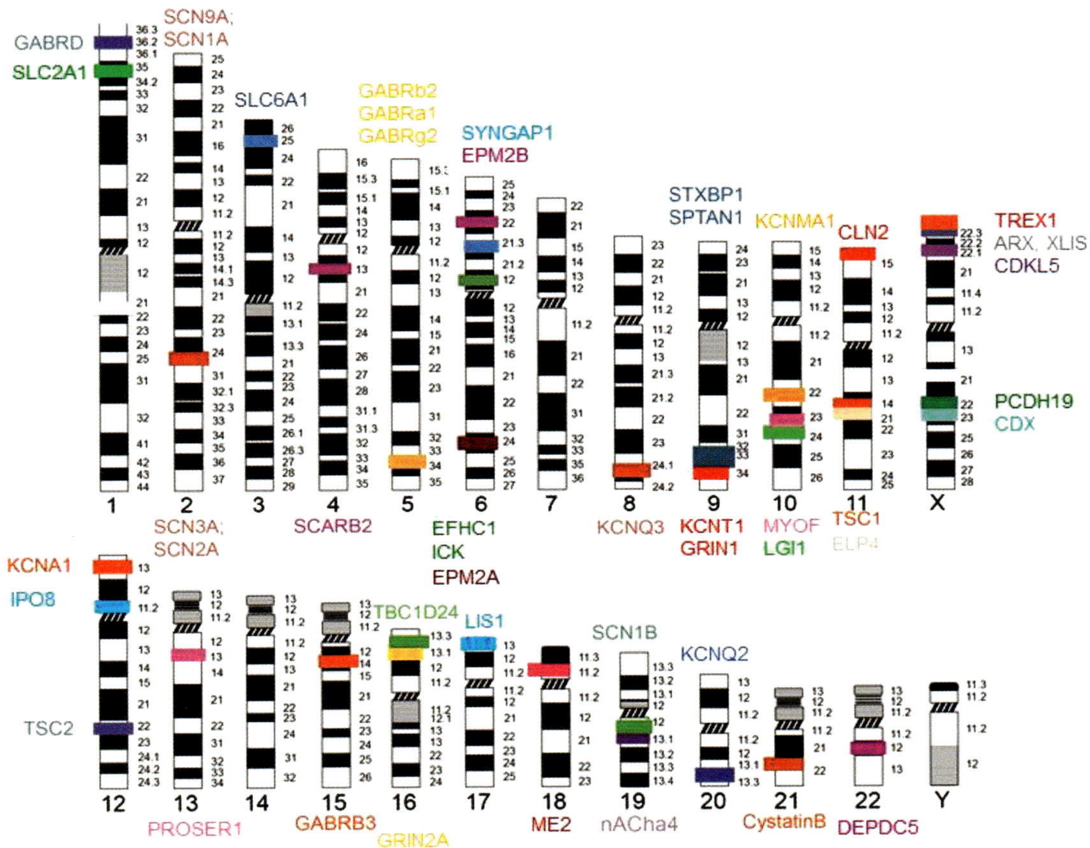

Figure 1

Genetic map (cartography of chromosome loci) of some human epilepsy genes for epileptic encephalopathies, some common epilepsies and progressive myoclonus epilepsies.

Table II Some genetic diseases whose phenotype includes epilepsy

Chromosome	Epilepsy gene
1p15	Late infantile neuronal ceroid lipofuscinoses
1p32	Infantile neuronal ceroid lipofuscinoses (Finnish type); Haltia-Santavuori disease; CLN1; palmitoyl-protein thiosterase recessive
1p34	Alpha-L-fucosidase-1/fucosidosis
1q21	Glucocerebrosidase/Gaucher's disease
2p21	Holoprosencephaly-2
3q25.2-q27	Cerebral cavernous malformations (CCM3)
3p26-p25	von Hippel-Lindau disease (VHL 1 and 2); type 1-retinal angiomas, CNS
3pter-3p21	Beta-galactosidase l/GMs gangliosidosis
6q25-qter	Fucosidosis; recessive; type 2; FUCA2
7p13-p15	Cerebral cavernous malformations (CCM2)
7q	Cavernous malformations of the brain; unknown gene
7q21-q22	Cerebral cavernous malformations (CCM1) (*Krit 1* gene)
7q36	Holoprosencephaly-3
8p23	Juvenile neuronal ceroid lipofuscinosis
11p15	Variant juvenile neuronal ceroid lipofuscinosis; Jansky-Bielschowsky disease; tripeptidyl peptidase (TPP1); (CLN2)
11p15.4-15.1	Niemann-Pick disease types A and B
11q21-q23	Desmin myopathy; alpha-beta-crystallin (CRY A-beta)
11q22	Charcot-Marie-tooth type 4B; myotubularin-related protein 2
11q22-q23	Dopamine D2 receptor; myoclonus-dystonia syndrome, dominant
11q22-23	Ataxia telangiectasia; ATM gene for regulation of cell cycle; mitogenic signal transduction and meiotic recombinantion
12q22-q24.2	Phenylalaninehydroxylase/phenylketonuria
13p22	Finnish late infantile neuronal ceroid lipofuscinosis
13q14.2-q21	Wilson's disease
13q21-q32	Late infantile neuronal ceroid-lipofuscinosis (Finnish type); *(CLN5)*; Novel transmembrane protein of unknown function; recessive
14q	Spastic paraparesis and epilepsy
14q11.1-q13	Holoprosencephaly-4
15q	Epilepsy, dysmorphic face, mental retardation, temporal lobe malformation; 15q trisomy (chromosome 12-15 translocation)
16p12	Batten's disease, juvenile neuronal ceroid lipofuscinosis; recessive; CLN-3; Novel transmembrane protein of unknown function

16q12.2-q21	Bilateral frontoparietal polymicrogyria (BFPP)
18q11-12	Niemann-Pick disease type C; intracellular cholesterol trafficking; NP-type Dis allelic
Xp22.1-p21.2	Glycine receptor, Rett syndrome
Xq26	Hypoxanthine-guaninephosphoribosyltransferase/Lesch-Nyhan syndrome
Xq27.3	Fragile X mental retardation syndrome; CGG repeats
Xq27.3-q28	Iduronate 2-sulfatase/Hunter's syndrome
Xq27-q28	Incontinentia pigmenti 2
Xq27-q28	Rett syndrome; methyl-CpG binding protein2 (MECP2); occurs almost exclusively in women
Xq28	Incontinentia pigmenti; NEMO/IKBKG
Xq28	Adrenoleukodystrophy, adrenoleukomyeloneuropathy
Xq28	Fragile X type E; GCC repeats
Xq28	Hydrocephalus aqueductal stenosis type

Concepts of genetic epilepsy syndromes

Ten genetic concepts of epilepsy syndromes as epilepsy diseases, based on the age-dependent genetic syndromes and their epilepsy causing pathogenic variants/mutations, can be summarized as follows:

- **Concept 1:** Epileptic encephalopathies of infancy and childhood can be genetic, as exemplified by *STXBP1/MUNC18-1* or *ARX or KCNQ2* mutations in Ohtahara syndrome (Kato *et al.*, 2007; Saitsu *et al.*, 2008; Weckhuysen *et al.*, 2012).

- **Concept 2:** Ion channelopathies such as *de novo SCN1A, SCN1B, SCN2A, SCN8A, SCN9A, KCNA2, KCNB1, KCNC1, KCNMA1, KCNQ2, KCNQ3, KCNT1*, pathogenic variants in EIEE or Dravet syndrome (Claes *et al.*, 2001; Dravet *et al.*, 2005; Harkin *et al.*, 2007; Wallace *et al.*, 1998, 2001, 2003; Hirose *et al.*, 2000) can cause simple febrile seizures and GEFS+ syndrome as well as benign neonatal, infantile epilepsy syndromes and epileptic encephalopathies (EE).

- **Concept 3:** Receptoropathies, *e.g.*, pathogenic variants in *nACH (CHRNA2, CHRNA4, CHRNB2)* or *GABR (GABRa1, GABRb1, GABRb2, GABRb3, GABRd, GABRg2)* can cause genetic focal epilepsies (ADNFLE) (Steinlein *et al.*, 1995; De Fusco *et al.*, 2000; Hirose *et al.*, 1999; Steinlein *et al.*, 1997) as well as genetic generalized epilepsies:
  – GEFS+ with absence epilepsies of childhood and adolescence (Baulac *et al.*, 2001; Cossette *et al.*, 2002);
  – *GRIN2A* gene in epilepsy plus aphasia spectrum disorder composed by Rolandic epilepsy, atypical benign partial epilepsy, epileptic encephalopathy of continuous spike-and-waves during slow-wave sleep and Landau-Kleffner syndrome;
  – *GRIN2B* in EIEE and *GRIN2D* in EIEE (Kearney, 2017; Dibbens *et al.*, 2004; Wallace *et al.*, 2001).

- **Concept 4:** Non-ion channel genes, *e.g.*, *myoclonin1/EFHC1*, Intestinal cell kinase *(ICK)*, Importin 8 *(IPO8), PROSER1, MYOFERLIN, BRD2, EL4, TBC1D24, CDKL5, STXBP1* and *MAG 12* can cause common epilepsies such as juvenile myoclonic epilepsy, Rolandic epilepsy, familial infantile myoclonic epilepsy and infantile spasms (Suzuki *et al.*, 2004; de Nijs *et al.*, 2009; Cavalleri *et al.*, 2007; Pal *et al.*, 2003; Lorenz *et al.*, 2006; Strug *et al.*, 2009; Falace *et al.*, 2010; Corbett *et al.*, 2010; Weaving *et al.*, 2004; Deprez *et al.*, 2010; Marshall *et al.*, 2008; Mei *et al.*, 2009).

- **Concept 5:** Some genes are transporters: *SLC1A2* (solute carrier family 1-glial high affinity glutamate transporter) in EIEE, *SLC12A5* (solute carrier family 12 – potassium/chloride transporter) in EIEE as well as IGE, *SLC13A5* (solute carrier family 13-sodium dependent citrate transporter) in EIEE, *SLC25A12* (solute carrier family 25,-mitochondrial carrier, aralar) in EIEE, *SLC25A22* (solute carrier family 25-mitochondrial carrier, glutamate) in EIEE, *SLC2A1 (solute carrier family 2-facilitated glucose transporter)* in IGE and *SLC6A1* (solute carrier family 6, neurotransmitter transporter, GABA) in myoclonic-atonic Doose syndrome.

- **Concept 6:** Genes involved in membrane trafficking and exocytosis: *STX1B* in GEFS+, *STXBP1* in EIEE; *SYNGAP1* (synaptic RAS-GTPase-activating protein) in EE plus autism spectrum.

• **Concept 7:** Cell adhesion molecules: *CNTN2* in FAME and *PCDH19* in Dravet syndrome.

• **Concept 8:** Genes involved in cell death in progressive myoclonus epilepsy, *e.g.*, *Laforin/DSP* and *cystatin B* (Minassian *et al.*, 1998; Serratosa *et al.*, 1999; Pennachio *et al.*, 1996), and the proteasome degradation pathways (malin/UbiquitinE3 ligase [Chen *et al.*, 2003]), as well as errors in glycogen metabolism (Turnbull *et al.*, 2011) can cause progressive myoclonus epilepsy.

• **Concept 9:** Specific developmental genes involved in cell proliferation (*e.g.*, *EMX2* homeobox gene in schizencephaly), migration (*e.g.*, *EFHC1*, *ICK* and *IPO8* in *JME; filamin 1* gene in periventri-cular nodular heterotopia; *US! gene* or *double cortin* gene in X-linked lissencephaly and subcortical band heterotopia) and differentiation (G *protein coupled receptor gene 6* or *GPR56* in bilateral frontoparietal polymicrogyria) cause epilepsies in malformations of the cerebral cortex (Guerrini & Marini, 2006).

• **Concept 10:** Microscopic rearrangements, microdeletions and chromosomal defects are common causes of epilepsy, dysmorphisms and mild mental retardation (Dibbens *et al.*, 2009; Helbig *et al.*, 2009) (*Table III*).

Clinical genetic testing (genotyping) and genetic counseling in the epilepsies

Clinical genetic testing (genotyping)

The neurology and epileptology practitioner rightfully asks: "When do we clinically test for these genetic epileptic syndromes? And what practical importance do results have? Do results affect treatment and prognosis? What are the risks or limitations of clinical genetic testing?" Genetic information can be provided by genotyping the symptomatic patient and family members even up to 4th degree relatives (see *www.genetests.org* sponsored by NIH).

Genetic counseling

When the neurologist/epileptologist plans to diagnose an epilepsy syndrome by genetic testing, genetic counseling should be offered before blood is drawn for the genotyping of a symptomatic patient or for the presymptomatic diagnosis of members of a family with epilepsy (Blandfort *et al.*, 1987; Ottman *et al.*, 2010) – see *www.nsqc.org* to find genetic counselors. The epilepsy patient and his/her family should be educated by the genetic counselor about what the test methods can reveal, the limitations of the test methods, what his/her own genetic material can reveal, and the "ripple effects" and impact of epilepsy genetic information on the patient and family members. The epilepsy patient should be given time to weigh the advantages and disadvantages of being genotyped. The neurological practitioner and genetic counselor should warn family members that he or she may feel sad or guilty or even angry as a consequence of test results. Genetic counselors should include discussions on risk estimates of the epilepsy syndrome for siblings or future offspring, if relevant, address reproductive consequences of having an epilepsy gene, and consider teratogenesis of antiepileptic drugs if the patient is female. Counseling should also include a discussion of the financial costs for genotyping and whether medical insurance will pay because financial costs can run into thousands of dollars. In the USA, although healthcare insurers sometimes cover genetic testing of symptomatic patients, co-pays can be cost prohibitive running into US$5,000 to US$10,000 or more (Blandfort *et al.*, 1987; Ottman *et al.*, 2010).

When and why to test?

Examples of why the neurological practitioner/epileptologist applies clinical genetic testing are: i) in order to make medical decisions in diagnosis and treatment of myoclonic epilepsies or grand mal-clonic-tonic-clonic convulsions in infancy, *e.g.*, clinch the diagnosis of *SCN1A* mutations in Dravet syndrome and avoid sodium channel blockers; ii) to obtain a diagnosis in drug resistant developmental and epileptic encephalopathies of infancy and early childhood; iii) to separate the various forms of ceroidlipofucsinoses in late infancy and childhood and offer intraventricular cerliponase alpha (Brineura) for Batten disease patients with *CLN2* variants (Schulz *et al.*, 2018); iv) to confirm the lack of GluN2A containing NMDA receptors *(GRIN2A)* in the epilepsy aphasia spectrum disorder; v) to separate the various genetic causes of absence epilepsy, *e.g.*, T-type-calcium-channel variants, *GABRa1, GABRb3, GABRg2, GABRb2* variants from *SLC2A1* variants (glucose transporter or *GLUT1* deficiency) and decide between AED *versus* ketogenic diet treament; vi) to separate JME variants from PME variants in adolescent onset grand mal-myoclonic-tonic-clonic convulsions and diagnose presymptomatic or early stage Lafora disease and offer early treatment, as metformin, an FDA approved "orphan drug" for Lafora disease; and vii) to test the carrier of an X-linked disorder in which females are often symptomatic, as in *protocadherin* 19 mutations in Dravet syndrome.

Family members have more personal reasons for genetic testing, such as life and family planning. Even if there is no treatment available for a fatal form of epilepsy, a family member or a parent may wish to know if he/she or an offspring is in a presymptomatic state. A newly married person may wish to be tested, asking if she is a carrier of an autosomal recessive epilepsy like Lafora disease or Unverricht-Lundborg disease. Carrier testing for at risk relatives and prenatal testing for pregnancies at increased risk are possible if both disease causing variant/mutations in a family is known. Rarely, has a person asked for genetic testing for prenatal diagnosis/preimplantation epilepsy diagnosis in our clinical practice.

The neurologist/epileptologist should know who will have access to results of genotyping and respect family confidentiality and the Genetic Information and Nondiscrimination Act of 2008 (see www.dnapolicy.org/gina) or equivalent policies in other parts of the world. It is worth repeating that the practitioner and genetic counselor should warn family members that he or she may feel sad or guilty or even angry as a consequence of test results in severe and fatal epilepsy syndromes. Thus, a mental health expert may need to be an important team member.

What are genetic variants?

Single nucleotide variants: a variation in a single base pair in the nucleotide sequence of a gene is called a "variant". Pathogenic variants previously known as "mutations" change the amino acid sequence of the encoded protein and cause havoc in the protein's functions. Such variants arise during "germ line" processing of the meiosis stage formation of oocytes or spermatocytes. This is the usual case for single gene epileptic disorders that are transmitted by one parent through several generations (vertical transmission by a heterozygous dominant) or by both parents into the offspring generation (horizontal transmission by homozygous recessive). When both parents do not harbor a variant, it is presumed to have arisen "*de novo*". When variations happen during embryonic development after the formation of the zygote, it is called "postzygotic mutation" or "somatic mutation". This occurs in cortical dysplasias, hemimegalencephaly and neurocutaneous syndromes with megalencephaly.

Structural variants such as copy number variations, deletions/duplications: structural variants are genetic mutations affecting more than 50 basepairs and include rearrangements such as duplications, deletions, new insertions, inversions and translocations. When variations involve a number of nucleotides to as large as around 20 kB, they are called copy number variations (CNVs). Such CNVs can happen as deletions or duplications. When deletions/duplications/insertions result in a shift in the reading frame of the gene and stop protein synthesis, it is called a truncated protein.

What genetic tests to use?

The practitioner should know what test methods are available for structural variants like CNVs, insertions, microdeletions/duplications and know the costs for such tests. If the epilepsy syndrome is accompanied by dysmorphic features, cognitive regression and autism-like features, one can start looking for structural variants like CNVs, deletion/duplication by array comparative genomic hybridization. Commercial genome companies use chromosomal microarray analysis which yield a success rate of 5% (see *Table IV* for definitions of some terms used in test results).

In single gene epileptic disorders, a specific gene may be targeted (*e.g.*, myoclonic epilepsy with ragged red fibers – MERRF – syndrome) or a panel of multiple genes associated with a specific phenotype in a so-called "platform" that can target 70 to 120 genes. Commercial genome companies actually perform what is more practical and execute whole exome sequencing and then target the 70 to 465 genes that emerge after whole exome sequencing (*e.g.*, various genes tested as a batch causing early infantile epileptic encephalopathy or infantile spasms, or progressive myoclonus epilepsy or Dravet syndrome or absence epilepsy syndromes). There are presently 8 commercial epilepsy gene panels and the neurologist/epileptologist/practitioner should check if the epilepsy syndrome suspected is ably screened by the commercial gene panel. Only the Athena 232 gene panel encompasses all the genes contained in the other commercial companies (Dunn *et al.*, 2018). Success in "hitting" on a specific and meaningful epilepsy variants range from 20% to 50%. When targeted sequencing does not yield a meaningful result, the rest of the genome can be searched for epilepsy genes that were not part of the targeted group, query for mosaicism and even new epilepsy genes.

Genetic test results impact treatment

At the present time, sensitivity, specificity and clinical utility of the screening epilepsy panels and whole exome sequencing enhances diagnosis and directs the practitioner towards the developing trends of treatment in a growing list of specific epilepsy syndromes. For many of these specific epilepsy syndromes, genotyping is the most direct, cost effective and accurate diagnostic test that can directly impact the choice of treatment. In the following examples of these specific epileptic syndromes, proof that certain agents aggravate or rescue seizures have come from multiple reports of single cases or actual prospective cohorts that justify future multicenter double blind randomized clinical trials.

Some examples where genotyping results impact treatment are: i) Dravet syndrome: separate *SCN1A* from *SCN2A* and *SCN8A* variants in repeating (5 or more) or prolonged (> 10 mins) febrile convulsions that start before 7 months of age; *SCN1A* variants worse with sodium channel blockers like carbamazepine or lamotrigine (Brunklaus *et al.*, 2012), better with stiripentol, and cannabidiol and fenfluramine (Chiron *et al.*, 2000; Ceulemans *et al.*, 2012; Devinsky *et al.*, 2017) while *SCN2A* and *SCN8A* variants respond to high dose phenytoin or carbamazepine (Wolff *et al.*, 2017; Boerma *et al.*, 2016; Barker *et al.*, 2016); ii) infantile spasms caused by genetic epileptic encephalopathies; separate various channelopathies like *KCNQ2* which responds to ezogabine, carbamezapine, phenytoin (Pisano *et al.*, 2015) from *PRRT2* which responds to carbamazepine (Ebrahimi-Fakhari *et al.*, 2015) and metabolic diseases (PLCB1, which responds to inositol; recessive variants of ALDH7A1 which responds to pyridoxine; PNPO which responds to pridoxal-5-phosphate); iii) malignant migrating focal epilepsies: quinidine or carbamezapine for gain of function KCNT1 variants (Abdelnour *et al.*, 2018); iv) epilepsy with speech disorder spectrum: memantine for GRIN2A variants (Pierson *et al.*, 2014); v) cortical dysplasias: genotypes of epilepsies with MRI proven cortical malformations can help separate tuberous sclerosis from disorders of migration and cell proliferation, also help decide surgery and prognosis; consider everolimus or other mTOR inhibitors for tuberous sclerosis and cortical dysplasias; vi) childhood and adolescent myoclonias and clonic-tonic-clonic seizures of JME and CAE from progressive myoclonus epilepsies; and vii) absence epilepsy of early childhood due to GLUT1 deficiency which responds to ketogenic diet (Kass *et al.*, 2016) should be separated from childhood absences associated with GABR subunit variants, *e.g.* GABRb3, GABRb2, GABRg2 variants which may respond to clobazam or clonazepam.

Presymptomatic genetic testing for the progressive myoclonus epilepsies can be justified since therapeutic agents can now be offered *e.g.*, in Lafora type PME when (a) IV gentamicin and the emerging premature stop-codon read-through drugs, such as PTC124, can be offered as "compassionate therapy" for nonsense mutations; and (b) metformin has now been approved by the FDA as an "orphan drug" for Lafora disease. Presymptomatic genetic testing in children of families with Lafora PME is justified because an abnormal genetic test results in 100% assurance that Lafora disease will develop and IV gentamicin can be started early in nonsense mutations or metformin for Lafora disease in general. Neurologist and epileptologists should not undertake this approach by themselves and should have a genetic counselor lead the pretest counseling.

How to tell a variant is pathogenic?

The practitioner should know how to interpret results of the genetic tests, what it means when the commercial lab reports a variant is "pathogenic" or "likely pathogenic" or a benign polymorphism. The first step is to familiarize oneself with the principles that underlie the guidelines of the National Human Genome Research Institute (NHGRI) (MacArthur *et al.*, 2014) for investigating disease causality of sequence variants in human disease and the evidentiary criteria recommended by the American College of Medical Genetics and Genomics and the Association for Molecular Pathology (ACMG–AMP) (Richards *et al.*, 2015) for classifying variants as "pathogenic" or "likely pathogenic" or "benign". The second step is to check how ClinVar, a public archive of human genetic variants maintained at NIH, interpret the significance of a variant reported to you by the commercial genome lab. ClinVar summarizes the properties of variants, and the supporting observations and evidences that make it "pathogenic" or "likely pathogenic" based on NHGRI and ACMG-AMP guidelines. (https://www.clinicalgenome.org/site/assets/files/1594/landrum_clinvar.pdf).

For the first step, the practitioner can use *Figure 2*, which depicts in the first column, the core guidelines used by the NHGRI to assign disease causality to variants. The NHGRI working group addresses rare germline variants with minor allele frequencies of < 0.01 that have relatively large effects on disease risk, variants that are "genetically implicated" as pathogenic in severe monogenic diseases and complex diseases (MacArthur *et al.*, 2014).

The concept of genetic implication

Since "unambiguous assignment of disease causality for sequence variants is often impossible," the NHGRI guidelines introduced the concept of ***"implication"*** – implicating by genetic evidence sequence variant(s) of a gene that is in the process of integrating and assessing experimental evidence for pathogenicity.

Because 27% of published severe disease mutations are either common polymorphisms or lack direct evidence for pathogenicity (MacArthur *et al.*, 2014) and even ClinVar has 11.5% of genetic disorders with inflation in pathogenic variant setups, (Shah *et al.*, 2018), the NHGRI guidelines emphasized the "critical primacy of strong robust statistical genetic support" for genetic implication such as co-inheritance in family studies, case control association studies, allele frequencies in (a) controls of ancestral origin similar to the ancestral origin of the person in whom the variants were discovered and (b) allele frequencies in public genome databases such as gnomAD and theoretical predictions for conservation and pathogenicity. Strong statistical genetic support for ***"implication"*** is then supplemented by variant specific experimental studies that demonstrate that a gene product is functionally disrupted by variants. The NHGRI guidelines value disease models that recapitulate the relevant pathology of human disease and that allows rescue of the phenotype when the molecular disease pathway is knocked out or eliminated. The ACMG-AMP guidelines, on the other hand (see columns 2 and 3 of *figure 2*), concerned more with reports of clinical genomic testing that impact medical decision making, took the evidentiary data recommended by NHGRI guidelines for assigning disease causality to variants, and rated their strengths as "very strong" "strong, "moderate" and "supportive". They then set rules for combining the strengths of these evidentiary data when classifying sequence variants into "pathogenic", "likely pathogenic", "uncertain significance", "likely benign" and "benign" *(Figure 2)*.

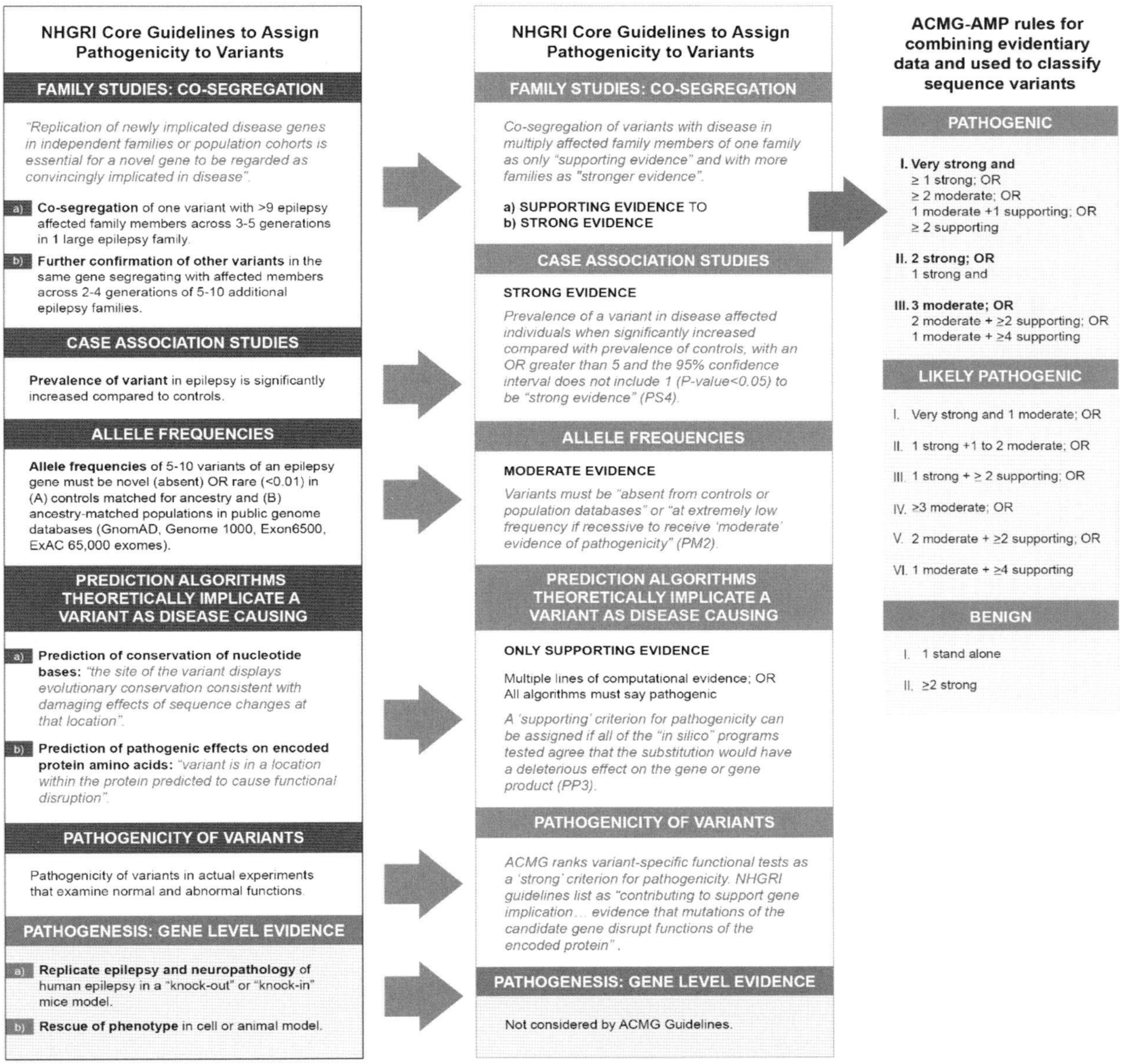

Figure 2

Assigning Disease causality to Sequence variants according to NHGRI and ACMG-AMP Guidelines.

Here, again, the practitioner should separate what an author claims or a commercial genome lab reports as "pathogenic" or "likely pathogenic" from what is "pathogenic or likely pathogenic" by ACMG-AMP guidelines and as annotated and summarized in ClinVar. When ACMG-AMP combinatorial criteria are used, the term "pathogenic" means over 95% chance of being disease producing and "likely pathogenic" means 90% chance of being disease producing.

Genetic testing for epileptic encephalopathies of infancy (EEI) and implications for treatment

Epileptic encephalopathies (EE) of infancy are conditions where sustained and recurrent epileptic activities are considered to be the major contributor to impaired motor, sensory and cognitive development. Combined neurodevelopmental disabilities and epileptic encephalopathies, now termed developmental and epileptic encephalopathies (DEE), recognize that an underlying etiology contribute to the encephalopathy in addition to the dire consequences of uncontrolled epileptic seizures. Genetic testing has helped separate and solidify these EE and DEE as true clinical entities and diseases. They appear in the neonatal period often with lethargy or coma due to epileptic seizures and include early myoclonic encephalopathy (EME) of Aicardi-Goutières with erratic myoclonus, early infancy epileptic encephalopathy (EIEE) of Ohtahara with tonic seizures, infantile spasms of West syndrome, Dravet syndrome, and malignant migrating partial seizures in infancy.

In a seminal contribution, Wolff *et al.* (2017) correlated response to sodium channel blockers in 66 patients with EE with loss or gain of function *SCN2A* mutations. Sodium channel blockers were often associated with clinically relevant seizure reduction or seizure freedom in early infantile epilepsies (< 3 months) with gain of function *SCN2A* mutations, whereas sodium channel blockers were rarely effective in epilepsies with later onset (≥ 3 months) and loss of function *SCN2A* mutations. The studies by Wolff *et al.* point to a trend supported by independent reports that gain of function mutations or loss of function mutations may influence response to channel blockers. Good response to phenytoin, a sodium channel blocker, in *SCN8A* gain of function mutations, has been observed by other investigators in EE in infancy (Boerma *et al.*, 2016; Barker, 2016).

Valproate and lamotrigine have been reported to make a rolandic epilepsy patient with gain of function *GluN2A* N447K variant seizure-free (Xu *et al.*, 2018). In which cell type and in which brain tissue a specific ion channel is expressed may also play a role in efficacy of seizure control by sodium channel blockers. *SCN1A* is expressed in GABAergic interneurons in cerebral cortex and in layer II stellate neurons of the medial entorhinal cortex while *SCN2A*, *SCN3A* and *SCN8A* are expressed in glutamergic pyramidal neurons. Sodium channel blockers can reduce seizures in *SCN2A* and *SCN8A* (EEI-13) neurodevelopmental disorders while aggravating seizures in *SCN1A* Dravet syndrome (Lai *et al.* presented in AES, 2017; Atkin *et al.*, 2018; Ottolini *et al.*, 2017). Phenytoin and carbamezepine have also been reported to be beneficial in retrospectively accumulated cohorts of KCNQ2 EE (Pisano, 2015). In general, disease-causing variants can be found in 23.5% and deletion/duplications in 9% of epileptic encephalopathies in infancy with the highest yield being *SCN1A* and *KCNQ2* variants (Lindy *et al.*, 2018). In over half of cases, the genotypes have driven the treatment.

Early myoclonic encephalopathy of Aicardi-Goutières

EME is a very rare genetic disorder characterized by erratic myoclonus, hypotonia, limited cognitive development, calcification of basal ganglia and EEG suppression-bursts. The syndrome is now considered an autoinflammatory disorder and has been associated with seven different genes encoding proteins implicated in the metabolism of nucleic acids, including *SAMHD1* which is a dNTP triphosphohydrolase (dNTPase) enzyme that controls the intracellular level of deoxyribonucleoside triphosphates (dNTPs) and plays a role in innate immune sensing and autoimmune disease. It inhibits infection of blood cells by retroviruses, including HIV, and prevents the development of the autoinflammatory Aicardi-Goutières syndrome. The inactive apo-SAMHD1 interconverts between monomers and dimers, and in the presence of dGTP the protein assembles into catalytically active tetramers (Ballana & Este, 2015).

Early infantile epileptic encephalopathy of Ohtahara

Most infants with Ohtahara syndrome have structural brain abnormalities as shown by brain MRI but a variety of pathogenic variants have been implicated and their disease mechanisms explained. Pathogenic variants in *SLC25A22* encoding a mitochondrial glutamate transporter were associated with EIEE and the accumulation of glutamate in astrocytes was hypothesized to result in seizures (Molinari *et al.*, 2006, 2009). Milh *et al.* (2007) then showed that inhibition of glutamate transporters in rat pups *"in vivo"* produced suppresion-burst patterns in the EEG. A hemizygous 33-bp duplication in exon 2 of aristaless-related homeobox gene *(ARX)* in Xp21.3 was first reported by Kato *et al.* (2007) in two unrelated patients with EIEE. ARX produces a transcription factor essential for development of cerebral interneurons. In 2010, Giordano *et al.* found missense variants in exon 5 of *ARX* in monozygotic twin sisters with EIEE. Saitsu *et al.*

(2010a, 2011) found *STXBP1/MUNC* 18-1 variants in chromosome 9q34 in 14 unrelated patients with EIEE, as well as paternal mosaicism. *STXBP1* is a regulatory component of the SNARE complex, which is involved in neuronal exocytosis and fusion steps during neurotransmitter release. Weckhuysen *et al.* (2012) first reported *de novo* mutations in *KCNQ2* in EIEE. Mutations in *SCN2A* have also been reported in EIEE (Liang *et al.*, 2017). Early infancy EE was reported to associate with *SCN8A* mutations in Chinese patients (Wang *et al.*, 2017).

Infantile spasms

When and what do you genotype in infantile spasms (West syndrome)?

When flexor or extensor or axial spasms are observed in an infant, an overnight 24 hours video-EEG is performed to demonstrate hypsarrythmia and document the semiology of infantile spasms. Brain imaging with MRI and 18fluoro 2 deoxyglucose (2FDG) PET scan should be done. A short trial with pyridoxine (100 mg IV) is followed by ACTH or viGABAtrin treatment. Sixty to 75% of infantile spasms are symptomatic, *e.g.* an evident associated underlying disorder (Jellinger, 1987; Riikonen, 2001, 2010; Pellock *et al.*, 2010). Brain imaging can display hypoxic-ischemic encephalopathy (33%), phacomatoses including tuberous sclerosis (16–25%), brain malformations including lissencephaly (4%), Down syndrome (6%), brain tumors, hydrocephalus and *in utero* infections. Structural lesions specific to tuberous scleroses or cortical dysplasias compel their respective genotyping panels. Diagnosing tuberous scleroses is important because a specific treatment for its disease pathways is now available, *e.g.*, rapamycin in addition to specific antiseizure medication (viGABAtrin) for its infantile spasms (Wong, 2010; Chiron *et al.*, 1997; Elterman *et al.*, 2001). Certain cortical dysplasias that can be treated surgically may not be detectable on MRI before 24 to 30 months of age and require 2FDG PET scan of the brain as well as fusion/coregistration of MRI and PET scans (Salamon *et al.*, 2008; Guerrini & Marini, 2006).

Twenty-five percent to 40% of infantile spasms are idiopathic and patients have a normal development before infantile spasms start. Forty percent of idiopathic infantile spasms patients, in turn, have a positive family history and suggest a genetic etiology *(Figure 2)*. *Thus, genotyping for genetic causes of infantile spasms should be done after brain imaging does not show structural disease.* After all, the best results of ACTH treatment are in the idiopathic variety and the most favorable results of vigabatrin treatment are in tuberous sclerosis (Lux *et al.*, 2004, 2005; Vigevano & Cilio, 1997). Trials with folinic acid for folinic acid sensitive infantile spasms (Gallagher *et al.*, 2009) or pyridoxine and vitamin B6 and for mutations in antiquitin for pyridoxine dependency infantile spasms (Mills *et al.*, 2006), biotine for biotinidase deficiency, serine for serine synthesis deficiency (Kalscheuer *et al.*, 2003), creatine for creatine deficiency and ketogenic diet for *de vivo* disease are all worth trying after proving their presence by genotyping idiopathic forms of infantile spasms. Over half of idiopathic infantile spasms develop normally.

In idiopathic infantile spasms where brain imaging is normal, metabolic disorders of lysosomes, peroxisomes and Golgi apparatus, energy metabolism, amino acid catabolism, synthesis/degradation of lipids and proteins, and non-ketotic hyperglycemia should be examined. Infantile spasms can result from excitotoxic mechanisms and reduction of ATP in disorders of pyruvate cycle, Krebs cycle and mitochondrial respiratory pathways.

Deletions of the MAGI2 gene at chromosome 7q11.23-q21.1 (Marshall *et al.*, 2008), X-linked cyclin dependent kinase like-5 (CDKL5/STK9) gene and interneuron related transcription factor Aristaless related homoebox gene (ARX) (Stromme *et al.*, 2002) should be screened for. Molecular cytogenetics and karyotyping are mandatory in these patients.

Many of the genetic causes of infantile spasms are forms of epileptic encephalopathies or EE. As mentioned earlier, Dravet syndrome was the first of the genetic forms of EE to be described. Since then, other epileptic infantile encephalopathies have been proven to be genetic. The difference with Dravet syndrome is that the phenotype more commonly consists of infantile spasms *(Table I and Figure 1)*. Such genetic epileptic encephalopathies can be caused by mutations in i) X linked cyclin dependent kinase like-5 (CDKL5/STK9) gene causing X linked infantile spasms, mental retardation and clinical features that overlap Rett and Angelman EE (Weaving *et al.*, 2004); ii) X linked interneuron related transcription factor ARX causing EE with West syndrome, infantile spasms, spasticity, Partington syndrome (mental retardation, ataxia and dystonia), EEG multifocal spikes, EEG electrodecremental episodes, lissencephaly, and mental retardation (Stromme *et al.*, 2002; Kitamura *et al.*, 2002); iii) Xq22 gene SPRX2 that produces rolandic seizures associated with oral and speech dyspraxia and mental retardation or bilateral perisylvian polymicrogyria (Roll *et al.*, 2006); iv) X linked protocadherin 19 gene (PCDH19) in female limited epilepsy and mental retardation (Dibbens *et al.*, 2008; Depienne *et al.*, 2009); v) syntaxin binding protein 1 or STXBP1(MUNC18-1) causing early EIEE (Ohtahara syndrome) (Saitsu *et al.*, 2008, 2011); vi) deletion in the MAG12 gene in chromosome 7q11.23-q21.11 as mentioned above (Marshall *et al.*, 2008); and vii) dominant-negative mutations in alpha II spectrin (Saitsu *et al.*, 2010b).

De novo, X-linked and gain of function variants in Infantile Spasms and Lennox-Gastaut Syndrome

In 2013, Epi4K and EPGP Investigators searched for *de novo* mutations in two "classic" forms of EE: Infantile Spasms (IS) or West Syndrome and Lennox-Gastaut Syndrome (LGS). Exomes of 264 trios

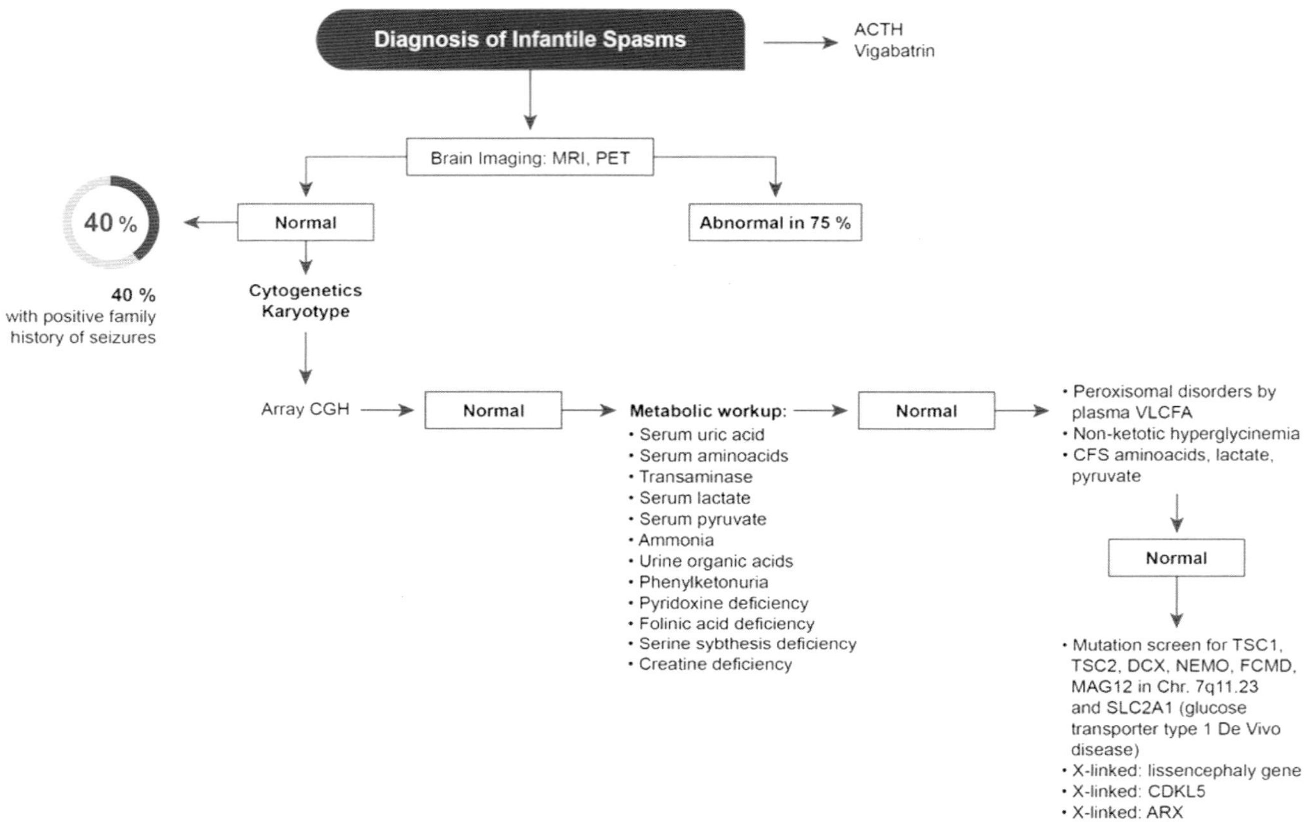

Figure 3

Diagnosis of infantile spasms.

were sequenced and 439 putative *de novo* mutations were identified. Sanger sequencing confirmed 329 *de novo* mutations. In these 264 trios, nine genes with *de novo* SNV mutations were present in two or more probands (*SCN1A* n = 7, *STXBP1* n = 5, *GABRB3* n = 4, *CDKL5* n = 3, *SCN8A* n = 2, *SCN2A n* = 2, *ALG13* n = 2, *DNM1 n* = 2, and *HDAC4* n = 2). Amongst these nine genes, *SCN1A*, *STXBP1*, *SCN8A*, *SCN2A*, and *CDKL5* have previously been associated with EE.[8]

Investigators claim that they had implicated, for the first time, "*GABRB* as a single gene cause of EE and provide the strongest evidence yet available for any epilepsy" based on i) four unique *de novo* mutations in *GABRB3*; ii) the absence of similar *de novo* mutations in 610 control exomes; iii) a computational modeling of these genes associated with EE having low tolerance for protein-disrupting mutations and producing adverse phenotypic consequences. They used the same reasoning to implicate *ALG13*, an X-linked gene encoding a subunit of the uridine diphosphate-N-acetylglucosamine transferase, which had been reported in two earlier studies of severe intellectual disability and seizures.

In 2017, Hamdan *et al.* combined three strategies during a search for *de novo* mutations in persons with develomental and epileptic encephalopathy (DEE): i) they identified candidate variants with *de novo* mutations during whole genome sequencing of 197 individuals with both epilepsy and intellectual disability; ii) they identified additional individuals with the same candidate variants in another series; iii) they combined several datasets of developmental and epileptic encephalopathy and intellectual disability. By combining these strategies, these authors suggested a causal link between DEE and *NTRK2*, *GABRB2*, *CLTC*, *DHDDS*, *NUS1*, *RAB11A*, *GABBR2*, and *SNAP25*. Overall, a molecular diagnosis was established in 63/197 (32%) of individuals who were whole genome sequenced.

The importance of *GABRB3 mutations with regards to causality in simple febrile seizures*, genetic epilepsies with febrile seizures plus, epilepsy with myoclonic-atonic seizures, West syndrome and other types of severe, early-onset epileptic encephalopathies were emphasized further by Moller *et al.* (2017) who identified 22 patients with heterozygous mutations in *GABRB3*, Electrophysiologic analysis of 7 *GABRB3*, mutations in Xenopus laevis oocytes, using coexpression of wild-type or mutant β_3, together with α_5 and γ_{2s} subunits and an automated 2-microelectrode voltage-clamp system, revealed reduced GABA-induced current amplitudes or GABA sensitivity for 5 of 7 mutations.

Epileptic seizure types, a varying degree of intellectual disability and developmental delay, sometimes with dysmorphic features or nystagmus have also been associated with variants in GABRA3 encoding the α3-subunit of the GABAA receptor of chromosome Xq28 (Niturad *et al.*, 2017).

Aristaless-related homeobox X-linked gene (ARX) which results in defective GABAergic interneuronal migration has also been observed in in infants with West syndrome (Katsarou *et al.*, 2017).

More recently, an autosomal–recessive DEE was associated with biallelic variants in PTPN23, which encodes a tyrosine phosphatase (Sowada *et al.*, 2017). Myers *et al.* (2017) identified six individuals with DEE harboring a *de novo* mutation in PPP3Ca, which encodes the alpha isoform of calcineurin (a calcium and calmodulin dependent serine/threonine phosphatase).

A cohort of 23 patients with epileptic encephalopathy carrying loss or gain of function *KCNA2* mutations was reported by Masnada *et al.* (2017). The more severe epilepsy, developmental problems and ataxia, and atrophy of the cerebellum or even the whole brain was observed in about half of the patients with gain-of-function mutations. Saitsu *et al.* (2016b) described the phenotypic spectrum of GNAO1 variants in epileptic encephalopathy with involuntary movements.

Malignant migrating partial seizures in infancy (MMPSI)

In 1995, Coppola et al. described healthy infants without cerebral dysplasia who develop within the first 6 months multifocal seizures that arise sequentially and independently from both cerebral hemispheres. Intractable seizures led to severe psychomotor retardation with 28% mortality. McTague et al. (2013) were the first to associate variants in sodium activated potassium channel or KCNT1 with two patients with MMPSI. Since then, pathogenic variants in KCNT1 have been reported in 50% of cases while single or two case series have been reported with *de novo* GABRB3 variants, SCN2A variants, SCN1A variants, and SMC1A (structural maintenance of chromosome 1A) variants in X chromosome, that encode a structural component of the cohesin complex. MMPS! has also been associated with compound heterozygous constellation consisting of a maternally inherited p.Ser399Leu and a *de novo* p.Arg880Leu in *SLC12A5*, which encodes the neuronal KCC2 cotransporter and compound heterozygous mutation of *TBC1D24* gene (p.Gln207*, p.Ala289Va). Saitsu *et al.* (2016a) sequenced whole exomes of ten sporadic and one familial case of MMPSI and observed compound heterozygous *SLC12A5* (encoding the neuronal K(+)-Cl(-) co-transporter *KCC2*) variants in two families: c.279 + 1G>C causing skipping of exon 3 in the transcript (p.E50_Q93del) and c.572 C>T (p.A191V) in individuals 1 and 2, and c.967T >C (p.S323P) and c.1243 A>G (p.M415V) in individual 3. Zhou *et al.* (2018) screened 70 patients with EE and found KCNT1, KCNQ2 and CLCN4 were most common in MMPSI. Milligan, (2014) studied Xenopus laevis oocyte transfected with 7 different MMPS! by single cell patch clamp and illustrated gain of function properties normalized by quinidine. Abdelnour (2018) reported four cases of MMPSI whose seizures were reduced by quinidine.

Dravet syndrome

***For repeating or prolonged febrile seizures in the first year of life, genotype for* SCN1A, SCN2A, SCN8A, SCN9A *and* PCDH19**

In the 1970s, Dravet and Bureau observed that some infants who presented with myoclonic seizures did not fulfill the criteria for the Lennox-Gastaut syndrome (LGS) (Dravet, 1965; Gastaut *et al.*, 1966). These patients had varying seizure phenotypes and an especially large spectrum of outcomes (Genton *et al.*, 2005). This led them to separate these infants from the LGS. They noted that most infants had repeated and prolonged febrile seizures in the first year of life, prolonged clonic seizures during sleep, and later myoclonus, plus a variety of other seizure types. By the second year, cognitive decline was evident often leading to mental deterioration and severe retardation. The patients did not have generalized tonic seizures, or drop attacks and the prominent sleep-related EEG changes (runs of rapid spikes and slow variety of diffuse spike waves) so characteristic of LGS. They called the syndrome "severe myoclonic epilepsy in infancy" or SMEI (Dravet, 1978; Dalla Bernardina *et al.*, 1982). Originally considered rare, SMEI was first reported to occur in 1 in 20,000 to 1 in 40,000 of the population (Yakoub *et al.*, 1992). By 1999, SMEI was found in 8% of seizures during the first year of life (Dravet *et al.*, 2005, 2005a; Hattori *et al.*, 2008).

When Claes *et al.* (2001) reported that *de novo* mutations in SCN1A caused a majority of isolated sporadic SMEI, it showed that sporadic epileptic encephalopathies of infancy can be genetic. Practitioners presently confirm the clinical diagnosis of Dravet's syndrome by the presence of *de novo* mutations in *SCN1A* (70%) (Claes *et al.*, 2001; Marini *et al.*, 2007), *SCN9A* (8%) (Singh *et al.*, 2009) and in proto-cadherin 19 gene or *PCDH19* (5%) (Dibbens *et al.*, 2008; Depienne *et al.*, 2009; Marini *et al.*, 2010) *(Table V)*. There are rare reports of mutations in *SCN1B* and *SCN2A* in Dravet syndrome. *SCN1A* is currently the most common epilepsy gene commercially screened because, for the community neurological practitioner, a mutation in *SCN1A* underpins the clinical diagnosis of Dravet syndrome. It remains perhaps the most important clinical advance in ion channelopathies because the mutation is *de novo*, and the epilepsy is sporadic and relatively frequent among channelopathies. Dravet syndrome is infrequently familial (5%).

"Targeted Sequencing" of *SCN1A* is the primary test as it detects mutations in 70–80% of Dravet syndrome. More than 630 novel mutations spread throughout the gene, and 95% are *de novo* (Mulley *et al.*, 2005; Ferraro *et al.*, 2006). Small chromosomal rearrangements involving *SCN1A* and contagious genes are also on record to be associated with Dravet syndrome. The alterations range from large deletions including *SCN1A* and several contiguous genes to single *SCN1A* exon deletions. *SCN1A* cryptic genomic deletions are rare and range from 607 kb to 4.7 Mb in size (Marini *et al.*, 2009; Wang *et al.*, 2008). Multiplex ligation-dependent probe amplification (MLPA) is a rapid, highly sensitive and relatively economical diagnostic tool that detects all copy number variations of *SCN1A* from the megabase range to one exon. Sequencing fails to detect a *SCN1A* mutation in about 10%. In the latter clinical situation, MLPA can be positive and clinch the diagnosis.

Nearly 300 *de novo* mutations in *SCN1A* have been described in other epilepsies but in Dravet syndrome, the variants are largely of paternal origin (Heron *et al.*, 2007). *SCN1A* has 26 exons in 100 kb genome. The *de novo* mutations in *SCN1A* include nonsense mutations and frameshifts (52–70%); 12–27% are missense mutations (Claes *et al.*, 2001; Fugiwara *et al.*, 2003, 2006; Ohmori *et al.*, 2002, 2003; Oguni *et al.* 2001, 2005; Nabbout *et al.*, 2003; Wallace *et al.*, 2003; Harkin *et al.*, 2007; Marini *et al.*, 2007). Nonsense and frameshift mutations cluster in the C terminus and loop between segments 5 and 6 of the first three domains of *SCN1A*. The 12–27% missense mutations occupy the voltage sensor of *SCN1A*. Ceulemans *et al.* (2004) and Kanai *et al.* (2004) observed that missense mutations around the pore-forming region and around the voltage sensor region were more likely to produce the most severe phenotype.

Kim *et al.* (2018) studied GABAergic neurons derived from induced pluripotent stem cells from fibroblasts of Dravet patients. Interestingly, a missense mutation, c.4261G-had more severe symptoms than a nonsense frameshift mutation, c.3576_3580 del TCAAA [GenBank: NM_006920.4]. Electrophysiologic recordings showed significantly lower sodium current density and reduced action potential frequency at strong current injection (> 60-pA) in GABAergic neurons derived from both Dravet patients.

Five percent of *SCN1A* mutations are also found in other family members. Such family members more commonly have the GEFS+ phenotypes; and less frequently they also have SMEI. Mosaic mutations of SCN1A have been rarely observed in several SMEI patients who manifest a milder form of the SMEI phenotype.

SCN9A *can cause or modify Dravet syndrome:* After finding a missense mutation (p.N641Y) in a highly conserved amino acid within the cytoplasmic loop between transmembrane domains I and II of *SCN9A* in 21 affected members of a large Utah family with febrile seizures, Singh *et al.* (2009) further analyzed 92 unrelated febrile seizure patients and found missense variants in 5% of patients. Singh *et al.* (2009) then extended their analyses to 109 Dravet syndrome patients and found missense variants in 9 patients (8%), all in highly conserved amino acids. Six of these 9 Dravet syndrome patients with *SCN9A* mutations also had missense or splice site mutations in *SCN1A*, providing for the first time mutational evidence for a modifying digenic mechanism for a human epilepsy. Three Dravet syndrome patients had only *SCN9A* mutations and no *SCN1A* mutation. These studies by Singh *et al.* (2009) provides evidence for SCN9A as a cause for febrile seizures, as a cause for Dravet syndrome, and as a modifying gene for *SCN1A* mutations *("two hit hypotheses")* in some Dravet syndrome patients. Until the reports by Singh *et al.* (2009), *SCN9A* had been previously classified as a peripheral nervous system channel-SCN9A encodes Nav1.7 which is primarily expressed in neurons of the dorsal root ganglion and brain. Disease associated mutations in *SCN9A* are observed in three inherited pain disorders, namely, autosomal dominant primary erytheromalgia, paroxysmal extreme pain disorder and autosomal recessive insensitivity to pain.

PCDH19, *the protocadherin 19 gene:* Dibbens *et al.* (2008) first reported X-linked PCDH19 as the disease causing gene for female limited epilepsy and cognitive impairment in six large families and one small family with two affected sib pairs. Independently, Depienne *et al.* (2009) observed point mutations in *PCDH19* in 11 unrelated females with clinical features similar to Dravet syndrome. Depienne *et al.* (2009) had initially identified a whole *PCDH19* gene deletion in a mosaic male patient with Dravet syndrome. The same authors (Depienne *et al.*, 2009) and others (Marini *et al.*, 2010) since calculate that mutations in PCDH19 could account for 5% of Dravet syndrome patients. Higurashi (2013) reduced clusters of seizures in PCDH19 Dravet syndrome by IV methylprednisolone while Lotte (2016) had some success (50% reduction) with clobazam in 68% of PCDH19 Dravet syndrome.

Aside from febrile seizure before 7 months of age, in what other clinical settings does the practitioner genotype* SCN1A, SCN9A *and* PCDH19*?

SCN1A and SCN9A should be genotyped by the community neurological practitioner in three clinical settings besides febrile seizures that start between 6 to 12 months of age and that are repeated or prolonged or evolve to convulsive status epilepticus. The three other settings include: i) when intractable grand mal tonic clonic or clonic tonic clonic seizures that start during infancy and into the second year of life (peripheral or borderline SMEI or SMEB) (Fugiwara *et al.*, 2003); ii) when an epileptic encephalo-pathy is blamed on vaccine encephalopathy as in post pertussis vaccine encephalopathy (Berkovic *et al.*, 2006); and iii) when the start and origins of refractory epilepsy and mild mental retardation in an adult can be traced to infancy and the early story during infancy is consistent with SMEI (adults with SMEI or SMEB) (Jansen *et al.*, 2006). In other words, when the practitioner suspect Dravet syndrome, genotype!

Because of early and correct diagnosis by genotyping of *SCN1A* or *SCN9A* mutations, the avoidance of sodium channel blockers as treatment, and aggressive treatment of prolonged convulsive status, there is hope that, in future, the Dravet syndrome may be less severe than observed in all past reports. Today, once the presence of *SCN1A* mutations are confirmed in the first year of life, sodium channel blockers, such as phenytoin, carbamazepine, oxcarbazepine and lamotrigine, should be avoided (Ceulemans *et al.*, 2004). These antiepileptic drugs are known to aggravate seizures and cause status epilepticus (Guerrini *et al.*, 1998). Status epilepticus, in turn, is suspected to contribute to if not cause the severity of mental retardation and death in Dravet's SMEI. Status epilepticus is listed as a cause of death in the series of Dravet (1992) and in the series of Sakauchi *et al.* (2011). Aggressive and acute seizure treatment with intravenous benzodiazepines, rigorous treatment of fever, prevention of hyperthermia, and maintenance of chronic treatment using combination antiepileptic drug treatment, such as valproate plus stiripentol (Chiron *et al.*, 2000) or valproate plus levetiracetam or valproate plus topiramate or valproate plus ketogenic diet (Guerrini *et al.*, 1998a, 1998b; Striano *et al.*, 2007; Ceulemans *et al.*, 2004; Korff *et al.*, 2007; Caraballo *et al.*, 2005) and most recently valproate plus cannabidiol (Devinsky *et al.*, 2017) are recommended. Since one-half to two-thirds of mutations are nonsense mutations, there is a 6% to 15.9% mortality rate (Dravet *et al.*, 1992; Sakauchi *et al.*, 2011) and all patients have some cognitive deficits by 2 years of age, a study trial with a premature stopcodon drug, such as IV gentamicin or oral "read through drugs like Exondys" that cross the blood brain barrier and even gene replacement therapy using adeno-associated virus serotype 9 should be conducted in the future.

Dravet syndrome cuts into the heterogeneous nature of febrile seizures in two ways: it proved the existence of genetic epileptic encephalopathies, and it gave practical importance to genotyping and separating Dravet syndrome from complex febrile seizures and GEFS+ syndrome. Between 1996 to the present, six separate chromosome loci have been reported for familial febrile seizures: FEB1 in 8q13–21, FEB2 in 19p, FEB3 in 2q23–24, FEB4 in 5q14-q15, FEB5 in 6q22–24 and FEB6 in 18p11. In 2009, Singh *et al.* identified the FEB3 gene to be *SCN9A*. These investigators further showed that 5% of unrelated febrile seizure patients from Utah had missense mutations in *SCN9A*.

After one of the children with febrile seizures later developed Dravet syndrome, they sequenced the *SCN1A* gene and found a heterozygous frameshift mutation. Further analyses of 109 Dravet syndrome patients found 8% to have missense mutations in *SCN9A*. Six Dravet syndrome patients had both *SCN9A* missense variants and missense or splice site *SCN1A* mutations.

GEFS+ and febrile seizures

More than 160 families have now been studied with GEFS, the acronym now standing for the newer term "Genetic Epilepsy with febrile seizures plus", as suggested by Schefer and Berkovic, who originally described the syndrome in 1997 (Zhang *et al.*, 2017). The latter authors recommend molecular genotyping for individuals with GEFS+ phenotypes. Thus, at present, we recommend genotyping for GEFS+ genes of major effects (*SCN1A*, *SCN2A*, *SCN1B*, *SCN9A*, *GABRg2* and *STX1B* are found in 31%) and GEFS+ susceptibility alleles (GABRD, CACNA1H, HCN2 719–722 de; PPP are found in 18%) because the genotype of GEFS+ may dictate its treatment. *SCN8A* mutation has been observed in a severely affected son with EE. The father had FS+ and was 13% mosaic for an SCN8A mutation.

The range of phenotypes within the GEFS+ spectrum has also been expanded. Afebrile generalized tonic-clonic seizures and focal seizures alone can occur in GEFS+ families although febrile seizures alone remain the most common GEFS+ seizure phenotype (44%). Febrile seizures plus is the second most common phenotype (27%). Febrile seizures or febrile seizures plus can occur with absence, myoclonic, or atonic seizures. MAE can be present in families with GEFS+.

In very specific circumstances where families want to confirm inheritance in family planning, screening for mutations in family members is an option during the early course of the illness in infancy. It helps separate the severe phenotype of Dravet syndrome from the generally favorable prognosis of GEFS+ and simple febrile seizures and other epilepsy syndromes rarely associated with *SCN1A* mutations (Colosimo *et al.*, 2007; Grosso *et al.*, 2007; Sugawara *et al.*, 2001, 2002).

Genetic testing for epilepsies in childhood and adolescence

Epilepsy in children with chromosome abnormalities

Why and when should physicians karyotype and test with array comparative genomic hybridization (Array-CGH) (Kim *et al.*, 2007; Singh *et al.*, 2002; Battaglia & Guerrini, 2005; Battaglia *et al.*, 1997; Bingham *et al.*, 1998; Macleod *et al.*, 2005; Schinzel & Niedrist, 2001)? Testing should be done when mental retardation is unexplained and/or when multiple dysmorphisms and anomalies are present.

Knowledge of the specific chromosome disorder (chromosomopathy) after genotyping when coupled with specific electroclinical syndromes improves the clinician's knowledge of the child's response to antiepileptic treatment as well as the child's prognosis and treatment outcomes *(Table III)*. This knowledge helps plan rational treatments and allows better genetic counseling of the families. These chromosome abnormalities are not a frequent cause of epilepsies, but specific chromosomopathies have higher risks for epilepsies, some with characteristic but not pathognomonic electroclinical presentations.

Table III lists some chromosome disorders that are associated with characteristic electroclinical patterns. Most notable are infantile spasms with high amplitude 8 to 20 Hz fast rhythms (not hypsarrythmia) associated with either a deletion in chromosome 17p13.3 or Miller Dieker syndrome (Dobyns *et al.*, 1993; Mantel *et al.*, 1994) or interstitial deletion of chromosome 14q with agenesis of corpus callosum (Ouertani *et al.*, 1995; Lippe & Sparkes, 1981). The combination of atypical absence status or nonconvulsive status epilepticus with diffuse 2–3 Hz slow wave/s and spikes of possible mesial frontal origin, behavioral restlessness and aggression, mild to moderate mental retardation appearing around 6 years of age, after an apparently normal development in the first 5 years, without dysmorphic features should point the practitioner to Ring chromosome 20 syndrome (Inoue *et al.*, 1997). In intellectually normal persons with the ring 20 syndrome, epilepsy is the usual presenting complaint. Fluorescent *in situ* hybridization with chromosome 20 specific probes show loss of telomeric regions in both arms of chromosome 20 which results in formation of the ring. All evidence indicates drug resistant seizures in all cases of ring chromosome 20 syndrome.

The appearance of focal motor and unilateral seizures and status epilepticus between the 6th and 12th months of age, often triggered by fever or hot baths, followed by atypical absences and myoclonias on eye closure, atypical slow spike wave complexes on EEGs and runs of sharp waves in centroparietal and occipital regions regions in profoundly retarded infants and children should suggest hemizygous deletion of distal short arm of chromosome 4p16.3 (Wolf-Hirschhorn syndrome) or deletion in chromosome 15q11–13 (Angelman syndrome). In both syndromes, deletions of chromosome regions harboring clusters of GABR subunits (alpha-2, alpha-4 and gamma1 in chromosome 4p16.3; and beta3, alpha-5 and gamma3 in chromosome 15q11–13) are thought to reduce GABA inhibition and produce the epilepsy phenotypes.

All developmentally delayed males must be screened for Fragile-X syndrome

At chromosome Xq27.3 are mutations in the FMR-1 gene due to expansion of a CGG trinucleotide repeat in exon 1 (Verkerk *et al.*, 1991). Learning disorders, delayed speech, hypotonic, hypere-lastic joints, macroorchidism, narrow, long face, large ears with small mandibles in a hyperactive or autistic child with focal epilepsy should point the clinician to the Fragile-X syndrome.

Mutations in the GABA transporter SLC6A1 cause epilepsy with myoclonic-atonic seizures (Doose syndrome)

Onset between 7 months and 6 years of age, the syndrome of myoclonic-astatic (also called myoclonic-atonic), absence, atonic and tonic seizures had been classified as a childhood idiopathic generalized epilepsy, partly derived from what was called Doose syndrome. In 2015, Carvill *et al.* identified six GABA transporter/SLC6A1 mutations in seven individuals with myoclonic atonic seizures when target sequencing 644 individuals with epileptic encephalopathies. Johannesen *et al.* (2018) reviewed the phenotypes of 34 persons with pathogenic SLC6A1 variants. The most common seizure phenotypes were absence, myoclonic and atonic seizures. Sixteen of 34 cases fulfilled diagnostic criteria of myoclonic-atonic epilepsy. Cognitive development was impaired in 97%; 28/34 had mild to moderate intellectual disability, with language impairment being the most common feature. Epilepsy was diagnosed in 31/34 cases with mean onset at 3.7 years. Palmer *et al.* (2016) described a ten-year-old girl with myoclonic-atonic seizures and a *de novo SLC6A1* mutation (c.491G>A; p.Cys164Tyr), who responded well to the ketogenic diet. These observations should rekindle the debate of whether the myoclonic atonic epilepsy should be called Doose syndrome.

Genetic testing in absence epilepsies (AE): Separate Glut1 (SLC2A1) variants and Glut2 (SLC45A1) from GABR and CaV2.1 (P/Q type) or CaV3.2 (T-type) variants to decide best treatment *(Table VI)*

Separating Glut1 (Glucose transporter type 1 gene or SLC2A1 for soluble carrier 2A1) and GLUT2 (Glucose transporter type 2 gene or SLC45A1 for soluble carrier 45A1) (Srour *et al.*, 2017) mutations from

GABR mutations and CaV2.1 or Cav3.2 mutations in (a) early childhood absence epilepsy (AE) that starts below 5 years of age, and (b) when absence is intractable to valproate and ethosuximide helps the clinician devise strategies for treatment. Absence epilepsy of all ages can also but rarely be an atypical presentation of the glucose transporter deficiency syndrome also called DeVivo syndrome (Wang *et al.*, 2002). Ten percent of early childhood AE is due to Glut1 deficiency (Suls *et al.*, 2009a,b; Chaix *et al.*, 2003) and AE may be the only complaint starting at 2 to 3 years of age. Most heterozygous mutations in SLC2A are *de novo* but may be transmitted as an autosomal dominant or recessive trait. SLC45A1 mutations were observed in two consanguineous multiple families with severe intellectual disability and epilepsy (Srour *et al.*, 2017). Aside from absence seizures, the child may have mild learning disabilities and mild motor delay. When mild gait problems are also present with rare to infrequent dystonia or paroxysmal exertion induced dyskinesia, the full spectrum of DeVivo syndrome comes to mind. In the full and typical spectrum of DeVivo syndrome, acquired microcephaly and spasticity is present with psychomotor delay starting from infancy. Affected infants appear normal at birth following uneventful pregnancy and delivery. Apneic episodes and abnormal episodic eye movements like opsoclonus may precede onset of absences.

Because of a failure to transport glucose across the blood brain barrier (BBB), CSF glucose measures usually less than 2.5 mM/liter or hypoglycorrhachia. A low CSF glucose with a decreased CSF lactate level indicates impairment of the glucose transporter gene. A lumbar puncture or the erythrocyte glucose uptake assay (Yang *et al.*, 2011) provides the diagnostic clue to Glut1 deficiency and can reduce diagnostic delay and allow the early start of ketogenic diet. Genotyping for the confirmatory diagnosis of Glut1 deficiency is therefore crucial because antiepileptic drug treament with valproate and ethosuximide is inadequate to stop seizures while the ketogenic diet or modified Adkin's diet is effective. Ketogenic diet stops seizures in 86%, reduces movement disorders in 48% to 71%, and helps psychomotor development (Ito *et al.*, 2008, 2011; Leen *et al.*, 2010; Wang *et al.*, 2002). Ketones provided by a high fat, low carbohydrate diet, serve as an alternative fuel to the brain. Novel compounds such as alpha-lipoic acid and triheptanoin are being studied as alternatives for ketogenic diet (Klepper, 2011). Failure to grow in height may be helped by growth hormone replacement in Glut1 deficiency because of severe growth hormone deficiency (Nakagama *et al.*, 2012).

Treatment for AE due to GABRalpha-1 (Cossette *et al.*, 2002), GABRgamma2 (Kananura *et al.*, 2002), GABRdelta and GABRbeta3 (Tanaka *et al.*, 2008) can start with clonazepam or clobazam while AE due to calcium channel mutations (CaV2.1) can start treatment with ethozuximide or valproate. Zhang, Lian and Xie (2017) identified a novel nonsense mutation (C.5G>A) in the exon 1 of GABRB3 Gene, associated with EOEE in a girl who developed multiple seizure types including myoclonic seizures, spasms, and absence seizures at 3 days of life. Through a 9-month follow up, the girl remained seizure-free with 0.5mgs of clonazepam orally. Kass, (2016) reported ketogenic diet caused 18 of 82 (46%) to be free of seizures and 66 of 83 (80%) > 90% reduction of seizures in SLC2A1 deficient patients with seizures.

For clarification of diagnosis, to separate nocturnal phenomenon and sleep disorders from autosomal dominant nocturnal frontal lobe epilepsy (ADNFLE), and clarify the genotyoe of familial focal epilepsies

In 1995, Steinlein *et al.* identified a missense mutation *(S248F)* that replaced serine with phenylalanine at codon 248 in the second transmembrane domain of neuronal nicotinic acetylcholine receptor alpha-4subunit (*CHRNA4* in chr.20q13.2) that segregated in 21 affected family members of a large Australian kindred with ADNFLE. It represented a turning point in understanding epilepsy since, for the first time, an idiopathic epilepsy was proven to have a genetic mutation. Since then, several more mutations *(776ins3, S252L,+L264, S256L, T265I)* in *CHRNA4* (Steinlein *et al.*, 1997) and three mutations *(V287L, V287M, I312M)* in *CHRNB2* (De Fusco *et al.*, 2000; Phillips *et al.*, 2001a, 2001b; Bertrand *et al.*, 2005; Diaz-Otero *et al.*, 2008), in *CHRNA2* and in the corticotrophin releasing hormone *(CRH)* and unidentified genes in four other chromosome loci (pericentromeric region of chromosome 1 (Gambardella *et al.*, 2000), chr. 15q24 (Phillipps *et al.*, 1998, 2000, 2001), chr 3p22–24 and chr. 8q11.2-q21.1 (Combi *et al.*, 2004) have been found in autosomal dominant nocturnal frontal lobe epilepsy. Physiological investigations of the receptor reconstituted with the mutated CH RNA4subunit or the mutated CHNRB2 show increased affinity to acetylcholine except for S256L and significantly lower permeability to calcium. This suggested that increasing CHRN alpha-4beta2 mediated glutamate release at central neuronal excitatory synapses is responsible for inducing seizures (Kuryatov *et al.*, 1997; Matsushima *et al.*, 2002; Rodrigues-Pinguet *et al.*, 2003).

Klaassen *et al.* (2006) engineered two mouse strains that harbored the ADNFLE *CHRNA4 S252F* and *+L264* mutant alleles and hypothesized an intriguing but opposite concept, namely, enhanced GABAergic inhibition as the basis of cortical synchrony, interictal spiking and spontaneous seizures in ADNFLE. Their data showed that both S252F and +L264 mutations were inherited as dominant mutations that caused cortical EEG abnormalities, spikes and spontaneous seizures in heterozygous mice. Whole cell voltage clamp recordings of spontaneous excitatory and inhibitory postsynaptic currents were obtained from layer II/III pyramidal tract cells. Low dose and non-convulsant doses of picrotoxin, a use-dependent antagonist of GABR, ameliorated EEG abnormalities and suppressed spontaneous seizures. Nicotine significantly increased both frequencies and amplitude of inhibitory postsynaptic currents in CHRNA4 S252F pyramidal tract cells while having no effects on wild type mice pyramidal tract cells. The observed increase in inhibitory currents is explained as an increased nicotine evoked GABA release from CHRNA4 S252 or +L264 expressing cortical interneurons that form synapses on soma, axon initial segments or dendrites of pyramidal cells.

In rare cases of drug resistant ADNFLE, these two hypotheses, namely, glutamate release *versus* enhanced GABA currents, should be considered by the clinician when designing a treatment strategy.

Since the first descriptions of ADNFLE, *KCNT1* has also been associated with ADNFLE and several more autosomal dominant focal epilepsies with their respective genotypes have been described namely familial temporal lobe epilepsy with auditory features or FTLE (neuronal secreted protein: LGI1-encoding protein), familial focal epilepsy with variable focio or FFEVF (mTOR–repressor DEPDC5: DEP domain-containing protein 5. DEPDC5 is now claimed to be the more common cause of inherited focal epilepsies, which include ADNFLE, FTLE and FFEVF.

Genetic testing in the epilepsy-aphasia spectrum disorder

The epilepsy-aphasia spectrum (EAS) is a continuum of genetic epilepsy syndromes with EEG focal sharp waves, and various speech and language disorders. At one end is the common Rolandic epilepsy (RE), frequently associated with speech and oromotor deficits, as well as reading disability, attention, and memory problems. Focal seizures commonly occur during sleep with blunt centrotemporal spikes. Atypical benign partial epilepsy is much more rare, have more severe seizures with regression of speech, motor skills and attention. The epileptic encephalopathy of continuous spike-and-waves during slow-wave sleep (ECSWS) and Landau-Kleffner syndrome (LKS) are both debilitating and more severe, and are at the less-frequent end of the spectrum. There is marked loss of receptive and expressive language in children who develop LKS.

The first reports of *GRIN2A* mutations in the Epilepsy-Aphasia Spectrum disorders came in 2012 from Szepetowski's group in Aix-Marseille University Inserm U901 (Lesca *et al.*, 2012). Replication of results came from Carvill and Mefford from Seattle and Scheffer from Australia in 2013 (Carvill *et al.*, 2013; von Stulpnagel *et al.*, 2017), who retrospectively, studied 19 patients with epilepsy and *GRIN2A* alteration emphasizing results of epilepsy treatment. Patients were treated with a mean of 5.6 AED. 4/5 patients with VPA had an improved seizure frequency (n = 3 with a truncation: n = 1 missense). 3/5 patients with STM reported an improvement of seizures (n = 2 truncation, n = 1 splicing). 3/5 CLB patients showed an improvement (n = 2: truncation; n = 1 splicing). Steroids were reported to have a positive effect on seizure frequency in 3/5 patients (n = 1 each truncation, splicing or deletion).

Genetic testing in genetically complex common epilepsies

To date, replication of genetic variants that contribute to epilepsy susceptibility of genetically complex epilepsies has been hard to find (Cavalleri *et al.*, 2007a, 2007b). The strongest case for SNP allele association with an epilepsy syndrome has been the *BRD2*-JME connection which could be an epigenetic phenomenon. Greenberg and collaborators have generated a murine model whose *Brd2* haploinsufficiency produces characteristics that typify the clinical hallmarks of human JME. No JME-related *BRD2* coding mutations have ever been found. Instead Greenberg's group investigated non-coding *BRD2* regions, like a CpG (C-phosphate-G dinucleotides) island (CpG76), "hotspot" for JME-associated epigenetic variants. Methylating promoter CpG sites causes gene silencing, often resulting in reduced gene expression. They tested differences in DNA methylation at 10 *BRD2* promoter CpG sites in lymphoblastoid cells from 3 different subgroups: i) JME patients *versus* their unaffected family members; ii) JME *versus* patients with other forms of GGE, and iii) Caucasian *versus* non-Caucasian JME patients. These investigators found that CpG76 is highly methylated in JME patients compared to unaffected family members. In families with non-JME GGE, they found no relationship between promoter methylation and epilepsy. In non-Caucasian JME families, promoter methylation was mostly not associated with epilepsy. This makes the *BRD2* promoter a JME-specific, ethnicity-specific, differentially methylated region (Pathak *et al.*, 2018).

Microdeletions in chromosome 15q13.3 genetically associate with 1% of patients with idiopathic generalized epilepsies (Dibbens *et al.*, 2009; Helbig *et al.*, 2009). How meaningful and practical this observation is in clinical management of idiopathic generalized epilepsies is presently unknown.

In clinical settings where the diagnosis is clear, where there is low clinical utility produced by heterogeneity, where test results offer little advantage over empiric risk assessment based on family history and where finding a mutation would not alter the course of treatment and would have little bearing on genetic and prognostic counseling, routine testing of patients with genetically complex familial idiopathic epilepsies, is not recommended. For examples, BRD2, ME2 and ELP4 have been genetically associated with JME and rolandic epilepsy but causative mutations did not segregate with affected members in multiple generations. Genotyping in these syndromes remain largely a research tool.

Genotyping separates progressive from non-progressive syndromes in late childhood and adolescent myoclonic epilepsy and help with choice of treatment

Genotyping adolescent myoclonic epilepsies will separate Lafora disease (LD or Lafora progressive myoclonus epilepsy or Lafora PME) (Serratosa, 1999; Minassian *et al.*, 1998; Chan *et al.*, 2003; Ganesh *et al.*, 2002; Tagliabracci *et al.*, 2008; Rao *et al.*, 2010) and Unverricht-Lundborg disease (ULD or UL PME) (Alakurtti *et al.*, 2005; deHaan *et al.*, 2004; Joensuu *et al.*, 2008; Lafrenierre *et al.*, 1997; Lalioti *et al.*, 1997a, 1997b; Pennachio *et al.*, 1996; Berkovic *et al.*, 2005) from juvenile myoclonic epilepsy (JME) (Suzuki *et al.*, 2004). Genotyping is especially indicated when myoclonias are stimuli-sensitive, when there is the possibility of consanguinity based on racial, ethnic and ancestral origin, when visual seizures are present or when EEG occipital spikes or hypometabolic occipital cortices are present on 2FDG PET scan of brain or when giant evoked potentials are recorded.

In their early and beginning stages, LD, ULD and JME can be clinically similar (Delgado-Escueta & Bourgeois, 2008). The identification of disease causing nonsense mutations in EPM2A or EPM2B of LD is important because nonsense mutations and their premature stop codon can be treated with premature stop codon readthrough drugs, such as IV gentamicin (Wagner *et al.*, 2001; Politano *et al.*, 2003; Welch *et al.*, 2007; Wilchanski *et al.*, 2003; Barton-Davis *et al.*, 1999; Brooks *et al.*, 2006; Clancy *et al.*, 2001). Theoretically, treatment in LD is best started when seizures are the only symptoms, before neurologic deterioration starts, and before ataxia and dementia set in, before independent daily living activities are lost, and certainly before the need for gastrostomy is realized. Approximately 25% of mutations in EPM2A (Laforin/DSP) and EPM2B (Malin/Ubiquitin E3 ligase) are nonsense mutations (Singh & Ganesh, 2009; Ianzano *et al.*, 2005).

An early diagnosis of JME due to myoclonin/EFHC1 means early use of valproate and avoidance of sodium channel blockers, such as phenytoin, carbamazepine, oxcarbazepine and lamotrigine (Biraben *et al.*, 2000; Carrazana & Wheeler, 2001). Mutations in SCARB2/LIMP-2 have been shown to be an important cause of PME resembling ULD (Berkovic *et al.*, 2008; Balreira *et al.*, 2008; Dibbens *et al.*, 2009). Separating SCARB2 or LIMB-2 mutation/ULD from cys-tatin B/ULD is important because the prognosis is worse in *SCARB2* mutations causing ULD than cystatin B mutations causing classical ULD (Dibbens *et al.*, 2009).

Can early Lafora PME and Unverricht-Lundborg PME be clinically distinguished from JME? Yes, a clinician experienced in PME can look for subtle clinical and EEG differences. However, genotyping will solidify and clarify diagnosis and also show if deletions, frameshifts, missense or nonsense mutations are present in Laforin/dual specificity phosphatase (Laforin/DSP) or Malin E3 Ubiquitin Ligase (Malin/E3UL) in Lafora PME. Genotyping is also crucial for early diagnosis in Lafora PME so treatment of nonsense mutations can begin early.

Genetic testing in sudden unexplained death in epilepsy

Sudden unexplained death refers to the sudden death of an otherwise healthy person with epilepsy usually occurring during or immediately after a tonic clonic seizure and often in sleep. It is the most frequent epilepsy related cause of death and is characterized by an absence of any identifiable cause of death at post-mortem, suggesting in many instances an inherited cardiac arrythmogenic predisposition. The risk of sudden unexplained death in epilepsy (SUDEP) is 20 times more than the risk of sudden unexplained death in the general population. Other mechanisms aside from cardiac arrhythmias suggested have been brain stem central respiratory depression, cerebral depression, and autonomic dysfunction (Aiba *et al.*, 2016). Risk factors that are statistically significant for SUDEP include frequent convulsions, polytherapy, epilepsy onset below 16 years of age, symptomatic/lesional cause and lamotrigine therapy (Hesdorfer *et al.*, 2011; Hirsch *et al.*, 2011).

When to genotype epilepsy patients for possible causes of SUDEP?

There are three clinical circumstances in which epilepsy patients should be genotyped to identify possible causes of SUDEP and reduce/prevent risks of same. The situations are as follows.

– *When the patient has epilepsy and a family history of sudden death or sudden infant death.*

When there is a family history of sudden infant death (autopsy negative sudden unexplained death prior to the first birthday) or sudden death after the first year of life or when the patient himself/herself has had repeated episodes of syncope or possible venricular fibrillation, then the patient should have an EKG and/or ECK Holter monitoring. Obtaining detailed history regarding cardiac events in the patient and his/her family members combined with the patient's standard 12 lead ECG with precise measurements of QT intervals and evaluation of T wave morphology is usually enough to recognize the congenital "long QT" syndrome. If necessary, ECG holter monitoring should be done. Cost analysis/effectiveness of screening the patient only *vs.* screening affected family members should be performed. The patient, then, and, subsequently, the other affected family members, if necessary, should be screened for the most frequent LTQS causing mutations (Tester *et al.*, 2005), such as *KCNQ1* (encodes alpha subunit of cardiac slowly activated delayed rectifier potassium channel) (Summers *et al.*, 2010), *KCNH2* (encodes the alpha subunit of the voltage gated potassium channel HERG, a rapid component of cardiac delayed rectifier potassium channel), *SCN5A* (encodes alpha-subunit of voltage gated sodium channel Nav1.5), *HCN2* and *HCN4* (hyperpolarization-activated cyclic nucleotide gated cation channels or HCN), and *KCNE1* and *KCNE2* (encodes auxilarry subunits of cardiac potassium channels), Rarely, LTQS causing mutations in CACNA1c (encodes L type calcium channel 1 c subunit), CAV3 (encodes caveolae 3, lipid rafts and membrane microdomains on cytoplasmic surface of sarcolemmal membrane where SCN5A localizes) (Vatta *et al.*, 2006), SCN4B (encodes auxillary beta 4 subunit of sodium channel) and Kir3.4 (encodes an inwardly rectifying potassium channel), can cause Brugada syndrome, long QT syndrome, catecholamineergic polymorphic ventricular tachycardia and short QT syndrome (Khan and Nair, 2004; Kaufman, 2009; Tu *et al.*, 2011; Shimizu & Horie, 2011; Kiehne & Kauferstein, 2007; Sakauchi *et al.* 2011; Medeiros-Domingo *et al.*, 2007; Vatta *et al.*, 2006; Crotti *et al.*, 2008; Gazzero *et al.*, 2011).

To treat epilepsy, sodium channel blockers, *e.g.*, phenytoin, carbamazepine, lamotrigine and oxcarbazepine, must be avoided since they can induce type I Brugada ECG patterns (QT prolongation and elevated ST segments in right precordial leads). Vagal nerve stimulators must also be avoided since it aggravates the ECG abnormalities. These patients must avoid really strenuous exercises. Molecular screening is now part of the diagnostic process for the LQTS. Treatment can begin with betablockers, unless contraindicated. If the patient has one more syncope despite full dosage of betablockers, an implantable cardioverter-defibrillator (ICD) should be considered with the final decision being based on individual patient characteristics that show high electrical instability. ICD is eventually the primary therapy (Crotti *et al.*, 2008). Anti-adrenergic therapy and quinidine may continue to be adjuncts. Levetiracetam, valproate and clobazam can be used to stop seizures.

– *When the patient has epilepsy and has survived an aborted cardiac arrest.*

This is not an unusual presentation for an epilepsy consultation, namely, a patient with epilepsy who has survived a cardiac arrest due to the long QT syndrome. The above list of more common LQTS causing mutations should be screened for Brugada syndrome, long QT syndrome, catecholaminergic polymorphic ventricular tachycardia and short QT syndrome. Similar precautions listed above, such as avoiding sodium channel blockers and vagal nerve stimulators and treatment with ICD, should be followed.

– *When the patient has Dravet syndrome.*

The incidence of sudden death and acute encephalopathy with status epilepticus in Dravet syndrome is 10% and peaks at 1 to 3 years of age and at 6 years of age. Because sudden death cause 50% of deaths in Dravet syndrome (Sakauchi *et al.*, 2011), a standard ECG, and if necessary ECG holter, should be performed, paying attention to heart rate variability and possible arrhythmias (Delogu *et al.*, 2011). In the presence of heart rate variability, or long QT syndrome, it is clinically prudent to screen for mutations in SCN5A or other more common LQTS causing mutations related to Brugada syndrome-long QT syndrome, catecholaminergic polymorphic ventricular tachycardia and short QT syndrome (Khan & Nair, 2004; Kaufman, 2009; Tu *et al.*, 2011; Shimizu & Horie, 2011; Kiehne & Kauferstein, 2007). The potential severity of the prognosis, namely, appearance of a cardiac asystole, justifies testing patients with Dravet syndrome with long QT intervals on the ECG and Holter monitor recording. Similar precautions listed above, such as avoiding sodium channel blockers and vagal nerve stimulators and treatment with ICD should be followed.

REFERENCES ▶

Abdelnour E, Gallentine W, McDonald M (2018): Does age affect response to quinidine in patients with KCNT1 mutations? Report of three new cases and review of the literature. *Seizure* 55: 1–3.

Aiba I, Wehrens XH, Noebels JL (2016): Leaky RyR2 channels unleash a brainstem spreading depolarization mechanism of sudden cardiac death. *Proc Natl Acad Sci USA* 113(33): E4895–903.

Alakurtti K, Weber E, Rinne R, *et al.* (2005): Loss of lysosomal association of cystatin B proteins representing progressive myoclonus epilepsy, EPM1, mutations. *Eur J Hum* Genet 13: 208–215.

Anangnostou ME, Ng YS Taylor RW, McFarland R (2016): Epilepsy due to mutations in the mitochondrial polymerase gamma (POLG) gene: A clinical and molecular genetic review. *Epilepsia* 57: 1531–1545.

Atkin TA, Maher CM, Gerlach AC, *et al.* (2018): A comprehensive approach to identifying repurposed drugs to treat SCN8A epilepsy. *Epilepsia* 59: 802–813.

Bailey JN, Patterson C, de Nijs L, *et al.* (2017): EFHC1 variants in juvenile myoclonic epilepsy: reanalysis according to NHGRI and ACMG guidelines for assigning disease causality. *Genet Med* 19: 144–156.

Bailey JN, de Nijs L, Bai D, *et al.* (2018): Variant Intestinal-Cell Kinase in Juvenile Myoclonic Epilepsy. *N Engl J Med* 15; 378: 1018–1028.

Bali B, Kull LL, Strug LJ, *et al.* (2007): Autosomal dominant inheritance of centrotemporal sharp waves in Rolandic epilepsy families. *Epilepsia* 48: 2266–2272.

Ballana E, Esté JA (2015). SAMHD1: at the crossroads of cell proliferation, immune responses, and virus restriction. *Trends Microbiol* 23: 680–692.

Balreira A, Gaspar P, Caiola D, *et al.* (2008): A nonsense mutation in the LIMP-2 gene associated with progressive myo-lonic epilepsy and nephritic syndrome. *Hum Mol* Genet 17: 2238–2243.

Barker RS, Ottolini M, Wagnon JL, *et al.* (2016): The SCN8A encephalopathy mutation p.Ile1327Val displays elevated sensitivity to the anticonvulsant phentyoin. *Epilepsia* 57: 1458–1466.

Barton-Davis ER, Cordier L, Shoturma DI, Leland SE, Sweeney HL (1999): Aminoglycoside antibiotics restore dystrophin function to skeletal muscles of mdx mice. *J Clin Invest* 104: 375–381.

Battaglia A, Guerrini R (2005): Chromosomal disorders associated with epilepsy. *Epileptic Disord* 7: 181–192.

Battaglia A, Gurrieri F, Bertini E, *et al.* (1997): The inv dup (15) syndrome: A clinically recognizable syndrome with altered behavior, mental retardation, and epilepsy. *Neurology* 48: 1081–1086.

Baulac S, Huberfeld G, Gourfinkel-An I, *et al.* (2001): First genetic evidence of GABAA receptor dysfunction in epilepsy: a mutation in the {gamma}2-subunit gene. *Nat Genet* 28: 46–48.

Berg AT, Berkovic SF, Brodie MJ, *et al.* (2010): Revised terminology and concepts for organization of seizures and epilepsies: reports of the ILAE commission on classification and terminology, 2005–2009. *Epilepsia* 51: 676–685.

Berkovic SF, Mazarib A, Walid S, *et al.* (2005): A clinical and molecular form of Unverricht-Lundborg disease localized by homozygosity mapping. *Brain* 128(pt 3): 652–658.

Berkovic SF, Harkin L, McMahon JM, *et al.* (2006): *De-novo* mutations of the sodium channel gene SCN1A in alleged vaccine encephalopathy: a retrospective study. *Lancet Neurol* 5: 488–492.

Berkovic SF, Dibbens LM, Oshlack A, *et al.* (2008): Array-based gene discovery with three unrelated subjects shows SCARB2/LIMP-2 deficiency causes myoclonus epilepsy and glome-rulosclerosis. *Am J Hum Genet* 82: 673–684.

Bertrand D, Elmslie F, Hughes E, *et al.* (2005): The CHRNB2 mutation I312M is associated with epilepsy and distinct memory deficits. *Neurobiol Dis* 20: 2799–2804.

Biervert C, Steinlein OK (1999): Structural and mutational analysis of KCNQ2, the major gene locus for benign familial neonatal convulsions. *Hum Genet* 104: 234–240.

Bievert C, Schroeder BC, Kubisch C, *et al.* (1998): A potassium channel mutation in neonatal human epilepsy. *Science* 279: 403–406.

Bingham PM, Lynch D, McDonald-McGinn D, Zackai E (1998): Polymicrogyria in chromosome 22 deletion syndrome. *Neurology* 51: 1500–1502.

Biraben A, Allain H, Scarabin JM, Schück S, Edan G (2000): Exacerbation of juvenile myoclonic epilepsy with lamotrigine. *Neurology* 55: 1758.

Blandfort ZM, Tsuboi T, Vogel F (1987): Genetic counseling in the epilepsies. I. Genetic risks. *Hum Genet* 76: 303–331.

Boerma RS, Braun KP, van den Broek MP *et al.* (2016): Remarkable phenytoin Sensitivity in 4 children with SCN8A-related epilepsy: A molecular neuropharmacological approach. *Neurotherapeutics* 13: 192–197.

Brooks DA, Muller VJ, Hopwood JJ (2006): Stop-codon read-through for patients affected by a lysosomal storage disorder. *Trends Mol Med* 12: 367–373.

Brunklaus A, Ellis R, Reavey E, Forbes GH, Zuberi SM (2012): Prognostic, clinical and demographic features in SCN1A mutation-positive Dravet syndrome. *Brain* 135: 2329–2336.

Burgener EB, Moss RB (2018): Cystic fibrosis transmembrane conductance regulator modulators: precision medicine in cystic fibrosis. *Curr Opin Pediatr* 30: 372–377.

Caraballo RH Cersosimo RO, Sakr D, Cresta A, Escobal N, Fejerman N (2005): Ketogenic diet in patients with Dravet syndrome. *Epilepsia* 46: 1539–1544.

Carrazana EJ, Wheeler SD (2001): Exacerbation of juvenile myoclonic epilepsy with lamotrigine. *Neurology* 56: 1424–1425.

Carvill GL, McMahon JM, Schneider A, *et al.* (2015): Mutations in the GABA Transporter SLC6A1 Cause Epilepsy with Myoclonic-Atonic Seizures. *Am J Hum Genet* 7;96: 808–815.

Cavalleri GL, Walley NM, Soranzo N, *et al.* (2007a): A multicenter study of BRD2 as a risk factor for juvenile myoclonic epilepsy. *Epilepsia* 48: 706–712.

Cavalleri GL, Weale ME, Shianna KV, *et al.* (2007b): Multicenter search for genetic susceptibility loci in sporadic epilepsy syndrome and seizure types: a case-control study. *Lancet Neurol* 6: 970–980.

Ceulemans B, Boel M, Claes L, *et al.* (2004): Severe myoclonic epilepsy in infancy: toward an optimal treatment. *Child Neurol* 19: 516–521.

Ceulemans B, Boel M, Leyssens, *et al.* (2012): Successful use of fenfluramine as an add-in treatment for Dravet syndrome. *Epilepsia* 53: 1131–1139.

Ceulemans B, Schoonjans AS, Marchau F *et al.* (2016): Five-year extended follow-up status of 10 patients with Dravet syndrome treated with fenfluramine. *Epilepsia* 57(7): e129–34. Erratum in: *Epilepsia* 2017 Mar; 58(3): 509–510.

Chaix Y, Daquin G, Monteiro F, Villeneuve N, Laguitton V, Genton P (2003): Absence epilepsy with onset before age three years: a heterogeneous and often severe condition. *Epilepsia* 44: 944–949.

Chan EM, Young EJ, Ianzano L, *et al.* (2003): Mutations in NHLRC1 cause progressive myoclonus epilepsy. *Nat Genet* 35: 125–127.

Charlier C, Singh NA, Ryan SG, *et al.* (1998): A pore mutation in a novel KQT-like potassium channel gene in an idiopathic epilepsy family. *Nat Genet* 18: 53–55.

Chen Y, Lu J, Pan H, *et al.* (2003): Association between genetic variation of CACNA1H and childhood absence epilepsy. *Ann Neurol* 54: 239–243.

Chiron C, Dumas C, Jambaque I, Mumford J, Dulac O (1997): Randomized trial comparing viGABAtrin and hydrocortisone in infantile spasms due to tuberous sclerosis. *Epilepsy Res* 26: 389–395.

Chiron C, Marchand MC, Tran A, *et al.* (2000): Stiripentol in severe myoclonic epilepsy in infancy: a randomized placebo-controlled syndrome-dedicated trial. *Lancet* 11;356 (9242): 1638–1642.

Claes L, Del-Favero J, Ceulemans B, Lagae L, Van Broeckhoven C, De Jonghe P (2001): *De novo* mutations in the sodium-channel gene SCN1A cause severe myoclonic epilepsy of infancy. *Am J Hum Genet* 68: 1327–1332.

Clancy JP, Bebök Z, Ruiz F, *et al.* (2001): Evidence that systemic gentamicin suppresses premature stop mutations in patients with cystic fibrosis. *Am J Respir Crit Care Med* 163: 1683–1692.

Clarke T, Strug LJ, Murphy PL, *et al.* (2007): High risk of reading disability and speech sound disorder in Rolandic epilepsy families: case control study. *Epilepsia* 48: 2258–2265.

Clarke T, Baskurt Z, Strug LJ, Pal DK (2009): Shared genetic risks factors for migraine and Rolandic epilepsy: family case-control study. *Epilepsia* 50: 2428–2433.

Colosimo E, Gambardella A, Mantegazza M, *et al.* (2007): Electroclinical features of a family with simple febrile seizrues and temporal lobe epilepsy associated with SCN1A loss-of-func-tion mutation. *Epilepsia* 48: 1691–1696.

Combi R, Dalprà L, Tenchini ML, Ferini-Strambi L (2004): Autosomal dominant nocturnal frontal lobe epilepsy-a critical overview. *J Neurol* 251: 923–934.

Commission on Classification and Terminology of the International League Against Epilepsy (1989): Proposal for revised classification of epilepsies and epileptic syndromes. *Epilepsia* 30: 389–399.

Coppola G. Plouin P, Chiron C, Robain O, Dulac O(1995): Migrating partial seizures in infancy: a malignant disorder with developmental arrest. *Epilepsia* 36: 1017–1024.

Corbett MA, Bahlo M, Jolly L, *et al.* (2010): A focal epilepsy and intellectual disability syndrome is due to a mutation in TBC1D24. *Am J Hum Genet* 87: 371–375.

Cossette P, Liu L, Brisebois K, *et al.* (2002): Mutation of GABRA1 in an autosomal dominant form of juvenile myo-clonic epilepsy. *Nat Genet* 31: 184–189.

Crotti L, Celano G, Dagradi F, Schwartz PJ (2008): Congenital long QT syndrome. *Orphanet J Rare Dis* 7(3): 18.

Dalla Bernardina BD, Capovilla G, Gattoni MB, Colamaria V, Bondavalli S, Bureau M (1982): Severe infant myoclonic epilepsy. *Rev Electroencephalogr Neurophysiol Clin* 12: 21–25.

De Fusco M, Becchetti A, Patrignani A, *et al.* (2000): The nicotinic β-receptor 2 subunit is mutant in nocturnal frontal lobe epilepsy. *Nat Genet* 26: 275–276.

de Haan GJ, Halley DJ, Doelman JC, *et al.* (2004): Unverricht-Lundborg disease: underdiagnosed in the Netherlands. *Epilepsia* 45: 1061–1063.

de Nijs L, Léon C, Nguyen L, *et al.* (2009): EFHC1 interacts with microtubules to regulate cell division and cortical development. *Nat Neurosci* 12: 1266–1274.

Delgado-Escueta AV, Bourgeois BG (2008): Debate: Does genetic information in humans help us treat patients? PRO – Genetic information in humans helps us treat patients. CON – Genetic information does not help at all. *Epilepsia* 49(S9): 13–24.

Delogu AB, Spinelli A, Battaglia D, *et al.* (2011): Electrical and autonomic cardiac function in patients with Dravet syndrome. *Epilepsia* 52(S2): 55–58.

Depienne C, Bouteiller D, Keren B, *et al.* (2009): Sporadic infantile epileptic encephalopathy caused by mutations in PCDH19 resembles Dravet syndrome but mainly affects females. *PLoS Genet* 5: e1000381.

Deprez L, Weckhuysen S, Holmgren P, *et al.* (2010): Clinical spectrum of early-onset epileptic encephalopathies associated with STXBP1 mutations. *Neurology* 75: 1159–1165.

Devinsky O, Cross JH, Laux L, *et al.* (2017): Trial of cannabidiol for drug-resistant seizures in the Dravet Syndrome. *N Eng J Med* 26,376: 2011–2020.

Diaz-Otero F, Quesada M, Morales-Corraliza J, *et al.* (2008): Autosomal dominant nocturnal frontal lobe epilepsy with mutation in the CHRNA gene. *Epilepsia* 49: 516–520.

Dibbens LM, Feng HJ, Richards MC, *et al.* (2004): GABRD encoding a protein for extra- or peri-synaptic GABAA receptors is a susceptibility locus for generalized epilepsies. *Hum Mol Genet* 13: 1315–1319.

Dibbens LM, Tarpey PS, Hynes K, *et al.* (2008): X-linked protocadherin 19 mutations cause female-limited epilepsy and cognitivie impairment. *Nat Genet* 40: 776–781.

Dibbens LM, Michellucci R, Gambardella A, *et al.* (2009): SCARB2 mutations in progressive myoclonus epilepsy (PME) without renal failure. *Ann Neurol* 66: 532–536.

Dibbens LM, Mullen S, Helbig I, *et al.* (2009a): Familial and sporadic 15q13.3 microdeletions in idiopathic generalized epilepsy: precedent for disorders with complex inheritance. *Hum Mol Genet* 18: 3626–3631.

Dobyns WB, Reiner O, Carrozzo R, Ledbetter DH (1993): Lissencephaly: A human brain malformation associated with deletion of the LIS1 gene located at chromosome 17p13. *JAMA* 270(23): 2838–2842.

Dravet C (1965): *Encéphalopathie épileptique de l'enfant avec Pointe-Onde lente diffuse (Petit Mal Variant)*. Thesis, Marseille.

Dravet C (1978): Les épilepsies graves de l'enfant. *Vie Med* 8: 543–548.

Dravet C, Bureau M, Guerrini R, Giraud N, Roger J (1992): Severe myoclonic epilepsy infants. In: Roger J, Bureau M, Dravet C, Dreifuss FE, Perret A, Wolf P (eds) *Epileptic Syndromes in Infancy, Childhood and Adolescence*, 2nd ed, pp. 75–88. London: John Libbey & Company Ltd.

Dravet C, Bureau M, Oguni H, Fukuyama Y, Cokar O (2005): Severe myoclonic epilepsy in infancy: Dravet syndrome. *Adv Neurol* 95: 71–102.

Dravet C, Bureau M, Oguni H, Fukuyama Y, Cokar O (2005a): Severe myoclonic epilepsy in infancy. In: Roger J, Bureau M, Dravet C, Genton P, Tassinari CA, Wolf P (eds) *Epileptic Syndromes in Infancy, Childhood and Adolescence*, 4th ed, pp. 89–113. Paris: John Libbey Eurotext.

Ebach K, Joos H, Doose H, *et al.* (2005): SCN1A mutation analysis in myoclonic astatic epilepsy and severe idiopathic generalized epilepsy of infancy with generalized tonic-clonic seizures. *Neuropediatrics* 36: 210–213.

Ebrahimi-Fakhari D, Saffari A, Wahlster L, *et al.* (2015): The evolving spectrum of PRRT2-associated paroxysmal diseases. *Brain* 138 (Pt 12): 3476–3495.

Edwards MJ, Hargreaves IP, Heales SJ, *et al.* (2002): N-acetylcysteine and Unverricht-Lundborg disease: variable response and possible side effects. *Neurology* 59: 1447–1449.

Eldridge R, Iivanainen M, Stern R, Koerber I, Wilder BJ (1983): "Baltic" myoclonus epilepsy: hereditary disorder of childhood made worse by phenytoin. *Lancet* ii: 838–842.

Elterman RD, Shields WD, Mansfield KA, Nakagawa J (2001): Randomized trial of viGABAtrin in patients with infantile spasms. *Neurology* 57: 1416–1421.

Epi4K Consortium; Epilepsy Phenome/Genome Project, Allen AS, *et al.* (2013): *De novo* mutations in epileptic encephalopathies. *Nature* 12;501(7466): 217–221.

Escayg A, MacDonald BT, Meisler MH, *et al.* (2000): Mutations of SCN1A, encoding a neuronal sodium channel in two families with GEFS+2. *Nat Genet* 24: 343–345.

Escayg A, Heils A, MacDonald BT, Haug K, Sander T, Meisler MH (2001): A novel SCN1A mutation associated with generalized epilepsy with febrile seizures plus and prevalence of variants in patients with epilepsy. *Am J Hum Genet* 68: 866–873.

Falace A, Filipello F, La Padula V, *et al.* (2010): TBC1D24, an ARF6-Interacting protein, is mutated in familial infantile myoclonic epilepsy. *Am J Hum Genet* 87: 365–370.

Ferraro TN, Dlugos DJ, Buono RJ (2006): Role of genetics in the diagnosis and treatment of epilepsy. *Expert Rev Neurother* 6: 1789–1800.

Fujiwara T (2006): Clinical spectrum of mutations in SCN1A gene: severe myoclonic epilepsy in infancy and related epilepsies. *Epilepsy Res* 70(S1): 223–230.

Fujiwara T, Sugawara T, Mazaki-Miyazaki E, *et al.* (2003): Mutations of sodium channel a subunit type 1 (SCN1A) in intractable childhood epilepsies with frequent generalized tonic clonic seizures. *Brain* 126: 531–546.

Gallagher RC, Van Hove JL, Scharer G, *et al.* (2009): Folinic acid-responsive seizures are identical to pyridoxine-dependent epilepsy. *Ann Neurol* 65: 550–556.

Gambardella A, Annesi G, De Fusco M, *et al.* (2000): A new locus for autosomal dominant nocturnal frontal lobe epilepsy maps to chromosome 1. *Neurology* 55: 1467–1471.

Ganesh S, Delgado-Escueta AV, Suzuki T, *et al.* (2002): Genotype-phenotype correlations for EPM2A mutations in Lafora's progressive myoclonus epilepsy: exon 1 mutations associate with an early-onset cognitive deficit subphenotype. *Hum Mol Genet* 11: 1263–1271.

Gastaut H (1969): Classification of the Epilepsies. Proposal for an International Classification. *Epilepsia* 10: S14-S21.

Gastaut H, Roger J, Soulayrol R, *et al.* (1966): Childhood epileptic encephalopathy with diffuse spike-waves (otherwise known as "petit mal variant") or Lennox syndrome. *Epilepsia* 7: 139–149.

Gazzerro E, Bonetto A, Minetti C (2011): Caveolinopathies: Translational implicatons of caveolin-3 in skeletal and cardiac muscle disorders. *Handb Clin Neurol* 101: 135–142.

Genton P, Roger J, Guerrini R, *et al.* (2005): History and classification of myoclonic epilepsies: from seizures to syndromes to diseases, Chapter 1. In: *Myoclonic Epilepsies*, Vol. 95 Advances in Neurology. Philadelphia: PA, Lippincott Williams and Wilkins.

Giordano L, Sartori S, Russo S, *et al.* (2010): Familial Ohtahara syndrome due to a novel ARX gene mutation. *Am J Med Genet A* 152A(12): 3133–7.

Greenberg DA, Cayanis E, Strug L, *et al.* (2005): Malic enzyme 2 may underlie susceptibility to adolescent-onset idiopathic generalized epilepsy. *Am J Hum Genet* 76: 139–146.

Grosso S, Orrico A, Galli L, Di Bartolo R, Sorrentino V, Balestri P (2007): SCN1A mutation associated with atypical Panayiotopoulos syndrome. *Neurology* 69: 609–611.

Guerrini R, Dravet C, Genton P, *et al.* (1998a): Antiepileptic drug worsening of seizures in children. *Epilepsia* 39(S3): 2–10.

Guerrini R, Dravet C, Genton P, Belmonte A, Kaminska A, Dulac O (1998b): Lamotrigine and seizure aggravation in severe myoclonic epilepsy. *Epilepsia* 39: 508–512.

Guerrini R, Bonanni P, Nardocci N, *et al.* (1999): Autosomal recessive Rolandic epilepsy with paroxysmal exercise-induced dystonia and writer's cramp: delineation of the syndrome and genetic mapping to chromosome 16p12–11.2. *Ann Neurol* 45: 344–352.

Guerrini R, Marini C (2006): Genetic malformations of cortical development. *Exp Brain Res* 173: 322–333.

Hamdan FF, Myers CT, Cossette P, *et al.* (2017): High Rate of Recurrent *De Novo* Mutations in Developmental and Epileptic Encephalopathies. *Am J Hum Genet* 101: 664–685.

Harkin LA, McMahon JM, IonaX, *et al.* (2007): The spectrum of SCN1A-related infantile epileptic encephalopathies. *Brain* 130(pt 3): 843–852.

Hattori J, Ouchida M, Ono J, *et al.* (2008): A screening test for the prediction of Dravet syndrome before one year of age. *Epilepsia* 49: 626–633.

Helbig I, Mefford HC, Sharp AJ, *et al.* (2009): 15q13.3 microdeletions increase risk of idiopathic generalized epilepsy. *Nat Genet* 41: 160–162.

Heron SE, Khosravani H, Verela D, *et al.* (2007): Extended spectrum of idiopathic generalized epilepsies associated with CAC-NA1H functional variants. *Ann Neurol* 62: 560–568.

Hesdorffer DC, Tomson T, Benn E, *et al.*, for the ILAE Commission on Epidemiology, Subcommission on Mortality (2011): Combined analysis of risk factors for SUDEP. *Epilepsia* 52: 1150–1159.

Higurashi N, Nakamura M, Sugai M, *et al.* (2013): PCDH19-related female-limited epilepsy: Further details regarding eaerly clinical features and therapeutic efficacy. *Epilepsy Research* 106: 191–199.

Hirose S, Iwata H, Akiyoshi H, *et al.* (1999): A novel mutation of CHRNA4 responsible for autosomal dominant nocturnal frontal lobe epilepsy. *Neurology* 53: 1749–1753.

Hirose S, Zenri F, Akiyoshi H, *et al.* (2000): A novel mutation of KCNQ3 (c.925T'C) in a Japanese family with benign familial neonatal convulsions. *Ann Neurol* 47: 822–826.

Hirsch LJ, Donner EJ, So EL, *et al.* (2011): Abbreviated report of the NIH/NINDS workshop on sudden unexpected death in epilepsy. *Neurology* 76: 1932–1938.

Huang X-J, Wang T, Wang JL, *et al.* (2015): Paroxysmal kinesigenic dyskinesia: Clinical and genetic analyses of 110 patients. *Neurology* 85: 1546–1553.

Hurd RW, Wilder BJ, Helveston WR, Uthman BM (1996): Treatment of four siblings with progressive myoclonus epilepsy of the Univerricht-Lundborg type with N-acetylcysteine. *Neurology* 47: 1264–1268.

Ianzano L, Zhang J, Chan EM, *et al.* (2005): Lafora progressive myoclonus epilepsy mutation database-EPM2A and NHLRC1 (EPM2B) genes. *Hum Mutat* 26: 397.

Imbrici P, Jaffe SL, Eunson LH, *et al.* (2004): Dysfunction of the brain calcium channel CaV2.1 in absence epilepsy and episodic ataxia. *Brain* 127: 2682–2692.

Inoue Y, Fujiwara T, Matsuda K, *et al.* (1997): Ring chromosome 20 and nonconvulsive status epilepticus: A new epileptic syndrome. *Brain* 120 (Pt 6): 939–953.

Ito S, Oguni H, Ito Y, Ishigaki K, Ohinata J, Osawa M (2008): Modified Atkins diet therapy for a case with glucose transporter type 1 deficiency syndrome. *Brain Dev* 30: 226–228.

Ito Y, Oguni H, Ito S, Oguni M, Osawa M (2011): A modified Atkins diet is promising as a treatment for glucose transporter type 1 deficiency syndrome. *Dev Med Child Neurol* 53: 658–663.

Jansen FE, Sadleir LG, Harkin LA, *et al.* (2006): Severe myoclonic epilepsy of infancy (Dravet syndrome): recognition and diagnosis in adults. *Neurology* 67: 2224–2226.

Jellinger K (1987): Neuropathological aspects of infantile spasms. *Brain Dev* 9: 349–357.

Joensuu T, Lehesjoki AE, Kopra O (2008): Molecular background of EPM1 – Univerricht-Lundborg disease. *Epilepsia* 49: 557–563.

Johannesen KM, Gardella E, Linnankivi T, *et al.* (2018): Defining the phenotypic spectrum of SLC6A1 mutations. *Epilepsia* 59: 389–402.

Kalachikov S, Evgrafov O, Ross B, *et al.* (2002): Mutations in LGI1 cause autosomal-dominant partial epilepsy with auditory features. *Nat Genet* 30: 335–341.

KalscheuerVM, Tao J, Donnelly A, *et al.* (2003): Disruption of the serine/threonine kinase 9 gene causes severe X-linked infantile spasms and mental retardation. *Am J Hum Genet* 72: 1401–1411.

Kanai K, Hirose S, Oguni H, *et al.* (2004): Effect of localization of missense mutations in SCN1A on epilepsy phenotype severity. *Neurology* 63: 329–334.

Kananura C, Haug K, Sander T, *et al.* (2002): A splice-site mutation in GABRG2 associated with childhood absence epilepsy and febrile convulsions. *Arch Neurol* 59: 1137–1141.

Kass HR, Winesett SP, Bessone SK, Turner Z, Kossoff EH (2016): Use of dietary therapies amongst patients with GLUT1 deficiency syndrome. *Seizure* 35: 106–110.

Kato M, Saitoh S, Kamei A, *et al.* (2007): A longer polyalanine expansion mutation in the ARX gene causes early infantile epileptic encephalopathy with suppression-burst pattern (Ohtahara syndrome). *Am J Hum Genet* 81: 361–366.

Katsarou AM, Moshé SL, Galanopoulou AS (2017): Interneuropathies and their role in early life epilepsies and neurodevelopmental disorders. *Epilepsia Open* 2(3): 284–306.

Kaufman ES (2009): Mechanisms and clinical management of inherited channelopathies: long QT syndrome, Brugada syndrome, catecholaminergic polymorphic ventricular tachycardia, and short QT syndrome. *Heart Rhythm* 6(S8): S51-S55.

Kearney JA (2017). Precision Medicine: NMDA Receptor-Targeted Therapy for GRIN2D Encepalopathy. *Epilepsy Curr* 17: 112–114.

Kerem E (2004): Pharmacologic therapy for stop mutations: how much CFTR activity is enough? *Curr Opin Pulm Med* 10: 547–552.

Khan IA, NairCK (2004): Brugada and longQT-3 syndromes: two phenotypes of the sodium channel disease. *Ann Noninvasive Electrocardiol* 9: 280–289.

Kiehne N, Kauferstein S (2007): Mutations in the SCN5A gene: evidence for a link between long QT syndrome and sudden death? *Forensic Sci Int Genet* 1(2): 170–174.

Kim HS, Yim SV, Jung KH, *et al.* (2007): Altered DNA copy number in patients with different seizure disorder type: by array-CGH. *Brain Dev* 29: 639–643.

Kitamura K, Yanazawa M, Sugiyama N, *et al.* (2002): Mutations of ARX causes abnormal development of fore-brain and testes in mice and X-linked lissencephaly with abnormal geni-talia in humans. *Nat Genet* 32: 359–369.

Klaassen A, Glykys J, Maguire J, Labarca C, Mody I, Boulter J (2006): Seizures and enhanced cortical GABAergic inhibition in two mouse models of human autosomal dominant nocturnal frontal lobe epilepsy. *Proc Natl Acad Sci USA* 103: 19152–19157.

Klepper J (2012): GLUT1 deficiency syndrome in clinical practice. Epilepsy Res [Epub ahead of print].

Ko A, Youn SE, Kim SH, *et al.* (2018): Targeted gene panel and genotype-phenotype correlation in children with developmental and epileptic encephalopathy. *Epilepsy Res* 141: 48–55. doi: 10.1016/j.eplepsyres.2018.02.003. Epub 2018 Feb 12.

Korff CM, Nordli DR Jr (2007): Diagnosis and management of nonconvulsive status epilepticus in children. *Nat Clin Pract Neurol* 3: 505–516.

Koskiniemi M, van Vleymen B, Hakamies L, Lamusuo S, Taalas J (1998): Piracetam relieves symptoms in progressive myoclonus epilepsy: a multicentre, randomized, double blind, crossover study comparing the efficacy and safety of three dosages of oral piracetam with placebo. *J Neurol Neurosurg Psychiatry* 64: 334–348.

Kugler SL, Bali B, Lieberman P, *et al.* (2008): An autosomal dominant genetically heterogeneous variant of Rolandic epilepsy and speech disorder. *Epilepsia* 49: 1086–1090.

Kuryatov A, Gerzanich V, Nelson M, Olale F, Lindstrom J (1997): Mutation causing autosomal dominant nocturnal frontal lobe epilepsy alters Ca2+ permeability, conductance, and gating of human alpha4beta2 nicotinic acetylcholine receptors. *J Neurosci* 17: 9035–9047.

Lafreniere RG, Rocheforg DL, Chretien N, *et al.* (1997): Unstable insertion in the 5′ flanking region of the cystatin B gene is the most common mutation in progressive myoclonus epilepsy type 1, EPM1. *Nat Genet* 15: 298–302.

Lalioti MD, Mirotsou M, Buresi C, *et al.* (1997a): Identification of mutations in cystatin B, the gene responsible for the Unverricht-Lundborg type of progressive myoclonus epilepsy (EPM1). *AmJ Hum Genet* 60: 342–351.

Lalioti MD, Scott HS, Buresi C, *et al.* (1997b): Dodecamer repeat expansion in cystatin B gene in progressive myoclonus epilepsy. *Nature* 386: 847–851.

Leen WG, KlepperJ, Verbeek MM, *et al.* (2010): Glucose transporter-1 deficiency syndrome: the expanding clinical and genetic spectrum of a treatable disorder. *Brain* 133: 655–670.

Lesca G, Rudolf G, Labalme A, *et al.* (2012): Epileptic encephalopathies of the Landau-Kleffner and continuous spike and waves during slow-wave sleep types: genomic dissection makes the link with autism. *Epilepsia* 53: 1526–1538.

Liang JS, Lin LJ, Yang MT, Wang JS, Lu JF (2017): The therapeutic implication of a novel SCN2A mutation associated early-onset epileptic encephalopathy with Rett-like features. *Brain Dev* 39: 877–881.

Lindy AS, Stosser MB, Butler E, *et al.* (2018): Diagnostic outcomes for genetic testing of 70 genes in 8565 patients with epilepsy and neurodevelopmental disorders. *Epilepsia* 59: 1062–1071.

Lippe BM, Sparkes RS (1981): Ring 14 chromosome: association with seizures. *Am J Med Genet* 9: 301–305.

Lorenz S, Taylor KP, Gehrmann A, *et al.* (2006): Association of BRD2 polymorphisms with photoparoxysmal response. *Neurosci Lett* 400: 135–139.

Lotte J, Bast T Borusiak P, Coppola A, Cross JH (2016): Effectiveness of antiepileptic therapy in patients with PCDH19 mutations. *Seizure* 35: 106–110.

Lux AL, Edwards SW, Hancock E, *et al.* (2004): The United Kingdom Infantile Spasms Study comparing viGABAtrin with prednisolone or tetracosactide at 14 days: a multicentre, randomized controlled trial. *Lancet* 364: 1773–1778.

Lux AL, Edwards SW, Hancock E, *et al.* (2005): The United Kingdom Infantile Spasms Study (UKISS) comparing hormone treatment with viGABAtrin on developmental and epilepsy outcomes to age 14 months: a multicentre randomized trial. *Lancet Neurol* 4: 712–717.

MacArthur DG, Manolio TA, Dimmock DP, *et al.* (2014): Guidelines for investigating causality of sequence variants in human disease. *Nature* 508: 469–476.

Macleod S, Mallik A, Tolmie JL, Stephenson JB, O'Regan ME, Zuberi SM (2005): Electro-clinical phenotypes of chromosome disorders associated with epilepsy in the absence of dysmorphism. *Brain Dev* 27: 118–124.

Mantel A, Leonard C, Husson B, Miladi N, Tardieu M, Landrieu P (1994): Submicroscopic deletions of 17p13.3 in type 1 lissencephaly. *Hum Genet* 94: 95–96.

Marini C, Mei D, Temudo T, *et al.* (2007): Idiopathic epilepsies with seizures precipitated by fever and SCN1A abnormalities. *Epilepsia* 48: 1678–1685.

Marini C, Scheffer IE, Nabbout R, *et al.* (2009): SCN1A duplications and deletions detected in Dravet syndrome: implications for molecular diagnosis. *Epilepsia* 50: 1670–1678.

Marini C, Mei D, Parmeggiani L, *et al.* (2010): Protocardherin 19 mutatons in girls with infantile-onset epilepsy. *Neurology* 75: 646–653.

Marshall CR, Young EJ, Pani AM, *et al.* (2008): Infantile spasms is associated with deletion of the MAG12 gene on chromosome 7q11.23-q21.11. *Am J Hum Genet* 83: 106–111.

Masnada S, Hedrich UBS, Gardella E, *et al.* (2017): Clinical spectrum and genotype-phenotype associations of KCNA2-related encephalopathies. *Brain* 1;140: 2337–2354.

Matsushima N, Hirose S, Iwata H, *et al.* (2002): Mutation (Ser284Leu) of neuronal nicotinic acetylcholine receptor alpha- 4 subunit associated with frontal lobe epilepsy causes faster desensitization of the rat receptor expressed in oocytes. *Epilepsy Res* 48: 181–186.

McTague A, Appleton R, Avula S, *et al.* (2013): Migrating partial seizures of infancy: Expansion of the electroclinical, radiological and pathological disease spectrum. *Brain* 136(Pt 5): 1578–91.

Medeiros-Domingo A, Kaku T, Tester DJ, *et al.* (2007): SCN4B-encoded sodium channel beta4 subunit in congenital long-QT syndrome. *Circulation* 116(2): 134–142.

Mei D, Marini C, Novara F, *et al.* (2010): Xp22.3 genomic deletions involving the CDKL5 gene in girls with early onset epileptic encephalopathy. *Epilepsia* 51: 647–654.

Mendell JR, Al-Zaidy S, Shell R, *et al.* (2017): Single-dose Gene-Replacement Therapy for Spinal Muscular Atrophy. *N Engl J Med* 377: 1713–1722.

Milh M, Becq H, Villeneuve N, Ben-Ari Y, Aniksztejn L (2007): Inhibition of glutamate transporters results in a "suppression-burst" pattern and partial seizures in the newborn rat. *Epilepsia* 48: 169–174.

Milligan CJ, Li M, Gazina EV, Heron SE? *et al.* (2014): KCNT1 Gain of Function in 2 Epilepsy Phenotypes is Reversed by Quinidine. *Ann Neurol* 75: 581–590.

Mills PB, Struys E, Jakobs C, *et al.* (2006): Mutations in antiquitin in individuals with pyridoxine-dependent seizures. *Nat Med* 12: 307–309.

Minassian BA, Lee JR, Herbrick JA, *et al.* (1998): Mutations in a gene encoding a novel protein tyrosine phospha-tase cause progressive myoclonus epilepsy. *Nat Genet* 20: 171–174.

Molinari F, Raas-Rothschild A, Rio M, *et al.* (2005): Impaired mitochondrial glutamate transport in autosomal recessive neonatal myoclonic epilepsy. *Am J Hum Genet* 76: 334–9.

Moller RS, Wuttke TV, Helbig I, *et al.* (2017): Mutations in GABRB3: From febrile seizures to epileptic encephalopathies. *Neurology* 88: 483–492.

Mulley JC, Scheffer IE, Petrou S, Dibbens LM, Berkovic SF, Harkin LA (2005): SCN1A mutations and epilepsy. *Hum Mutat* 25: 535–542.

Murthy JM, Yangala R, Srinivas M (1998): The syndromic classification of the International League Against Epilepsy: a hospital-based study from South India. *Epilepsia* 39: 48–54.

Myers CT, Stong N, Mountier EI, *et al.* (2017): *De Novo* Mutations in PPP3CA Cause Severe Neurodevelopmental Disease with Seizures. *Am J Hum Genet* 101: 516–524.

Nabbout R, Gennaro E, Dalla Bernardina B, *et al.* (2003): Spectrum of SCN1A mutations in severe myoclonic epilepsy of infancy. *Neurology* 60: 1961–1967.

Nakagama Y, Isojima T, Mizuno Y, Takahashi N, Kitanaka S, Igarashi T. Growth hormone deficiency: a possible complication of glucose transporter 1 deficiency? *Acta Paediatr* 101: e259–262.

Niturad CE, Lev D, Kalscheuer VM, *et al.* (2017): Rare GABRA3 variants are associated with epileptic seizures, encephalopathy and dysmorphic features. *Brain* 140: 2879–2894.

Oguni H, Hayashi K, Awaya Y, *et al.* (2001): Severe myoclonic epilepsy in infants – A review based on the Tokyo Women's medical university series of 84 cases. *Brain Dev* 23: 736–748.

Oguni H, Hayashi K, Osawa M, *et al.* (2005): Severe myoclonic epilepsy in infancy: clinical analysis and relation to SCN1A mutations in a Japanese cohort. *Adv Neurol* 95: 103–117.

Ohmori I, Ouchida M, Ohtsuka Y, Oka E, Shimizu K (2002): Significant correlation of the SCN1A mutations and severe myoclonic epilepsy in infancy. *Biochem Biophys Res Commun* 295: 17–23.

Ohmori I, Ohtsuka Y, Ouchida M, *et al.* (2003): Is phenotype difference in severe myoclonic epilepsy in infancy related to SCN1A mutations? *Brain Dev* 27: 488–493.

Ottman R, Hirose S, Jain S, *et al.* (2010): Genetic testing in the epilepsies – Report of the ILAE genetics commission. *Epilepsia* 51: 655–670.

Ouertani I, Chaabouni M, Turki I, *et al.* (2009): A 24-Mb deletion in 14q in a girl with corpus callosum hypoplasia. *Eur J Med Genet* 52(4): 256–259.

Pal DK, Evgrafov OV, Tabares P, Zhang F, Durner M, Greenberg DA (2003): BRD2 (RING3) is a probable major susceptibility gene for common juvenile myoclonic epilepsy. *Am J Hum Genet* 73: 261–270.

Palmer EE, Schofield D, Shrestha R, *et al.* (2018): Integrating exome sequencing into a diagnostic pathway for epileptic encephalopathy: Evidence of clinical utility and cost effectiveness. *Mol Genet Genomic Medicine* 6: 186–199.

Pathak S, Miller J, Morris EC, Stewart WCL, Greenberg DA (2018): DNA methylation of the BRD2 promoter is associated with juvenile myoclonic epilepsy in Caucasians. *Epilepsia* 59: 1011–1019.

Pellock JM, Hrachovy R, Shinnar S, *et al.* (2010): Infantile spasms: a US consensus report. *Epilepsia* 51: 2175–2189.

Pennachio LA, Lehesjoki AE, Stone NE, *et al.* (1996): Mutations in the gene encoding cystatin B in progressive myoclonus epilepsy (EPM1). *Science* 271: 1731–1734.

Phillips HA, Marini C, Scheffer IE, *et al.* (2000): A *de novo* mutation in sporadic nocturnal frontal lobe epilepsy. *Ann Neurol* 48: 264–267.

Phillips HA, Favre I, Kirkpatrick M, *et al.* (2001a): CHRNB2 is the second acetylcholine receptor subunit associated with autosomal dominant nocturnal frontal lobe epilepsy. *Am J Hum* Genet 68: 225–231.

Phillips HA, Favre I, Kirkpatrick M, *et al.* (2001b): CHRNB2 is the second acetylcholine receptor subunit associated with autosomal dominant nocturnal frontal lobe epilepsy. *Am J Hum Genet* 68: 225–231.

Pierson TM, Yuan H, Marsh ED, *et al.* (2014): *GRIN2A* mutation and early-onset epileptic encephalopathy: personalized therapy with memantine. *Ann Clin Transl Neurol* 1: 190–198.

Pisano T, Numis AL,Heavin SB, *et al.* (2015): Early and effective treatment of KCNQ2 encephalopathy. *Epilepsia* 56: 685–691.

Politano L, Nigro G, Nigro V, *et al.* (2003): Gentamicin administration in Duchenne patients with premature stop codon. Preliminary results. *Acta Myol* 22: 15–21.

Ramalho AS, Beck S, Meyer M, Penque D, Cutting GR, Amaral MD (2002): Five percent of normal cystic fibrosis transmembrane conductance regulator mRNA ameliorates the severity of pulmonary disease in cystic fibrosis. *AmJRespir Cell Mol Biol* 27: 619–627.

Rao SN, Maity R, Sharma J, *et al.* (2010): Sequestration of chaperones and proteasome into Lafora bodies and proteasomal dysfunction induced by Lafora disease-associated mutations of malin. *Hum Mol Genet* 19: 4726–4734.

Richards S, Aziz N, Bale S, *et al.* (2015): Standards and guidelines for the interpretation of sequence variants: a joint consensus recommendation of the American College of Medical Genetics and Genomics and the Association for Molecular Pathology. *Genet Med* 17: 405–423.

Riikonen R (2001): Epidemiological data of West syndrome in Finland. *Brain Dev* 23: 539–541.

Riikonen RS (2010): Favorable prognostic factors with infantile spasms. *Eur J Paediatr Neurol* 14: 13–18.

Rodrigues-Pinguet N, Jia L, Li M, *et al.* (2003): Five ADNFLE mutations reduce the Ca2+ dependence of the mammalian a4b2 acetylcholine response. *J Physiol (Lond)* 550: 11–26.

Roger J, Dravet C, Bureau M, Dreifuss FE, Wolf P (1985): *Epileptic Syndromes in Infancy*, Childhood *and Adolescence*, 1st ed. London: John Libbey.

Roll P, Rudolf G, Pereira S, *et al.* (2006): SRPX2 mutations in disorders of language cortex and cognition. *Hum Mol Genet* 15: 1195–1207.

Saitsu H, Kato M, Mizuguchi T, *et al.* (2008): *De novo* mutations in the gene encoding STXBP1 (MUNC18-1) cause early infantile epileptic encephalopathy. *Nat Genet* 40: 782–788.

Saitsu H, Kato M, Okada I, *et al.* (2010a): STXBP1 mutations in early infantile epileptic encephalopathy with suppression-burst pattern. *Epilepsia* 51: 2397–405.

Saitsu H, Tohyama J, Kumada T, *et al.* (2010b): Dominant-negative mutations in alpha-II spectrin cause West syndrome with severe cerebral hypomyelination, spastic quadriplegia, and developmental delay. *Am J Hum Genet* 86: 881–891.

Saitsu H, Hoshino H, Kato M, *et al.* (2011): Paternal mosaicism of an STXBP1 mutation in OS. *Clin Genet* 80: 484–488.

Saitsu H, Watanabe M, Akita T, *et al.* (2016a): Impaired neuronal KCC2 function by biallelic SLC12A5 mutations in migrating focal seizures and severe developmental delay. *Sci Rep* 6: 30072.

Saitsu H, Fukai R, Ben-Zeev B, *et al.* (2016b): Phenytoin spectrum of GNAO1 variants: Epileptic encephalopathy to involuntary movements with severe developmental delay. *Eur J Hum Genet* 24: 129–134.

Sakauchi M, Oguni H, Kato I, *et al.* (2011): Mortality in Dravet syndrome: search for risk factors in Japanese patients. *Epilepsia* 52(S2): 50–54.

Salamon N, Kung J, Shaw SJ, *et al.* (2008): FDG-PET/MRI coregistration improves detection of cortical dysplasia in patients with epilepsy. *Neurology* 71: 1594–1601.

Scheffer IE, Berkovic SF (1997): Generalised epilepsy with febrile seizures plus. A genetic disorder with heterogeneous clinical phenotypes. *Brain* 120: 479–490.

Schinzel A, Niedrist D (2001): Chromosome imbalances associated with epilepsy. *Am J Med Genet* 106: 119–124.

Schulz A, Ajayi T, Specchio N, *et al.* (2018): Study of intraventricular cerliponase Alfa for CLN2 Disease. *N Engl J Med* 378: 1898–1908.

Serratosa JM, Gomez-Garre P, Gallardo ME, *et al.* (1999): A novel protein tyrosine phosphatase gene is mutated in progressive myoclonus epilepsy of the Lafora type (EPM2).*Hum Mol Genet* 8: 345–352.

Shah N, Hou YC, Yu HC, *et al.* (2018): Identification of Misclassified ClinVar Variants *via* Disease Population Prevalence. *Am J Hum Genet* 102: 609–619. doi: 10.1016/j.ajhg.2018.02.019.

Shimizu W, Horie M (2011): Phenotypic manifestations of mutations in genes encoding subunits of cardiac potassium channels. *Ore Res* 109(1): 97–109.

Singh S, Ganesh S (2009): Lafora progressive myoclonus epilepsy: a meta-analysis of reported mutations in the first decade following the discovery of the EPM2A and NHLRC1 genes. *Hum Mutat* 30: 715–723.

Singh NA, Charlier C, Stauffer D, *et al.* (1998): A novel potassium channel gene, KCNQ2, is mutated in an inherited epilepsy of newborns. *Nat Genet* 18: 25–29.

Singh R, Gardner RJ, Crossland KM, Scheffer IE, Berkovic SF (2002): Chromosomal abnormalities and epilepsy: a review for clinicians and gene hunters. *Epilepsia* 43: 127–140.

Singh NA, Pappas C, Dahle EJ, *et al.* (2009): A role of SCN9A in human epilepsies, as a cause of febrile seizures and as a potential modifier of Dravet syndrome. *PLoS Genet* (9): e 10000649.

Sowada N, Hashem MO, Yilmaz R, *et al.* (2017): Mutations of PTPN23 in developmental and epileptic encephalopathy. *Hum Genet* 136(11–12): 1455–1461.

Srour M, Shimokawa N, Hamdan FF (2017:. Dysfunction of the Cerebral Glucose Transporter SLC45A1 in Individuals with Intellectual Disability and Epilepsy. *Am J Hum Genet* 100: 824–830.

Steinlein O, Mulley JC, Propping P, *et al.* (1995): A missense mutation in the neuronal nicotinic acetylcholine receptor alpha 4 subunit is associated with autosomal dominant nocturnal frontal lobe epilepsy. *Nat Genet* 11: 201–203.

Steinlein OK, Mgnusson A, Stoodt J, *et al.* (1997): An insertion mutation of the CHRNA4 gene in a family with autosomal dominant nocturnal frontal lobe epilepsy. *Hum Mol Genet* 6: 943–947.

Striano P, Coppola A, Pezzella M, *et al.* (2007): An open-label trial of levetiracetam in severe myoclonic epilepsy of infancy. *Neurology* 69: 250–254.

Stromme P, Mangelsdorf ME, Shaw MA, *et al.* (2002): Mutations in the human ortholog of Aristaless cause X-linked mental retardation and epilepsy. *Nat Genet* 30: 441–445.

Strug LJ, Clarke T, Chiang T, *et al.* (2009): Centrotemporal sharp wave EEG trait in Rolandic epilepsy maps to Elon-gator Protein Complex 4 (ELP4). *Eur J Hum Genet* 17: 1171–1181.

Sugawara T, Mazaki-Miyazaki E, Fukushima K, *et al.* (2002): Frequent mutations of SCN1A in severe myoclonic epilepsy in infancy. *Neurology* 58: 1122–1124.

Sugawara T, Tsurubuchi Y, Agarwala KL, *et al.* (2001): A missense mutation of the Na+ channel alpha II subunit gene Na(v)1.2 in a patient with febrile and afebrile seizures causes channel dysfunction. *Proc Natl Acad Sci USA* 98: 6384–6389.

Suls A, Kedeken P, Goffin K, *et al.* (2008): Paroxysmal exercise-induced dyskinesia and epilepsy is due to mutations in SLC2A1, encoding the glucose transporter GLUT1. Brain 131: 1831–1844.

Suls A, Mullen SA, Weber YG, *et al.* (2009): Early onset absence epilepsy caused by mutations in the glucose transporter GLUT1. *Ann Neurol* 66: 415–419.

Summers KM, Bokil NJ, Lu FT, *et al.* (2010): Mutations at KCNQ1 and an unknown locus cause long QT syndrome in a larger Australian family: Implications for genetic testing. *Am J Med Genet* 152A(3): 613–621.

Suzuki T, Delgado-Escueta AV, Aguan K, *et al.* (2004): Mutations in EFHC1 cause juvenile myoclonic epilepsy. *Nat Genet* 36: 842–849.

Tagliabracci VS, Girard JM, Segvich D, *et al.* (2008): Abnormal metabolism of glycogen phosphate as a cause for Lafora disease. *J Biol Chem* 283: 33816–33825.

Tanaka M, Olsen RW, Medina MT, *et al.* (2008): Hyperglycosylation and reduced GABA currents of mutated GABRB3 polypeptide in remitting childhood absence epilepsy. *Am J Hum Genet* 82: 1249–1261.

Tester DJ, Will ML, Haglund CM, Ackerman MJ (2005): Compendium of cardiac channel mutations in 541 consecutive unrelated patients referred for long QT syndrome genetic testing. *Heart Rhythm* 2: 507–517.

Tu E, Bagnall RD, Duflou J, Semsarian C (2011a): Post-mortem review and genetic analysis of sudden unexpected death in epilepsy (SUDEP) cases. *Brain Pathol* 21: 201–208.

Tu E, Waterhouse L, Duflou J, Bagnall RD, Semsarian C (2011b): Genetic analysis of hyperpolarisation-activated cyclic nucleotide-gated cation (HCN) channels in sudden unexpected death in epilepsy (SUDEP) cases. *Brain Pathol* 21: 692–698.

Turnbull J, DePaoli-Roach AA, Zhao X, *et al.* (2011): PTG depletion removes Lafora bodies and rescues the fatal epilepsy of Lafora disease. *PLos Genet* 7(4): e1002037

Unverricht H (1891): *Die Myoklonie*. Leipzig, Vienna: Franz Deuticke.

Vatta M, Ackerman MJ, Ye B, *et al.* (2006): Mutant caveolin-3 induces persistent late sodium current and is associated with long-QT syndrome. *Circulation* 114: 2104–2112.

Verkerk AJ, Pieretti M, Sutcliffe JS, *et al.* (1999): Identification of a gene (FMR-1) containing a CGG repeat coincident with a breakpoint cluster region exhibiting length variation in fragile X syndrome. *Cell* 65: 905–914.

Vigevano F, Cilio MR (1997): ViGABAtrin *versus* ACTH as first-line treatment for infantile spasms: a randomized, prospective study. *Epilepsia* 38: 1270–1274.

von Stülpnagel C, Ensslen M, Møller RS, *et al.* (2017): Epilepsy in patients with GRIN2A alterations: Genetics, neurodevelopmental, epileptic phenotype and response to anticonvulsive drugs. *Eur J Paediatr Neurol* 21: 530–541.

Wagner KR, Hamed S, Hadley DW, *et al.* (2001): Gentamicin treatment of Duchenne and Becker muscular dystrophy due to nonsense mutations. *Ann Neurol* 49: 706–711.

Wallace RH, Wang DW, Singh R, *et al.* (1998): Febrile seizures and generalized epilepsy associated with a mutation in the Na+ channel?1 subunit gene SCN1B. *Nat Genet* 19: 366–370.

Wallace RH, Marini C, Petrou S, *et al.* (2001): Mutant GABA(A) receptor gamma2-subunit in childhood absence epilepsy and febrile seizures. *Nat Genet* 28: 49–52.

Wallace RH, Scheffer IE, Barnett S, *et al.* (2001a): Neuronal sodium-channel 1-subunit mutations in generalized epilepsy with febrile seizures? plus. *Am J Hum Genet* 68: 859–865.

Wallace RH, Hodgson BL, Grinton BE, *et al.* (2003): Sodium channel a1 -subunit mutations in severe myoclonic epilepsy of infancy and infantile spasms. *Neurology* 61: 765–679.

Wang D, Pascual JM, De Vivo D (2009): Glucose transporter type 1 deficiency syndrome. In: Pagon RA, Bird TD, Dalon CR, Stephens K, Adams MP (eds) Gene Reviews [Internet]. Seattle: University of Washington.

Wang J, Lin Z-J, Liu L, *et al.* (2016): Epilepsy-Associated genes. *Seizure*44: 11–20.

Wang JW, Kurahashi H, Ishii A, *et al.* (2008): Microchromosomal deletions involving SCN1A and adjacent genes in severe myoclonic epilepsy of infancy. *Epilepsia* 49: 1528–1534.

Wang D, Pascual JM, De Vivo D (2018): Glucose Transporter Type 1 Deficiency Syndrome. In: Adam MP, Ardinger HH, Pagon RA, Wallace SE, Bean LJH, Stephens K, Amemiya A, editors. *Gene Reviews* [Internet]. Seattle (WA): University of Washington, Seattle; 1993–2018.

Weaving LS, *et al.* (2004): Mutations of CDKL5 cause a severe neurodevelopmental disorder with infantile spasms and mental retardation. *Am J Hum Genet* 75: 1079–1093.

Weckhuysen S, Mandebtam S, Suls A, *et al.* (2012): KCNQ2 encephalopathy: emerging phenotype of a neonatal epileptic encephalopathy. *Ann Neurol* 71: 15–25.

Welch EM, Barton ER, Zhuo J, *et al.* (2007): PTC 124 targets genetic disorders caused by nonsense mutations. *Nature* 447: 88–93.

Wilschanski M, *et al.* (2003): Gentamicin-induced correction of CFTR function in patients with cystic fibrosis and CFTR stop mutations. *N Engl J Med* 349: 1433–1441.

Wolff M, Johannessen KM, Hedrich UBS, *et al.* (2017): Genetic and phenotypic heterogeneity suggest therapeutic implications in SCN2A-related disorders. *Brain* 140: 1316–1336.

Wong M (2010): Mammalian target of rapamycin (mTOR) inhibition as a potential antiepileptogenic therapy: from tuberous sclerosis to common acquired epilepsies. *Epilepsia* 51: 27–36.

Xu XX, Liu XR, Fan CY, *et al.* (2018): Functional Investigation of a GRIN2A Variant Associated with Rolandic *Epilepsy Neurosci Bull* 34: 237–246.

Yakoub M, Dulac O, Jambaque I, Chrion C, Plouin P (1992): Early diagnosis of severe myoclonic epilepsy in infancy. *Brain Dev* 14: 299–303.

Yang H, Wang D, Engelstad K, Bagay L, Wei Y, Rotstein M, *et al.* (2011): Glut1 deficiency syndrome and erythrocyte glucose uptake assay. *Ann Neurol* 70: 996–1005.

Yang Y, Yang Y, Liang B, *et al.* (2010): Identification of a Kir3.4 mutation in congenital long QT syndrome. *Am J Hum Genet* 86: 872–880.

Zara F, Labuda M, Garofalo PG, *et al.* (1998): Unusual EEG pattern linked to chromosome 3p in a family with idiopathic generalized epilepsy. *Neurology* 51: 493–498.

Zeng LH, Xu L, Gutmann DH, Wong M, Crino PB (2008): Rapamycin prevents epilepsy in a mouse model of tuberous sclerosis complex. *Ann Neurol* 63: 444–453.

Zhang Y, Lian Y, Xie N (2017): Early onset epileptic encephalopathy with a novel GABRB3 mutation treated effectively with clonazepam: A case report. *Medicine* (Baltimore) 96(50): e9273.

Zhang YH, Burgess R, Malone JP, *et al.* (2017): Genetic epilepsy with febrile seizures plus: Refining the spectrum. *Neurology* 89: 1210–1219.

Zhou P, He N, Zhang JW, *et al.* (2018): Novel mutations and phenotypes of epilepsy-associated genes in epileptic encephalopathies. *Genes Brain Behav* 17: e1245.

CHAPTER 3
ANIMAL MODELS OF EPILEPTIC SYNDROMES

Aristea S. Galanopoulou[1], Valerio Conti[2], Solomon L. Moshé[1,3] and Astrid Nehlig[4]

[1] Saul R. Korey Department of Neurology, Dominick P. Purpura Department of Neuroscience, Laboratory of Development Epilepsy, Montefiore/Einstein Epilepsy Management Center, Albert Einstein College
of Medicine and Montefiore Medical Center, Bronx, New York, USA
[2] Pediatric Neurology, Neurogenetics and Neurobiology Unit and Laboratories, Neuroscience Department, A. Meyer Children's Hospital, Florence, Italy
[3] Department of Pediatrics, Albert Einstein College of Medicine and Montefiore Medical Center, Bronx, New York, USA
[4] Inserm U1129, Pediatric Neurology, Necker-Enfants Malades Hospital, Paris-Descartes University, Paris, France

Introduction

There are numerous types of epileptic syndromes in the pediatric population, recognized by specific electroclinical characteristics. The age-dependent specificity of these syndromes may reflect a combination of events: i) the increased susceptibility to seizures of the developing brain as it relates to the maturation of neuronal communication and glia (Moshé *et al.*, 1995); ii) genetic factors that may first be expressed during early development; and iii) epigenetic influences that are more likely to occur early in life (trauma, asphyxia, infections, etc.). There is an even greater diversity in etiologies (including structural, metabolic, genetic, infectious/inflammatory). Their impact and consequences may differ depending on age, gender, epigenetic or biological factors, further increasing the richness of the phenotypic variability of these syndromes. To understand the pathophysiology of these developmental syndromes, it is important to have relevant models. In this chapter, we describe models of early life epilepsies and epileptic encephalopathies, including genetic epilepsies and epilepsies due to inflammatory/immune etiologies, and developmental models of temporal lobe epilepsy (TLE), a condition that may occur at any age with variable consequences. We also discuss the models relevant to brain malformations and the kindling model which offered insights in early life epileptogenesis.

Brain development across species

There are significant differences across species that have challenged the creation of a system to accurately compare developmental stages across species (Galanopoulou & Moshe, 2011). In rodents, postnatal days 8–13 (PN8-10) rodents are equivalent to full term newborn human infants, based on crude measures of brain growth, DNA and water content (Dobbing & Sands,1979). The first postnatal week is considered as equivalent to a premature newborn, while puberty begins around PN32-36 in female and PN35-45 in male rodents; adulthood is reached around PN60 (Akman *et al.*, 2014). However, rodent pups develop the ambulatory ability during the first two weeks of life, and can explore the environment around the 3rd week, when both ambulation and eye opening (around PN12-15) have matured (Scantlebury *et al.*, 2010). Considering therefore the third postnatal week as "infantile stage" for rodents may not reflect the fact that the ambulatory abilities are already more developed than in humans. Each developmental process (*e.g.*, motor milestones, cell migration, neurotransmitter expression or signaling responses, synaptogenesis, brain growth) follows its own temporal rhythm of maturation that may also differ across brain regions, cell types, and sexes (Avishai-Eliner *et al.*, 2002; Galanopoulou & Moshe, 2011; Akman *et al.*, 2014).

Animal models of early life epilepsies

Early infantile encephalopathy with suppression-burst: Ohtahara syndrome

Ohtahara syndrome or early infantile epileptic encephalopathy (EIEE) typically begins in the first month of life, tonic seizures dominate over the myoclonic with a burst suppression EEG background, has poor prognosis and is due to either structural, genetic (including *STXBP1* or

MUNC18-1, SLC25A22, CDKL5, ARX, SPTAN1, PCDH19, KCNQ2, SCN2A) or metabolic etiologies. Some of these infants may subsequently progress into West or Lennox-Gastaut syndromes. A zebrafish model with homozygous *stxbp1b* (syntaxin binding protein 1) loss of function mutations demonstrates seizures with burst-suppression patterns and shows reduced locomotor activity in response to dark flash visual stimulus (Grone *et al.*, 2016). The *Munc18-1* knockout mice (KO) (*Munc18-1*$^{-/-}$) are not viable beyond birth due to paralysis that impairs respiration (Verhage *et al.*, 2000). Haploinsufficiency of *Munc18-1* in mice causes anxiety but no seizures (Hager *et al.*, 2014). Mice with *Arx* (aristaless related X-linked homeobox) defects are being discussed in the West syndrome section. Sodium channel 2A (*Scn2A*) mutations in mice leading to epilepsy have been reported, yet these are observed in adult mice with unclear relevance to Ohtahara syndrome (Kearney *et al.*, 2001). Double *Scn2a/Kcnq2* mutants demonstrated severe early onset epilepsy in mice (onset ~PN12) with generalized tonic clonic seizures and early lethality, although the EEG background has not been described (Kearney *et al.*, 2006).

Animal models of West syndrome (infantile spasms)

West syndrome (West, 1841) is an epileptic encephalopathy that typically manifests during the first year of life with at least two of the following three features: (a) a characteristic seizure type called infantile or epileptic spasms (IS) (flexion or extension brief tonic spasms, often in clusters) which can have ictal electrodecremental response (EDR) EEG correlates, (b) hypsarrhythmia (high amplitude, chaotic, multifocally epileptiform EEG), and (c) intellectual disabilities (Pellock *et al.*, 2010). The treatment options include hormonal (adrenocorticotropic hormone (ACTH) and high dose glucocorticoids) and the GABA aminotransferase inhibitor vigabatrin, particularly for IS due to tuberous sclerosis complex (TSC) (Pellock *et al.*, 2010; Mytinger *et al.*, 2012; Hancock *et al.*, 2013). Ketogenic diet or pyridoxine trial in case IS are pyridoxine-sensitive are also used. The prognosis is overall poor with high mortality and increased risk of persistent epilepsy and intellectual and behavioral deficits, even if IS remit. Genetic etiologies can be found in 14.4% of patients, genetic-structural in 10%, structural congenital in 10.8%, structural-acquired in 22.4%, metabolic in 4.8%, and infectious in 2%, while in a third of the patients an etiology cannot be found (Wirrell *et al.*, 2015). An increasing number of gene variants have been linked to IS (Paciorkowski *et al.*, 2011; EuroEPINOMICS-RES Consortium *et al.*, 2014; Galanopoulou & Moshe, 2015). Efforts to develop animal models of IS, with the hope to identify pathogenic mechanisms and therapies (Stafstrom *et al.*, 2006), have produced acute models of IS, manifesting spasms only during the immediate post-induction period, and chronic models which also demonstrate chronic features of West syndrome (Galanopoulou & Moshe, 2015).

Acute models of spasms

N-methyl-D-aspartate *(NMDA) model and variants with perinatal predisposing conditions*: Administration of NMDA, which activates NMDA receptors (NR), induces status epilepticus (SE) in both immature and adult rodents (Hirayasu & Wada, 1992; Stafstrom & Sasaki-Adams, 2003). The recognition of a distinct seizure, *"emprosthotonus"* (forward flexion spasm), occurring preferentially in PN7-19 rats, and not in adults, proposed this as an acute model of IS (Mares & Velisek 1992). NMDA spasms respond to valproic acid but paradoxically become exacerbated by hydrocortisone, while pyridoxine increases epileptic discharges (Kabova *et al.*, 1999). NMDA spasms were initially proposed as models for ACTH-resistant spasms based on the ineffectiveness of $ACTH_{1-24}$ or rat synthetic $ACTH_{1-39}$ (Velisek *et al.*, 2007), yet independent studies showed that higher doses of porcine $ACTH_{1-39}$ suppressed NMDA spasms in Wistar rats or C57 mice (Wang *et al.*, 2012; Shi *et al.*, 2015). There is no report of subsequent development of spontaneous recurrent seizures (SRS) in this model, while NMDA-induced SE in PN12-20 rats resulted in spatial memory deficits and increased susceptibility to pentylenetetrazol (PTZ) seizures in adulthood (Stafstrom & Sasaki-Adams, 2003).

Modifications of the model introduce earlier interventions that (a) simulate elements of prenatal stress, like prenatal betamethasone injections (Velisek *et al.*, 2007) or prenatal restrain stress (Yum *et al.*, 2012) at gestational day 15 (G15), (b) disrupt the stress response, like postnatal adrenalectomy at PN10 (Wang *et al.*, 2012), or (c) predispose to brain malformations, like injections of methylazoxymethanol acetate (MAM) at G15 (Kim *et al.*, 2017). These interventions have been shown to exacerbate NMDA-induced spasms. ACTH responsiveness of NMDA-induced spasms is improved in the prenatal betamethasone (Velisek *et al.*, 2007) but not in the prenatal MAM model (Kim *et al.*, 2017) and is preserved in the postnatal adrenalectomy model (Wang *et al.*, 2012). Pretreatment with vigabatrin, ganaxolone (enhances $GABA_AR$ activity) or repetitive, high doses of methylprednisolone reduce NMDA spasms in the prenatal betamethasone model (Chachua *et al.*, 2011). Repeated pretreatment with the mTOR (mechanistic target of rapamycin) inhibitor rapamycin had no effect on NMDA spasms, although the relevance of mTOR overactivation in this model is unclear (Chachua *et al.*, 2012). Neonatal pretreatment with estradiol benzoate also had no effect (Chachua *et al.*, 2016). No epilepsy has been reported.

These models implicate NR signaling in the ictogenesis of spasms. NR2D or NR2B (GRIN2B) or NR1 (GRIN1) genetic variants have been associated with IS patients (Epi4K Consortium *et al.*, 2013; Lemke *et al.*, 2014).

Down syndrome Ts65Dn model of spasms

There is relatively high incidence of IS in patients with Down syndrome (0.6–13%), suggesting shared predisposing pathways (Cortez *et al.*, 2009; Sanmaneechai *et al.*, 2013; Beatty *et al.*, 2017). The Ts(17^{16})65Dn (Ts65Dn) mouse model of Down syndrome, overexpresses $GABA_B$ receptors ($GABA_BR$) and the $GABA_BR$-associated GIRK2 protein (inward rectifying K^+ channel) that is associated with the $GABA_BR$. Injections of gamma-butyrolactone (GBL) (prodrug of gamma-hydroxybutyrate, $GABA_BR$ agonist) elicit more acute extensor spasms with facial myoclonias and EDRs in Ts65Dn than in wild type mice. GBL also exacerbates the spontaneous spike wave discharges (SWDs) seen in the naïve Ts65Dn mice (Cortez *et al.*, 2009). These GBL-induced spasms can be induced in both sexes between 1 week till 2 months old, lacking the age-specificity of the syndrome. Spasms are suppressed by vigabatrin, valproic acid and $ACTH_{1-24}$, but not by porcine $ACTH_{1-39}$, while ethosuximide paradoxically also suppressed spasms (Cortez *et al.*, 2009). Pre-treatment with the $GABA_BR$ inhibitor CGP35348 and genetic or pharmacologic knockdown of GIRK2 rescued from the GBL-induced spasms (Cortez *et al.*, 2009; Joshi *et al.*, 2016). $GABA_BR$ genetic variants were described in one patient with IS and 3 patients with Lennox Gastaut syndrome (LGS) (Epi4K Consortium *et al.*, 2013; EuroEPINOMICS-RES Consortium *et al.*, 2014).

Chronic models of spasms

Tetrodotoxin (TTX) model: TTX is a sodium channel blocker which is infused chronically in the right cerebral cortex and/or hippocampus of PN10-40 rats resulting in chronic appearance of spasms and EDRs, from PN16-20 through adulthood. The EEG background in sleep resembles hypsarrhythmia (Lee *et al.*, 2008). Even though the model lacks the expected age-specificity, it allows for more extensive EEG electrode coverage since EEGs are done in older or adult rats, permitting the determination of hypsarrhythmia. Ictal EEG recordings also showed high frequency oscillations (HFOs) from areas contralateral to the induced lesion (Frost *et al.*, 2011). Hypsarrhythmia determination has not been possible in models that show spasms in the first 2 weeks of life due to the small size and fragility of the skull. Spasms, hypsarrhythmia and pathological HFOs in the TTX model are responsive to vigabatrin (Frost *et al.*, 2015). Long-term cognitive outcomes have not been done in this model. It represents a model of structural etiology spasms, having a lesion and encephalomalacia at the cortical and hippocampal regions ipsilateral to the TTX infusion (Frost *et al.*, 2015).

ARX models

ARX is a transcription factor involved in the migration and differentiation of interneuronal progenitors that has been implicated in several types of epileptic encephalopathies, including West and Ohtahara syndromes (Friocourt & Parnavelas, 2010). The term "interneuronopathy" was initially introduced to describe the defective tangential migration of interneurons in ARX-linked disorders (Kato & Dobyns, 2005). There are several mouse models with *Arx* gene defects but only two of them have reported seizures.

The *Arx* conditional KO (*Arx* cKO) at Dlx5/6 ganglionic eminence interneuronal progenitors manifests spasms with EDR in adulthood but stage 5 (Racine scale) seizures at ~PN14 (Marsh *et al.*, 2009). The interneuronal deficit in the male PN14 $Arx^{-/Y}$ cKO mice consists of reduced hippocampal calbindin and parvalbumin cells, reduced cortical Neuropeptide Y (NPY) cells and increased cortical parvalbumin cells (Marsh *et al.*, 2016). In adulthood, there are fewer cortical calretinin and calbindin interneurons and hippocampal calbindin neurons (Marsh *et al.*, 2016).

The *Arx* knockin (KI) mouse model with extension of the first polyalanine repeat ($Arx^{(CGG)10+7}$) manifests spasms between PN7-11, seizures with behavioral arrest, limbic or generalized tonic clonic seizures that are observed in older ages (Price *et al.*, 2009). The $Arx^{(CGG)10+7}$ model has reduced calbindin interneurons in the cortex, hippocampus and striatum and reduced cholinergic and NPY interneurons in striatum, but no deficits in parvalbumin or calretinin neurons. Low anxiety and impaired associative learning and social interactions have been reported. Neonatal administration of 17β-estradiol between PN3-10, prevented spasms and rescued from interneuronopathy suggesting a disease-modifying effect (Olivetti *et al.*, 2014). The same treatment protocol has not however shown efficacy in the prenatal betamethasone/postnatal NMDA (Chachua *et al.*, 2016) and the multiple-hit model (Galanopoulou *et al.*, 2017), which could suggest that this could possibly be an etiology-specific treatment.

Multiple-hit rat model of spasms due to structural lesion

This model was designed to model IS due to structural lesion. The induction method includes right intracerebroventricular (i.c.v) doxorubicin (cytotoxic) and right intracortical lipopolysaccharide (causes white matter injury and inflammation) injections on PN3 followed by p-chlorophenylalanine on PN5 (Scantlebury *et al.*, 2010). Spasms and EDRs are evident between PN4-13, the interictal EEG has abundant epileptic discharges bilaterally, and other types of seizures emerge while spontaneous motor seizures can be detected through adulthood (Akman *et al.*, 2012). There is a structural lesion around the infusion sites (right neocortex and hippocampus, right periventricular sites) (Briggs *et al.*, 2014; Jequier Gygax *et al.*, 2014). Interneuronopathy has also been documented in the multiple-hit rat model (Katsarou *et al.*, 2017).

The multiple-hit model has been extensively used to identify new therapy targets and treatments for IS utilizing a screening method that is clinically relevant, by introducing treatments after spasms' onset. Spasms in this model are ACTH-resistant but partially responsive to vigabatrin, reminiscent of the more refractory course or IS due to structural lesions (Scantlebury *et al.*, 2010). Spasms, as expected, do not respond to phenytoin (Ono *et al.*, 2011). Acute reduction of spasms was achieved with carisbamate (Ono *et al.*, 2011). CPP-115, a new high affinity vigabatrin analog with lower risk for retinal toxicity in preclinical studies, showed a better efficacy/tolerability profile than vigabatrin in the multiple hit model (Briggs *et al.*, 2014). Both carisbamate and CPP-115 have been since designated by the U.S. Food and Drug Administration (FDA) as orphan drugs with indication for IS. CPP-115 has already been tried in an infant with IS with significant clinical improvement after the transition from vigabatrin to CPP-115 treatment (Doumlele *et al.*, 2016). Using a pulse three day treatment with rapamycin, at doses that prevent the pathologic overactivation of mTOR pathway, spasms stopped and learning improved between PN16-19, suggesting disease modification (Raffo *et al.*, 2011). Despite the fact that this is a chemically induced model, these findings are reminiscent of the involvement of mTOR pathways in IS due to TSC, focal cortical dysplasias or brain malformations from genetic defects in pathways intersecting with mTOR (Galanopoulou *et al.*, 2012), raising the possibility that this is a pathogenic pathway shared across various etiologies. Unlike the Ts65Dn mouse model, CGP35348 had no therapeutic effect on spasms in the multiple-hit model and unlike the *Arx*$^{(CGG)10+7}$ KI model, neonatal estradiol had no therapeutic effect (Galanopoulou *et al.*, 2017). These demonstrate the challenges in across model comparisons and validation, particularly in disorders with heterogeneous etiologies and pathologies. Other investigative drugs tested in the multiple-hit included the NAX 5055, a galanin receptor 2 analog, and the VX-765 caspase 1 inhibitor, which failed to show an effect (Jequier Gygax *et al.*, 2014; Galanopoulou *et al.*, 2017).

Adenomatous polyposis coli (Apc) cKO mouse model

APC is a tumor suppressor protein that is involved in the ubiquitination of β-catenin; APC inactivation promotes cell proliferation. Although gene associations of *Apc* with IS have not been reported, APC signaling interacts with pathways involved in neurodevelopmental disorders and epilepsies. *Apc* cKO in excitatory forebrain neurons manifests spasms in PN9 mice and spontaneous seizures in adulthood (Pirone *et al.*, 2017). Comorbidities and drug effects on spasms have not yet been reported in this model.

Tuberous sclerosis (Tsc1$^{+/-}$) model

TSC is a common genetic etiology of spasms, whereas IS have been reported in ~38% of TSC patients (Chu-Shore *et al.*, 2010; Galanopoulou *et al.*, 2012). Spasms had not yet been reported in any of the existing models of TSC until a report of electrographic patterns resembling EDRs (high amplitude spikes followed by fast activity) in PN12-16 *Tsc1*$^{+/-}$ mice appeared (Gataullina *et al.*, 2016). *In vivo* characterization and electroclinical correlation of these patterns is still needed.

Chronic early life stress model

An early hypothesis proposed that exaggerated stress response predisposes certain infants to IS (Baram, 1993). Intracerebral injection (cortex or hippocampus) of corticotropin releasing hormone (CRH) demonstrated its proconvulsant effect in PN5-10 rats, yet the induced seizures responded to phenytoin but not to ACTH and were considered as limbic seizures but not spasms (Baram & Schultz 1995). More recently, chronic early life stress, by disrupting the nesting and bedding in the cages, was reported to induce spasm-like behaviors associated with spikes and low voltage EEG (Dube *et al.*, 2015).

Other genetic early life epilepsies

For more extensive review of these animal models we refer the reader to references (Galanopoulou & Moshe, 2015; Katsarou *et al.*, 2017; Pitkanen *et al.*, 2017).

KCNQ2 and KCNQ3 early onset epilepsies: Kcnq2 or *Kcnq3* potassium channel mutations have been associated with self-limited neonatal convulsions but also with more severe encephalopathies (Serino *et al.*, 2013). In mice, *Kcnq2*$^{A306T/+}$ or *Kcnq3*$^{G311V/+}$ mutations result in early onset epilepsy and early mortality (Singh *et al.*, 2008). Mice which survive through adulthood manifest generalized tonic-clonic seizures without associated hippocampal sclerosis. Genetic substrate influences the severity of the phenotype. The age-specific expression of self-limited seizures has been proposed to be due to either the early presence of depolarizing $GABA_AR$ signaling (Uchida *et al.*, 2017) or to age-specific expression patterns of KCNQ2 and KCNQ3 (Kanaumi *et al.*, 2008).

SCN8A related epilepsies

Mutations in *SCN8A* may also cause epilepsy and and developmental regression. Mice with the *Scn8A*^{N1768D} mutation have ataxia, generalized tonic-clonic seizures and early mortality (Wagnon *et al.*, 2015). The age-specificity of symptoms was attributed to compensatory expression of other SCNs.

Dravet syndrome

Dravet syndrome or severe myoclonic epilepsy of infancy (SMEI) has been linked to genetic defects in SCNs (SCN1A in 70–80% of patients; SCN1B) and rarely to $GABA_AR$ mutations (GABRG2) (Galanopoulou & Moshe 2015). In the *Scn1a* KO mouse model, the homozygous *Scn1a*$^{-/-}$ mice display ataxia and seizures beginning on PN9 and die on PN15. Heterozygous *Scn1a*$^{+/-}$ mice exhibit spontaneous seizures at around PN21-27 and sporadic death after PN21. Seizures begin with stereotypic behaviors such as myoclonic jerks and hindlimb flexions, progress to forelimb clonus and head bobbing and finish with relaxed muscle tone. The seizure duration is typically 20 sec (Yu *et al.*, 2006). Other *Scn1a* rodent models of Dravet syndrome include the *Scn1a cKO* mouse with deletion of exon 25 in GABAergic interneurons (Cheah *et al.*, 2012), the R1407X *Scn1a* KI mouse (Ogiwara *et al.*, 2007; Auerbach *et al.*, 2013), the *Scn1a* cKO mice with exon 7 deletions either in inhibitory interneurons or in excitatory forebrain neurons (Ogiwara *et al.*, 2013), and a rat *Scn1a*^{N1417H} model (for reviews see references (Galanopoulou & Moshe 2015; Katsarou *et al.*, 2017)). These models have suggested the importance of GABAergic interneurons for the development of the epilepsy phenotype (Ogiwara *et al.*, 2013). Furthermore, they offered the opportunity to test various treatments for their efficacy, including clonazepam, tiagabine, stiripentol, methylphenidate, ketogenic diet (Dutton *et al.*, 2011; Cao *et al.*, 2012; Han *et al.*, 2012; Oakley *et al.*, 2013; Ohmori *et al.*, 2014). Genetic ablation of tau protein also improved mortality and epilepsy in the R1407X KI mouse (Gheyara *et al.*, 2014). High throughput drug screening in a zebrafish model *(scn1aLab)* identified clemizole as promising treatment for Dravet syndrome seizures (Baraban *et al.*, 2013). *In addition, Scn1b* KO (Chen *et al.*, 2004) and *Scn1b KI*^{C121W} (Reid *et al.*, 2014) mouse models of Dravet syndrome have also been developed.

Genetic epilepsies with febrile seizures plus (GEFS+)

SCN1A and SCN1B have also been implicated in GEFS+ which shows a genetic susceptibility to a variety of focal or generalized, febrile and afebrile seizures (Wallace *et al.*, 1998; 2001). R1648H KI mouse models for GEFS+ may exhibit either more severe kainate-induced seizures or SRS (Tang *et al.*, 2009; Martin *et al.*, 2010).

Progressive myoclonus epilepsy (PME) type 1 (EPM1)

The PMEs are diseases characterized by tonic-clonic seizures, myoclonus and progressive neurological dysfunction, including dementia and ataxia (Berkovic *et al.*, 1986). Unverricht-Lundborg disease (EPM1) is an autosomal recessive inherited disorder due to a mutation in a gene that encodes for cystatin B (CSTB), a cysteine protease inhibitor. Symptoms start around 6–15 years and include myoclonic and tonic-clonic seizures. A *CstB* KO mouse model of EPM1 has been developed. *Cstb*-deficient mice are developmentally normal and fertile, but exhibit widespread granule cell loss in the cerebellum, myoclonic seizures during sleep and mild signs of ataxia at six months that worsen with age. However, mutant mice do not develop tonic-clonic seizures, photosensitivity or SWDs which have been reported in patients. Whether these differences indicate additional contributing factors in humans, or reflect the differences between human and mouse biology, brain development or a background strain effect, remains to be investigated (Pennacchio *et al.*, 1998).

Early life epilepsies due to immune/inflammatory etiologies

Rasmussen's encephalitis (RE): RE is characterized by refractory epilepsy that usually begins in the first decade of life leading to progressive degeneration of one cerebral hemisphere. The progressive worsening of the unilateral seizures is accompanied by evolving atrophy of the affected hemisphere and neurological symptoms. The etiology and pathogenesis are incompletely understood. A humoral autoimmune mechanism appears to contribute to the pathogenesis. Indeed, the immunization of rabbits with the glutamate receptor subunit GLUR3 results in epileptic seizures, with neurological deficits and histopathology of the cortex (Rogers *et al.*, 1994). Accordingly, a subset of patients with RE has circulating anti-GLUR3 IgG. Importantly, in some patients, seizure severity and frequency are reduced after plasmapheresis of IgG-selective immunoadsorption, in parallel with reduction of GLUR3 antibody titers (Rogers *et al.*, 1994; Andrews & McNamara 1996; Antozzi *et al.*,1998).

In this model, repeated subcutaneous injections of a GLUR3 protein linked to glutathione-S-transferase (GST) were given to white New Zealand male rabbits (He *et al.*, 1998). Two weeks after the second immunization, 2/5 animals developed motor incoordination while ambulating and epileptic seizures (repetitive tonic or clonic movements of the four paws). Subsequently animals developed persistent obtundation and failure to thrive. Immunization of rabbits with other GLURs and nicotinic acetylcholine receptor (nAChR) subunits did not induce this disorder. Multifocal inflammatory abnormalities are observed consisting of microglial nodules and perivascular lymphocytic cuffing, mainly in cerebral cortex and meninges. In contrast with the humans, the pathology occurs bilaterally (He *et al.*, 1998). Anti-GLUR3 IgG stained cortical neurons were present in two ill rabbits but not in healthy GLUR3 immunized rabbits. Limitations of this model are the cost for purchasing and maintaining of rabbits and the lack of reagents for this species.

Autoimmune encephalitides

Few studies have stereotactically injected patient intracerebroventricular auto-antibodies in adult rodents, but might shed insight in pediatric cases of autoimmune encephalitides. Anti-NR1 patients' auto-antibodies in the CA1 region cortical regions of adult rats increased extracellular glutamate (Manto *et al.*, 2010). Anti-NR1 auto-antibodies injections in 2 month old female rats impaired long term potentiation, action potential firing, excitatory post-synaptic potentials from hippocampal dentate granule neurons and also learning (Wurdemann *et al.*, 2016). No spontaneous seizures were observed and no change in susceptibility to chemically (gabazine, 8mM K^+, low Mg^{++}) induced epileptiform activity. However, a different study reported increased number of seizures and epileptic activity in adult mice injected with anti-NR autoantibodies, following PTZ challenge (Wright *et al.*, 2015). In utero (IU) exposure of mice to CASPR2 auto-antibodies predisposed them to sociability deficits in adulthood, disrupted the localization of glutamatergic neurons and formation of glutamatergic synapses, and increased microglia in the prefrontal and somatosensory cortices (Coutinho *et al.*, 2017).

Animal modes of absence epilepsy

Chronic models of atypical absence epilepsy (presumed to reflect a component of LGS)

The repeated administration over the first three postnatal weeks in rats of AY-9944 that inhibits the reduction of 7-dehydrocholesterol to cholesterol (Cenedella, 1980) leads to absence-like seizures starting at PN21. They are associated with abnormal cognitive outcome and persist into adulthood. Onset and offset of seizures are gradual and the animals maintain their ability to move purposefully as children with atypical absences. Valproate and ethosuximide reduce while phenytoin and GABA agonists exacerbate seizure frequency (Cortez *et al.*, 2001).

In a second model, MAM is administered on G15 leading to neuronal migration disorders. Then pups receive the AY-9944 treatment over the first three weeks, and develop spontaneous, recurrent, atypical absence seizures characterized by bilaterally synchronous slow 4–6 Hz SWDs. Seizures are refractory to ethosuximide and valproate, mimicking refractory atypical absence seizures that might occur in children with brain dysgenesis (Serbanescu *et al.*, 2004).

The overexpression of the $GABA_BR1a$ subtype in forebrain results in spontaneous atypical absence seizures. The $GABA_BR1a^{tg}$ mutant mouse shows all features of atypical absence seizures, including impaired hippocampal plasticity and impaired learning abilities, and hippocampal involvement in slow SWDs characteristic of this epilepsy (Wu *et al.*, 2007). The $GABA_BR1b$ transgenic mouse is a less severe model of this epilepsy (Stewart *et al.*, 2009).

Genetic models of absence epilepsy in rats (presumed to be models of CAE)

Two models of spontaneous occurrence of SWDs evocative of absence seizures have been described in untreated rats. Genetic absence epilepsy rats from Strasbourg (GAERS) were selected from Wistar colonies displaying spontaneous SWDs on routine cortical EEG. Breeding selected pairs for three or four generations produced a strain with 100% of rats displaying SWDs (Vergnes *et al.*, 1982). Concurrently, the fully inbred Wistar albino Glaxo strain of rats expressing cortical SWDs was discovered in Nijmegen and kept in Rijswijk (WAG/Rij) (van Luijtelaar & Coenen 1986).

In both strains, SWDs (7–11 Hz, 300–1,000 μV, 0.5–7.5 sec) start and end abruptly on normal, low amplitude desynchronized EEG background and are accompanied by behavioral arrest, staring and sometimes twitching of the vibrissae. Apart from epileptic episodes, these rats show normal behavior including feeding, exploration, social interaction, and learning. SWDs are expressed bilaterally in a thalamocortical pathway. In GAERS SWDs can last from 15 to 60 sec and occur about every minute (Danober *et al.*, 1998) In WAG/Rij, SWDs last only about 5 sec mainly during the dark period of the cycle. In both models, the seizures share many common features with human CAE. They are suppressed by antiepileptic medication effective in humans (ethosuximide, trimethadione, valproate, benzodiazepines, lamotrigine) and worsened by carbamazepine, phenytoin and all GABAergic drugs that aggravate human symptoms (Danober *et al.*, 1998; Jarre *et al.*, 2017b). They represent excellent predictive models for the response of the disease to new drugs in humans.

The main difference between the two models and human features is the ontogenetic development. In GAERS, the first SWDs are detected around PN30, about 30% of the rats are affected at PN40 and 100% by 3 months (Vergnes *et al.*, 1986). In WAG/Rij, the first SWDs occur by PN60-80 and only 50% of the rats display SWDs at 3 months, all rats being epileptic by 6 months (Coenen & Van Luijtelaar, 1987). Epileptogenesis progresses from oscillatory discharges, to oscillations and spike-waves and subsequently mature to well organized SWDs (Jarre *et al.*, 2017a; Jarre *et al.*, 2017b).

SWDs in GAERS and WAG/Rij are genetically determined by autosomal dominant inheritance (Marescaux *et al.*, 1992; Peeters *et al.*, 1992) of polygenic origin (Gauguier *et al.*, 2004; Rudolf *et al.*, 2004). No overt morphological modification was observed in the models. Glial fibrillary acidic protein (GFAP) expression was increased in cortex and thalamus of PD20 and adult GAERS, suggesting the presence of reactive astrocytes expressing interleukin-1β (IL-1β) and hence inflammation (Vezzani *et al.*, 2012) before the onset of absences (Dutuit *et al.*, 2000).

There are limited discrepancies between rat models and human absence epilepsy. The frequency of SWDs in humans is 3 Hz, compared to 7–11 Hz in rats. This could be species-dependent. Likewise, SWDs in GAERS and WAG/Rij occur when brain maturation is finished and last throughout the animals' life, while in humans they start during childhood and usually disappear at adolescence.

In mice and rats, spontaneous mutants display SWDs and absence epilepsy features. The mutation of over 20 genes is linked to this seizure phenotype. The mutations affect mainly calcium channels, glutamate- and GABA-receptor related channels. In addition, there are some monogenic models (Noebels, 2017). Some of the mutants are the tottering (tg) mouse with a mutation on a P/Q type calcium channel alpha subunit, the lethargic (lh) mouse with a mutation on the calcium channel beta 4 subunit, the ducky (du) mouse with a mutation on an alpha2-delta2 calcium channel subunit, the stargazer (stg) mouse with a mutation on the gamma2 calcium channel subunit, the SWE (swe) mouse with a mutation on the sodium hydrogen exchanger, the Mocha2j (mh) mouse with a mutation on the delta subunit AP3 adaptor protein and the Coloboma (Cm) mouse with a microdeletion including SNA25 and phospholipase C isoform β1. In most models, multiple abnormalities in network synchronization and excitability were found (Noebels, 2017).

Several transgenic mice with SWDs have been engineered, one with the deletion of the pacemaker channel HCN2 (Ludwig *et al.*, 2003) and one with the deletion a1G T-type calcium channel (Song *et al.*, 2004). A KI mouse for the $GABA_A$ receptor γ2 subunit point mutation (R43Q) was built based on a mutation found in an affected Australian family. Homozygous mice die before PN18. Heterozygous mice exhibit behavioral arrest associated with 6–7 Hz SWDs appearing with abrupt onset at PD20, corresponding to human childhood. These EEG abnormalities are suppressed by ethosuximide (Tan *et al.*, 2007).

In humans, the complex pattern of inheritance suggests the involvement of a large number of susceptibility genes (Hempelmann *et al.*, 2006). A polymorphism in the promoter of the $GABA_A$ and $GABA_B$ receptor subunit genes *GABRB3*, *GABRG3* and *GABRA5* (Robinson *et al.*, 2002; Urak *et al.*, 2006) and variants in the T-type calcium channel gene *CACNA1H* have been associated with CAE. Genes coding for voltage-gated calcium channels, including *CACNG3* (Robinson *et al.*, 2002; Everett *et al.*, 2007b) and the chloride channel gene *CLCN2* (Everett *et al.*, 2007a) may also be susceptibility loci. A homozygous, missense, single nucleotide mutation in *Cacna1h* was found in GAERS. This mutation segregates with seizure number and time in seizure activity. There are two major thalamic *Cacna1h* splice variants leading to a gain-of-function mutation, the one reported in GAERS depending on exonic splicing for functional expression (Powell *et al.*, 2009).

Animal models of epilepsy following early life SE

TLE is a common cause of complex partial seizures that most often originate in mesial temporal structures where lesions are often observed. Retrospective studies have shown that a large proportion of patients with TLE underwent an "initial precipitating injury" (IPI) occurring often before 4 years. The IPI is most frequently prolonged complex febrile seizures, SE, trauma, encephalopathy (Mathern *et al.*, 1997). This early event is followed by a latent phase free of any overt clinical or EEG signs. Spontaneous seizures usually start occurring around 10–15 years and become frequently medically intractable after a few years, requiring surgery of the epileptic focus (Engel, 1995).

However, the causal relationship between the IPI and subsequent TLE has not yet been established. Prospective clinical studies reported that seizures occurring early in life rarely result in hippocampal sclerosis (Shinnar, 1998; Berg *et al.*, 1999). According to VanLandigham *et al.* (VanLandingham *et al.*, 1998) and reviewed by Cendes (Cendes, 2004), only human infants having a preexisting hippocampal lesion or a genetic predisposition and experiencing an acute injury will develop hippocampal sclerosis and TLE. In rats also, prior exposure to a freeze lesion increases to 86% the percentage of immature rats that will develop epilepsy if subjected to febrile seizures (Scantlebury *et al.*, 2005). On the same line, in rats exposed to MAM-induced neuronal migration disorders, the dysplasias render the immature brain more sensitive to a further episode of seizures induced by hyperthermia at PN14 (Germano *et al.*, 1996), bicuculline or kainate at PN15 (de Feo *et al.*, 1995).

In animal models of TLE, the IPI is most often an episode of SE chemically induced by pilocarpine, lithium-pilocarpine or kainate, or electrically by stimulation of a limbic region like amygdala. About 100% of adult rats undergoing SE develop spontaneous recurrent seizures (SRS) after a mean latency of about two weeks (Turski *et al.*, 1989; Sperk, 1994; Curia *et al.*, 2008). SRS are usually motor stage 3–5 seizures involving myoclonic movements of the head, fore- and hindpaws, rearing and falling. On the EEG, seizures start with very rapid low amplitude activities followed by larger amplitude rapid spikes concurrent with myoclonic movements. After 30–60 sec the amplitude decreases and the postictal trace is characterized by synchronous discharges on a low amplitude background.

In younger rats, the severity, clinical expression and outcome of SE is different. In the kainate model, SE induction in PN15-18 male rats caused severe seizures, no detectable brain injury, no deoxyglucose (DG) uptake in the substantia nigra pars reticulata (SNR), no synaptic re-organization (mossy fiber sprouting) in the supragranular layer of the dentate gyrus, and did not increase the susceptibility to amygdala kindled seizures in adulthood (Albala *et al.*, 1984; Okada *et al.*, 1984; Sperber *et al.*, 1991). In contrast, kainate-induced SE in in PN33-37 and adult male rats caused less severe seizures, necrotic lesions, mossy fiber sprouting in the dentate gyrus, and increased DG uptake in the SNR. In PN4-6 rats exposed to repetitive kainate-induced SE, no FluoroJadeB stained cells were noted in the brain, no SRS were seen in adulthood, but sex-specific differences were reported in learning and $GABA_AR$ signaling after the SE (Galanopoulou, 2008; Akman *et al.*, 2015).

In the lithium-pilocarpine model, SE at PN10 does not lead to cell loss, SRS or change in seizure susceptibility in adulthood (Nehlig *et al.*, 2002). Only the repetition of pilocarpine SE on three consecutive days, PN7-9, leads to electrographic seizures accompanied by behavioral arrest followed sometimes by masticatory and orofacial automatisms. In 10% of animals, spontaneous clonic seizures are recorded in rats over PN60. These animals suffer from severe cognitive deficits and present persistent hyperexcitability in CA1 despite any major long-term neuronal loss (dos Santos *et al.*, 2000).

The occurrence of SRS is observed in ~30% of rats that experience SE at PN12-14 and in 50–70% of rats with SE at PN21-25 (Sankar *et al.*, 1998; Kubova *et al.*, 2004; Auvin *et al.*, 2010). At 3 months after SE, only non-convulsive seizures (freezing and/or automatisms like chewing, licking, vibrissae twitching) are recorded in rats with SE at PN12-14 (Kubova *et al.*, 2004; Suchomelova *et al.*, 2006; Auvin *et al.*, 2010; Kubova & Mares, 2013). A clonic motor component in SRS appears in 75–100% of the rats subjected to SE at 3–4 postnatal weeks (Priel *et al.*, 1996; Sankar *et al.*, 1998; Dube *et al.*, 2000; 2001; Kubova & Mares, 2013).

The induction of SE at PN14 leads to cell loss in CA1 while in PN18-24 rats, moderate neuronal loss is observed in the CA3, dentate gyrus hilus, entorhinal and piriform cortices and lateral thalamus, and mossy fiber sprouting (Priel *et al.*, 1996; Sankar *et al.*,1998; Cilio *et al.*, 2003). In the lithium-pilocarpine model applied in PN12 and PN25 rats, both the severity and incidence of SRS tend to progress with time, together with worsening of the loss of hilar neurons (Kubova & Mares 2013).

SE at PN12 leads to decreased performance on the rotarod, hypoactivity in the open field (Kubova *et al.*, 2000) and deficits in visual-spatial memory and water maze in adulthood (Cilio *et al.*, 2003). The cognitive/behavioral impairment is observed as early as 2 days after SE translating into ultrasonic vocalization at PN14 and memory impairment in rats that performed worse than controls when tested in the water maze at between PN20 and PN50 (Rutten *et al.*, 2002; Lopez-Meraz *et al.*, 2010). This cognitive involvement can be partially restored by enriched environment but this improvement is unrelated to EEG and histology that were not affected (Rutten *et al.*, 2002).

The use of MRI showed that, in adult rats subjected to lithium-pilocarpine SE, piriform and entorhinal cortices undergo rapid activation which appears only secondarily in the hippocampus (Roch *et al.*, 2002a). In PN21 rats, in which only a subset of animals subjected to SE becomes epileptic, the occurrence of a visible or measurable signal in piriform and entorhinal cortices at 24–48 h after SE is predictive of the later development of SRS and represents a surrogate marker to discriminate as soon as 24 h after SE whether rats will become epileptic or not (Roch *et al.*, 2002b).

Animal models of epilepsy following early life hypoxia/ischemia

Approximately 60% of neonatal seizures are associated with a hypoxic-ischemic event (Tekgul *et al.*, 2006; Ronen *et al.*, 2007). Survivors of neonatal hypoxic-ischemic encephalopathy often develop brain injury and neurologic disabilities such as cognitive deficits and epilepsy in later life (Bergamasco *et al.*, 1984; Robertson & Finer, 1988). Neonatal seizures occurring during hypoxic encephalopathy are usually prolonged and refractory to conventional antiepileptic drug therapy.

A model of perinatal seizures induced by hypoxia has been developed in rats (Jensen *et al.*, 1991). The model consists of a 15 min exposure to graded global hypoxia (7–4% O_2 in N_2) in an airtight chamber. A strict control of the body temperature is maintained with a heating pad. Seizures appear after 3–7 min and only during a specific age window (PN10-12). The model is easy to develop and mortality is extremely low (Jensen *et al.*, 1991). Acute seizures occur in more than 95% pups within 2–6 min after hypoxia onset, and are characterized by head bobbing, wet-dog shakes, and tonic-clonic movements. On the EEG, trains of rapid spike discharges associated with tonic-clonic body movements appear. The tonic-clonic seizures become progressively longer and can occur up to 4 days after the hypoxic episode. The EEG is isoelectric in adulthood (PN50). There is no overt cell loss or gliosis but hypoxia-induced seizures in pups lead to significant increases in CA3 mossy fiber sprouting later in life (Rakhade *et al.*, 2011; Lippman-Bell *et al.*, 2013).

These seizures are blocked by systemic administration of the AMPA receptor antagonist, NBQX (2,3-Dioxo-6-nitro-1,2,3,4-tetrahydrobenzo[*f*]quinoxaline-7-sulfonamide) and other agents that inhibit the AMPA receptor such as topiramate, talampanel and levetiracetam (Koh & Jensen 2001; Aujla *et al.*, 2009; Talos *et al.*, 2012). They do not respond to NR antagonists, $GABA_AR$ agonists or phenytoin (Jensen *et al.*, 1995). This model of hypoxia-induced seizures (Sun *et al.*, 2016) leads to mTOR pathway upregulation, long-term epilepsy and autistic-like social behavior deficits. These effects are blocked by early treatment with the mTOR inhibitor rapamycin (Talos *et al.*, 2013). Transient mTOR pathway activation is also suppressed by brief NBQX administration during the 48 h post-seizure in PN10 rats. NBQX or topiramate treatment reduces also spontaneous recurrent seizures, social preference deficits, and mossy fiber sprouting (Koh & Jensen, 2001; Lippman-Bell *et al.*, 2013). Rats that experience hypoxia induced seizures at PN10 show a long term increase in susceptibility to seizures induced by PTZ, flurothyl or kainate (Jensen *et al.*, 1992).

Mouse hypoxia models have also been developed. On one hand, acute seizures were evoked during intermittent global hypoxia in PN9 C57BL/6 mice (Rakhade *et al.*, 2012). Oxygen concentration is lowered sequentially to 9%, 6%, 5.5% and 5% for 5 min periods with 5 min intervals lasting 40 min before termination of hypoxia. Acute seizures are observed in more than 85% mice during hypoxia. These seizures are characterized by pawing, myoclonic jerks, head shaking, and loss of posture. In this model, acute changes in hippocampal neuronal excitability and glutamate receptor alterations are recorded in the mice (Rakhade *et al.*, 2012). On the other hand, hypoxic seizures in immature mice can be induced during the phase of reoxygenation. Typical electrographic seizures are reliably evoked within 2 min of reoxygenation after exposing PN7–8 mice to global hypoxia (3–4% O_2) for 4 min (Zanelli *et al.*, 2014). On the EEG, rhythmic spike activity starting as low amplitude polyspikes is recorded. Both approaches recapitulate a panel of clinical features of human neonatal seizures but it is not yet known whether these mice will develop spontaneous seizures later in life.

Animal models of epilepsy associated with fever/hyperthermia

Febrile seizures (FS) are commonly affecting about 3–5% of infants and young children (Smith *et al.*, 1996). The mechanisms responsible for the occurrence of FS are still not fully understood.

FS models have been mainly developed in rats and mice. In rats, the highest susceptibility to hyperthermia-induced seizures is found in PN10-13 pups. The best characterized FS model in rats was developed by Baram *et al.* (Baram *et al.*, 1997). Core and brain temperature is slowly increased in PN10-11 rats by a stream of heated hair and seizures occur at a threshold temperature of 40.9° C. The brain temperature increases by 2° C/min until seizure onset. The latency to seizure onset is usually 2–4 min and hyperthermia is maintained for 30 min (Dube *et al.*, 2000). Afterwards, pups are hydrated orally and transferred to a cool surface until their core temperature reaches 32–34° C. Mouse FS models have also been used to facilitate studies on genetically mutant strains (Dube *et al.*, 2005; van Gassen *et al.*, 2008).

Acute FS seizures start with sudden freezing followed by oral automatisms (chewing, biting) and often forelimb clonic movements followed by tonic body flexion (Dube *et al.*, 2004). The EEG activity shows trains of spikes and SWDs of progressively increasing amplitude in hippocampus and amygdala that coincide with immobility and oral automatisms. There is a progression to the cortex where the EEG is unchanged or just flattening (Dube *et al.*, 2006). SRS develop in adulthood in about 35% of rats and interictal spiking occur in about 88% of the rats (Dube & Baram, 2006). An i.c.v. injection of IL-1β lowers the threshold for hyperthermic seizures in mouse pups. A high-dose i.c.v. injection of IL-1β is even capable of inducing seizures without a thermal trigger (Dube *et al.*, 2005). Likewise, in rats, intranasal administration of IL-1β results in lower temperature seizure threshold (Fukuda *et al.*, 2009).

Hyperthermia-induced seizures do not lead to any acute or delayed neuronal death in hippocampus (Bender *et al.*, 2003), although transient neuronal injury is detectable over two weeks in hippocampus, amygdala and perirhinal cortex (Toth *et al.*, 1998). Prolonged hyperthermic seizures and hyperthermia-induced SE (HSE) lead to strong astrocytic and mild microglial activation 6 h after seizure onset. At 24 h, IL-1β is produced in hippocampus (Dube *et al.*, 2010). The T2 MRI hypersignal seen in hippocampus and amygdala after HSE is predictive of epilepsy correlating with increased proinflammatory cytokines expression (Patterson *et al.*, 2015).

Schuchmann *et al.* (2006) chose to induce hyperthermia by placing the pups in a chamber heated at about 48° C. The rise in body temperature is slower than in the Baram's group model. Hyperthermia-induced seizures start at about 30 min from hyperthermia exposure onset (Schuchmann *et al.*, 2006). This work highlighted that heat-induced respiratory alkalosis is a key factor for hyperthermic seizure occurrence in both the heated chamber and the hot air convection system (Schuchmann *et al.*, 2008). Hyperthermia-induced seizures are rapidly suppressed by a low (5%) level of ambient CO_2 (Schuchmann *et al.*, 2006).

Hyperthermic seizures have also been induced in larval zebrafish (Hunt *et al.*, 2012) and one tentative was made *in vitro* (Tancredi *et al.*, 1992).

Animal models of epilepsy associated with brain malformations

Malformations of cortical development (MCD) represent a wide spectrum of pathological abnormalities of the brain whose classification scheme is based on the stage at which cortical development is first disrupted (Barkovich *et al.*, 2012). However, there is considerable overlap between different types of MCD, and some may result from defects in multiple stages of cortical development (Wong & Roper, 2016). Epilepsy associated with MCD is typically severe, often with onset of seizures in early childhood or infancy, and frequently intractable or resistant to available anti-seizure medications (Aronica *et al.*, 2012; Guerrini & Dobyns, 2014). Several models of MCD have been generated to help researchers in clarifying basic mechanisms underlying these conditions. In some cases, these models offered many advantages for investigating cellular and molecular features of human cortical malformations associated with epilepsy (Wong & Roper, 2016).

Examples of genetic models

ARX models. Mutations in this gene cause malformative as well as non-malformative phenotypes (Kato *et al.*, 2004; Shoubridge *et al.*, 2010). Mice lacking this gene exhibit small brains and aberrant migration and differentiation of GABAergic interneurons, recapitulating some of the clinical features of X-linked lissencephaly with abnormal genitalia (XLAG), and die within the first postnatal day (Kitamura *et al.*, 2002). See also the section on chronic models of infantile spasms.

Doublecortin (DCX) models. DCX mediates neuronal migration by regulating the organization and stability of microtubules (Gleeson *et al.*, 1999). Knockdown (KD) of *Dcx* in rat embryos brains through *IU*-RNA interference (IU-RNAi) causes subcortical band heterotopia (SBH), increased propensity to convulsant-induced seizures at juvenile ages, and spontaneous focal, absence-like seizures in adulthood, recapitulating the phenotype observed in patients with *DCX* mutations (Ackman *et al.*, 2009; Lapray *et al.*, 2010).

Filamin A (FlnA) models. FLNA is a widely expressed actin-binding protein involved in regulating the reorganization of the actin cytoskeleton. *FlnA* KO mice, which die during mid-gestation, do not exhibit periventricular nodular heterotopia (PNH) or misplaced neurons (Feng *et al.*, 2006; Hart *et al.*, 2006). Conversely, IU-RNAi-based *Flna* KD in rat embryos brains impairs cell-cycle progression and neuronal migration by disrupting the organization of radial glia, leading to a PNH phenotype that partially recapitulates that observed in patients carrying *FLNA* mutations (Fox *et al.*, 1998; Sheen *et al.*, 2001; Parrini *et al.*, 2006; Carabalona *et al.*, 2012). Juvenile *FlnA* KD rats also exhibit a higher susceptibility to PTZ-induced seizures, although a correlation between seizure occurrence and the extent of PNH has not been demonstrated (Carabalona *et al.*, 2012). These observations are in line with clinical observations that no correlation is feasible between the extent of PNH and epilepsy severity (Parrini *et al.*, 2006).

Tsc1 models. By interacting with TSC2, TSC1 inhibits the activity of mTOR pathway (Caban *et al.*, 2017). Conditional KO of *Tsc1* in selected neuronal populations and at precise developmental timepoints results in white matter heterotopic nodules and discrete tuber-like lesions resembling those observed in patients with TSC (Feliciano *et al.*, 2011). Although these cKO mice do not develop SRS, they exhibit 25% reduction in seizure latency compared to control littermates after PTZ treatment (Feliciano *et al.*, 2011).

Phosphatase and tensin homolog (PTEN) models. PTEN antagonizes the mTOR pathway through its lipid phosphatase activity (Pezzolesi *et al.*, 2007). Homozygous deletion of *PTEN* results in early embryonic lethality in rodents (Stambolic *et al.*, 1998; Suzuki *et al.*, 1998). Mice with targeted inactivation of *Pten* in neurons of the cerebral cortex and hippocampus show macrocephaly and abnormal social interaction, resembling in part the phenotype observed in patients with autism spectrum disorders (Kwon *et al.*, 2006). These mice also exhibit neuronal hypertrophy, hypertrophic dendrites and axon tracts with increased synapses. Spontaneous seizures with repetitive spike and wave patterns, sometimes accompanied by rhythmic slow activity and continuous spike and wave bursting have been observed in about 10% of *Pten* cKO mice (Kwon *et al.*, 2006). Selective deletion of *Pten* in adult granule cells in mice results in spontaneous seizures beginning 4–6 weeks after gene deletion (Pun *et al.*, 2012). Granule cells from these mice developed abnormally, exhibiting morphological features indicative of increased excitatory input (LaSarge *et al.*, 2015).

MTOR models. MTOR controls many basic cellular functions including protein synthesis, energy metabolism, cell size, and autophagy. In the brain, it is involved in neuronal development, synaptic plasticity, and cognition (Bockaert & Marin 2015). By using IU electroporation, Lim and collaborators demonstrated that mice expressing the p.Leu247Pro *mTOR* mutation, which in humans is associated with focal cortical dysplasia type II and intractable epilepsy, exhibited neuronal migration disruption and cytomegalic neurons (Lim *et al.*, 2015). In addition, more than 90% of these mice exhibited SRS with epileptic discharges comprising high-voltage spikes and low voltage fast activities (Lim *et al.*, 2015). Notably, epileptic and histopathological phenotypes observed in p.Leu247Pro mice were almost completely rescued by rapamycin treatment (Lim *et al.*, 2015).

Examples of physical and chemical models

Ibotenate models. Ibotenate is an agonist of the NR. Intracerebral injection of ibotenate in mice, rats and hamsters produces excitotoxic brain lesions mimicking human neuronal migration disorders including polymicrogyria, PNH and SBH (Takano *et al.*, 2004). Although epileptic seizures have not so far been described in these models (Luhmann, 2016), electrophysiological recordings of evoked field potentials in slice preparations from adult rats treated with ibotenate at day of birth revealed hyperexcitability in widespread cortical regions surrounding the dysplasia (Redecker *et al.*, 1998).

MAM models. MAM is a potent cytotoxic agent that induces a time-specific aberrant DNA methylation and alkylation, leading to abnormal patterns of cell formation and migration. (Luhmann, 2016). In the brain of ferrets treated with MAM, the migration speed and exploratory behavior of migrating neurons is significantly reduced (Abbah & Juliano, 2014). MAM administration causes alterations in hippocampal and neocortical regions, as well as neuronal heterotopia along the walls of lateral ventricles which resembles human PNH (Luhmann, 2016). Subcortical heterotopic nodules exhibit abnormal intrinsic firing properties with sustained repetitive bursts of action potentials (Colacitti *et al.*, 1999).

Freeze lesion models. The freeze lesion model can be easily established by applying stainless or copper probes cooled in liquid nitrogen on the exposed calvarium above the cortical region of interest for 8–10 sec (Luhmann, 2016). The severity and type of cortical malformation generated is directly related to the number and duration of freeze lesions, indicating that a single pathophysiological event of variable severity at a specific developmental stage can induce different brain malformations (Rosen & Galaburda, 2000). The most consistent result of focal cortical freeze in newborn rodents is the formation of a four layered microgyrus (Luhmann, 2016). Electrophysiological studies demonstrated that freeze-lesioned rats exhibit a pronounced hyperexcitability in the subcortical region surrounding the microgyrus, indicating that the neocortical region adjacent to the microgyrus, and not the microgyrus itself, is the generator of the epileptiform activity (Luhmann, 2016). Andresen and collaborators demonstrated that one-week treatment with gabapentin immediately after freeze lesioning prevented the development of hyperexcitabilty *in vitro* and *in vivo* and may have therapeutic potential to minimize epileptogenic processes associated with developmental cortical malformations (Andresen *et al.*, 2014).

Kindling in developing rodents

Kindling is the progressive development of seizures in response to a subconvulsant stimulus administered at regular intervals (Goddard *et al.*, 1969). Traditionally kindling has been performed using brief, low intensity trains of electrical stimulation (electrical kindling), but kindling can be obtained also using chemicals. Kindling is an epilepsy model of complex partial seizures with secondary generalization (McIntyre, 1970). Electrical kindling represents the best model of age-specific patterns of seizure propagation and is considered a reliable method of assessing seizure susceptibility in the developing brain. Once induced it persists into adulthood. Kindling was the first model to document increased seizure susceptibility *via* amygdala stimulation in infantile pups (Moshe, 1981).

The kindling phenomenon has been studied in rats starting at the end of the first postnatal week (Baram *et al.*, 1993). Seizure propagation from the stimulation site occurs faster during the first three weeks of life than in mature animals (Moshe, 1981). Immature rats spend less time in kindling stages marking the focal seizure origin (stages 1–2) compared to older rats. Focal afterdischarges are not easily confined to the stimulated focus and kindled seizures recurring at short time intervals develop rapidly (Moshe, 1981; Moshe & Albala 1983; Moshe *et al.*, 1983; Baram *et al.*, 1993). At PN7-9, kindled rats rarely develop bilateral clonic seizures or rearing and progress from unilateral clonic seizures to tonic seizures. At PN15-17, pups are also more prone to develop recurrent kindled seizures (Moshe & Albala 1983). Likewise, more severe seizures such as explosive jumping and tonic seizures (stages 6–7) require less than 30 stimulations in immature rats (Haas *et al.*, 1990;1992) compared to about 100 stimulations in adult rats (Pinel & Rovner 1978). Alternating stimulations of two sites in immature rats leads to the development of seizures from both sites and accelerates kindling at both sites (Haas *et al.*, 1990;1992) while in adult rats kindling antagonism develops (Burchfiel *et al.*, 1986). This observation suggests that in pups, the circuits for seizure control are not mature. One of these circuits involves the SNR and its output system (Moshe, 1987). These kindling data suggest that in the immature brain, the refractory period that follows a seizure is very short compared to the long refractory period observed in adulthood and this may underlie the propensity of the immature brain for faster progression of seizures and development of SE (Moshe & Albala 1983). In immature rats, kindling of limbic structures leads to persistent alterations in the brain. Kindled PN15-18 rats can be rekindled faster during adulthood, whether the stimulation is applied ipsilaterally or contralaterally (Moshe & Albala 1983). These rats do not show any significant cell loss at CA3 or CA1, or mossy fiber sprouting, demonstrating that the permanent kindling phenomenon occurs without any underlying histological change (Ackermann *et al.*, 1989; Haas *et al.*, 2001).

Diazepam (Albertson *et al.*, 1982), gabapentin (Lado *et al.*, 2001) and ACTH (Holmes & Weber, 1986) inhibit the development of kindling in immature rats. Progesterone has no effect on kindling in adult while in immature rats the hormone markedly inhibits kindling, preventing generalization of seizures (Holmes & Weber, 1984).

Conclusions

The immature brain is not a miniature version of the adult brain. Indeed, its maturation is based on careful sequences of cell birth, proliferation, formation of synapses and pruning and, at times, cell death. These events have time specific windows and are influenced by genetic and epigenetic factors including sex hormones. In the past 40 years, there has been much progress in developing animal models depicting human epileptic syndromes that have their onset early in life. We have reached a better understanding of the pathophysiology of seizure onset and propagation as well as the consequences and potential therapeutic paradigms for the epileptic disorders that occur in infancy and childhood. Treatment discovery has already started shifting towards using syndrome-specific animal models of pediatric epilepsies and seizures to identify better treatments for these syndromes. Nevertheless, there is a continuing need to develop effective translational approaches in order to prevent, treat or cure the progressive syndromes that may have long term effects on brain development and the life of the individual. It is necessary to identify the best possible models to screen for the efficacy of putative agents to stop ongoing seizures and, when appropriate, prevent the creation of a permanent epileptic state without disturbing the delicate steps underlying brain maturation.

Acknowledgements

ASG has been supported by research grants from NINDS-NS91170, NINDS-1U54NS100064, Department of Defense (W81XWH-13-1-0180 and W81XWH-18-1-0612), an IDDRC pilot grant from the Rose F. Kennedy IDDRC NICHD grant 5U54HD090260-03, and the Infantile Spasms Initiative from CURE (Citizens United for Research in Epilepsy), and acknowledges also research funding from the Heffer Family and the Segal Family Foundations and the Abbe Goldstein/Joshua Lurie and Laurie Marsh/Dan Levitz families. She is Editor-in-Chief of Epilepsia Open. She has received honoraria for participation at scientific advisory boards for Mallinckrodt and Eisai and royalties from Elsevier for publications. There are no conflicts in regards to this manuscript.

SLM is the Charles Frost Chair in Neurosurgery and Neurology and partially funded by grants from NIH U54 NS100064 and NS43209, US Department of Defense (W81XWH-13-1-0180 and W81XWH-18-1-0612), CURE Infantile Spasms Initiative and the Heffer Family and the Segal Family Foundations and the Abbe Goldstein/Joshua Lurie and Laurie Marsh/Dan Levitz families. He is serving as Associate Editor of *Neurobiology of Disease* and is on the editorial board of *Brain and Development*, *Pediatric Neurology and Physiological Research*. He receives from Elsevier an annual compensation for his work as Associate Editor in *Neurobiology of Disease* and royalties from 2 books he co-edited. He received a consultant fee from Mallinkrodt and UCB. He has no conflicts on interest in regards to this article.

AN has been supported by continuous INSERM grants (U272, U398, U666, U1129) and grants from the Fondation pour la Recherche Médicale and Fondation Française pour la Recherche en Epilepsie.

REFERENCES

Abbah J, Juliano SL (2014): Altered migratory behavior of interneurons in a model of cortical dysplasia: the influence of elevated GABAA activity. *Cereb Cortex* 24: 2297–2308.

Ackermann RF, Moshe SL, Albala BJ (1989): Restriction of enhanced [2–14C]deoxyglucose utilization to rhinencephalic structures in immature amygdala-kindled rats. *Exp Neurol* 104: 73–81.

Ackman JB, Aniksztejn L, Crepel V, *et al.* (2009): Abnormal network activity in a targeted genetic model of human double cortex. *J Neurosci* 29: 313–327.

Akman O, Briggs SW, Galanopoulou AS (2012). Long-term follow up of the multiple-model of symptomatic infantile spasms. *American Epilepsy Society annual meeting*, San Diego, CA, American Epilepsy Society.

Akman O, Moshe SL, Galanopoulou AS (2014): Sex-specific consequences of early life seizures. *Neurobiol Dis* 72 Pt B: 153–166.

Akman O, Moshe SL, Galanopoulou AS (2015): Early life status epilepticus and stress have distinct and sex-specific effects on learning, subsequent seizure outcomes, including anticonvulsant response to phenobarbital. *CNS Neurosci Ther* 21: 181–192.

Albala BJ, Moshe SL, Okada R (1984): Kainic-acid-induced seizures: a developmental study. *Brain Res* 315: 139–148.

Albertson TE, Bowyer JF, Paule MG (1982): Modification of the anticonvulsant efficacy of diazepam by Ro-15-1788 in the kindled amygdaloid seizure model. *Life Sci* 31: 1597–1601.

Andresen L, Hampton D, Taylor-Weiner A, *et al.* (2014): Gabapentin attenuates hyperexcitability in the freeze-lesion model of developmental cortical malformation. *Neurobiol Dis* 71: 305–316.

Andrews PI, McNamara JO (1996): Rasmussen's encephalitis: an autoimmune disorder? *Curr Opin Neurol* 9: 141–145.

Antozzi C, Granata T, Aurisano N, *et al.* (1998): Long-term selective IgG immuno-adsorption improves Rasmussen's encephalitis. *Neurology* 51: 302–305.

Aronica E, Becker AJ, Spreafico R (2012): Malformations of cortical development. *Brain Pathol* 22: 380–401.

Auerbach DS, Jones J, Clawson BC, *et al.* (2013): Altered cardiac electrophysiology and SUDEP in a model of Dravet syndrome. *PLoS One* 8: e77843.

Aujla PK, Fetell MR, Jensen FE (2009): Talampanel suppresses the acute and chronic effects of seizures in a rodent neonatal seizure model. *Epilepsia* 50: 694–701.

Auvin S, Mazarati A, Shin D, Sankar R (2010): Inflammation enhances epileptogenesis in the developing rat brain. *Neurobiol Dis* 40: 303–310.

Avishai-Eliner S, Brunson KL, Sandman CA, Baram TZ (2002): Stressed-out, or in (utero)? *Trends Neurosci* 25: 518–524.

Baraban SC, Dinday MT, Hortopan GA (2013): Drug screening in SCN1A zebrafish mutant identifies clemizole as a potential Dravet syndrome treatment. *Nat Commun* 4: 2410.

Baram TZ (1993): Pathophysiology of massive infantile spasms: perspective on the putative role of the brain adrenal axis. *Ann Neurol* 33: 231–236.

Baram TZ, Gerth A, Schultz L (1997): Febrile seizures: an appropriate-aged model suitable for long-term studies. *Brain Res Dev Brain Res* 98: 265–270.

Baram TZ, Hirsch E, Schultz L (1993): Short-interval amygdala kindling in neonatal rats. *Brain Res Dev Brain Res* 73: 79–83.

Baram TZ, Schultz L (1995): ACTH does not control neonatal seizures induced by administration of exogenous corticotropin-releasing hormone. *Epilepsia* 36: 174–178.

Barkovich AJ, Guerrini R, Kuzniecky RI, Jackson GD, Dobyns WB (2012): A developmental and genetic classification for malformations of cortical development: update 2012. *Brain* 135: 1348–1369.

Beatty CW, Wrede JE, Blume HK (2017): Diagnosis, treatment, and outcomes of infantile spasms in the Trisomy 21 population. *Seizure* 45: 184–188.

Bender RA, Dube C, Gonzalez-Vega R, Mina EW, Baram TZ (2003): Mossy fiber plasticity and enhanced hippocampal excitability, without hippocampal cell loss or altered neurogenesis, in an animal model of prolonged febrile seizures. *Hippocampus* 13: 399–412.

Berg AT, Shinnar S, Levy SR, Testa FM (1999): Childhood-onset epilepsy with and without preceding febrile seizures. *Neurology* 53: 1742–1748.

Bergamasco B, Benna P, Ferrero P, Gavinelli R (1984): Neonatal hypoxia and epileptic risk: a clinical prospective study. *Epilepsia* 25: 131–136.

Berkovic SF, Andermann F, Carpenter S, Wolfe LS (1986): Progressive myoclonus epilepsies: specific causes and diagnosis. *N Engl J Med* 315: 296–305.

Bockaert J, Marin P (2015): mTOR in Brain Physiology and Pathologies. *Physiol Rev* 95: 1157–1187.

Briggs SW, Mowrey W, Hall CB, Galanopoulou AS (2014): CPP-115, a vigabatrin analogue, decreases spasms in the multiple-hit rat model of infantile spasms. *Epilepsia* 55: 94–102.

Burchfiel JL, Applegate CD, Konkol RJ (1986): Kindling antagonism: A role for norepinephrine in seizure suppresion. *Kindling 3*. Wada JA (ed). New York, Raven Press: 213–229.

Caban C, Khan N, Hasbani DM, Crino PB (2017): Genetics of tuberous sclerosis complex: implications for clinical practice. *Appl Clin Genet* 10: 1–8.

Cao D, Ohtani H, Ogiwara I, Ohtani S, *et al.* (2012): Efficacy of stiripentol in hyperthermia-induced seizures in a mouse model of Dravet syndrome. *Epilepsia* 53: 1140–1145.

Carabalona A, Beguin S, Pallesi-Pocachard E, *et al.* (2012): A glial origin for periventricular nodular heterotopia caused by impaired expression of Filamin-A. *Hum Mol Genet* 21: 1004–1017.

Cendes F (2004): Febrile seizures and mesial temporal sclerosis. *Curr Opin Neurol* 17: 161–164.

Cenedella RJ (1980): Concentration-dependent effects of AY-9944 and U18666A on sterol synthesis in brain. Variable sensitivities of metabolic steps. *Biochem Pharmacol* 29: 2751–2754.

Chachua T, Di Grazia P, Chern CR, *et al.* (2016): Estradiol does not affect spasms in the betamethasone-NMDA rat model of infantile spasms. *Epilepsia* 57: 1326–1336.

Chachua T, Poon KL, Yum MS, *et al.* (2012): Rapamycin has age-, treatment paradigm-, and model-specific anticonvulsant effects and modulates neuropeptide Y expression in rats. *Epilepsia* 53: 2015–2025.

Chachua T, Yum MS, Veliskova J, Velisek L (2011): Validation of the rat model of cryptogenic infantile spasms. *Epilepsia* 52: 1666–1677.

Cheah CS, Yu FH, Westenbroek RE, *et al.* (2012): Specific deletion of NaV1.1 sodium channels in inhibitory interneurons causes seizures and premature death in a mouse model of Dravet syndrome. *Proc Natl Acad Sci USA* 109: 14646–14651.

Chen C, Westenbroek RE, Xu X, *et al.* (2004): Mice lacking sodium channel beta1 subunits display defects in neuronal excitability, sodium channel expression, and nodal architecture. *J Neurosci* 24: 4030–4042.

Chu-Shore CJ, Major P, Camposano S, Muzykewicz D, Thiele EA (2010): The natural history of epilepsy in tuberous sclerosis complex. *Epilepsia* 51: 1236–1241.

Cilio MR, Sogawa Y, Cha BH, Liu X, Huang LT, Holmes GL (2003): Long-term effects of status epilepticus in the immature brain are specific for age and model. *Epilepsia* 44: 518–528.

Coenen AM, Van Luijtelaar EL (1987): The WAG/Rij rat model for absence epilepsy: age and sex factors. *Epilepsy Res* 1: 297–301.

Colacitti C, Sancini G, DeBiasi S, *et al.* (1999): Prenatal methylazoxymethanol treatment in rats produces brain abnormalities with morphological similarities to human developmental brain dysgeneses. *J Neuropathol Exp Neurol* 58: 92–106.

Cortez MA, McKerlie C, Snead OC, 3rd (2001): A model of atypical absence seizures: EEG, pharmacology, and developmental characterization. *Neurology* 56: 341–349.

Cortez MA, Shen L, Wu Y, *et al.* (2009): Infantile spasms and Down syndrome: a new animal model. *Pediatr Res* 65: 499–503.

Coutinho E, Menassa DA, Jacobson L, *et al.* (2017): Persistent microglial activation and synaptic loss with behavioral abnormalities in mouse offspring exposed to CASPR2-antibodies in utero. *Acta Neuropathol* 134: 567–583.

Curia G, Longo D, Biagini G, Jones RS, Avoli M (2008): The pilocarpine model of temporal lobe epilepsy. *J Neurosci Methods* 172: 143–157.

Danober L, Deransart C, Depaulis A, Vergnes M, Marescaux C (1998): Pathophysiological mechanisms of genetic absence epilepsy in the rat. *Prog Neurobiol* 55: 27–57.

de Feo MR, Mecarelli O, Ricci GF (1995): Seizure susceptibility in immature rats with micrencephaly induced by prenatal exposure to methylazoxymethanol acetate. *Pharmacol Res* 31: 109–114.

Dobbing J, Sands J (1979): Comparative aspects of the brain growth spurt. *Early Hum Dev* 3: 79–83.

dos Santos NF, Arida RM, Filho EM, Priel MR, Cavalheiro EA (2000): Epileptogenesis in immature rats following recurrent status epilepticus. *Brain Res Brain Res Rev* 32: 269–276.

Doumlele K, Conway E, Hedlund J, Tolete P, Devinsky O (2016): A case report on the efficacy of vigabatrin analogue (1S, 3S)-3-amino-4-difluoromethylenyl-1-cyclopentanoic acid (CPP-115) in a patient with infantile spasms. *Epilepsy Behav Case Rep* 6: 67–69.

Dube C, Boyet S, Marescaux C, Nehlig A (2000): Progressive metabolic changes underlying the chronic reorganization of brain circuits during the silent phase of the lithium-pilocarpine model of epilepsy in the immature and adult Rat. *Exp Neurol* 162: 146–157.

Dube C, Boyet S, Marescaux C, Nehlig A (2001): Relationship between neuronal loss and interictal glucose metabolism during the chronic phase of the lithium-pilocarpine model of epilepsy in the immature and adult rat. *Exp Neurol* 167: 227–241.

Dube C, Richichi C, Bender RA, Chung G, Litt B, Baram TZ (2006): Temporal lobe epilepsy after experimental prolonged febrile seizures: prospective analysis. *Brain* 129: 911–922.

Dube C, Vezzani A, Behrens M, Bartfai T, Baram TZ (2005): Interleukin-1beta contributes to the generation of experimental febrile seizures. *Ann Neurol* 57: 152–155.

Dube C, Yu H, Nalcioglu O, Baram TZ (2004): Serial MRI after experimental febrile seizures: altered T2 signal without neuronal death. *Ann Neurol* 56: 709–714.

Dube CM, Baram TZ (2006): Complex febrile seizures – An animal model in rodents. *Book Complex febrile seizures – An animal model in rodents*, pp. 333–340. San Diego: Elsevier.

Dube CM, Molet J, Singh-Taylor A, Ivy A, Maras PM, Baram TZ (2015): Hyper-excitability and epilepsy generated by chronic early-life stress. *Neurobiol Stress* 2: 10–19.

Dube CM, Ravizza T, Hamamura M, *et al.* (2010): Epileptogenesis provoked by prolonged experimental febrile seizures: mechanisms and biomarkers. *J Neurosci* 30: 7484–7494.

Dutton SB, Sawyer NT, Kalume F, *et al.* (2011): Protective effect of the ketogenic diet in Scn1a mutant mice. *Epilepsia* 52: 2050–2056.

Dutuit M, Didier-Bazes M, Vergnes M, *et al.* (2000): Specific alteration in the expression of glial fibrillary acidic protein, glutamate dehydrogenase, and glutamine synthetase in rats with genetic absence epilepsy. *Glia* 32: 15–24.

Engel J, Jr. (1995): Critical evaluation of animal models for localization-related epilepsies. *Ital J Neurol Sci* 16: 9–16.

Epi4K Consortium, Epilepsy Phenome/Genome P, Allen AS, Berkovic SF, Cossette P, *et al.* (2013): *De novo* mutations in epileptic encephalopathies. *Nature* 501: 217–221.

EuroEPINOMICS-RES Consortium, Epilepsy Phenome/Genome Project and Epi4K Consortium (2014): *De novo* mutations in synaptic transmission genes including DNM1 cause epileptic encephalopathies. *Am J Hum Genet* 95: 360–370.

Everett K, Chioza B, Aicardi J, *et al.* (2007a): Linkage and mutational analysis of CLCN2 in childhood absence epilepsy. *Epilepsy Res* 75: 145–153.

Everett KV, Chioza B, Aicardi J, *et al.* (2007b): Linkage and association analysis of CACNG3 in childhood absence epilepsy. *Eur J Hum Genet* 15: 463–472.

Feliciano DM, Su T, Lopez J, Platel JC, Bordey A (2011): Single-cell Tsc1 knockout during corticogenesis generates tuber-like lesions and reduces seizure threshold in mice. *J Clin Invest* 121: 1596–1607.

Feng Y, Chen MH, Moskowitz IP, *et al.* (2006): Filamin A (FLNA) is required for cell-cell contact in vascular development and cardiac morphogenesis. *Proc Natl Acad Sci USA* 103: 19836–19841.

Fox JW, Lamperti ED, Eksioglu YZ, *et al.* (1998): Mutations in filamin 1 prevent migration of cerebral cortical neurons in human periventricular heterotopia. *Neuron* 21: 1315–1325.

Friocourt G, Parnavelas JG (2010): Mutations in ARX Result in Several Defects Involving GABAergic Neurons. *Front Cell Neurosci* 4: 4.

Frost JD, Jr., Le JT, Lee CL, Ballester-Rosado C, Hrachovy RA, Swann JW (2015): Vigabatrin therapy implicates neocortical high frequency oscillations in an animal model of infantile spasms. *Neurobiol Dis* 82: 1–11.

Frost JD, Jr., Lee CL, Hrachovy RA, Swann JW (2011): High frequency EEG activity associated with ictal events in an animal model of infantile spasms. *Epilepsia* 52: 53–62.

Fukuda M, Suzuki Y, Ishizaki Y, *et al.* (2009): Interleukin-1beta enhances susceptibility to hyperthermia-induced seizures in developing rats. *Seizure* 18: 211–214.

Galanopoulou AS (2008): Dissociated gender-specific effects of recurrent seizures on GABA signaling in CA1 pyramidal neurons: role of GABA(A) receptors. *J Neurosci* 28: 1557–1567.

Galanopoulou AS, Gorter JA, Cepeda C (2012): Finding a better drug for epilepsy: the mTOR pathway as an antiepileptogenic target. *Epilepsia* 53: 1119–1130.

Galanopoulou AS, Moshe SL (2011): In search of epilepsy biomarkers in the immature brain: goals, challenges and strategies. *Biomark Med* 5: 615–628.

Galanopoulou AS, Moshe SL (2015): Pathogenesis and new candidate treatments for infantile spasms and early life epileptic encephalopathies: A view from preclinical studies. *Neurobiol Dis* 79: 135–149.

Galanopoulou AS, Mowrey WB, Liu W, Li Q, Shandra O, Moshe SL (2017): Preclinical Screening for Treatments for Infantile Spasms in the Multiple Hit Rat Model of Infantile Spasms: An Update. *Neurochem Res* 42: 1949–1961.

Gataullina S, Lemaire E, Wendling F, *et al.* (2016): Epilepsy in young Tsc1(+/-) mice exhibits age-dependent expression that mimics that of human tuberous sclerosis complex. *Epilepsia* 57: 648–659.

Gauguier D, van Luijtelaar G, Bihoreau MT, *et al.* (2004): Chromosomal mapping of genetic loci controlling absence epilepsy phenotypes in the WAG/Rij rat. *Epilepsia* 45: 908–915.

Germano IM, Zhang YF, Sperber EF, Moshe SL (1996): Neuronal migration disorders increase susceptibility to hyperthermia-induced seizures in developing rats. *Epilepsia* 37: 902–910.

Gheyara AL, Ponnusamy R, Djukic B, *et al.* (2014): Tau reduction prevents disease in a mouse model of Dravet syndrome. *Ann Neurol* 76: 443–456.

Gleeson JG, Lin PT, Flanagan LA, Walsh CA (1999): Doublecortin is a microtubule-associated protein and is expressed widely by migrating neurons. *Neuron* 23: 257–271.

Goddard GV, McIntyre DC, Leech CK (1969): A permanent change in brain function resulting from daily electrical stimulation. *Exp Neurol* 25: 295–330.

Grone BP, Marchese M, Hamling KR, *et al.* (2016): Epilepsy, Behavioral Abnormalities, and Physiological Comorbidities in Syntaxin-Binding Protein 1 (STXBP1) Mutant Zebrafish. *PLoS One* 11: e0151148.

Guerrini R, Dobyns WB (2014): Malformations of cortical development: clinical features and genetic causes. *Lancet Neurol* 13: 710–726.

Haas KZ, Sperber EF, Moshe SL (1990): Kindling in developing animals: expression of severe seizures and enhanced development of bilateral foci. *Brain Res Dev Brain Res* 56: 275–280.

Haas KZ, Sperber EF, Moshe SL (1992): Kindling in developing animals: interactions between ipsilateral foci. *Brain Res Dev Brain Res* 68: 140–143.

Haas KZ, Sperber EF, Opanashuk LA, Stanton PK,Moshe SL (2001): Resistance of immature hippocampus to morphologic and physiologic alterations following status epilepticus or kindling. *Hippocampus* 11: 615–625.

Hager T, Maroteaux G, Pont P, Julsing J, van Vliet R, Stiedl O (2014): Munc18-1 haploinsufficiency results in enhanced anxiety-like behavior as determined by heart rate responses in mice. *Behav Brain Res* 260: 44–52.

Han S, Tai C, Westenbroek RE, *et al.* (2012): Autistic-like behaviour in Scn1a+/- mice and rescue by enhanced GABA-mediated neurotransmission. *Nature* 489: 385–390.

Hancock EC, Osborne JP, Edwards SW (2013): Treatment of infantile spasms. *Cochrane Database Syst Rev*: CD001770.

Hart AW, Morgan JE, Schneider J, *et al.* (2006): Cardiac malformations and midline skeletal defects in mice lacking filamin A. *Hum Mol Genet* 15: 2457–2467.

He XP, Patel M, Whitney KD, Janumpalli S, Tenner A, McNamara JO (1998): Glutamate receptor GluR3 antibodies and death of cortical cells. *Neuron* 20: 153–163.

Hempelmann A, Taylor KP, Heils A, *et al.*(2006): Exploration of the genetic architecture of idiopathic generalized epilepsies. *Epilepsia* 47: 1682–1690.

Hirayasu Y, Wada JA (1992): Convulsive seizures in rats induced by N-methyl-D-aspartate injection into the massa intermedia. *Brain Res* 577: 36–40.

Holmes GL, Weber DA (1984): The effect of progesterone on kindling: a developmental study. *Brain Res* 318: 45–53.

Holmes GL,Weber DA (1986): Effects of ACTH on seizure susceptibility in the developing brain. *Ann Neurol* 20: 82–88.

Hunt RF, Hortopan GA, Gillespie A, Baraban SC (2012): A novel zebrafish model of hyperthermia-induced seizures reveals a role for TRPV4 channels and NMDA-type glutamate receptors. *Exp Neurol* 237: 199–206.

Jarre G, Altwegg-Boussac T, Williams MS, *et al.* (2017a): Building Up Absence Seizures in the Somatosensory Cortex: From Network to Cellular Epileptogenic Processes. *Cereb Cortex* 27: 4607–4623.

Jarre G, Guillemain I, Deransart C, Depaulis A (2017b). Genetic Models of Absence epilepsy in rats and mice. In: Pitkänen A, Buckmaster PS, Galanopoulou AS and Moshé SL. *Models of Seizures and Epilepsy*. San Diego, Elsevier: 455–471.

Jensen FE, Applegate CD, Holtzman D, Belin TR, Burchfiel JL (1991): Epileptogenic effect of hypoxia in the immature rodent brain. *Ann Neurol* 29: 629–637.

Jensen FE, Blume H, Alvarado S, Firkusny I, Geary C (1995): NBQX blocks acute and late epileptogenic effects of perinatal hypoxia. *Epilepsia* 36: 966–972.

Jensen FE, Holmes GL, Lombroso CT, Blume HK, Firkusny IR (1992): Age-dependent changes in long-term seizure susceptibility and behavior after hypoxia in rats. *Epilepsia* 33: 971–980.

Jequier Gygax M, Klein BD, White HS, Kim M, Galanopoulou AS (2014): Efficacy and tolerability of the galanin analog NAX 5055 in the multiple-hit rat model of symptomatic infantile spasms. *Epilepsy Res* 108: 98–108.

Joshi K, Shen L, Michaeli A, *et al.* (2016): Infantile spasms in down syndrome: Rescue by knockdown of the GIRK2 channel. *Ann Neurol* 80: 511–521.

Kabova R, Liptakova S, Slamberova R, Pometlova M, Velisek L (1999): Age-specific N-methyl-D-aspartate-induced seizures: perspectives for the West syndrome model. *Epilepsia* 40: 1357–1369.

Kanaumi T, Takashima S, Iwasaki H, Itoh M, Mitsudome A, Hirose S (2008): Developmental changes in KCNQ2 and KCNQ3 expression in human brain: possible contribution to the age-dependent etiology of benign familial neonatal convulsions. *Brain Dev* 30: 362–369.

Kato M, Das S, Petras K, *et al.* (2004): Mutations of ARX are associated with striking pleiotropy and consistent genotype-phenotype correlation. *Hum Mutat* 23: 147–159.

Kato M, Dobyns WB (2005): X-linked lissencephaly with abnormal genitalia as a tangential migration disorder causing intractable epilepsy: proposal for a new term, "interneuronopathy". *J Child Neurol* 20: 392–397.

Katsarou AM, Moshé SL,Galanopoulou AS (2017): Interneuronopathies and their role in early life epilepsies and neurodevelopmental disorders. *Epilepsia Open* 2: 284–306.

Kearney JA, Plummer NW, Smith MR, *et al.* (2001): A gain-of-function mutation in the sodium channel gene Scn2a results in seizures and behavioral abnormalities. *Neuroscience* 102: 307–317.

Kearney JA, Yang Y, Beyer B, *et al.* (2006): Severe epilepsy resulting from genetic interaction between Scn2a and Kcnq2. *Hum Mol Genet* 15: 1043–1048.

Kim EH, Yum MS, Lee M, Kim EJ, Shim WH, Ko TS (2017): A New Rat Model of Epileptic Spasms Based on Methylazoxymethanol-Induced Malformations of Cortical Development. *Front Neurol* 8: 271.

Kitamura K, Yanazawa M, Sugiyama N, *et al.* (2002): Mutation of ARX causes abnormal development of forebrain and testes in mice and X-linked lissencephaly with abnormal genitalia in humans. *Nat Genet* 32: 359–369.

Koh S, Jensen FE (2001): Topiramate blocks perinatal hypoxia-induced seizures in rat pups. *Ann Neurol* 50: 366–372.

Kubova H, Haugvicova R, Suchomelova L, Mares P (2000): Does status epilepticus influence the motor development of immature rats? *Epilepsia* 41 (Suppl 6): S64–69.

Kubova H, Mares P (2013): Are morphologic and functional consequences of status epilepticus in infant rats progressive? *Neuroscience* 235: 232–249.

Kubova H, Mares P, Suchomelova L, Brozek G, Druga R,Pitkanen A (2004): Status epilepticus in immature rats leads to behavioural and cognitive impairment and epileptogenesis. *Eur J Neurosci* 19: 3255–3265.

Kwon CH, Luikart BW, Powell CM, *et al.* (2006): Pten regulates neuronal arborization and social interaction in mice. *Neuron* 50: 377–388.

Lado FA, Sperber EF, Moshe SL (2001): Anticonvulsant efficacy of gabapentin on kindling in the immature brain. *Epilepsia* 42: 458–463.

Lapray D, Popova IY, Kindler J, *et al.* (2010): Spontaneous epileptic manifestations in a DCX knockdown model of human double cortex. *Cereb Cortex* 20: 2694–2701.

LaSarge CL, Santos VR, Danzer SC (2015): PTEN deletion from adult-generated dentate granule cells disrupts granule cell mossy fiber axon structure. *Neurobiol Dis* 75: 142–150.

Lee CL, Frost JD, Jr., Swann JW, Hrachovy RA (2008): A new animal model of infantile spasms with unprovoked persistent seizures. *Epilepsia* 49: 298–307.

Lemke JR, Hendrickx R, Geider K, *et al.* (2014): GRIN2B mutations in West syndrome and intellectual disability with focal epilepsy. *Ann Neurol* 75: 147–154.

Lim JS, Kim WI, Kang HC, *et al.* (2015): Brain somatic mutations in MTOR cause focal cortical dysplasia type II leading to intractable epilepsy. *Nat Med* 21: 395–400.

Lippman-Bell JJ, Rakhade SN, Klein PM, *et al.* (2013): AMPA receptor antagonist NBQX attenuates later-life epileptic seizures and autistic-like social deficits following neonatal seizures. *Epilepsia* 54: 1922–1932.

Lopez-Meraz ML, Wasterlain CG, Rocha LL, Allen S, Niquet J (2010): Vulnerability of postnatal hippocampal neurons to seizures varies regionally with their maturational stage. *Neurobiol Dis* 37: 394–402.

Ludwig A, Budde T, Stieber J, *et al.* (2003): Absence epilepsy and sinus dysrhythmia in mice lacking the pacemaker channel HCN2. *EMBO J* 22: 216–224.

Luhmann HJ (2016): Models of cortical malformation – Chemical and physical. *J Neurosci Methods* 260: 62–72.

Manto M, Dalmau J, Didelot A, Rogemond V, Honnorat J (2010): *In vivo* effects of antibodies from patients with anti-NMDA receptor encephalitis: further evidence of synaptic glutamatergic dysfunction. *Orphanet J Rare Dis* 5: 31.

Mares P, Velisek L (1992): N-methyl-D-aspartate (NMDA)-induced seizures in developing rats. *Brain Res Dev Brain Res* 65: 185–189.

Marescaux C, Vergnes M, Depaulis A (1992): Genetic absence epilepsy in rats from Strasbourg – a review. *J Neural Transm Suppl* 35: 37–69.

Marsh E, Fulp C, Gomez E, *et al.* JA (2009): Targeted loss of Arx results in a developmental epilepsy mouse model and recapitulates the human phenotype in heterozygous females. *Brain* 132: 1563–1576.

Marsh ED, Nasrallah MP, Walsh C, *et al.* (2016): Developmental interneuron subtype deficits after targeted loss of Arx. *BMC Neurosci* 17: 35.

Martin MS, Dutt K, Papale LA, *et al.* (2010): Altered function of the SCN1A voltage-gated sodium channel leads to gamma-aminobutyric acid-ergic (GABAergic) interneuron abnormalities. *J Biol Chem* 285: 9823–9834.

Mathern G, Babb T, Armstrong D (1997). Mesial temporal lobe epilepsy. *Epilepsy: a Comprehensive Textbook*. Engel JJ and Pedley TA. New York, Lippincott-Raven.

McIntyre DC (1970): Differential amnestic effect of cortical *vs.* amygdaloid elicited convulsions in rats. *Physiol Behav* 5: 747–753.

Moshé SL (1981): The effects of age on the kindling phenomenon. *Dev Psychobiol* 14: 75–81.

Moshé SL (1987): Epileptogenesis and the immature brain. *Epilepsia* 28 Suppl 1: S3–15.

Moshé SL, Albala BJ (1983): Maturational changes in postictal refractoriness and seizure susceptibility in developing rats. *Ann Neurol* 13: 552–557.

Moshé SL, Albala BJ, Ackermann RF, Engel J, Jr. (1983): Increased seizure susceptibility of the immature brain. *Brain Res* 283: 81–85.

Moshé SL, Shinnar S, Swann JW (1995): Partial (focal) seizures in the developing brain. In: Schwartzkroin PA, Moshé SL, Noebels JL and Swann JW. *Brain Development and Epilepsy*. New York, Oxford University Press: 34–65.

Mytinger JR, Joshi S and Pediatric Epilepsy Research Consortium SoIS (2012): The current evaluation and treatment of infantile spasms among members of the Child Neurology Society. *J Child Neurol* 27: 1289–1294.

Nehlig A, Dube C, Koning E (2002): Status epilepticus induced by lithium-pilocarpine in the immature rat does not change the long-term susceptibility to seizures. *Epilepsy Res* 51: 189–197.

Noebels JL (2017): Spontaneous and gene-directed epilepsy mutations in the mouse. In: Pitkänen A, Buckmaster PS, Galanopoulou AS, Moshé SL (eds). *Models of Seizures and Epilepsy, 2nd ed.* Cambridge: Academic Press, pp. 763-776.

Oakley JC, Cho AR, Cheah CS, Scheuer T, Catterall WA (2013): Synergistic GABA-enhancing therapy against seizures in a mouse model of Dravet syndrome. *J Pharmacol Exp Ther* 345: 215–224.

Ogiwara I, Iwasato T, Miyamoto H, *et al.* (2013): Nav1.1 haploinsufficiency in excitatory neurons ameliorates seizure-associated sudden death in a mouse model of Dravet syndrome. *Hum Mol Genet* 22: 4784–4804.

Ogiwara I, Miyamoto H, Morita N, *et al.* (2007): Nav1.1 localizes to axons of parvalbumin-positive inhibitory interneurons: a circuit basis for epileptic seizures in mice carrying an Scn1a gene mutation. *J Neurosci* 27: 5903–5914.

Ohmori I, Kawakami N, Liu S, *et al.* (2014): Methylphenidate improves learning impairments and hyperthermia-induced seizures caused by an Scn1a mutation. *Epilepsia* 55: 1558–1567.

Okada R, Moshe SL, Albala BJ (1984): Infantile status epilepticus and future seizure susceptibility in the rat. *Brain Res* 317: 177–183.

Olivetti PR, Maheshwari A, Noebels JL (2014): Neonatal estradiol stimulation prevents epilepsy in Arx model of X-linked infantile spasms syndrome. *Sci Transl Med* 6: 220ra212.

Ono T, Moshe SL, Galanopoulou AS (2011): Carisbamate acutely suppresses spasms in a rat model of symptomatic infantile spasms. *Epilepsia* 52: 1678–1684.

Paciorkowski AR, Thio LL, Dobyns WB (2011): Genetic and biologic classification of infantile spasms. *Pediatr Neurol* 45: 355–367.

Parrini E, Ramazzotti A, Dobyns WB, *et al.* (2006): Periventricular heterotopia: phenotypic heterogeneity and correlation with Filamin A mutations. *Brain* 129: 1892–1906.

Patterson K, Brennan G, Curran M, Kinney-Lang E, Dube C, Rashid F (2015): Rapid, coordinate inflammatory responses after experimental febrile status epilepticus: Implication for epileptogenesis. *Book Rapid, coordinate inflammatory responses after experimental febrile status epilepticus: Implication for epileptogenesis*. eNeuro 2.

Peeters BW, Kerbusch JM, Coenen AM, Vossen JM, van Luijtelaar EL (1992): Genetics of spike-wave discharges in the electroencephalogram (EEG) of the WAG/Rij inbred rat strain: a classical mendelian crossbreeding study. *Behav Genet* 22: 361–368.

Pellock JM, Hrachovy R, Shinnar S, *et al.* (2010): Infantile spasms: a U.S. consensus report. *Epilepsia* 51: 2175–2189.

Pennacchio LA, Bouley DM, Higgins KM, Scott MP, Noebels JL, Myers RM (1998): Progressive ataxia, myoclonic epilepsy and cerebellar apoptosis in cystatin B-deficient mice. *Nat Genet* 20: 251–258.

Pezzolesi MG, Zbuk KM, Waite KA, Eng C (2007): Comparative genomic and functional analyses reveal a novel cis-acting PTEN regulatory element as a highly conserved functional E-box motif deleted in Cowden syndrome. *Hum Mol Genet* 16: 1058–1071.

Pinel JP, Rovner LI (1978): Experimental epileptogenesis: kindling-induced epilepsy in rats. *Exp Neurol* 58: 190–202.

Pirone A, Alexander J, Lau LA, *et al.* (2017): APC conditional knock-out mouse is a model of infantile spasms with elevated neuronal beta-catenin levels, neonatal spasms, and chronic seizures. *Neurobiol Dis* 98: 149–157.

Pitkänen A, Buckmaster PS, Galanopoulou AS, Moshé SL (2017): *Animal Models of Seizures and Epilepsy*. Cambridge: Academic Press.

Powell KL, Cain SM, Ng C, *et al.* (2009): A Cav3.2 T-type calcium channel point mutation has splice-variant-specific effects on function and segregates with seizure expression in a polygenic rat model of absence epilepsy. *J Neurosci* 29: 371–380.

Price MG, Yoo JW, Burgess DL, *et al.* (2009): A triplet repeat expansion genetic mouse model of infantile spasms syndrome, Arx(GCG)10+7, with interneuronopathy, spasms in infancy, persistent seizures, and adult cognitive and behavioral impairment. *J Neurosci* 29: 8752–8763.

Priel MR, dos Santos NF, Cavalheiro EA (1996): Developmental aspects of the pilocarpine model of epilepsy. *Epilepsy Res* 26: 115–121.

Pun RY, Rolle IJ, Lasarge CL, *et al.* (2012): Excessive activation of mTOR in postnatally generated granule cells is sufficient to cause epilepsy. *Neuron* 75: 1022–1034.

Raffo E, Coppola A, Ono T, Briggs SW, Galanopoulou AS (2011): A pulse rapamycin therapy for infantile spasms and associated cognitive decline. *Neurobiol Dis* 43: 322–329.

Rakhade SN, Fitzgerald EF, Klein PM, *et al.* (2012): Glutamate receptor 1 phosphorylation at serine 831 and 845 modulates seizure susceptibility and hippocampal hyperexcitability after early life seizures. *J Neurosci* 32: 17800–17812.

Rakhade SN, Klein PM, Huynh T, *et al.* (2011): Development of later life spontaneous seizures in a rodent model of hypoxia-induced neonatal seizures. *Epilepsia* 52: 753–765.

Redecker C, Lutzenburg M, Gressens P, Evrard P, Witte OW, Hagemann G (1998): Excitability changes and glucose metabolism in experimentally induced focal cortical dysplasias. *Cereb Cortex* 8: 623–634.

Reid CA, Leaw B, Richards KL, *et al.* SF (2014): Reduced dendritic arborization and hyperexcitability of pyramidal neurons in a SCN1B-based model of Dravet syndrome. *Brain* 137: 1701–1715.

Robertson CM, Finer NN (1988): Educational readiness of survivors of neonatal encephalopathy associated with birth asphyxia at term. *J Dev Behav Pediatr* 9: 298–306.

Robinson R, Taske N, Sander T, *et al.* (2002): Linkage analysis between childhood absence epilepsy and genes encoding GABAA and GABAB receptors, voltage-dependent calcium channels, and the ECA1 region on chromosome 8q. *Epilepsy Res* 48: 169–179.

Roch C, Leroy C, Nehlig A, Namer IJ (2002a): Magnetic resonance imaging in the study of the lithium-pilocarpine model of temporal lobe epilepsy in adult rats. *Epilepsia* 43: 325–335.

Roch C, Leroy C, Nehlig A, Namer IJ (2002b): Predictive value of cortical injury for the development of temporal lobe epilepsy in 21-day-old rats: an MRI approach using the lithium-pilocarpine model. *Epilepsia* 43: 1129–1136.

Rogers SW, Andrews PI, Gahring LC, *et al.* (1994): Autoantibodies to glutamate receptor GluR3 in Rasmussen's encephalitis. *Science* 265: 648–651.

Ronen GM, Buckley D, Penney S, Streiner DL (2007): Long-term prognosis in children with neonatal seizures: a population-based study. *Neurology* 69: 1816–1822.

Rosen GD, Galaburda AM (2000): Single cause, polymorphic neuronal migration disorders: an animal model. *Dev Med Child Neurol* 42: 652–662.

Rudolf G, Bihoreau MT, Godfrey RF, *et al.* (2004): Polygenic control of idiopathic generalized epilepsy phenotypes in the genetic absence rats from Strasbourg (GAERS). *Epilepsia* 45: 301–308.

Rutten A, van Albada M, Silveira DC, *et al.* (2002): Memory impairment following status epilepticus in immature rats: time-course and environmental effects. *Eur J Neurosci* 16: 501–513.

Sankar R, Shin DH, Liu H, Mazarati A, Pereira de Vasconcelos A, Wasterlain CG (1998): Patterns of status epilepticus-induced neuronal injury during development and long-term consequences. *J Neurosci* 18: 8382–8393.

Sanmaneechai O, Sogawa Y, Silver W, Ballaban-Gil K, Moshe SL, Shinnar S (2013): Treatment outcomes of West syndrome in infants with Down syndrome. *Pediatr Neurol* 48: 42–47.

Scantlebury MH, Galanopoulou AS, Chudomelova L, Raffo E, Betancourth D, Moshe SL (2010): A model of symptomatic infantile spasms syndrome. *Neurobiol Dis* 37: 604–612.

Scantlebury MH, Gibbs SA, Foadjo B, Lema P, Psarropoulou C, Carmant L (2005): Febrile seizures in the predisposed brain: a new model of temporal lobe epilepsy. *Ann Neurol* 58: 41–49.

Schuchmann S, Schmitz D, Rivera C, *et al.* (2006): Experimental febrile seizures are precipitated by a hyperthermia-induced respiratory alkalosis. *Nat Med* 12: 817–823.

Schuchmann S, Tolner EA, Marshall P, Vanhatalo S, Kaila K (2008): Pronounced increase in breathing rate in the "hair dryer model" of experimental febrile seizures. *Epilepsia* 49: 926–928.

Serbanescu I, Cortez MA, McKerlie C, Snead OC, 3rd (2004): Refractory atypical absence seizures in rat: a two hit model. *Epilepsy Res* 62: 53–63.

Serino D, Specchio N, Pontrelli G, Vigevano F, Fusco L (2013): Video/EEG findings in a KCNQ2 epileptic encephalopathy: a case report and revision of literature data. *Epileptic Disord* 15: 158–165.

Sheen VL, Dixon PH, Fox JW, *et al.* (2001): Mutations in the X-linked filamin 1 gene cause periventricular nodular heterotopia in males as well as in females. *Hum Mol Genet* 10: 1775–1783.

Shi XY, Yang XF, Tomonoh Y, *et al.* (2015): Development of a mouse model of infantile spasms induced by N-methyl-D-aspartate. *Epilepsy Res* 118: 29–33.

Shinnar S (1998): Prolonged febrile seizures and mesial temporal sclerosis. *Ann Neurol* 43: 411–412.

Shoubridge C, Fullston T, Gecz J (2010): ARX spectrum disorders: making inroads into the molecular pathology. *Hum Mutat* 31: 889–900.

Singh NA, Otto JF, Dahle EJ, *et al.* (2008): Mouse models of human KCNQ2 and KCNQ3 mutations for benign familial neonatal convulsions show seizures and neuronal plasticity without synaptic reorganization. *J Physiol* 586: 3405–3423.

Smith RA, Martland T, Lowry MF (1996): Children with seizures presenting to accident and emergency. *J Accid Emerg Med* 13: 54–58.

Song I, Kim D, Choi S, Sun M, Kim Y, Shin HS (2004): Role of the alpha1G T-type calcium channel in spontaneous absence seizures in mutant mice. *J Neurosci* 24: 5249–5257.

Sperber EF, Haas KZ, Stanton PK, Moshe SL (1991): Resistance of the immature hippocampus to seizure-induced synaptic reorganization. *Brain Res Dev Brain Res* 60: 88–93.

Sperk G (1994): Kainic acid seizures in the rat. *Prog Neurobiol* 42: 1–32.

Stafstrom CE, Moshe SL, Swann JW, Nehlig A, Jacobs MP, Schwartzkroin PA (2006): Models of pediatric epilepsies: strategies and opportunities. *Epilepsia* 47: 1407–1414.

Stafstrom CE, Sasaki-Adams DM (2003): NMDA-induced seizures in developing rats cause long-term learning impairment and increased seizure susceptibility. *Epilepsy Res* 53: 129–137.

Stambolic V, Suzuki A, de la Pompa JL, *et al.* (1998): Negative regulation of PKB/Akt-dependent cell survival by the tumor suppressor PTEN. *Cell* 95: 29–39.

Stewart LS, Wu Y, Eubanks JH, *et al.* (2009): Severity of atypical absence phenotype in GABAB transgenic mice is subunit specific. *Epilepsy Behav* 14: 577–581.

Suchomelova L, Baldwin RA, Kubova H, Thompson KW, Sankar R, Wasterlain CG (2006): Treatment of experimental status epilepticus in immature rats: dissociation between anticonvulsant and antiepileptogenic effects. *Pediatr Res* 59: 237–243.

Sun H, Juul HM, Jensen FE (2016): Models of hypoxia and ischemia-induced seizures. *J Neurosci Methods* 260: 252–260.

Suzuki A, de la Pompa JL, Stambolic V, *et al.* (1998): High cancer susceptibility and embryonic lethality associated with mutation of the PTEN tumor suppressor gene in mice. *Curr Biol* 8: 1169–1178.

Takano T, Sawai C, Takeuchi Y (2004): Radial and tangential neuronal migration disorder in ibotenate-induced cortical lesions in hamsters: immunohistochemical study of reelin, vimentin, and calretinin. *J Child Neurol* 19: 107–115.

Talos DM, Chang M, Kosaras B, *et al.* (2013): Antiepileptic effects of levetiracetam in a rodent neonatal seizure model. *Pediatr Res* 73: 24–30.

Talos DM, Sun H, Zhou X, *et al.* (2012): The interaction between early life epilepsy and autistic-like behavioral consequences: a role for the mammalian target of rapamycin (mTOR) pathway. *PLoS One* 7: e35885.

Tan HO, Reid CA, Single FN, *et al.* (2007): Reduced cortical inhibition in a mouse model of familial childhood absence epilepsy. *Proc Natl Acad Sci USA* 104: 17536–17541.

Tancredi V, D'Arcangelo G, Zona C, Siniscalchi A, Avoli M (1992): Induction of epileptiform activity by temperature elevation in hippocampal slices from young rats: an *in vitro* model for febrile seizures? *Epilepsia* 33: 228–234.

Tang B, Dutt K, Papale L, *et al.* (2009): A BAC transgenic mouse model reveals neuron subtype-specific effects of a Generalized Epilepsy with Febrile Seizures Plus (GEFS+) mutation. *Neurobiol Dis* 35: 91–102.

Tekgul H, Gauvreau K, Soul J, *et al.* (2006): The current etiologic profile and neurodevelopmental outcome of seizures in term newborn infants. *Pediatrics* 117: 1270–1280.

Toth Z, Yan XX, Haftoglou S, Ribak CE, Baram TZ (1998): Seizure-induced neuronal injury: vulnerability to febrile seizures in an immature rat model. *J Neurosci* 18: 4285–4294.

Turski L, Ikonomidou C, Turski WA, Bortolotto ZA, Cavalheiro EA (1989): Review: cholinergic mechanisms and epileptogenesis. The seizures induced by pilocarpine: a novel experimental model of intractable epilepsy. *Synapse* 3: 154–171.

Uchida T, Lossin C, Ihara Y, *et al.* (2017): Abnormal gamma-aminobutyric acid neurotransmission in a Kcnq2 model of early onset epilepsy. *Epilepsia* 58: 1430–1439.

Urak L, Feucht M, Fathi N, Hornik K, Fuchs K (2006): A GABRB3 promoter haplotype associated with childhood absence epilepsy impairs transcriptional activity. *Hum Mol Genet* 15: 2533–2541.

van Gassen KL, Hessel EV, Ramakers GM, *et al.* (2008): Characterization of febrile seizures and febrile seizure susceptibility in mouse inbred strains. *Genes Brain Behav* 7: 578–586.

van Luijtelaar EL, Coenen AM (1986): Two types of electrocortical paroxysms in an inbred strain of rats. *Neurosci Lett* 70: 393–397.

VanLandingham KE, Heinz ER, Cavazos JE, Lewis DV (1998): Magnetic resonance imaging evidence of hippocampal injury after prolonged focal febrile convulsions. *Ann Neurol* 43: 413–426.

Velisek L, Jehle K, Asche S, Veliskova J (2007): Model of infantile spasms induced by N-methyl-D-aspartic acid in prenatally impaired brain. *Ann Neurol* 61: 109–119.

Vergnes M, Marescaux C, Depaulis A, Micheletti G, Warter JM (1986): Ontogeny of spontaneous petit mal-like seizures in Wistar rats. *Brain Res* 395: 85–87.

Vergnes M, Marescaux C, Micheletti G, *et al.* (1982): Spontaneous paroxysmal electroclinical patterns in rat: a model of generalized non-convulsive epilepsy. *Neurosci Lett* 33: 97–101.

Verhage M, Maia AS, Plomp JJ, *et al.* (2000): Synaptic assembly of the brain in the absence of neurotransmitter secretion. *Science* 287: 864–869.

Vezzani A, Auvin S, Ravizza T,Aronica E (2012): Glia-neuronal interactions in ictogenesis and epileptogenesis: role of inflammatory mediators. In: Noebels JL, Avoli M, Rogawski MA, Olsen RW, Delgado-Escueta AV (eds). *Jasper's Basic Mechanisms of the Epilepsies (Internet), 4th ed.* Bethesda: National Center for Biotechnology Information (US).

Wagnon JL, Korn MJ, Parent R, *et al.* (2015): Convulsive seizures and SUDEP in a mouse model of SCN8A epileptic encephalopathy. *Hum Mol Genet* 24: 506–515.

Wallace RH, Scheffer IE, Barnett S, *et al.* (2001): Neuronal sodium-channel alpha1-subunit mutations in generalized epilepsy with febrile seizures plus. *Am J Hum Genet* 68: 859–865.

Wallace RH, Wang DW, Singh R, *et al.* (1998): Febrile seizures and generalized epilepsy associated with a mutation in the Na+-channel beta1 subunit gene SCN1B. *Nat Genet* 19: 366–370.

Wang YJ, Zhang Y, Liang XH, Yang G, Zou LP (2012): Effects of adrenal dysfunction and high-dose adrenocorticotropic hormone on NMDA-induced spasm seizures in young Wistar rats. *Epilepsy Res* 100: 125–131.

West WJ (1841): On a peculiar form of infantile convulsions. *Lancet* 35: 724–725.

Wirrell EC, Shellhaas RA, Joshi C, *et al.* (2015): How should children with West syndrome be efficiently and accurately investigated? Results from the National Infantile Spasms Consortium. *Epilepsia* 56: 617–625.

Wong M, Roper SN (2016): Genetic animal models of malformations of cortical development and epilepsy. *J Neurosci Methods* 260: 73–82.

Wright S, Hashemi K, Stasiak L, *et al.* (2015): Epileptogenic effects of NMDAR antibodies in a passive transfer mouse model. *Brain* 138: 3159–3167.

Wu Y, Chan KF, Eubanks JH, *et al.* (2007): Transgenic mice over-expressing GABA(B)R1a receptors acquire an atypical absence epilepsy-like phenotype. *Neurobiol Dis* 26: 439–451.

Wurdemann T, Kersten M, Tokay T, *et al.* (2016): Stereotactic injection of cerebrospinal fluid from anti-NMDA receptor encephalitis into rat dentate gyrus impairs NMDA receptor function. *Brain Res* 1633: 10–18.

Yu FH, Mantegazza M, Westenbroek RE, *et al.* (2006): Reduced sodium current in GABAergic interneurons in a mouse model of severe myoclonic epilepsy in infancy. *Nat Neurosci* 9: 1142–1149.

Yum MS, Chachua T, Veliskova J, Velisek L (2012): Prenatal stress promotes development of spasms in infant rats. *Epilepsia* 53: e46–49.

Zanelli S, Goodkin HP, Kowalski S, Kapur J (2014): Impact of transient acute hypoxia on the developing mouse EEG. *Neurobiol Dis* 68: 37–46.

CHAPTER 4

EEG TRAITS AND EPILEPTIC SYNDROMES

Guido Rubboli[1,2], Elena Gardella[1,3] and Carlo Alberto Tassinari[4]

[1] Danish Epilepsy Center, Epilepsihospitalet, Dianalund, Filadelfia, Denmark
[2] University of Copenhagen, Copenhagen, Denmark
[3] Syddansk Universitet, Odense, Denmark
[4] University of Bologna, Bologna, Italy

Introduction

The EEG is still the most useful and dependable laboratory technique in epilepsy investigation and management, providing evidence of functional markers of abnormal electrical brain activity, either ictal and interictal, relevant for the diagnosis of this pathologic condition. The recognition and correct interpretation of the wide variety of interictal and ictal EEG abnormalities that can be associated with an "epileptic disorder" may be crucial for a precise diagnosis of an epileptic syndrome. The corollary of this assumption is that the EEG contribution is still highly dependent on the skill and expertise of the EEG reader. The diagnostic yields of the EEG for the diagnosis of epilepsy may furtherly increase when the EEG assessment, coupled with an epilepsy expert consultation, is performed temporally close to the ictal event, allowing even in first-seizure patients a correct diagnosis of epilepsy up to a syndromic level (King *et al.*, 1998).

In the management of patients with established epilepsy, the definition of epilepsy syndromes based on age at onset, seizure types, EEG findings and aetiology has been an important advance. In particular, the recognition of clusters of EEG features (such as, for instance, the background activity, the morphology and topography of epileptiform graphoelements, the response to activation procedures, the influence of sleep on epileptiform abnormalities), associated with a clinically defined epileptic condition has significantly contributed to the introduction of the "electroclinical concept" of epilepsy syndrome. In this respect, the EEG has been a crucial and essential tool for the classification of seizures and epilepsies since the very first attempts of the ILAE on classification (Commission on Classification and Terminology of the ILAE, 1969) and the consolidation of the first (and last) ILAE classifications of 1981/1989 (Commission on Classification and Terminology of the ILAE 1981; 1989). In reestablishing the concept of electroclinical syndrome, the 2005–2009 ILAE Report of the ILAE Commission on Classification and Terminology (Berg *et al.*, 2010) has reaffirmed the role of the EEG to identify specific EEG features that permit a specific diagnosis. This role is maintained in the recent Position Paper on classification of the epilepsies by the ILAE Commission for Classification and Terminology, by including EEG among the clusters of features that contribute to a syndromic diagnosis (Scheffer *et al.*, 2017). Finally, the contribution of the EEG in the diagnosis and classification of the epilepsy syndromes has been detailed in two recent comprehensive papers (Koutroumanidis *et al.*, 2017a, b).

In this chapter, we will briefly overview and discuss some EEG features that, when occurring together, can represent the "EEG trait" of some syndromic groups as defined by previous ILAE Proposals (Commission on Classification and Terminology of the ILAE, 1989; Berg *et al.*, 2010).

EEG traits in genetic/idiopathic generalized epilepsies (GGE/IGE)

The 2017 ILAE Proposal (Scheffer *et al.*, 2017) has suggested to replace the term "idiopathic generalized epilepsies" (IGE) with the term "genetic generalized epilepsies (GGE)" for those condition in which there is sufficient evidence for a genetic background. The term "idiopathic" has been considered as still applicable for the well-recognized syndromes of childhood absence epilepsy (CAE), juvenile absence epilepsy (JAE), juvenile myoclonic epilepsy (JME) and generalized tonic-clonic seizures alone (GTCSa) (Scheffer *et al.*, 2017), encompassed in the former group of IGE. Since several former IGE syndromes, including some not yet officially recognized, sharing with CAE, JAE, JME and GTCSa some features (such as the typical 3 Hz generalized spike and wave discharge (GSWD), which is an acknowledged genetic marker), have possibly a genetic substrate, the terms GGE and IGE will be used together as GGE/IGE (see also Koutroumanidis *et al.*, 2017a; www.epilepsydiagnosis.org).

The main EEG features, common to the different syndromes included in GGE/IGE and that delineate the "EEG trait" of this group of epilepsies, are normal for age background activity and a variety of either interictal or ictal epileptiform generalized abnormalities. *The GSWD is* the cardinal element of the "EEG trait" characterizing GGE/IGE. This pattern is observed in GGE/IGE with onset in childhood or adolescence, but it can persist, almost unmodified, in IGE persisting in adult life (Gastaut *et al.*, 1986; Panayiotopoulos *et al.*, 1992; Michelucci *et al.*, 1996; Michel *et al.*, 2011). Moreover, it is observed in those forms of IGE in development, at the boundaries of recognized GGE/IGE syndromes (such as, for instance, GGE/IGE with absences of early childhood and GGE/IGE with phantom absences) (Panayiotopoulos, 2005; Rubboli *et al.*, 2009; Koutroumanidis *et al.*, 2017a). Finally, the same EEG pattern has been also described in GGE/IGE with adult-onset, indistinguishable from the EEG features of GGE/IGE with classic childhood-adolescent onset, (Yeniun *et al.*, 2003; Pimentel *et al.*, 2018), suggesting that this EEG trait can be considered a biologic marker of GGE/IGE, with a genetic aetiology (Marini *et al.*, 2003).

The morphology of the "typical" 3 c/sec generalized spike and wave complex, as observed in CAE, has been described in detail since Weir (1965). More or less typical 3 c/sec generalized spike-and-waves complexes have been described also in other childhood absence epilepsy related syndromes, such as epilepsy with perioral myoclonia and absences and eyelids myoclonia with absences as well as in JAE, JME and GTCSa, encompassed in the group of GGE/IGE (see chapter 15 in this book) *(Figure 1)*. In addition, a quite typical 3 c/sec spike-and-wave complex has been reported in the syndrome of myoclonic absences (MAE - myoclonic absence epilepsy) (Tassinari *et al.*, 1969; Medina *et al.*, see chapter 15). Myoclonic absences seizures are characterized by 3 c/sec generalized spike-and wave discharges with anterior predominance, associated with myoclonic jerks time-locked to the spike-wave complex, that involve the face and, mainly proximally, the upper limbs *(Figure 2)*. According to 1989 Classification Proposal (Commission on Classification and Terminology of the ILAE,

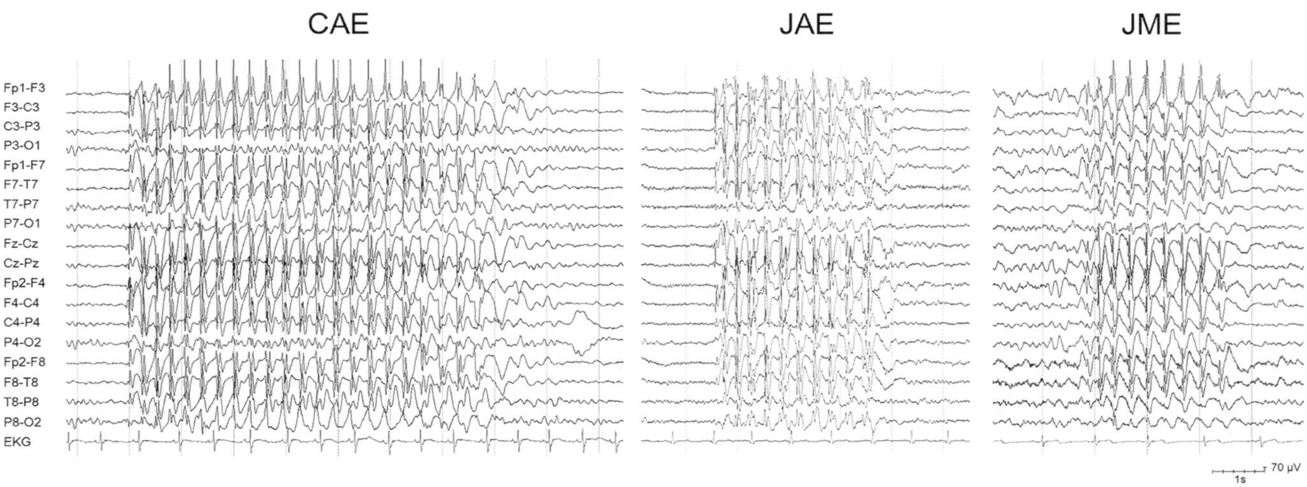

Figure 1

Typical 3 Hz generalized spike-and-wave discharge (GSWD) with homogenous features in GGE/IGE such as childhood absence epilepsy, juvenile absence epilepsy and juvenile myoclonic epilepsy.

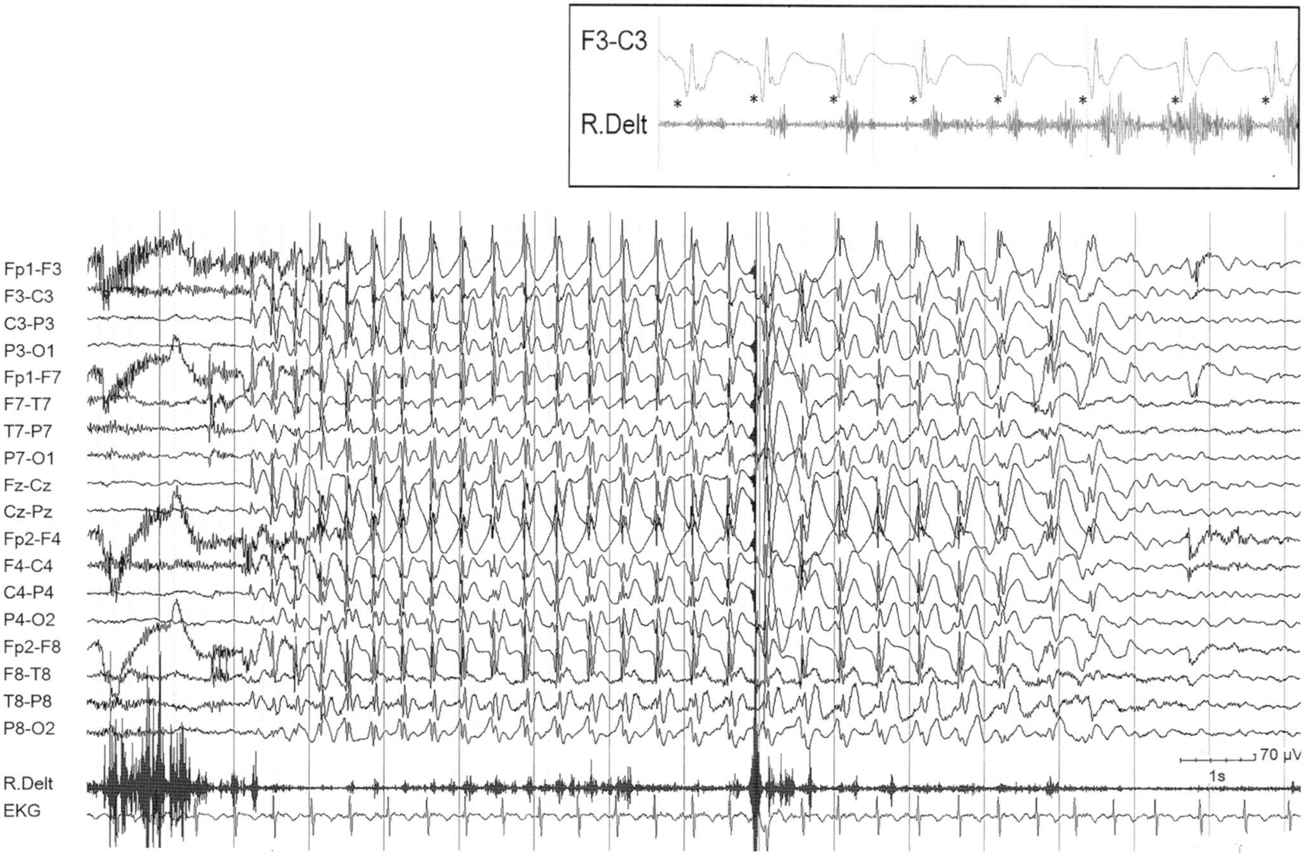

Figure 2

3 Hz GSWD associated with rhythmic myoclonia in the right deltoid in a myoclonic absence seizure. A progressive tonic contraction, over which the myoclonia are superimposed, appears during the evolution of the seizures. In the insert above, a strict relationship between the positive transient (asterisk) of the spike-wave complex and the myoclonia is shown. The myoclonia and the following post-myoclonic silent period fragments the ensuing tonic contraction.

1989), MAE is classified among the "generalized cryptogenic or symptomatic epilepsies". Indeed, the prognosis of MAE may not be as favourable as in most of GGE/IGE. Bureau & Tassinari (2005) distinguished two forms of MAE, one with simple absences as the only seizure type associated with myoclonic absence seizures and with a benign prognosis, the other with associated numerous generalized tonic-clonic seizures and a poor prognosis. Tassinari *et al.* (1969; 1971), analyzing the morphology of the 3 c/sec spike-complex of MAE, pointed out that the positive transient, identified by Weir (1965) in between the spike component and the slow wave of the "typical" spike-wave complex, is particularly prominent in myoclonic absence seizures. Indeed, the positive transient and its amplitude appeared to be directly related to the appearance and amplitude of the myoclonic jerks that characterize myoclonic absences *(Figure 2)*. The relationships between a cortical positive transient and myoclonic jerks has been described in other conditions, such as JME (Panzica *et al.*, 2001), whereas a negative transient has been demonstrated to be related to "epileptic negative myoclonus" (Tassinari *et al.*, 1998, 2010). Various types of myoclonic manifestations, involving face and neck muscles, associated with typical 3 c/sec spike-and wave discharges have been observed also in children presenting with CAE, with excellent prognosis (Capovilla *et al.*, 2001). Current evidences are insufficient to demonstrate whether the features of the spike-wave discharges of this latter group of CAE with overt myoclonic manifestations and those of the myoclonic absence seizures show significant differences. A distinguishing clinical feature between the myoclonic manifestations in typical CAE and MAE is the association in MAE of myoclonic jerks with a tonic contraction that involve proximally the upper limbs, causing the elevation of the arms. The superposition of myoclonia to a tonic contraction might depend on the ictal involvement of mesial supplementary motor areas, as shown in other types of epilepsies by means of subdural recordings (Ikeda *et al.*, 1999). It can be hypothesized that MAE encompasses the EEG trait of GGE/IGE, however multiple additional factors, genetic and/or environmental, might contribute to modify the overall course of this syndrome, bearing, at variance with GGE/IGE, a variable and less favourable prognosis. Finally, commenting the relevance of the analysis of the spike-and-wave features, it is worth to note that historically the description of the morphology of the spike-wave complex was the basis of the distinction between "typical" "fast" spike-and-wave at 3 c/sec of "petit mal" absences and the slow spike-and-wave discharges that helped to define the "Petit Mal variant", later on identified as Lennox-Gastaut syndrome (Gastaut *et al.*, 1966).

Brief bursts of generalized spike-wave discharges associated with normal background activity can be observed at the very initial stages of some forms of progressive myoclonus epilepsies, that are classified among the "symptomatic generalized epilepsies of specific aetiologies" (Commission on Classification and Terminology of the ILAE, 1989). In Unverricht-Lundborg disease, at the onset when no neurological impairment is evident, the occurrence of generalized tonic-clonic or myoclonic seizures may lead to a misdiagnosis of IGE; in fact, initially the differential diagnosis from JME may be a puzzling issue. Similarly, Lafora disease and the described PME associated with SCARB2 mutations, at the onset may present EEG features reminiscent of the IGE trait (Tassinari *et al.*, 1978; Rubboli *et al.*, 2011). Indeed, at the onset of Lafora disease, "the EEG tracings display normal background activity, generalized fast spike-and-wave discharges, facilitated by intermittent photic stimulation, that are identical to those of primary generalized epilepsies" (Tassinari *et al.*, 1978) *(Figure 3a and 3b)*. These observations might suggest that, at least in some PMEs, clinical and EEG traits of GGE/IGE are incorporated in these complex disorders, recognizable at disease onset, then disappearing during the disease course because of the more or less severe progressive neurological impairment, the occurrence of other seizure types and the EEG deterioration, caused by the different pathophysiological mechanisms (*i.e.*, genetic and/or metabolic) underlying PMEs.

The generalized "EEG trait" requires evidence of *"generalized"* SW complexes, defined as a "generalized, bilateral, synchronous, symmetrical" discharge (Commission on Classification and Terminology of

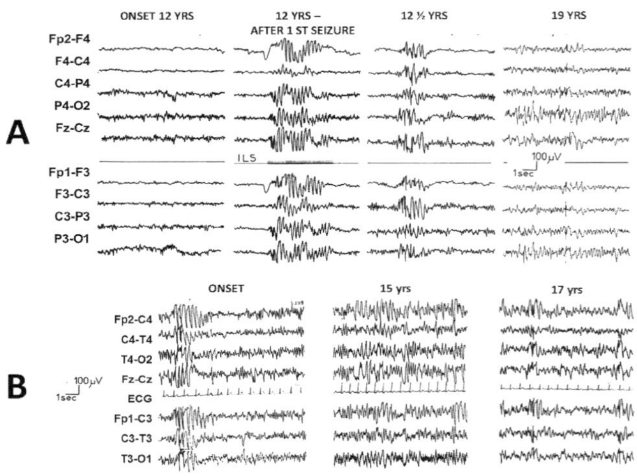

Figure 3 **Evolution of the EEG tracings in two brothers (A and B) suffering from Lafora disease. In both subjects, at the onset of the disease (first panel on the left in A and B) background activity is normal, with some bursts of fast generalized spike-and-wave discharges (second panel from left in A, first panel on the left in B). During the course of the disease, slow activity increases and background activity progressively slows down (last panels on the right in A and B), and spikes and sharp waves appear in the posterior regions (last panel on the right in A). (Modified from Tassinari *et al.*, 1978).**

the ILAE, 1989). However, reports showing an asynchronous, asymmetric or regional, more often frontal, onset of the 3 c/sec generalized spike-wave discharges associated with childhood absences were first reported since a long time ago (Jewesbury & Parsonage, 1949), demonstrating inter-hemispheric differences of the onset of the spike-and-wave discharge of up to 20 ms (Ogden *et al.*, 1956). A fronto-temporal spike-wave onset or predominance has been reported to occur in about 60% of the children with CAE and no relapse (Lombroso, 1997; Yoshinaga *et al.*, 2004; Ma *et al.*, 2011; Mariani *et al.*, 2011). Accordingly, a focal or bilateral anterior onset has been noted in 16–60% of typical absences (Holmes *et al.*, 1987). Such asymmetric onsets have been accepted within the concept of IGE, even in well recognized syndromes such as CAE, provided that the asymmetric/focal EEG onset was not consistent from one seizure to another, suggesting therefore an equipotentiality of the two hemispheres in triggering the spike-wave discharge. In analogy, on clinical grounds, the 2010 ILAE proposal admits that in generalized epileptic seizures "although individual seizure onsets can appear localized, the location and lateralization are not consistent from one seizure to another. Generalized seizure can be asymmetric" (Report of the ILAE Commission on Classification and Terminology, 2005–2009, Berg *et al.*, 2010). On the other hand, arguments favouring the existence of a subset of "absence" seizures with a focal onset, based on asymmetric EEG onsets of the generalized spike and wave discharges and atypical clinical features, have been proposed (Lagae *et al.*, 2001; Jocic-Jakubi *et al.*, 2009). The role of the frontal lobe in generating typical absence seizures (that could explain the usually anteriorly predominant onset of the 3 c/sec spike and wave discharge) and the so-called *cortical focus theory* have been reviewed in the light of recent experimental evidences in animal models (Meeren *et al.*, 2002, Unterberger *et al.*, 2018) and further data in humans (Stefan & Snead 1997; Craiu *et al.*, 2006), and following the contribution of new methods of investigation such as EEG-MEG correlations (Stefan *et al.*, 2009; Amor *et al.*, 2009; Westmijse *et al.*, 2009; Sakurai *et al.*, 2010), and EEG-functional MRI studies. These latter investigations were performed mainly in typical CAE and showed a cortical deactivation related to slow waves, possibly contrasted by a thalamic activation. The variable impairment of consciousness is related to the slow waves whereas motor symptoms are related to the spike component of the 3 Hz GSWD. This abnormal sequence might be triggered by an initial abnormality in arousal mechanisms (Moeller *et al.*, 2010; Benuzzi *et al.*, 2012). It remains to be elucidated whether these pathophysiological mechanisms can be translated in all different GGE/IGE syndromes, or whether and which eventual variations of these mechanisms may account for the different phenotypes and prognosis.

The "Rolandic" EEG trait

The "Rolandic" spike observed in benign epilepsy with centro-temporal spikes is a focal negative diphasic slow spike followed by a slow wave component distributed over the "Rolandic" centro-temporal regions (Dalla Bernardina *et al.*, 2005; Demirbilek *et al.*, see chapter 13). This "Rolandic" EEG trait can be detected in other idiopathic focal epilepsies of childhood (Dalla Bernardina *et al.*, 2005) as well as to common developmental disorders (speech dyspraxia, attention deficit hyperactivity disorders, developmental coordination disorders) (Echenne *et al.*, 1992; Holtmann *et al.*, 2003; Scabar *et al.*, 2006). In addition, the "Rolandic" EEG trait has been described in subjects presenting fragile X syndrome, with and without epileptic seizures (Musumeci *et al.*, 1988). Finally, Rolandic spikes have been reported in non-epileptic children, followed up until adolescence without appearance of seizures (Eeg-Olofsson *et al.*, 1971; Cavazzuti *et al.*, 1980; Danielsson & Petermann, 2009). Overall, these findings have suggested that the EEG "Rolandic" trait might not be specific to epilepsy, but it could possibly be a biologic marker for an underlying subtle but widespread abnormality of neurodevelopment. Based on EEG evidences, a genetic background has been hypothesized since several decades by Bray and Wiser (1964, 1965), and then supported by linkage and association studies (Neubauer *et al.*, 1998; Strug *et al.*, 2009; Pal *et al.*, 2010). Further support has been provided by several reports showing the association of the "Rolandic" spike with GSWD, which has been reported in about one third of children with idiopathic occipital epilepsy (Gastaut & Zifkin, 1987; Caraballo *et al.*, 2008) and one fourth of patients with Panayiotopoulos syndrome (Ohtsu *et al.*, 2003; Specchio *et al.*, 2010), in whom some reports observed at the onset only GSWD (Caraballo *et al.*, 2015). However, at present, conclusive evidence for primary genetic aetiology of this trait is still elusive (Vadlamudi *et al.*, 2014). Genetic investigations have excluded that the Rolandic EEG trait is linked to the fragile X region (Rees *et al.*, 1993). Data have shown that the EEG "Rolandic" trait maps to Elongator Protein Complex 4 (ELP4), a component of the elongator complex involved in transcription and tRNA modification, and whose depletion can result in altered actin cytoskeleton production, impaired cell motility and abnormal neuronal migration during development (Strug *et al.*, 2009). Such mechanisms could explain the wide spectrum of developmental disorders associated with "Rolandic" spikes. Additional, presumably genetic, factors likely acting in combination with ELP4 locus have to be invoked to explain the occurrence of focal epileptic seizures.

EEG features orienting to specific electro-clinical conditions

A number of EEG features, when properly recognized, may be reminiscent of specific syndromic entities, therefore orienting the diagnosis.

Hypsarrhythmia is the characteristic pattern associated with infantile spasms and West syndrome (WS), although infants presenting with epileptic spasms without hypsarrhythmia have been described (Dulac & Tuxhorn, 2005; Fusco *et al.*, see chapter 8). Recent data in patients with WS suggest that the investigation of fast oscillations (20–100 Hz) might be a EEG localization biomarker in lesional WS (Kim *et al.*, 2018). The *suppression-burst EEG patterns* (SBP), characterized by a succession of bursts of epileptiform abnormalities separated by episodes of flat or low-amplitude tracing is relatively common in neonatal encephalopaties, particularly when associated with seizures. SBP is the EEG hallmark of early infantile epileptic encephalopathy with suppression bursts or Ohtahara syndrome and of early neonatal myoclonic encephalopathy (Aicardi & Ohtahara, 2005; Mizrahi & Milh, see chapter 7). However, other aetiologically heterogeneous conditions with SBP include neonatal hypoxic encephalopathy, structural brain damage and metabolic disorders, especially non-ketotic hyperglicinemia. Finally, SBP can be observed in Ohtahara syndrome associated with various mutations (*ARX*, mitochondrial glutamate transporter, *SL-C25A22*, *STXBP1*, *SCNA2*) (Weyckhusen & Korff, 2014). Some variation in the presentation of SBP that might more specifically orient to a specific diagnosis (for instance, Ohtahara syndrome *versus* early myoclonic encephalopathy or *versus* neonatal seizures with serious brain damage) have been described (Yamamoto *et al.*, 2011). In any case, the SBP bears per se a poor prognostic significance. Asymmetric and asynchronous abnormal EEG activity, in hypsarrhythmic or SBP tracings, either during wakefulness or sleep, are characteristic features of Aicardi syndrome.

Angelman syndrome (AS) displays peculiar EEG characteristics such as high amplitude rhythmic 2–3 Hz activity predominantly over the frontal regions with superimposed interictal epileptiform discharges; in children under 12 years of age, high amplitude rhythmic 4–6 Hz activity with spikes, prominent in the occipital regions, that can be facilitated by eye closure, are often seen. There is no difference in EEG findings in AS patients with or without epileptic seizures. AS patients with a deletion of chromosome 15q11–13 have more prominent EEG abnormalities than patients with other genetic disturbances related to chromosome 15 region (Laan & Vein, 2005). These EEG findings are highly suggestive of AS when observed in the appropriate clinical context and can help to identify AS patients at an early age when genetic counselling may be particularly useful (Leyser *et al.*, 2014). Some of the AS EEG features can be observed also in *4p-syndrome* (Sgrö *et al.*, 1995) and *Rett syndrome* (RS). Interestingly, data showed genetic and phenotypic similarities in RS, AS and autism (Jedele, 2007), suggesting that overlapping molecular pathways might be disregulated in these disorders; in particular, the involvement of *GABRB3* receptor subunit gene in the sharing of the epileptic/EEG phenotype in RT and AS has been postulated (Hogart *et al.*, 2007).

Miller-Dieker lissencephaly shows quite recognizable interictal EEG features represented by abnormal high-amplitude fast activities, mainly in the alpha and beta band, persisting on eyes opening, and not modified by sleep (Gastaut *et al.*, 1987). Indeed, this EEG pattern is specific of Miller-Dieker lissencephaly when it is observed before the age of one year.

An abnormal EEG pattern characterized by long bursts or trains of rhythmic theta waves, sharply contoured or with a notched morphology has been described in the *ring chromosome 20 syndrome* (Inoue *et al.*, 1997; Canevini *et al.*, 1998). This EEG pattern associated with a clinical picture of recurrent non convulsive status, atypical absences or other seizure types, and mild to moderate mental retardation can suggest the correct diagnosis. In a recent report, the detection of the typical EEG pattern, associated with drug-resistant frontal lobe seizures and recurrent nonconvulsive status epilepticus has been showed to be highly predictive ring chromosome 20 (Gago-Veiga *et al.*, 2018). EEG-fMRI studies have demonstrated a peculiar pattern characterized by BOLD increment in the perisylvian network and the decrease of the default mode network (DMN) and dorsal attention network (DAN) that could be related to the cognitive and behavioural derangements observed in this syndrome. This pattern is not dissimilar to the ones observed in other epileptic encephalopathies, suggesting that dysfunctions in similar brain networks might underlie neurobehavioral regression in different epileptic disorders (Vaudano *et al.*, 2014).

Extreme activation of epileptiform abnormalities during slow sleep is one of the main diagnostic criteria suggestive of *encephalopathy with status epilepticus during sleep* (ESES) (see Tassinari *et al.*, chapter 14). Clinically, ESES is associated with epilepsy with different seizure types and with neuropsychological impairment with various degrees of cognitive regression, including acquired aphasia (*i.e.*, Landau-Kleffner syndrome). Importantly, the huge increment of EEG epileptiform abnormalities during sleep is postulated to be directly implicated in the cognitive impairment that occurs in ESES syndromes, by altering the processes of learning and memory consolidation that take place during normal sleep in infancy and childhood (Tassinari & Rubboli, 2006; Tassinari *et al.*, 2009; Rubboli *et al.*, 2018; Tassinari *et al.*, this book). These interferences in sleep-related plastic brain processes underlying normal cognitive development might also occur in other conditions with extreme activation of epileptiform abnormalities during sleep, such as for instance benign partial epilepsy of childhood (Cantalupo *et al.*, 2011; Urbain *et al.*, 2011). In this respect, the status epilepticus during sleep might be the common EEG trait of different clinical conditions characterized by abnormal increment of epileptiform EEG activities during sleep and concomitant appearance of neuropsychological derangement (Tassinari & Rubboli, 2018).

In *eyelids myoclonia with absences or Jeavons syndrome* (Jeavons, 1977), the eyelids myoclonia, appearing as an eyelid flutter following eye closure are associated with EEG high-amplitude generalized polyspikes or polyspike-waves, often followed by brief discharges (3–6 seconds or less) or rhythmic spike- or polyspike-wave complexes at 3 or more c/sec. These epileptiform activities are triggered by active eye-closure (and not eyeblink), and occur right after closing the eyes (Striano *et al.*, 2009). Recent studies have emphasized the occurrence of posterior focal interictal and ictal abnormalities preceding the generalized epileptic discharge, further suggesting that the ictogenic process in EMA originates in the occipital cortex (Viravan *et al.*, 2012; Dragoumi *et al.*, 2018). With age, absence seizures and photosensitivity usually decline, whereas the eyelids myoclonia may persist, associated with short runs of EEG polyspike/polyspike-wave complexes.

Isolated or brief runs of fast spikes in the vertex regions, spreading bilaterally to central regions, during REM sleep have been reported in various conditions characterized by *action myoclonus*, such as Lance-Adams syndrome (Tassinari *et al.*, 1973), Lafora disease (Tassinari *et al.*, 1978) Unverricht-Lundborg disease (previously labelled as Ramsay-Hunt syndrome; Tassinari *et al.*, 1974), MERRF (Roger *et al.*, 1991); PME associated with *SCARB2* mutations (Rubboli *et al.* 2011). In addition, also the polygraphic features of action myoclonus in these different forms are strikingly similar (Tassinari *et al.*, 1995). Deep neurophysiological phenotyping has shown that an aberrant subcortical or cortical loop (possibly short-cutting the somatosensory cortex) is involved in generating the prominent action myoclonus in Unverricht-Lundborg disease, whereas in Lafora disease, this type of myoclonus might depend on sustained hyperexcitability of the sensorimotor cortex in response to afferent stimuli, which suggest a more severe impairment of inhibitory mechanisms (Canafoglia *et al.*, 2004; Avanzini *et al.*, 2016). Moreover, a peculiar pattern of brief bursts of rhythmic myoclonia at rest, of increasing amplitude, at a frequency around 20 Hz, associated with a rhythmic EEG activity in the contralateral centro-parietal regions has been observed in PMEs of different aetiologies and in post-hypoxic myoclonus *(Figure 4)*. In PMEs, this finding might be related to an abnormal hyperexcitability of the motor cortex due to reduced GABA-mediated intracortical inhibition as shown by TMS studies (Valzania *et al.*, 1999; Badawy *et al.*, 2010).

The occurrence of brief focal fast rhythmic EEG discharges is suggestive of an underlying *focal cortical dysplasia* (Gambardella *et al.*, 1996); indeed, this EEG finding is highly specific of this type of lesion, and usually it corresponds topographically to the epileptogenic area, thus it may be helpful to orient the MRI investigation.

Conclusions

In modern epileptology, EEG can still provide information of paramount importance either for a correct syndromic diagnosis or for assessing the clinical relevance (ictal? interictal? subclinical?) of paroxysmal EEG discharges (particularly when EEG is coupled with additional recording parameters such as polygraphic channels). In the era of genetics and neuroimaging, a detailed EEG characterization of a given epileptic condition can contribute to a more precise phenotyping that can be undoubtely useful to perform genetic investigations, as well as it can reveal specific EEG epileptiform patterns and their topography (for instance, fast rhythmic discharges associated with focal cortical dysplasias) that can be helpful to carry out an adequate MRI study.

In the future, the more and more widespread application of new digitized techniques of EEG collection and analysis (such as dense array recordings, source analysis of EEG generators, computerized processing of EEG and polygraphic signals, analysis of high frequencies EEG activities - ripples and fast ripples -) will hopefully provide a new wealth of information relevant for pathophysiological speculations as well as for diagnostic and classification purposes.

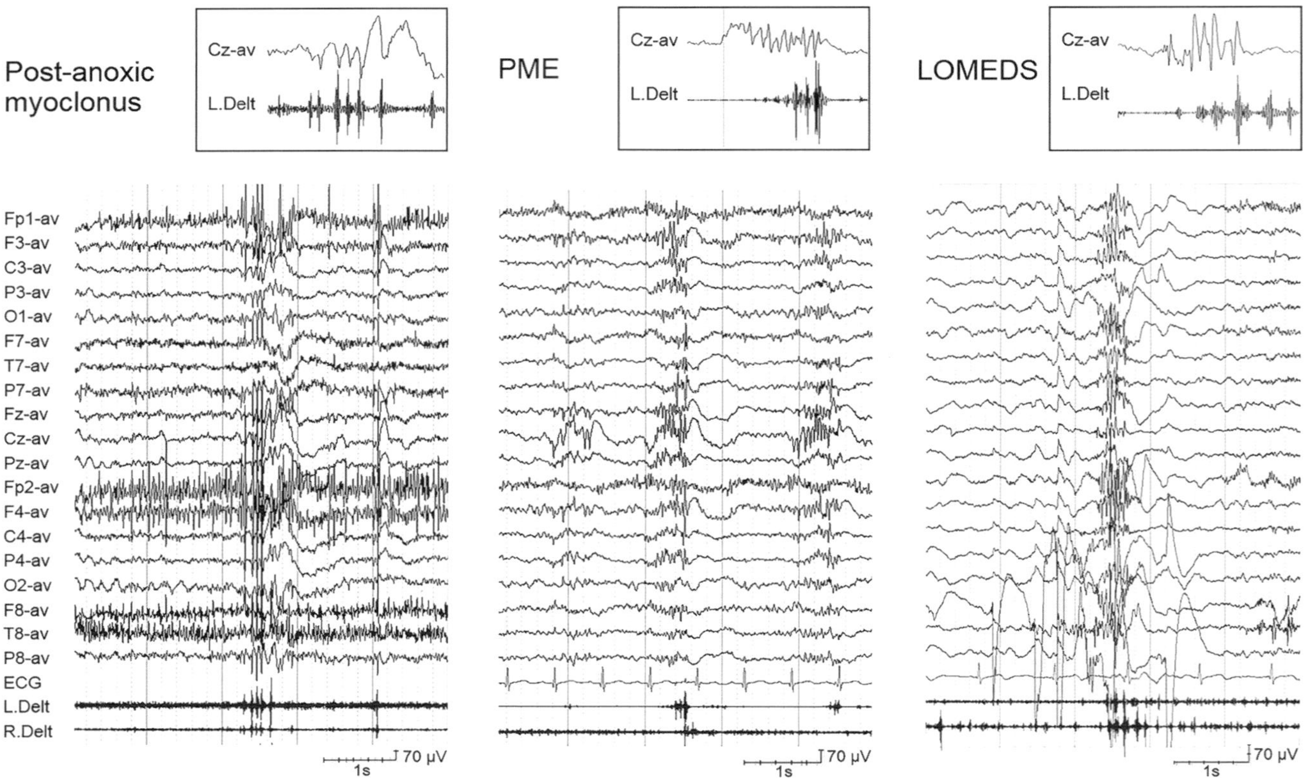

Figure 4

Fragments of polygraphic recording in three epileptic syndromes with action myoclonus, *i.e.* post-hypoxic action myoclonus, progressive myoclonus of undetermined aetiology and late-onset myoclonic epilepsy in Down syndrome (De Simone *et al.*, 2010). At rest, brief bursts of myoclonic potentials are associated with an EEG rhythmic activity at the same frequency (around 20 Hz) in the vertex and contralateral central regions.

REFERENCES ▶

Aicardi J, Ohtahara S (2005): Severe neonatal epilepsies with suppression-burst pattern. In: Roger J, Bureau M, Dravet C, Genton P, Tassinari CA, Wolf P (eds) *Epileptic Syndromes in Infancy, Childhood and Adolescence*, 4th ed, pp. 39–50. Paris: John Libbey Eurotext Ltd.

Amor F, Baillet S, Navarro V, Adam C, Martinerie J, Quyen MV. (2009): Cortical local and long-range synchronization interplay in human absence seizure initiation. *NeuroImage* 45: 950–962.

Avanzini G, Shibasaki H, Rubboli G, *et al.* (2016): Neurophysiology of myoclonus and progressive myoclonus epilepsies. *Epileptic Disord* 18: 11–27.

Badawy RA, Macdonell RA, Jackson GD, Berkovic SF (2010): Can changes in cortical excitability distinguish progressive from juvenile myoclonic epilepsy? *Epilepsia* 51: 2084–2088.

Benuzzi F, Mirandola L, Pugnaghi M, *et al.* (2012): Increased cortical BOLD signal anticipates generalized spike and wave discharges in adolescents and adults with idiopathic generalized epilepsies. *Epilepsia* 53: 622–630.

Berg AT, Berkovic SF, Brodie MJ, *et al.* (2010): Revised terminology and concepts for organization of seizures and epilepsies: report of the ILAE Commission on Classification and Terminology, 2005–2009. *Epilepsia* 51: 676–685.

Bray PF, Wiser WC (1964): Evidence for a genetic etiology of temporal-central abnormalities in focal epilepsy. *N Engl J Med* 271: 926–933.

Bray PF, Wiser WC (1965): The relation of focal to diffuse epileptiform EEG discharges in genetic epilepsy. *Arch Neurol* 13: 223–237.

Canafoglia L, Ciano C, Panzica F, *et al.* (2004): Sensorimotor cortex excitability in Unverricht-Lundborg disease and Lafora body disease. *Neurology* 63: 2309–2315.

Canevini MP, Sgro V, Zuffardi O, *et al.* (1998): Chromosome 20 ring: a chromosomal disorder associated with a particular electroclinical pattern. *Epilepsia* 39: 942–951.

Cantalupo G, Rubboli G, Tassinari CA (2011): Night-time unravelling of the brain web: impaired synaptic downscaling in ESES - the Penelope syndrome. *Clin Neurophysiol* 122: 1691–1692.

Capovilla G, Rubboli G, Beccaria F, *et al.* (2001): A clinical spectrum of the myoclonic manifestations associated with typical absences in childhood absence epilepsy. A video-polygraphic study. *Epileptic Disord* 3: 57–62.

Caraballo RH, Cersosimo RO, Fejerman N (200). Childhood occipital epilepsy of Gastaut: a study of 33 patients. *Epilepsia* 49: 288–297.

Cavazzuti GB, Cappella L, Nalin A (1980): Longitudinal study of epileptiform EEG patterns in normal children. *Epilepsia* 21: 43–55.

Commission on Classification and Terminology of the International League Against Epilepsy (1969): Clinical and electroencephalographic classification of epileptic seizures. *Epilepsia* 10 (Suppl): S2–S13.

Commission on Classification and Terminology of the International League Against Epilepsy (1981): Proposal for revised classification of epilepsies and epileptic syndromes. *Epilepsia* 22: 489–501.

Commission on Classification and Terminology of the International League Against Epilepsy (1989): Proposal for revised classification of epilepsies and epileptic syndromes. *Epilepsia* 30: 389–399.

Craiu D, Magureanu S, van Emde Boas W (2006): Are absences truly generalized seizures or partial seizures originating from or predominantly involving the pre-motor areas? Some clinical and theoretical observations and their implications for seizure classification. *Epilepsy Res* 70 (Suppl 1): S141–S155.

Dalla Bernardina B, Sgro V, Fejerman N (2005): Epilepsy with centro-temporal spikes and related syndromes. In: Roger J, Bureau M, Dravet C, Genton P, Tassinari CA, Wolf P (eds) *Epileptic Syndromes in Infancy, Childhood and Adolescence, 4th ed*, pp. 203–225. Montrouge: John Libbey Eurotext Ltd.

Danielsson J, Petermann F (2009): Cognitive deficits in children with benign Rolandic epilepsy of childhood or Rolandic discharges: a study of children between 4 and 7 years of age with and without seizures compared with healthy controls. *Epilepsy Behav* 16: 646–651.

Dragoumi P, Emery J, Chivers F, *et al.* (2018): Crossing the lines between epilepsy syndromes: a myoclonic epilepsy variant with prominent eyelid myoclonia and atonic components. *Epileptic Disord* 20: 35–41.

Dulac O, Tuxhorn I (2005): Infantile spasms and West syndrome. In: Roger J, Bureau M, Dravet C, Genton P, Tassinari CA, Wolf P (eds). *Epileptic Syndromes in Infancy, Childhood and Adolescence*, 4th ed, pp. 53–72. Montrouge: John Libbey Eurotext Ltd.

Echenne B, Cheminal R, Rivier F, Negre C, Touchon J, Billiard M (1992): Epileptic electroencephalographic abnormalities and developmental dysphasias: a study of 32 patients. *Brain Dev* 14: 216–225.

Eeg-Olofsson O, Petersén I, Selldén U (1971): The development of the electroencephalogram in normal children from the age of 1 through 15 years. Paroxysmal activity. *Neuropadiatrie* 2: 375–404.

Gago-Veiga AB, Toledano R, García-Morales I, Pérez-Jiménez MA, Bernar J, Gil-Nagel A (2018): Specificity of electroclinical features in the diagnosis of ring chromosome 20. *Epilepsy Behav* 80: 215–220.

Gambardella A, Palmini A, Andermann F, *et al.* (1996): Usefulness of focal rhythmic discharges on scalp EEG of patients with focal cortical dysplasia and intractable epilepsy. *Electroencephalogr Clin Neurophysiol* 98: 243–249.

Gastaut H, Zifkin BG (1987): Benign epilepsy of childhood with occipital spike and wave discharges. In: Andermann F, Lugaresi E, eds. *Migraine and Epilepsy*. Boston: Butterworths: pp. 47–81.

Gastaut H, Roger J, Soulayrol R, *et al.* (1966): Childhood epileptic encephalopathy with diffuse slow spike-waves (otherwise known as "petit mal variant"): or Lennox syndrome. *Epilepsia* 7: 139–179.

Gastaut H, Zifkin BG, Mariani E, Puig JS (1986): The long-term course of primary generalized epilepsy with persisting absences. *Neurology* 36: 1021–1208.

Gastaut H, Pinsard N, Raybaud C, Aicardi J, Zifkin B. (1987): Lissencephaly (agyria-pachygyria): clinical findings and serial EEG studies. *Dev Med Child Neurol* 29: 167–180.

Hogart A, Nagarajan RP, Patzel KA, Yasui DH, Lasalle JM. (2007): 15q11–13 GABAA receptor genes are normally biallelically expressed in brain yet are subject to epigenetic dysregulation in autism-spectrum disorders. *Hum Mol Genet* 16: 691–703.

Holmes GL, McKeever M, Adamson M (1987): Absence seizures in children: clinical and electroencephalographic features. *Ann Neurol* 21: 268–273.

Holmes GL (1992): Rolandic epilepsy: clinical and electoencepahalographic features. *Epilepsy Res* 6 (Suppl 2): 29–43.

Holtmann M, Becker K, Kentner-Figura B, Schmidt MH (2003): Increased frequency of Rolandic spikes in ADHD children. *Epilepsia* 44: 1241–1244.

Ikeda A, Nagamine T, Kunieda T, *et al.* (1999): Clonic convulsion caused by epileptic discharges arising from the human supplementary motor area as studied by subdural recording. *Epileptic Disord* 1: 21–26.

Inoue Y, Fujiwara T, Matsuda K, *et al.* (1997): Ring chromosome 20 and nonconvulsive status epilepticus. A new epileptic syndrome. *Brain* 120: 939–953.

Jeavons PM (1977): Nosological problems of myoclonic epilepsies in childhood and adolescence. *Dev Med Child Neurol* 19: 3–8.

Jedele KB (2007): The overlapping spectrum of Rett and Angelman syndromes: a clinical review. *Semin Pediatr Neurol* 14: 108–117.

Jewesbury EC, Parsonage MJ (1949): Observations on the wave and spike complex in the electro-encephalogram. *J Neurol Neurosurg Psychiatry* 12: 239–245.

Jocic-Jakubi B, Jovanovic M, Jankovic DS, Lagae L (2009): Frontal-onset absences in children: associated with worse outcome? A replication study. *Seizure* 18: 275–278.

Kim MJ, Yum MS, Yeh HR, Ko TS (2018): Fast oscillation dynamics during hypsarrhythmia as a localization biomarker. *J Neurophysiol* 119: 679–687.

King MA, Newton MR, Jackson GD, *et al.* (1998): Epileptology of the first-seizure presentation: a clinical, electroencephalographic, and magnetic resonance imaging study of 300 consecutive patients. *Lancet* 352: 1007–1011.

Koutroumanidis M, Arzimanoglou A, Caraballo R, *et al.* (2017a): The role of EEG in the diagnosis and classification of the epilepsy syndromes: a tool for clinical practice by the ILAE Neurophysiology Task Force (Part 1). *Epileptic Disord* 19: 233–298.

Koutroumanidis M, Arzimanoglou A, Caraballo R, *et al.* (2017b): The role of EEG in the diagnosis and classification of the epilepsy syndromes: a tool for clinical practice by the ILAE Neurophysiology Task Force (Part 2). *Epileptic Disord* 19: 385–437.

Lagae L, Pauwels J, Monté CP, Verhelle B, Vervisch I (2001): Frontal absences in children. *EurJ Paediatr Neurol* 5: 243–251.

Laan LA, Vein AA (2005): Angelman syndrome: is there a characteristic EEG? *Brain Dev* 27: 80–87.

Leyser M, Penna PS, de Almeida AC, Vasconcelos MM, Nascimento OJ (2014): Revisiting epilepsy and the electroencephalogram patterns in Angelman syndrome. *Neurol Sci* 35: 701–705.

Lombroso CT (1997): Consistent EEG focalities detected in subjects with primary generalized epilepsies monitored for two decades. *Epilepsia* 38: 797–812.

Ma X, Zhang Y, Yang Z, *et al.* (2011): Childhood absence epilepsy. Electroclinical features and diagnostic criteria. *Brain Dev* 33: 114–119.

Mariani E, Rossi LN, Vajani S (2011): Interictal paroxysmal EEG abnormalities in childhood absence epilepsy. *Seizure* 20: 299–304.

Marini C, King MA, Archer JS, Newton MR, Berkovic SF (2003): Idiopathic generalised epilepsy of adult onset: clinical syndromes and genetics. *J Neurol Neurosurg Psychiatry* 74: 192–196.

Meeren HK, Pijn JP, Van Luijtelaar EL, Coenen AM, Lopes da Silva FH (2002): Cortical focus drives widespread corticothalamic networks during spontaneous absence seizures in rats. *J Neurosci* 22: 1480–1495.

Michel VH, Sebban C, Debray-Meignan S, *et al.* (2011): Electroclinical features of idiopathic generalized epilepsies in the elderly: a geriatric hospital-based study. *Seizure* 20: 292–298.

Michelucci R, Rubboli G, Passarelli D, *et al.* (1996): Electroclinical features of idiopathic generalised epilepsy with persisting absences in adult life. *J Neurol Neurosurg Psychiatry* 61: 471–477.

Moeller F, LeVan P, Muhle H, *et al.* (2010): Absence seizures: individual patterns revealed by EEG-fMRI. *Epilepsia* 51: 2000–2010.

Musumeci SA, Colognola RM, Ferri R, *et al.* (1988): Fragile-X syndrome: a particular epileptogenic EEG pattern. *Epilepsia* 29: 41–47.

Neubauer BA, Fiedler B, Himmelein B, *et al.* (1998): Centrotemporal spikes in families with rolandic epilepsy: linkage to chromosome 15q14. *Neurology* 51: 1608–1612.

Ogden TE, Aird RB, Garoutte BC (1956): The nature of bilateral and synchronous cerebral spiking. *Acta Psychiatrica Scandinavica* 31: 273–284.

Ohtsu M, Oguni H, Hayashi K, Funatsuka M, Imai K, Osawa M (2003): EEG in children with early-onset benign occipital seizure susceptibility syndrome: Panayiotopoulos syndrome. *Epilepsia* 44: 435–442.

Pal DK, Li W, Clarke T, Lieberman P, Strug LJ (2010): Pleiotropic effects of the 11p13 locus on developmental verbal dyspraxia and EEG centrotemporal sharp waves. *Genes Brain Behav* 9: 1004–1012.

Panayiotopoulos CP, Chroni E, Daskalopoulos C, Baker A, Rowlinson S, Walsh P (1992): Typical absence seizures in adults: clinical, EEG, video-EEG findings and diagnostic/syndromic considerations. *J Neurol Neurosurg Psychiatry* 55: 1002–1008.

Panayiotopoulos CP (2005): Syndromes of idiopathic generalized epilepsies not recognized by the International League Against Epilepsy. *Epilepsia* 46 (Suppl 9): 57–66.

Panzica F, Rubboli G, Franceschetti S, *et al.* (2001): Cortical myoclonus in Janz syndrome. *Clin Neurophysiol* 112: 1803–1809.

Pimentel J, Varanda S, Guimarães P, Lopes da Silva F (2018): Idiopathic generalised epilepsies of adult onset: a reappraisal and literature review. *Epileptic Disord* 20: 169–177.

Rees M, Diebold U, Parker K, Doose H, Gardiner RM, Whitehouse WP (1993): Benign childhood epilepsy with centrotemporal spikes and the focal sharp wave trait is not linked to the fragile X region. *Neuropediatrics* 24: 211–213.

Roger J, Bureau M, Dravet C, Genton P, Tassinari CA, Michelucci R (1991): The role of mitochondrial encephalopathies in progressive myoclonus epilepsy. *Rev Neurol* 147: 480–490.

Rubboli G, Gardella E, Capovilla G (2009): Idiopathic generalized epilepsy (IGE): syndromes in development: IGE with absences of early childhood, IGE with phantom absences, and perioral myoclonia with absences. *Epilepsia* 50 (Suppl 5): 24–28.

Rubboli G, Franceschetti S, Berkovic SF, *et al.* (2011): Clinical and neurophysiological features of progressive myoclonus epilepsy without renal failure caused by SCARB2 mutations. *Epilepsia* 52: 2356–2363.

Rubboli G, Huber R, Tononi G, Tassinari CA (2018): Encephalopathy related to status epilepticus during sleep: a link with sleep homeostasis? *Epil Disord* [Epub ahead of print].

Sakurai K, Takeda Y, Tanaka N, *et al.* (2010): Generalized spike-wave discharges involve a default mode network in patients with juvenile absence epilepsy: a MEG study. *Epilepsy Res* 89: 176–184.

Scabar A, Devescovi R, Blason L, Bravar L, Carrozzi M (2006): Comorbidity of DCD and SLI: significance of epileptiform activity during sleep. *Child Care Health Dev* 32: 733–739.

Scheffer IE, Berkovic S, Capovilla G, *et al.* (2017): ILAE classification of the epilepsies: Position paper of the ILAE Commission for Classification and Terminology. *Epilepsia* 58: 512–521.

Sgro V, Riva E, Canevini MP, *et al.* (1995): 4p(-): syndrome: a chromosomal disorder associated with a particular EEG pattern. *Epilepsia* 36: 1206–1214.

Specchio N, Trivisano M, Di Ciommo V, *et al.* (2010). Panayiotopoulos syndrome: a clinical, EEG, and neuropsychological study of 93 consecutive patients. *Epilepsia* 51: 2098–2107.

Stefan H, Snead OC III (1997): Absence seizures. In Engel JJ, Pedley TA (eds) *Epilepsy: A Comprehensive Textbook*, pp. 579–590. Philadelphia: Lippincott-Raven Publishers.

Stefan H, Paulini-Ruf A, Hopfengartner R, Rampp S (2009): Network characteristics of idiopathic generalized epilepsies in combined MEG/EEG. *Epilepsy Res* 85: 187–198.

Striano S, Capovilla G, Sofia V, *et al.* (2009): Eyelid myoclonia with absences (Jeavons syndrome): a well-defined idiopathic generalized epilepsy syndrome or a spectrum of photosensitive conditions? *Epilepsia* 50 (Suppl 5): 15–19.

Strug LJ, Clarke T, Chiang T, *et al.* (2009): Centrotemporal sharp wave EEG trait in Rolandic epilepsy maps to Elongator Protein Complex 4 (ELP4): *EurJ Hum Genet* 17: 1171–1181.

Tassinari CA, Lyagoubi S, Santos V, *et al.* (1969): Study on spike and wave discharges in man. II. Clinical and electroencephalographic aspects of myoclonic absences. *Rev Neurol* 121: 379–383.

Tassinari CA, Lyagoubi S, Gambarelli F, Roger J, Gastaut H (1971): Relationships between EEG discharges and neuromuscular phenomena. *Electroencephalogr Clin Neurophysiol* 31: 176.

Tassinari CA, Coccagna G, Mantovani M, Bernardina BD, Roger J (1973): Polygraphic study of dyssynergia cerebellaris myoclonica (Ramsay-Hunt syndrome): and of the intention myoclonus (Lance-Adams syndrome) during sleep. *Eur Neurol* 9: 105–120.

Tassinari CA, Bureau-Paillas M, Dalla Bernardina B, Grasso E, Roger J (1974): Étude électroencéphalographique de la dyssinergie cérébelleuse myoclonique avec épilepsie (syndrome de Ramsay-Hunt). *Rev EEG Neurophysiol* 4: 407–428.

Tassinari CA, Bureau-Paillas M, Dalla Bernardina B, *et al.* (1978): La maladie de Lafora. *Rev EEEG Neurophysiol* 8: 107–122.

Tassinari CA, Rubboli G, Parmeggiani L, *et al.* (1995): Epileptic negative myoclonus. In: Fahn S, Hallett M, Luders HO, Marsden CD (eds) *Negative motor phenomena, Adv Neurol*, vol. 67, pp. 181–197. New York: Raven Press.

Tassinari CA, Rubboli G, Shibasaki H (1998): Neurophysiology of positive and negative myoclonus. *Electroencephalogr Clin Neurophysiol* 107: 181–195.

Tassinari CA, Rubboli G (2006): Cognition and paroxysmal EEG activities: from a single spike to electrical status epilepticus during sleep. *Epilepsia* 47 (Suppl 2): 40–43.

Tassinari CA, Cantalupo G, Rios-Pohl L, Giustina ED, Rubboli G (2009): Encephalopathy with status epilepticus during slow sleep: "the Penelope syndrome". *Epilepsia* 50 (Suppl 7): 4–8.

Tassinari CA, Cantalupo G, Rubboli G (2010): Polygraphic recordings of epileptic seizures. In: Panayiotopoulos CP (ed) *The Atlas of Epilepsies*, pp. 723–740. London: Springer-Verlag.

Tassinari CA, Rubboli G (2018): Encephalopathy related to Status Epilepticus During Slow Wave Sleep. Current concepts and future perspectives. *Epil Disord* [Epub ahead of print].

Urbain C, Di Vincenzo T, Peigneux P, Van Bogaert P (2011): Is sleep-related consolidation impaired in focal idiopathic epilepsies of childhood? A pilot study. *Epilepsy Behav* 22: 380–384.

Unterberger I, Trinka E, Kaplan PW, Walser G, Luef G, Bauer G (2018): Generalized nonmotor (absence) seizures-What do absence, generalized, and nonmotor mean? *Epilepsia* 59: 523–529.

Vadlamudi L, Milne RL, Lawrence K, *et al.* (2014): Genetics of epilepsy: the testimony of twins in the molecular era. *Neurology* 83: 1042–1048.

Valzania F, Strafella AP, Tropeani A, Rubboli G, Nassetti SA, Tassinari CA (1999): Facilitation of rhythmic events in progressive myoclonus epilepsy: a transcranial magnetic stimulation study. *Clin Neurophysiol* 110: 152–157.

Vaudano AE, Ruggieri A, Vignoli A, *et al.* (2014) Epilepsy-related brain networks in ring chromosome 20 syndrome: an EEG-fMRI study. *Epilepsia* 55: 403–413.

Viravan S, Go C, Ochi A, Akiyama T, Carter Snead O 3rd, Otsubo H (2011): Jeavons syndrome existing as occipital cortex initiating generalized epilepsy. *Epilepsia* 52: 1273–1279.

Weir B (1965): The morphology of the spike-wave complex. *Electroenceph Clin Neurophysiol* 19: 284–290.

Westmijse I, Ossenblok P, Gunning B, van LG (2009): Onset and propagation of spike and slow wave discharges in human absence epilepsy: A MEG study. *Epilepsia* 50: 2538–2548.

Weckhuysen S, Korff CM (2014): Epilepsy: old syndromes, new genes. *Curr Neurol Neurosci Rep* 14: 447.

Yamamoto H, Okumura A, Fukuda M (2011): Epilepsies and epileptic syndromes starting in the neonatal period. *Brain Dev* 33: 213–220.

Yenjun S, Harvey AS, Marini C, Newton MR, King MA, Berkovic SF (2003): EEG in adult-onset idiopathic generalized epilepsy. *Epilepsia* 44: 252–256.

Yoshinaga H, Ohtsuka Y, Tamai K, *et al.* (2004): EEG in childhood absence epilepsy. *Seizure* 13: 296–302.

CHAPTER 5
SYNDROMES AND ANTIEPILEPSY DRUGS

Pierre Genton[1], Natalio Fejerman[2] and Philippe Gélisse[3]

[1] Centre Saint-Paul, Henri-Gastaut Hospital, Marseille, France
[2] Hospital de Pediatrica "Juan P. Garrahan", Buenos Aires, Argentina
[3] Epilepsy Unit, Montpellier, France

This paper is a tribute to Prof. Natalio Fejerman, who contributed with his usual dedication and skill to the previous edition of this book. He will be fondly remembered.

Introduction

The recent classification proposal of seizures and epilepsies (Scheffer *et al.*, 2017) does not mention specific pharmacologic treatment procedures for seizures, epilepsies or epileptic syndromes; the previous classification (Commission, 1989), and subsequent proposals and schemes (Engel, 2001), did mention the fact that some syndromes are easily controlled, while others are usually therapy-resistant. They did not, however, point to specific efficacy of individual antiepileptic drugs (AED) in the various syndromes, nor do they mention the fact that patients may be aggravated by anticonvulsants, with more and different seizures occurring as a consequence of antiepileptic therapy (Genton & McMenamin, 1998). Controlled drug trials are usually performed in patients presenting with drug-resistant focal seizures, but some recent studies have been designed to address more specific issues, *e.g.*, drug efficacy in specific syndromes or even epileptic diseases. Indeed, there is a longstanding and lingering discrepancy between the theoretical body of knowledge that associates AEDs with efficacy in given seizure types and real-life practice that makes us select drugs and treatment strategies according to "syndromic" situations. This fact has been highlighted by widely circulated recommendations and guidelines on the use of AEDs in practical situations, most of which rely on opinion polls among experienced epileptologists (Trost *et al.*, 2005; Wheless *et al.*, 2005, 2007) and on the review of published data, which is usually rated in terms of "quality", the highest ratings going to controlled studies, and the lowest to anecdotal reports (Glauser *et al.*, 2006; NICE guidelines, 2004, 2018). Very few reviews have focused on evidence-based recommendations in a syndromic context, *e.g.*, in idiopathic generalized epilepsy (IGE) (Bergey, 2005; Camfield & Camfield, 2005).

One may qualify as *anecdotal* the evidence based on personal experience and on open studies. However, the highly regarded *controlled* studies are often biased by their sponsorship: not all AEDs have been studied equally, and in all possible indications. Moreover, in spite of a long history of converging reports on AED-induced seizure aggravation, there is still no consensus on the fact that this major problem should influence the AED choice in given epilepsy syndromes.

Among the factors that determine the choice of an AED, and besides the economic considerations that may play a major part in some settings, the main determinants are: patient profile, seizure type, and epileptic syndrome. A syndromic approach to the diagnosis and management of epilepsy may be possible at the very onset of the seizures (King *et al.*, 1998) and is usually considered easier in children than in adults. It is the aim of this chapter to review the existing evidence that the epilepsy syndrome is the major determinant of a rational drug and treatment program choice: the evidence specifically includes rational and/or controlled studies of individual AEDs in epilepsy syndromes, and the description of paradoxical seizure aggravation. The international abbreviations used for the AEDs are listed on *Table I*.

Table I **Conventional abbreviations used for antiepileptic drugs**

AED	Antiepileptic drug(s)
BZP	Benzodiazepines
BRV	Brivaracetam
CLB	Clobazam
CBD	Cannabidiol
CBZ	Carbamazepine
ESL	Eslicarbazepine
ESM	Ethosuximide
FBM	Felbamate
GBP	Gabapentin
LEV	Levetiracetam
LCM	Lacosamide
LTG	Lamotrigine
OXC	Oxcarbazepine
PB	Phenobarbital
PER	Perampanel
PGN	Pregabalin
PHT	Phenytoin
PRM	Primidone
RFN	Rufinamide
STP	Stiripentol
STM	Sulthiame
TGB	Tiagabine
TPM	Topiramate
VGB	Vigabatrin
VPA	Valproate or valproic acid
ZNS	Zonisamide

Controlled *vs.* open studies of AEDs in epilepsy syndromes

In this section we will focus on the problems of AED trials in children, emphasizing the concept that recognition of epileptic syndromes may be more important than the seizure approach. Large population studies demonstrated that syndromic classification is successful in a vast majority of patients evaluated in qualified epilepsy centers. In Italy, a multicenter group (Osservatorio Regionale per l'Epilessia, 1997) studied 3,469 patients with ages between 4 and 80 years, and in France, the CAROLE study evaluated 1,016 patients aged over 1 month with recent diagnosis of epilepsy (Jallon *et al.*, 2001). In both studies, in only around 10% of the patients, specific epilepsy syndromes could not be identified.

"We live in the age of the Clinical Guideline" was the title of a critical editorial comment (Shorvon, 2006) and there are several treatment guidelines based on the analysis and meta-analysis of controlled randomized trials (CRT). Most of them refer to adults and seizures and not to children and syndromes (French *et al.*, 2004; Marson *et al.*, 2007). An already mentioned study spanned six seizure types in different age groups and only two epileptic syndromes, one of them a typical childhood epileptic syndrome (Glauser *et al.*, 2006). Despite the strict criteria to categorize types of CRT and levels of evidence, many experts find these conclusions not convincing in relation to their clinical experience.

AED trials in children imply specific age-related difficulties:

- reluctance to recruit children has provoked selection of more severe cases in children than in adults (Shinnar & Pellock, 2005);
- in studies comparing high and low doses of an AED, non-convenient extremes may be elected in children (Pina-Garza *et al.*, 2005);
- the following considerations should be taken into account: i) to limit as much as possible the size of the sample; ii) to quantify not only the reduction in the frequency of seizures but also the potential increase in frequency; iii) to reduce the duration of the double-blind period due to risk of cognitive impairment; iv) to evaluate interictal EEG activity because it may contribute to cognitive deterioration; and v) to consider cognitive evaluation as an efficacy criterion;
- there are several ways to reduce the number of children in a CRT without diminishing the statistic power. When a homogeneous subpopulation with only one epileptic syndrome or only one etiology is included, demonstration of the effect is facilitated. For instance, a sample of 41 children with Dravet syndrome was enough to demonstrate the efficacy of stiripentol (Chiron *et al.*, 2000). In the same line, randomization of 22 patients with infantile spasms associated with tuberous sclerosis was enough to demonstrate superiority of vigabatrin over steroids (Chiron *et al.*, 1997);
- besides, trials in children oblige to consider: i) age-specific toxicities; ii) concern regarding AED and health in the child; iii) impact of AEDs on learning and behavior; iv) comorbidities.

There are several reviews on published trials of AED in children (Sankar, 2004; Caldwell *et al.*, 2004; Shinnar & Pellock, 2005; Glauser *et al.*, 2006; Chiron *et al.*, 2008; Hwang & Kim, 2008). The need to practice CRT in children has received special attention from the governments of the United States and the European Union which will surely be of help to solve our problem as pediatric neurologists (National Institute of Health, 1998; European Medicines Agency, 2007).

Infantile spasms/West syndrome

The association of infantile spasms (IS) and hypsarrhythmia constitutes a characteristic epileptic encephalopathy in infancy. It is really difficult to categorize the different drug trials performed in these patients, and practically all AED have been tried. However, the two accepted alternatives are now ACTH or steroids and vigabatrin (VGB).

A clear demonstration of superiority of high doses natural ACTH over prednisone was provided in the 1990s (Baram *et al.*, 1996). In the same decade, a comparison between VGB and ACTH was published (Vigevano & Cilio, 1997) and a randomized trial comparing VGB and hydrocortisone in IS ascertained the superiority of VGB in children with tuberous sclerosis (Chiron *et al.*, 1997).

In 2000, one of us reported a multicenter prospective open study of VGB as first choice drug in the treatment of 116 children with West syndrome. Followed up for 17–40 months, patients became seizure-free in 61.8% of cryptogenic cases and 29.5% of symptomatic cases. All seizure-free cryptogenic cases showed normal neuropsychological development. The most effective dose of VGB was 150 mg/kg/day (Fejerman *et al.*, 2000a).

Later came the time of consensus on therapeutic trials (Osborne & Lux, 2001; Mackay *et al.*, 2004; Pellock *et al.*, 2010). In the US consensus report it is stated that at this time "ACTH and vigabatrin are the only drugs with proven efficacy to suppress clinical spasms and the hypsarrhythmic EEG". Interestingly, one of the letters to the editor in the same issue of *Epilepsia* stresses the difference in therapeutic responses in relation to etiologies and opens the spectrum of durations of treatment comparing patients with Down syndrome, periventricular leukomalacia, or cryptogenic West syndrome (Dulac *et al.*, 2010). Another CRT compared the ketogenic diet (KD) and high-dose ACTH, and, in spite of the comparatively small number in each group (16 and 16) concluded that the KD and ACTH had similar efficacy, while the KD was better tolerated (Dressler *et al.*, 2019).

A recent review (Song *et al.*, 2017) noted that there had been only 9 controlled trials in West syndrome and that further studies were necessary to assess the indications for valproate, topiramate, zonisamide, benzodiazepines, and the KD or its variants. Cannabidiol has been the subject or recent interest (Hussain, 2018).

Dravet syndrome (DS)

Most of the classic AEDs except valproic acid are not useful in the treatment of DS. Add-on open studies showed certain results with bromides, clobazam (CLB), TPM and zonisamide (ZNS) (Dravet & Guerrini, 2011). KD was shown as a useful alternative treatment (Caraballo & Fejerman, 2006). In a series of 24 patients treated with KD, 16 (66.6%) remained on the diet after achieving significant improvement (Caraballo, 2011). Two drugs have been subjected to controlled trials. The efficacy of stiripentol (STP) was demonstrated in two multicenter randomized double-blind, placebo-controlled add-on trials (Chiron *et al.*, 2000; Guerrini *et al.*, 2002b). Long-term efficacy and safety of STP were reported (Than *et al.*, 2002). Comparable results with European studies were published in an open-level multicenter study in Japan (Inoue *et al.*, 2009). This almost syndrome-specific characteristic of STP moved the European Medicines Agency to consider STP as an "orphan" drug (review in Chiron, 2019). Cannabidiol (CBD) has also shown efficacy in a placebo-controlled study, but is associated with significant side-effects (Devinsky *et al.*, 2017).

Lennox-Gastaut syndrome (LGS)

The felbamate (FBM) study group paper (1993) was a CRT comparing add-on FBM with placebo in 73 patients who had LGS. Beneficial effects, especially on atonic seizures, were clearly demonstrated. The authors stated that the types and frequency of side effects were similar in the two treatment groups, and it took time to recognize the severe adverse effects of FBM which led to the practical avoidance of this drug in the treatment of epilepsies. Lamotrigine (LTG) and topiramate (TPM) showed effectiveness in double blind, placebo-controlled add-on trials (Motte *et al.*, 1997; Sachdeo *et al.*, 1999). Add-on rufinamide (RFN) also showed effectiveness for generalized seizures in a CRT including 74 patients with LGS. It was most useful in "drop attacks" (Glauser *et al.*, 2008). A review article on the use of RFN in children and adults with LGS compared studies done in the United States and Europe (Resnick *et al.*, 2011). A retrospective observational study conducted in Germany and Austria documented the clinical course of 31 patients with LGS. A long-term follow-up with good results was reported (Kluger *et al.*, 2009, 2010). Another long-term open-label add-on study of RFN in 43 patients recruited from 11 centers in Italy showed that 60.5% of the cases were responders (Coppola *et al.*, 2010). As in Dravet syndrome, cannabidiol (CBD) has also shown efficacy, especially against drop attacks (Devinsky *et al.*, 2018).

Childhood absence epilepsy (CAE)

A double-blind CRT study in 453 children with newly diagnosed CAE compared efficacy, tolerability and neuropsychological effects of ethosuximide (ESM) (156 children), LTG (149 patients), or

VPA (148 children). ESM and VPA showed to be more effective than LTG. ESM is associated with fewer adverse attentional effects (Glauser *et al.*, 2010).

After this thorough analysis of the mentioned three drugs usually used in the treatment of so many children with CAE, it sounds strange to remind an open study of 5 patients with refractory absence seizures who were evaluated with serial video-EEG studies after the administration of the VPA-ESM combination therapy. All 5 children became seizure free (Rowan *et al.*, 1983). An expert opinion research also recommended ESM, followed by VPA and LTG on the treatment of CAE, whereas valproic was considered the drug of first choice in juvenile absence epilepsy (Wheless *et al.*, 2005).

Benign childhood epilepsy with centrotemporal spikes (BECTS)

Carbamazepine (CBZ) was the classic AED elected for treatment in children with BECTS. Gabapentin (GBP) was tried in a double-blind placebo controlled study of 225 patients with BECTS, preliminary report showing good results (Bourgeois *et al.*, 1998). Oxcarbazepine (OXC) monotherapy in an open study of 70 newly diagnosed patients with BECTS was considered effective in preventing seizures and normalizing EEGs (Tzitiridou *et al.*, 2005). A non-controlled study on monotherapy with levetiracetam (LEV) in 21 children showed that it is effective and well tolerated (Verrotti *et al.*, 2007). An open label, parallel group comparative trial of LEV or OXC evaluated LEV monotherapy in 21 children with BECTS and OXC monotherapy in 18 other patients. Both drugs seemed to be effective and well tolerated (Coppola *et al.*, 2007). Benzodiazepines (BZP) had been repeatedly recommended for the treatment of children with BECTS, and it is well known that they do not worsen EEG discharges as it may occur with classic AEDs. At present, the use of CLB at night is one of the first choices in those children who only have seizures during sleep (Fejerman *et al.*, 2007a; Fejerman 2008a, 2009).

However, an old drug such as sulthiame (STM) is still considered the drug of choice for those children with BECTS who present atypical features with neuropsychological impairments (Fejerman *et al.*, 2007b). In a double blind, placebo control study, 66 children with BECTS were randomized either to STM or placebo during a 6-month-trial. STM was found to be not only remarkably effective in preventing seizures (Rating *et al.*, 2000), but also clearly superior to placebo in normalizing EEGs (Bast *et al.*, 2003). An open study compared 38 children with BECTS who received CBZ with 18 children treated with STM. Normalization of interictal epileptiform discharges was seen more often following treatment with STM (71%) than with CBZ (42%) (Kramer *et al.*, 2002.) Deterioration in cognitive function in six children treated with STM was reported (Wirrell *et al.*, 2008), but the interpretation was questioned in a letter to the editor (Deonna *et al.*, 2010).

Juvenile myoclonic epilepsy (JME)

An expert opinion research published in 2005 rated VPA as the drug of choice in the treatment of patients with JME, placing LTG and TPM in second and third place. However, the ILAE Treatment Guidelines failed to recognize adequate CRT for patients with JME (Glauser *et al.*, 2006). In a randomized controlled trial of TPM *vs.* VPA conducted in a small number of patients with JME, TPM showed to be an effective and well-tolerated alternative (Levisohn & Holland, 2007). In a multicenter CRT, TPM was considered effective for JME (Biton *et al.*, 2005), but a recent literature survey did not find evidence of its superiority compared to VPA (Liu *et al.*, 2019). An open-label, long term treatment with LEV study was performed with 48 JME patients with good results (Specchio *et al.*, 2006). In a randomized, double-blind, placebo-controlled multicenter trial of adjunctive treatment with LEV including mainly patients with JME, LEV was found to be effective for previously uncontrolled patients (Noachtar *et al.*, 2008). The analysis of two other studies of add-on LEV done with similar methodology reached the same conclusions regarding the use of LEV in JME (Rosenfeld *et al.*, 2009). Perampanel is increasingly used in IGE, and shows promising efficacy in JME, but only open and retrospective reports have been published (Villanueva *et al.*, 2018).

AED-induced worsening of epilepsy syndromes

The risk of seizure aggravation has increased with the number of AEDs (Genton & McMenamin, 1998). IGE are primary candidates for a pharmacodynamic aggravation but we must keep in mind that a paradoxical, unpredictable aggravation can be observed with all AEDs, and even on vagus nerve stimulation (review in Arhan *et al.*, 2018). This is confirmed by modern controlled trials in refractory focal epilepsies with aggravation in a minority of cases without any evidence explanation. Epilepsy is a waxing and waning condition and it is sometime difficult to differentiate the natural course of the disease (spontaneous worsening) and the effect of the drug. In this paragraph, we would like to give some general rules using a syndromic approach.

Idiopathic generalized epilepsies

Animal models

It is accepted that two genetic models in rats (WAG/Rij and Genetic Absence Epilepsy Rats from Strasbourg [GAERS]) are considered predictive of human absence epilepsy. ESM, VPA, BZP are effective against spike-wave discharges. CBZ, phenytoin (PHT), GBP, VGB, tiagabine (TGB) worsen spiking (Depaulis & van Luijtelaar, 2006). Phenobarbital (PB) had a biphasic effect. It is suppressive at low dose but not at 20 mg/kg. However, there are exceptions. LTG has no effects on these two models but it is active against absences in human. TPM, LEV, pregabalin (PGN) suppressed spike-wave discharges in animals (Depaulis & van Luijtelaar, 2006) but not necessarily in humans.

Aggravation in absence epilepsies

Many antiepileptic drugs such as CBZ, OXC, GBP, VGB, TGB may aggravate absence epilepsies (Parker *et al.*, 1998; Genton, 2000; Gélisse *et al.*, 2004; Thomas *et al.*, 2006) *(Figure 1)*. PHT seems to be less aggravating for absences (Genton, 2000). PB may have a dual effect (increasing absences at high doses, decreasing them at low dosages) (Genton, 2000). There is one paper which reports aggravation of absence seizures in 8 cases within days of VPA introduction. All improved after VPA discontinuation. In five, VPA was reintroduced resulting in new seizure aggravation (Lerman-Sagie *et al.*, 2001). An aggravation of absence seizures was reported in three adolescents with juvenile absence epilepsy at a daily dose more than 1,750 mg/day (Auvin *et al.*, 2011).

Aggravation in myoclonic epilepsies

In myoclonic-astatic epilepsy, CBZ and VGB should be avoided as they may be responsible for paradoxical aggravation of seizures, resulting at times in myoclonic status (Lortie *et al.*, 1993; Guerrini *et al.*, 2002a, 2005). Talwar *et al.* (1994) reported aggravation in two patients treated with CBZ. A presumed diagnosis of cryptogenic partial epilepsy was made before a correct diagnosis of myoclonic-astatic epilepsy was made.

In a series of 19 patients with JME, 16 experienced increased myoclonic jerks with CBZ monotherapy, and four also experienced absences (Sozuer *et al.*, 1996). Among 28 consecutive JME patients treated with CBZ alone or in association, 68% had aggravated symptoms including myoclonic status in two whereas 14% were improved (two in monotherapy, one in association with VPA, and one in association with VPA and PB) (Genton *et al.*, 2000). No effect was seen in the remaining five cases (one in monotherapy, three in association with VPA, and one in association with PB). OXC was also found to provoke a clear aggravation in four JME patients: aggravation of myoclonic jerks in all, increase in generalized tonic-clonic seizure frequency in three and absence seizures in two (Gélisse *et al.*, 2004). However, there is a discrepancy with the study published by Carignani & Rosso (1997). They used OXC (doses < 45 mg/kg/day) in six JME patients with clinical and EEG asymmetries. The authors mentioned that exacerbation of spike-wave activity and myoclonic jerks did not

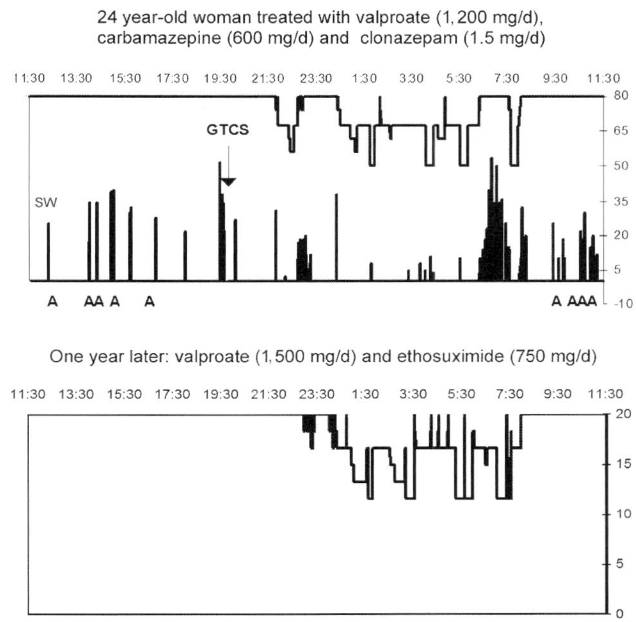

Figure 1 **24 year-old woman with juvenile absence epilepsy. Onset of epilepsy at age 14 with typical absences and rare generalized tonic-clonic seizures (GTCS). She had been misdiagnosed as having focal epilepsy due to asymmetric EEG changes. Top: 24-hr ambulatory EEG on admission. Numerous spike-wave (SW) discharges, absences (A) and one GTCS. At this time, she was treated with valproate, carbamazepine and clonazepam. Bottom: control 24-h ambulatory EEG performed one year later after she was switched to valproate and ethosuximide. Full remission since the change of treatment. All SW discharges and absences disappeared.**

occur in their cases and they "were surprised by the good response obtained with this drug". The main problem of this study is the characterization of the epilepsy. The authors also mentioned that some patients had hemitonic or hemiclonic seizures at the onset of the disorder, which is a very atypical presentation for JME.

In the earlier studies on JME, it was noted that PB and primidone (PRM) were much more efficient than PHT (Janz & Christian, 1957). Kivity & Rechtman (1995) reported that PHT at high dose is highly toxic in JME patients and Sozuer *et al.* (1996) reported that PHT exacerbated MJ in four of six JME patients. In the Genton *et al.* study (2000), PHT aggravated symptoms in 38%, 12% were improved but the others (50%) did not notice a change in seizure frequency.

LTG can exacerbate myoclonic seizures in JME (Biraben *et al.*, 2000) but it was also reported *de novo* appearance of myoclonic jerks in juvenile IGE: 5.4% according to Crespel *et al.* (2005). These authors highlighted two distinct profiles: i) a dose-related aggravation of myoclonic jerks during or at the end of LTG titration that may respond to LTG dosage reduction by 25 to 50%; ii) a severe aggravation of myoclonic jerks occurring several months after LTG titration and evolving into myoclonic status, requiring cessation of LTG.

Status epilepticus due to inappropriate drug choice in IGE

LTG was ascribed to provoke myoclonic status epilepticus in juvenile IGE (Crespel *et al.*, 2005) but this condition seems to be very rare (see above). There is one published case of absence status epilepticus occuring several months after the introduction of LTG in a 10-year-old girl with a history of absence seizures who became seizure-free following LTG cessation (Hasan *et al.*, 2006). On the other hand, CBZ, VGB and PHT play a crucial role in aggravation. Thomas *et al.* (2006) collected over 8 years 14 patients (CAE: 2 cases; JAE: 6 cases; JME: 4 cases; epilepsy with grand mal on awakening: 2 cases). All had aggravation several months before referral. Indeed, they were misdiagnosed either as cryptogenic partial epilepsy (8 cases) or cryptogenic generalized epilepsy (4 cases) and all were treated with CBZ. Seven had polytherapy with PHT, VGB or GBP. At admittance, five had typical absence status, five had atypical absence status, three had atypical myoclonic status and one had typical myoclonic status epilepticus. Potential precipitating factors for absence status were increase of CBZ or of CBZ and PHT; initiation of CBZ, VGB or GBP and decrease of PB. Following change of treatment including withdrawal of the aggravating drugs and adjustment of medication, all but one became seizure free. One had persisting rare absences due to poor compliance. The use of lacosamide has provoked the occurrence of absence status in a patient with JME (Akos Szabo *et al.*, 2019).

Idiopathic focal epilepsies

Benign epilepsy with centrotemporal spikes

It is known that in a small percentage of cases, BECTS is not really "benign" (Lerman, 1986), including several cases of Landau-Kleffner syndrome and continuous spike-and-wave during slow sleep (CSWS) (Fejerman *et al.*, 2000b, 2007b). In many cases of atypical evolutions of BECTS, the appearance of spike-and-waves during slow sleep was apparently associated with AEDs. In two children with BECTS who developed atypical benign partial epilepsy of childhood after treatment with CBZ, discontinuation of this drug was followed by clear clinical and EEG improvement (Caraballo *et al.*, 1989). Guerrini *et al.* (1995) reported three cases of atypical BECTS in which the administration of CBZ in two and PB in one aggravated epileptic negative myoclonus and triggered subcontinuous unilateral or bilateral central spike-and-wave activity. EEG discharge morphology in these patients apparently indicated that CBZ-induced epileptic negative myoclonus was in only in those BECTS patients who had Rolandic spike-and-waves and not in those with only Rolandic sharp waves (Guerrini *et al.*, 1998a).

Other old and new AEDs also may be a cause of worsening seizures (Perucca *et al.*, 1998; Guerrini *et al.*, 1998a). Six patients with classic BECTS evolved atypically with CSWS and neuropsychologic abnormalities, 4 in association with CBZ and 2 with VPA (Prats *et al.*, 1998). In one series of 26 patients with atypical evolutions of BECTS, 16 of them were taking CBZ before worsening (Fejerman *et al.*, 2000b). PB-induced atypical absences in patients with BECTS were also reported (Hamano *et al.*, 2002). Two of us have reported a retrospective study of 98 patients with BECTS and found only one with electroclinical aggravation among 40 children who received CBZ and another among 14 receiving PB (Corda *et al.*, 2001). In a larger series of 39 cases of atypical evolutions in patients with BECTS exposed to different AEDs, significant changes were obtained switching those drugs to BZD, ESM, or STM (Fejerman *et al.*, 2007b). Watemberg *et al.* (2009) reported 5 cases of BECTS and epileptic negative myoclonus only. One patient experienced myoclonus aggravation with CBZ which was not seen in the others cases who were treated with either VPA, TPM, LEV or STM. Gélisse *et al.* (2011) reported a 5-year-old boy with BECTS with proximal negative myoclonus as the only seizure type who experienced severe aggravation of seizures when LTG (25 mg/d) was added to VPA (400 mg/d). Previously, Catania *et al.* (1999) and Cerminara *et al.* (2004) reported a deleterious effect of LTG in cotherapy with VPA, resulting in increased seizure frequency, transient cognitive impairment and in the case of Cerminara *et al.* (2004) the appearance of negative myoclonus. Yang *et al.* (2009) published the cases of 14 patients with epileptic negative myoclonus and atypical benign partial epilepsy of childhood and reported that in some patients, changes in AED regimen where related to the apparition of epileptic negative myoclonus: add-on therapy with CBZ, OXC, PB or withdrawal of VPA. A case of aggravation after use of TPM has also been reported (Montenegro & Guerreiro, 2002). LEV was associated with induction of CSWS syndrome in two children, but they were not cases of BECTS (Caraballo *et al.*, 2010).

Other idiopathic focal epilepsies

Clinical and EEG aggravation was also seen in a few children with Panayiotopoulos syndrome (Caraballo *et al.*, 2001; Ferrie *et al.*, 2002; Kikumoto *et al.*, 2006; Fejerman, 2008b). At least in one of the patients the EEG and seizure exacerbation was induced by CBZ.

Epileptic encephalopathies

Infantile spasms do not represent a homogenous syndrome. Various AEDs have been used. There are few reports of aggravation but no conclusions can be made. Talwar *et al.* (1994) reported aggravation in 3 patients with cryptogenic infantile spasms. Orally administered BZP have been reported to worsen spasms or to provoke short tonic seizures (Otani *et al.*, 1991). On the other hand, DS represents nowadays a well-defined entity. LTG should be used only with utmost care. This drug aggravates more than 80% of the patients at any stage of the condition (Guerrini *et al.*, 1998b). The same phenomenon has been noted for CBZ (Horn *et al.*, 1986; Wakai *et al.*, 1996) but according to Dravet *et al.* (2005) it is not so obvious. Both drugs act on Na channels, which are implicated in the pathophysio-pathology of the DS. In the LGS, intravenous injections of BZP can worsen or induce tonic status epilepticus especially in patients with numerous spike-waves discharges in their EEG (Martin, 1970; Tassinari *et al.*, 1972). GBP may aggravate atypical absences and myoclonic seizures in the LGS (Vossler, 1996). Myoclonic status epilepticus can be exacerbated in LGS syndrome with increased dosages of LTG (Guerrini *et al.*, 1999). Cuzzola *et al.* (2010) observed paradoxical aggravation in three consecutive LGS patients with lacosamide (LCM). At onset of LCM, patients experienced an increase in the frequency of tonic seizures and one patient had a tonic status epilepticus. In ESES, it is recommended to avoid overmedication (Tassinari *et al.*, 2005). A detrimental effect of CBZ has been reported (Caraballo *et al.*, 1989). The same phenomenon was observed with VGB. However, when this syndrome occurs in a child with an extensive cortical dysplasia (micropolygyria), VGB may on the contrary be effective (Genton, 2000). It was also shown that LEV had provoked seizure aggravation in a patient with a cryptogenic focal epilepsy who experienced negative myoclonus associated with ESES (Caraballo *et al.*, 2010). According to Tassinari *et al.* (2005), PHT, CBZ and PB are ineffective in the Landau-Kleffner syndrome or can even worsen the condition.

Practical considerations and conclusions

What we know about the relationship between epilepsy syndromes and AEDs reflects the general state of our knowledge about epilepsy. Epilepsy syndromes vary greatly in terms of severity, homogeneity, etiologies and mechanisms (when they are known); AEDs are very heterogenous in terms of mechanisms of action: with few exceptions, preclinical, experimental and premarketing studies do not provide data on specific efficacy in any given epilepsy syndrome. AED choice will thus result from a compound decision taking into account pharmacological data (pertaining to the AED), clinical data (pertaining to the seizure and epilepsy types) and the patient profile. Applying one given AED to a patient with a given type of epilepsy syndrome may have variable results: in most cases, the choice provides seizure relief. In quite a few cases, there will be no beneficial effect, and some patients will even experience AED-induced "aggravation".

There are, fortunately, a number of instances where a fairly consensual attitude is shared by all well-informed practitioners, and the relationship between epilepsy syndrome and AED seems to be very close. A good example is childhood absence epilepsy, with a limited choice of adequate drugs (VPA and ESM, with LTG as an option). However, convincing observations of typical absence aggravated by VPA have been reported. These observations constitute a very small minority, and it may be hypothetized that these unusual patients differ from the flock by a most unusual individual sensitivity, probably related to rare genetic polymorphism.

In other instances, the relationship between AED and syndrome is looser. This may be the case in most non-syndromic situations, *e.g.*, in most acquired, lesional focal epilepsies: most drugs will help and the risk of seizure aggravation is small, but a minority of patients are not satisfactorily controlled. In severe, encephalopathic epilepsies, with multiple seizure types (*e.g.*, LGS or DS), a few drugs may produce aggravation in most (but may help in a small subset of patients), a few drugs are highly recommended, but these only rarely produce satisfactory seizure control.

There are even numerous situations in which there is no apparent bond between syndrome and AED. This is for instance the case in idiopathic focal epilepsies of childhood: many AEDs may help, but many (including those with a beneficial effect in some patients) may cause aggravation, and the "no treatment" option has to be seriously considered in most patients. A study detected SCN1A mutations in isolated cases of partial epilepsy with antecedent febrile seizures and seizure aggravation by AEDs, the authors stated that the mutants cause loss of function of sodium channel Nav l.l, suggesting a potential relationship between dysfunction of Nav l.l and seizure aggravation by sodium channel blocking AEDs (Liao *et al.*, 2010).

In spite of the fact that the mechanisms of action of AEDs are nowadays better understood, and in spite of the increasing knowledge about the seizure-inducing mechanisms responsible for human epilepsies, the relationship between AEDs and epilepsy syndrome is still very much empirical and pragmatic. We have no evidence that allows us to be dogmatic about the treatment of epilepsy syndromes, we should continue to gather knowledge about the basic mechanisms related to epilepsy syndromes and to look for the chemical compound that will correct the biological anomaly and control seizures. Given the complexity of mechanisms involved, and the fact that the correction of one single contributor is most unlikely to bring about perfectly normal function, this goal seems to be still far away. One may even wonder at the excellent results obtained in the control of epileptic seizures in so many patients with our present tools. Future generations will probably look back on us with some irony. But the best we can do today, in terms of epilepsy treatment, means already a lot for a majority of our patients.

AEDs are obviously purely "symptomatic" agents, *i.e.* they prevent seizures or seizure spread, but do not influence the course of the condition. This consideration is contradicted, however, by several studies that showed how anticonvulsants may prevent the establishment of chronic epilepsy: they may thus indeed have an antiepileptic effect, and not solely exhibit anticonvulsant potential. The next step in this direction is represented by the present interest for "precision" medicine (EpiPM consortium, 2015): ideally, treatment indicated in a patient with epilepsy should be specifically tailored to the patients genetic configuration, and to the intimate, precisely defined mechanisms of epilepsy in his case. However, this "precision", etiologically-based therapeutic approach, is not fully secure or efficient (Mullen *et al.*, 2018). Perhaps the first step of this era of "precision" treatment is already, to some extent, available: it is represented by a rational choice of drug and overall treatment strategy based, whenever possible, on the epilepsy syndrome (Sharma *et al.*, 2019).

REFERENCES ▶

Ákos Szabó C, Morgan LC, Sonnenberg S, Karkar KM (2019): Absence status induced by lacosamide adjunctive therapy. *Epileptic Disord* 21: 97–101.

Arhan E, Serdaroğlu A, Hirfanoğlu T, Kurt G (2018): Aggravation of seizures and status epilepticus after vagal nerve stimulation therapy: the first pediatric case and review of the literature. *Childs Nerv Syst* 34: 1799–1801.

Auvin S, Chhun S, Berquin P, Ponchel E, Delanoë C, Chiron C (2011): Aggravation of absence seizure related to levetiracetam. *Eur J Paediatr Neurol* 15: 508–511.

Baram TZ, Mitchell WG, Tournay A, Snead OC, Hanson RA, Horton EJ (1996): High-dose corticotropin (ACTH) *versus* prednisone for infantile spasms: a prospective, randomized, blinded study. *Pediatrics* 97: 375–379.

Bast T, Völp A, Wolf C, Rating D; Sulthiame Study Group (2003): The influence of sulthiame on EEG in children with benign childhood epilepsy with centrotemporal spikes (BECTS). *Epilepsia* 44: 215–220.

Bergey GK (2005): Evidence-based treatment of idiopathic generalized epilepsies with new antiepileptic drugs. *Epilepsia* 46 (Suppl 9): 161–168.

Biraben A, Allain H, Scarabin JM, *et al.* (2000): Exacerbation of juvenile myoclonic epilepsy with lamotrigine. *Neurology* 55: 1758.

Biton V, Bourgeois BF, YTC/YTCE Study Investigators (2005): Topiramate in patients with juvenile myoclonic epilepsy. *Arch Neurol* 62: 1705–1708.

Bourgeois B, Brown W, Pellock JM, *et al.* (1998): Gabapentin (Neurontin) monotherapy in children with benign childhood epilepsy with centrotemporal spikes (BECTS): A 36-week, double blind, placebo-controlled study. *Epilepsia* 39 (Suppl 6): 163.

Caldwell PH, Murphy SB, Butow PN, Craig JC (2004): Clinical trials in children. *Lancet* 364 (9436): 803–811.

Camfield C, Camfield P (2005): Management guidelines for children with idiopathic generalized epilepsy. *Epilepsia* 46 (Suppl 9): 112–116.

Caraballo RH (2011): Nonpharmacologic treatments of Dravet syndrome: focus on the ketogenic diet. *Epilepsia* 52 (Suppl 2): 79–82.

Caraballo R, Fontana E, Michelizza B, *et al.* (1989): Carbamazepina, "assenze atipiche", "crisi atoniche" e stato di PO continua del sonno (POCS). *Boll Lega It Epil* 66/67: 379–381.

Caraballo RH, Astorino F, Cersosimo R, Soprano AM, Fejerman N (2001): Atypical evolution in childhood epilepsy with occipital paroxysms (Panayiotopoulos type). *Epileptic Disord* 3: 157–162.

Caraballo RH, Fejerman N (2006): Dravet syndrome: a study of 53 patients. *Epilepsy Res* 70 (Suppl 1): S231-S238.

Caraballo RH, Cersosimo R, De los Santos C (2010): Levetiracetam-induced seizure aggravation associated with continuous spikes and waves during slow sleep in children with refractory epilepsies. *Epileptic Disord* 12: 146–150.

Carignani M, Rosso D (1997): To the editor. *Epilepsia* 38: 258.

Catania S, Cross H, de Sousa C, Boyd S (1999): Paradoxic reaction to lamotrigine in a child with benign focal epilepsy of childhood with centrotemporal spikes. *Epilepsia* 40: 1657–1660.

Cerminara C, Montanaro ML, Curatolo P, Seri S (2004): Lamotrigine-induced seizure aggravation and negative myoclonus in idiopathic Rolandic epilepsy. *Neurology* 63: 373–375.

Chiron C, Dumas C, Jambaqué I, *et al.* (1997): Randomized trial comparing vigabatrin and hydrocortisone in infantile spasms due to tuberous sclerosis. *Epilepsy Res* 26: 389–395.

Chiron C, Marchand MC, Tran A, *et al.* (2000): Stiripentol in severe myoclonic epilepsy in infancy: a randomised placebo-controlled syndrome dedicated trial. STICLO study group. *Lancet* 356 (9242): 1638–1642.

Chiron C (2019): Stiripentol for the treatment of seizures associated with Dravet syndrome. *Expert Rev Neurother [Epub ahead of print]*.

Commission on Classification and Terminology of the International League Against Epilepsy (1989): Proposal for revised classification of epilepsies and epileptic syndromes. *Epilepsia* 30: 389–399.

Coppola G, Franzoni E, Verrotti A, *et al.* (2007): Levetiracetam oroxcarbazepine as monotherapy in newly diagnosed benign epilepsy of childhood with centrotemporal spikes (BECTS): an open-label, parallel group trial. *Brain Dev* 29: 281–284.

Coppola G, Grosso S, Franzoni E, *et al.* (2010): Rufinamide in children and adults with Lennox-Gastaut syndrome: first Italian multicenter experience. *Seizure* 19: 587–591.

Corda D, Gélisse P, Genton P, Dravet C, Baldy-Moulinier M (2001): Incidence of drug-induced aggravation in benign epilepsy with centro-temporal spikes. *Epilepsia* 42: 754–759.

Crespel A, Genton P, Berramdane M, *et al.* (2005): Lamotrigine associated with exacerbation or *de novo* myoclonus in idiopathic generalized epilepsies. *Neurology* 65: 762–765.

Cuzzola A, Ferlazzo E, Italiano D, Calabro RS, Bramanti P, Genton P (2010): Does lacosamide aggravate Lennox-Gastaut syndrome? Report on three consecutive cases. *Epilepsy Behav* 19: 650–651.

Deonna T, Roulet-Perez E, Cronel-Ohayon S, Mayor-Dubois C (2010): Correspondence on "deterioration in cognitive function in children with benign epilepsy of childhood with central temporal spikes treated with sulthiame". *J Child Neurol* 25: 127–128.

Depaulis A, Van Luijteaar G (2006): Genetic models of absence epilepsy in the rat. In: Pitkänen A, Schwartzkroin PA, Moshé SL (eds) *Models of Seizures and Epilepsy*, pp. 233–248. Burlington: Elsevier Academic Press.

Devinsky O, Cross JH, Laux L, *et al.* (2017): Trial of Cannabidiol for Drug-Resistant Seizures in the Dravet Syndrome. *N Engl J Med* 376: 2011–2020.

Devinsky O, Patel AD, Cross JH, *et al.* (2018): Effect of cannabidiol on drop seizures in the Lennox-Gastaut syndrome. *N Engl J Med* 378: 1888–1897.

Dravet C, Bureau M, Oguni H, Fukuyama, Cokar O (2005): Severe myoclonic epilepsy in infancy (Dravet syndrome). In: Roger J, Bureau M, Dravet C, Genton P, Tassinari CA, Wolf P (eds) *Epileptic Syndromes in Infancy, Childhood and Adolescence*, 4th ed, pp. 89–113. Paris: John Libbey Eurotext.

Dravet C, Guerrini R (2011): Dravet Syndrome. Paris: John Libbey Eurotext.

Dressler A, Benninger F, Trimmel-Schwahofer P, *et al.* (2019): Efficacy and tolerability of the ketogenic diet *versus* high-dose adrenocorticotropic hormone for infantile spasms: A single-center parallel-cohort randomized controlled trial. *Epilepsia* 60: 441–451.

Dulac O, Bast T, Dalla Bernardina B, Gaily E, Neville B (2010): Infantile spasms: toward a selective diagnostic and therapeutic approach. *Epilepsia* 51: 2218–2219.

Engel J Jr (2001): A proposed diagnostic scheme for people with epileptic seizures and with epilepsy: report of the ILAE Task Force on Classification and Terminology. *Epilepsia* 42: 796–803.

EpiPM Consortium, Berkovic SF, Scheffer IE, Petrou S, *et al.* (2015): A roadmap for precision medicine in the epilepsies. *Lancet Neurol* 14: 1219–1228.

European Medicines Agency (2007): Committee for Medicinal Products for Human Use: guideline on clinical trials in small populations [online]. http://www.emea.europa.eu/pdfs/human/epw/8356105en.pdf

Fejerman N (2008a): Benign childhood epilepsy with centrotemporal spikes. In: Engel J, Pedley TA (eds) *Epilepsy. A Comprehensive Textbook* (2nd ed) pp. 2369–2378. Philadelphia: Lippincott, Williams & Wilkins.

Fejerman N (2008b): Early-onset benign childhood occipital epilepsy (Panayiotopoulos type). In: Engel J, Pedley TA (eds) Epilepsy. *A Comprehensive Textbook* (2nd ed) pp. 2379–2386. Philadelphia: Lippincott, Williams & Wilkins.

Fejerman N (2009): Atypical Rolandic epilepsy. *Epilepsia* 50 (Suppl 7): 9–12.

Fejerman N, Cersosimo R, Caraballo R, *et al.* (2000a): Vigabatrin as a first-choice drug in the treatment of West syndrome. *J Child Neurol* 15: 161–165.

Fejerman N, Caraballo R, Tenembaum S (2000b): Atypical evolutions of benign localization-related epilepsies in children: are they predictable? *Epilepsia* 41: 380–390.

Fejerman N, Caraballo RH, Dalla Bernardina B (2007a): Benign childhood epilepsy with centrotemporal spikes. In: Fejerman N, Caraballo RH (eds) *Benign Focal Epilepsies in Infancy, Childhood and Adolescence*, pp. 77–113. Paris: John Libbey Eurotext.

Fejerman N, Caraballo RH, Dalla Bernardina B (2007b): Atypical evolutions of benign focal epilepsies in childhood (BFEC), or syndromes related to BFEC? In: Fejerman N, Caraballo RH (eds) *Benign Focal Epilepsies in Infancy, Childhood and Adolescence*, pp. 179–219. Paris: John Libbey Eurotext.

Ferrie CD, Koutroumanidis M, Rowlinson S, Sanders S, Panayiotopoulos CP (2002): Atypical evolution of Panayiotopoulos syndrome: a case report. *Epileptic Disord* 4: 35–42.

French J, Kanner AM, Bautista J, *et al.* (2004): Efficacy and tolerability of the new antiepileptic drugs 1: treatment of new onset epilepsy: report of the Therapeutics and Technology Assesment Subcommittee and the Quality Standards Subcommittee of the American Academy of Neurology and the American Epilepsy Society. *Neurology* 62: 1252–1260.

Gélisse P, Genton P, Kuate C, *et al.* (2004): Worsening of seizures by oxcarbazepine in juvenile idiopathic generalized epilepsies. *Epilepsia* 45: 1282–1286.

Gélisse P, Genton P, Velizarova R, Serafini A, Crespel A (2012): Worsening of negative myoclonus by lamotrigine in a case of idiopathic focal epilepsy of children with long-term follow-up. *Brain Dev* 34: 248–250.

Genton P (2000): When antiepileptic drugs aggravate epilepsy. *Brain Dev* 22: 75–80.

Genton P, McMenamin J (1998): Summary: aggravation of seizures by antiepileptic drugs: what to do in clinical practice. *Epilepsia* 39 (Suppl 3): 26–29.

Genton P, Gélisse P, Thomas P, Dravet C (2000): Do carbamazepine and phenytoin aggravate juvenile myoclonic epilepsy? *Neurology* 55: 1106–1109.

Glauser T, Ben-Menachem E, Bourgeois B, *et al.* (2006): ILAE treatment guidelines: evidence-based analysis of antiepileptic drug efficacy and effectiveness as initial monotherapy for epileptic seizures and syndromes. *Epilepsia* 47: 1094–1120.

Glauser T, Kluger G, Sachdeo R, Krauss G, Perdomo C, Arroyo S (2008): Rufinamide for generalized seizures associated with Lennox-Gastaut syndrome. *Neurology* 70: 1950–1958.

Glauser TA, Cnaan A, Shinnar S, *et al.* (2010): Childhood Absence Epilepsy Study Group. Ethosuximide, valproic acid, and lamotrigine in childhood absence epilepsy. *N EnglJ Med* 4: 790–799.

Guerrini R, Belmonte A, Strumia S, *et al.* (1995): Exacerbation of epileptic negative myoclonus by carbamazepine or phenobarbital in children with atypical benign Rolandic epilepsy. *Epilepsia* 36 (Suppl 3): 65.

Guerrini R, Belmonte A, Genton P (1998a): Antiepileptic drug-induced worsening of seizures in children. *Epilepsia* 39 (Suppl 3): 2–10.

Guerrini R, Dravet C, Genton P, Belmonte A, Kaminska A, Dulac O (1998b): Lamotrigine and seizure aggravation in severe myoclonic epilepsy. *Epilepsia* 39: 508–512.

Guerrini R, Belmonte A, Parmeggiani L, Perucca E (1999): Myoclonic status epilepticus following high-dosage lamotrigine therapy. *Brain Dev* 21: 420–424.

Guerrini R, Bonanni P, Rothwell J, Hallett M (2002a): Myoclonus and epilepsy. In: Guerrini R, Aicardi J, Andermann F, Hallett M (eds) *Epilepsy and Movement Disorder*, pp. 165–210. Cambridge: Cambridge University Press.

Guerrini R, Tonnelier S, D'Athis P, *et al.* (2002b): Stiripentol in severe myoclonic epilepsy in infancy (SMEI): A placebo-controlled trial. *Epilepsia* 43 (Suppl 9): S155.

Guerrini R, Parmeggiani L, Bonanni P, Kaminska A, Dulac O (2005): Myoclonic astatic epilepsy. In: Roger J, Bureau M, Dravet C, Genton P, Tassinari CA, Wolf P (eds) *Epileptic Syndromes in Infancy, Childhood and Adolescence* (4th ed) pp. 115–124. Paris: John Libbey Eurotext.

Hamano S, Mochizuki M, Morikawa T (2002): Phenobarbital-induced atypical absence seizure in benign childhood epilepsy with centrotemporal spikes. *Seizure* 11: 201–204.

Hasan M, Lerman-Sagie T, Lev D, Watemberg N (2006): Recurrent absence status epilepticus (spike-and-wave stupor) associated with lamotrigine therapy. *J Child Neurol* 21: 807–809.

Horn CS, Ater SB, Hurst DL (1986): Carbamazepine-exacerbated epilepsy in children and adolescents. *Pediatr Neurol* 2: 340–345.

Hussain SA (2018): Treatment of infantile spasms. *Epilepsia* Open 3(Suppl 2): 143–154.

Hwang H, Kim KJ (2008): New antiepileptic drugs in pediatric epilepsy. *Brain Dev* 30: 549–555.

Inoue Y, Ohtsuka Y, Oguni H, Tohyama J, Baba H, Fukushima K, *et al.* (2009): Stiripentol open study in Japanese patients with Dravet syndrome. *Epilepsia* 50: 2362–2368.

Jallon P, Loiseau P, Loiseau J (2001): Newly diagnosed unprovoked epileptic seizures: presentation at diagnosis in CAROLE study. Coordination Active du Réseau Observatoire Longitudinal de l'Épilepsie. *Epilepsia* 42: 464–475.

Janz D, Christian W (1957): Impulsiv Petit-Mal. *Dtsch Z Nervenheilk* 176: 346–386.

Kikumoto K, Yoshinaga H, Oka M, *et al.* (2006): EEG and seizure exacerbation induced by carbamazepine in Panayiotopoulos syndrome. *Epileptic Disord* 8: 53–56.

King MA, Newton MR, Jackson GD, *et al.* (1998): Epileptology of the first-seizure presentation: a clinical, electroencephalographic, and magnetic resonance imaging study of 300 consecutive patients. *Lancet* 352: 1007–1011.

Kivity S, Rechtman E (1995): Juvenile myoclonic epilepsy: serious consequences due to pitfalls in diagnosis and management. *Epilepsia* 36 (Suppl 3): 66.

Kluger G, Kurlemann G, Haberlandt E, *et al.* (2009): Effectiveness and tolerability of rufinamide in children and adults with refractory epilepsy: first European experience. *Epilepsy Behav* 14: 491–495.

Kluger G, Glauser T, Krauss G, Seeruthun R, Perdomo C, Arroyo S (2010): Adjunctive rufinamide in Lennox-Gastaut syndrome: a long-term, open-label extension study. *Acta Neurol Scand* 122: 202–208.

Kramer U, Shahar E, Zelnik N, *et al.* (2002): Carbamazepine *versus* sulthiame in treating benign childhood epilepsy with centrotemporal spikes. *J Child Neurol* 17: 914–916.

Lerman P (1986): Seizures induced or aggravated by anticonvulsants. *Epilepsia* 27: 706–710.

Lerman-Sagie T, Watemberg N, Kramer U, Shahar E, Lerman P (2001): Absence seizures aggravated by valproic acid. *Epilepsia* 42: 941–943.

Levisohn PM, Holland KD (2007): Topiramate or valproate in patients with juvenile myoclonic epilepsy: a randomized open-label comparison. *Epilepsy Behav* 10: 547–552.

Liao WP, Shi YW, Long YS, *et al.* (2010): Partial epilepsy with antecedent febrile seizures and seizure aggravation by antiepileptic drugs: Associated with loss of function of Nav l.l *Epilepsia* 51: 1669–1678.

Lortie A, Chiron C, Mumford J, Dulac O (1993): The potential for increasing seizure frequency, relapse, and appearance of new seizure types with vigabatrin. *Neurology* 43 (Suppl 5): 24–27.

Liu J1, Wang LN, Wang YP (2019): Topiramate for juvenile myoclonic epilepsy. Cochrane *Database Syst Rev.* 1: CD010008.

Mackay MT, Weiss SK, Adams-Weber T, *et al.* (2004): Practice parameter: medical treatment of infantile spasms: report of the American Academy of Neurology and the Child Neurology Society. *Neurology* 62: 1668–1681.

Marson AG, Al-Kharusi AM, Alwaidh M, *et al.*, SANAD Study group (2007): The SANAD study of effectiveness of valproate, lamotrigine, or topiramate for generalized and unclassifiable epilepsy: an unblinded randomized controlled trial. *Lancet* 369: 1016–1026.

Martin D (1970): Intravenous nitrazepam (Mogadon) in the treatment of epilepsy. *Neuropediatrie* 2: 27–37.

Montenegro MA, Guerreiro MM (2002): Electrical status epilepticus of sleep in association with topiramate. *Epilepsia* 43: 1436–1440.

Motte J, Trevathan E, Arvidsson JF, *et al.* (1997): Lamotrigine for generalized seizures associated with the Lennox-Gastaut syndrome. Lamictal Lennox-Gastaut Study Group. *N Engl J Med* 337: 1807–1812.

National Institutes of Health (1998): NIH policy and guidelines on the inclusion of children as participants in research involving human subjects. http://grants.nih.gov/grants/guide/notice-files/not98-024.html

Mullen SA, Carney PW, Roten A, *et al.* (2018) : Precision therapy for epilepsy due to KCNT1 mutations: A randomized trial of oral quinidine. *Neurology* 90: e67-e72.

NICE guideline (2004): Clinical Guideline 20. The epilepsies. The diagnosis and management of the epilepsies in adults and children in primary and secondary care. http://www.nice.org.uk/CG020NICEguideline.

NICE (2018): Epilepsies; diagnosis and management. ttps://www.nice.org.uk/Guidance/cg137

Noachtar S, Andermann E, Meyvisch P, *et al.*, N166 (2008): Levetiracetam Study Group. Levetiracetam for the treatment of idiopathic generalized epilepsy with myoclonic seizures. *Neurology* 70: 607–616.

Osborne JP, Lux A (2001): Towards an international consensus on definitions and standardised outcome measures for therapeutic trials (and epidemiological studies) in West syndrome. *Brain Dev* 23: 677–682.

Osservatorio Regionale per l'Epilessia (OREp), Lombardy (1997): The contribution of tertiary centers to the quality of the diagnosis and treatment of epilepsy. *Epilepsia* 38: 1338–1343.

Otani K, Tagawa T, Futagi Y, Okamoto N, Yabuuchi H (1991): Induced microseizures in West syndrome. *Brain Dev* 13: 196–199.

Parker APJ, Agathonikou A, Robinson RO, Panayiotopoulos CP (1998): Inappropriate use of carbamazepine and vigabatrin in typical absence seizures. *Dev Med Child Neurol* 40: 517–519.

Pellock JM, Hrachovy R, Shinnar S, Baram TZ, Bettis D, Dlugos DJ, *et al.* (2010): Infantile spasms: a US consensus report. *Epilepsia* 51: 2175–2189.

Perucca E, Gram L, Avanzini G, *et al.* (1998): Antiepileptic drugs as a cause of worsening seizures. *Epilepsia* 39: 5–17.

Pina-Garza JE, Espinoza R, Nordli D, *et al.* (2005): Oxcarbazepine adjunctive therapy in infants and young children with partial seizures. *Neurology* 65: 1370–1375.

Prats J, Garaizar C, Garcia-Nieto M, Madoz P (1998): Antiepileptic drugs and atypical evolution of idiopathic partial epilepsy. *Pediatr Neurol* 18: 402–406.

Rating D, Wolf C, Bast T (2000): Sulthiame as monotherapy in children with benign childhood epilepsy with centrotemporal spikes: a 5 month randomized, double-blind, placebo-controlled study. Sulthiame Study Group. *Epilepsia* 41: 1284–1288.

Resnick T, Arzimanoglou A, Brown LW, *et al.* (2011): Rufinamide from clinical trials to clinical practice in the United States and Europe. *Epileptic Disord* 13 (Suppl 1): S27-S43.

Rosenfeld WE, Benbadis S, Edrich P, Tassinari CA, Hirsch E (2009): Levetiracetam as add-on therapy for idiopathic generalized epilepsy syndromes with onset during adolescence: analysis of two randomized, double-blind, placebo-controlled studies. *Epilepsy Res* 85: 72–80.

Rowan AJ, Meijer JW, de Beer-Pawlikowski N, *et al.* (1983): Valproate-ethosuximide combination therapy for refractory absence seizures. *Arch Neurol* 40: 797–802.

Sachdeo RC, GlauserTA, Ritter F, *et al.* (1999): A double blind, randomised trial of topiramate in Lennox-Gastaut syndrome. Topiramate YI. Study Group. *Neurology* 52: 1882–1887.

Sankar R (2004): Initial tretment of epilepsy with antiepileptic drugs: pediatric issues. *Neurology* (63/10 Suppl 4): S30-S39.

Scheffer IE, Berkovic S,Capovilla G *et al.* (2017): ILAE classification of the epilepsies: Position paper of theILAE Commission for Classification and Terminology. *Epilepsia* 58: 512–521.

Sharma P, Hussain A, Greenwood R (2019): Precision in pediatric epilepsy. *F1000Res:* Feb 6; 8.

Shinnar S, Pellock JM (2005): The trials and tribulations of pediatric drug trials. *Neurology* 65: 1348–1349.

Shorvon S (2006): We live in the age of the Clinical Guideline. *Epilepsia* 47: 1091–1093.

Song JM, Hahn J, Kim SH, Chang MJ (2017): Efficacy of Treatments for Infantile Spasms: A Systematic Review. *Clin Neuropharmacol* 40: 63–84.

Sozuer DT, Atakli D, Atay T, *et al.* (1996): Evaluation of various antiepileptic drugs in juvenile myoclonic epilepsy. *Epilepsia* 37 (Suppl 4): 77.

Specchio LM, Gambardella A, Giallonardo AT, *et al.* (2006): Open label, long-term, pragmatic study on levetiracetam in the treatment of juvenile myoclonic epilepsy. *Epilepsy Res* 71: 32–39.

Talwar D, Arora MS, Sher PK (1994): EEG changes and seizure exacerbation in young children treated with carbamazepine. *Epilepsia* 35: 1154–1159.

Tassinari CA, Dravet C, Roger J, Cano JP, Gastaut H (1972): Tonic status epilepticus precipitated by intravenous benzodiazepine in five patients with Lennox-Gastaut syndrome. *Epilepsia* 13: 421–435.

Tassinari CA, Rubboli G, Volpi L, Billard C, Bureau M (2005): Electrical status epilepticus during slow sleep (ESES or CSWS) including acquired epileptic aphasia (Landau-Kleffner syndrome). In: Roger J, Bureau M, Dravet C, Genton P, Tassinari CA, Wolf P (eds) *Epileptic Syndromes in Infancy, Childhood and Adolescence* (4th ed) pp. 295–314. Paris: John Libbey Eurotext.

Thanh TN, Chiron C, Dellatolas G, *et al.* (2002): Long-term efficacy and tolerance of stiripentaol in severe myoclonic epilepsy of infancy (Dravet syndrome). *Arch Pediatr* 9: 1120–1127.

The Felbamate Study Group in Lennox-Gastaut Syndrome (1993): Efficacy of felbamate in childhood epileptic encephalopathy (Lennox-Gastaut syndrome). *N Engl J Med* 328: 29–33.

Thomas P, Valton L, Genton P (2006): Absence and myoclonic status epilepticus precipitated by antiepileptic drugs in idiopathic generalized epilepsy. *Brain* 129: 1281–1292.

Trost LF 3rd, Wender RC, Suter CC, *et al.*; National Epilepsy Management Pane (2005): Management of epilepsy in adults. Treatment guidelines. *Postgrad Med* 118: 29–33.

Tzitiridou M, Panou T, Ramantani G, *et al.* (2005): Oxcarbazepine monotherapy in benign childhood epilepsy with centrotemporal spikes: A clinical and cognitive evaluation. *Epilepsy Behav* 7: 458–467.

Verrotti A, Coppola G, Manco R, *et al.* (2007): Levetiracetam monotherapy for children and adolescents with benign Rolandic seizures. *Seizure* 16: 271–275.

Vigevano F, Cilio MR (1997): Vigabatrin *versus* ACTH as first-line treatment for infantile spasms: a randomized, prospective study. *Epilepsia* 38: 1270–1274.

Villanueva V, Montoya J, Castillo A, *et al.* (2018): Perampanel in routine clinical use in idiopathic generalized epilepsy: The 12-month GENERAL study. *Epilepsia* 59: 1740–1752.

Vossler DG (1996): Exacerbation of seizures in Lennox-Gastaut syndrome by gabapentin. *Neurology* 46: 852–853.

Wakai S, Ikehata M, Nihira H, *et al.* (1996): "Obtundation status (Dravet)" caused by complex partial status epilepticus in a patient with severe myoclonic epilepsy in infancy. *Epilepsia* 37: 1020–1022.

Watemberg N, Leitner Y, Fattal-Valevski A, Kramer U (2009): Epileptic negative myoclonus as the presenting seizure type in Rolandic epilepsy. *Pediatr Neurol* 41: 59–64.

Wheless JW, Clarke DF, Carpenter D (2005): Treatment of pediatric epilepsy: expert opinion, 2005. J Child Neurol 20 (Suppl 1): 1–56.

Wheless JW, Clarke DF, Arzimanoglou A, Carpenter D (2007): Treatment of pediatric epilepsy: European expert opinion, 2007. *Epileptic Disord* 9: 353–412.

Wirrell E, Sherman EM, Vanmastrigt R, Hamiwka L (2008): Deterioration in cognitive function in children with benign epilepsy of childhood with central temporal spikes treated with sulthiame. *J Child Neurol* 23: 14–21.

Yang Z, Liu X, Qin J, *et al.* (2009): A study on epileptic negative myoclonus in atypical benign partial epilepsy of childhood. *Brain Dev* 31: 274–281.

Epileptic Syndromes in Infancy, Childhood and Adolescence (6th ed), M. Bureau, P. Genton, C. Dravet, A. V. Delgado-Escueta, R. Guerrini, C.A. Tassinari, P. Thomas & P. Wolf

WITH VIDEO SUPPLEMENTS

CHAPTER 6

BENIGN NEONATAL AND INFANTILE SEIZURES AND EPILEPSIES

Federico Vigevano[1], Paola De Liso[1], Michelle Bureau[2], Perrine Plouin[3], Bernd A. Neubauer[4] and Marina Trivisano[1]

[1] Department of Neurosciences, Bambino Gesù Children's Hospital, IRCCS, Rome, Italy
[2] Centre Saint-Paul, Henri-Gastaut Hospital, Marseille, France
[3] Clinical Neurophysiology Unit, Necker Enfants Malades Hospital, Paris, France
[4] Department of Neuropediatrics, University Hospital Giessen and Marburg (UKGM), Giessen, Germany

Afebrile seizures with onset within the first year of life are often associated with metabolic disorders, structural brain lesions, genetic diseases and are often followed by epileptic encephalopathies (Matsumoto *et al.*, 1983). However, seizures may manifest in newborns and infants with normal neurologic or metabolic status and family history of early onset seizures. Three epileptic conditions have been so far delineated, accounting for predominant focal to bilateral tonic-clonic seizures, benign outcome, and autosomal dominant mode of inheritance. These conditions are differentiated mainly on the basis of the age of onset: typically before the 5th day of life in benign familial neonatal seizures (BFNS) (Rett & Teubel, 1964), between 2 days and 6 months of age in benign familial neonatal-infantile seizures (BFNIS) (Kaplan & Lacey, 1983), and between 3 and 8 months of age in benign familial infantile seizures (BFIS) (Vigevano *et al.*, 1992).

These three epileptic entities have many elements in common, as they have an autosomal dominant mode of inheritance and are characterized by the occurrence of seizures self-limited in a very brief period of life in newborns and infants without other etiological factors. The patients present clusters of focal motor seizures evolving to bilateral tonic-clonic, staring, and apnea. Typical and diagnostic interictal EEG trait are not described. The developmental outcome in the majority of patients is normal and other type of seizures or epilepsies are very rare. In some patients non-epileptic paroxysmal disorders can appear later on. These three entities are differentiated not only for the age of onset, but also because due to different gene mutations: *KCNQ2* mutations are the major cause of BFNS and BFNIS, *PRRT2* of BFIS, but this is not exclusive. Other genes can cause similar epileptic conditions as *KCNQ3*, *SCN2A*, *SCN8A* and *CHRNA2*. The same genes can provoke also severe forms of epilepsy.

As above-mentioned, these three epileptic entities have in common the occurrence of seizures just in a very brief period of life in newborns and infants. For this reason, some authors proposed the terms "Self-limited neonatal or infantile epilepsy". Nevertheless, although this is more appropriate, it is not currently included in the glossary of epileptic syndromes and for this reason, we preferred in this chapter to continue to use the generic term of "benign". Lastly, the distinction between the familial and sporadic forms, that was considered in the past, is not more currently used as there are not significant differences in clinical features and mutations (Zara *et al.*, 2013).

Benign familial and non-familial neonatal seizures

Rett and Teubel (1964) reported the first BFNS family, with eight cases over 3 generations. On the 3rd day of life the male proband developed an initial tonic phase with cyanosis followed by clonic movements of the whole body including the face and eye muscles, and he had 15–20 seizure events on the following day. A brother born 16 months later had a similar experience. The authors noted the familial history, the normality of the interictal EEG and the favourable outcome. Later on, a second family of 14 members in 5 generations with similar clinical histories was reported (Bjerre & Corelius, 1968). After a normal delivery, seizures (sometimes with cyanosis) usually started on the 3rd day of life but stopped within 1 month. A few seizures were observed up to 7 months in 3 children and up to 10 years in 2 others. In 1979, Quattlebaum reported a family in which 11 had seizures that started on or before 3 days of age, one at 3 weeks and 3 others at 3 months.

Most had seizures until 6 or 8 months, but all were otherwise normal. These kinships demonstrate the autosomal dominant pattern of inheritance that has been confirmed in basically all later reports. Only Schiffmann *et al.* (1991) reported on a family with an autosomal recessive inheritance pattern.

The family reported by Quattlebaum (1979), including 19 individuals, was suitable candidate for linkage analysis. In 1989, Leppert *et al.* established linkage of the gene for BFNS to the long arm of chromosome 20, the first linkage to be reported for an epilepsy syndrome. That conclusion was soon confirmed in a Newfoundland family with 69 affected (Ronen *et al.*, 1993), in a Northern European family (Ryan *et al.*, 1991), and in six French families (Malafosse *et al.*, 1992). The BFNS syndrome that maps to chromosome 20q has been designated EBN1.

Linkage to D20S19 and D20S20 was excluded; however, in a three-generation Mexican-American family (Ryan *et al.*, 1991), suggesting locus heterogeneity. Further study of this and other families (Lewis *et al.*, 1993; Steinlein *et al.*, 1995) demonstrated linkage to a locus on 8q. (The BFNS syndrome on 8q is designated EBN2.) In other families no linkage could be found on either 20q or 8q (Lewis *et al.*, 1996). These linkage studies led to the identification of mutations in the voltage-gated potassium channel genes *KCNQ2* and *KCNQ3*, (Singh *et al.*, 1998; Biervert *et al.*, 1998; Charlier *et al.*, 1998) respectively encoding for the potassium channels Kv7.2 and Kv7.3. Most detected mutations in BFNS are localized in the *KCNQ2* gene (~ 95%), residing in the carboxy-terminal domain of the Kv7.2 channel protein (Singh *et al.*, 2003). Most detected mutations exert their effect by haplo-insufficiency. Some mutations with a dominant negative effect are also reported (Volkers *et al.*, 2009). Usually this does not affect the phenotype. There is no explanation as yet for the very small number of Q3 mutations in BFNS. During brain development in the mouse, *KCNQ3* is expressed later than *KCNQ2* (Tinel *et al.*, 1998), but this has not been confirmed in humans.

The early onset and spontaneous remission of seizures in BFNS have long been matters of interest (Tinel *et al.*, 1998; Jentsch, 2000). In 2003 Okada *et al.* proposed that these clinical features have a basis in age-specific expression of the ion channels, and that possible development-specific appearance of other channels may compensate for the loss of function of the channel that has the mutation. They studied the effect of inhibitors of KCNQ-channels, and GABA – and glutamate – receptors on neuronal-excitability and neurotransmitter release, using rat hippocampus from day of birth (P0) to postnatal day 56. They found that during the first week of life, KCNQ2 channels were a predominant inhibitory system whereas, after P7, GABAergic transmission switched from excitatory to inhibitory function. On the other hand glutamatergic-transmission acquired an excitatory function from P0. Hence, a small reduction in KCNQ related M – current resulting from deficient KCNQ – channels in BFNS may lead to convulsions only during neonatal age (= 0.008). These data on functional switching in GABAergic transmission in neonates were later confirmed in other studies on mouse models (Kanaumi *et al.*, 2008). In families with BFNS sequence analysis in *KCNQ2* and *KCNQ3* will detect mutations in about 60–70% of cases. Estimates of sporadic cases vary from 4 to 38% of NNS, this large scatter probably reflecting differences in patients' referral and recruitment: intensive care units, maternity clinics, departments of neonatology or paediatric neurology. *KCNQ2* mutations are the most common, with > 80 different mutations described (Bellini *et al.*, 2013), whereas *KCNQ3* mutations are rare (Zara *et al.*, 2013). Now we know that *KCNQ2* mutations are the major cause of benign familial neonatal-infantile seizures too.

The smaller the families, or the number of affected, the lower the yield. Germline mosaicism was reported in at least one case (Sadewa *et al.*, 2008). In families with BFNS and a negative sequence analysis genomic microdeletions and rarely also microduplications (which are undetectable by classic sequence analysis) may be disclosed (Heron *et al.*, 2007). In some patients these microdeletions also include the neighbouring *CHRNA4* gene (known to be associated with autosomal dominant frontal lobe epilepsy in some families). Amazingly that did not seem to change the phenotype (Kurahashi *et al.*, 2009). The detection rate of the copy number variants is difficult to assess due to low numbers in the reported series, however it may be in the order of magnitude of 20%, but about 10% of BFNS families still remain without a genetic cause (Zara *et al.*, 2013).

Clinical features

Patients with benign familial and non-familial neonatal seizures typically have neonatal onset of seizures, usually on the second or third day of life, and spontaneous remission by 6 months of age. As already discussed, actually the previous distinction the familiar and sporadic cases is not so far considered as there are no differences in clinical features between cases with inherited of *de novo* mutation.

Birth is at full-term (except for three cases of Ronen *et al.*, 1993), with normal birthweight and an APGAR score above 7 at the first minute of life. None of these neonates was in an intensive care unit.

There was always a free interval between birth and occurrence of seizures. However, seizures onset is mostly within the first week of life. The sex-ratio shows an equal distribution between boys and girls.

In 80% of cases seizures start on the second or third day of life, but some infants start having seizures later, during the first month of life or even up to the third month. Ronen *et al.* (1993), in their wide family, report that two of the individuals in whom seizures started at 1 month of age, were premature. Premature babies could not be able to have seizures before having reached full-term neurological state: this point is important considering the strict age-dependence of this syndrome.

The neurological state of the babies remains normal in most cases and they can drink their bottle between seizures; a mild hypotonia that may be transitory is noticed in some cases. Then the infants recover a normal neurological state.

Seizures are focal with different motor manifestations, mainly clonic, never tonic. They are often lateralized, starting on one side then affecting the other side, and rarely of a bilateral tonic-clonic type. They lasted from 1–3 min. They were frequently repeated, leading to a status epilepticus. The mean duration of status epilepticus was about 20 hours, but could be shorter (2 hours) or longer (up to 3 days).

In the first reported families, before the use of video-EEG monitoring, seizures were described as clonic, sometimes with apneic spells. Tonic seizures were reported in two cases. Clonic or tonic seizures were short (lasting 1–3 min), frequently repeated over 7 days, whereas isolated seizures could occur in some cases during the following weeks. In previous reports seizures had already been described (Giacoia, 1982; Crispen & Kelly 1985; Shevell *et al.*, 1986; Camfield *et al.*, 1991), but there was no evidence in these cases for a homogeneous presentation. Ronen *et al.* (1993) have listed all the clinical components of the 70 seizures they analysed in their wide family. They concluded that most of the time, seizures started with tonic, autonomic or oculo-facial features, being of a mixed type. Hirsch *et al.* (1993) recorded 14 seizures in three neonates with video-EEG monitoring. All seizures started with a tonic phase, with a right or left maximum, varying from one seizure to the next in a one given baby, always accompanied by tachycardia and a short apnea. The clonic phase (focal or generalized) was introduced by vocalization or chewing. We had the opportunity to record seizures in three cases with video-EEG monitoring (unreported families): seizures were stereotyped, starting with a diffuse hypertonia and a short apnea, followed by autonomic or oculo-facial features and symmetrical or asymmetrical clonic movements of the limbs. In 1994, Bye reported a new case of BFNS with two seizures recorded and video-taped. Both seizures started with an arousal, but in one groping and clonic movements of the limbs remained localized on the left side, whereas in the second these movements were generalized. From these different video recordings it appears that in most cases seizures start with a diffuse tonic component, followed by various autonomic and motor changes, which can be uni-or bilateral, symmetrical or not. The only cases without an initial tonic component are those of Bye (1994).

No myoclonic seizure has been reported, no spasm either, nor in fact true generalized tonic-clonic seizure.

Long-term outcome is characterized by a normal development. Febrile or afebrile seizures can occur later in life in approximately 15% of cases (Grinton *et al.*, 2015). Febrile seizures, rolandic seizures and generalized tonic clonic seizures are reported (*e.g.*, Singh *et al.*, 2003). In a retrospective analysis of families with Rolandic epilepsy and the associated EEG trait (*i.e.*, centrotemporal spikes) benign neonatal seizures were clearly overrepresented (6%) (Doose *et al.*, 1997).

EEG findings

When described, interictal EEG was normal, discontinuous with focal or multifocal abnormalities or with "theta pointu alternant" pattern. Actually an interictal EEG pattern considered as pathognomonic of BFNS has never been described. Interictal patterns such as a paroxysmal, inactive or suppression-burst EEG were never reported and are considered suggesting of a poor prognosis (Weckhuysen *et al.*, 2013).

The ictal pattern (Ronen *et al.*, 1993; Hirsch *et al.*, 1993) is characterized by a generalized flattening of the background activity followed by focalized or bilateral spikes or slow waves lasting as long as the clinical manifestations. A prolonged flattening of the EEG could follow the seizures. Hirsch *et al.* (1993) studied very carefully the ictal EEG and found that the length of the flattening could vary from 5 to 19 s and the complete seizure lasted from 59 to 155 s.

The electroclinical presentation of these seizures suggests that they are of a generalized type. Aso & Watanabe (1992) discussed this point because they recorded a unilateral seizure in a 3-month-old infant having had BFNS. However, the publication of Hirsch *et al.* (1993) emphasizes that the initial flattening of the EEG is generalized from the onset and that the successive symptoms occurring during a seizure (tonic, apnea, clonic phases) are identical to those reported in generalized tonic-clonic seizures in children and adults. The same authors suggest that the asymmetrical character of some clinical and EEG signs during the tonic or the clonic phase could be related to the absence of maturation of the corpus callosum during the first weeks of life (Bardovick & Kjos, 1988). Bye (1994) discussed again the place of BFNS among idiopathic generalized epilepsies: at the time the classification was adopted (1989) no video tape of BFNS existed, whereas nowadays it appears that some focal seizures may be present, with or without an evolution to bilateral tonic-clonic, but most of them are of a generalized type. When a focal onset is recognizable, seizures can be localized in any area but are more frequently present in the rolandic areas *(Figure 1)*.

Electroclinical seizures or subclinical discharges (so-called electrical seizures) can be recorded; clinical seizures without EEG modifications have also been reported. At the beginning of the status epilepticus, seizures are clinical and/or electroclinical, but at the end subclinical discharges may persist up to several hours.

Treatment

Familial and non-familial neonatal seizures were termed "benign" to reflect that they are self-limited conditions in most affected individuals, independently form the treatment. Nevertheless, seizures may be difficult to control in the neonatal period, and patients were often treated with loading doses of intravenous anti-epileptic drugs (AEDs), such as phenobarbital and benzodiazepines, which may necessitate cardiorespiratory support and lead to prolonged and unnecessary hospitalization.

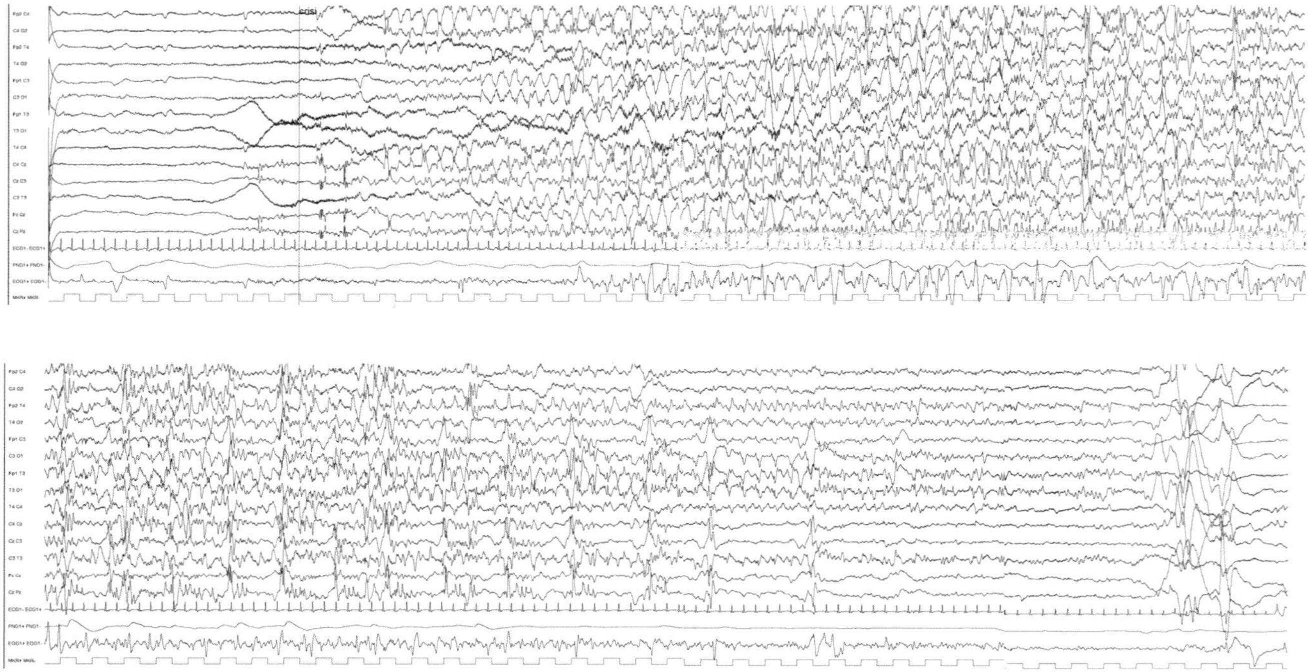

Figure 1

A 20 day-old boy affected by a non-familial form of BNS, due to KCNQ2 missense variant. The EEG shows a lateralized spike, and spike and waves in the left fronto-central areas, a focal discharge characterized by a recruiting rhythm of increasing amplitude, spreading over the same contralateral region and later to the entire brain. This baby presents with a slow deviation of head and eyes to the left side and asymmetric tonic contraction of limbs. In the same patient the side of the head and eye deviation sometimes changed from seizure to seizure, and also during the same seizure.

Currently, the use of sodium-channel blocker AEDs, such as carbamazepine and phenytoin, are preferred. They have been demonstrated to be effective in seizures caused by *KCNQ2* mutations as they are loss-of-function variants (Pisano *et al.*, 2015; Sands *et al.*, 2016) and avoid sedation and hypotonia associated with loading doses of intravenous PB, which delays establishment of oral feeding and consequently pro-longs the NICU stay of these otherwise healthy babies. *Vice-versa*, the response to carbamazepine can confirm the diagnostic suspicion of this electroclinical phenotype early in the clinical course, before the genetic results are available.

Clinical entities associated to the same gene mutations

Spectrum of phenotypes associated with *KCNQ2* and *KCNQ3* mutations and *KCNQ2* gene variants have been also associated to different epileptic phenotypes, from self- limited to drug-resistant epilepsy associated with developmental delay. Among the self-limited phenotype, patients with benign epilepsy with centro-temporal spikes (BECTS) have been reported. They were described within large families (Maihara *et al.*, 1999; Coppola *et al.*, 2003) with a BFNS as well as sporadic cases. On the other hand, *KCNQ2* mutations have been associated with severe phenotype characterized by early-onset developmental and epileptic encephalopathy (DEE). The first description dates back to 2003 (Dedek *et al.*, 2003) when a neonate with drug-resistant epilepsy starting on day 3 was described. The EEG showed several focal seizures of mainly frontal origin. By 2.5 years the seizures decreased but his psychomotor development was delayed. More recently the epileptic phenotype of KCNQ2-DEE, has been refined: seizures at onset typically consisted of tonic posturing often associated with focal clonic jerking, and were accompanied by apnea with desaturation. Moderate to severe intellectual disability usually characterizes the outcome even if a good seizure control is gained with the use of sodium-channel blockers AEDs (Weckhuysen *et al.*, 2013; Pisano *et al.*, 2015).

More recently the phenotype of KCNQ2-related DEE has been distinguished into two clinical phenotypes due to the different impact of the mutation on the channel functionality (gain or loss of function) (Pisano *et al.*, 2015; Mulkey *et al.*, 2017). Variants that cause the loss of function cause the neonatal onset epileptic encephalopathy, while variants that cause a gain of function of the potassium channel cause a DEE with an infantile onset with epileptic spasms followed by drug-resistant focal epilepsy and the occurrence of non-epileptic myoclonus during the first months of life (Mulkey *et al.*, 2017).

Finally, mutations in *KCNQ2* have been associated with BFNS and myokymia. Dedek *et al.* (2001) reported on a family with all affected members suffering from BFNS and myokymia. The affected carried a mutation (R207W) that neutralized a charged amino acid in the S4 voltage-sensor segment of *KCNQ2*. Four members had continuous myokymic muscle activity, preceded or accompanied by myalgia, while the mother had myokymia only. Her twin daughters had neonatal convulsions (at 7 and 30 days in one and at 10 days in the other) and grand mal seizures at 2 and 12 years (some with fever). A half-sister of the twins had convulsions at day 4. The son of one of the twins had convulsions at days 3, 30, 45, and 47 but only EMG discharges (no myokymia). All affected members carried a nucleotide exchange mutation in the S4 voltage-sensor segment of *KCNQ2* which, together with the myokymia, suggested to the authors that at least some motoneurons express KCNQ2/3 channels.

Benign familial neonatal-infantile seizures (BFNIS)

The first report of BFNIS onset dates back 1983 (Kaplan & Lacey). In this form, the onset of seizures varies from 2 days to 3.5 months. Later on, in 2002, Heron (Heron *et al.*, 2002) described 2 families with afebrile secondarily generalized partial seizures occurring between 1.9 and 3.8 months of life and having *SCN2A* missense mutations, encoding the voltage-gated sodium channel Nav1.2, with an autosomal dominant mode of inheritance. The role of *SCN2A* was afterwards confirmed in 2004 (Berkovic *et al.*, 2004) in other 5 families with similar phenotype and other authors (Striano *et al.*, 2006; Zara *et al.*, 2013) and also sporadic cases have been identified. The semiology of the seizures was characterized by a predominant focal motor manifestation, with head and eye deviation followed by tonic and clonic movements. Interictal EEGs were normal, or showed some epileptiform discharges in the posterior areas. All patients had a normal development before and after the seizure occurrence. As for *KCNQ2* gene, mutations in *SCN2A* have been associated with a spectrum of epilepsies and neurodevelopmental disorders, other than self-limited forms (Wolff *et al.*, 2017).

Different epileptic phenotypes according to the age at onset have been described: severe epileptic phenotypes with early infantile onset (< 3 months) include early-onset DEE, Ohtahara syndrome and epilepsy of infancy with migrating focal seizures, epilepsies with infantile/childhood onset (> 3 months of age) including West syndrome, myoclonic-atonic epilepsy, Lennox-Gastaut syndrome, focal epilepsies with an electrical status epilepticus during slow sleep (ESES) and intellectual disability or autism without epilepsy (Wolff *et al.*, 2017). Current models of *SCN2A* pathophysiology demonstrated that gain-of-function variants potentiate glutamatergic neuronal excitability, leading to infantile-onset seizure phenotypes (both benign and DEE), whereas loss-of-function variants impair excitability, leading to autism spectrum disorder (ASD) and/or intellectual disability (ID). Seizure severity is correlated with the degree of gain-of-function, with variants that cause the most excitability leading to DEE, while milder variants lead to benign infantile seizures (Sanders *et al.*, 2018).

Benign familial and non-familial infantile seizures

In 1963, Fukuyama reported cases occurring in the first 2 years of life that were characterized by generalized tonic-clonic seizures, absence of aetiologic factors, normal psychomotor development, normal EEG and benign outcome. Later, other reports of this clinical entity studied the localization and semiology of seizures (Watanabe *et al.*, 1987, 1990, 1993), the prognosis (Sugiura *et al.*, 1983), and the presence or absence of familial occurrence (Vigevano *et al.*, 1990, 1992, 1994; Vigevano, 2005). In particular, Watanabe *et al.* on several occasions described cases with partial seizures of a different type, proposing the term benign partial epilepsy in infancy with complex partial seizures (BPE with CPS) and benign partial epilepsy in infancy with secondarily generalized seizures (BPE with SGS). Most of these cases were not familial. Vigevano *et al.* directed attention to the presence of cases with a family history of convulsions with benign outcome during infancy, with autosomal dominant inheritance, suggesting the term "benign infantile familial convulsions" and later on "benign familial infantile seizures" (BFIS). Just as benign seizures with neonatal onset were distinguished in familial and non-familial forms, benign infantile seizures are thus also divided into familial and non-familial forms, even though now we know that the two forms overlap.

In 1997, Szepetowski described the association between BFIS and variably expressed paroxysmal choreo-athetosis (Szepetowski *et al.*, 1997). Following the identification of a specific marker on chromosome 16p12-q12, this entity constitutes a variant of the familial forms, called infantile convulsions and choreo-athetosis (ICCA). By combining classic linkage analysis with whole-exome sequencing, mutations in the *PRRT2* gene have been identified as the cause of paroxysmal kinesigenic dyskinesia (PKD) (Wang *et al.*, 2011) and infantile convulsions and choreoathetosis (ICCA) (Heron *et al.*, 2012; Lee *et al.*, 2012) and benign familial infantile epilepsy (BFIE) (Heron *et al.*, 2012; Ono *et al.*, 2012). In 2012, Specchio *et al.* showed that *PRRT2* is mutated in familial and non-familial benign infantile seizures. PRRT2 mutations currently represent the major cause of familial and non-familial benign infantile seizures, associated or not at PKD (Zara *et al.*, 2013).

PRRT2 is located at chromosomal region 16p11.2 and encodes a membrane protein that seems to interact with synaptosomal-associated protein 25 kDa (SNAP- 25). The c.649_650insC mutation is the most commonly reported mutation: it is a hot spot mutation consisting of a cytosine (C) base insertion in a homopolymer of 9 C bases adjacent to 4 guanine bases. This mutation has been associated with different phenotypes, familial and non-familial cases of BFIS, with or without PKD, and migraine (Marini *et al.*, 2012; Specchio *et al.*, 2012).

Other that *PRRT2*, also mutations in *SCN2A* and *KCNQ2-3* genes have been reported in BFIS, with an overall yield of about 90%. Ten percent of BFIS families still remain without a genetic diagnosis. There is a description of single family with different genes involved as *CHRNA2* in BFIS (Trivisano *et al.*, 2015), and further studies will be necessary to definitively fill this gap.

Clinical and EEG manifestations

This clinical entity is characterized by focal seizures that occur in clusters, with subacute onset in children in the first or second year of life, without clear etiological factors, and with completely normal psychomotor development. Age at onset has been described from 3 to 20 months of age, but in the familial forms it occurs mostly between the 4th and 7th months. History of pregnancy and delivery is unremarkable. All the aetiological investigations, especially metabolic and neuroimaging tests, provide normal results.

Familial cases include first- and second-degree relatives who have convulsions during infancy without subsequent development of other forms of epilepsy. The incidence in these families of other idiopathic epilepsies and febrile convulsions does not differ from that of the general population and there were no reports of convulsions in the neonatal period (Grinton *et al.*, 2015). The disorder is transmitted with autosomal dominant inheritance. Greater incidence among females was reported for the familial forms, but this prevalence was not confirmed among the relatives (Vigevano *et al.*, 1992). After the first description in 1992, a lot of similar cases have been described over the world; Gally *et al.* in 2016 found that benign familial and non-familial infantile epilepsy has an incidence in the first year of life more common than previously suggested, between the epileptic syndromes second only to West syndrome.

All children have absolutely normal psychomotor development before seizures onset. An almost constant characteristic is the occurrence of seizures in a cluster: mostly brief, successive seizures, maximum of 8–10 daily, which does not reach a true status epilepticus. The interictal clinical condition is normal, with occasional sopor that could be attributed mostly to drug treatment. Isolated seizures in the 10–15-day period before the cluster are reported in about one third of the cases. Seizures are usually longer in the beginning, lasting 2–5 minutes, and became shorter as treatment took effect. The cluster could last 1–3 days.

Concerning the semiology of seizures, it is difficult to say if there are real differences between the sporadic and familial forms. Elements common to both forms include motor arrest, impairment of consciousness, staring and convulsive movements. Watanabe stressed the presence of limb or oral and facial automatisms in cases described as BPE with CPS (Watanabe *et al.*, 1990), and of prompt generalization with tonic-clonic manifestations in cases described as BPE with SGS (Watanabe *et al.*, 1993). On the other hand, in addition to the symptoms already described, Vigevano documented the presence during the seizures of slow deviation of head and eyes to one side, diffuse hypertonia, cyanosis and unilateral limb jerks which became bilateral and were synchronous or asynchronous (Vigevano *et al.*, 1992). The side of the head and eye deviation sometimes changed from seizure to seizure in the same patient.

When described, the waking and sleep interictal EEG before and after the cluster is normal. Vigevano described lateralized slow waves and spikes in the occipito-parietal areas in the interictal EEG performed during a cluster of seizures. In the presence of secondary generalization, the ictal EEG disclosed a focal discharge characterized by recruiting rhythm of increasing amplitude spreading over the hemisphere and involving the entire brain *(Figure 2)*. The site of origin of the seizures seems to be a distinguishing characteristic. According to Watanabe, the site of origin in the cases described as BPE with CPS (Watanabe *et al.*, 1990) is most frequently the temporal area, while the site varies in cases described as BPE with SGS (Watanabe *et al.*, 1993). In familial cases, the seizures originate in the parieto-occipital area, with the side varying from one seizure to another (Vigevano *et al.*, 1992).

Treatment

Seizures are well responsive to antiepileptic drugs. Carbamazepine is the drug of choice and dosages that are much lower than those used to treat epilepsy are usually sufficient.

Several antiepileptic drugs may be effective, including specially carbamazepine, as reported by Ebrahimi-Fakhari *et al.* in 2015. In untreated cases, isolated or brief clusters can occur before the age of one year. These children have normal psychomotor development and do not present other forms of epilepsy in later life. In cases associated with paroxysmal choreoathetosis, the clinical picture of infantile seizures is the same as already described. Choreoathetoid movements start during infancy, childhood or adolescence; they are of a dystonic type, occur at rest or can be induced by exertion or anxiety (Szepetowski *et al.*, 1997). Also this kind of movement disorder is particularly sensitive to carbamazepine as well as seizures. Because outcome is benign, it is theoretically possible not to treat these patients. In practice, however, withholding treatment is not easy for various reasons. Most patients have recurring seizures (seizures every 2–3 hours); patients not treated after the first cluster of seizures can have other seizures or clusters; diagnosis is not simple at onset, except for the familial forms. In familial cases, the decision to withhold treatment can be made more easily.

Differential diagnosis

In the neonatal period BFNS and BINS must be differentiated from non-epileptic paroxysmal events (NEPE) of neonates and from other aetiologies of new-onset neonatal seizures (NNS). Tremulations and benign sleep myoclonus are frequent NEPE among neonates: they can be easily recognized. Tremor occur in normal neonates during wakefulness and sleep: they can be of great amplitude, very frequent, increased when babies are crying; the main characteristic is that they can be stopped by restraining the limb involved in the phenomenon. The EEG remains normal between and during these events.

Benign neonatal sleep myoclonus occurs only during quiet sleep and is never present during wakefulness and active sleep. Rhythmic myoclonia involving the limbs may last up to 1 or 2 min without any other symptom. The EEG is strictly normal between and during the fits. This phenomenon disappears spontaneously by some days or some weeks and the baby develops in a normal way (Di Capua & Vigevano, 1993).

Other conditions such as hyperekplexia do not share the same electroclinical characteristics, and tonic fits associated with gastro-oesophageal reflux are linked to feeding. Symptomatic NNS are the most frequent, secondary to hypoxic-ischemic encephalopathy, to metabolic disturbances, structural brain abnormalities or infectious process. These aetiologies can be assessed by different diagnostic tools and the seizures do not have the same clinical presentation: day of onset, clinical type, duration and repetition. The neurological state is rarely normal. Interictal and ictal EEG present with different abnormal patterns. The outcome depends on the aetiology, the duration of the status epilepticus, the interictal EEG pattern, and the number of antiepileptic drugs necessary to stop the seizures.

In the first year of life, familial convulsions may be caused by pyridoxine dependency or deficiency (Bankier *et al.*, 1983). However, in this disorder, convulsions that are therapy-resistant appear in the first days of life and the clinical condition is always severe.

Again BFNS and BINS remain as diagnosis by exclusion, as we know that many neonates may present with cryptogenic convulsions associated with an uncertain outcome

Diagnosing BFIS is still difficult (Okumura *et al.*, 2000). Early diagnosis is possible only in the familial forms. In the sporadic forms with either complex partial or secondarily generalized seizures,

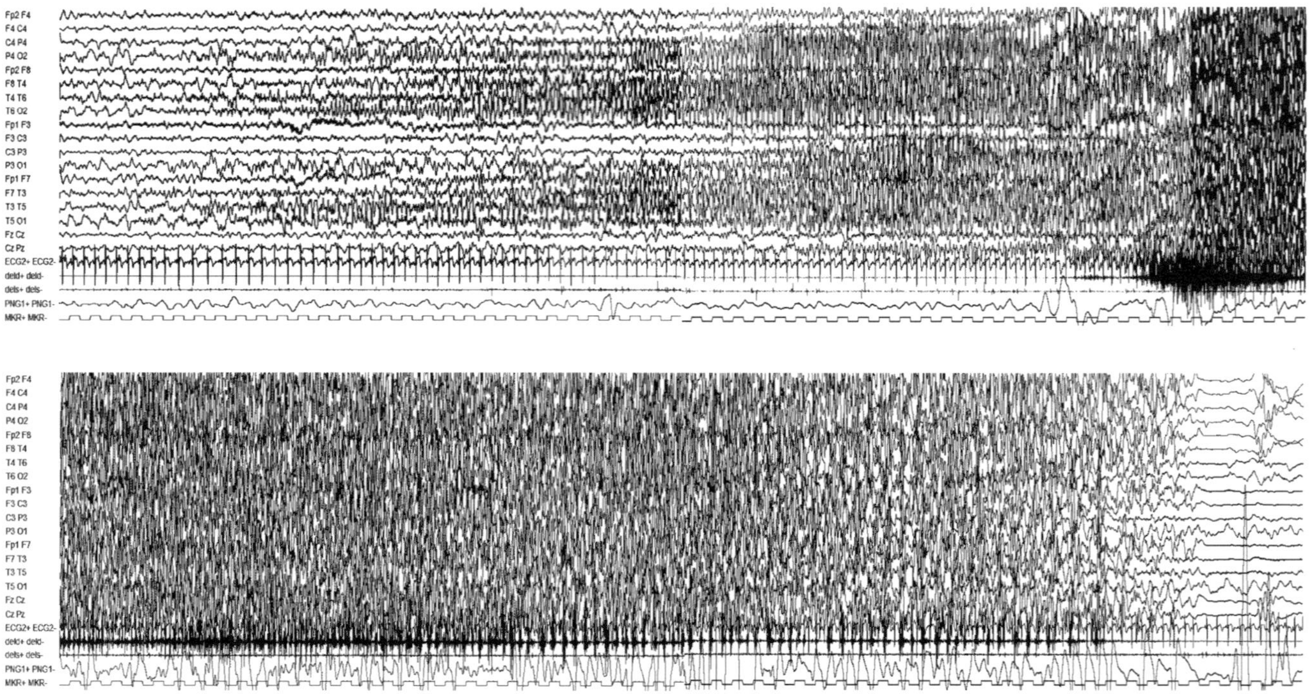

Figure 2

Video-polygraphic recording of a focal seizure in an 8-month-old girl with PRRT2 mutation showing a rhythmic ictal discharge originating from the left parieto-tempo-occipital region (A), rapidly involving the contralateral same region involve, and within 40 seconds from its onset, the whole bilateral hemispheres The seizure ends 2 minutes after onset. The discharge is followed by small-amplitude asymmetric slow activity, corresponding to the postictal phase. Clinically the patient is unresponsive and stares for 10 seconds, then becomes stiff, manifesting some clonic, asynchronous jerking of the limbs.

diagnosis can be suspected on the basis of the criteria presented above, with exclusion of any possible etiologic factor. Also in the sporadic cases genetic test can be very useful for the diagnosis.

As mentioned before, reported cases associated with choreoathetosis are due to PRRT2 mutation. Very similar cases with *SCN8A* mutation have been described by Gardella *et al.* in 2016; 16 patients from 3 families presented afebrile focal seizures during the first-second year of life with benign evolution; 5 of them developed later on paroxysmal dystonic attacks triggered by stretching, motor initiation, emotional stimuli. There have been reports of very similar clinical pictures closely associated with episodes of diarrhea and gastroenteritis. First description of this peculiar entity called "benign infantile seizures associated with mild gastroenteritis" dates back to 1982 in Japan (Morooka *et al.*, 1982). It is characterized by non-febrile generalized seizures associated with symptoms of gastroenteritis in previously healthy patients between the age of 6 months and 3 years. Seizures often occur in cluster, and laboratory examination results, including blood and CSF glucose, are normal. Interictal EEG is normal in all patients, and all of them had an excellent outcome.

Seizures are mostly brief, focal to bilateral, and mainly occur within the first 5 days of the gastroenteritis episode. The rotavirus antigens are reported in 40–50% of cases (Uemura *et al.*, 2002) and noravirus in about 67% of case which results negative to rotavirus (Kim *et al.*, 2018).

Seizure recurrence, also without prophylactic antiepileptic treatment, has been reported in few cases when an infant has repeated episodes of gastroenteritis. Many studies looked for genetic basis of these seizures. Particularly, *PRRT2* gene mutations, as they are responsible of BFIS, have been looked for, however without significant results (Ishii *et al.*, 2013).

Concerning the so called "benign partial epilepsy in infancy and early childhood with vertex or central spikes and waves during sleep", described by Bureau & Maton (1998), Bureau *et al.* (1998) and Capovilla & Beccaria (2000), many elements indicate that this could be an idiopathic form: family history of epilepsy in about 30% of the cases, peculiar EEG pattern and benign spontaneous outcome. This form is distinguished from the category of BFIS by a slightly later onset, absence of seizures in clusters, presence of characteristic EEG anomalies and multifactorial genetic predisposition. Some features of this form evoke benign epilepsy of childhood with centro-temporal spikes (BECTS), although there are differences in age at onset, ictal semiology and EEG pattern. In BECTS, onset is later; there is only one type of seizure while in the cases with vertex or central SW the ictal manifestations are variable. On the other hand, the EEG pattern constitutes in both forms a marker of benignity, perhaps the same at different ages.

REFERENCES ▶

Aso K, Watanabe K (1992): Benign familial neonatal convulsions: generalized epilepsy? *Ped Neurol* 8: 226–228.

Bankier A, Turner M, Hopkins J (1983): Pyridoxine-dependent seizures: a wider clinical spectrum. *Arch Dis Child* 58: 415–418.

Bardovick AJ, Kjos BO (1988): Normal post-natal development of the corpus callosum as demonstrated by MR imaging. *AmJ Neurol Radiol* 3: 497–491.

Bellini G, Miceili F, Soldovieri MV, *et al. KCNQ2*-Related Disorders Genereviews – NCBI Bookshelf (2013): GeneReviews. Available at: http://www.ncbi.nlm.nih.gov/bookshelf/br.fcgi?book=gene&-part=bfns. Accessed November 17, 2014.

Berkovic SF, Heron SE, Giordano L, *et al.* (2004): Benign familial neonatal-infantile seizures: characterization of a new sodium channelopathy. *Ann Neurol* 55: 550–557.

Biervert C, Schroeder BC, Kubisch C, *et al.* (1998): A potassium channel mutation in neonatal human epilepsy. *Science* 279: 403–404.

Bjerre I, Corelius E (1968): Benign neonatal familial convulsions. *Acta Paediat Scand* 57: 557–561.

Bureau M, Cokar O, Maton B, Genton P, Dravet C (2002): Sleep-related, low voltage Rolandic and vertex spikes: an EEG marker of benignity in infancy-onset focal epilepsies. *Epileptic Disord* 4: 15–22.

Bureau M, Kaleli O, Maton B, Dravet C (1998): EEG correlates of benign focal epilepsy in early childhood. *Epilepsia* 39 (Suppl 2): 91–92.

Bureau M, Maton B (1998): Valeur de l'EEG dans le pronostic précoce des épilepsies partielles non idiopathiques de l'enfant. In: Bureau M, Kahane P, Munari C (eds) *Épilepsies partielles graves pharmaco-résistantes de l'enfant: stratégies diagnostiques et traitements chirurgicaux*, pp. 67–78. Paris: John Libbey Eurotext.

Bye AME (1994): Neonate with benign familial neonatal convulsions: recorded generalized and focal seizures. *Ped Neurol* 10: 164–165.

Camfield PR, Dooley J, Gordon K, Orlik P (1991): Benign familial neonatal convulsions are epileptic. *J Child Neurol* 6: 340–342.

Capovilla G, Beccaria F (2000): Benign partial epilepsy in infancy and early childhood with vertex spikes and waves during sleep: a new epileptic form. *Brain Dev* 22: 93–99.

Caraballo R, Pavek S, Lemainque A, *et al.* (2001): Linkage of benign familial convulsions to chromosome 16p12-q12 suggests allelism to the infantile convulsions and choreoathetosis syndrome. *Am J Hum Genet* 68: 764–788.

Charlier C, Singh NA, Ryan SG, *et al.* (1998): A pore mutation in a novel KQT-like potassium channel gene in an idiopathic epilepsy family. *Nat Genet* 18: 53–55.

Commission on Classification and Terminology of the International League Against Epilepsy (1989): Proposal for revised classification of epilepsies and epileptic syndromes. *Epilepsia* 30: 389–399.

Contino MF, Lebby T, Arcinue EL (1994): Rotavirus gastrointestinal infection causing afebrile seizures in infancy and childhood. *Am J Emerg Med* 12: 94–95.

Coppola G, Castaldo P, Miraglia del Giudice E, *et al.* (2003): A novel KCNQ2 K+ channel mutation in benign neonatal convulsions and centrotemporal spikes. *Neurology* 61: 131–134.

Crispen C, Kelly T (1985): Benign familial neonatal convulsions. *Iowa Medical* 75: 397–401.

Dedek K, Fusco L, Teloy N, Steinlein OK (2003): Neonatal convulsions and epileptic encephalopathy in an Italian family with a missense mutation in the fifth transmembrane region of KCNQ2. *Epilepsy Res* 54: 21–27.

Dedek K, Kunath B, Kananura C, Reuner U, Jentsch TJ, Steinlein OK (2001): Myokymia and neonatal epilepsy caused by a mutation in the voltage sensor of the KCNQ2 K+ channel. *PNAS* 98: 12273–12277.

Di Capua M, Vigevano F (1993): Benign neonatal sleep myoclonus. *Mov Dis* 812: 191–194.

Doose H, Brigger-Heuer B, Neubauer B (1997): Children with focal sharp waves: Clinical and genetic aspects. *Epilepsia* 38: 788–796.

Ebrahimi-Fakhari D, Saffari A, Westenberger A, Klein C (2015): The evolving spectrum of PRRT2-associated paroxysmal diseases. *Brain* 138 (Pt 12): 3476–3495.

Flesler S, Sakr D, Cersosimo R, Caraballo R (2011): Benign infantile focal epilepsy with midline spikes and waves during sleep: a new epileptic syndrome or a variant of benign focal epilepsy? *Epileptic Disord* 12: 205–211.

Fukuyama Y (1963): Borderland of epilepsy with special reference to febrile convulsions and so-called infantile convulsions. Seishing-Igaku. *Seishing-Igaku (Clin Psychiatry)* 5: 211–223.

Gaily E, Lommi M, Lapatto R, Lehesjoki AE (2016): Incidence and outcome of epilepsy syndromes with onset in the first year of life: A retrospective population-based study. *Epilepsia* 57: 1594–1601.

Gardella E, Becker F, Møller RS, *et al.* (2016): Benign infantile seizures and paroxysmal dyskinesia caused by an SCN8A mutation. *Ann Neurol* 79: 428–436.

Giacoia GP (1982): Benign familial neonatal convulsions. *Southern Med J* 5: 629–630.

Grinton BE, Heron SE, Pelekanos JT, *et al.* (2015): Familial neonatal seizures in 36 families: Clinical and genetic features correlate with outcome. Epilepsia. 56: 1071–1080.

Heron SE, Cox K, Grinton BE, *et al.* (2007): Deletions or duplications in KCNQ2 can cause benign familial neonatal seizures. *J Med Genet* 44 (12): 791–796.

Heron SE, Crossland KM, Andermann E, *et al.* (2002): Sodium-channel defects in benign familial neonatal-infantile seizures. *Lancet* 360: 851–852.

Heron SE, Grinton BE, Kivity S, *et al.* (2012): PRRT2 mutations cause benign familial infantile epilepsy and Infantile convulsions with choreoathosis syndrome. *Ann J Hum Genet* 90: 152–160.

Hirsch E, Velez A, Sellal F, Maton B, Grinspan A, Malafosse A, Marescaux C (1993): Electroclinical signs of benign neonatal familial convulsions. *Ann Neurol* 134: 835–841.

Imai K, Otani K, Yanagihara K, *et al.* (1999): Ictal Video-EEG recording of three partial seizures in a patient with the benign infantile convulsions associated with mild gastroenteritis. *Epilepsia* 40: 1455–1458.

Ishii A, Yasumoto S, Ihara Y, *et al.* (2013): Genetic analysis of PRRT2 for benign infantile epilepsy, infantile convulsions with choreoathetosis syndrome, and benign convulsions with mild gastroenteritis. *Brain Dev* 35: 524–530.

Itou J, Takahashi Y, Kusunoki Y, Oki J, Chou K (1988): Convulsions associated with mild acute diarrhea. *Shounika-Rinsho Jpn J Pediatr* 41: 2011–2015.

Jentsch TJ (2000): Neuronal KCNQ potassium channels: physiology and role in disease. *Neuroscience* 1: 21–30.

Kanaumi T, Takashima S, Iwasaki H, Itoh M, Mitsudome A, Hirose S (2008): Developmental changes in KCNQ2 and KCNQ3 expression in human brain: possible contribution to the age-dependent etiology of benign familial neonatal convulsions. *Brain Dev* 30: 362–369.

Kaplan RE, Lacey DJ (1983): Benign familial neonatal-infantile seizures. *Am J Med Genet* 16: 595–599.

Kim BR, Choi GE, Kim YO, Kim MJ, Song ES, Woo YJ (2018): Incidence and characteristics of norovirus-associated benign convulsions with mild gastroenteritis, in comparison with rotavirus ones. *Brain Dev* 40: 699–706.

Kurahashi H, Wang JW, Ishii A, *et al.* (2009): Deletions involving both KCNQ2 and CHRNA4 present with benign familial neonatal seizures. *Neurology* 73: 1214–1217.

Lee HY, Huang Y, Bruneau N, *et al.* (2012): Mutations in the gene PRRT2 cause paroxysmal kinesigenic dyskinesia with infantile convulsions. *Cell Rep* 1 (1): 2–12.

Leppert M, Anderson VE, Quattlebaum T, *et al.* (1989): Benign familial neonatal convulsions linked to genetic markers on chromosome 20. *Nature* 337: 647–648.

Lewis TB, Leach RJ, Ward K (1993): Genetic heterogeneity in benign familial neonatal convulsions: identification of a new locus on chromosome-8q. *Am J Hum Gen* 53: 670–675.

Lewis TB, Shevell MI, Andermann E, Ryan SG, Leach RJ (1996): Evidence of a third locus for benign familial convulsions. *J Child Neurol* 11: 211–214.

Maihara T, Tsuji M, Higuchi Y, Hattori H (1999): Benign familial neonatal convulsions followed by benign epilepsy with centro-temporal spikes in two siblings. *Epilepsia* 40: 110–113.

Malafosse A, Leboyer M, Dulac O, *et al.* (1992): Confirmation of linkage of benign familial neonatal convulsions to D20S19 and D20S20. *Hum Gen* 89: 54–58.

Marini C, Conti V, Mei D, *et al.* (20012): PRRT2 mutations in familial infantile seizures, paroxysmal dyskinesia, and hemiplegic migraine. *Neurology* 79: 2109–2114.

Matsumoto A, Watanabe K, Sugiura M, Negoro T, Takaesu E, Iwase K (1983): Long-term prognosis of convulsive disorders in the first year of life: mental and physical development and seizure persistence. *Epilepsia* 24: 321–329.

Miles KD, Holmes GL (1990): Benign neonatal seizures. *J Clin Neurophysiol* 7: 369–379.

Morooka K (1982): Convulsions and mild diarrhea [in Japanese]. Shonika (Tokyo). 23: 131–137.

Mulkey SB, Ben-Zeev B, Nicolai J, *et al.* (2017): Neonatal nonepileptic myoclonus is a prominent clinical feature of KCNQ2 gain-of-function variants R201C and R201H. *Epilepsia* 58: 436–445.

Okada M, Zhu G, Hirose S, Ito KI, Murakami T, Wakui M, Kaneko S (2003): Age-dependent modulation of hippocampal excitability by KCNQ-channels. *Epilepsy Res* 53: 81–94.

Okumura A, Hayakawa F, Kato T, Kuno K, Negoro T, Watanabe K (2000): Early recognition of benign partial epilepsy in infancy. *Epilepsia* 41: 714–717.

Ono S, Yoshiura K, Kinoshita A, Kikuchi T, Nakane Y, Kato N, *et al.* (2012): Mutations in PRRT2 responsible for paroxysmal kinesigenic dyskinesias also cause benign familial infantile convulsions. *Am J Hum Genet* 57: 338–341.

Pisano T, Numis AL, Heavin SB, *et al.* (2015): Early and effective treatment of KCNQ2 encephalopathy. *Epilepsia* 56: 685–91.

Plouin P (1985): Benign neonatal convulsions (familial and nonfamilial). In: Roger J, Dravet C, Bureau M, Dreifuss FE, Wolf P (eds) *Epileptic Syndromes in Infancy Childhood and Adolescence*, pp. 2–11. London: John Libbey.

Quattlebaum TG (1979): Benign familial convulsions in the neonatal period and early infancy. *J Pediatr* 95: 257–259.

Rett A R, Teubel R (1964): Neugeborenenkrämpfe im Rahmen einer epileptisch belasten Familie. *Wien Klin Wschr* 76: 609–613.

Ronen GM, Rosales TO, Connolly ME, Anderson VE, Leppert M (1993): Seizure characteristics in chromosome 20 benign familial neonatal convulsions. *Neurology* 43: 1355–1360.

Rose AL, Lombroso CT (1970): Neonatal seizure states. A study of clinical pathology and EEG features in 137 full-term babies with a long term follow-up. *Pediatrics* 45: 405–425.

Rundfeldt C, Netzer R (2000): Retigabine stabilizes neuronal cell activity in epileptic patients by activating KCNQ2/3 channels and its mutation. *Abst Soc Neurosci* 26: 662.

Ryan SG, Wiznitzer M, Hollman C, Torres C, Szekeresova M, Schneider S (1991): Benign familial neonatal convulsions: evidence for clinical and genetic heterogeneity. *Ann Neurol* 29: 469–473.

Sadewa AH, Sasongko TH, Gunadi, Lee MJ, Daikoku K, Yamamoto A, *et al.* (2008): Germ-line mutation of KCNQ2, p.R213W, in a Japanese family with benign familial neonatal convulsion. *Pediatr Int* 50 (2): 167–171.

Sanders SJ, Campbell AJ, Cottrell JR, *et al.* (2018): Progress in Understanding and Treating SCN2A-Mediated Disorders. *Trends Neurosci* 41 (7): 442–456.

Sands TT, Balestri M, Bellini G, *et al.* (206): Rapid and safe response to low-dose carbamazepine in neonatal epilepsy. *Epilepsia* 57: 2019–2030.

Schiffmann R, Shapira Y, Ryan G (1991): An autosomal recessive form of benign familial neonatal seizures. *Clin Genet* 40: 467–470.

Shevell MI, Sinclair DB, Metrakos K (1986): Benign familial neonatal seizures: clinical and electroencephalographic characteristics. *Ped Neurol* 2: 272–275.

Singh NA, Charlier C, Stauffer D, *et al.* (1998): A novel potassium channel gene, KCNQ2, is mutated in an inherited epilepsy of newborns. *Nat Genet* 18: 23–29.

Singh NA, Westenskow P, Charlier C, *et al.* (2003): KCNQ2 and KCNQ3 potassium channel genes in benign familial neonatal convulsions: expansion of the functional and mutation spectrum. *Brain* 126: 2726–2737.

Specchio N, Terracciano A, Trivisano M, *et al.* (2013): PRRT2 is mutated in familial and non-familial benign infantile seizures. *Eur J Paediatr Neurol* 17: 77–81.

Steinlein O, Schuster V, Fischer C, Häussler M (1995): Benign familial neonatal convulsions: Confirmation of genetic heterogeneity and further evidence for a second locus on chromosome 8q. *Hum Genet* 95: 411–415.

Striano P, Bordo L, Lispi ML, Specchio N, Minetti C, Vigevano F, Zara F (2006): A novel SCN2A mutation in family with benign familial infantile seizures. *Epilepsia* 47: 218–220.

Sugiura M, Matsumoto A, Watanabe K, Negoro T, Takaesu E, Iwase K (1983): Long-term prognosis of generalized convulsions in the first year of life, with special reference to benign infantile convulsions. *Jpn J Epil Soc* 1: 116–121.

Szepetowski P, Rochette J, Berquin P, Piussan C, Lathrop GM, Monaco AP (1997): Familial infantile convulsions and paroxysmal choreoathetosis: a new neurological syndrome linked to the pericentromeric region of human chromosome 16. *Am J Hum Genet* 61: 889–898.

Tinel N, Lauritzen I, Chouabe C, Lazdunski M, Borsotto M (1998): The KCNQ2 Trivisano M, Terracciano A, Milano T, *et al.* (2015): Mutation of CHRNA2 in a family with benign familial infantile seizures: Potential role of nicotinic acetylcholine receptor in various phenotypes of epilepsy. *Epilepsia* 56 (5): e53–7.

Uemura N, Okumura A, Negoro T, Watanabe K (2002): Clinical features of benign convulsions with mild gastroenteritis. *Brain Dev* 24: 745–749.

Vigevano F (2005): Benign familial infantile seizures. *Brain Dev* 27: 172–177.

Vigevano F, Di Capua M, Fusco L, Ricci S, Sebastianelli R, Lucchini P (1990): Sixth-month benign familial convulsions. *Epilepsia* 31: 613.

Vigevano F, Fusco L, Di Capua M, Ricci S, Sebastianelli R, Lucchini P (1992): Benign infantile familial convulsions. *Eur J Pediatr* 151: 608–612.

Vigevano F, Sebastianelli R, Fusco L, *et al.* (1994): Benign infantile familial convulsions. In: Malafosse A, Genton P, Hirsch E, Marescaux C, Broglin D, Bernasconi R (eds) *Idiopathic Generalized Epilepsies: Clinical, Experimental and Genetic Aspects*, pp. 45–49. London: John Libbey.

Vigevano F, Specchio N, Caraballo R, Watanabe K (2008): Benign familial and nonfamilial seizures. In: Engel J, Pedley P (eds) *Epilepsy. A Comprehensive Textbook*, 2nd ed, pp. 2313–2321. Philadelphia: Lippincott Williams and Wilkins.

Volkers L, Rook MB, Das JH, *et al.* (2009): Functional analysis of novel KCNQ2 mutations found in patients with benign familial neonatal convulsions. *Neurosci Lett* 462 (1): 24–29.

Wang JL, Cao L, Li XH, *et al.* (2011): Identification of PRRT2 as the causative gene of paroxysmal kinesigenic dyskinesias. *Brain* 134 (Pt 12): 3493–3501.

Watanabe K, Negoro T, Aso K (1993): Benign partial epilepsy with secondarily generalized seizures in infancy. *Epilepsia* 34: 635–638.

Watanabe K, Yamamoto N, Negoro T, Takaesu E, Aso K, Furune S, Takahashi I (1987): Benign complex partial epilepsies in infancy. *Pediatr Neurol* 3: 208–211.

Watanabe K, Yamamoto N, Negoro T, Takahashi I, Aso K, Maehara M (1990): Benign infantile epilepsy with complex partial seizures. *J Clin Neurophysiol* 7: 409–416.

Weckhuysen S, Ivanovic V, Hendrickx R, *et al.* (2013): Extending the KCNQ2 encephalopathy spectrum: clinical and neuroimaging findings in 17 patients. *Neurology* 81: 1697–703.

Wolff M, Johannesen KM, Hedrich UBS, *et al.* (2017): Genetic and phenotypic heterogeneity suggest therapeutic implications in SCN2A-related disorders. *Brain* 140: 1316–1336.

Zara F, Specchio N, Striano P, *et al.* (2013): Genetic testing in benign familial epilepsies of the first year of life: clinical and diagnostic significance. Epilepsia. 54: 425–436.

WITH VIDEO SUPPLEMENTS

CHAPTER 7

EARLY SEVERE NEONATAL AND INFANTILE EPILEPSIES

Eli M. Mizrahi[1] and Mathieu Milh[2]

[1] Peter Kellaway Section of Neurophysiology, Department of Neurology, Section of Pediatric Neurology, Department of Pediatrics, Baylor College of Medicine, Houston, USA
[2] Inserm U910, Faculté de Médecine de la Timone, Department of Paediatric Neurology, Hôpital Timone-Enfants, Marseille, France

Introduction

In the fourth edition of *Epileptic Syndromes in Infancy, Childhood and Adolescences* Aicardi and Ohtahara together discussed and provided valuable perspectives concerning two syndromes of severe neonatal epilepsy with suppression-burst pattern (Aicardi & Ohthara, 2005). These syndromes are early myoclonic encephalopathy (EME) originally described by Aicardi and Goutières (1978) and early infantile epileptic encephalopathy (EIEE) first described by Ohtahara and colleagues (Ohtahara *et al.*, 1976). In the subsequent edition, the discussion of these syndromes was extended utilizing both their insights as well as new findings with a focus on pathophysiology and the genetic basis of these disorders (Mizrahi & Milh, 2012). The current chapter continues to build on the previous discussions to develop a more uniform understanding of these two distinct, but overlapping, epileptic syndromes.

The International League Against Epilepsy (ILAE) described two age-dependent electroclinical syndromes characterized by encephalopathy which occur in the neonatal period (Berg *et al.*, 2009): early myoclonic encephalopathy (EME) and Ohtahara syndrome (OS), also known as early infantile epileptic encephalopathy (EIEE). Each of these syndromes are characterized by a specific clinical seizure type, clinical signs of encephalopathy and a suppression-burst (SB) pattern on the electroencephalogram (EEG). While age of onset, underlying etiology, associated secondary clinical seizure types, co-morbidities and aspects of immediate and long-term outcome may vary within and between each syndromic category, both EME and EIEE share some common features which contribute to the high incidence of neurological impairment in affected infants. The recent ILAE operational classification of seizure types (Fisher *et al.*, 2017) reaffirmed the clinical semiology for these syndromes and the recent ILAE classification of epilepsies (Scheffer *et al.*, 2017) provided a framework to consider seizure type, syndrome and etiology which can be applied to the consideration of EME and EIEE.

Historically, each syndrome had been first identified and discussed separately (Ohthara *et al.*, 1976; Aicardi and Goutières, 1978). However, over time there has been discussion that the two clinical syndromes may represent variants of a single disorder with overlapping features (Aicardi and Ohthara, 2005; Djukic *et al.*, 2006; Yamamoto *et al.*, 2011). Whether these are two distinct syndromes or representation of a spectrum of one, a detailed description of each is critical in understanding diagnosis and management of these age-dependent epileptic encephalopathies. In this chapter, some common features of the two syndromes will be described followed by a discussion of the specific features of each which make them distinct. This is followed by a return to the discussion of whether or not these syndromes represent a continuum of a single disorder.

Common features of early epileptic encephalopathies

Discussing EME and EIEE is at times made more difficult by efforts to group them into a single syndromic category. For example, they may be included in the groups such as neonatal epileptic encephalopathy, neonatal/infantile epileptic encephalopathy, early onset epileptic encephalopathies with SB, and developmental epileptic encephalopathies. These groupings may be helpful in describing larger populations of at risk infants, but is limited in comparing and contrasting EME and EIEE. The concept of epileptic encephalopathy is challenged in these forms of very early epilepsy. Indeed, it is very difficult to distinguish between the role of the developmental disorder, and the role of seizures and EEG abnormalities, in the relatively poor outcome of some of these affected children. Increasingly, the term "developmental encephalopathy with epilepsy" is used, reflecting the fact that there are often, and above all, serious and early developmental disorders, with epilepsy. While there are important features which differentiate EME and EIEE there are also some features which the two syndromes have in common. The clinical features of each syndrome may first appear in the neonatal period (the first 28 days of life, or 46 weeks post menstrual age), although EIEE may also present later. Infants in each group have some degree of neurological impairment, including altered consciousness (lethargy or coma) at onset and may also demonstrate abnormalities of muscle tone. In addition, all infants present with some type of clinical seizures, erratic myoclonus predominating in EME and tonic spasms in EIEE. However, these seizure types are not exclusive to the respective syndromes and may be present as secondary seizure types in each group. Most notably tonic spasms may be present at onset in EIEE and later in the course of EME. As the syndrome evolves in both groups, affected infants may experience continuous developmental delay, further neurological impairment, persistent seizures, and the emergence of epileptic spasms and hypsarrhythmia on EEG (although the latter is transient with EME and tends to be persistent in EIEE).

An important common feature in both groups is the finding of a SB pattern on EEG as part of the diagnostic criteria for both EME and EIEE (Auvin *et al.*, 2016). A SB pattern may be observed in a number of conditions in the neonate (Lombroso, 1990). However, when the pattern is associated with clinical seizures and signs of encephalopathy, the disorders of EME and EIEE are initially considered, depending upon predominant seizure type. There has been some discussion concerning specific features of the particular SB patterns associated with either syndrome and these differences will be discussed below. These differences relate to the degree of persistence of the pattern in wakefulness and sleep (most often persistent in EIEE) and the degree of generalized flattening during the periods of suppression (greatest in EME).

Early myoclonic encephalopathy

Early neonatal myoclonic encephalopathy (EME) was first described by Aicardi and Goutières (1978). Other reports have referred to this syndrome as myoclonic encephalopathy with neonatal onset (Cavazzuti *et al.*, 1978), early myoclonic encephalopathy (Murakami *et al.*, 1993), neonatal myoclonic encephalopathy (Aicardi, 1978; Vigevano *et al.*, 1981) and early myoclonic encephalopathy with epilepsy (Dalla Bernardina *et al.*, 1982). The clinical, electroencephalographic, etiologic and outcome features are listed in *Table I* and compared to EIEE.

Neurological features at onset

Onset of the disorder is almost always within the first month of life and as such is considered a neonatal epileptic syndrome (Berg *et al.*, 2009). The neurological status of the affected infant is abnormal at birth or at the time of onset of seizures. This is characterized by altered consciousness, limited reactivity and limited cognitive development. In addition, there may be abnormalities of muscle tone. The infants may be hypotonic or there may be hypertonia to varying degrees with greatest severity reported to be associated with trismus (Schlumberger *et al.*, 1992). Infants may also demonstrate clinical and laboratory signs of peripheral neuropathy (Aicardi, 1992). Females and males are affected equally. Familial cases have been reported, most likely based upon the inheritance of the underlying etiology. Typically, prenatal and perinatal histories are unremarkable.

Seizure semiology

The predominant clinical ictal manifestation is fragmentary, segmental or erratic myoclonus. These movements may involve the face and limbs; usually distal more than proximal regions. The muscle groups involved may be very confined or may involve the entire limb or face. The individual jerking movements may be isolated and randomly distributed over time and across body region. The movements may be repeated, sustained or almost continuous. Most often the movements shift from one region of the body to another and may occur simultaneously, but asynchronously in various regions. The jerking movements may be very obvious to even the casual observer or may be brief and with minimal muscle excursions so as to be missed, even with careful surveillance. The myoclonus may be present during wakefulness and may persist in sleep (Dalla Bernardina *et al.*, 1982, 1983). There may also be prominent partial seizures and/or epileptic spasms. Late in the course of the disorder, tonic spasms may be present (Aicardi & Ohtahara, 2005). Other seizure types may also be present in infants with EME. Partial seizures may occur at the time of onset of erratic myoclonus (Dalla Bernardina *et al.*, 1982, 1983) or soon after (Aicardi & Ohtahara, 2005). Eventually, most infants who survive the neonatal period with this disorder develop tonic spasms, typically between 3 and 4 months of age (Aicardi & Ohtahara, 2005).

Electroencephalography

The hallmark EEG pattern associated with EME is SB (*Figure 1*). There has been discussion concerning the character and variability of the periods of suppression and periods of bursting.

Table I **Comparison of features of severe epileptic syndromes in infancy**

	Early myoclonic encephalopathy (EME)	Early Infantile epileptic encephalopathy (EIEE)	Infantile spasms (IS)
Predominant seizure type	Erratic myoclonus	Tonic spasms (early)	Spasms in clusters
Other possible seizure type	Generalized myoclonus	Partial seizures	Partial seizures associated with spasms
	Partial seizures	Generalized myoclonus (rare)	
	Tonic spasms (late)	No erratic myoclonus	
Neurological examination	Abnormal	Abnormal	Variable
	Hypotonia	Asymmetrical findings in case of brain structural abnormalities	
EEG Features	S-B with short paroxysmal bursts and longer periods of suppression	S-B with longer periods of bursts and shorter periods of suppression	Hypsarrhythmia
	S-B enhanced in sleep (perhaps only found in sleep)	S-B occurs in wakefulness and sleep	Modified hypsarrhythmia
	S-B may persist for variable durations	S-B may be asymmetric	
Evolution	Spasms and hypsarrhythmia	IS with hypsarrhythmia or EEG and epilepsy improvement	Variable
Etiology	Metabolic disorders	CNS structural abnormalities	Variable symptomatic
	Genetic	Genetic	Genetic
Prognosis	Early death	Mental retardation	Etiology dependent
	Progressive deterioration in survivors	Severe neurological impairment	
	Vegetative state in survivors	Variable epilepsy outcome	
		Static encephalopathy	

Ohtahara *et al.* (1997) characterize the bursts as lasting between 1 and 5 seconds in duration alternating with periods of suppression lasting 3 to 10 seconds. Schlumberger *et al.* (1992) also noted the brevity of the bursts. Both groups of investigators also emphasized the marked depression of amplitude of the suppression periods: the interburst flattening. In addition both groups indicated that the SB pattern is present during sleep. However, Schlumberger *et al.* (1992) suggest that the pattern is always present during both wakefulness and sleep with no differentiation of the pattern during either state, while Ohtahara *et al.* (1997) suggest the pattern may be state dependent, observing that the pattern may be only present during sleep or may be most prominent during this state. The SB pattern most often evolves over time to patterns described as atypical hypsarrhythmia or multifocal recordings between 3 to 5 months of age. Ohtahara *et al.* (1997) suggest the atypical hysarrhythmia may be transient with the SB pattern returning, while Aicardi has observed that the hypsarrhythmia is persistent once it appears (Aicardi & Ohtahara, 2005).

Etiology

Two etiologic factors have received the most attention: genetic disorders and inborn errors of metabolism. For familial cases, it has been suggested that the mode of inheritance is autosomal

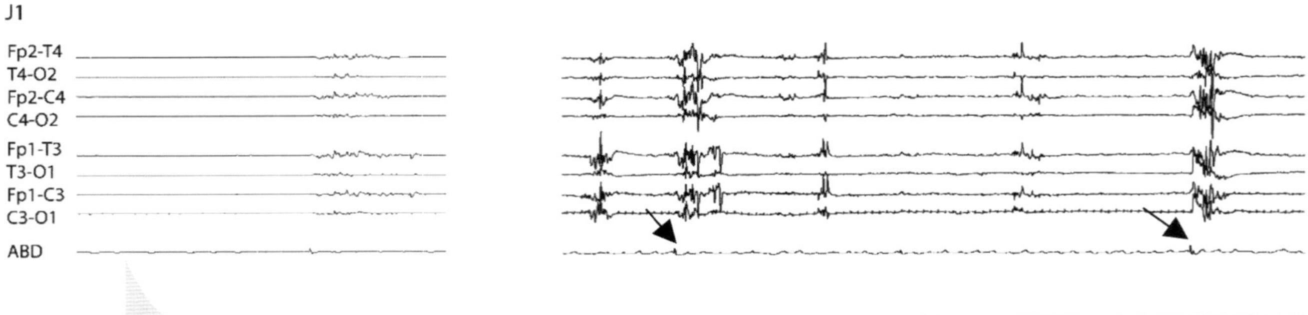

Figure 1 **Suppression-bursts recorded in a neonate at 1 day of life. The accelerometer of the abdomen shows very low amplitude movements due to the myoclonic jerks associated to the bursts.**

recessive (Aicardi & Ohtahara, 2005). Aicardi reported that four of twelve families with infants with EME had genetic histories of this disorder (Aicardi, 1992). Other investigators have also reported familial cases (Dalla Bernardina *et al.*, 1983; Schlumberger *et al.*, 1992; Wang *et al.*, 1998). There has also been a more focused investigation of genetic mutations in EME. Kojima *et al.* (2018) and Ishii *et al.* (2017) recently summarized reported genetic causes of EME to include involvement of *ERBB4*, *SIK1*, *SLC24A22*, and *GABRB2*. Ohba and colleagues (2014) also reported finding a *de novo* mutation of *SCN8A* in EME. Mignon-Ravix *et al.* (2018) described a patient with EME and bi-allelic mutation in *UBA5*.

The case of a patient with a Schinzel–Giedion syndrome displaying epileptic and EEG features of EME has been reported (Watanabe *et al.*, 2011). Schinzel-Giedion syndrome is a very rare disorder characterized by severe mental retardation, distinctive facial features and multiple congenital malformations, in association with *de novo* mutations in *SETBP1* gene (Hoischen *et al.*, 2010).

Inborn errors of metabolism have been described in several cases of EME and appear to, as a group, represent an important etiology of this disorder. The most commonly reported disorder is nonketotic hyperglycinemia (Lombroso, 1990; Aicardi, 1992; Ohtahara *et al.*, 1998; Wang *et al.*, 1998; Rossi *et al.*, 2009). Other reported metabolic disorders include: hyperglycinemia, D-glyceric acidemia, methylmalonic acidemia, hyperammonemia due to carbamyl phosphate synthetase (Lombroso, 1990), propionic acidemia (Vigevano *et al.*, 1982; Lombroso, 1990), and urinary secretion of abnormal oligosaccharides (Michalski *et al.*, 1984; Schlumberger *et al.*, 1992). One report describes the finding in an infant with EME of a reciprocal translocation t(2;6)(q34;p25.3), disrupting the tyrosine kinase receptor ErbB4 (erythroblastic leukemia viral oncogene homolog 4) (Backx *et al.*, 2009).

Because of the expanding concern that genetic factors may underly EME diagnostic approaches to these infants now include current genetic testing and screening (Gursoy and Ercal, 2016). Olson *et al.* (2017) performed genetic screening on a group of infants described as "early onset epileptic encephalopathies with burst suppression" (which included EME and EIEE) without previously identified molecular diagnosis and identified genetic mutations in 17 of 28 (61%). Numerous cases of pyridoxine dependent seizures mimicking EME have been described and a pyridoxine trial is recommended in such conditions (Mills *et al.*, 2010). Similarly Pearl (2016) has emphasized that EME (and EIEE) may be vitamin-dependent disorders.

Pathophysiology

The pathophysiology of early onset epileptic encephalopathies with a SB is still unknown. Using SPECT with a technetium-99m–labeled ethyl cysteinate dimer and PET with [18F]-fluoro-D-deoxyglucose positron emission tomography (FDG-PET), Hirose *et al.* (2010) showed interictal hypoperfusion/hypometabolism of bilateral basal ganglia, thalami, and the right parietooccipital cortices in one case of EME. Ictal SPECT obtained at repetitive tonic spasms showed hyperperfusion of bilateral cortices. The authors suggest that functional deafferentation of the cortex from subcortical structures may characterize EME, and that these imaging abnormalities may provide insight into the pathophysiology of the SB pattern in EME.

Ishii *et al.* (2017) further noted that three of the reported genes associated with EME were either oncogenes (*ERBB4* and *SIK1*) or encoded a mitochondrial solute carrier (*SLC25A22*), therefore without obvious association with neuronal excitability or inhibition (in contrast to EIEE associated genes which have a more direct impact on neuronal function). This suggests different mechanisms of the disorders.

Galanopoulou & Moshe (2015) and Auvin *et al.* (2016) suggest that further investigations of animal models of both EME and EIEE, grouped as neonatal and infantile epileptic encephalopathies, may provide additional advances in understanding the physiologic basis of these disorders.

Treatment

Treatment is usually directed at controlling the various seizure types in the hope that their control may coincide with improvement in developmental outcome. Unfortunately such treatment has not been effective. Antiepileptic drugs and hormonal therapy (corticosteroids or ACTH) have been used with little success. However, Nakano *et al.* (2013) reported success in the treatment of EME with lidocaine and carbamazepine. Because of the diffuse, rather that persistently focal nature of the intractable seizures, epilepsy surgery is not considered a therapeutic option.

Non-antiepileptic drug therapy is most often directed toward the underlying etiology associated with the syndrome – particularly inborn errors of metabolism and other metabolic disturbances. For example, dextromethorphan and benzoate have been used to treat nonketotic hyperglycinemia (Hamosh *et al.*, 1992). The N-methyl-d-aspartate receptor antagonist ketamine has also been reported to suppress seizures (Suzuki *et al.*, 2010). In addition, there is now a group of neonatal metabolic disorders associated with epilepsy which are considered treatable (Pearl, 2009; Pearl, 2016). Wang *et al.* (1998) described an infant with EME and atypical SB pattern with pyridoxine-dependency and recovery after treatment with pyridoxine. Guerin *et al.* (2015) reported similar findings in neonatal epileptic encephalopathy. This has prompted some to advocate for an empirical trial of pyridoxine in all infants with EME (Aicardi & Ohtahara, 2005), with the caution that the case reported by Wang and colleagues (1998) was transient and atypical. The use of gamma-aminobutryic acid (GABA) analogue vigabatrin in two infants with EME secondary to non-ketotic hyperglycinemia has been reported to be associated with progressive deterioration of the infants, manifested by worsening encephalopathy (Tekgul *et al.*, 2006).

Prognosis

The long-term outcome of infants with EME is typically poor. Approximately half affected infants die within the first year of life. Neurological development, which is usually significantly delayed at the time of diagnosis, is limited or non-existent. While there are limited studies of long-term follow-up, it has been reported that all survivors were considered to be in a vegetative state (Aicardi & Ohtahara, 2005). The erratic myoclonus may resolve after weeks or months, however the partial seizures may persist and become intractable to medical management.

Early infantile epileptic encephalopathy

Early infantile epileptic encephalopathy (EIEE) was initially reported and then more completely described as an age-dependent epileptic encephalopathy by Ohtahara and colleagues (Ohtahara *et al.*, 1976; Ohtahara, 1978; Ohtahara *et al.*, 1987, 1992, 1997; Yamatogi and Ohtahara, 2002; Ohtahara and Yamatogi, 2003). The disorder is characterized by onset in infancy, tonic spasms and a SB pattern on EEG. The disorder is rare. In 2005, it was reported that 36 cases had been described in the literature and that it was estimated that the incidence of EIEE compared to West syndrome was 1:40. (Aicardi & Ohtahara, 2005; Yamatogi & Ohtahara, 2002). The clinical, electroencephalographic, etiologic and outcome features are listed in *Table I* comparing the features of EIEE to EME and to West syndrome.

Neurological features at onset

Onset of the disorder, heralded by seizures, is within the first 3 months of life, typically within the first month, although the seizures may occur within the first few weeks (Hirata *et al.*, 1985; Miller *et al.*, 1998). There have been rare reports of familial incidence (Giordano *et al.*, 2010). Even though some of the cases of EIEE may occur within the neonatal period, it is classified as an epileptic syndrome of infancy (Berg *et al.*, 2009). Infants show altered consciousness or responsiveness. The interictal motor examination is also typically abnormal with hypotonia or hypertonia which may be manifest as spasticity. There may be focal features on neurological examination with the motor examination being asymmetric.

Seizure semiology

Tonic spasms represent the predominant seizure type. These may occur in isolation or in clusters and typically may be present both during wakefulness and sleep. The duration of a spasm may be up to 10 seconds with the interval between spasms from 5 to 15 seconds (Aicardi & Ohtahara, 2005). While tonic spasms predominate, other seizure types may be present. Partial seizures with variable focality or hemiconvulsive seizures have been reported to occur in between one-third and one-half of cases (Aicardi and Ohtahara, 2005). An important clinical distinction between EIEE and EME is that in EIEE myoclonic seizures are rare (Ohtahara *et al.*, 1997, 2003) and erratic or fragmentary myoclonus is not present (Schlumberger *et al.*, 1992).

Electroencephalography

The SB pattern has been described in detail by Ohtahara and colleagues (1992; 1998). The bursts last from 2 to 6 seconds and are characterized by high voltage slow waves mixed with multifocal and generalized spike discharges. The interburst intervals range from 5 to 10 seconds *(Figure 2)*. The SB pattern is considered unchanging in appearance in both wakefulness and sleep (Ohtahara *et al.*, 1992, 1998), particularly if the recordings are made before the evolution to hypsarrhythmia. Then, SB is present mostly during sleep. Other investigators have suggested that the SB pattern may be present only during sleep in some of their reported cases (Schlumberger *et al.*, 1992). The electrical correlate of the tonic spasm is diffuse desynchronization. At times, the seizure onset coincides with a generalized high-amplitude slow sharp wave (Martin *et al.*, 1981) or generalized fast activity (Yamatogi & Ohtahara, 1981). A report indicates that there may be subclinical focal electrographic ictal discharges recorded during both prolonged suppressions and bursts in EIEE (Al-Futaisi *et al.*, 2005), although this is a rare finding.

Etiology

Although genetic factors have been most recently intensively investigated in EIEE, structural brain abnormalities still represent the most important etiologic factor in EIEE, making detailed neuroimaging a critical component of the evaluation of these infants. Reported structural brain abnormalities include: Aicardi syndrome, porencephaly, hydrocephalus, hemimegalencephaly, lissencephaly, dentate-olivary dysplasia, and cerebral dysgenesis (Martin *et al.*, 1981; Harding and Boyd, 1991; Schlumberger *et al.*, 1992; Robain and Dulac, 1992; Bermjeo *et al.*, 1992; Ogihara *et al.*, 1993; Ohtsuka *et al.*, 1999; Fusco *et al.*, 2001). In addition, some cases of migrational disorders of cerebral cortex have been identified on autopsy in EIEE infants with no MRI findings (Miller *et al.*, 1998). Metabolic disorders have been reported to occur in only a few cases of EIEE including: nonketotic hyperglycinemia (Clarke *et al.*, 1987), cytochrome oxidase deficiency (Williams *et al.*, 1998). In addition, some cases have been reported in association with Leigh's encephalopathy (Tatsuno *et al.*, 1984; Miyake *et al.*, 1987). Despite thorough evaluations, some infants with EIEE have no known etiology associated with their disorder.

There has been a more recent focus on the relationship between EIEE and mitochrondrial disorders. Several authors have reported cases of EIEE associated with mitochondrial respiratory chain deficiency. One case of cytochrome C oxidase activity reduction (complex 4) was firstly described in 1998 (Williams *et al.*, 1998). Two cases of EIEE have been reported in infants with complex 1 deficiency (Castro-Cago

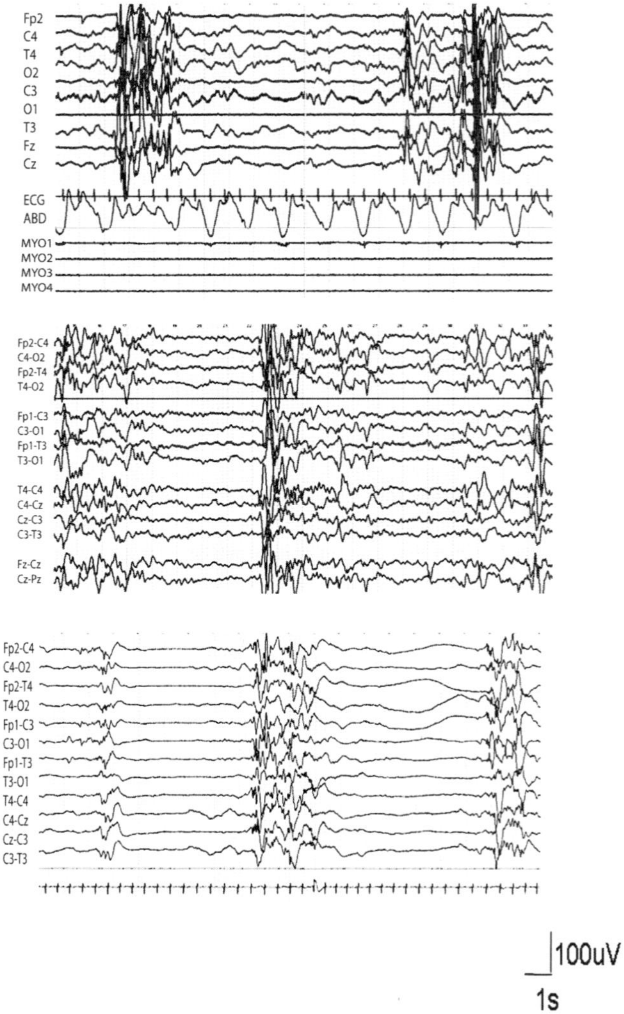

Figure 2 **Representative examples of suppression-burst EEG patterns in three conditions: right hemimegalencephaly** (top); **unknown aetiology with normal brain MRI** (middle); **and mutation of *STXBP1*** (bottom). **The three patients had an Ohtahara syndrome and the EEGs were recorded at one month of age.**

et al., 2009; Seo *et al.*, 2010). These cases show that respiratory chain deficiency is a possible mechanism to explain the occurrence of EIEE, however, no DNA mutations were found in these patients.

There has been a growing literature describing genetic mutations in EIEE. In a recent review Pearl (2018) listed genes which have thus far been associated with EIEE: *CDKL5, SLC25A22, STXBP1, KCNQ2*, and *SCN2A*. Mutations in aristaless-related homeobox gene (*ARX*) may also be associated with EIEE. *ARX* is located in the human chromosome Xp21.3 region and provides instructions for producing a protein transcription factor that is essential for the development of cerebral interneurons. A hemizygous 33-bp duplication in exon 2 was firstly described in two unrelated patients with Ohtahara syndrome (Kato *et al.*, 2007). The infant had early onset of brief tonic seizures beginning during the first weeks of life followed by a transition from EIEE to West syndrome and severe developmental delay. Giordano *et al.* (2010) reported the finding of the same missense mutation in exon 5 of *ARX* in monozygotic twin sisters with EIEE and Fullston and colleagues (2010) reported a family with ARX protein truncation mutation.

Mutations in the *SLC25A22* gene encoding a mitochondrial glutamate carrier were identified in two families with a neonatal encephalopathy with SB (Molinari *et al.*, 2006, 2009). This gene is located in the inner mitochondrial membrane and catalyzes a glutamate/H+ transport into the mitochondria. Patients presented with epileptic spasms and focal seizures from the first few days of life, with acquired microcephaly, severe hypotonia and lack of any psychomotor development. EEG showed a persistent SB pattern. Both patients had abnormal ERG recordings. Brain MRI showed cerebellar hypoplasia, callosal dysmorphia and abnormal gyration of temporoparietal regions. Analysis of glutamate transport of the mutated proteins showed that glutamate could not enter into the patient's mitochondria. This could result in the accumulation of glutamate in the astrocytes and lead to a dysregulation of glutamate homeostasis and neurotransmission.

Mutations/deletions of *STXBP1/MUNC18-1* have also been reported to be a possible aetiology of EIEE (Saitsu *et al.*, 2008). *STXBP1/MUNC18-1* is a regulatory component of the SNARE complex that is placed in a late step of neuronal/exocytic fusion (Shen *et al.*, 2007). The human *STXBP1* gene contains 20 exons and has been mapped to 9q34.1 (Swanson *et al.*, 1998). Exon 19 is alternatively spliced, the shorter isoform being expressed in all tissues examined and the longer isoform containing exon 19 being expressed in the brain and retina (Swanson *et al.*, 1998). Saitsu *et al.* reported *STXBP1* mutations in 14 unrelated patients, from a cohort of 43 patients with EIEE in two distinct papers (Saitsu *et al.*, 2008, 2010). The patients displayed early onset seizures, typically frequent epileptic spasms, SB pattern on EEG, transition to West syndrome after a few to several months in most cases, and severe developmental delay. The authors showed that mutant STXBP1 proteins were degraded and they concluded that STXBP1/MUNC18-1 haploinsufficiency could be a major molecular marker of EIEE. Milh *et al.* (2011) screened this gene in 51 patients with early onset epileptic encephalopathy, of which 37 had Ohtahara syndrome. They found a mutation in 5 patients with Ohtahara syndrome (13%). The epilepsy began during the first week of age for 4 patients, and at 1 month for one patient. Two patients had initially clonic seizures. During the first three months, the main type of seizure was epileptic spasms in all cases. Spasms were associated with other types of seizures: clonic seizures, tonic seizures and partial seizures. Interestingly, the 5 patients became seizure free during the second half of the first year of life. Initial EEG was discontinuous in two cases, before showing a SB pattern. SB pattern was recorded from the beginning in the 3 remaining cases. Then, EEG turned to be more and more continuous. At 6 months, activity was made of generalized and asynchronous spikes and slow waves. Surprisingly, paroxysmal activity disappeared in each case before the age of one year, giving place to a continuous activity with occurrence of fast rhythms in the posterior regions. All patients had frequent dyskinetic non-epileptic movements that still persisted after epilepsy remission. More rarely, *STXBP1* may be found mutated in other epileptic syndromes (West syndrome) and in several developmental encephalopathies with epilepsy that do not fit with any recognized syndrome (Di Meglio *et al.*, 2016; Stamberger *et al.*, 2016). Overall, approximatively one third of patients carrying a mutation in *STXBP1* display EIEE.

STXBP1 has also been implicated in other early onset epilepsies that either do not fit with any recognizable syndrome, or can be classified as early onset epileptic spasms (Deprez *et al.*, 2010; Otsuka *et al.*, 2010).

Weckhuysen *et al.* (2012) screened *KCNQ2* and *KCNQ3* in a cohort of early onset epileptic encephalopathy. Surprisingly, they found a mutation of *KCNQ2* (already known to be associated with benign familial neonatal seizures [BFNS]) in 10% of patients, more than half of them displaying features of Ohtahara syndrome. Most of the mutations occurred *de novo* and were all different from those observed in BFNS.

KCNQ2 now appears as the major EIEE gene; it is involved in about 1/4 of the EIEEs (Olson *et al.*, 2017). The initial features are highly stereotyped: very early onset (first week); numerous tonic asymmetric seizures with cyanosis, sometimes poorly tolerated, very little sensitive to phenobarbital. EEG typically shows a SB pattern. In half of cases, it can be either asynchronous between hemispheres, or with very short periods of silence. The evolution is more heterogeneous;

half of patients rapidly become seizure free but still have major neurological impairment; half of them continue to experience seizures, and some can have epileptic spasms around 6 months (Milh *et al.*, 2013).

Within increasing interest in EIEE there have been additional genetic mutations associated with the syndrome. A patient with herozygotous deletion of *SPRGAP2* and EEG pattern compatible with Ohtahara syndrome was also described in a case report (Saitsu *et al.*, 2010). The clinical spectrum of *SCN2A* mutation has been expanded to include EIEE (Nakamura *et al.*, 2013; Wolff *et al.*, 2017) and a *de novo SCN8A* mutation has also been associated with EIEE (Ohba *et al.*, 2014). However, *SCN8A* may not be frequently found in patients with EIEE and a SB pattern (Olson *et al.*, 2017). A *de novo* variant in *ZEB2* was identified by exome sequencing (Babkina *et al.*, 2016). A mutation in *GABRB3* has suggested to Papandreaou and colleagues (2016) that this should be considered a new cause of EIEE.

Fung and colleagues (2017) applied high-throughput sequencing to investigate the genetic causes of non-syndromic cryptogenic neonatal/infantile epileptic encephalopathy in 31 patients with seizure onset before 24 months with a diagnostic rate of 29%. While the study does not specify EIEE (or EME) it does emphasize the value – as does the previously cited study of Olson and colleagues (2017) – of genetic screening of otherwise undiagnosed infants with early onset seizures.

Overall, among the dozens of genes associated with EIEEs and EMEs, three seem to play a major role and represent half of the cases: *KCNQ2*, *STXBP1* and *SCN2A*.

Pathophysiology

Although many of the infants with EIEE have structural brain abnormalities implicated as etiology, a main focus of investigations concerning pathophysiology of EIEE has been on associated genetic mutations. In animal models of ARX alterations, epilepsy is due to the absence or decrease of certain subtypes of GABAergic interneurons. Kato *et al.* (2007) hypothesized that an error of GABAergic system could be critical to the SB pattern on EEG in infants with EIEE *via* dysfunction of interneurons due to the ARX mutation. Alternatively, Milh *et al.* (2007) have shown that the inhibition of the glutamate transporters in rat pups *in vivo* resulted in the generation of an abnormal EEG pattern, with bursts of paroxysmal activity alternating with periods of silence. The EEG resembled what is observed in patients with a SB pattern. Injection of a NMDA receptor antagonist (ketamine) ameliorated the SB trace. *In vitro* experiments showed that blockade of glutamate transporters led to an overactivation of NMDA receptor. They proposed that a common mechanism of generation of a SB pattern could be an alteration of glutamate homeostasis (synthesis, exocytosis, clearance, glutamate receptor properties). In accordance with this hypothesis, two genes that have been described to be altered in EIEE are directly implicated in glutamate homeostasis: *GC1/SLC25A22*, a mitochondrial glutamate transporter implicated in glutamate clearance; and *GRIN2A*, an NMDA receptor subunit implicated in glutamate post-synaptic effect (Endele *et al.*, 2010). More generally, in the setting of normal brain architecture, early onset epileptic encephalopathies could be the result of any alteration of the GABAergic or glutamatergic neurotransmission.

Functionnal analysis of several severe *KCNQ2* mutations have revealed that mutations could have several consequences and lead to a relatively similar phenotype: negative impact on IM (dominant negative action [Orhan *et al.*, 2014]), positive impact on IM (gain of function [Micelli *et al.*, 2015]), or little impact, but alteration of the distribution of IM at the cell surface (Abidi *et al.*, 2015). It is very intriguing to see that three different consequences can lead to a similar clinical presentation. It is likely that much remains to be done to better understand the pathophysiology of EIEEs.

Treatment

Because focal structural brain lesions represent such an important etiologic factor in this disorder, some affected infants have undergone epilepsy surgery with some reported improvement. This has included hemispherectomy (Pedespan *et al.*, 1995; Fusco *et al.*, 2001; Tharp, 2002; Hamiwka *et al.*, 2007) and focal resection for focal cortical dysplasia (Komaki *et al.*, 1999). Thus, epilepsy surgery may be discussed in the presence of focal or hemispheric lesion.

The therapy of EIEE without a focal lesion has, historically, been considered disappointing (Aicardi & Ohtahara, 2005) with limited newer encouraging data.

There is no controlled study considering the rarity of the pathology, but interest in sodium channel blockers (SCB) deserves to be emphasized. Indeed, several investigative teams have shown that KCNQ2-related EIEE is remarkably sensitive to carbamazepine and sodium blockers in general (Pisano *et al.*, 2015; Abidi *et al.*, 2017). More recently, it has been shown that *SCN2A*-related EIEEs also statistically better respond to SCBs (Wolff *et al.*, 2017).

Interestingly, mutation of *STXBP1* seems to impact *KCNQ2* in a negative manner (Devaux *et al.*, 2018). Thus, it may be that SCBs are effective in patients carrying a mutation of *KCNQ2*, *SCN2A* or *STBP1*, representing half of the cases. Thus, SCBs may probably be considered very early in cases of EIEE with normal brain MRI.

Most often ACTH or corticosteroids are used, with variable success in seizure control and improvement of development outcome (Ohtahara *et al.*, 1987; Yamatogi & Ohtahara, 2002). Other therapies have included pyridoxine, valproate, thyrotropin releasing hormone, chloral hydrate (Kresk *et al.*, 2002), high-dose phenobarbital (Ozawa *et al.*,

2002) and ketogentic diet with limited success (Aicardi & Ohtahara, 2005). There is only emerging experience with newer antiepileptic drugs such as zonisamide (Ohno *et al.*, 2000; Yamatogi & Ohtahara, 2002). However, there have been some reports of successful treatment. Dilena and colleagues (2017) described successful treatment in *SCN2A* associated EIEE with carbamazepine and Foster and colleagues (2017) reported *SCN2A* associated EIEE responsive to oral mexiletine after treatment with lidocaine.

Prognosis

The long-term outcome of infants with EIEE is poor. There is a high incidence of death, with significant neurological impairment and developmental disabilities in survivors. Radaelli and colleagues (2018) recently conducted a systemic review of causes of mortality of reported EIEE. The mean age of seizure onset was 19.6 days ± 33 days with mean age at death 12.9 ± 14.1 months. Most infants survived less than one year with the cause of death described only in eight (47%) patients (either pneumonia/respiratory illness or sudden unexpected death in epilepsy).

Ohtahara *et al.* have emphasized that EIEE represents one of the age-dependent epileptic encephalopathies that include West sydrome and Lennox-Gastaut syndrome. While clinically distinct, they may evolve from one to the next with advancing years (Ohtahara & Yamatogi, 2003). Thus some EIEE patients who survive infancy may subsequently develop the signs and symptoms of these syndromes. For those that do not, other seizure types may be present including multifocal partial seizures. In general, seizures, regardless of type, are intractable to medical management.

Controversies and conclusions

There has been discussion in the literature questioning whether or not EME and EIEE are two distinct syndromes or whether they represent a continuum of a single syndrome (Lombroso, 1990; Wang *et al.*, 1998; Djukic *et al.*, 2006). Aicardi & Ohtahara addressed this issue in the fourth edition of *Epileptic Syndromes* (Aicardi & Ohtahara, 2005). Both syndromes are characterized by a SB pattern on EEG that may persist beyond the neonatal period. Tonic spasms may be present in both, although more prominent and appearing earlier in the course of the disorder in EIEE. In both syndromes the infants have severe and persistent neurological and cognitive abnormalities. While EME is most often associated with metabolic disorders and EIEE with structural brain abnormalities, there is some overlap of underlying etiologies. Prognosis is poor in both.

Aicardi & Ohtahara (2005) comment that although the syndromes of EME and EIEE are well-defined, a number of cases remain difficult to classify because of a lack of precision in the clinical and electroencephalographic features of many of the reported cases. This may be due to either the differences in diagnostic criteria used by different authors or by the atypical characteristics of some cases (Aicardi & Ohtahara, 2005). They also point out that some authors consider some etiologies syndrome-specific while others believe there is an overlap. Diagnostic criteria may vary because of the lack of precise characterizations of myoclonus found in some infants. It may also vary with time, some patients evolving from one syndrome to another with time.

In addition, there is some controversy concerning the features of SB: whether the pattern is persistent during wakefulness and sleep or present only in sleep and whether these findings are the same or different in the two syndromes. In addition, the discussion by Aicardi and Ohtahara (2005) focused primarily on the common finding of SB on EEG and its pathophysiologic and clinical implications. It has been emphasized that the pattern does not have etiologic specificity, but may have common mechanisms of action. On the other hand, seizure types may suggest specific pathophysiologic mechanisms. Fragmentary and erratic myoclonus, a major characteristic of EME, is seen mostly in infants without obvious structural lesions, in infants with metabolic or unknown etiologies. On the other hand, tonic seizures suggest the presence of gross brain abnormalities, with the asymmetry of the events consistent with lateralizing lesions, even though the majority of patients carrying a pathogenic mutation of *KCNQ2* display tonic seizures initially (Milh *et al.*, 2013), while MRI does not show any malformation.

Alternatively, Djukic *et al.* (2006) hypothesize that EIEE and EME represent a continuum with the presence *versus* absence of tonic seizures indicating the severity of brainstem pathology or dysfunction at the time of the presentation of the syndrome. They suggest that brainstem dysfunction is already present in EIEE infants at birth, but may be initially less severe in EME infants. Over time, the brainstem disease burden increases as a result of a kindling process increasing seizure susceptibility. These investigators believe that the presence or absence of myoclonic or tonic seizures is an epiphenomenon of brainstem disease burden, not a phenotype specific to one syndrome or another. They suggest that EIEE and EME represent a continuum in the sense that both syndromes result from underlying brainstem injury and that the differences in onset and evolution of each syndrome is related to the extent and progress of brainstem injury present from birth.

They propose further animal work to substantiate this hypothesis (Galanopoulou & Moshe, 2015). Growing genetic data regarding early epileptic encephalopathies with SB may allow the generation of animal models, so the pathophysiologies of EME and EIEE may be further delineated (Ishii *et al.*, 2017).

Both EME and EIEE represent two well-defined syndromes in their purest form. Whether they represent two aspects of a continuum of one disorder remains an open question. The study of cases which are carefully defined from a clinical, electroencephalographic, radiological and genetic perspective and with well-studied pathology is still useful to better classify and understand early onset epilepsies with a SB pattern.

REFERENCES ▶

Abidi A, Devaux JJ, Molinari F, *et al.* (2015): A recurrent KCNQ2 pore mutation causing early onset epileptic encephalopathy has a moderate effect on M current but alters subcellular localization of Kv7 channels. *Neurobiol Dis* 80: 80–92.

Aicardi J, Goutières F (1978): Encéphalopathie myoclonique néonatale. *Rev EEG Neurophysiol* 8: 99–101.

Aicardi J (1992): Early myoclonic encephalopathy (neonatal myoclonic encephalopathy). In: Roger J, Bureau M, Dravet C, Dreifuss FE, Perret A, Wolf P (eds) *Epileptic Syndromes in Infancy, Childhood and Adolescence* (2nd ed), pp. 13–22. London: John Libbey.

Aicardi J, Ohtahara S (2005): Severe neonatal epilepsies with suppression-burst. In: Roger J, Bureau M, Dravet Ch, Genton P, Tassinari CA, Wolf P (eds). *Epileptic Syndromes in Infancy, Childhood and Adolescence*, 4th ed, pp. 39–50. Paris: John Libbey Eurotext.

Al-Futaisi A, Banwell B, Ochi A, *et al.* (2005): Hidden focal EEG seizures during prolonged suppressions and high-amplitude bursts in early infantile epileptic encephalopathy. *Clin Neurophysiol* 116: 1113–1117.

Auvin S, Cilio MR, Vezzani A (2016): Current understanding and neurobiology of epileptic encephalopathies. *Neurobiol Dis* 92(Pt A): 72–89.

Babkina N, Deignan JL, Lee H, *et al.* (2016): Early Infantile Epileptic Encephalopathy with a *de novo* variant in ZEB2 identified by exome sequencing *Eur J Med Genet* 59: 70–74.

Backx L, Ceulemans B, Vermeesch JR, Devriendt K, Van Esch H (2009): Early myoclonic encephalopathy caused by a disruption of the neuregulin-1 receptor ErbB4. *Eur J Hum Genet* 17: 378–382.

Bermejo AM, Martin VL, Arcas J, Perez-Higueras A, Morales C, Pascual-Castroviejo I (1992): Early infantile epileptic encephalopathy: a case associated with hemimegalencephaly. *Brain Dev* 14: 425–428.

Berg A, Berkovic SF, Brodie J, *et al.* (2010): Revised terminology and concepts for organization of seizures and epilepsies: Report of the ILAE Commission on Classification and Terminology, 2005–2009. *Epilepsia* 51: 679–685.

Castro-Gago M, Blanco-Barca MO, Eirís-Puñal J (2009): Epilepsy and respiratory chain defects in children. *Neuropediatrics* 40: 152.

Cavazzuti GB, Nalin A, Ferrai F, Grandori L, Beghini GE (1978): Encefalopatia epilettica and insorgenza neonatale. *Clin Pediatric* 60: 239–246.

Dalla Bernardina B, Dulac O, Bureau M, Dravet C, Del Zotti F, Roger J (1982): Encephalopathie myoclonique precoce avec épilepsie. *Rev EEg Neurophysiol* 12: 8–14.

Dalla Bernardina B, Dulac O, Fejerman N, Dravet C, Capovilla G, Bondavilli S (1983): Early myoclonic epileptic encephalopathy (EMEE). *Eur J Pediatr* 140: 248–252.

Di Meglio C, Lesca G, Villeneuve N, *et al.* (2015): Epileptic patients with *de novo* STXBP1mutations: Key clinical features based on 24 cases. *Epilepsia* 56: 1931–1940.

Deprez L, Weckhuysen S, Holmgren P, *et al.* (2010): Clinical spectrum of early-onset epileptic encephalopathies associated with *STXBP1* mutations. *Neurology* 75: 1159–1165.

Devaux J, Abidi A, Roubertie A, *et al.* (2016): A Kv7.2 mutation associated with early onset epileptic encephalopathy with suppression-burst enhances Kv7/M channel activity. *Epilepsia* 57: e87–e93.

Djukic A, Lado FA, Shinnar S, Moshe SL (2006): Are early myoclonic encephalopathy (EME) and the Ohtahara syndrome (EIEE) independent of each other? *Epilepsy Res* 70 (Suppl 1): S68–S76.

Endele S, Rosenberger G, Geider K, *et al.* (2010): Mutations in *GRIN2A* and *GRIN2B* encoding regulatory subunits of NMDA receptors cause variable neurodevelopmental phenotypes. *Nat Genet* 42: 1021–1026.

Fisher RS, Cross JH, French JA, *et al.* (2017): Operational classification of seizure types by the International League Against Epilepsy: Position paper of the ILAE Commission for Classification and Terminology. *Epilepsia* 58: 522–530.

Foster LA, Johnson MR, MacDonald JT, *et al.* (2017): Infantile epileptic encephalopathy associated with *SCN2A* mutation responsive to oral mexiletine. *Pediatr Neurol* 66: 108–111.

Fullston T, Brueton L, Willis T, *et al.* (2010): Ohtahara syndrome in a family with an ARX protein truncation mutation (c.81C>G/p.Y27X). *Eur J Hum Genet* 18: 157–162.

Fusco L, Pachatz C, Di Capua M, Vigevano F (2001): Video EEG/aspects of early-infantile encephalopathy with suppression-bursts (Ohtahara syndrome). *Brain Dev* 23: 708–714.

Galanopoulou AS, Moshé SL (2015): Neonatal and Infantile Epilepsy: Acquired and Genetic Models. *Cold Spring Harb Perspect Med* 6: a022707.

Giordano L, Sartori S, Russo S, *et al.* (2010): Familial Ohtahara syndrome due to a novel ARX gene mutation. *Am J Med Genet* 152A: 3133–3137.

Guerin A, Aziz AS, Mutch C, Lewis J, Go CY, Mercimek-Mahmutoglu S (2015): Pyridox(am)ine-5-Phosphate Oxidase Deficiency Treatable Cause of Neonatal Epileptic Encephalopathy With Burst Suppression: Case Report and Review of the Literature. *J Child Neurol* 30: 1218–1225.

Gürsoy S, Erçal D (2016): Diagnostic Approach to Genetic Causes of Early-Onset Epileptic Encephalopathy. *J Child Neurol* 31: 523–532.

Hamiwka L, Duchowny M, Alfonso I, Liu E (2007): Hemispherectomy in early infantile epileptic encephalopathy. *J Chil Neurol* 22: 41–44.

Hamosh A., McDonal JW, Valle D, Francomano CA, Niedermeyer E, Johnston MV (1992): Dextromethorphan and high-dose benzoate therapy for non-ketotic hyperglycinemia in an infant. *J Pediatr* 121: 131–135.

Harding BN, Boyd SG (1991): Intractable seizures from infancy can be associated with dentate-olivary dysplasia. *J Neurol Sci* 104: 157–165.

Hirata Y, Lishikawa A, Somiya K (1985): A case of linear nevus sebaceous syndrome associated with early infantile epileptic encephalopathy with suppression-burst (EIEE). *No To Hattatsu* 17: 577–582.

Hirose M, Haginoya K, Yokoyama H, *et al.* (2010): Functional cortical deafferentation from the subcortical structures in a patient with early myoclonic encephalopathy: a functional neuroimaging study. *Epilepsia* 51: 699–702.

Hoischen A, van Bon BW, Gilissen C, *et al.* (2010): *De novo* mutations of *SETBP1* cause Schinzel-Giedion syndrome. *Nat Genet* 42: 483–485.

Ishii A, Kang JQ, Schornak CC, *et al.* (2017): A *de novo* missense mutation of *GABRB2* causes early myoclonic encephalopathy. *J Med Genet* 54: 202–221.

Kato M, Saitoh S, Kamei A, *et al.* (2007): A longer polyalanine expansion mutation in the ARX gene causes early infantile epileptic encephalopathy with suppression-burst pattern (Ohtahara syndrome). *Am J Hum Genet* 81: 361–366.

Kojima K, Shirai K, Kobayashi M, *et al.* (2018): A patient with early myoclonic encephalopathy (EME) with a *de novo KCNQ2* mutation. *Brain Dev* 40: 69–73.

Komaki H, Sugai K, Maehara T, Shimizu J (2001): Surgical treatment of early-infantile epileptic encephalopathy with suppression-burst associated with focal cortical dysplasia. *Brain Dev* 23: 727–731.

Kresk P, Sebronova V, Prochazka T, Maulisova A, Komarek V (2002): Successful treatment of Ohtahara syndrome with chloral hydrate. *Pediatr Neurol* 27: 388–391.

Lombroso CT (1990): Early myoclonic encephalopathy, early epileptic encephalopathy, and benign and severe infantile myoclonic epilepsies: A critical review and personal contributions. *J Clin Neurophysiol* 7: 380–408.

Martin HJ, Deroubbaix-Tella P, Thellie PH (1981): Encéphalopathie épileptique néonatale à bouffées périodiques. *Rev EEG Neurophysiol* 11: 397–403.

Melani F, Mei D, Pisano T, *et al.* (2011): *CDKL5* gene-related epileptic encephalopathy: electroclinical findings in the first year of life. *Dev Med Child Neurol* 53: 354–360.

Miceli F, Soldovieri MV, Ambrosino P, *et al.* (2013): Genotype-phenotype correlations in neonatal epilepsies caused by mutations in the voltage sensor of K(v)7.2 potassium channel subunits. *Proc Natl Acad Sci USA* 110: 4386–4391.

Michalski JC, Bouquelet S, Montreuil J, Strecker G, Dulac O, Munnich A (1984): Abnormal galactoside excretion in urine of a patient with early myoclonic epileptic encephalopathy. *Clin Chem Acta* 137: 43–51.

Mignon-Ravix C, Milh M, Kaiser CS, *et al.* (2018): Abnormal function of the UBA5 protein in a case of early developmental and epileptic encephalopathy with suppression-burst. *Hum Mutat* 39: 934–938.

Miller SP, Dilenge ME, Meagher-Villenure K, *et al.* (1998): Infantile epileptic encephalopathy (Ohtahara syndrome) and migrational disorder. *Pediatr Neurology* 19: 50–54.

Milh M, Becq H, Villeneuve N, Ben-Ari Y, Aniksztejn L (2007): Inhibition of glutamate transporters results in a "suppression-burst" pattern and partial seizures in the newborn rat. *Epilepsia* 48: 169–174.

Milh M, Villeneuve N, Chouchane M, *et al.* (2011): Epileptic and nonepileptic features in patients with early onset epileptic encephalopathy and *STXBP1* mutations. *Epilepsia* 52: 1828–1834.

Milh M, Boutry-Kryza N, Sutera-Sardo J, Mignot C, *et al.* (2013): Similar early characteristics but variable neurological outcome of patients with a *de novo* mutation of KCNQ2. *Orphanet J Rare Dis* 22: 80.

Mills PB, Footitt EJ, Mills KA, *et al.* (2010): Genotypic and phenotypic spectrum of pyridoxine-dependent epilepsy (ALDH7A1 deficiency). *Brain* 133: 2148–2159.

Miyake S, Yamashita S, Yamada M, Iwamoto H (1987): Therapeutic effect of ACTH and gamma-globulin in 8 cases with the early infantile epileptic encephalopathy with suppression-burst (EIEE). *Shonika Rinsho* (Tokyo) 40: 1681–1688 [in Japanese].

Mizrahi EM, Clancy RR (2000): Neonatal seizures: Early-onset seizure syndromes and their consequences for development. *Ment Retard Dev Disabil Res Rev* 6: 229–241.

Mizrahi EM, Milh M (2012): Early severe neonatal and infantile epilepsies. In: Bureau M, Genton P, Delgado-Escueta A, Tassinari CA, Thomas P, Wolf P (eds) *Epilepsy Syndromes in Infancy, Childhood and Adolescence* (5th ed), pp. 89–98. London: John Libbey Eurotext Ltd.

Molinari F, Raas-Rothschild A, Rio M, *et al.* (2005): Impaired mitochondrial glutamate transport in autosomal recessive neonatal myoclonic epilepsy. *Am J Hum Genet* 76: 334–339.

Murakami N, Ohtsuka Y, Ohtahara S (1993): Early infantile epileptic syndromes with suppression-bursts: early myoclonic encephalopathy *vs.* Ohtahara syndrome. *J Pyschiatr Neurol* 47: 197–200.

Nakamura K, Kato M, Osaka H, *et al.* (2013): Clinical spectrum of SCN2A mutations expanding to Ohtahara syndrome. *Neurology* 81: 992–998.

Nakano K, Kobayashi K, Maniwa S, Kodani N, Ohtsuka Y (2013): Successful treatment of early myoclonic encephalopathy using lidocaine and carbamazepine. *Epil Disord* 15: 352–357.

Ogihara M, Kinoue K, Takamiya H, *et al.* (1993): A case of early infantile epileptic encephalopathy (EIEE) with anatomical cerebral asymmetry and myoclonus. *Brain Dev* 15: 133–139.

Ohba C, Kato M, Takahashi S, *et al.* (2014): Early onset epileptic encephalopathy caused by *de novo* SCN8A mutations. *Epilepsia* 55: 994–1000.

Ohno M, Shimotsuji Y, Abe J, Shimada M, Tamiya H (2000): Zonisamide treatment of early infantile epileptic encephalopathy. *Pediatr Neurol* 23: 341–344.

Ohtahara S (1978): Clinico-electrical delineation of epileptic encephalopathies in childhood. *Asian Med J* 21: 499–509.

Ohtahara S, Ishida T, Oka E, *et al.* (1976): On the specific age-dependent epileptic syndromes: the early-infantile epileptic encephalopathy with suppression-burst. *No To Hattatsu* 8: 270–280.

Ohtahara S, Ohtsuka Y, Erba G (1998): Early epileptic encephalopathy with suppression-burst. In: Engel J Jr, Pedley T (eds) *Epilepsy: A Comprehensive Textbook*, vol. 3. pp. 2257–2261. Philadephia: Lippincott-Raven.

Ohtahara S, Ohtsuka Y, Yamatogi Y, *et al.* (1987): The early infantile epileptic encephalopathy with suppression-burst: developmental aspects. *Brain Dev* 9: 371–376.

Ohtahara S, Ohtsuka Y, Yamatogi Y, *et al.* (1992): Early epileptic encephalopathy with suppression-bursts. In: Roger J, Bureau M, Dravet C, Dreifuss FE, Perret A, Wolf P (eds) *Epileptic Syndromes in Infancy, Childhood and Adolescence* (2nd ed), pp. 25–34, London: John Libbey.

Ohtahara S. Yamatogi Y (2003): Epileptic encephalopathies in early infancy with suppression-burst. *J Clin Neurophysiology* 20: 398–407.

Ohtahara S. Yamatogi Y (2006): Ohtahara syndrome: with special reference to its developmental aspects for differentiating from early myoclonic encephalopathy. *Epil Res* 70S: S58–S67.

Ohtsuka Y, Ohno S, Oka E (1999): Electroclinical characteristics of hemimegalencephaly. *Pediatr Neurol* 20: 390–393.

Olson HE, Kelly M, LaCoursiere CM, *et al.* (2017): Genetics and genotype-phenotype correlations in early onset epileptic encephalopathy with burst suppression. *Ann Neurol* 81: 419–429.

Orhan G, Bock M, Schepers D, *et al.* (2014): Dominant-negative effects of KCNQ2 mutations are associated with epileptic encephalopathy. *Ann Neurol* 75: 382–394.

Otsuka M, Oguni H, Liang JS, *et al.* (2010): STXBP1 mutations cause not only Ohtahara syndrome but also West syndrome-Result of Japanese cohort study. *Epilepsia* 51: 2449–2452.

Ozawa H, Kawada Y, Noma S, Sugai K. (2002): Oral high-dose Phenobarbital therapy for early infantile epileptic encephalopathy. *Pediatr Neurol* 26: 222–224.

Papandreou A, McTague A, Trump N, *et al.* (2016): GABRB3 mutations: a new and emerging cause of early infantile epileptic encephalopathy. *Dev Med Child Neurol* 58: 416–420.

Pearl PL (2009): New treatment paradigms in neonatal metabolic epilepsies. *J Inherit Metab Dis* 32: 204–213.

Pearl PL (2016): Amenable Treatable Severe Pediatric Epilepsies. *Semin Pediatr Neurol* 23: 158–166.

Pearl PL (2018): Epilepsy Syndromes in Childhood. *Continuum (Minneap Minn).* 24 (1, Child Neurology): 186–209.

Pedespan JM, Loiseau H, Vital A, *et al.* (1995): Surgical treatment of an early epileptic encephalopathy with suppression-bursts and focal cortical dysplasia. *Epilepsia* 36: 37–40.

Pisano T, Numis AL, Heavin SB, *et al.* (2015): Early and effective treatment of *KCNQ2* encephalopathy. *Epilepsia* 56: 685–691.

Radaelli G, de Souza Santos F, Borelli WV, *et al.* (2018): Causes of mortality in early infantile epileptic encephalopathy: A systematic review. *Epilepsy Behav* 85: 32–36.

Robain O, Dulac O (1992): Early epileptic encephalopathy with suppression-bursts and olivary-dentate dysplasia. *Neuropediatrics* 23: 162–164.

Rossi S, Daniele I, Bastrenta P, Mastrangelo M, Lista G (2009): Early myoclonic encephalopathy and nonketotic hyperglycinemia. *Pediatr Neurol* 41: 371–374.

Saitsu H, Kato M, Mizuguchi T, *et al.* (2008): *De novo* mutations in the gene encoding *STXBP1* (MUNC18-1) cause early infantile epileptic encephalopathy. *Nat Genet* 40: 782–788.

Saitsu H, Kato M, Okada I, *et al.* (2010): *STXBP1* mutations in early infantile epileptic encephalopathy with suppression-burst pattern. *Epilepsia* 51: 2397–2405.

Scheffer IE, Berkovic S, Capovilla G, *et al.* (2017): ILAE classification of the epilepsies: Position paper of the ILAE Commission for Classification and Terminology. *Epilepsia* 58: 512–521.

Schlumberger E, Dulac O, Plouin P (1992): Early infantile syndrome(s) with suppression-burst: nosological considerations. In: Roger J, Bureau M, Dravet C, Dreiffus FE, Perret A, Wolf P (eds) *Epileptic Syndromes of Infancy, Childhood and Adolescence*, 2nd ed, pp. 35–42. London: John Libbey.

Seo JH, Lee YM, Lee JS, Kim SH, Kim HD (2010): A case of Ohtahara syndrome with mitochondrial respiratory chain complex I deficiency. *Brain Dev* 32: 253–257.

Shen J, Tareste DC, Paumet F, Rothman JE, Melia TJ (2007): Selective activation of cognate SNAREpins by Sec1/Munc18 proteins. *Cell* 128: 183–195.

Stamberger H, Nikanorova M, Willemsen MH, *et al.* (2016): STXBP1encephalopathy. *Neurology* 86: 954–962.

Suzuki Y, Kure S, Oota M, Hino H, Fukuda M (2010): Nonketotic hyperglycinemia: proposal of a diagnostic and treatment strategy. *Pediatr Neurol* 43: 221–224.

Swanson DA, Steel JM, Valle D (1998): Identification and characterization of the human ortholog of rat *STXBP1*, a protein implicated in vesicle trafficking and neurotransmitter release. *Genomics* 48: 373–376.

Tatsuno M, Hayashi M, Iwamoto H, *et al.* (1984): Leigh's encephalopathy with wide lesions and early infantile epileptic encephalopathy with suppression-burst pattern: an autopsy case. *No To Hattatsu* 16: 68–75.

Tekgul H, Serdargoulu G, Karapinar B, *et al.* (2006). Vigabatrin caused rapidly progressive deterioration in two cases with early myoclonic encephalopathy associated with nonketotic hyperglycinemia. *J Child Neurol* 21: 82–84.

Tharp BR (2002): Neonatal seizures and syndromes. *Epilepsia* 43 (Suppl 3): 2–10.

Vigevano F, Maccagnani F, Bertini E, *et al.* (1982): Encefalopatia mioclonia precoce associata ad alti livelli di acido propionico nel siero. *Boll Lega It Epil* 39: 181–182.

Watanabe S, Murayama A, Haginoya K, *et al.* (2012): Schinzel-Giedion syndrome: A further cause of early myoclonic encephalopathy and vacuolating myelinopathy. *Brain Dev* 34: 151–155.

Williams AN, Gray RG, Poulton K, *et al.* (1998): A case of Ohtahara syndrome with cytochrome oxidase deficiency. *Dev Med Child Neurol* 40: 568–570.

Wolff M, Johannesen KM, Hedrich UBS, *et al.* (2017): Genetic and phenotypic heterogeneity suggest therapeutic implications in SCN2A and related disorders. *Brain* 140: 1316–1336.

Yamatogi Y, Ohtahara S (1981): Age-dependent epileptic encephalopathy: a developmental study. *Folia Psychiatr Neurol Jpn* 35: 321–332.

Yamatogi Y, Ohtahara S (2002): Early-infantile epileptic encephalopathy with suppression-bursts. Ohtahara syndrome. Its overview referring to our 16 cases. *Brain Dev* 24: 13–23.

Yamatogi Y, Ohtahara S (2003): Severe epilepsy with multiple independent spike foci. *J Clin Neurophysiol* 20: 442–448.

Yamamoto H, Okumura A, Fukuda M (2011): Epilepies and epileptic syndromes starting in the neonatal period. *Brain Dev* 33: 213–220.

WITH VIDEO SUPPLEMENTS

CHAPTER 8

INFANTILE SPASMS

Lucia Fusco[1], Catherine Chiron[2], Marina Trivisano[1], Federico Vigevano[1] and Harry T. Chugani[3]

[1] Department of Neuroscience and Neurorehabilitation, Bambino Gesù Children's Hospital, Rome, Italy
[2] Inserm U663, University Paris-Descartes, Necker Hospital, Paris, France
[3] Departments of Pediatrics and Neurology, Nemours A.I. duPont Hospital for Children, Wilmington, DE and Thomas Jefferson University, Philadelphia, USA

Introduction

Infantile spasms (IS) syndrome is an age-dependent epileptic syndrome, characterized by epileptic spasms and chaotic EEG abnormalities, frequently associated with modification of behavior or cognitive decline. The diagnosis of IS syndrome is often preferred when the EEG does not show the classical picture of hypsarrhythmia. However, the diagnosis of West syndrome is customarily used when onset of IS is in the first year of life. West syndrome is a well-recognized syndrome, although it should be noted that there has never been a formal classification of syndromes by the ILAE (Berg *et al.*, 2010). Actually IS syndrome and West syndrome are synonymous as each differentiation is often artificial and useless (Lux & Osborne, 2004).

Epileptic spasm is the type of seizure which characterizes IS syndrome and West syndrome. Epileptic spasms were not mentioned as types of seizures in 1981 (Commission on Classification and Terminology of the International League Against Epilepsy, 1981) and 1989 classifications (Commission on Classification and Terminology of the International League Against Epilepsy, 1989) in which they were considered as integral part of West syndrome. They were classified as generalized seizures and named "spasms" in the 2001 classification (Engel, 2001), then "epileptic spasms" in the 2006 classification (Engel, 2006), in which they were recognized as a distinctive type of seizure. In the 2010 classification, epileptic spasms were confirmed as a type of seizure, defined as unknown if generalized or partial (Berg *et al.*, 2010). Lastly, in the current classification (Fischer *et al.*, 2017), epileptic spasms, which were previously described only as seizures of unknown origin, were recognized to have also a generalized or focal onset. Therefore, they are seizures represented in focal, generalized, and unknown onset categories. Moreover, the term "epileptic" is recommended to be explicitly stated for epileptic spasms, because of the ambiguity of the single word "spasms" in neurologic use (Fischer *et al.*, 2017). Epileptic spasms historically belong to West syndrome. It was recognized as a distinctive age-dependent epileptic syndrome in the late 1950s and included in the first classification of epilepsies and epileptic syndromes in 1989 (Commission on Classification and Terminology of the International League Against Epilepsy, 1989). However, in the last decade many papers regarding IS and West syndrome have been published supporting the idea that they are extraordinarily heterogeneous syndromes according to etiology and evolution, ranging from the normal child with only genetic predisposition (Specchio *et al.*, 2010) to severe epileptic encephalopathy due to metabolic or genetic disorders (Mei *et al.*, 2010; El Sabbagh *et al.*, 2010).

After describing the essential clinical and EEG picture of the IS syndrome, and its heterogeneous etiology, we will highlight the new diagnostic and therapeutic options.

General features

The incidence of IS syndrome ranges between 2.9 (Trevathan *et al.*, 1999) and 4.3 (Riikonen, 2001) per 10,000 live births. Despite the increasing number of preterm or extremely low-birth-weight infants in the last decade, the incidence has not changed during the past 30 years (Riikonen, 2001).

The age of onset of epileptic spasms peaks between 3 and 9 months. An earlier beginning and a later onset have been reported, usually associated with a symptomatic etiology. Genetic, metabolic or diffuse cerebral malformative etiology have been described mainly for the early onset forms of IS, and focal cortical malformations or a cryptogenic etiology for the late onset form of IS (Eisermann *et al.*, 2006, Mei *et al.*, 2010; El Sabbagh *et al.*, 2010; Auvin *et al.*, 2010).

Clinical and EEG features of epileptic spasms

Clinical semiology of epileptic spasms

Epileptic spasms are sudden and brief contractions of axial (neck and trunk) and proximal limb muscles. A variety of patterns of muscle contraction can be observed, ranging from the typical rhombus appearance (Fusco & Vigevano, 1993) to a more prolonged tonic contraction. Epileptic spasms may involve flexor or extensor muscles, and both patterns can be present in the same child depending on whether the child is sitting or in a supine position. Actually, epileptic spasms manifest with a very rough pattern, affecting poorly specialized muscles, mainly axial or bilaterally proximal. Differing from motor seizures that are derived from specialized cerebral cortical motor areas, signs such as head or eye deviation, one side facial or limb, hand or foot contractions, are rarely observed during the epileptic spasm. When present, they suggest a contralateral cerebral cortical involvement, often on the side of an underlying pathogenetic lesion. For this reason, according to the last ILAE classification, epileptic spasms are considered to have focal or generalized onset (Fischer *et al.*, 2017). A careful study of a video-EEG may be necessary to clarify this issue.

Epileptic spasms usually occur in cluster, mainly on awakening or during transition from slow NREM sleep to REM sleep (Plouin *et al.*, 1987). A cluster is characterized by many spasms at different intensity, usually mild at the onset and the end, and of major intensity in the middle part of the cluster. In different children or in different clusters in the same child, the intensity of muscle contraction and the amount of muscle groups involved, can vary significantly. Epileptic spasms may be subtle and consist of upward eye deviation or slight shoulder elevation only, isolated or in cluster.

The length of muscle contraction may also varies: most epileptic spasms are characterized by a phasic contraction, polymyographically with rhombus or half-rhombus appearance, lasting 1 to 2 seconds *(Figure 1A and B)*. Others may have the same initial phasic component, followed by a less intense but more sustained tonic contraction of variable duration, lasting up to 10 seconds. In this case the event should be named spasm-tonic seizure *(Figure 1C)*.

Epileptic spasms are usually symmetric, but a variety of asymmetric or focal signs can be observed during the event. Asymmetric epileptic spasms are easily recognizable by one side flexor and other side extensor contraction and usually the EEG counterpart is also asymmetric. Asymmetric spasms can be asynchronous, one side contracting earlier than the other. Asymmetric and asynchronous spasms, usually, imply an asymmetry in the function of the two hemispheres and often bilateral asymmetric lesions (Fusco & Vigevano, 1993). The presence of focal signs during the epileptic spasm is a further element which suggests a symptomatic etiology. Signs such as one side eye deviation and one side hand fist during the spasm are suggestive elements of a contralateral cerebral cortical lesion.

However, EMG recordings of different muscle groups during an epileptic spasm, usually show a more complex picture of what one might expect (Bisulli *et al.*, 2002). A large latency variability in different muscle groups and the pattern of activation, which is not clear either

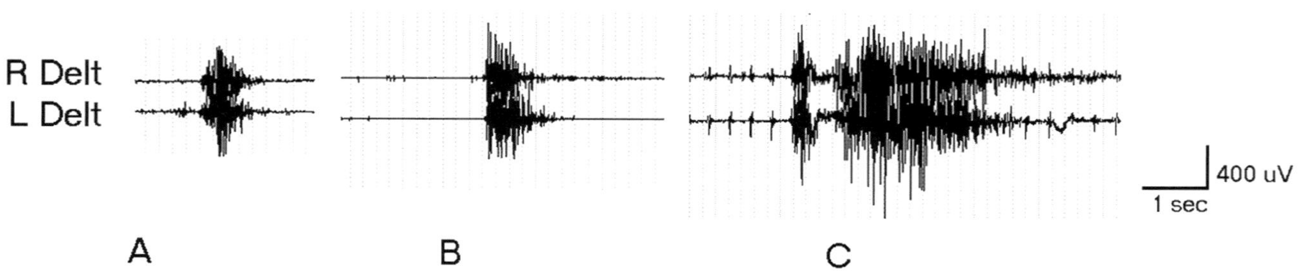

Figure 1

Diverse EMG appearance of epileptic spasms. A: typical phasic spasm with rhombus appearance. B: less typical spasm with abrupt and massive onset. C: spasm-tonic seizure, characterized by a spasm followed by sustained tonic contraction.

rostro-caudal or propriospinal, suggest an important participation of subcortical structures, while the stereotyped clinical manifestation could suggest involvement of central pattern generators (Bisulli *et al.*, 2002).

Ictal EEG

Nowadays, we can assume that most of the ictal EEG of epileptic spasms will show high amplitude slow wave (Fusco &Vigevano, 1993; Haga *et al.*, 1995), which is usually diffuse. The diffuse slow waves may show a predominance over one hemisphere, depending on the functional balance of the two sides of the brain *(Figure 2A and B)*. A brief beta activity, called spindle-like (Fusco & Vigevano, 1993), fast (Panzica *et al.*, 1999) or very fast rhythmic (Kobayashi *et al.*, 2004) activity, has also been described as EEG counterpart of epileptic spasms. These beta activities are variably associated with the high amplitude slow waves. Fast activity usually precedes and then is superimposed on the slow waves, at least in its ascending part *(Figure 2C)*. Fast activity can be focal or diffuse, independently of the etiology. Focal fast activity during stereo-EEG suggests an underlying epileptogenic lesion and focal cortical dysplasia. Most of the reports published in the second part of the last century, starting with the masterpiece by Kellaway *et al.* (1979), describe the EEG counterpart of the epileptic spasms as variable, characterized by more than ten different ictal pattern, (high voltage slow wave, sharp wave, voltage attenuation and so on). When looking only at motor epileptic spasms, the same authors found mostly high voltage generalized slow-wave transients. The lack of simultaneous ictal clinical, polymyographic and EEG recordings of epileptic spasms in most of the published papers, can be the reason why there are so many different interpretations. It is difficult to correlate the EEG and associated clinical phenomenon, if the ictal epileptic spasm is not myographically recorded. "Even though beta activities appear simultaneous with diffuse high voltage slow waves, the possibility that low voltage fast activities may have a role in triggering the epileptic spasm is not excluded."

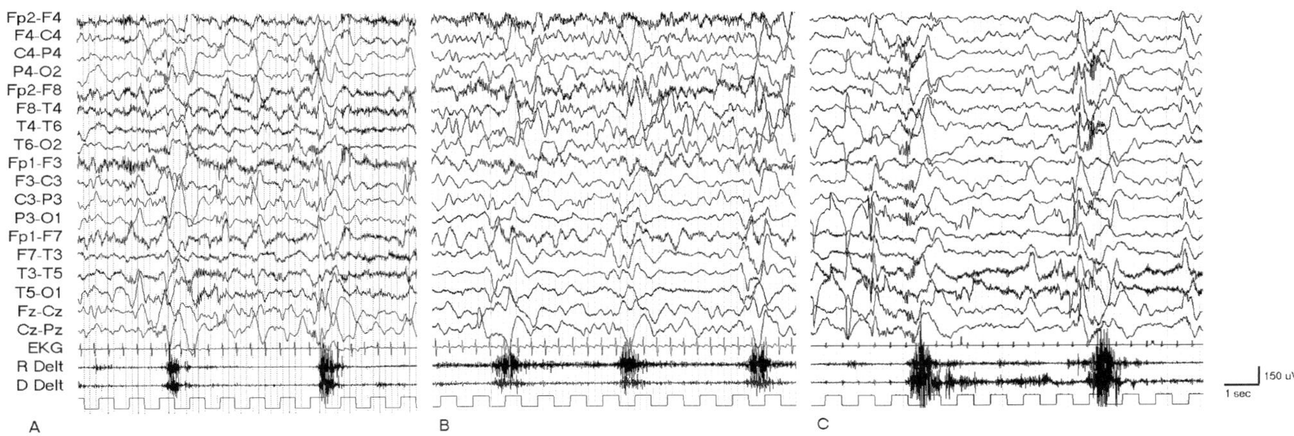

Figure 2

Ictal pattern of epileptic spasms.
A: a 6 month-old child, idiopathic etiology, the EEG counterpart is a high amplitude diffuse slow wave, the EMG pattern is characterized by a symmetric and synchronous contraction. B: epileptic spasms in a child who underwent neonatal surgery for left temporal giant cavernoma. Epileptic spasms appeared at 9 months, the EEG counterpart was characterized by an asynchronous slow wave with more amplitude over the left hemisphere, the EMG pattern shows an asymmetry in the contraction of the right and left deltoid, more sustained and with more amplitude on the right side. C: perinatal hypoxic-ischemic encephalopathy, child aged 5 months, the EEG counterpart of the spasms is a high amplitude slow wave preceded by fast rhythm lasting less than a second, diffuse or prevalent over the right hemisphere.

Panzica *et al.*, in 1999 reported that autoregressive analysis of the 500 ms EEG epochs preceding spasm onset revealed, in 13 of the 18 studied cases, the presence of a short discharge of fast activity, restricted to a narrow frequency band (17.5 ± 2.1 Hz). The fast discharge had rather low inter-hemispheric coherence values and asymmetric amplitude on homologous EEG derivations, with a rather long inter-hemispheric time difference (more than 10 ms). The asymmetric EEG pattern and the long inter-hemispheric time difference, led the authors to hypothesize a localized cortical origin of the more diffuse ictal discharge associated with the epileptic spasm. Moreover, in a following paper, the same authors demonstrated the consistency between the side of earliest appearance of EEG fast activity and the side of focal epileptiform EEG discharges, occurring in 10 of those patients, during the follow-up (Panzica *et al.*, 2007). The authors made the reasonable assumption, among others, that epileptic spasms could result from the activation of an archaic brainstem circuit by unilateral cortical descending input (Avanzini *et al.*, 2007). The similarity of epileptic spasms with a startle reaction (Koch, 1999) or Moro reflex (Gobbi *et al.*, 1987), already known as a brainstem phenomenon, supports this hypothesis (Avanzini *et al.*, 2007).

Epileptic spasms can be associated with a partial seizure in a single ictal event (Pachatz *et al.*, 2003). Regarding the temporal association of the two phenomena, different seizure patterns have been described: partial seizures followed by epileptic spasms or appearing during a cluster of epileptic spasms without interrupting the cluster *(Figure 3)*. This association of partial seizures and epileptic spasms as a single ictal event can be related to different etiologies and should not be considered distinctive for cortical malformations or severe brain damage.

Interictal EEG

When epileptic spasms appear in the first year of life, they are usually associated with EEG hypsarrhythmia. EEG hypsarrhythmia is a chaotic cerebral activity, characterized by asynchronous, arrhythmic, high-voltage slow-waves variably intermingled with multifocal spikes. Hypsarrhythmia is the most common EEG pattern associated with epileptic spasms in the first year of life. At this age, epileptic spasms, hypsarrhythmia and developmental regression or stagnation, are the three elements which characterize IS and West

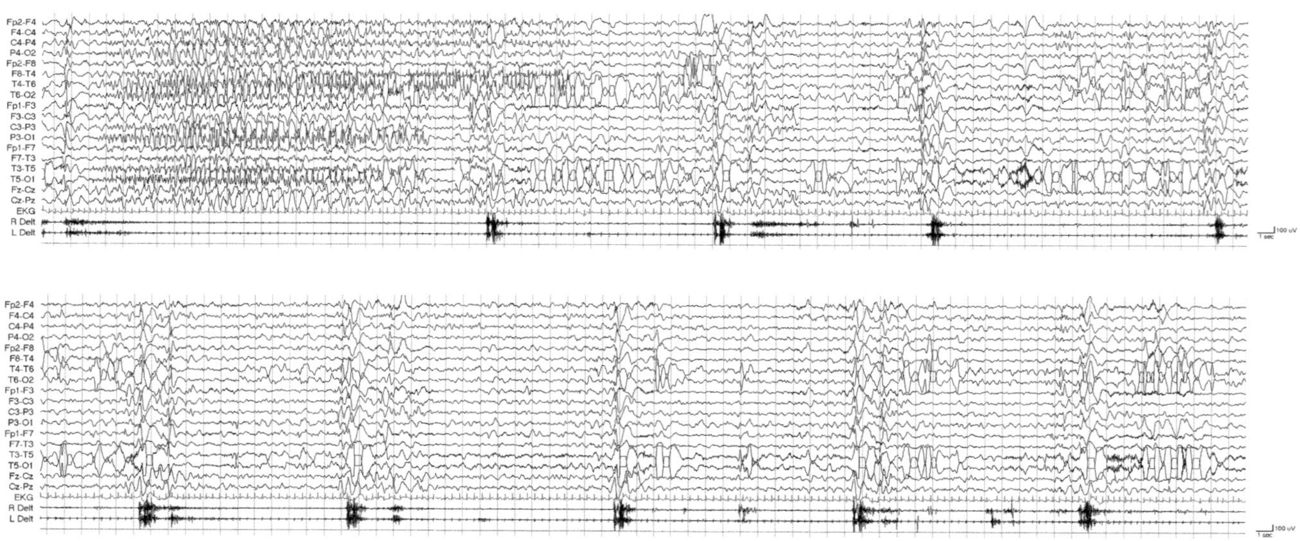

Figure 3

A partial seizure involving left and then right temporal regions, intermingled and followed by a cluster of epileptic spasms in a single event. Patient with tuberous sclerosis, 4 months old.

syndrome. The main feature of hypsarrhythmia is the presence of very high voltage slow activity, which appears diffuse or with some unilateral predominance, variably associated with diffuse or multifocal spikes.

Hypsarrhythmia is usually a wakefulness pattern *(Figure 4A)*. During NREM sleep, EEG abnormalities break up into diffuse irregular arrhythmic spike-wave discharges, lasting 1–3 seconds, which alternate with a lower theta-beta activity, delineating a typical paroxysmal alternating pattern *(Figure 4B)*. At times, a pattern of multifocal random attenuation can be observed, especially in symptomatic cases. During REM sleep the EEG pattern is very similar to what is observed during wakefulness. Many variant patterns of hypsarrhythmia have been described. Asymmetric hypsarrhythmia is one in which the true hypsarrythmic pattern is observed mostly over one hemisphere or completely lateralized (Watanabe *et al.*, 1993) *(Figure 4C and D)*, Hypsarrhythmia can have a predominance of focal slow activity (Parmeggiani *et al.*, 1990) or have persisting focal spikes, especially during REM sleep *(Figure 4E and F)*. All these variants are suggestive of symptomatic etiology. However, in many cases focal epileptiform abnormalities show a predominance over the posterior areas regardless of the region of the underlying lesion (Oka *et al.*, 2004) and even in the idiopathic cases *(Figure 4A)*. More than focal spikes on the interictal EEG, the localization of spikes on the inter-spasms EEG interval has been found to coincide with the underlying focal cortical lesion, as shown by MRI, or with the focus of associated partial seizures (Oka *et al.*, 2004).

Some authors wonder if hypsarrhythmia is an interictal or ictal pattern (Lux, 2007). The severe disturbance of cerebral activity, as shown by the EEG, certainly interferes with behavior and cognition, so much so that West syndrome has been included in the ILAE classification under epileptic encephalopathies. Accordingly, Epileptic encephalopathies are conditions where the epileptic activity itself contributes to severe cognitive and behavioral impairments above and beyond what might be expected from the underlying pathology alone (Scheffer *et al.*, 2017). Defining hypsarrhythmia as an ictal pattern is somehow simplistic, as hypsarrhythmia is a more chronic and profound dysfunction than a seizure or a status epilepticus.

Epileptic spasms without EEG hypsarrhythmia

Several papers have reported infants with clusters of epileptic spasms without EEG hypsarrhythmia, neither at the onset nor throughout the clinical course of the condition (Caraballo *et al.*, 2003; Oguni *et al.*, 2005; Caraballo *et al.*, 2011). Etiology was mainly not known or consistent with focal cortical dysplasia and age at onset showed a wider range than classical West syndrome, ranging from 2 to 82 months (Oguni *et al.*, 2005). Even in this group of patients the response to common antiepileptic drugs was poor whereas ACTH gave best results.

Etiology of infantile spasms

According to the ILAE classification (Scheffer *et al.* 2017), the etiology of IS is classified as structural, genetic, infectious, metabolic, immune, unknown. The term "symptomatic" of the previous classification (Engel, 2001) has been replaced by the different categories above mentioned, and the term "cryptogenic" corresponds to the cases of unknown origin.

Some authors identified a small group of patients with no proven etiology except for a genetic predisposition to epilepsy (Dulac *et al.*, 1993; Vigevano *et al.*, 1993; Riikonen, 2010; Specchio *et al.*, 2010). In these patients IS have a particular good outcome, with complete recovery from seizures and normal cognitive development suggesting an "idiopathic" etiology. However, the definition of an idiopathic etiology is based on the latter outcome and cannot be definite at the time epileptic spasms present or at the time of diagnosis (Riikonen, 2010). Despite this term is still widely used, the new Classification has removed the term "idiopathic" from the nomenclature, as it could be replaced by "genetic" or "with unknown etiology" (Scheffer *et al.* 2017). In this chapter we still use the term "idiopathic" for this small group.

In symptomatic IS, a clearly and defined cause is identified and/or a significant developmental delay is present before the onset of spasms suggesting the presence of an underlying disorder (Riikonen, 2010).

When known, causes could be classified, according to the time of appearance of the etiology, whether prenatal, perinatal or postnatal, or according to the context in which the brain lesion occurs (neonatal infections, strokes, hypoxic ischemic or metabolic diseases) (Michaud *et al.*, 2014).

Genetic etiology represents about 25% of prenatal etiologies of IS (Michaud *et al.*, 2014). Several chromosomal abnormalities have been reported in about a fourth of spasms of genetic etiology and the most frequent are trisomy 21, XXY, 17p13.3 microdeletion, 1p36 del (Greco *et al.*, 2018), del 1q36 1ptel, inv/dup15 (Matricardi *et al.*, 2018). CNVs variants are responsible of about 7% of epileptic spasms with genetic etiology and this high rate supports the use of CGH-Array as one of the first-line screening tools in patients with unexplained cause (Michaud *et al.*, 2014). Moreover, mutations in X-linked genes have been described such as *CDKL5*, particularly in female, and *ARX*, usually in male patients (Mei *et al.*, 2010; Shoubridge *et al.*, 2010). Other gene mutations (*SCN1A*, *MAG12*, *CACNA1A*) have also been reported (Auvin *et al.*, 2009).

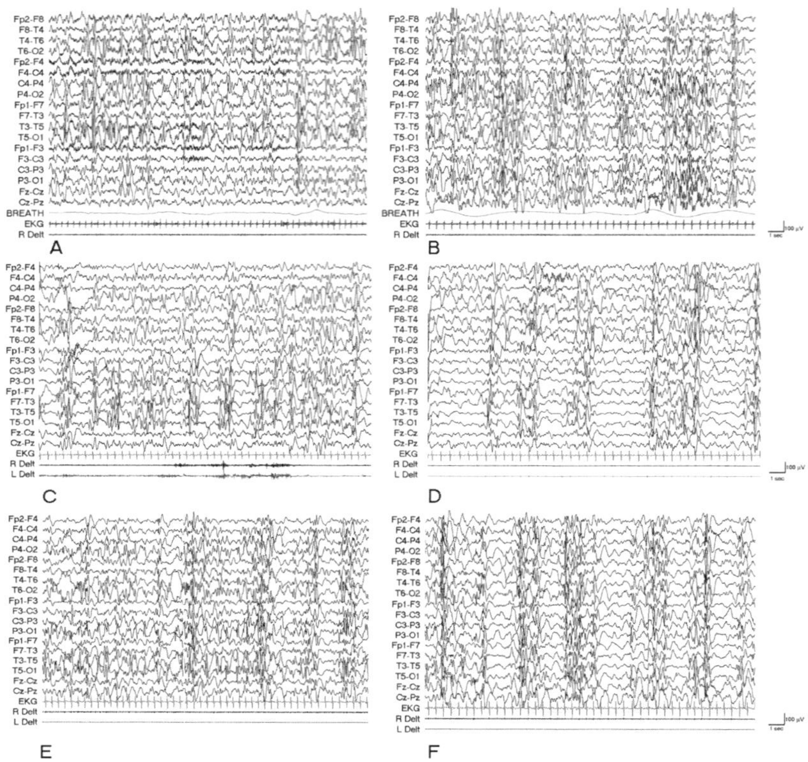

Figure 4

A and B: idiopathic etiology. In A: Wakefulness EEG, very high amplitude background activity, high amplitude slow waves intermingled with spikes are evident mainly over the central and posterior region with asynchronous trend. In B: During NREM sleep abnormalities tend to cluster in diffuse discharges lasting several seconds alternating with low voltage diffuse activity. No asymmetry nor clear focal abnormalities are evident.
C and D: symptomatic etiology. In C: Wakefulness EEG, other than a slowing down of diffuse background activity, a clearcut slow waves are evident over the left temporal and central regions, intermingled with several spikes with temporal predominance. In D: Sleep EEG, an asymmetry in sleep synchronization is evident with less synchronization over the left hemisphere, where more spikes are recorded in the temporal regions. Slow and spike wave are clustering in diffuse discharges. Sleep spindles are evident only over the healthy right hemisphere. E and F: Symptomatic etiology. In E: Wakefulness EEG, very slow background activity is evident over the posterior and central regions with asynchronous trend, in association to several spikes with multifocal or diffuse trend. In F: Sleep EEG, clustering of spikes and slow wave in brief and diffuse discharges alternating with brief and diffuse low voltage activity.

More recently, thanks to the next generation sequencing techniques, other genes have been associated with epileptic spasms. Epileptic spasms appear genetically heterogeneous as they can result from a disruption of several fundamental neurodevelopmental processes. In fact, *de novo* variants have been identified in genes involved in a wide spectrum of functions such as gene transcription or protein translation, neurogenesis, neuronal differentiation, guidance and/or cellular or neuronal migration (*i.e.*, *ARX*), synaptic transmission, (*i.e.*, *STXBP1*, *CASK*), protein modification or degradation (*i.e.*, *ALG13* and other glycosylation defects) (Michaud *et al.*, 2014).

Cerebral malformations are a major cause of IS, which usually start early, in the first year of life. Among cerebral malformations, disorders of abnormal neurogenesis, neuronal migration and neuronal organization resulting in different pictures like cortical dysplasia, microcephaly, hemimegalencephaly, agyria/polygyria, schizencephaly and heterotopias, have been reported (Osborne *et al.*, 2010). Cerebral midline developmental anomalies such as agenesis of the corpus callosum and holoprosencephaly can manifest with IS and often they are associated with a facial phenotype characterized by major anomalies (cyclopia) or more frequently by minor malformations (median cleft lip, cleft palate, hypotelorism, flat nose). In these cases endocrinological dysfunction, such as diabetes insipidus, and idiopathic hyper- or hyponatremia, can be associated (Levey *et al.*, 2010).

Other cerebral malformations, with a recognized genetic etiology, manifest with IS such as tuberous sclerosis complex, neurofibromatosis, incontinentia pigmenti, hypomelanosis of Ito.

All vascular accidents, either ischemic or hemorrhagic, due to vascular disease such as a cerebral artery disease or stroke, can cause IS in the first year of life. Vascular accidents can occur in the prenatal period, at birth or later on. Hypoxic-ischemic encephalopathy, following full-term or preterm delivery, is still a major cause of IS. Prognosis is usually worse in the infants following full-term delivery probably due to cortical rather than white matter damage (Dulac *et al.*, 2010).

Other structural etiologies include cerebral infections. They occur during pregnancy and more frequently are due to cytomegalovirus, herpes viruses and toxoplasmosis that cause cerebral epileptogenic malformations. Also infections at birth or in the post-natal period (meningitis, encephalitis and cerebral abscess) are associated with IS. Although rare, even brain neoplasms (benign or malignant) have been reported to be the cause.

As regards metabolic or endocrine diseases, usually these diseases have already been known before epileptic spasms start. Among metabolic etiologies, hypoglycemia, phenylketonuria, organic acidurias, amino acidurias, enzyme deficiencies such as pyridoxine dependency, or mitochondrial disorders have been reported (El Sabbag *et al.*, 2010). Also Congenital Deficit of Glycosylation (CDG) disorders can be associated with epileptic spasms showing particular features, such as absence of hypsarrhythmia and an unusual combination of epileptic spasms with myoclonus (Pereira *et al.*, 2017).

In about 20% of IS, the underlying cause is unknown. This group continues to decrease as diagnostic methods become more refined. In fact, the increased numbers of recognized cerebral malformations due to improving neuroradiological techniques, and the discovery of novel mutated genes associated with epileptic spasms have both been responsible for reducing the number of epileptic spasms classified as cryptogenic IS.

Among the group without any recognized etiological factors, approximately 5–6% of patients have an "idiopathic" etiology. They have a pure genetic predisposition to epilepsy, which causes a functional cerebral dysfunction that manifest in a short temporal window (Riikonen, 2010; Specchio *et al.*, 2010). This group of patients was firstly recognized by Vigevano and Dulac (Vigevano *et al.*, 1993, Dulac *et al.*, 1993) and later supported by case reports on the simultaneous occurrence of idiopathic West syndrome in siblings of two families (Reiter *et al.*, 2000) and on the occurrence of childhood absence epilepsy in two patients with previously idiopathic IS (Specchio *et al.*, 2010). Patients with IS due to idiopathic etiology recover completely, with no residual dysfunction. Diagnosis could be better defined during the follow-up, as slight mental retardation could manifest during childhood, still suggesting an unrecognized genetic cause. Even though from the beginning we can suspect an idiopathic etiology, further studies are certainly warranted to better delineate the early clinical and neurophysiological characteristics of these patients.

European researchers (Dulac *et al.*, 2010) have stressed the need to identify early the underlying etiology, in each patient with IS, as this epileptic manifestation *per se* "is all but a disease". The authors reinforce the thought that "epileptic spasms are a manifestation of a final common pathway of various diseases within a specific age range and express transient (although eventually prolonged) hyperexcitability of the brain". If we consider IS a transient phenomenon of different diseases and we recognize the underlying etiology, we will "treat the disease itself and not merely a transient phenomenon" (Dulac *et al.*, 2010).

Metabolic and functional neuroimaging

One of the most important developments in the management and prognosis of patients with IS and West syndrome over the past two decades has been the rapid advances in neuroimaging, such as MRI, PET and SPECT scanning. Based on these neuroimaging results, we now recognize that malformations of cortical development, even when not readily seen on MRI, are the most common underlying etiology of otherwise cryptogenic (with unknown etiology in the present terminology) epileptic spasms. These advances, together with detailed analysis of EEG activity, have also led to an evolution from prior concepts of IS as primary generalized seizures to the current thinking that IS have a *focal* onset with a pattern of secondary generalization that is age-specific (Chugani *et al.*, 1990, 1992). Indeed, neuroimaging is largely responsible for new treatment approaches aimed at intractable IS, such as focal cortical resection.

Glucose metabolism PET and perfusion SPECT scans

Although MRI is unarguably the primary imaging modality in patients with IS, PET scans of glucose metabolism and SPECT scans of cerebral blood flow often disclose abnormalities even when the MRI scan is normal. Four different types of PET abnormalities have been observed in patients with *cryptogenic* IS (Chugani & Conti, 1996) *(Figure 5)*, so that the term "cryptogenic" becomes less meaningful. It should, however, be cautioned that glucose metabolism PET scans should not be performed when the child is on ketogenic diet as the results are difficult to interpret. Since these abnormalities can also be seen on SPECT scans *(Figure 6)* (Chiron *et al.*, 1993; Haginoya *et al.*, 2001; Hamano *et al.*, 2010), patients who are unable to come off the ketogenic diet should perhaps have SPECT scans instead of PET.

When a single region of abnormal glucose metabolism (or SPECT hypoperfusion) is present, and there is good concordance with the focus identified on the EEG (characterized by ictal or interictal focal epileptiform activity, or focal background slowing), surgical removal of the epileptogenic region (often a previously unsuspected area of cortical dysplasia) results not only in seizure control but also in complete or partial reversal of the associated developmental delay (Chugani *et al.*, 1993; Asarnow *et al.*, 1997; Jonas *et al.*, 2005). Indeed, on electrocorticography, there appears to be a close correlation between localization of the spasms characterized by a "leading spike" followed by fast-wave bursts and localization from PET hypometabolism (Asano *et al.*, 2005). Therefore, we suggest that all patients with *cryptogenic* IS resistant to conventional medical treatment should have a PET scan of glucose metabolism (or SPECT scan) in order to uncover potential surgical candidates. The "ideal surgical candidate" is the patient with a single MRI lesion or PET hypometabolism not involving motor or visual cortex. The extent of the epileptogenic or "nociferous" cortex is typically underestimated by the MRI and a lesionectomy may be insufficient to achieve an optimum seizure and developmental outcome *(Figure 7)*. Even when an MRI lesion is present, the extent of functional disturbances on PET serves as a useful guide for subdural electrode placements to ensure a more comprehensive evaluation of potential epileptogenic zones (Asano *et al.*, 2005).

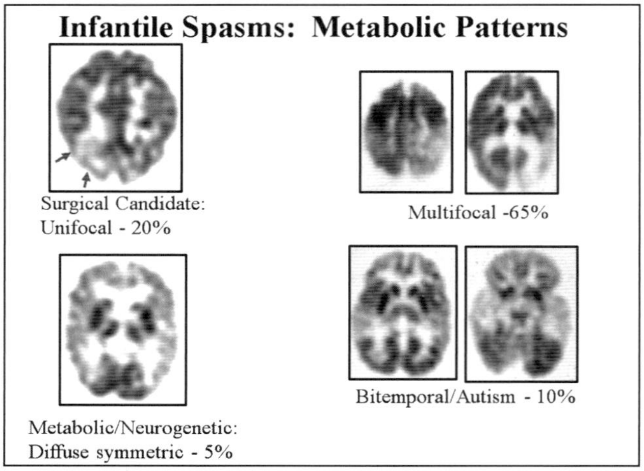

Figure 5 **Four patterns of glucose metabolism in so-called cryptogenic cases of infantile spasms. The term "cryptogenic" becomes less meaningful after PET scanning. Ideal surgical candidates comprise only about 20% of patients originally classified as cryptogenic.**

Unfortunately, about 65% of patients with cryptogenic epileptic spasms are not "ideal" candidates because they show more than one area of cortical hypometabolism on the PET scan (often representing multifocal cortical dysplasias). However, even some of these children may benefit from a "palliative" cortical resection in order to improve their quality of life provided that the majority of their seizures arise from one focus (Ilyas *et al.*, 2014).

About 10% of all patients with cryptogenic IS will show bilateral temporal lobe hypometabolism on the PET scan *(Figure 8)*. These children show a distinct clinical phenotype characterized by severe developmental delay (particularly in the language domain) and autism spectrum disorder (Chugani *et al.*, 1996). Hypometabolism may also be seen in the frontal and parietal lobes in the autism group (Dilber *et al.*, 2013). Finally, in about 5% of cryptogenic cases, the glucose metabolism PET scan may reveal bilateral symmetric or generalized cortical hypometabolism, with or without associated cerebellar

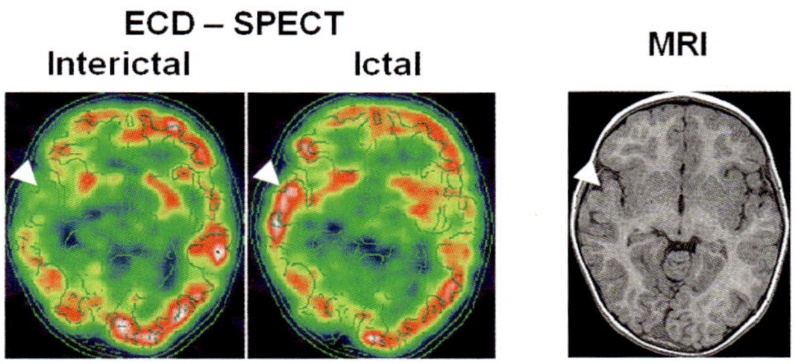

Figure 6 **SPECT scan in a 2-year-old girl with focal seizures and epileptic spasms. Interictal SPECT showed hypoperfusion in the right temporal pole (arrow) and ictal SPECT (injection of the tracer 10 seconds after the onset of a focal seizure) showed hyperfusion in the same area (arrow). MRI was initially considered negative, but proved to disclose a subtle anomaly of the right temporal pole (arrow). The child underwent surgical exeresis of the right temporal pole without any intracranial EEG. Pathology: focal cortical dysplasia of Taylor type. Surgical outcome: seizure free for more than 6 years.**

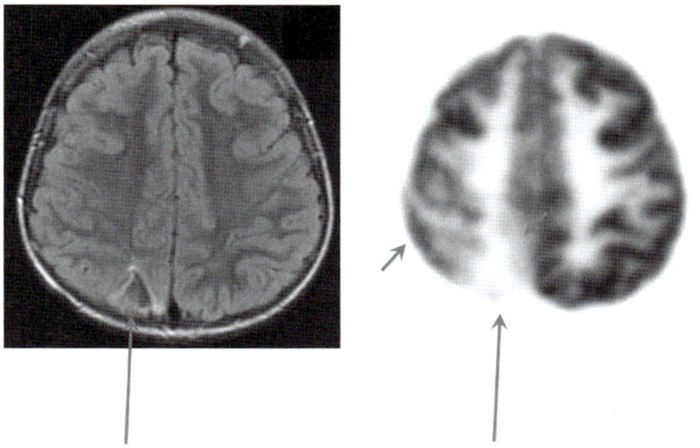

Figure 7 **MRI and FDG PET in a 6-year-old boy with a history of focal seizure and epileptic spasms as a single ictal event. MRI showed a cortical lesion in the right parietal region (arrow). FDG PET showed severe hypometabolism of the MRI lesion (long arrow) and mild hypometabolism in the surrounding area (short arrows), including medial parietal cortex. Chronic subdural EEG recording showed seizure onset arising from the hypometabolic cortex seen on PET. Pathology: dysembryoplastic neuroepithelial tumor, scattered abnormal neurons in surrounding hypercellular cortex. Surgical outcome: seizure-free following removal of the right parietal-occipital cortex including the tumor.**

involvement. Clearly, this pattern does not hint to an underlying lesional etiology or a surgical option. Rather, it may indicate that an underlying genetic/metabolic condition should be pursued.

Several studies using glucose metabolism PET have reported that focal cortical hypometabolism in patients with newly diagnosed IS may be a transient phenomenon. In one such study, the investigators reported transient focal cortical hypometabolism and suggested that the hypometabolism may not necessarily be related to structural lesions, but neuropathological data were not available and therefore this suggestion remains speculative (Metsahonkala *et al.*, 2002). They also found the absence of correlation between hypometabolism and prognosis. In contrast, another group of investigators reported that although PET may show transient hypometabolism, it appears to be a useful prognostic tool in patients with cryptogenic IS (Watanabe, 1998; Itomi *et al.*, 2002). A more recent study confirmed that PET hypometabolism may not always be permanent and, if present after initial treatment, confers poor seizure and developmental prognosis (Natsume *et al.*, 2014). Despite initial controversy, surgical resection of focal cortical regions guided in part by anatomical or functional neuroimaging is now widely accepted and carried in many centers worldwide. Many of these cases have revealed focal cortical dysplasias, even when anatomical neuroimaging showed subtle findings at best. In a study of 65 patients with epileptic spasms who underwent cortical resection, PET scan was abnormal in almost all patients [61/63 (97%) with lateralizing/localizing findings in 56/61 (92%) patients. Although ILAE class-1 outcomes were higher (79%) in patients with MRI lesions, still 50% of patients with normal MRI but focal PET achieved class-1 outcomes, attesting to the value of PET in this population (Chugani *et al.*, 2015). Often, the epileptogenic zone is quite large, involving the whole hemisphere such that a hemispherectomy or a "subtotal" hemispherectomy (*i.e.*, sparing only sensory-motor-cortex) is performed with excellent results including the 11 patients with epileptic spasms (Chugani *et al.*, 2014).

Glucose metabolism PET scans have also been used to further elucidate the pathophysiology of IS. Ictal PET scans of glucose metabolism performed during prolonged clusters of spasms or during frequent

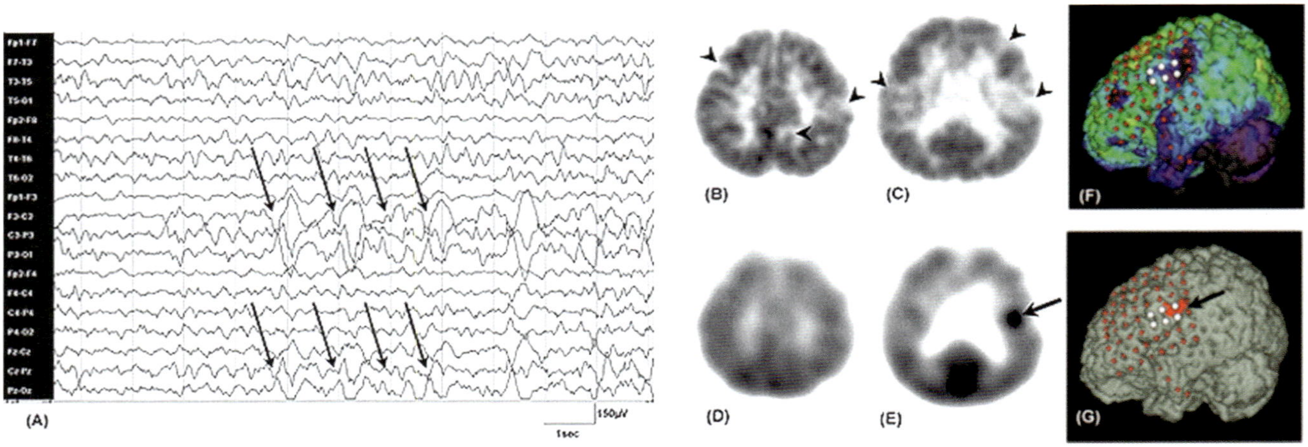

Figure 8

A 1-year-old boy with tuberous sclerosis, medically-refractory partial epilepsy and infantile spasms. A: scalp EEG showed ictal onset arising from the left central-parietal region. B and C: FDG PET showed nodular hypometabolic regions, each of which represents the location of cortical tuber. D and E: AMT PET demonstrated increased tracer uptake in the cortical tuber in the lateral surface of the left central-parietal region (arrow). F: Subdural electrodes were placed over the left hemisphere; nodular glucose hypometabolic areas (dark purple) are noted in the left central-parietal and frontal regions. G: Increased AMT uptake was noted only in the lateral surface of left central-parietal region (red). Chronic subdural EEG recording demonstrated that ictal onset (white electrodes) arose from the cortex overlying the tuber showing increased AMT uptake.

interictal spiking on the EEG have shown bilateral symmetric *hypermetabolism* of the lenticular nuclei and brainstem, in addition to focal area of cortical hypo- or hypermetabolism, thus suggesting that the spasms are initiated by a primary cortical epileptic focus that interacts with subcortical and brainstem structures (Chugani *et al.*, 1992). In other words, during a critical stage of brain development (beginning at about 3 months, when cortical maturation becomes evident on glucose metabolism PET scans), the primary cortical focus interacts through its epileptic discharges with brainstem structures, particularly the raphe nuclei, which have strong cortical projections. The raphe-cortical and cortico-cortical propagation may be responsible for the EEG feature of hypsarrhythmia. The raphe nuclei also have projections to the striatal region (bilateral putamen), and these pathways may activate descending spinal pathways bilaterally to result in the bilateral and relatively symmetric clinical semiology of epileptic spasms (Chugani *et al.*, 1992).

This proposed mechanism of seizure propagation has found some support from other investigations. For example, ictal SPECT studies performed during spasms in patients with epileptic cortical lesions have revealed increased perfusion not only in the cortical lesion but also in the bilateral basal ganglia (Mori *et al.*, 2007). In another study, patients with daily clusters of IS and hypsarrhythmia showed decreased diffusion in the pallidi and posterior brainstem on MRI diffusion weighted imaging; some patients also showed decreased diffusion in the thalamus and dentate nuclei (Desguerre *et al.*, 2008). Interestingly, when the hypsarrhythmia had resolved but not the spasms, these diffusion changes were no longer the same pattern. In yet another study, using subtraction ictal SPECT, one group of investigators found a good correlation between ictal cortical hyperperfusion and ictal EEG findings and, in addition, hyperperfusion of subcortical structures and a tight cortico-subcortical perfusion relationship (Kakisaka *et al.*, 2009). Together, these studies nicely illustrate the capability of advanced neuroimaging towards improving our understanding of the mechanisms involved in the generation and propagation of IS.

PET scans using ligands

In addition to studies of glucose metabolism in children with IS, PET has also been applied using various ligands. The most frequently applied of these ligands is alpha-[11 C]methyl-L-tryptophan (AMT) in patients with tuberous sclerosis (TSC) and IS. In these patients, interictal AMT PET can identify the epileptogenic tuber in about 65% of cases, revealing an increased uptake in the vicinity of the epileptogenic tuber *(Figure 8)*, but decreased uptake in the remaining tubers (Chugani *et al.*, 1998; Asano *et al.*, 2000).

In a large study of 191 TSC patients who had AMT PET scans, there was excellent correlation between seizure focus lateralization/localization and AMT PET findings of increased uptake and was sometimes the only test to show the seizure focus (Chugani *et al.*, 2013). This approach has been used in the surgical approach of TSC patients whose seizures have been refractory (Kagawa *et al.*, 2005; Chugani *et al.*, 2013). Other than AMT, there are isolated reports of various ligands being used to study patients with IS, but the value of such studies remains to be shown. Certainly, there is great potential for ligand PET investigations to enhance our understanding of the underlying basic mechanisms of IS. Finally, the recent technological advance of hybrid PET/MRI scanners with simultaneous acquisition of PET and MRI datasets will facilitate both clinical and research studies on children with IS.

Treatment of IS

IS are most often highly refractory. The complete cessation of seizures and the disappearance of hypsarrhythmia are the two goals of treatment. Hormonal treatment (ACTH or corticosteroids) and vigabatrin are now considered as the two standard first line therapies. Combining both seems beneficial (O'Callaghan *et al.*, 2017). Earlier the diagnosis and earlier the treatment, better the developmental outcome as measured at 4 years of age (O'Callaghan *et al.*, 2011).

Conventional AEDs are less efficient than standard therapy (Knupp *et al.*, 2016a; Demarest *et al.*, 2017), most of them being tested through open trials. Valproate and clonazepam control about 25% to 30% of the cases, but relapse rate is very high. Nitrazepam was as effective as ACTH in a randomized study, but there were life-threatening side-effects (Dreifuss *et al.*, 1986). Pyridoxine may be useful and is still extensively used in Japan. Immunoglobulins have been proposed, but were rather disappointing. Despite a positive placebo-controlled trial on 37 patients, sulthiame remains limited to Germany (Debus & Kurlemann, 2004). Worsening has been observed using carbamazepine.

New AEDs other than vigabatrin provide preliminary open data. Lamotrigine, topiramate, zonisamide, and felbamate may occasionally be helpful as add-on therapy and levetiracetam and zonisamide as first line. Ketogenic diet controlled 37% of 104 patients with refractory IS (Hong *et al.*, 2010). Some patients with symptomatic IS benefited from surgery, either by resection in case of unifocal lesion or by complete callosotomy in multifocal cases. The earlier the surgery, the better the developmental outcome (Jonas *et al.*, 2005).

ACTH and corticosteroids

ACTH has been extensively used as IS therapy for a long time, but the dose and the duration of ACTH regimen still remain under discussion. Daily low-doses (1–2 IU/kg) for 2 weeks prove to be as efficient as the high regimen of 40 IU (3–6 IU/kg) previously recommended and control seizures in about 75% of the patients (Ito *et al.*, 2002; Hrachovy *et al.*, 1983). Extremely low-doses were also used with some success in Japan (Oguni *et al.*, 2006). Adding magnesium did better than ACTH alone (Zou *et al.*, 2010). Relapse rates range around 55% and a second course of therapy produces a 74% response rate. However, the incidence of cushingoid adverse events approaches 100%. Other common adverse effects include infections, increased arterial blood pressure, gastritis and hyperexcitability. These are often reported as severe, and the mortality rate is between 2% and 5%.

Oral steroids are less extensively prescribed, although they are cheaper and better tolerated than ACTH (Kossoff *et al.*, 2009). In a randomized study, the efficacy of prednisone (2 mg/kg/day) was inferior to that of ACTH at very high doses (150 IU/day) but similar to that of ACTH administered at lower doses (Baram *et al.*, 1996; Hrachovy *et al.*, 1983). Uncontrolled data are available with hydrocortisone (15 mg/kg/day for 2 weeks): 74% were responders, 18% of them relapsed but 90% were further controlled by tetracosactide (Schlumberger & Dulac, 1994). The same applies to oral prednisolone (40–60 mg/day for 2 weeks): 67% were responders, a proportion similar to that previously obtained with ACTH in the same center (Kossoff *et al.*, 2009).

Vigabatrin

The efficacy of vigabatrin was firstly suggested 20 years ago as adjunctive therapy in an open labeled study showing complete control of spasms at short term in 43% of 70 patients with refractory IS (Chiron *et al.*, 1991). Soon after, vigabatrin was advocated for first-line monotherapy (Appleton & Montiel-Viesca, 1993) and was largely used in routine clinical practice. Long term effect is satisfactorily maintained with 42% having epilepsy and intellectual delay in the largest cohort reported (180 patients followed for a mean of 10 years) (Djuric *et al.*, 2014). Overall, there are five randomized studies with vigabatrin as first-line monotherapy in IS.

Despite a higher responder rate on ACTH (74%) than vigabatrin (48%) at short term in the whole population of 42 patients, vigabatrin did better in those with tuberous sclerosis and ACTH in those with perinatal anoxo-ischemia, whereas both drugs did the same in cryptogenic cases (Vigevano & Cilio, 1997).

In a trial dedicated to IS due to TSC, a sample of 22 patients was enough to definitely establish the superiority of vigabatrin (150 mg/kg/d) over hormonal treatment (oral hydrocortisone at 15 mg/kg/d). In this sub-population of 22 patients with TSC, 100% and 45% were responders to vigabatrin and hormonal treatment, respectively, at one month therapy ($p < 0.01$) (Chiron *et al.*, 1997). In addition, vigabatrin acted more rapidly and was better tolerated ($p = 0.006$) than hydrocortisone.

A dose-ranging study on 221 patients proved that high doses of vigabatrin (100–150 mg/kg/day) produced better results than doses under 40 mg/kg/d at 2 weeks. Vigabatrin had a relatively low rate of relapse (23%) up to 3 years and a high rate (72%) of these patients achieved control of seizures once more with reinstitution of vigabatrin (Elterman *et al.*, 2010).

By contrast, a study of 40 infants with IS that was not due to TSC, failed to demonstrate a significant superiority of vigabatrin over placebo, with 35% and 10% responders respectively (Appleton *et al.*, 1999).

Similarly, there were more responders at 2 weeks of prednisolone or tetracosactide treatment (73%) than there were with vigabatrin treatment (54%) ($p < 0.04$) in the UKISS trial. This trial had 107 patients left after TSC had been excluded (Lux *et al.*, 2004). However, this difference of having more responders on prednisone or tetracosactide disappeared in the long term. A similar efficacy (about 75%) after 1 and 4 years of treatment was allocated to hormonal treatment and to vigabatrin treatment (Darke *et al.*, 2010; Lux *et al.*, 2005).

The most preoccupying side effect of vigabatrin is its retinal toxicity that induces irreversible visual field loss (VFL). Toxicity involves the peripheral vision but visual functions may occasionally be affected. Vigabatrin attributed VFL was less frequent in children (20%) than in adults (34%) in a large prospective study on 734 patients with focal epilepsy (Wild *et al.*, 2009), and it was not observed in children having received less than 15 months of vigabatrin (Vanhatalo *et al.*, 2002). A systematic review including 11 pediatric series concluded that vigabatrin increases the risk of VFL fourfold, with age and exposure as predicting factors (Maguire *et al.*, 2010). Focusing on school-aged children previously treated for infantile spasms with vigabatrin, VFL rates of 6% (1/16) and 34% (11/32) were reported, related to cumulative dose and treatment duration (Gaily *et al.*, 2009; Riikonen *et al.*, 2015). Diagnosing such toxicity before the age of 6 years is challenging since visual field examination is not possible. Electroretinogram (30-Hz ERG flicker amplitude) provides an alternative to detect vigabatrin retinal damage in very young and/or non-cooperative patients: abnormalities were identified in 21% out of 146 infants on vigabatrin, whose prevalence rose with treatment duration (Westall *et al.*, 2014) and are still persisting 10 years after discontinuation of vigabatrin (Wright *et al.*, 2017).

MRI hypersignals on T2/FLAIR and restricted diffusion-weighted imaging have also been reported within deep brain structures in 20–30% of infants vigabatrin-treated for IS, based on retrospective studies (Dracopoulos *et al.*, 2010; Pearl *et al.*, 2009; Mihl *et al.*, 2009; Wheless *et al.*, 2009). These abnormalities are usually asymptomatic, transient, and they resolve even in subjects who remain on vigabatrin therapy. Doses over 200 mg/kg/d and concomitant hormonal therapy do expose to symptomatic forms (Hussain *et al.*, 2017).

Prognosis

Prognosis of IS is highly variable, ranging from complete recovery with no residual neurological dysfunction, to drug-resistant epilepsy associated with severe developmental delay (Watanabe, 1998). Prognosis is generally poor, with only 15% to 25% of individuals having a normal developmental outcome (Riikonen, 1982).

The most important factor affecting prognosis is aetiology. In general symptomatic cases do worse than cryptogenic cases and structural abnormalities including TSC, Down syndrome, cortical malformations, hypoxic ischemic encephalopathy, and central nervous system infection (Riikonen, 2010).

IS of unknown cause comprises cases previously referred to as either cryptogenic or idiopathic. The so called "idiopathic" cases have the best outcome in terms of seizures and cognitive outcome. A meta-analysis of IS suggested that 54% of the cryptogenic IS subgroup had favorable neurodevelopment outcomes (Widjaja *et al.*, 2015).

Among patients with unknown cause, poor prognosis and subsequent seizures are common. Normal development prior to IS and response to first line therapy are predictors of more favourable outcomes, as well as initiation of treatment within one month of IS onset. On the contrary, predictors of worse outcome include younger age of IS onset, seizures prior to IS, and refractory IS (Gul Mert *et al.*, 2017; Yuskaitisa *et al.*, 2018; Widjaja *et al.*, 2015).

Current practice and future directions

There are variations around the world in the choice of first line therapy for IS mainly depending on the local use, but clearly etiology is the major factor both for spasm cessation and cognitive outcome: vigabatrin is more effective in TSC and dysplasia whereas hormonal therapy is in anoxo-ischemic and cryptogenic forms. On another hand, both therapies have side effects, although different in potential severity: vigabatrin induces peripheral visual field loss in about 20% of cases and transient hypersignals on MRI, and hormonal therapy carries a mortality rate up to 5%.

Based on open data showing that more than one third of infants will respond to a second standard drug after the first one has failed (Knupp *et al.*, 2016b), the recent ICISS trial compared first line hormonal therapy with vigabatrin to hormonal therapy alone in 377 patients (TSC excluded). Combined treatment resulted in more responders (72%) (seizure free between days 14 and 42) than hormonal monotherapy (57%, $p < 0.002$) (O'Callaghan *et al.*, 2017).

Reducing vigabatrin toxicity is therefore a key question. Since the risk of visual field loss is exposure dependent, treatment duration and maintenance dose should be reduced to the minimum, but the risk of intractable relapse of spasms after premature withdraw is still unpredictable (Kroll-Seger *et al.*, 2007) and the minimal effective dose is not formally testable. Optimizing the pediatric formulation, testing in humans the retinal protective effect of taurine reported in rodents (Jammoul *et al.*, 2009; Jammoul *et al.*, 2010) and developing new targets on the new animal models of infantile spasms (Kubova & Mares, 2010; Scantlebury *et al.*, 2010; Briggs *et al.*, 2014) are promising strategies.

REFERENCES ▶

Appleton RE, Montiel-Viesca F (1993): Vigabatrin in infantile spasms-why add on? *Lancet* 341: 962.

Appleton RE, Peters AC, Mumford JP, Shaw DE (1999): Randomized, placebo-controlled study of vigabatrin as first-line treatment of infantile spasms. *Epilepsia* 40: 1627–1633.

Asano E, Chugani DC, Muzik O, *et al.* (2000): Multimodality imaging for improved detection of epileptogenic lesions in children with tuberous sclerosis complex. *Neurology* 54: 1976–1984.

Asano E, Juhasz C, Shah A, *et al.* (2005): Origin and propagation of epileptic spasms delineated on electrocorticography. *Epilepsia* 46: 1086–1097.

Asarnow RF, LoPresti C, Guthrie D, *et al.* (1997): Developmental outcomes in children receiving resection surgery for medically intractable infantile spasms. *Dev Med Child Neurol* 39: 430–440.

Auvin S, Lamblin MD, Andrieux J (2009): Array-CGH detection of a *de novo* 0.7-Mb deletion in 19p13.13 including CACNA1A associated with mental retardation and epilepsy with infantile spasms. *Epilepsia* 50: 2501–2503.

Auvin S, Lamblin MD, Pandit F, Vallée L, Bouvet-Mourcia A (2010): Infantile epileptic encephalopathy with late-onset spasms: report of 19 patients. *Epilepsia* 51: 1290–1296.

Avanzini G, Panzica F, Franceschetti S (2007): West syndrome revised. In: Guzzetta F, Dalla Bernardina B, Guerrini R (eds) *Progress in Epileptic Spasms and West Syndrome*, pp. 15–22. Paris: John Libbey Eurotext.

Baram TZ, Mitchell WG, Tournay A, Snead OC, Hanson RA, Horton EJ (1996): High-dose corticotropin (ACTH) *versus* prednisone for infantile spasms: a prospective, randomized, blinded study. *Pediatrics* 97: 375–379.

Berg AT, Berkovic SF, Brodie MJ, *et al.* (2010): Revised terminology and concept for organization of seizures and epilepsies: report of the ILAE Commission on Classification and Terminology, 2005–2009. *Epilepsia* 51: 676–685.

Bisulli F, Volpi L, Meletti S, *et al.* (2002): Ictal pattern of EEG and muscular activation in symptomatic infantile spasms: a videopolygraphic and computer analysis. *Epilepsia* 43: 1559–1563.

Briggs SW, Mowrey W, Hall CB, Galanopoulou AS (2014): CPP-115, a vigabatrin analogue, decreases spasms in the multiple-hit rat model of infantile spasms. *Epilepsia* 55: 94–102.

Caraballo R, Fejerman N, Dalla Bernardina B, *et al.* (2003): Epileptic spasms in clusters without hypsarrhythmia. *Epilepsia* 5: 109–113.

Caraballo R, Ruggieri V, Gonzalez G, *et al.* (2011): Infantile spasms without hypsarrhythmia: a study of 16 cases. *Seizure* 20: 197–202.

Chiron C, Dulac O, Beaumont D, Palacios L, Pajot N, Mumford J (1991): Therapeutic trial of vigabatrin in refractory infantile spasms. *J Child Neurol* 6 (Suppl 2): S52-S59.

Chiron C, Dulac O, Bulteau C, *et al.* (1993): Study of regional cerebral blood flow in West syndrome. *Epilepsia* 34: 707–715.

Chiron C, Dumas C, Jambaque I, Mumford J, Dulac O (1997): Randomized trial comparing vigabatrin and hydrocortisone in infantile spasms due to tuberous sclerosis. *Epilepsy Res* 26: 389–395.

Chugani HT, Conti JR (1996): Etiologic classification of infantile spasms in 140 cases: role of positron emission tomography. *J Child Neurol* 11: 44–48.

Chugani HT, Shields WD, Shewmon DA, Olson DM, Phelps ME, Peacock WJ (1990): Infantile spasms: I. PET identifies focal cortical dysgenesis in cryptogenic cases for surgical treatment. *Ann Neurol* 27: 406–413.

Chugani HT, Shewmon DA, Sankar R, Chen BC, Phelps ME (1992): Infantile spasms: II. Lenticular nuclei and brainstem activation on positron emission tomography. *Ann Neurol* 31: 212–219.

Chugani HT, Shewmon DA, Shields WD, *et al.* (1993): Surgery for intractable infantile spasms: neuroimaging perspectives. *Epilepsia* 34: 764–771.

Chugani HT, Da Silva E, Chugani DC (1996): Infantile spasms: III. Prognostic implications of bitemporal hypometabolism on positron emission tomography. *Ann Neurol* 39: 643–649.

Chugani DC, Chugani HT, Muzik O, *et al.* (1998): Imaging epileptogenic tubers in children with tuberous sclerosis complex using alpha-[11C]methyl-L-tryptophan positron emission tomography. *Ann Neurol* 44: 858–866.

Chugani HT, Luat AF, Kumar A, Govindan R, Pawlik K, Asano E (2013): Alpha-[11C]-methyl-L-tryptophan PET in 191 patients with tuberous sclerosis complex. *Neurology* 81: 674–680.

Chugani HT, Asano E, Juhasz C, Kumar A, Kupsky WJ, Sood S (2014): "Subtotal" hemispherectomy in children with intractable focal epilepsy. *Epilepsia* 55: 1926–1933.

Chugani HT, Ilyas M, Kumar A, Juhasz C, Kupsky WJ, Sood S, Asano E (2015): Surgical treatment for refractory epileptic spasms: The Detroit series. *Epilepsia* 56: 1941–1949.

Commission on Classification and Terminology of the International League Against Epilepsy. (1981): Proposal for revised clinical and electrographic classification of epileptic seizures. *Epilepsia* 22: 489–501.

Commission on Classification and Terminology of the International League Against Epilepsy. (1989): Proposal for revised classification of epilepsies and epileptic syndromes. *Epilepsia* 30: 389–399.

Darke K, Edwards SW, Hancock E, *et al.* (2010): Developmental and epilepsy outcomes at age 4 years in the UKISS trial comparing hormonal treatments to vigabatrin for infantile spasms: a multi-centre randomized trial. *Arch Dis Child* 95: 382–386.

Debus O, Kurlemann G (2004): Sulthiame in the primary therapy of West syndrome: A randomized double-blind placebo-controlled add-on trial on baseline pyridoxine medication. *Epilepsia* 45: 103–108.

Demarest ST, Shellhaas RA, Gaillard WD, *et al.* (2017): Pediatric Epilepsy Research Consortium. The impact of hypsarrhythmia on infantile spasms treatment response: Observational cohort study from the National Infantile Spasms Consortium. *Epilepsia*. 58: 2098–2103.

Desguerre I, Marti I, Valayannopoulos V, *et al.* (2008): Transient magnetic resonance diffusion abnormalities in West syndrome: the radiological expression of non-convulsive status epilepticus? *Dev Med Child Neurol* 50: 112–116.

Dilber C, Caliskan M, Sonmezoglu K, *et al.* (2013): Positron emission tomography findings in children with infantile spasms and autism. *J Clin Neurosci* 20: 373–376.

Djuric M, Kravljanac R, Tadic B, Mrlje-Popovic N, Appleton RE (2014): In response to: Long-term outcome in children with infantile spasms treated with vigabatrin: A cohort of 180 patients. *Epilepsia*. 56: 809–810.

Dracopoulos A, Widjaja E, Raybaud C, Westall CA, Snead OC III. (2010): Vigabatrin-associated reversible MRI signal changes in patients with infantile spasms. *Epilepsia* 51: 1297–1304.

Dreifuss F, Farwell J, Holmes G, *et al.* (1986): Infantile spasms. Comparative trial of nitrazepam and corticotropin. *Arch Neurol* 43: 1107–1110.

Dulac O, Plouin P, Jambaqué I (1993): Predicting favorable outcome in idiopathic West syndrome. *Epilepsia* 34: 747–756.

Dulac O, Bast T, Dalla Bernardina B, Gaily E, Neville B (2010): Infantile spasms: toward a selective diagnostic and therapeutic approach. *Epilepsia* 51: 2218–2219.

Eisermann M, Ville D, Soufflet C, *et al.* (2006): Cryptogenic late-onset epileptic spasms: an overlooked syndrome of early childhood. *Epilepsia* 47: 1035–1042.

El Sabbagh S, Lebre AS, Bahi-Buisson N, *et al.* (2010): Epileptic phenotypes in children with respiratory chain disorders. *Epilepsia* 51: 1225–1235.

Elterman RD, Shields WD, Bittman RM, Torri SA, Sagar SM, Collins SD (2010): Vigabatrin for the treatment of infantile spasms: final report of a randomized trial. *J Child Neurol* 25: 1340–1347.

Engel J Jr (2001): A proposed diagnostic scheme for people with epileptic seizures and with epilepsy: Report of the ILAE task force on classification and terminology. *Epilepsia* 42: 769–803.

Engel J Jr (2006): Report of the ILAE classification core group. *Epilepsia* 47: 1558–1568.

Fisher RS, Cross JH, French JA, *et al.* (2017): Operational classification of seizure types by the International League Against Epilepsy: Position Paper of the ILAE Commission for Classification and Terminology. *Epilepsia* 58: 522–530.

Fusco L, Vigevano F (1993): Ictal clinical electroencephalographic findings of spasms in West syndrome. *Epilepsia* 34: 671–678.

Gaily E, Jonsson H, Lappi M (2009): Visual fields at school-age in children treated with vigabatrin in infancy. *Epilepsia* 50: 206–216.

Gul Mert G, Herguner MO, Incecik F, Altunbasak S, Sahan D, Unal I (2017): Risk factors affecting prognosis in infantile spasm. *Int J Neurosci* 127: 1012–1018.

Gobbi G, Bruno L, Pini A, Giovanardi Rossi P, Tassinari CA (1987): Periodic spasms: an unclassified type of epileptic seizures in childhood. *Dev Med Child Neurol* 29: 766–775.

Greco M, Ferrara P, Farello G, Striano P, Verrotti A (2018): Electroclinical features of epilepsy associated with 1p36 deletion syndrome: A review. *Epilepsy Res* 139: 92–101.

Haga Y, Watanabe K, Negoro T, *et al.* (1995): Do ictal, clinical and electroencephalographic features predict outcome in West syndrome? *Pediatr Neurol* 13: 226–229.

Haginoya K, Munakata M, Yokoyama H, *et al.* (2001): Mechanism of tonic spasms in West syndrome viewed from ictal SPECT findings. *Brain Dev* 23: 496–501.

Hamano S, Higurashi N, Koichihara R, *et al.* (2010): Interictal cerebral blood flow abnormality in cryptogenic West syndrome. *Epilepsia* 51: 1259–1265.

Hong AM, Turner Z, Hamdy RF, Kossoff EH (2010): Infantile spasms treated with the ketogenic diet: prospective single-center experience in 104 consecutive infants. *Epilepsia* 51: 1403–1407.

Hrachovy RA, Frost JD Jr, Kellaway P, Zion TE (1983): Double-blind study of ACTH *vs.* prednisone therapy in infantile spasms. *J Pediatr* 103: 641–645.

Hussain SA, Tsao J, Li M, *et al.* (2017): Risk of vigabatrin-associated brain abnormalities on MRI in the treatment of infantile spasms is dose-dependent. *Epilepsia* 58: 674–682.

Ito M, Aiba H, Hashimoto K, *et al.* (2002): Low-dose ACTH therapy for West syndrome: Initial effects and long-term outcome. *Neurology* 58: 110–114.

Ilyas M, Sivaswamy L, Asano E, Sood S, Zidan M, Chugani H. (2014): Seizure control following palliative resective surgery for intractable epilepsy-a pilot study. *Pediatr Neurol* 51 : 330–335.

Itomi K, Okumura A, Negoro T, *et al.* (2002): Prognostic value of positron emission tomography in cryptogenic West syndrome. *Dev Med Child Neurol* 44: 107–111.

Jammoul F, Wang Q, Nabbout R, *et al.* (2009): Taurine deficiency is a cause of vigabatrin-induced retinal phototoxicity. *Ann Neurol* 65: 98–107.

Jammoul F, Degardin J, Pain D, *et al.* (2010): Taurine deficiency damages photoreceptors and retinal ganglion cells in vigabatrin-treated neonatal rats. *Mol Cell Neurosci* 43: 414–421.

Jonas R, Asarnow RF, LoPresti C, *et al.* (2005): Surgery for symptomatic infant-onset epileptic encephalopathy with and without infantile spasms. *Neurology* 64: 746–750.

Kagawa K, Chugani DC, Asano E, *et al.* (2005): Epilepsy surgery outcome in children with tuberous sclerosis complex evaluated with alpha-[11C]methyl-L-tryptophan positron emission tomography (PET). *J Child Neurol* 20: 429–438.

Kakisaka Y, Haginoya K, Ishitobi M, *et al.* (2009): Utility of subtraction ictal SPECT images in detecting focal leading activity and understanding the pathophysiology of spasms in patients with West syndrome. *Epilepsy Res* 83: 177–183.

Kellaway P, Hrachovy RA, Frost JD, Zion T (1979): Precise characterization and quantification of infantile spasms. *Ann Neurol* 6: 214–218.

Knupp KG, Coryell J, Nickels KC, *et al.* (2016a): Pediatric Epilepsy Research Consortium. Response to treatment in a prospective national infantile spasms cohort. *Ann Neurol* 79: 475–484.

Knupp KG, Leister E, Coryell J, *et al.* (2016b): Pediatric Epilepsy Research Consortium. Response to second treatment after initial failed treatment in a multicenter prospective infantile spasms cohort. *Epilepsia* 57: 1834–1842.

Kobayashi K, Oka M, Akiyama T, *et al.* (2004): Very fast rhythmic activity on scalp EEG associated with epileptic spasms. *Epilepsia* 45: 488–496.

Koch M (1999): The neurobiology of startle. *Progr Neurobiol* 59: 107–128.

Kossoff EH, Hartman AL, Rubenstein JE, Vining EP (2009): High-dose oral prednisolone for infantile spasms: an effective and less expensive alternative to ACTH. *Epilepsy Behav* 14: 674–676.

Kroll-Seger J, Kaminska A, Moutard ML, *et al.* (2007): Severe relapse of epilepsy after vigabatrin withdrawal: for how long should we treat symptomatic infantile spasms? *Epilepsia* 48: 612–613.

Kubova H, Mares P (2010): Vigabatrin but not valproate prevents development of age-specific flexion seizures induced by N-methyl-D-aspartate (NMDA) in immature rats. *Epilepsia* 51: 469–472.

Levey EB, Stashinko E, Clegg NJ, Delgado MR (2010): Management of children with holoprosencephaly. *Am J Med* Genet C *Semin Med* Genet 154C: 183–190.

Lux AL (2007): Is hypsarrhythmia a form of non-convulsive status epilepticus in infants? *Acta Neurol Scand* 186: 37–44.

Lux AL, Osborne JP (2004): A proposal for case definitions and outcome measures in studies of infantile spasms and West syndrome: consensus statement of the West Delphi Group. *Epilepsia* 45: 1416–1428.

Lux AL, Edwards SW, Hancock E, *et al.* (2004): The United Kingdom Infantile Spasms Study comparing vigabatrin with prednisolone or tetracosactide at 14 days: A multicentre, randomised controlled trial. *Lancet* 364: 1773–1778.

Lux AL, Edwards SW, Hancock E, *et al.* (2005): The United Kingdom Infantile Spasms Study (UKISS) comparing hormone treatment with vigabatrin on developmental and epilepsy outcomes to age 14 months: a multicentre randomized trial. *Lancet Neurol* 4: 712–717.

Maguire MJ, Hemming K, Wild JM, Hutton JL, Marson AG (2010): Prevalence of visual field loss following exposure to vigabatrin therapy: a systematic review. *Epilepsia* 51: 2423–2431.

Matricardi S, Darra F, Spalice A, *et al.* (2018): Electroclinical findings and long-term outcomes in epileptic patients with inv dup (15). *Acta Neurol Scand* 137: 575–581.

Mei D, Marini C, Novara F, *et al.* (2010): Xp22.3 genomic deletions involving the CDKL5 gene in girls with early onset epileptic encephalopathy. *Epilepsia* 51: 647–656.

Metsahonkala L, Gaily E, Rantala H, *et al.* (2002): Focal and global cortical hypometabolism in patients with newly diagnosed infantile spasms. *Neurology* 58: 1646–1651.

Michaud JL, Lachance M, Hamdan FF, *et al.* (2014): The genetic landscape of infantile spasms. *Hum Mol Genet* 23: 4846–4858.

Milh M, Villeneuve N, Chapon F, *et al.* (2009): Transient brain magnetic resonance imaging hyperintensity in basal ganglia and brain stem of epileptic infants treated with vigabatrin. *J Child Neurol* 24: 305–315.

Mori K, Toda Y, Hashimoto T, *et al.* (2007): Patients with West syndrome whose ictal SPECT showed focal cortical hyperperfusion. *Brain Dev* 29: 202–209.

Natsume J, Maeda N, Itomi K, *et al.* (2014): PET in infancy predicts long-term outcome during adolescence in cryptogenic West syndrome. *AJNR Am J Neuroradiol* 35: 1580–1585.

O'Callaghan FJ, Lux AL, Darke K, *et al.* (2011): The effect of lead time to treatment and of age of onset on developmental outcome at 4 years in infantile spasms: evidence from the United Kingdom Infantile Spasms Study. *Epilepsia*. 52: 1359–1364.

O'Callaghan FJ, Edwards SW, Alber FD, *et al.* (2017): Safety and effectiveness of hormonal treatment *versus* hormonal treatment with vigabatrin for infantile spasms (ICISS): a randomised, multicentre, open-label trial. *Lancet Neurol* 16: 33–42.

Oguni H, Funatsuka M, Sasaki K, *et al.* (2005): Effect of ACTH therapy for epileptic spasms without hypsarrhythmia. *Epilepsia* 46: 709–715.

Oguni H, Yanagaki S, Hayashi K, *et al.* (2006): Extremely low-dose ACTH step-up protocol for West syndrome: maximum therapeutic effect with minimal side effects. *Brain Dev* 28: 8–13.

Oka M, Kobayashi K, Akiyama T, Ogino T, Oka E (2004): A study of spike-density on EEG in West syndrome. *Brain Dev* 26: 105–112.

Osborne JP, Lux AL, Edwards SW, *et al.* (2010): The underlying etiology of infantile spasms (West syndrome): information from the United Kingdom Infantile Spasms Study (UKISS) on contemporary causes and their classification. *Epilepsia* 51: 2168–2174.

Pachatz C, Fusco L, Vigevano F (2003): Epileptic spasms and partial seizures as a single ictal event. *Epilepsia* 44: 693–700.

Parmeggiani A, Plouin P, Dulac O (1990): Quantification of diffuse and focal delta activity in hypsarrhythmia. *Brain Dev* 12: 310–315.

Panzica F, Franceschetti F, Binelli S, Canafoglia L, Granata T, Avanzini G (1999): Spectral properties of EEG fast activity ictal discharges associated with infantile spasms. *Clin Neurophysiol* 110: 593–603.

Panzica F, Binelli S, Granata T, Freri E, Visani E, Franceschetti S (2007): Ictal fast EEG discharges in infantile spasms, from onset to outcome. *Clin Neurophysiol* 117 (Suppl 1): S144-S145.

Pearl PL, Vezina LG, Saneto RP, McCarter R, Molloy-Wells E, Heffron A (2009): Cerebral MRI abnormalities associated with vigabatrin therapy. *Epilepsia* 50: 184–194.

Pereira AG, Bahi-Buisson N, Barnerias C, *et al.* (2017): Epileptic spasms in congenital disorders of glycosylation. *Epileptic Disord* 19: 15–23.

Plouin P, Jalin C, Dulac O, Chiron C (1987): Enregistrement ambulatoire de l'EEG pendant 24 heures dans les spasmes infantiles épileptiques. *Rev EEG Neurophysiol Clin* 17: 309–318.

Reiter E, Tiefenthaler M, Freillinger M, Bernert G, Seidl R, Hauser E (2000): Familial idiopathic West syndrome. *J Child Neurol* 15: 249–252.

Riikonen R. (1982): A long-term follow-up study of 214 children with the syndrome of infantile spasms. *Neuropediatrics* 13: 14–23.

Riikonen R (2001): Epidemiological data of West syndrome in Finland. *Brain Dev* 23: 539–541.

Riikonen RS (2010): Favorable prognostic factors with infantile spasms. *Eur J Paediatr Neurol* 14: 13–18.

Riikonen R, Rener-Primec Z, Carmant L, Dorofeeva M, Hollody K, Szabo I (2015): Does vigabatrin treatment for infantile spasms cause visual field defects? An international multicentre study. *Dev Med Child Neurol* 57: 60–67.

Scantlebury MH, Galanopoulou AS, Chudomelova L, Raffo E, Betancourth D, Moshe SL (2010): A model of symptomatic infantile spasms syndrome. *Neurobiol Dis* 37: 604–612.

Scheffer IE, Berkovic S, Capovilla G, *et al.* (2017): ILAE classification of the epilepsies: Position paper of the ILAE Commission for Classification and Terminology. *Epilepsia* 58: 512–521.

Schlumberger E, Dulac O (1994): A simple, effective and well-tolerated treatment regime for West syndrome. *Dev Med Child Neurol* 36: 863–872.

Shoubridge C, Fullston T, Gécz J (2010): ARX spectrum disorders: making inroads into the molecular pathology. *Hum Mutat* 31: 889–900.

Specchio N, Trivisano M, Vigevano F, Fusco L (2010): Idiopathic West syndrome followed by childhood absence epilepsy. *Seizure* 19: 383–393.

Trevathan E, Murphy CC, Yeargin-Allsopp M (1999): The descriptive epidemiology of infantile spasms among Atlanta children. *Epilepsia* 40: 748–751.

Vanhatalo S, Nousiainen I, Eriksson K, *et al.* (2002): Visual field constriction in 91 Finnish children treated with vigabatrin. *Epilepsia* 43: 748–756.

Vigevano F, Fusco L, Cusmai R, Claps D, Ricci S, Milani L (1993): The idiopathic form of West syndrome. *Epilepsia* 34: 743–746.

Vigevano F, Cilio MR (1997): Vigabatrin *versus* ACTH as first-line treatment for infantile spasms: a randomized, prospective study. *Epilepsia* 38: 1270–1274.

Watanabe K (1998): West syndrome: etiological and prognostic aspects. *Brain Dev* 20: 1–8.

Watanabe K, Negoro T, Aso K, Matsumoto A (1993): Reappraisal of interictal electroencephalograms in infantile spasms. *Epilepsia* 34: 679–685.

Westall CA, Wright T, Cortese F, Kumarappah A, Snead OC. 3rd, Buncic JR (2014): Vigabatrin retinal toxicity in children with infantile spasms: An observational cohort study. *Neurology* 83: 2262–2268.

Wheless JW, Carmant L, Bebin M, Conry JA, Chiron C, Elterman RD (2009): Magnetic resonance imaging abnormalities associated with vigabatrin in patients with epilepsy. *Epilepsia* 50: 195–205.

Widjaja E, Go C, McCoy B, Snead OC (2015): Neurodevelopmental outcome of infantile spasms: a systematic review and meta-analysis. *Epilepsy Res* 109: 155–162.

Wild JM, Chiron C, Ahn H, *et al.* (2009): Visual field loss in patients with refractory partial epilepsy treated with vigabatrin: final results from an open-label, observational, multicentre study. *CNS Drugs* 23: 965–982.

Wright T, Kumarappah A, Stavropoulos A, Reginald A, Buncic JR, Westall CA (2017): Vigabatrin toxicity in infancy is associated with retinal defect in adolescence: A Prospective Observational Study. *Retina* 37: 858–866.

Yuskaitisa CJ, Ruzhnikovb MRZ, Howellc KB, *et al.* (2018): Infantile Spasms of Unknown Cause: Predictors of Outcome and Genotype-Phenotype Correlation. *Pediatric Neurol*: 1–9.

Zou LP, Wang X, Dong CH, Chen CH, Zhao W, Zhao RY (2010): Three-week combination treatment with ACTH + magnesium sulfate *versus* ACTH monotherapy for infantile spasms: A 24-week, randomized, open-label, follow-up study in China. *Clin Ther* 32: 692–700.

WITH VIDEO SUPPLEMENTS

CHAPTER 9

FEBRILE SEIZURES AND GENETIC EPILEPSY WITH FEBRILE SEIZURES PLUS (GEFS+)

Peter R. Camfield[1], Carol S. Camfield[1], Nancy A. McNamara[2], Renee A. Shellhaas[2], Carla Marini[3] and Ingrid E. Scheffer[4]

[1] Department of Pediatrics, IWK Health Centre and Dalhousie University, Halifax, Nova Scotia, Canada
[2] Department of Pediatrics, University of Michigan, Ann Arbor, Michigan, USA
[3] Child Neurology Unit, Children's Hospital A. Meyer, Florence, Italy
[4] Epilepsy Research Centre, Department of Medicine, the University of Melbourne, Austin Health, Department of Paediatrics, the University of Melbourne, Royal Children's Hospital, Florey and Murdoch Children's Research Institutes, Melbourne, Australia

Introduction

Febrile seizures are the most common convulsive event in humans. The lifetime risk of a seizure of any kind is estimated at 8% - half of these events will be febrile seizures (Hauser & Kurland, 1975). Overall, 4–5% of the population will have at least one febrile seizure (Nelson & Ellenberg, 1978; Verity *et al.*, 1985), but estimates of 6–14% are made for Finland, Japan and Pacific islands (Sillanpaa *et al.*, 2008, Stanhope, 1972; Tsuboi, 1984).

Based on a massive literature (4,806 articles listed in PubMed in 2017) there is consensus about the following. Febrile seizures do not cause brain damage or intellectual decline. The risk of subsequent epilepsy is only 2–5% and the risk of a recurrent febrile seizure after a first is about 30–40%. Children with febrile seizures when compared with controls have the same school performance, academic achievement, personality, behavior and later use of healthcare resources. Children with febrile seizures do not have an increased risk of premature death (Vestergaard & Christensen, 2009).

There has been controversy about how "benign" febrile seizures are arising from the tension between primary care physicians who clearly see the benign outcome and neurologists who focus on patients who develop severe epilepsies and developmental delay. In terms of etiology, febrile seizures are the archetype of a gene-environment interaction, but little is understood regarding the mechanisms involved. Nonetheless, many of the issues were settled by large, robust studies reported 30–40 years ago. This chapter is largely devoted to areas where a controversy persists.

Definition

In 1980 an influential Consensus Conference in the USA defined febrile seizures as "an event in infancy or childhood, usually occurring between 3 months and 5 years of age, associated with fever but without evidence of intracranial infection or defined cause" (Consensus Development Panel, 1980). The event in question is typically a brief generalized tonic-clonic seizure (GTCS), although focal seizures are noted in about 8% and seizures longer than 20 minutes are seen in about 5% (Annegers *et al.*, 1987; Nelson & Ellenberg, 1976). The temperature is usually high, typically greater than 38.5° C. Since frantic parents are the only witnesses of most febrile seizures, and they often believe that their child is dying when they witness a febrile seizure, the details about the seizure, such as the duration and focality, may be inaccurate. Other events that occur with fever must be carefully excluded. Rigors, febrile delirium, febrile myoclonus (Rajakumar & Bodensteiner, 1996) and syncope triggered by illness are most important (Stephenson, 1990).

Of particular interest are "illness-related" seizures without fever (Lee & Ong, 2004; Zerr *et al.*, 2005; Verrotti *et al.*, 2014). Many of these seizures are related to diarrheal illnesses. The seizures are similar to febrile seizures – typically brief and the age range is the same. Many of these children subsequently experience febrile seizures and approximately 7% later develop epilepsy.

Two related epileptic syndromes may present with febrile seizures and initially be difficult to distinguish from febrile seizures: Dravet syndrome (previously called severe myoclonic epilepsy of infancy) and Febrile seizures Plus (FS+) (often seen in a family with the Genetic Epilepsy with Febrile Seizures Plus (GEFS+) spectrum). In Dravet syndrome prolonged focal or generalized febrile seizures in the first year of life (typically beginning at about 6 months of age) are followed by devastating intractable epilepsy and intellectual disability. This disorder is uncommon and is discussed in detail in Chapter 10. GEFS+ is discussed in detail at the end this chapter.

Etiology

The biologic basis of febrile seizures remains unsolved, but is related to several main features: immature brain, fever, inflammation, trace elements and blood gases, and genetic predisposition.

Brain maturation

Because febrile seizures rarely occur before age 6 months or after age 5 years, there is a clear relationship with brain maturation. The nature of this maturation process is unclear but could be related to increasing myelination, "dying back" of excessive neurons, and/or increasing synaptic complexity. Animal studies have demonstrated enhanced neuronal excitability during normal brain maturation (Jenssen & Baram, 2000), which may contribute to the age-related susceptibility of children to febrile seizures.

Infection

In previous decades the causes of fever associated with febrile seizures included upper respiratory tract infection or pharyngitis (38%), otitis media (23%), pneumonia (15%), gastroenteritis (7%), roseola infantum (5%), and noninfectious illness (12%) (Nelson & Ellenberg 1978; Lewis *et al.*, 1979). As a result of current vaccines there are now fewer infections from *Haemophilus Influenzae*, varicella, peumococcus and meningococcus. Viral infections predominate (Millichap & Millichap, 2006) especially influenza A (Chung & Wong 2007; Hara *et al.*, 2007), human corona virus HKU1 (Lau *et al.*, 2006) and human herpes virus type 6 (HHV6) (Suga *et al.*, 2000) which causes roseola, a common infection of infants and toddlers typically with high fever. In a systematic review and meta-analysis, HHV6 virus was found in 119/592 (21%) of febrile seizure cases (Mohammadpour-Touserkani, 2017). It is postulated that direct viral invasion of the brain by HHV6, combined with fever, causes the initial febrile seizure. Reactivation of the virus by fever during subsequent illnesses may cause recurrent febrile seizures.

Vaccines

About 10% of febrile seizures occur within 2 weeks of receipt of a vaccination (Francis, 2016). The mechanism seems to be the induction of fever by the vaccine products. The most infamous of these vaccines is whole cell diphtheria-pertussis-tetanus (DPT). The frequency of febrile seizures after whole cell DPT is estimated at 6–9 per 100,000 children and after measles vaccine 24–25 per 100,000 children. The newer routinely used acellular pertussis vaccines rarely induce a febrile reaction, which in Canada led to a 79% decrease in DPT vaccine related febrile seizures (Le Saux *et al.*, 2003).

Combinations of vaccines have been studied and there is good evidence that coadministration of influenza vaccine with pneumococcal conjugate and DTP leads to a slight increase in the risk of febrile seizures. There were 30 more febrile seizures per 100,000 vaccinated children with these combinations compared with giving these vaccines on separate days (Duffy *et al.*, 2016). With measles, mumps, rubella (MMR) combined vaccines, the incidence of febrile seizures may be up to 70 per 100,000 (Jacobsen *et al.*, 2009; Vestergaard & Christensen 2009) and when MMR is combined with varicella vaccine (MMRV), there is an estimated one additional febrile seizure for every ~2,500 children in the febrile seizure age range compared with separate MMR and varicella vaccine administration (Klein *et al.*, 2010; Ma *et al.*, 2015; Committee on Infectious Diseases, 2011).

It appears that most vaccine related febrile seizures should be regarded as "ordinary febrile seizures" triggered by fever induced by the vaccine (Hirtz *et al.*, 1983a). Their subsequent clinical course is identical to other febrile seizures (Hirtz *et al.*, 1983b), with no increased risk for subsequent afebrile seizures or abnormal neurologic development (Barlow *et al.*, 2001; Sun *et al.*, 2012; Tartof *et al.*, 2014). The significant benefit from these highly effective and lifesaving vaccines should be weighed against the very minor risk of a febrile seizure (Maglione *et al.*, 2014).

In contrast to other vaccines, there is convincing evidence that children who receive rotavirus vaccine have a lower risk of febrile seizures (Sheridan *et al.*, 2016). This vaccine rarely causes fever itself; therefore, the net effect of the vaccine is to reduce the number of febrile episodes in the febrile seizure age range by decreasing rotavirus infections.

Cytokines

Activation of the cytokine network has been postulated to play a role in febrile seizures. Studies have indicated that this is a complex relationship. Increased susceptibility to febrile seizures has been associated with specific interleukin alleles (Tsai *et al.*, 2002; Virta *et al.*, 2002; Kanemoto *et al.*, 2003; Kira *et al.*, 2005; Serdaroglu *et al.*, 2001); whereas, other alleles may be protective (Ishizaki *et al.*, 2009). A specific polymorhphism of the TNF-A (tumor necrosis factor) gene has shown an association with febrile seizures (Zare-Shahbadi, 2015). It has been suggested that circulating toxins and immune reaction products modulate neuronal excitability. One study showed that in the presence of viral RNA, the leukocytes of children who had febrile seizures produced more interleukin-1β than those of healthy controls (Matsuo *et al.*, 2006), and interleukin-1β may promote hyperthermia-induced seizures in young rats (Fukuda *et al.*, 2009, and summarized in Gallentine *et al.*, 2017). However, others have reported no significant role of interleukin-1β, interleukin-1α, or interleukin-1Ra in the pathogenesis of febrile seizures (Haspolat *et al.*, 2005; Tomoum *et al.*, 2007). The varying results of individual studies were summarized in a recent systematic review that highlighted the possibility that inflammatory mediators of temporal lobe epilepsy may differ from those of febrile seizures (de Vries *et al.*, 2016).

IL-1β plays an important role in fever and inflammation and there have been a number of studies associating certain IL-1β polymorphisms with febrile seizures. In 2012 Wu provided a careful meta-analysis of the association of the polymorphism IL-1β -511 C/T with febrile seizures and concluded that there was an important association in Asia but not in Europe (Wu *et al.*, 2012) The authors suggested that different genetic backgrounds may influence the febrile seizure tendency.

Cytokines might influence the febrile seizure tendency by increasing fever (some cytokines are endogenous pyrogens) or by influencing brain development. A recent study (Kim *et al.*, 2017) compared seven serum cytokine levels in four groups of toddlers presenting to an emergency room: i) fever and febrile seizure; ii) fever and remote history of febrile seizures; iii) fever with no history of febrile seizures; or iv) no fever but recent afebrile seizure. They found that "pro-inflammatory cytokines, including IFN-γ, IL-6, and IL-8 and anti-inflammatory cytokines (including IL-1Ra and IL-10) were increased in children with febrile seizures." They also reported that anti-inflammatory cytokines (IL-10 and IL- 1Ra) were increased which suggested to the authors that these compounds played a role in protecting from or limiting the severity of febrile seizures. The ratio of specific interleukins may be more important than the absolute serum or CSF levels. For example, lower IL-1β to IL-IRA ratios are thought to result in decreased systemic/brain inflammation and increased seizure threshold, and a large imbalance between IL-1RA and IL-6 is hypothesized to be a risk factor for acute hippocampal injury associated with febrile status epilepticus (Gallentine *et al.*, 2017).

Finally, there has been an association reported between transforming growth factor beta (TGFB) and febrile seizures (Shahrokhi *et al.*, 2015). TGFB is of particular interest because it plays a role in cellular differentiation and proliferation but also may be part of the inflammatory reaction that occurs with seizures (Vezzani *et al.*, 2013).

We conclude that inflammatory cytokines likely have a role in a child's susceptibility to febrile seizures but exactly which cytokines are most important remains uncertain.

Trace metals and anemia

Zn^{2+} is essential for a number of biological functions. Much of the Zn^{2+} in the brain is protein-bound; however, a noteworthy proportion of free Zn^{2+} is found in synaptic vesicles and is released in an activity-dependent manner. Based on a meta-analysis, it appears that there is a strong association between low blood and/or CSF levels of Zn^{2+} and an increased risk of febrile seizures (Saghazadeh *et al.*, 2015). A recent paper (Reid *et al.*, 2017) reviewed several clinical studies which demonstrate that Zn^{2+} levels are significantly lower in blood and cerebrospinal fluid of children experiencing a febrile seizure. Likewise, several animal models demonstrate that low levels of brain Zn^{2+} increase seizure susceptibility. A recent publication (Hildebrand *et al.*, 2015) provides "human genetic evidence that disruption of brain Zn^{2+} homeostasis at the level of the synapse" is associated with increased seizure susceptibility.

Low blood selenium levels have been found in three case controlled studies in children with febrile seizures compared with controls (Mahyar *et al.*, 2010; Akbayram *et al.*, 2012; Khoshdel *et al.*, 2013). The connection between low selenium and seizures is not simple. It is postulated that low selenium leads to a reduction in glutathione peroxidase which is important in antioxidative defence. The link between antioxidative defense and febrile seizures is unclear.

Iron deficiency anemia has been reported to be associated with febrile seizures. A meta-analysis that included 17 studies with 2,416 patients with febrile seizures and 2,387 controls concluded that there was a reasonably strong relationship between febrile seizures and iron deficiency anemia (OR, 1.98; 95% CI, 1.26–3.13; P = 0.003), although the relationship was primarily related to iron deficiency assessed by serum ferritin rather than by serum iron (Kwak *et al.*, 2017). A second meta-analysis also found an association between febrile seizures and iron deficiency anemia. Iron deficiency was 1.5 times more common in those with febrile seizures than controls (Habibian *et al.*, 2014). Not surprisingly, the association was most impressive in populations with mild-moderate rates of iron deficiency compared with populations with high rates of iron deficiency. When many subjects and controls are anemic, it is difficult to distinguish a difference related to another factor. On the other hand, this meta-analysis found that serum ferritin levels were not associated with febrile seizures; however, they did point out that ferritin blood levels vary with fever, so the timing of blood samples related to a febrile seizure might be a very important confounder. Overall, we are of the opinion that iron deficiency anemia is indeed associated with febrile seizures.

Therefore, it appears that the febrile tendency is increased with reductions in body zinc, selenium and iron. It remains unclear how important these associations are in determining how likely an individual child is to have febrile seizures and what other factors are necessary for a febrile seizure to result.

Respiratory alkalosis

In both rat pups and children a fever may lead to respiratory alkalosis from hyperventilation which causes increased cortical pH. This in turn appears to increase neuronal excitability and the likelihood of seizures (Schuchmann *et al.*, 2006; Schuchmann *et al.*, 2011). This observation lead to a case controlled study of 213 children with febrile seizures compared to a similarly febrile group of 220 children with gastroenteritis. Capillary pH was higher and blood pCO_2 lower in the febrile seizures group. The authors acknowledge that systemic and brain acidosis is common during seizures and that their febrile seizure patients were studied in the postictal period. Therefore, the role of respiratory alkalosis in the genesis of febrile seizures remains unclear.

Thermoregulation

Immaturity of thermoregulatory mechanisms (McCaughran & Schechter 1982) may contribute to susceptibility for febrile seizures. Gordon *et al.* (2009) studied children presenting to an emergency room and concluded that those with febrile seizures had higher temperatures than those presenting with febrile illness but no seizure. Holtzman *et al.* (1981) suggested that children with febrile seizures had a limited capacity to increase cellular energy metabolism at elevated temperatures.

Genetics of febrile seizures (see *Table I*)

There is a very important genetic predisposition for febrile seizures. Most febrile seizures follow complex inheritance where multiple genes are involved with an environmental contribution. Evidence for a genetic basis is drawn from classical twin and family studies. Monozygotic twins have high concordance with estimates ranging from 0.1–0.8 as compared with dizygotic twins with estimates ranging from 0.03–0.32 (Saghazadeh *et al.*, 2014). Autosomal recessive inheritance is unlikely, as there is an excess of affected parents and the risk to siblings is approximately 25% (Nelson & Ellenberg 1978). The mode of inheritance could be polygenic or even autosomal dominant with reduced penetrance in some families (Annegers *et al.*, 1982; Tsuboi & Endo, 1991; Maher & McLachlan 1997). When a child has a first degree relative with febrile seizures, the risk of febrile seizures is about 10–15% (Bethune *et al.*, 1993; van Esch *et al.*, 1998).

Multiple genes have been identified as causal for epilepsy syndromes in which febrile seizures play a major role (Winawer & Hesdorffer, 2004; Zhang *et al.*, 2017). In addition, at least 11 chromosomal loci have been associated with febrile seizures (see Saghazadeh *et al.*, 2014 for review), consistent with locus heterogeneity as expected in such a common disorder.

Because many of the gene alterations associated with FS are also associated with GEFS+, they are reviewed together at the end of this chapter following the definition and clinical features of GEFS+.

Clinical factors associated with a first febrile seizure (see *Table II*)

Factors that predict a first febrile seizure are: delayed neonatal hospital discharge, slow neurologic development as judged by parents, a parent or sibling with febrile seizures, an uncle or aunt with febrile seizures, and attendance at day care (Forsgren *et al.*, 1991; Bethune *et al.*, 1993; van Esch *et al.*, 1998). Based on the case controlled study of Bethune (75 cases and 300 controls), each of these factors is associated with a risk of 6–10% for a first febrile seizure. In the general population, only about 3% of children have two or more of these factors; however, this select group has an impressive risk of about 28% (95% confidence interval, 20–73%) for a first febrile seizure. These risk factors demonstrate the complex interactions that lead up to a febrile seizure. The child is born with an apparent genetic predisposition, which may be enhanced by other brain problems (as suggested by delayed neonatal discharge or developmental delay). Fever must occur at a critical age and day care attendance may increase the risk of infection.

Distinction between simple and complex febrile seizures

An arbitrary division of febrile seizures into simple and complex is pragmatic, but when closely examined the clinical distinction may be less precise. About 60–70% of febrile seizures are simple

Table I Molecular genetic findings of FS and GEFS+

Location	Gene	Phenotype	Relevance	Reference
8q13-q21	–	FS only	Unkown	Saghazadeh *et al.*, 2014 for review
19p	–	FS only	Unkown	
6q22-q24	–	FS only	Unkown	
18p11	–	FS only	Unkown	
21q22	–	FS only	Unkown	
3p24	–	FS only	Unkown	
5q14-q15	*GPR98*	FS only	only 1 patient	
2q24.3	*SCN1A*	FS and GEFS+	20% GEFS+	Zhang *et al.*, 2017 for review
19q13	*SCN1B*	FS+, GEFS+, TLE	5% GEFS+	
2q24.3	*SCN2A*	EE, GEFS+, FS	to be confirmed	Sugawara *et al.*, 2001; Shi *et al.*, 2012
12q13.13	*SCN8A*	EE, GEFS+	to be confirmed	Makinson *et al.*, 2016
2q24.3	*SCN9A*	FS and GEFS+	to be confirmed	Zhang *et al.*, 2017 for review
5q34	*GABRG2*	FS, CAE, GEFS+	5% GEFS+	Zhang *et al.*, 2017 for review
5q34	*GABRA1*	GEFS+, other EE	few patients	Johannesen *et al.*, 2016
15q12	*GABRB3*	FS, GEFS+, other EE	few patients	Moller *et al.*, 2017
16p11.2	*STX1B*	GEFS+	< 1% GEFS+	Schubert *et al.*, 2014
8q13	*CPA6*	FS and TLE	Unknown	Salzmann *et al.*, 2012
Xq26	*FGF13*	GEFS+	Unknown	Rigbye *et al.*, 2016
19p13.3	HCN2	GEFS+	Unknown	Dibbens *et al.*, 2010
16p13.3	CACNA1H	GEFS+	Unknown	Heron *et al.*, 2007

FS only: febrile seizures only; FS+: febrile seizures plus (see text for explanation); GEFS+: genetic epilepsy with febrile seizures plus; TLE: temporal lobe epilepsy; CAE: childhood absence epilepsy; EE: epileptic encephalopathy

Table II Febrile seizure prediction: the first event, a recurrent febrile seizure and epilepsy

	Predicting a first febrile seizure	Predicting recurrence after a first febrile seizure	Predicting epilepsy after a first febrile seizure
Family history of febrile seizures in a first degree relative	+	+	-
Developmental delay or neurologic problems	+	-	+
Complex febrile seizure (focal, prolonged, repeated)		-	+
Age of onset < 18 months		+	-
Level of temperature at first seizure		+	-
Duration of illness before seizure		+	-
Attendance at day care	+	+ (possible)	-
Family history of epilepsy			+

and 30–40% complex (Nelson & Ellenberg, 1976; Berg & Shinnar, 1996). Simple febrile seizures are generalized and brief with a single seizure per illness. Complex febrile seizures are defined by at least one of the following: focal features, prolonged duration or repeated seizures in the same illness. A Todd's paresis (transient focal postictal weakness) occurs in 0.4% of seizures (Nelson & Ellenberg, 1978). In a prospective cohort study of first febrile seizures, 35% of 428 children had one or more features of a complex febrile seizure (Berg & Shinnar, 1996). A retrospective study from Singapore reported similar findings (Lee & Ong, 2004). Postictal unconsciousness lasting more than 30 minutes, although rare, has been associated with seizures that are focal and/or last longer than five minutes (Okumura *et al.*, 2004).

For clinical practice, it may be worthwhile to emphasize that the assessment of complex *versus* simple febrile seizures may be challenging. Parents are terrified, especially with witnessing their child's first febrile seizure. We suspect that during this fright "time stands still" and an estimate of the duration of the seizure is often exaggerated. Likewise focal features may not be noted. With very careful history taking, one study reported that 81 of 106 (75%) febrile seizures had focal features (Takasu *et al.*, 2017), while most epidemiological studies have estimated the chance of focality to be only ~10%. Therefore, the length of the seizure and focal features may not be accurately reported by parents, and many "simple" febrile seizures may actually be "complex" and vice versa.

The duration of a febrile seizure to be classified as prolonged has also been explored. A sample of 158 consecutive patients presenting to a US emergency department were carefully interviewed (Hesdorffer *et al.*, 2011). There seemed to be two groupings of febrile seizure duration. For 82% the length of the seizures was estimated as ≤ 3.8 minutes while 18% had a mean seizure duration of 39.8 minutes. The cut point between these two populations was 10 minutes suggesting that a seizure longer than 10 minutes should define the duration of a prolonged febrile seizure. Patients in the prolonged group were much more likely to show "developmental delay".

Simple febrile seizures are followed by epilepsy in about 2% of cases, while complex febrile seizures have a 4–12% risk of subsequent epilepsy (Nelson & Ellenberg, 1976; Annegers *et al.*, 1987). In Rochester, Minnesota, a long term follow-up of 687 children with febrile seizures showed that only 32 (4.7%) developed epilepsy (or at least one unprovoked afebrile seizure). When epilepsy followed a simple febrile seizure, it usually was a generalized epilepsy syndrome, while complex febrile seizures tended to be followed by focal epilepsies (Annegers *et al.*, 1987). Caution about these results is warranted based on the small sample size.

It should be emphasized that if a child has a complex febrile seizure the risk of later epilepsy remains small. For example, a child with a focal, prolonged febrile seizure that repeats within the same illness still has about an 85% chance of not developing epilepsy (Nelson & Ellenberg, 1976). When febrile seizures of any kind are followed by epilepsy, the majority of preceding febrile seizures are simple.

When children with epilepsy are considered, about 15% have a preceding history of febrile seizures without much variation between epilepsy types. If anything, "idiopathic" (genetic) epilepsies are more likely to be preceded by febrile seizures than focal epilepsies (Sofijanov, 1982; Rocca *et al.*, 1987a, b, c; Camfield *et al.*, 1994; Hamati-Haddad & Abou- Khalil, 1998).

We conclude that the distinction between simple and complex febrile seizures is of great epidemiological interest but is insufficiently precise to determine the investigation, management and outcome of the majority of individual patients.

Roughly 40% of children with a first febrile seizure will have at least one recurrence. Two risk factors have been consistent – young age at the time of the first febrile seizure (< 15–18 months) and a family history of febrile seizures (Knudsen, 1985a, b; Rantala & Uhari, 1994; Berg *et al.*, 1997). Two additional predictive factors are important, low temperature at the time of the seizure and short duration of illness prior to the seizure. Berg *et al.* (1997) followed 428 children who presented to an urban emergency room with a first febrile seizure. Over the next two years 32% had febrile seizure recurrence. The recurrence risk for those with none of the above four risk factors was 14%, with one factor 23%, with two 32%, with three 62% and with all four 76%. We note that complex febrile seizures and neurologic dysfunction have not been consistent predictors of recurrence.

After a first febrile seizure, the risk factors for subsequent epilepsy have been replicated in several studies (Nelson & Ellenberg, 1976; Annegers *et al.*, 1987). The most important are the factors that define a complex febrile seizure - focal seizure, prolonged seizure, repeated seizures within a single illness. Developmental delay or neurologic dysfunction also increases the risk of epilepsy as does a family history of epilepsy. Most studies do not find a relationship between the number of febrile seizures and subsequent epilepsy. Children with no risk factors have only a 2% chance of developing epilepsy. Each of the risk factors increases the chance by about 5%. Children with two or more risk factors have about a 15% risk of subsequent epilepsy, still a modest risk. Again, most children at increased risk do not develop epilepsy.

The value of identifying predictive factors for subsequent epilepsy or recurrent febrile seizures has not been well studied. Does it matter to a family if the risk of a recurrent seizure is increased from 15 to 45%? If a family knows there is a 98% chance of their child not developing epilepsy, is this really any different than an 88% of not developing epilepsy? It is unlikely that identification of prediction of risk factors will lead to an alteration in overall management.

Children followed for 7 years after a first "simple" febrile seizure have the same health care utilization (*i.e.* physician visits, hospital admissions) as age matched febrile and afebrile controls, except for a minor increase in referrals to ENT services shortly after the febrile seizure (Gordon *et al.*, 2000). A febrile seizure does not appear to be a "red flag" to families indicating the child is overly vulnerable to illness. In addition, throughout the following years they do not use physician's services more than their afebrile controls. Apparently the fright of the first febrile seizure does not have a long lasting effect. A Finnish study came to the same conclusion (Forsgren *et al.*, 1997).

Prolonged febrile seizures and mesial temporal sclerosis

The pioneering observations of Falconer based on a series of 100 children who had surgery for intractable temporal lobe epilepsy suggested two main ideas (Falconer *et al.*, 1964). First, the etiology of temporal lobe epilepsy often appeared to be mesial temporal sclerosis (MTS) - in 41 of his 100 cases it was the only pathology. Second, a significant proportion of those with MTS had preceding prolonged febrile seizures (30% in the MTS-only group compared with 6% in the group with other pathologies). A cause and effect relationship was postulated and further confirmation came from work with status epilepticus in adolescent baboons (Meldrum *et al.*, 1974). Very severe status seemed to damage mesial temporal structures. Studies in immature rats subjected to prolonged febrile seizures showed that some of the experimental rats later developed subtle but definite spontaneous complex partial seizures (focal impaired awareness seizures). Others found an increased susceptibility to convulsive drugs suggesting that the febrile status permanently lowered their seizure threshold (Dube *et al.*, 2000).

The sequence of febrile status followed by intractable temporal lobe epilepsy is rare when seen from a population perspective - about once in 150,000 children (Camfield *et al.*, 1994). The association is more complicated than simple cause and effect, because many patients show "dual pathology" in the temporal lobe (*i.e.* a small area of malformation plus MTS [Ho *et al.*, 1998]). So far, published MRI studies in children with febrile status have only included a few children who were completely neurologically normal with no perinatal difficulties and who had febrile status with initial unilateral hippocampal swelling followed by volume loss in mesial temporal structures (Lewis *et al.*, 2014; French & Kuzniecky 2014). Other investigators have found that following febrile status, a more common finding is bilateral hippocampal swelling which most often resolves completely (Scott *et al.*, 2003). We are not aware of any prospective studies documenting the sequence of a prolonged febrile seizure, unilateral hippocampal swelling, then MTS and finally intractable temporal lobe epilepsy.

An American prospective multicenter study named the Consequences of Prolonged Febrile Seizures in Childhood (FEBSTAT) was designed to address this issue. A total of 199 children, aged 1 month to 6 years of age, who presented with a febrile seizure lasting longer than 30 minutes in duration, were enrolled (Hesdorffer *et al.*, 2012). Comparisons were made to a control group of children who had simple febrile seizures. An MRI and EEG were performed within 72 hours of the presenting seizure and the children had subsequent baseline developmental assessments as well. A total of 22 (11.5%) had temporal lobe findings on their initial MRI, most commonly increased T2 FLAIR signal (Shinnar *et al.*, 2012). Surprisingly, 10.5% of the cohort had concurrent temporal lobe abnormalities such as hippocampal malrotation (*versus* 2.1% in control group).

After 1 year, 14 of the 22 with T2 FLAIR changes underwent a repeat MRI. Ten of the 14 had developed hippocampal sclerosis following febrile status epilepticus, whereas only 1 of the 116 subjects with normal hippocampal signal immediately after febrile status epilepticus went on to develop abnormal signal on follow-up MRI (Lewis *et al.*, 2014). Hippocampal malrotation was found in higher prevalence in children with a history of febrile status epilepticus (8.8%) *versus* normal controls (2.1%), but this finding is of unclear pathological or clinical significance (Chan *et al.*, 2015). There was no relationship between the side of the malrotation and the T2 FLAIR changes.

The children in the FEBSTAT study are being followed to evaluate if these MRI findings are predictors of later development of epilepsy. An additional aim of the FEBSTAT study is to assess risk factors associated with the development of MTS following febrile status.

No matter how rare or complicated, there is little doubt that the syndrome of prolonged febrile seizures associated with MTS and intractable temporal lobe epilepsy is a privileged one in terms of outcome from seizure surgery - about 80% have an excellent outcome (Abou-Khalil *et al.*, 1993). It is interesting that specialized epilepsy centres are finding fewer patients with MTS without dual pathology. This suggests that the more aggressive approach to treatment of febrile status epilepticus beginning in the 1970's has prevented this unfortunate outcome (Butler *et al.*, 2015).

Evaluation of children with febrile seizures

A thorough history from a reliable witness and a careful pediatric and neurologic examination are essential for the initial workup of a febrile seizure. When the cause of fever is identified and the child presents no disturbance of consciousness, it is usually not necessary to obtain further laboratory evaluation. A practice parameter from the American Academy of Pediatrics was based on peer-reviewed publications about simple febrile seizures (Provisional Committee on Quality Improvement, Subcommittee on febrile seizures, 1996). The evidence reviewed supports very little investigation.

Routine blood work

Routine blood work has not been shown to be of value (Yousefichaijan *et al.*, 2015). Several studies have suggested that low serum sodium after a first febrile seizure is associated with a significant risk of a recurrent febrile seizure within that illness (Hugan *et al.*, 1995; Kiviranta & Airaksinen, 1995), although one other study failed to confirm this association (Thoman *et al.*, 2004). Because rates of bacteremia (2%) and other serious bacterial illnesses are low (2%), blood cultures and complete blood count are not routinely necessary.

Lumbar puncture

The value of a lumbar puncture (LP) remains contentious. About 15% of children with meningitis will have seizures; however, virtually none are neurologically normal shortly after the seizure (Gerber & Berliner 1981). Once a febrile seizure has stopped, excluding meningitis/encephalitis becomes a critical task for the physician. Vaccines against varicella, *Hemophilus influenza, pneumococcus, and meningococcus* have decreased the number of bacterial/viral meningitis cases markedly, although other organisms such as streptococcus still exist.

While meningitis in infants may be associated with fever and seizures, the child under 12 months may only have minimal symptoms/signs of meningitis and may not appear otherwise ill (Wears *et al.*, 1986). The American Academy of Pediatrics Committee on Quality Improvement Practice Parameter (2011) states: "The clinical evaluation of young febrile children requires skills that vary among examiners. In all children younger than 12 months, performance of a lumbar puncture should be strongly considered." In the slightly older child, the practice parameter maintains: "In a child between 12 to 18 months of age, a lumbar puncture should be considered because clinical signs and symptoms of meningitis may be subtle".

Meningitis is even more unlikely in an > 18 month-old child who appears well shortly after a febrile seizure. For this reason The American Academy of Pediatrics Committee on Quality Improvement also states, "In a child older than 18 months, although a lumbar puncture is not routinely warranted, it is recommended in the presence of meningeal signs and symptoms. In addition, if the child has previously been treated with antibiotics, the clinician should be aware that the signs and symptoms of CNS infection may become masked, and lumbar puncture should be strongly considered in such cases."

In one series, of 503 children with meningitis, none had a simple febrile seizure (Green *et al.*, 1993). In a study of 839 patients presenting to a Paris emergency room with a complex febrile seizure there were 5 cases of bacterial meningitis, all of whom had clinical findings "suggesting meningitis or encephalitis" beyond the seizure itself (Guedj *et al.*, 2017). Most authors have suggested that children under about 6–12 months of age with a febrile seizure are of special concern because the signs of meningitis may be very subtle. Offringa *et al.* (1992) studied 309 children who had a lumbar puncture after presenting to an emergency department with a seizure associated with fever. Ten cases had meningitis (bacterial or viral) and all had major signs pointing to serious illness. Six other children had the same signs but did not have meningitis. Therefore, only 16/309 "needed" an LP to exclude a CNS infection. An older study by Lorber & Sunderland (1980) suggests that an experienced paediatrician could avoid many lumbar punctures without missing a case of meningitis. Such a selective approach implies that the physician assessing the child is experienced with the symptoms that are associated with meningitis in children. The judgment is based on either "the child appeared more ill than the physical signs suggested; had photophobia, neck stiffness, or a positive Kernig's sign; had continuing pyrexia without obvious cause; or deteriorated in hospital" (Offringa *et al.*, 1992). The contention that "lack of experience by junior doctors does not justify routine lumbar puncture" needs to be tempered by what is realistically possible. We suggest following the practice parameter recommendation (noted above) to perform a lumbar puncture if the child is less than 12 months of age, unless an experienced paediatrician is available to assist.

Neuroimaging

Neuroimaging studies are not of proven benefit for simple (American Academy of Pediatrics, 2011) or complex febrile seizures, but should be reserved "only when an underlying structural lesion is suspected" (Hirtz, 1997). It is unclear what should lead to such suspicion but presumably includes focal neurologic abnormalities, significant developmental delay, neurocutaneous lesions or abnormal head circumference.

Anxiety about complex febrile seizures does not justify routine imaging, especially considering that this group involves 30–40% of all first febrile seizures. Studies of CT and MRI have not lead to changes in management (Hampers *et al.*, 2006; Teng *et al.*, 2006; Hesdorffer *et al.*, 2008). We find it an uphill battle to persuade families and physicians that neuroimaging is not indicated even when the technology is readily available. Radiation dosage from head CT is of particular concern in this age group and MRI usually requires sedation, which also is not without risk.

EEG

Routine EEG is not justified following simple or complex febrile seizures. Older literature clearly indicated that routine EEG after a febrile seizure does not predict febrile seizure recurrence or subsequent epilepsy (Frantzen *et al.*, 1968; Sofijanov *et al.*, 1992). Despite strong evidence, many neurologists continue to request an EEG after an initial febrile seizure (Millichap & Colliver, 1991; Sofijanov *et al.*, 1992).

A number of studies have addressed the more specific question of the role of EEG after a complex febrile seizure. A retrospective Canadian study reviewed EEGs in 175 children with a complex febrile seizure (Joshi *et al.*, 2005). Forty percent were abnormal. Rather predictably, abnormalities were more common in those > 3 years of age, those recorded within a week of the seizure, and those with neurological abnormalities. The authors wisely questioned the value of such findings. A US study examined 154 children with a complex febrile seizure who had an EEG and at least two years of follow up (Harini *et al.*, 2015). Twenty percent of those who developed epilepsy had an "epileptiform" EEG, compared with 13% who did not develop epilepsy (p = 0.48). The positive predictive value of an epileptiform EEG was only 15%. A Cochrane Review concluded that there are no high-quality studies to support or refute the role of EEG or the timing of EEG after complex febrile seizures (Shah *et al.*, 2015).

A special feature of the EEG after a febrile seizure is hypnagogic spike-wave. Short bursts of irregular high voltage delta with a few buried spikes are seen as the child drifts off to sleep. Hypnagogic spike-wave has a peak expression at about 3–4 years of age (long after the peak age of febrile seizures), but apparently appears in the majority of children with febrile seizures (Tsuboi & Endo, 1977; Alvarez *et al.*, 1983; Sofijanov *et al.*, 1992). Some authorities view hypnagogic spike-wave as an expression/marker of the febrile seizure tendency. In any case, it carries no long-term negative connotations.

Treatment of febrile seizures

Most febrile seizures last only a few minutes and are over before the child presents to the health care system. If a child presents during a seizure, the duration is almost always longer than 20 minutes. Stopping an ongoing seizure is nearly always accomplished with rectal diazepam (0.5 mg/kg), rectal lorazepam (0.1 mg/kg) or buccal/nasal midazolam 0.2 mg/kg (Knudsen, 1979; Appleton *et al.*, 1995). Once the seizure has stopped, physicians need to remember that most parents think that their child is dying during a first febrile seizure (Rutter & Metcalfe, 1978; Balslev, 1991; Van Stuijvenberg *et al.*,1999; Kolahi & Tahmooreszadeh (2009). Dealing with this fear directly is prudent.

The cause of the fever is the second management issue with meningitis to be excluded clinically or with a lumbar puncture in very selected patients. After this step there is little "medical" intervention that is of proven value. No study has demonstrated that any form of treatment for febrile seizures alters the rate of subsequent epilepsy.

A recent meta-analysis finds that very few medications have been demonstrated to have any effectiveness in febrile seizures (Offringa *et al.*, 2017). In addition, "We found reduced recurrence rates for children with febrile seizures for intermittent diazepam and continuous phenobarbitone, with adverse effects in up to 30%. Apparent benefit for clobazam treatment in one trial needs to be replicated to be judged reliable."

Daily phenobarbital (4–5 mg/kg/day as a single daily dose) may be effective if compliance is excellent; however, the side effects of phenobarbital with behavioural change and intellectual dulling make it hard to justify (Wolf *et al.*, 1977; Wolf & Forsythe, 1978; Camfield *et al.*, 1979, 1980; Newton, 1988). A large USA randomized, double-blind, placebo controlled trial of 217 children with complex febrile seizures compared daily phenobarbital with placebo (Farwell *et al.*, 1990). Medication compliance was problematic but phenobarbital was not effective in reducing recurrence (46% recurrence phenobarbital, 38% placebo). The original publication suggested that Phenobarbital was associated with an IQ decrement of 7 points compared with placebo; however, a later correction suggested a 4 point difference in IQ which was not statistically significant (Farwell *et al.*, 1992). Daily phenytoin and carbamazepine appear ineffective (Bacon *et al.*, 1981; Camfield *et al.*, 1982; Anthony & Hawke, 1983). Daily valproic acid may be effective although the risk of toxic, fatal hepatitis appears high in this age range (Dreifuss *et al.*, 1987).

Benzodiazepines given at the time of illness/fever do reduce the incidence of recurrent febrile seizures. Rectal liquid diazepam 0.5 mg/kg every 12 hours when the child was ill appeared equally effective to phenobarbital in one important study (Knudsen & Vestermark, 1978). Oral diazepam at the time of illness was marginally effective in a randomized study of 406 children (Rosman *et al.*, 1993). The children received placebo or oral diazepam, 0.3 mg/kg/dose, at the time of illness. Over the next three years, 31% taking placebo and 23% taking diazepam had a recurrent febrile seizure. To prevent one febrile seizure, it was necessary to treat 14 children. Thirty% of those treated with diazepam had significant side effects with somnolence or ataxia - side effects that are of special concern in a febrile child when meningitis must be excluded. Another large randomized, placebo controlled trial (n = 185) used oral diazepam at a lower dose (0.5 mg/kg, then 0.2 mg/kg every 12 h) at the time of temperature 38° C (Autret *et al.*, 1990). Side effects were reduced, but the drug was ineffective. Finally, Uhari and colleagues (Uhari *et al.*, 1995) randomized 180 children with a first febrile seizure to receive placebo or diazepam 0.2 mg/kg three times/day during fever. There was no reduction in recurrence with diazepam. In summary, we do not recommend intermittent oral diazepam treatment.

Diazepam 0.5 mg/kg can be given rectally at the time of a febrile seizure (Knudsen, 1979). A randomized trial in an emergency room compared intravenous diazepam (0.3 mg/kg) with buccal Midazolam (0.2 mg/kg) for 47 children with prolonged febrile seizures (Lahat *et al.*, 2000). The overall effectiveness (safety and efficacy) was identical. Based on this study it seems likely that buccal midazolam could be used at home to shorten prolonged febrile seizures, although there are no publications so far evaluating this approach. The advantages of buccal midazolam would be ease and discretion of administration.

Oral intermittent clobazam has also been studied in one randomized, clinical trial in India. Patients with a history of a first febrile seizure were randomized to receive oral clobazam (n = 37) or oral diazepam (n = 35) at the time of fever (Khosroshahi *et al.*, 2011). The two regimes seemed to be equally effective in terms of febrile seizure recurrence but the clobazam group had fewer side effects. An observational study from Bangladesh came to similar conclusions (Sattar *et al.*, 2014). The benefit of an intermittent treatment is to limit the duration of the febrile seizure and give frightened parents a sense of being in control. We endorse this approach for selected families, although we acknowledge that it has not been subjected to a randomized trial with family anxiety as an outcome variable (Camfield & Camfield 2014).

Antipyretics

There is a convincing literature that obsessional use of antipyretics does not reduce the rate of recurrent febrile seizures. In a randomized double-blind trial of acetaminophen *versus* placebo in 180 children following a first febrile seizure, Uhari found no reduction in febrile seizure recurrences (Uhari *et al.*, 1995). Intense antipyretic instruction in the placebo arm of a double-blind trial of phenobarbital for simple febrile seizures (n = 79) did not reduce recurrences (Camfield *et al.*, 1980). In a consecutive series of 89 febrile seizure patients, Rutter noted that 50% had received an appropriate dose of antipyretic medication within an hour prior to the seizure (Rutter & Metcalfe, 1978). An Israeli study randomized 104 children admitted with a febrile seizure to continuous acetaminophen every 4 hours *versus* the same medication only if the temperature was about 37.9° C (Schnaiderman *et al.*, 1993). Four children in each group recurred during their hospitalization.

A Dutch study randomized 230 children with a first febrile seizure plus a risk factor for recurrence to receive ibuprofen or placebo during subsequent illnesses (van Stuijvenberg *et al.*, 1998). Over the next year, 32% on ibuprofen recurred compared with 34 percent on placebo. A final Finnish study randomized rectal placebo *vs.* rectal diclofenac followed by oral placebo *vs.* acetaminophen compared with ibuprofen for fever control and showed no efficacy in prevention of febrile seizures (Strengell *et al.*, 2009).

A very old approach to fever control is to sponge the child with cold water. A Canadian study showed this technique to be ineffective (Newman, 1985).

Therefore, antipyretic medication has no effect at all in the prevention of febrile seizure recurrences. Antipyretics may render a febrile child more comfortable but that is their only role in treatment of febrile seizures.

Long term cognitive and behavioral outcome

Two massive febrile seizure cohorts have proven that febrile seizures are benign. In the National Perinatal Collaborative Study in the USA, more than 50,000 babies were identified prenatally and followed to age 7 years (Nelson & Ellenberg, 1976). There were 1706 with at least one febrile seizure. Of these, 431 children had a sibling without febrile seizures. At age 7, the intelligence and school performance of those with febrile seizures was the same as their unaffected siblings (Ellenberg & Nelson, 1978). The British Child Health and Education Study followed a cohort of 16,163 infants and at age 10 years, 14,676 were available for follow-up - 381 had febrile convulsions (Verity *et al.*, 1998). An extensive battery of tests showed that children with febrile seizures had the same academic progress, intellect and behaviour as other children.

Chang and colleagues (Chang *et al.*, 2001) used a prospective, population-based, case-control method to assess the learning, spatial, and sequential working memory of 87 school-aged children with a previous febrile seizure and 87 randomly selected age-matched control subjects. The febrile seizure group performed significantly and consistently better than control subjects on mnemonic capacity and had more flexible mental processing abilities than their age-matched controls.

Finally, in Denmark a population-based study identified 507 men aged 18–20 years who had a history of febrile seizures but no other seizure types. They were evaluated by the military draft board and compared with 17,769 controls without febrile seizures. There were no differences in intelligence on standard tests (Norgaard *et al.*, 2009).

Parental quality of life

Several studies indicate that parents are very upset at the time of a first febrile seizure often fearing that their child might die. There are surprisingly few longer term studies that assess the impact of a febrile seizure. Huang and colleagues (Huang *et al.*, 2010) randomized a group of Taiwanese parents with a child with a febrile seizure to receive a pamphlet about febrile seizures (n = 87) or attend a 2-hour group session (n = 122) that offered information about febrile seizures, fever management and group discussion. There was a prompt reduction in negative scores which focused on anxiety and febrile seizures in the group session parents and gradual further improvement over 2 years. The pamphlet group gradually improved over 2 years, but they always remained considerably more concerned than the group session parents.

The FEBSTAT study looked at a series of family quality of life measures one month after the febrile status and one year later and compared them with families with a child with a simple febrile seizure (Shinnar *et al.*, 2017). Rather surprisingly, at one month families with a child with a simple febrile seizure reported higher parental stress scores than those with febrile status. These differences vanished by one year. At one year, parents of a child with developmental problems had the lowest quality of life scores. As mentioned previously, a Nova Scotia study indicated that after a simple febrile seizure the children did not consume excess health resources over the next 7 years suggesting that they adapted to their fright and anxiety fairly promptly (Gordon *et al.*, 2000).

GEFS + (Genetic Epilepsy with Febrile Seizures Plus)

Febrile seizures are a key component and the most frequent phenotype within the familial epilepsy syndrome of Genetic Epilepsy with Febrile Seizures Plus (GEFS+). GEFS+ was first coined "Generalized Epilepsy with Febrile Seizures Plus" by Scheffer and Berkovic (1997), when it was recognized in large families with autosomal dominant inheritance of seizures, with a predominance of febrile seizures. The heterogeneous spectrum of GEFS+ phenotypes ranges from typical simple febrile seizures, as described above, to mild seizure disorders such as Febrile Seizures Plus (FS+) to developmental and epileptic encephalopathies such as Epilepsy with Myoclonic-Atonic Seizures (MAE) and Dravet syndrome (Scheffer & Berkovic, 1997; Singh *et al.*,1999, 2001). GEFS+ phenotypes also include focal seizures, with or without preceding febrile seizures. Hence the acronym GEFS+ was changed to Genetic (not generalized) Epilepsy with Febrile Seizures Plus (Zhang *et al.*, 2017).

GEFS+ phenotypic spectrum

The change in name from "generalized" to "genetic" was based on the observation by many groups that focal seizures are part of the GEFS+ spectrum. Both temporal lobe and frontal lobe epilepsies have been reported in GEFS+ families and these individuals have been shown to carry familial GEFS+ gene mutations (Abou-Khalil *et al.*, 2001; Baulac *et al.*, 2001; Sugawara *et al.*, 2001). In individual patients focal epilepsy may follow febrile seizures or FS+ or may occur without febrile seizures. Although MTS has been observed in some cases, most patients with GEFS+ and temporal lobe epilepsy do not have MTS, indicating that the preceding febrile seizures were not causative (Scheffer *et al.*, 2007). Interestingly one patient without MTS and refractory temporal lobe epilepsy in the setting of GEFS+ with a sodium channel gene *(SCN1B)* mutation was rendered seizure free by anterior temporal lobectomy (Scheffer *et al.*, 2007).

Epilepsy with myoclonic-atonic seizures, formerly called myoclonic-astatic epilepsy (MAE) (see Chapter 11), was originally described by Doose as a genetic disorder with a polygenic basis. Doose reported that one third of probands had a family history of early childhood febrile and afebrile seizures, consistent with the GEFS+ spectrum. Detailed family studies of many MAE probands show GEFS+ phenotypes in their relatives (Singh *et al.*, 1999). We note, however, that the majority of MAE patients have a "sporadic" disorder without a family history of GEFS+ and without mutations in the GEFS+ genes.

Dravet syndrome (see Chapter 10) is a rare developmental and epileptic encephalopathy found in some GEFS+ families (Singh *et al.*, 2001; Veggiotti *et al.*, 2001). Most often Dravet syndrome occurs sporadically without familial antecedents. There are a few reported cases with a familial sodium channel gene *(SCN1A)* mutation in which one family member has Dravet syndrome and the remaining family members have mild GEFS+ phenotypes (Fujiwara *et al.*, 2003, Nabbout *et al.*, 2003). Such mutations are typically missense mutations and the family member with Dravet syndrome and the same SCN1A mutation presumably has other modifier genes leading to the more severe phenotype.

When siblings are born with Dravet syndrome and a *SCN1A* mutation, they may have a parent who is mosaic for the *SCN1A* mutation; the parent may be unaffected or have a mild phenotype such as FS consistent with the GEFS+ spectrum (Marini *et al.*, 2006). An elegant French study of 19 autosomal dominant families with Dravet syndrome, GEFS+ and *SCN1A* mutations found that the mutation was inherited in 12 families from a parent who was mosaic for the *SCN1A* mutation (Depienne *et al.*, 2010). They found that if the parents were > 42% mosaic for the mutation, they were affected with a greater phenotypic severity correlating with higher mosaicism rates (up to 85% in their study). Parents with < 43% mosaicism were unaffected.

An analysis of 60 large and small families with GEFS+ has emphasized the wide range of phenotypes (Zhang *et al.*, 2017). Families were included if there were one of two scenarios: 1) There were ≥ 2 individuals with a GEFS+ phenotype with ≥ 1 having FS+ (see below for definition of FS+) or 2) There was no one with FS+; however, ≥ 3 had GEFS+ phenotype such as FS or MAE. Families with only FS were excluded. Of the 409 affected individuals, the most common phenotype was FS (44%). The second most frequent phenotype was Febrile Seizures Plus (FS+) which occurred in 27%.

FS+ patients had febrile seizures that persisted beyond the typical ages of febrile seizures (3 months to six years) and/or had afebrile GTCS. These afebrile GTCS occurred during the typical FS age or appeared after the FS had stopped. The EEG in FS+ patients was normal or showed irregular generalized spike wave discharges. The remaining 29% of patients with GEFS+ had a remarkable spectrum of phenotypes including FS followed by absence seizures, FS followed by GTCS, classic generalized genetic epilepsies (such as JME), FS plus focal epilepsy, focal epilepsy without febrile seizures, myoclonic astatic epilepsy (MAE), Dravet syndrome and "complex phenotypes". Overall, 9% had focal epilepsy.

Although GEFS+ was originally recognized through the study of large multiplex families with many affected individuals, it most frequently follows complex inheritance where several genes play a role, possibly with an environmental contribution. There is growing information that susceptibility genes (*i.e.* contribute to the complex inheritance pattern) include rare variants in genes that encode the GABA receptor subunit *GABRD*, *HCN2*, *CACNA1A* and *STX1B* (Dibbens *et al.*, 2004; 2010; Heron *et al.*, 2004; Schubert *et al.*, 2014). It is likely that further susceptibility gene variants will emerge.

Given the wide variation in phenotypic expression and the many causative gene mutations, it is not easy to offer simple recommendations for drug treatment for GEFS+. In general when the cause is a sodium channel mutation, "sodium channel" drugs such as carbamazepine and phenytoin may make seizures worse and are best avoided. Otherwise the drug treatment follows the usual approach for the individual epilepsy syndromes.

Genetics of Febrile Seizures and Genetic Epilepsy with Febrile Seizures Plus

The epilepsy syndromes of Febrile Seizures (FS) and Genetic Epilepsy with Febrile Seizures Plus (GEFS+) are both considered genetic in origin based on clinical genetic studies. Confirmation of their genetic etiology has been obtained through the discovery of pathogenic mutations in an array of genes, albeit in a minority of patients to date, with molecular overlap discovered between FS and GEFS+ (Wallace *et al.*, 1998). This is unsurprising as it reflects that the most common phenotype within the GEFS+ spectrum is typical FS (Scheffer & Berkovic, 1997; Zhang *et al.*, 2017). Some genes implicated in GEFS+, such as the sodium channel gene *SCN1A*, cause both FS and also more complex GEFS+ phenotypes ranging from Febrile Seizures Plus (FS+) to a range of developmental and epileptic encephalopathies (DEE) (Scheffer *et al.*, 2017), such as Dravet syndrome (Singh *et al.*, 1999; Claes *et al.*, 2001).

Clinical genetic studies, familial aggregation and twin studies suggest that FS follow a complex genetic architecture where multiple genes are involved with a minor environmental contribution (Annegers *et al.*, 1982; Tsuboi & Endo, 1991; Maher & McLachlan, 1997).

As noted above monozygotic twin studies of classical FS show high concordance ranging from 0.1–0.8 compared with dizygotic twins who have much lower concordance ranging from 0.03–0.32 (Saghazadeh *et al.*, 2014). The risk of FS in a first degree relative of a patient with FS increases from the background incidence of 3% to about 10–15% (Bethune *et al.*, 1993; van Esch *et al.*, 1998). These data confirm that genetic factors play an important etiological role.

GEFS+ was originally recognized through the study of large multiplex families with many affected individuals who had a spectrum of heterogeneous phenotypes following an autosomal dominant inheritance pattern (Scheffer & Berkovic, 1997; Singh *et al.*, 1999). Recently, rare small families with recessive inheritance have been reported (Brunklaus *et al.*, 2015). Yet, subsequent clinical genetic studies suggest that smaller GEFS+ families may follow complex inheritance where several genes interact, possibly with an environmental contribution. More recently, *de novo* mutations have explained sporadic patients with GEFS+ phenotypes showing that GEFS+ is not always familial (Myers *et al.*, 2017).

Molecular genetics of FS and GEFS+

Although FS and GEFS+ often follow complex or polygenic inheritance, there are families with several affected individuals across different generations in whom molecular genetic studies have identified mutations in single genes. Both GEFS+ and FS show marked genetic heterogeneity.

To date, molecular genetic studies for common FS have not been very rewarding in identifying genes causing FS-only phenotypes. Several chromosomal loci have been associated with FS-only (see Saghazadeh *et al.*, 2014 for review), suggesting locus heterogeneity yet no gene mutations have been identified (see *Table I*).

Molecular genetic studies of GEFS+ families with predominant monogenic inheritance have instead been more gratifying. To date, at least 6 genes of major effect that, when mutated, cause GEFS+ phenotypes have been reported including *SCN1A, SCN2A, SCN9A* and *SCN1B, GABRG2*, and *STX1B*, altogether accounting for about 30% of families and patients (Zhang *et al.*, 2017).

First, the gene coding for the auxiliary subunit of the neuronal sodium channel *SCN1B* was identified, some 20 years ago (Wallace *et al.*, 1998). Next emerged the most important and frequently recognized genetic cause of FS and GEFS+, *SCN1A*, encoding the pore-forming alpha 1 subunit of the neuronal sodium channel, accounting for more than 20% of families (Escayg *et al.*, 2000). The neuronal sodium channel comprises an alpha pore-forming subunit with 4 transmembrane domains, associated with two auxiliary beta subunits responsible for channel gating and localization at the cell membrane. Mutations have been reported most frequently in the alpha 1 subunit gene, *SCN1A*, and next most frequently in the beta 1 subunit gene, *SCN1B* (Wallace *et al.*, 1998; Escayg *et al.*, 2000). Mutations in GEFS+ are usually missense in nature and associated with loss of function. In contrast, mutations in the sodium channel genes *SCN2A* and *SCN9A* in GEFS+ require confirmation as they have been reported in single families (Sugawara *et al.*, 2001; Singh *et al.*, 2009). A mosaic mutation of *SCN8A*, coding for the alpha 8 subunit of the sodium channel, has recently been found in a father with FS+ whose son had a severe DEE (Zhang *et al.*, 2017). It is not clear if the *SCN8A* mutation is contributing to the FS+ phenotype in the father and thus, this observation requires confirmation.

Much of remaining 10% of GEFS+ individuals with a known genetic etiology carry mutations in the gene coding for the gamma 2 subunit of the $GABA_A$ receptor, *GABRG2*. Functional studies of the *GABRG2* mutations are consistent with loss of function. The net effect of these mutations has been to decrease chloride conductance and decrease inhibition, although to date only 6 *GABRG2* mutations has been associated with FS, GEFS+, and Childhood Absence Epilepsy (CAE) (Baulac *et al.*, 2001; Wallace *et al.*, 2001; Harkin *et al.*, 2002). Recent next generation sequencing genetic technologies including whole exome and whole genome sequencing and gene panels, allow the concomitant screening of many epilepsy genes. These approaches are being applied to large cohorts of patients with heterogeneous epilepsies. Such studies have uncovered mutations in additional $GABA_A$ subunit genes including alpha1 *(GABRA1)* and beta 3 *(GABRB3)* in a few patients with GEFS+ (Johannesen *et al.*, 2016; Moller *et al.*, 2017). *GABRD*, coding for the delta subunit of the $GABA_A$ receptor, is currently regarded as a susceptibility gene rather than a causative gene; it has only been reported in a single family and requires confirmation in other individuals (Dibbens *et al.*, 2004).

Finally, a small number of families have mutations in *STX1B* which encodes for syntaxin-1B (Schubert *et al.*, 2014). The *STX1B* gene encodes a protein that plays a major role in the regulation of neurotransmitter synaptic transmission.

HCN2 and *CACNA1H* are also considered to be susceptibility genes for GEFS+ (Dibbens *et al.*, 2010; Heron *et al.*, 2007). Variants in these genes contribute, but are likely to not be sufficient alone to cause the seizure phenotype; their role awaits confirmation. How these susceptibility genes contribute to complex inheritance still needs to be elucidated.

As the commonest phenotype in GEFS+ families is FS, it is not surprising that there are families who have FS exclusively and carry mutations in GEFS+ or other epilepsies genes *(Table I)*. One such family has been reported with a *SCN1A* mutation whilst another has a *GABRG2* mutation (Mantegazza *et al.*, 2005; Audenaert *et al.*, 2006). In these families, the gene appears to cause FS but each gene is known in a broader context as a gene for GEFS+. Sporadic cases with GEFS+ phenotypes with *de novo SCN1A* mutations have been identified, highlighting that GEFS+ phenotypes do not always occur in a familial setting.

In conclusion, no genes account for the majority of patients with GEFS+ or FS. Nor has phenotypic heterogeneity been explained at the molecular level for the broad range of phenotypes that occur within the GEFS+ spectrum.

Conclusions about febrile seizures

Febrile seizures are common. The aetiology remains unknown although there is evidence for important genetic and environmental influences. Only rarely are they followed by epilepsy. Usually clinical assessment is sufficient, without any laboratory, EEG or neuroimaging studies. It is possible to predict recurrent febrile seizures and subsequent epilepsy but not accurately enough to be of major clinical use. Fortunately, it is rare for prolonged febrile seizures to be followed by intractable temporal lobe epilepsy. Drug treatment is not indicated to attempt to prevent recurrences and antipyretic treatment is ineffective. After the initial shock of observing their own child having a seizure, most parents seem to successfully adapt and allow their children to develop normally. Education about febrile seizures may be helpful for families, especially if delivered in a group setting.

Conclusions about GEFS+

GEFS+ is a well-recognized, complex familial epilepsy syndrome in which a minimum of two family members have GEFS+ phenotypes to satisfy the familial diagnosis. Most GEFS+ phenotypes have a good prognosis and, when indicated, are readily treated with conventional antiepileptic therapy. GEFS+ often follows complex inheritance, but insights into its genetic basis have been gained from large and small family studies in which it has been possible to identify dominant mutations of ion channel genes and other genes affecting synaptic transmission. Originally this disorder was called Generalized Epilepsy with Febrile Seizures Plus; however, with the observations that ~10% of affected individuals have focal epilepsies, the name has evolved to Genetic Epilepsy with Febrile Seizures Plus. Understanding the interaction of multiple genes and environment components continues to be a major challenge.

REFERENCES ▶

Abou-Khalil B, Andermann E, Andermann F, Olivier A, Quesney LF (1993): Temporal lobe epilepsy after prolonged febrile convulsion: excellent outcome after surgical treatment. *Epilepsia* 34: 878–883.

Abou-Khalil B, Ge Q, Desai R, *et al.* (2001): Partial and generalized epilepsy with febrile seizures plus and a novel SCN1A mutation. *Neurology* 57: 2265–2272.

Akbayram S, Cemek M, Buyukben A, *et al.* (2012): Major and minor bioelement status in children with febrile seizure. *Bratisl Les Listy* 113: 421–423.

Alvarez N, Lombroso CT, Medina C, Cantlon B (1983): Paroxysmal spike and wave activity in drowsiness in young children: its relationship to febrile convulsions. *Electroencephalogr Clin Neurophysiol* 56: 406–413.

American Academy of Pediatrics; Subcommittee on Febrile Seizures (2011): Neurodiagnostic evaluation of the child with a simple febrile seizure. *Pediatrics* 127: 389–394.

Annegers JF, Hauser WA, Anderson VE, Kurland LT (1982): The risks of seizure disorders among relatives of patients with childhood onset epilepsy. *Neurology* 32: 174–179.

Annegers JF, Hauser WA, Shirto S, Kurland LT (1987): Factors prognostic of unprovoked seizures after febrile convulsions. *N Engl J Med* 316: 493–498.

Anthony J, Hawke S (1983): Phenobarbital compared with carbamazepine in prevention of recurrent febrile convulsions. *Am J Dis Child* 137: 892–895.

Appleton R, Sweeney A, Choonara I, Borson J, Molyneux E (1995): Lorazepam *versus* diazepam in the acute treatment of epileptic seizures and status epilepticus. *Dev Med Child Neurol* 37: 682–688.

Audenaert D, Schwartz E, Claeys KG, *et al.* (2006): A novel GABRG2 mutation associated with febrile seizures. *Neurology* 67: 687–690.

Autret E, Billard C, Bertrand P, *et al.* (1990): Double-blind, randomized trial of diazepam *versus* placebo for prevention of recurrence of febrile seizures. *J Pediatr* 117: 490–494.

Bacon C, Mucklow J, Rawlins M, *et al.* (1981): Placebo-controlled study of phenobarbitone and phenytoin in the prophylaxis of febrile convulsions. *Lancet* 11: 600–603.

Balslev T (1991): Parental reactions to a child's first febrile convulsion. *Acta Paediatr Scand* 80: 466–469.

Barlow WE, Davis RL, Glasser JW, *et al.* (2001): The risk of seizures after receipt of whole-cell pertussis or measles, mumps, and rubella vaccine. *N Engl J Med* 345: 656–661.

Baulac S, Huberfeld G, Gourfinkel-An I, *et al.* (2001): First genetic evidence of GABA(A) receptor dysfunction in epilepsy: a mutation in the gamma2-subunit gene. *Nat Genet* 28: 46–48.

Berg AT, Shinnar S (1996): Complex febrile seizures. *Epilepsia* 37: 126–133.

Berg AT, Shinnar S, Darefsky AF, *et al.* (1997): Predictors of recurrent febrile seizures. A prospective cohort study. *Arch Pediatr Adolesc Med* 151: 371-378.

Bethune P, Gordon KG, Dooley JM, Camfield CS, Camfield PR (1993): Which child will have a febrile seizure? *Am J Dis Child* 147: 35–39.

Brunklaus A, Ellis R, Stewart H, Aylett S, *et al.* (2015): Homozygous mutations in the SCN1A gene associated with genetic epilepsy with febrile seizures plus and Dravet syndrome in 2 families. *Eur J Paediatr Neurol* 2015;19: 484–488.

Butler TA, Dugan P, French J (2015): Why is mesial temporal lobe epilepsy with Ammon's horn sclerosis becoming less common? *Eur J Neurol* 22: e12.

Camfield CS, Chaplin S, Doyle AB, Shapiro SH, Cummings C, Camfield PR (1979): Side effects of phenobarbital in toddlers: behavioural and cognitive aspects. *J Pediatr* 95: 361–365.

Camfield PR, Camfield CS, Shapiro S, Cummings C (1980): The first febrile seizure - Antipyretic instruction plus either phenobarbital or placebo to prevent a recurrence. *J Pediatr* 97: 16–21.

Camfield PR, Camfield CS, Tibbles JAR (1982): Carbamazepine does not prevent febrile seizures in phenobarbital failures. *Neurology* 32: 288–299.

Camfield PR, Camfield CS, Gordon K, Dooley JM (1994): What types of epilepsy are preceded by febrile seizures? A population based study of children. *Dev Med Child Neurol* 36: 887–892.

Camfield P, Camfield C (2014): Are febrile seizures an indication for intermittent benzodiazepine treatment, and if so, in which cases? *Epileptic Disord* 16 (Suppl. 1): S84–88.

Chan S, Belllo JA, Shinnar S, *et al.* (2015): Hippocampal malrotation is associated with prolonged febrile seizures: Results of the FEBSTAT Study. *Am J Roentgenol* 205: 1064–1068.

Chang YC, Guo NW, Wang ST, Huang CC, Tsai JJ (2001): Working memory of school-aged children with a history of febrile convulsions: a population study. *Neurology* 57: 37–42.

Chung B, Wong V (2007): Relationship between five common viruses and febrile seizure in children. *Arch Dis Child* 92: 589–593.

Claes L, Del-Favero J, Ceulemans B, Lagae L, Van Broeckhoven C, De Jonghe P (2001): *De novo* mutations in the sodium-channel gene SCN1A cause severe myoclonic epilepsy of infancy. *Am J Hum Genet* 68: 1327–1332.

Committee on Infectious Diseases. Policy Statement – Prevention of Varicella (2011): Update of recommendations for use of quadrivalent and monovalent varicella vaccines in children. *Pediatrics* 128: 630–632.

Consensus Development Panel (1980): Febrile seizures: long-term management of children with fever-associated seizures. *Pediatrics* 66: 1009–1012.

Depienne C, Trouillard O, Gourfinkel-An I, *et al.* (2010): Mechanisms for variable expressivity of inherited SCN1A mutations causing Dravet Syndrome. *J Med Genet* 47: 404–410.

De Vries EE, van den Munckhof B, Braun KP, *et al.* (2016): Inflammatory mediators in human epilepsy: a systematic review and meta-analysis. *Neurosci Biobehav* 63: 177–190.

Dibbens LM, Feng HJ, Richards MC, *et al.* (2004): GABRD encoding a protein for extra- or peri-synaptic GABAA receptors is a susceptibility locus for generalized epilepsies. *Hum Mol Genet* 13: 1315–1319.

Dibbens LM, Reid CA, Hodgson B, *et al.* (2010): Augmented currents of an HCN2 variant in patients with febrile seizure syndromes. *Ann Neurol* 67: 542–546.

Dreifuss FE, Santilli N, Langer DH, Sweeney KP, Moline KA, Menander KB (1987): Valproic acid hepatic fatalities: a retrospective review. *Neurology* 37: 379–385.

Dube C, Chen K, Eghbal-Ahmadi M, Brunson K, Soltesz I, Baram TZ (2000): Prolonged febrile seizures in the immature rat model enhance hippocampal excitability long term. *Ann Neurol* 47: 336–444.

Duffy J, Weintraub E, Hambidge SJ, *et al.* (2016): Vaccine Safety Datalink. Febrile Seizure Risk After Vaccination in Children 6 to 23 Months. *Pediatrics* 138(1). pii: e20160320.

Ellenberg JH, Nelson KB (1978): Febrile seizures and later intellectual performance. *Arch Neurol* 35: 17–21.

Escayg A, MacDonald BT, Meisler MH, *et al.* (2000): Mutations of SCN1A, encoding a neuronal sodium channel, in two families with GEFS+2. *Nat Genet* 24: 343–345.

Falconer MA, Serafetinides EA, Corsellis JA (1964): Etiology and pathogenesis of temporal lobe epilepsy. *Arch Neurol* 10: 233–248.

Farwell J, Lee YJ, Hirtz DG, Sulzbacher S, Ellenberg JH, Nelson KB (1990): Phenobarbital for febrile seizures - effects on intelligence and on seizure recurrence. *N Engl J Med* 322: 364–369.

Farwell J, Lee YJ, Hirtz DG, Sulzbacher S, Ellenberg JH, Nelson KB (1992): Corrections *Engl J Med* 326: 144.

Forsgren L, Sidenvall R, Blomquist HM, Heijbel J, Nystrom L (1991): Pre- and perinatal factors in febrile convulsions. *Acta Paediatr Scand* 80: 218–225.

Forsgren L, Heijbel J, Nyström L, Sidenvall RA (1997): Follow-up of an incident case-referent study of febrile convulsions seven years after the onset. *Seizure* 6: 21–26.

Francis JR, Richmond P, Robins C, *et al.*(2016): Observational study of febrile seizures: the importance of viral infection and immunization. *BMC Pediatr* 16: 202–206.

Frantzen E, Lennox-Buchthal M, Nygaard A, Stene J (1968): Longitudinal EEG and clinical study of children with febrile convulsions. *Electroencephalogr Clin Neurophysiol* 24: 197–212.

French JA, Kuzniecky R (2014): Can febrile status cause hippocampal sclerosis? *Ann Neurol* 75: 173–174.

Fujiwara T, Sugawara T, Mazaki-Miyazaki E, *et al.* (2003): Mutations of sodium channel alpha subunit type 1 (SCN1A) in intractable childhood epilepsies with frequent generalized tonic-clonic seizures. *Brain* 126: 531–546.

Fukuda M, Suzuki Y, Ishizaki Y, *et al.* (2009): Interleukin-1beta enhances susceptibility to hyperthermia-induced seizures in developing rats. *Seizure* 18: 211–214.

Gallentine WB, Shinnar S, Hersdorfer DC, *et al.* (2017): Plasma cytokines associated with febrile status epilepticus in children: a potential biomarker for acute hippocampal injury. *Epilepsia* 58: 1102–1111.

Gerber MA, Berliner BC (1981): The child with a "simple" febrile seizure. Appropriate diagnostic evaluation. *Am J Dis Child* 135: 431–433.

Gordon KE, Camfield PR, Camfield CS, *et al.* (2000): Children with febrile seizures do not consume excess health care resources. *Arch Pediatr Adolesc Med* 154: 594–597.

Gordon KE, Dooley JM, Wood EP, *et al.* (2009): Is temperature regulation different in children susceptible to febrile seizures? *Can J Neurol Sci* 36: 192–195.

Green SM, Rothrock SG, Clem KJ (1993): Can seizures be the sole manifestation of meningitis in febrile children? *Pediatrics* 92: 527–534.

Guedj R, Chappuy H, Titomanlio L, *et al.* (2017): Do All Children Who Present With a Complex Febrile Seizure Need a Lumbar Puncture? *Ann Emerg Med* 70: 52–62.

Habibian N, Alipour A, Rezaianzadeh A (2014): Association between Iron Deficiency Anemia and Febrile Convulsion in 3- to 60-Month-Old Children: A Systematic Review and Meta-Analysis. *Iran J Med Sci* 39: 496–505.

Hamati-Haddad A, Abou Khalil B (1998): Epilepsy diagnosis and localization in patients with antecedents of febrile convulsions. *Neurology* 50: 917–922.

Hampers LC, Thompson DA, Bajaj L, Tseng BS, Rudolph JR (2006): Febrile seizure: measuring adherence to AAP guidelines among community ED physicians. *Pediatr Emerg Care* 22: 465–469.

Hara K, Tanabe T, Aomatsu T, *et al.* (2007): Febrile seizures associated with influenza A. *Brain Dev* 29: 30–38.

Harini C, Nagarajan E, Kimia AA, *et al.* (2015): Utility of initial EEG in first complex febrile seizure. *Epilepsy Behav* 52: 200–204.

Harkin LA, Bowser DN, Dibbens LM, *et al.* (2002): Truncation of the GABA(A)-receptor gamma2 subunit in a family with generalized epilepsy with febrile seizures plus. *Am J Hum Genet* 70: 530–536.

Haspolat S, Baysal Y, Duman O, Coskun M, Yegin O (2005): Interleukin-1alpha, interleukin-1beta, and interleukin-1Ra polymorphisms in febrile seizures. *J Child Neurol* 20: 565–568.

Hauser WA, Kurland LT (1975): The epidemiology of epilepsy in Rochester, Minnesota, 1935 through 1967. *Epilepsia* 16: 1–66.

Heron SE, Phillips HA, Mulley JC, *et al.* (2004): Genetic variation of CACNA1H in idiopathic generalized epilepsy. *Ann Neurol* 55: 595–596.

Heron SE, Khosravani H, Varela D, *et al.* (2007): Extended spectrum of idiopathic generalized epilepsies associated withCACNA1H functional variants. *Ann Neurol* 62: 560–568.

Hesdorffer DC, Chan S, Tian H, *et al.* (2008): Are MRI-detected brain abnormalities associated with febrile seizure type? *Epilepsia* 49: 765–771.

Hesdorffer DC, Benn EK, Bagillia E, *et al.* (2011): Distribution of febrile seizure duration and associations with development. *Ann Neurol* 70: 93–100.

Hesdorffer DC, Shinnar S, Lewis DV, *et al.* (2012): Design and phenomenology of the FEBSTAT Study. *Epilepsia* 53: 1471–1480.

Hildebrand MS, Phillips AM, Mullen SA, *et al.* (2015): Loss of synaptic Zn2+ transporter function increases risk of febrile seizures. *Sci Rep* 5: 17816.

Hirtz DG (1997). Febrile seizures. *Pediatr Rev* 18: 5–8.

Hirtz DG, Nelson KB (1983a): The natural history of febrile seizures. *Ann Rev Med* 134: 453–471.

Hirtz DG, Nelson KB, Ellenberg JH (1983b): Seizures following childhood immunizations. *J Pediatr* 120: 14–18.

Ho SS, Kuzniecky RI, Gilliam F, Faught E, Morawetz R (1998): Temporal lobe developmental malformations and epilepsy: Dual pathology and bilateral hippocampal abnormalities. *Neurology* 50: 748–754.

Holtzman D, Obana K, Olson J (1981): Hyperthermia-induced seizures in the rat pup: a model for febrile convulsions in children. *Science* 213: 1034–1036.

Huang MC, Liu CC, Chi YC, Huang CC, Cain K (2010): Parental concerns for the child with febrile convulsion: long-term effects of educational interventions. *Acta Neurol Scand* 103: 288–293.

Hugan CAC, Oudesluys-Murphy Am, Hopp WCJ (1995): Serum sodium levels and probability of recurrent febrile seizures. *Eur J Pediatr* 154: 403–405.

Ishizaki Y, Kira R, Fukuda M, Torisu H, *et al.* (2009): Interleukin-10 is associated with resistance to febrile seizures: genetic association and experimental animal studies. *Epilepsia* 50: 761–767.

Jacobsen SJ, Ackerson BK, Sy LS, *et al.* (2009): Observational safety study of febrile convulsion following first dose MMRV vaccination in a managed care setting. *Vaccine* 27: 4656–4661.

Jennsen F, Baram T (2000): Developmental seizures induced by common early-life insults: short- and long-term effects on seizure susceptibility. *Ment Retard Dev Disabil Res Rev* 6: 253–257.

Johannesen K, Marini C, Pfeffer S, *et al.* (2016): Phenotypic spectrum of GABRA1: From generalized epilepsies to severe epileptic encephalopathies. *Neurology* 13: 1140–1151.

Joshi C, Wawrykow T, Patrick J, Prasad (2005): Do clinical variables predict an abnormal EEG in patients with complex febrile seizures? *Seizure* 14: 429–434.

Kanemoto K, Kawasaki J, Yuasa S, *et al.* (2003): Increased frequency of interleukin-1 beta-511T allele in patients with temporal lobe epilepsy, hippocampal sclerosis, and prolonged febrile convulsion. *Epilepsia* 44: 796–799.

Khoshdel A, Parvin N, Abbasi M (2013): Selenium and leptin levels in febrile seizure: a case-control study in children. *Korean J Pediatr* 56: 80–85.

Khosroshahi N, Faramarzi F, Salamati P, Haghighi SM, Kamrani K (2011): Diazepam *versus* clobazam for intermittent prophylaxis of febrile seizures. *Indian J Pediatr* 78: 38–40.

Kim K, Kwak B, Kwon A, *et al.* (2017): Analysis of plasma multiplex cytokines and increased level of IL-10 and IL-1Ra cytokines in febrile seizures. *J Neuroinflammation* 14: 200–205.

Kira R, Torisu H, Takemoto M, *et al.* (2005): Genetic susceptibility to simple febrile seizures: interleukin-1beta promoter polymorphisms are associated with sporadic cases. *Neurosci Lett* 384: 239–244.

Kiviranta T, Airaksinen EM (1995): Low serum sodium levels are associated with subsequent febrile seizures. *Acta Ped* 84: 1372–1374.

Klein NP, Fireman B, Yih WK, *et al.* (2010): Vaccine Safety Datalink. Measles-mumps-rubella-varicella combination vaccine and the risk of febrile seizures. *Pediatrics* 126: e1–8.

Knudsen FU (1979): Rectal administration of diazepam in solution in the acute treatment of convulsions in infants and children. *Arch Dis Child* 54: 855–857.

Knudsen FU (1985a): Effective short term diazepam prophylaxis in febrile convulsions. *J Pediatr* 106: 487–490.

Knudsen FU (1985b): Recurrence risk after first febrile seizure and effect of short-term diazepam prophylaxis. *Arch Dis Child* 60: 1045–1049.

Knudsen FU, Vestermark S (1978): Prophylactic diazepam or phenobarbitone in febrile convulsions: a prospective controlled study. *Arch Dis Child* 53: 660–663.

Kolahi AA, Tahmooreszadeh S (2009): First febrile convulsions: inquiry about the knowledge, attitudes and concerns of the patients' mothers. *Eur J Pediatr* 168: 167–171.

Kwak BO, Kim K, Kim SN, Lee R (2017): Relationship between iron deficiency anemia and febrile seizures in children: A systematic review and meta-analysis. *Seizure* 52: 27–34.

Lahat E, Goldman M, Barr J, Bistritzer T, Berkovitch M (2000). Comparison of intranasal midazolam with intravenous diazepam for treating febrile seizures in children: prospective randomised study. *BMJ* 321: 83–86.

Lau SK, Woo PC, Yip CC, *et al.* (2006): Coronavirus HKU1 and other coronavirus infections in Hong Kong. *J Clin Microbiol* 44: 2063–2071.

Lee W, Ong H (2004): Afebrile seizures associated with minor infections: Comparison with febrile seizures and unprovoked seizures *Pediatr Neurol* 3: 157–164.

Lewis HM, Parry JV, Parry RP, *et al.* (1979): Role of viruses in febrile convulsions. *Arch Dis Child* 54: 869–876.

Lewis DV, Shinnar S, Hesdorffer DC, *et al.* (2014): FEBSTAT Study Team. Hippocampal sclerosis after febrile status epilepticus: the FEBSTAT study. *Ann Neurol* 75: 178–185.

Le Saux N, Barrowman N, Moore D, Whiting S, Scheifele D, Halperin S (2003): Decrease in hospital admissions for febrile seizures and reports of hypotonic-hyporesponsive episodes presenting to hospital emergency departments since switching to acellular pertussis vaccine in Canada: a report from IMPACT. *Pediatrics* 112; e348.

Lorber J, Sunderland R (1980): Lumbar puncture in children with convulsions associated with fever. *Lancet* 1: 785–786.

Ma SJ, Xiong YQ, Jiang LN, Chen Q (2015): Risk of febrile seizures after measles-rubella-varicella vaccine: a systematic review and meta-analysis. *Vaccine* 33: 3636–3649.

Maglione MA, Das L, Raaen L, *et al.* (2014): Safety of vaccines used for routine immunization of US children: a systematic review. *Pediatrics* 134: 325–337.

Maher J, McLachlan RS (1997): Febrile convulsions in selected large families: a single-major-locus mode of inheritance? *Dev Med Child Neurol* 39: 79–84.

Mahyar A, Ayazi P, Fallahi M, Javadi A (2010): Correlation between serum selenium level and febrile seizures. *Pediatr Neurol* 2010: 43: 331–334.

Makinson CD, Dutt K, Lin F, Papale LA, *et al.* (2016): An Scn1a epilepsy mutation in Scn8a alters seizure susceptibility and behavior. *Exp Neurol* 275 Pt 1: 46–58.

Mantegazza M, Gambardella A, Rusconi R, *et al.* (2005): Identification of Nav1.1 sodium channel (SCN1A) loss-of-function mutation associated with familial simple febrile seizures. *Proc Natl Acad Sci* USA 102: 1817–1882.

Marini C, Mei D, Cross HJ, Guerrini R (2006): Mosaic SCN1A mutation in familial severe myoclonic epilepsy of infancy. *Epilepsia* 47: 1737–1740.

Matsuo M, Sasaki K, Ichimaru T, Nakazato S, Hamasaki Y (2006): Increased IL-1beta production from dsRNA-stimulated leukocytes in febrile seizures. *Pediatr Neurol* 35: 102–106.

McCaughran JA Jr, Schechter N (1982): Experimental febrile convulsions: long-term effects of hyperthermia-induced convulsions in the developing rat. *Epilepsia* 23: 173–183.

Meldrum BS, Horton RW, Brierley JB (1974): Epileptic brain damage in adolescent baboons following seizures induced by allylglycine. *Brain* 97: 407–418.

Millichap JG, Colliver JA (1991): Management of febrile seizures: Survey of current practice and phenobarbital usage. *Pediatr Neurol* 7: 243–248.

Millichap JG and Millichap JJ (2006): Role of viral infections in the etiology of febrile seizures. *Pediatr Neurol* 35: 165–172.

Mohammadpour Touserkani F, Gaínza-Lein M, Jafarpour S, *et al.* (2017): HHV-6 and seizure: A systematic review and meta-analysis. *J Med Virol* 89: 161–169.

Møller RS, Wuttke TV, Helbig I, *et al.* (2017): Mutations in GABRB3: From febrile seizures to epileptic encephalopathies. *Neurology* 88: 483–492.

Myers KA, Burgess R, Afawi Z, *et al.* (2017): *De novo* SCN1A pathogenic variants in the GEFS+ spectrum: Not always a familial syndrome. *Epilepsia* 58: e26-e30.

Nabbout R, Gennaro E, Dalla Bernardina B, *et al.* (2003): Spectrum of SCN1A mutations in severe myoclonic epilepsy of infancy. *Neurology* 60: 1961–1967.

Nelson KB, Ellenberg JH (1976): Predictors of epilepsy in children who have experienced febrile seizures. *N Engl J Med* 295: 1029–1033.

Nelson KB, Ellenberg JH (1978): Prognosis in children with febrile seizures. *Pediatrics* 61: 720–727.

Newman J (1985): Evaluation of sponging to reduce body temperature in febrile children. *Can Med Assoc J* 132: 641–642.

Newton RW (1988): Randomized controlled trials of phenobarbitone and valproate in febrile convulsions. *Arch Dis Child* 63: 1189–1191.

Nørgaard M, Ehrenstein V, Mahon BE, Nielsen GL, Rothman KJ, Sørensen HT (2009): Febrile seizures and cognitive function in young adult life: a prevalence study in Danish conscripts. *J Pediatr* 155: 404–409.

Offringa M, Beishuizen A, Derksin-Lubsen G (1992): Seizures and fever: can we rule out meningitis on clinical grounds alone? *Clin Pediatr* 31: 514–522.

Offringa M, Newton R, Cozijnsen MA, Nevitt SJ. (2017): Prophylactic drug management for febrile seizures in children. *Cochrane Database Syst Rev* 2: CD003031.

Okumura A, Uemura N, Suzuki M, Itomi K, Watanabe K (2004): Unconsciousness and delirious behavior in children with febrile seizures. *Pediatr Neurol* 30: 316–319.

Provisional committee on quality improvement, subcommittee on febrile seizures (1996): Practice parameter: the neurodiagnostic evaluation of the child with a first simple febrile seizure. *Pediatrics* 97: 769–775.

Rajakumar K, Bodensteiner JB (1996): Febrile myoclonus: A survey of pediatric neurologists. *Clin Ped* 22: 331–332.

Rantala H, Uhari M (1994): Risk factors for recurrence of febrile convulsions. *Acta Neurol Scand* 90: 207–210.

Reid CA, Hildebrand MS, Mullen SA, *et al.* (2017): Synaptic Zn(2)(+) and febrile seizure susceptibility. *Br J Pharmacol* 174: 119–125.

Rigbye KA, van Hasselt PM, Burgess R, *et al.* (2016): Is FGF13 a major contributor to genetic epilepsy with febrile seizures plus? *Epilepsy Res* 128: 48–51.

Rocca WA, Sharbrough FW, Hauser WA, Annegers JF, Schoenberg BS (1987a): Risk factors for absence seizures: a population-based case-control study in Rochester, Minnesota. *Neurology* 37: 1309–1314.

Rocca WA, Sharbrough FW, Hauser WA, Annegers JF, Schoenberg BS (1987b): Risk factors for generalized tonic-clonic seizures: a population-based case control study in Rochester, Minnesota. *Neurology* 37: 1315–1322.

Rocca WA, Sharbrough FW, Hauser WA, Annegers JF, Schoenberg BS (1987c): Risk factors for complex partial seizures: A population-based case-control study. *Ann Neurol* 21: 22–31.

Rosman NP, Colton T, Labazzo J, Gilbert PL, Gardella NB, Kay EM (1993): A controlled trial of diazepam administered during febrile illnesses to prevent recurrence of febrile seizures. *N Engl J Med* 329: 79–84.

Rutter N, Metcalfe DH (1978): Febrile convulsions - What do parents do? *Brit Med J* 2: 1345–1346.

Saghazadeh A, Mastrangelo M, Rezaei N (2014): Genetic background of febrile seizures. *Rev Neurosci* 25: 129–161.

Saghazadeh A, Mahmoudi M, Meysamie A, *et al.* (2015): Possible role of trace elements in epilepsy and febrile seizures: a meta-analysis. *Nutr Rev* 2015;73: 760–779.

Salzmann A, Guipponi M, Lyons PJ, *et al.* (2012): Carboxypeptidase A6 gene (CPA6) mutations in a recessive familial form of febrile seizures and temporal lobe epilepsy and in sporadic temporal lobe epilepsy. *Hum Mutat* 33: 124–135.

Sattar S, Saha SK, Parveen F, *et al.* (2014): Intermittent prophylaxis of recurrent febrile seizures with clobazam *versus* diazepam. *Mymensingh Med* J 23: 676–685.

Scheffer IE, Berkovic SF (1997): Generalized epilepsy with febrile seizures +: a genetic disorder with heterogeneous clinical phenotypes. *Brain* 120: 479–490.

Scheffer IE, Harkin LA, Grinton BE, *et al.* (2007): Temporal lobe epilepsy and GEFS+ phenotypes associated with SCN1B mutations. *Brain* 130(Pt 1); 100–109.

Scheffer IE, Berkovic S, Capovilla G, *et al.* (2017): ILAE classification of the epilepsies: Position paper of the ILAE Commission for Classification and Terminology. *Epilepsia* 58: 512–521.

Schnaiderman D, Lahat E, Sheffer T, Aladjem M (1993): Antipyretic effectiveness of acetaminophen in febrile seizures: ongoing prophylaxis *versus* sporadic usage. *Eur J Pediatr* 152: 747–749.

Schubert J, Siekierska A, Langlois M *et al.* (2014): Mutations in STX1B, encoding a presynaptic protein, cause fever-associated epilepsy syndromes. *Nat Genet* 46: 1327–1332.

Schuchmann S, Schmitz D, Rivera C (2006): Experimental febrile seizures are precipitated by a hyperthermia-induced respiratory alkalosis. *Nat Med* 12: 817–823.

Schuchmann S, Hauck S, Henning S, *et al.* (2011): Respiratory alkalosis in children with febrile seizures. *Epilepsia* 52: 1949–1955.

Scott RC, King MD, Gadian DG, Neville BG, Connelly A (2003): Hippocampal abnormalities after prolonged febrile convulsion: a longitudinal MRI study. *Brain* 126: 2551–2560.

Serdaroglu G, Alpman A, Tosun A, *et al.* (2001): Febrile seizures: interleukin 1β and interleukin-1 receptor antagonist polymorphisms. *Pediatr Neurol* 40: 113–116.

Shah PB, James S, Elayaraja S, (2015): EEG for children with complex febrile seizures. *Cochrane Database Syst Rev* 12: CD009196.

Shahrokhi A, Zare-Shahabadi A, Soltani S, *et al.* (2015): Association of TGFB, but not IL10, single nucleotide polymorphisms with febrile seizures. *Seizure* 29: 148–152.

Sheridan SL, Ware RS, Grimwood K, Lambert SB (2016): Febrile Seizures in the era of Rotavirus vaccine. *J Pediatric Infect Dis Soc* 5: 206–209.

Shi X, Yasumoto S, Kurahashi H, Nakagawa E, Fukasawa T, Uchiya S, Hirose S (2016): Clinical spectrum of SCN2A mutations. *Brain Dev* 34: 541–545.

Shinnar RC, Shinnar S, Hesdorffer DC, *et al.* (2017): Parental stress, pediatric quality of life, and behavior at baseline and one-year follow-up: Results from the FEBSTAT study. *Epilepsy Behav* 69: 95–99.

Shinnar S, Bello JA, Chan S, *et al.* (2012): MRI abnormalities following febrile status epilepticus in children: The FEBSTAT Study. *Neurology* 79: 871–877.

Sillanpää M, Camfield P, Camfield C, *et al.* (2008): Incidence of febrile seizures in Finland: prospective population-based study. *Pediatr Neurol* 38: 391–394.

Singh NA, Pappas C, Dahle EJ, *et al.* (2009): A role of SCN9A in human epilepsies, as a cause of febrile seizures and as a potential modifier of Dravet syndrome. *PLoS Genet* 5: e1000649.

Singh R, Scheffer IE, Crossland K, Berkovic SF (1999): Generalized epilepsy with febrile seizures plus: A common childhood-onset genetic syndrome. *Ann Neurol* 45: 75–81.

Singh R, Andermann E, Whitehouse WP, *et al.* (2001): Severe myoclonic epilepsy of infancy: extended spectrum of GEFS+? *Epilepsia* 42: 837–844.

Sofijanov NG (1982): Clinical evolution and prognosis of childhood epilepsies. *Epilepsia* 23: 61–69.

Sofijanov NG, Emoto S, Kuturec M, *et al.* (1992): Febrile seizures: Clinical characteristics and initial EEG. *Epilepsia* 33: 52–57.

Stanhope JM, Brody JA, Brink E, Morris CE (1972): Convulsions among the Chamarro people of Guam, Mariana islands, II: febrile convulsions. *Am J Epidemiol* 95: 299–304.

Stephenson JBP (1990): *Fits and Faints*. Oxford: MacKeith Press.

Strengell T, Uhari M, Tarkka R, *et al.* (2009): Antipyretic agents for preventing recurrences of febrile seizures: randomized controlled trial. *Arch Pediatr Adolesc Med* 163: 799–804.

Suga S, Suzuki K, Ihira M, *et al.* (2000): Clinical characteristics of febrile convulsions during primary HHV-6 infection. *Arch Dis Child* 82: 62–66.

Sugawara T, Mazaki-Miyazaki E, Ito M, *et al.* (2001): Nav1.1 mutations cause febrile seizures associated with afebrile partial seizures. *Neurology* 57: 703–705.

Sun Y, Christensen J, Hviid A, *et al.* (2012): Risk of febrile seizures and epilepsy after vaccination with diphtheria, tetanus, acellular pertussis, inactivateoliovirus, and Haemophilus Influenzae type b. *JAMA* 307: 823–831.

Takasu M, Kubota T, Tsuji T, *et al.* (2017): The semiology of febrile seizures: Focal features are frequent. *Epilepsy Behav* 73: 59–63.

Tartof SY, Tseng HF, Liu IL, *et al.* (2014): Inpatient admission for febrile seizure and subsequent outcomes do not differ in children with vaccine-associated *versus* non-vaccine associated febrile seizures. *Vaccine* 32: 6408–6414.

Teng D, Dayan P, Tyler S, *et al.* (2006): Risk of intracranial pathologic conditions requiring emergency intervention after a first complex febrile seizure episode among children. *Pediatrics* 117: 304–308.

Thoman J, Duffner P, Shucard J (2004): Do serum sodium levels predict recurrent febrile seizures within 24 hours? *Pediatr Neurol* 31: 342–344.

Tomoum HY, Badawy NM, Mostafa AA, Harb MY (2007): Plasma interleukin-1beta levels in children with febrile seizures. *J Child Neurol* 22: 689–692.

Tsai FJ, Hsieh YY, Chang CC, Lin CC, Tsai CH (2002): Polymorphisms for interleukin 1 beta exon 5 and interleukin 1 receptor antagonist in Taiwanese children with febrile convulsions. *Arch Pediatr Adolesc Med* 156: 545–548.

Tsuboi T (1984): Epidemiology of febrile and afebrile convulsions in children in Japan. *Neurology* 34: 175–181.

Tsuboi T, Endo S (1977): Febrile convulsions followed by nonfebrile convulsions. A clinical, electroencephalographic and follow-up study. *Neuropadiatrie* 8: 209–223.

Tsuboi T, Endo S (1991): Genetic studies of febrile convulsions: analysis of twin and family data. *Epilepsy Res* (Suppl): 119–128.

Uhari M, Rantala H, Vainionpaa L, Kurttila R (1995): Effect of acetaminophen and of low dose intermittent diazepam on prevention of recurrences of febrile seizures. *J Pediatr* 126: 991–995.

Van Esch A, Steyerberg EW, van Duijn CM, *et al.* (1998): Prediction of febrile seizures in siblings: a practical approach. *Neuropediatrics* 157: 340–344.

Van Stuijvenberg M, Derksen-Lubsen G, Steyerberg EW, Habbema JD, Moll HA (1998): Randomized, controlled trial of ibuprofen syrup administered during febrile illnesses to prevent febrile seizure recurrences. *Pediatrics* 102: e51.

Van Stuijvenberg M, de Vos S, Tjiang GC, *et al.* (1999): Parents' fear regarding fever and febrile seizures. *Acta Paediatr* 88: 618–622.

Veggiotti P, Cardinali S, Montalenti E, Gatti A, Lanzi G (2001): Generalized epilepsy with febrile seizures plus and severe myoclonic epilepsy in infancy: a case report of two Italian families. *Epileptic Disord* 3: 29–32.

Verity CM, Butler NR, Golding J (1985): Febrile convulsions in a national cohort followed up from birth. II. Medical history and intellectual ability at 5 years of age. *Br Med J* 290: 1311–1315.

Verity CM, Greenwood R, Golding J (1998): Long-term intellectual and behavioural outcomes in children with febrile convulsions. *N Engl J Med* 338: 1723–1728.

Verrotti A, Moavero R, Vigevano F, *et al.* (2014): Long-term follow-up in children with benign convulsions associated with gastroenteritis. *Eur J Paediatr Neurol* 18: 572–577.

Vezzani A, Friedman A, Dingledine RJ (2013): The role of inflammation in epileptogenesis. *Neuropharmacology* 69: 16–24.

Vestergaard M, Christensen J (2009): Register-based studies on febrile seizures in Denmark. *Brain Dev* 31: 372–377.

Virta M, Hurme M, Helminen M (2002): Increased plasma levels of pro- and anti-inflammatory cytokines in patients with febrile seizures. *Epilepsia* 43: 920–923.

Wallace RH, Wang DW, Singh R, *et al.* (1998): Febrile seizures and generalized epilepsy associated with a mutation in the Na+-channel beta1 subunit gene SCN1B. *Nat Genet* 19: 366–370.

Wallace RH, Marini C, Petrou S, *et al.* (2001): Mutant GABA(A) receptor gamma2-subunit in childhood absence epilepsy and febrile seizures. *Nat Genet* 28: 49–52.

Wears RL Luten RC, Lyons RG (1986): Which laboratory tests should be performed on children with apparent febrile confusions: An analysis and review of the literature. *Pediatr Emerg Care* 2: 191–196.

Winawer M, Hesdorffer D (2004): Turning on the heat: the search for febrile seizure genes. *Neurology* 63: 1770–1771.

Wolf SM, Carr A, David DC, (1977): The value of phenobarbital in the child who has had a single febrile seizure: A controlled prospective study. *Pediatrics* 59: 378–385.

Wolf SM, Forsythe A (1978): Behaviour disturbance, phenobarbital and febrile seizures. *Pediatrics* 61: 728–731.

Wu ZQ, Sun L, Sun YH, *et al.* (2012): Interleukin 1 beta -511 C/T gene polymorphism and susceptibility to febrile seizures: a meta-analysis. *Mol Biol Rep* 39: 5401–5407.

Yousefichaijan P, Dorreh F, Abbasian L, Pakniyat AG (2015): Assessing the prevalence distribution of abnormal laboratory tests in patients with simple febrile seizure. *J Pediatr Neurosci* 10: 93–97.

Zare-Shahabadi A, Ashrafi MR, *et al.* (2015): Single nucleotide polymorphisms of TNF-α gene in febrile seizures. *J Neurol Sci* 356: 153–156.

Zerr DM, Blume HK, Berg AT, *et al.* (2005): Nonfebrile illness seizures: a unique seizure category. *Epilepsia* 46: 952–955.

Zhang YH, Burgess R, Malone JP, *et al.* (2017): Genetic epilepsy with febrile seizures plus: Refining the spectrum. *Neurology* 89: 1210–1219.

WITH VIDEO SUPPLEMENTS

CHAPTER 10

DRAVET SYNDROME (PREVIOUSLY SEVERE MYOCLONIC EPILEPSY IN INFANCY)

Charlotte DRAVET[1], Michelle BUREAU[2], Hirokasu OGUNI[3], Özlem ÇOKAR[4] and Renzo GUERRINI[5]

[1] Centre Saint-Paul, Henri-Gastaut Hospital, Marseille, France; Infantile Neuropsychiatric Unit, Fondazionze Policlinico Universitario A. Gemelli, IRCCS, Catholic University Sacro Cuore, Rome, Italy
[2] Centre Saint-Paul, Henri-Gastaut Hospital, Marseille, France
[3] Tokyo Women's Medical University, Department of Pediatrics, Tokyo, Japan
[4] Department of Neurology, Haseki Educational and Research Hospital, Health Sciences University, Istanbul, Turkey
[5] Pediatric Neurology Unit and Laboratories, Children's Hospital A. Meyer and University of Florence, Florence, Italy

History

Dravet syndrome (DS) was initially described as "severe myoclonic epilepsy of infancy" (SMEI), in order to distinguish it from the Lennox-Gastaut syndrome (LGS) (Dravet, 1978, Dravet *et al.*, 1982). Many children have since been reported to have symptoms similar to SMEI but without myoclonus (Sugama *et al.*, 1987; Ogino *et al.*, 1989; Kanazawa, 1992; Yakoub *et al.*, 1992; Dravet *et al.*, 1992). These patients also had variable electroencephalographic (EEG) features but they shared the same course and outcome as those with myoclonic jerks and were included in the same syndrome as *borderline forms* (SMEB). This view was supported by the genetic studies which have discovered *SCN1A* gene mutations in patients with and without myoclonic manifestations (Fukuma *et al.*, 2004). It also appeared that epilepsy was not limited to infancy and childhood and persisted in adulthood. For these reasons, it was proposed to change the syndrome name, first to "severe polymorphic epilepsy of infants" (Aicardi, 1994) and then to the eponym "Dravet syndrome" (Engel, 2001). Two main forms are recognized: the typical/complete form and the atypical/incomplete form, the latter referring to patients without myoclonic seizures and often a milder phenotype and referred to as *borderline* forms. In the scheme proposed by the ILAE (Berg *et al.*, 2010) DS is considered as an "epileptic encephalopathy", defined as "a condition in which the epileptic activity itself may contribute to severe cognitive and behavioral impairment above and beyond what might be expected from the underlying pathology alone (*e.g.*, cortical malformation) and that these can worsen over time". In 2017, the ILAE classification Commission (Scheffer *et al.*, 2017) refined this definition by recognizing that factors other than epilepsy can be at the origin of the cognitive and behavioral impairment, for example genetic factors, and distinguished three types of encephalopathy: i) *developmental encephalopathy* where there is only developmental impairment without frequent epileptic activity; ii) *epileptic encephalopathy* where there is no preexisting developmental delay and the genetic mutation is not thought to cause cognitive slowing in its own right; iii) *developmental and epileptic encephalopathy* where both factors play a role. DS is perhaps the best example of this third type in which "often it may not be possible to disentangle whether the epileptic or developmental component is more important in contributing to a patient's presentation".

Definition

DS is actually a neurogenetic disease characterized by epilepsy, cognitive decline, behavior disorders and motor impairment, in which both epilepsy and genetic alterations contribute to the encephalopathic features.

According to the 1989 ILAE classification (Commission 1989), the typical DS is characterized by "febrile and afebrile generalized and unilateral, clonic or tonic clonic, seizures that occur in the first year of life in an otherwise normal infant and are later associated with myoclonus, atypical absences, and partial seizures. All seizure types are resistant to antiepileptic drugs (AEDs). Developmental delay becomes apparent within the second year of life and is followed by definite cognitive impairment and personality disorders." Later on, other criteria appeared: frequent convulsive/non convulsive epileptic status, progressive motor impairment, normal neuro-imaging, possible photo and pattern-sensitivity (42%), possible family history of epilepsy or febrile seizures (25-71%).

Since 2001 (Claes *et al.*, 2001) it is known that a mutation or deletion of the *SCN1A* gene, encoding the voltage-gated sodium channel Nav1.1, is associated with the syndrome and it has become progressively clear that this association can be demonstrated in almost all the patients

Epidemiology

DS is a rare disorder and is classified as ORPHA 33069 in the Orphanet classification. An incidence of probably less than 1 per 40,000 was reported in 1990 in the USA (Hurst, 1990). In 1992, the incidence in France was estimated between 1/20,000 and 1/30,000 (Yakoub *et al.*, 1992). More recent studies consider genetic criteria.

The first population-based study reports an incidence of mutation-positive DS of at least 1/40,900 births in the UK (Brunklaus *et al.*, 2012) but the authors believe this figure is underestimated. Other European studies found a higher incidence of 1/22,000 in Denmark, including only mutation-positive patients (Bayat *et al.*, 2015) and 1/33,000 in Sweden, 88% mutation-positive (Rosander & Hallböök, 2015). In the USA, the incidence was estimated at 1/22,000 births for patients carrying a *SCN1A* mutation, and 1/15, 700 when patients without mutation were included (Wu *et al.*, 2015). Durà-Travé *et al.* (2007) found 1.4% of patients with DS in a hospital population aged from one month to less than 15 years. The rate of DS among patients with seizure onset in the first year of life or before the age of three was estimated to be between 3% and 7% (Caraballo *et al.*, 1997; Yakoub *et al.*, 1992; Dalla Bernardina *et al.*, 1983; Dravet *et al.*, 1992). A slight predominance of males appears (54%) in the total number of 300 patients in three population-based studies (Brunklaus *et al.*, 2012; Bayat *et al.*, 2015; Rosander & Hallbook, 2015), but lower in a large survey of 802 patients (Skluzacek *et al.*, 2011) with only 51% of males.

Clinical and EEG description

Some authors considered that the course of DS can be divided in three stages: a "febrile phase", in the first year, then a "catastrophic phase", of variable duration, and a "sequel phase" (Lambarri San Martin *et al.*, 1997). We agree with this description but will not use this distinction because the age limits between the second and the third phases are unclear. Instead the onset and steady state are considered in this chapter and there is a separate section for long-term outcome.

Onset

Age at onset

Occurrence of the first seizure in the first year of life is part of the definition and has been recently confirmed (Cetica *et al.*, 2017). A later onset should question the diagnosis of DS. All the authors give a mean onset age between five and eight months.

Personal antecedents and associated pathology

The infants usually do not have a personal pathological history. However, pathologic antecedents during pregnancy and delivery were noted in some series, varying from 22% to 66% (Dravet *et al.*,1992; Ragona *et al.*, 2010; Giovanardi-Rossi *et al.*, 1991). This variability seems to be linked to the different considerations with which reported events were deemed as relevant. Associated diseases are rare, and anecdotal: Rud Syndrome, epidermal naevus syndrome, type I neurofibromatosis, hemophilia (one case each), growth hormone deficit (two cases), congenital cardiac defects (4.6%, Skluzacek *et al.*, 2011). Development is apparently normal, even in patients with an associated pathological history.

Large genomic deletions involving *SCN1A* and the sodium gene cluster located on chromosome 2, are associated with a phenotype in which DS features are associated to other traits not belonging to the syndrome (Madia *et al.*, 2006; Marini *et al.*, 2009). These patients should not be diagnosed as DS.

Clinical semiology at onset

To describe seizure types we will use the newly introduced seizure terminology (Fisher *et al.*, 2017) as long as we found it adequate to correctly describe the at times peculiar seizure types in the syndrome. We group the generalized/unilateral clonic and tonic-clonic seizures and the tonic seizures under the word "convulsive" seizures. The first seizure is typically convulsive, clonic, generalized or unilateral, triggered by fever but often longer than a simple febrile seizure (FS). Several Japanese authors (Sugama *et al.*, 1987; Fujiwara *et al.*, 1990) underlined the triggering effect of a Japanese-style hot water immersion, causing increased body temperature (see below). However, variations in the mode of onset have been observed by many authors. Convulsive seizures can occur without fever, from 28% (Ohki *et al.*, 1997) to 61% (Ragona *et al.*, 2010) of the children. In our series (Dravet *et al.*, 1992), these afebrile seizures usually occurred after a vaccination or during an infectious episode, or after a hot bath. These seizures, with or without fever, are most often long, lasting more than twenty minutes, and may evolve to status epilepticus

(SE). The initial seizure can be focal. In some patients, isolated episodes of focal myoclonic jerking are observed, even in the absence of fever, either some weeks or days before the first convulsive seizure, and remain isolated, or occur in the hours preceding the first convulsive seizure. Focal seizures with impaired awareness, with or without motor symptoms (alias complex partial seizures) are rarely observed (Dravet *et al.*, 2005a; Oguni *et al.*, 2001; Ohki *et al.*, 1997). Focal seizures with ictal vomiting have been reported (Hino-Fukuyo *et al.*, 2009).

EEG semiology at onset

At onset, background activity while awake is usually normal. In some cases a 4-5-Hz rhythmic theta activity is noted over the rolandic and vertex areas (Dalla Bernardina *et al.*, 1982; Giovanardi-Rossi *et al.*, 1991). The sleep EEG shows normal organization. Diffuse or unilateral slowing of the background activity may be observed if the EEG is recorded shortly after a prolonged seizure.

Generalized spike waves elicited by intermittent photic stimulation, a most unusual finding in infants, have been reported with variable frequency (Specchio *et al.*, 2011; Ragona *et al.*, 2010; Caraballo & Fejerman, 2006; Dalla Bernardina *et al.*, 1982; Dravet *et al.*, 1992).

Steady state

The first seizure is often considered as a FS, few investigations are performed and, usually, no treatment is given. But shortly after other febrile and afebrile seizures occur. Between one and four years old, different seizure types appear, simultaneously with a slowing in the psychomotor development and the picture becomes characteristic of a steady state.

Steady state: seizures

Patients with DS have multiple seizure types during the course, including generalized motor onset, either clonic (GCS) or tonic clonic (GTCS), and alternating unilateral clonic, rarely tonic, seizures, grouped as "convulsive seizures"; generalized or focal onset myoclonic seizures; generalized non motor onset seizures such as atypical absences; focal onset seizures with either retained or impaired awareness, with or without motor, autonomic symptoms, with or without tonic clonic bilateralization; unclassified seizures we have named "obtundation status".

The following description is based on one study conducted in Marseille on 60 patients whose seizures were carefully analyzed by video-polygraphic-EEG recordings.

Convulsive seizures

They are present all along in all the patients. In our study most clonic seizures were recorded during sleep, at various stages of the course, usually after the age of three.

We distinguished several forms including apparently true generalized clonic or tonic-clonic seizures, unilateral seizures, "falsely generalized" seizures, "unstable seizures", and tonic seizures. They can be associated in the same patient. The distinction between "falsely generalized" and "unstable" is somewhat artificial as these seizures have in common the focal onset and rapid spread to the adjacent areas or to the opposite hemisphere.

Generalized motor onset seizures, clonic (GCS) or tonic-clonic (GTCS). The EEG discharge is bilateral, synchronous from the onset (*Figure 1*). GTCS are shorter than in adults, with a very brief tonic phase, few autonomic symptoms, a transient postictal flattening quickly replaced by diffuse delta waves. In some seizures the initial tonic phase is almost immediately mixed with clonic jerks, giving a vibratory aspect, as documented by Ogihara *et al.* (1994). We did not record seizures described as clonic-tonic-clonic convulsions by Fujiwara *et al.* (1992) and also reported by others (Ohki *et al.*, 1997).

Unilateral seizures. True hemiclonic seizures (Gastaut *et al.*, 1974), have been recorded only in two young children (16 months and 3 years) in our series. They become rare when patients are older (Ohki *et al.*, 1997). Ragona *et al.* (2010) reported them to have occurred in 14/37 patients in the first year of life. Other types of unilateral seizures have different characteristics including shorter duration, association of contralateral changes in muscle tonus, ictal EEG abnormalities limited to one hemisphere. In all cases there is postictal EEG asymmetry and, often, postictal transient hemiparesis. These seizures can be on either side in the same patient, this alternating pattern being rather typical for DS (*Figures 2 and 3*). Two patients with DS and hemiclonic SE followed by permanent hemiparesis and cerebral hemiatrophy are on record (Caraballo & Fejerman, 2006; Sakakibara *et al.*, 2009). This situation realizes the hemiconvulsion-hemiplegia (HH) syndrome (Gastaut *et al.*, 1974) which is, overall, rarely observed in DS.

"Falsely generalized seizures". These seizures are described as GTCS by the parents but have instead a complex semiology with some degree of discrepancy between clinical and EEG phenomena. They usually consist of a bilateral, asymmetric, tonic contraction, leading to variable postures (extension of one limb, flexion of another), with impaired awareness. The ensuing clonic phase is asymmetric and asynchronous, often lasting more than one minute. The autonomic symptoms are milder than in a GTCS (*Figure 4 and video*). The EEG discharge is always bilateral but often asymmetric (Ogino, 1986; Kanazawa, 1992).

"Unstable seizures". They are characterized by topographic changes of the ictal EEG discharge that involves different parts of the brain irregularly, in the course of the same seizure. The clinical manifestations are close to those of the "falsely generalized" seizures with

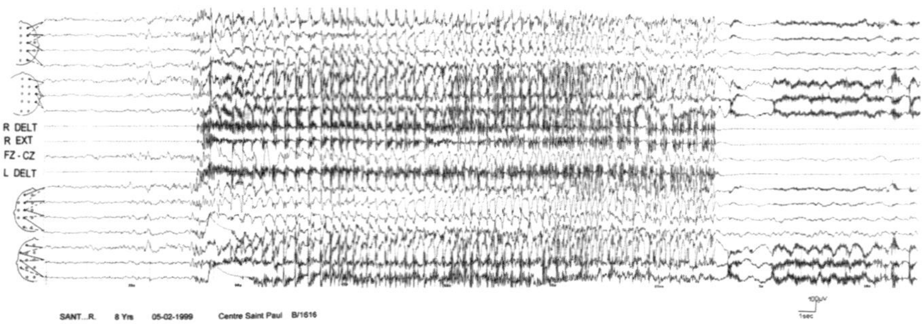

Figure 1

A generalized tonic-clonic seizure in an 8-year-old boy. At onset: brief burst of fast activity (less than 1 s) progressively intermixed with slow waves. End of the seizure: brief flattening followed by theta activity. On the EMG (two deltoids): tonic contraction followed by sustained myoclonias that become irregular and very fast, with a vibratory aspect.

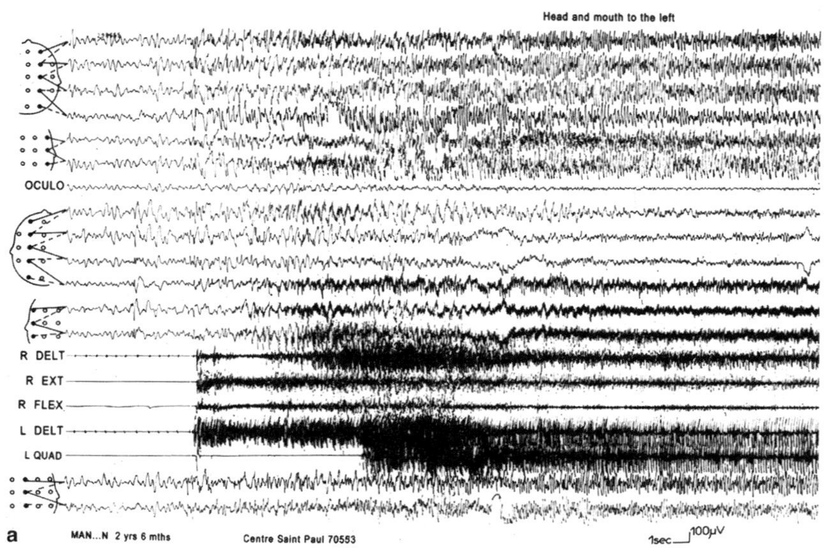

Figure 2

A left hemiclonic seizure recorded in a 2-year-6-month-old boy. On the right hemisphere, spikes and slow waves during 5 sec, followed by rapid, high voltage spikes and slow waves on the frontocentral area, followed by a low-voltage rapid activity.

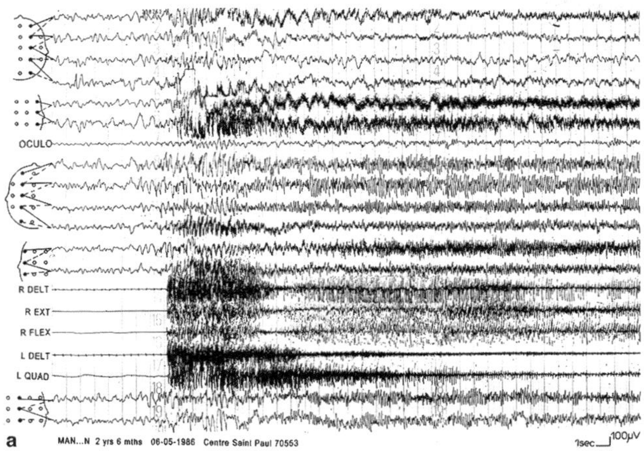

Figure 3 **A right hemiclonic seizure in a 2-year-6-month-old boy during a status.**

On the left hemisphere, slow waves and spikes followed by high-voltage fast activity. On the right hemisphere theta activity with muscular artefacts over the temporal area due to the head and mouth deviation to the right. On the polygraphy, at onset diffuse tonic contraction, then vibratory phase on the right muscles.

asymmetric and asynchronous tonic and clonic movements, sometimes predominant on one side or shifting from one side to the other. As in the falsely generalized seizures, the EEG discharge involves different parts of the brain irregularly *(Figure 5)*. Relationship between clinical events and accompanying EEG is not always clear.

Tonic seizures. These seizures are unusual in this syndrome but have been mentioned in the literature (Dulac & Arthuis, 1982; Dravet *et al.*, 1992; Lambarri San Martin *et al.*, 1997; Ohmori *et al.*, 2001; Caraballo & Fejerman, 2006; Nabbout *et al.*, 2008; Losito *et al.*, 2017). and we recorded them too *(Figure 6)*. They have variable electroclinical features resembling the axial tonic seizures of the LGS, sometimes with a myoclonic component, but are usually sporadic and only in a few patients they were repeated in cluster during the same recording, as in the LGS. Losito *et al.* (2017) observed tonic and tonic-clonic seizures in 35.6% of 73 patients, occurring in clusters during the night, not responsive to treatment and persisting from late childhood to adulthood.

With the exception of tonic seizures all these convulsive seizures can be prolonged (more than 30 minutes) or repeated, realizing SE, requiring intravenous drug administration and, often, respiratory support. Most authors mention the frequency of convulsive status, mainly in the first years, which occur in around 75–80% of the patients (Oguni *et al.*, 2001; Fontana *et al.*, 2004; Akiyama *et al.*, 2010; Ragona *et al.*, 2010, 2011; Brunklaus *et al.*, 2012; Nabbout *et al.*, 2013). Most episodes are not followed by neurological sequel. However, febrile SE are at times intractable and may evolve to an acute encephalopathy resulting in severe neurological sequelae or death (Sakauchi *et al.*, 2011a, b). Rhabdomyolisis with renal failure and liver dysfunction has also been reported by Sato *et al.* (1995).

Myoclonic seizures

We distinguish ictal and interictal myoclonus. Ictal myoclonus, or a myoclonic seizure, is accompanied by a paroxysmal EEG discharge, whereas interictal myoclonic jerks do not have an EEG correlate.

Myoclonic seizures appear between the ages of one and five years, rarely earlier (Caraballo & Fejerman, 2006; Dravet *et al.*, 2005a, b; Oguni *et al.*, 2001; Ohki *et al.*, 1997). They can be massive, involving the whole body, particularly axial muscles, leading to hurling of objects held by the child, and to falling. But their intensity is variable, and they are sometimes barely discernible. When they are attenuated they can involve only the axial muscles (head and trunk), causing a small movement forward or backward. Some parents describe sudden falls to the ground without apparent myoclonic jerk and several authors reported atonic seizures which have never been recorded with polygraphy. We never observed or recorded such atonic drop attacks but documented an atonic component associated with myoclonus *(Figure 7)*. Myoclonic seizures can be either isolated or grouped in two or three jerks. They occur several times a day, sometimes incessantly, but in some children are observed only on awakening or in the minutes or hours preceding a seizure. They persist during drowsiness and disappear during slow sleep, can be initiated by photic stimulation, variation in light intensity, closure of the eyes and fixation on patterns. They do not seem to be accompanied by changes in awareness, except when they occur at very close intervals.

The polygraphic EEG recordings demonstrate generalized spike-waves (SWs) or multiple SWs, at 3 Hz or more *(Figure 8)*. Their duration is usually brief (1–3 s) but can sometimes be longer (up to 10 s). In one video-polygraphic study, myolonic seizures in DS were different from those in benign myoclonic epilepsy in infancy and myoclonic-atonic epilepsy with respect to frequency of spike-wave (3.2 Hz *vs.* 1.3–1.5 Hz) and duration of myoclonus (< 100 msec. *vs.* 250 msec) and resembled to those in juvenile myoclonic epilepsy (Hirano *et al.*, 2009). A neurophysiological study of these myoclonic jerks

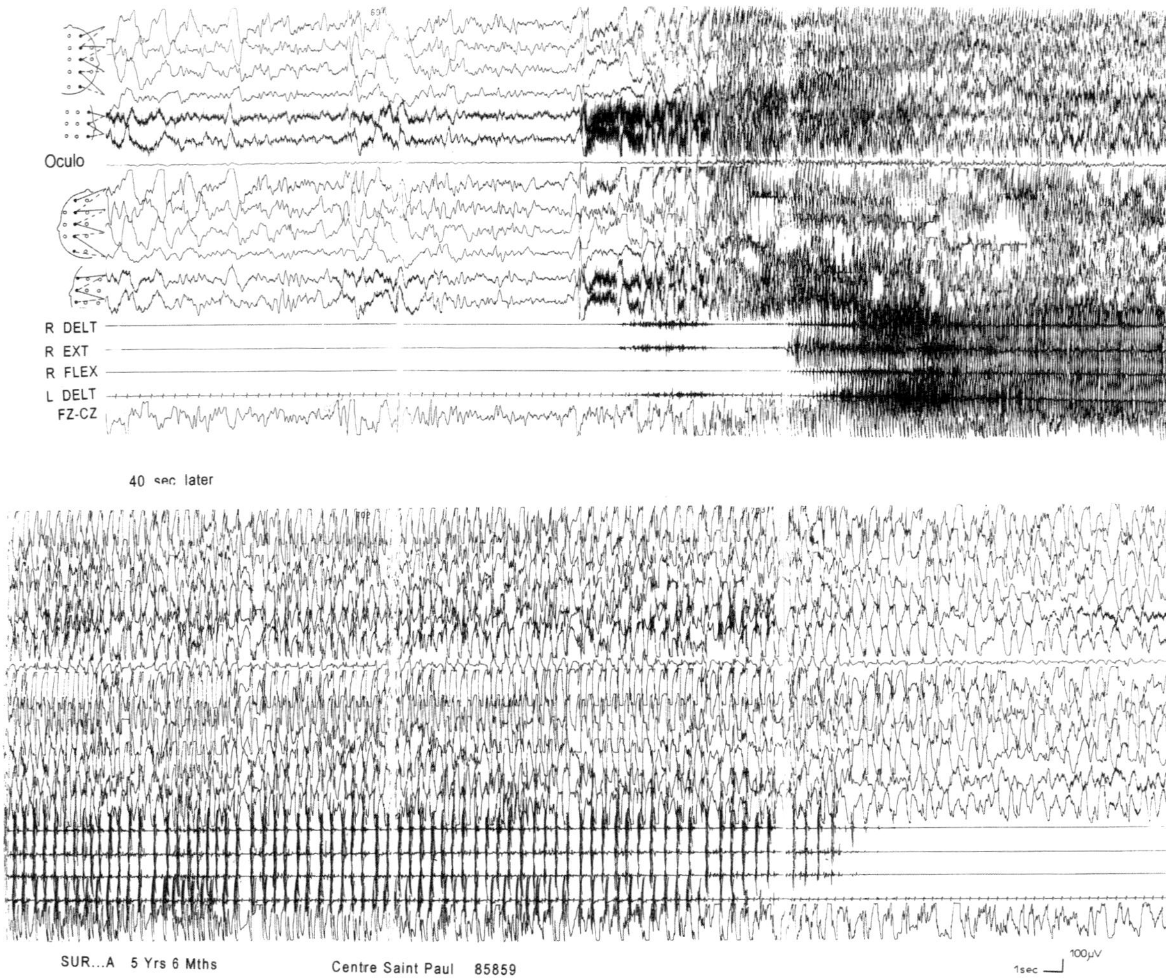

Figure 4

A "falsely generalized seizure" occurring in NREM sleep in a 5-year 6-month-old boy.
Top: **At onset a generalized slow spike followed by a low voltage theta activity, then bilateral fast activity of higher voltage over the left hemisphere. Note on the EMG recording that a slight bilateral tonic contraction begins 2 seconds after the EEG onset, remits, then is followed by an irregular tonic contraction associated with a vibratory aspect.**
Bottom: **40 sec later: diffuse SW associated with bilateral myoclonias which become progressively asynchronous and stop on the left deltoid before they stop on the right muscles. At the end of the seizure note the absence of a flattening but the presence of high-voltage delta waves.**

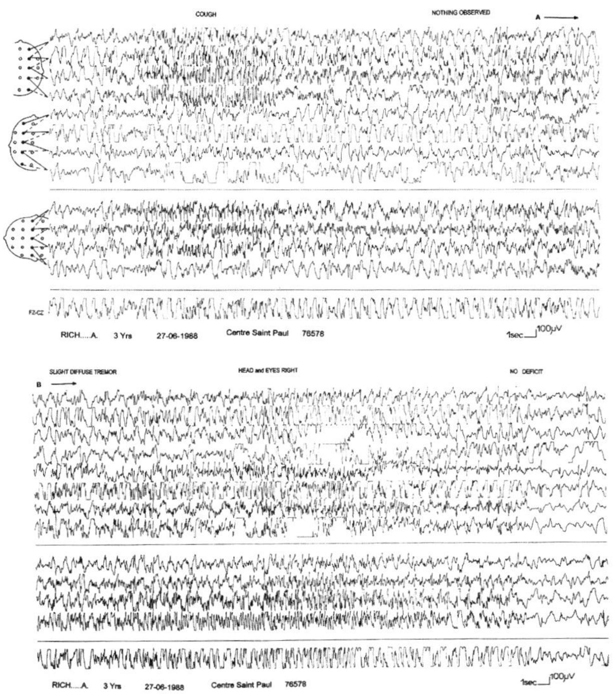

Figure 5 **An unstable seizure occurring during NREM sleep in a 3-year-old boy.**
Top: **brief diffuse lowering of voltage intermixed on the right hemisphere with fast activity, then spikes and slow waves evident only on the right hemisphere during 10 seconds followed by a more or less rhythmic activity around 10 Hz on the right centro-parietal area. 20 seconds after the onset of that activity a similar activity appears on the left fronto-centro-temporal region.**
Bottom: **continuation of the seizure: the activity is progressively associated with slow waves on the left hemisphere, becoming slower at the end of the seizure.**

demonstrated that the generalized jerks are caused by the spreading of cortical activity that originates independently from multiple cortical areas (Guerrini *et al.*, 2005).

In our series, the occurrence of myoclonic status is rare *(Figure 9)*, but in many cases the recurrence in clusters can culminate into a convulsive seizure. Other authors also describe these episodes of status in their patients, sometimes lasting even days (Dalla Bernardina *et al.*, 1987; Yakoub *et al.*, 1992).

Atypical absence seizures

They can appear at different ages, either between one and three years, together with myoclonic attacks, or later up to age 12 years. Earlier occurrence has been reported (Ohki *et al.*, 1997; Tsuda *et al.*, 2013). There may be, inconstantly, a myoclonic component. They last from 3–10 s up to 20 s (Tsuda *et al.*, 2013). Eyelid myoclonia and nodding can be observed. When the myoclonic component is pronounced, it is difficult to differentiate these atypical absences from myoclonic attacks as also underlined by Oguni *et al.* (2005). In fact, both are probably the expression of the same epileptic process with different intensity and duration. Only one patient was reported to exhibit true myoclonic absences (Myers & Scheffer, 2017). In the EEG both seizure types correspond to generalized, irregular SWs at 2–3.5 Hz *(Figure 10)* that can be preceded by a focal discharge, either in the occipital or in the frontal and temporal regions (Ohmori *et al.*, 2001; Tsuda *et al.*, 2013). Occasionally, absences with rhythmic, generalized SWs at 3 Hz, similar to those observed in

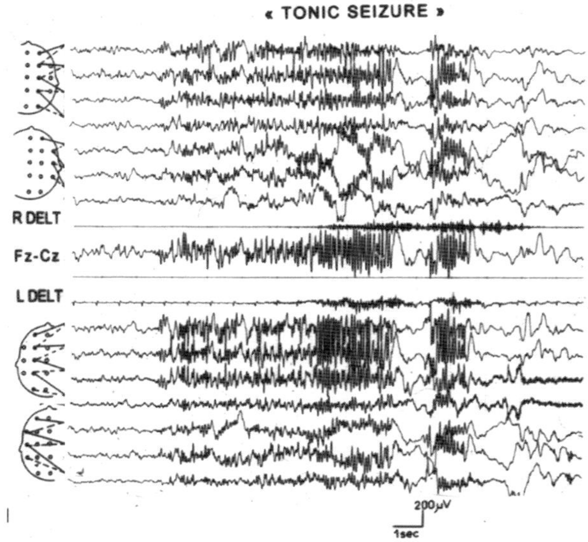

Figure 6 **A tonic seizure in a 11-year-7-month-old girl occurring during NREM sleep. Onset by polyspikes followed high voltage fast activity intermixed by a brief flattening.**

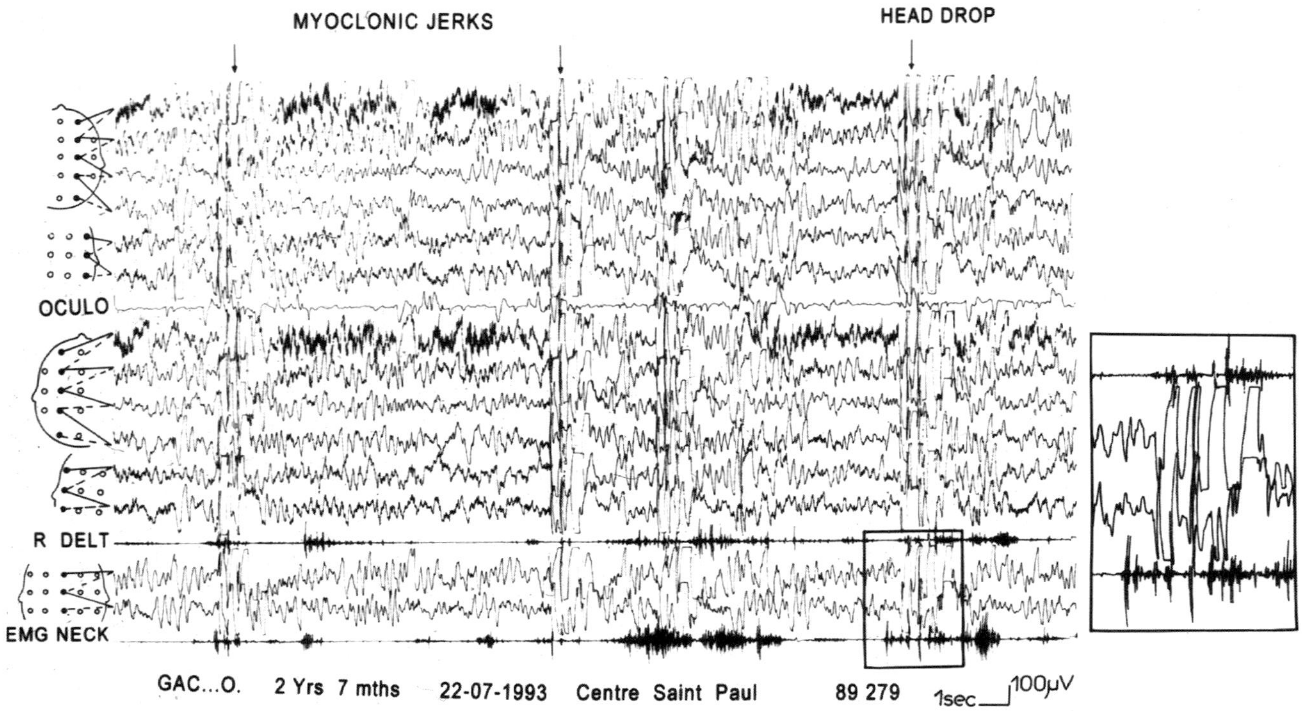

Figure 7

A series of myoclonic-atonic seizures in a 2-year-7-month-old boy.
Four discharges of rapid, high voltage, generalized SW, during one second, accompanied once by a brief head drop. On the right, the enlargement of the image shows the postmyoclonic atonia responsible for the clinical event.

childhood absence epilepsy, were recorded (Dulac & Arthuis,1982) *(Figure 11)*. Rarely, absence status can be observed (Bureau & Dalla Bernardina, 2011). This status appears progressively as impairment of consciousness of fluctuating intensity, without motor manifestations. EEG is characterized by diffuse, subcontinuous sequences of slow polySWs, fluctuating in amplitude. Episodes of absence status are long-lasting, they can disappear spontaneously during sleep, but can reappear upon awakening.

Obtundation status

They represent a relatively characteristic manifestation, distinct from absence status, reported in around 40% of patients in several series (Dalla Bernardina *et al.*, 1987; Oguni *et al.*, 2001; Fontana *et al.*, 2004; Dravet *et al.*, 2005a, b). However, they are not reported in three series (Ohki *et al.*, 1997; Caraballo & Fejerman, 2006; Ragona *et al.*, 2010). Their clinical and EEG features do not suggest a generalized or focal nature. We recorded 18 obtundation status in 11 patients age 2 to 19 years. They consist of an impairment of consciousness, variable in intensity, with fragmentary and segmental, erratic myoclonus, of low amplitude, involving the limbs and face, sometimes associated with drooling and a slight increase in the muscle tone. Randomly recurrent massive jerks are intercalated. Patients can or cannot react to stimuli, perform simple activities, interrupted by short episodes of complete unresponsiveness and staring. Strong sensory stimulations can interrupt the status but never

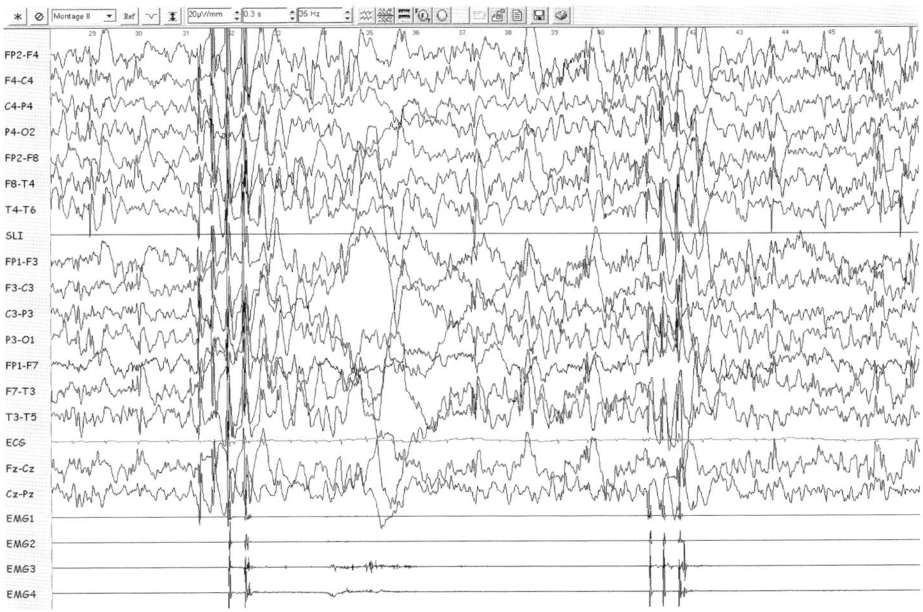

Figure 8

Typical awake EEG in a 5-year-old girl.
2 bursts of generalized SW accompanied by generalized myoclonic jerks and independent multifocal spikes over the fronto-central and parieto-occipital areas.

definitively. Myoclonic jerks may build up into brief synchronous fits. Convulsive seizures can either follow (Yasuda *et al.*, 1989), initiate, occur during, or terminate these episodes that can be prolonged for hours, even days, and favored by environmental light stimuli, eye closure and pattern fixation. EEG is usually characterized by diffuse dysrhythmia of slow waves, intermingled with focal and diffuse spikes *(Figure 12)*, sharp waves and SWs, of higher voltage in anterior and vertex regions, without temporal relationship between spikes and myoclonic jerks, except during major myoclonic fits as also described by Ohmori *et al.*, 2001). Intravenous or rectal diazepam attenuated but did not stop this status. Other EEG aspects were described: pseudorhythmic diffuse high-amplitude, irregular slow waves, occasionally notched with small spikes (Oguni *et al.*, 2005) and continuous focal, posterior discharge corresponding to a focal non motor onset status (Wakai *et al.*, 1996a; Oguni *et al.*, 2001).

Focal seizures

Focal aware motor onset (previously simple partial seizures, SPS) and focal non motor onset with impaired awareness and prominent autonomic symptoms (previously complex partial seizures, CPS) occur in 43-78.6% of patients in the largest series (Oguni *et al.*, 2001; Ohmori *et al.*, 2001; Caraballo & Fejerman, 2006; Ragona *et al.*, 2010). They can appear early, from four months to four years (Ohki *et al.*, 1997). In our series (Dravet *et al.*, 2005a, b) they were reported in 32 patients (53%), four with only SPS, 17 with only CPS and 11 with both. SPS were either versive seizures, or clonic jerks limited to a limb or one hemiface, or a combination of the two. CPS were characterized by unresponsiveness, autonomic phenomena (pallor, cyanosis, rubefaction, respiratory changes, drooling, sweating), oral automatisms, hypotonia, rarely stiffness, sometimes with eyelid or distal myoclonus *(Figure 13)*. These two seizure types could evolve to tonic-clonic bilateralization. Ictal EEG is a focal discharge usually

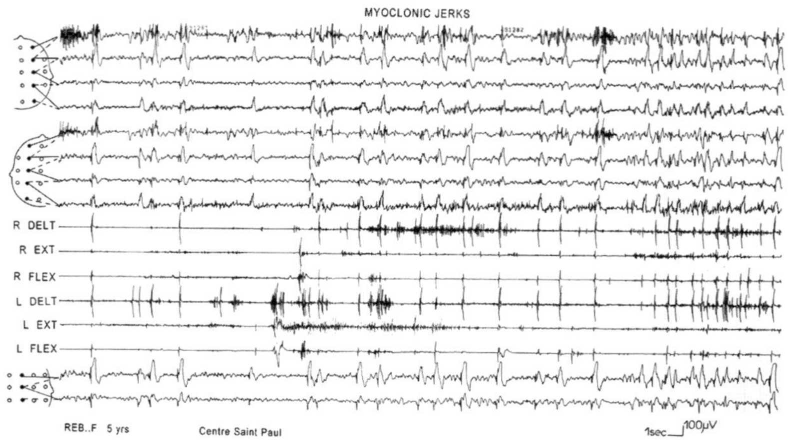

Figure 9

Myoclonic status in a 5-year-old boy.
Rapid high-voltage arhythmic generalized fast SW accompanied by myoclonic jerks more important on the deltoid muscles, sometimes associated with a tonic contraction.

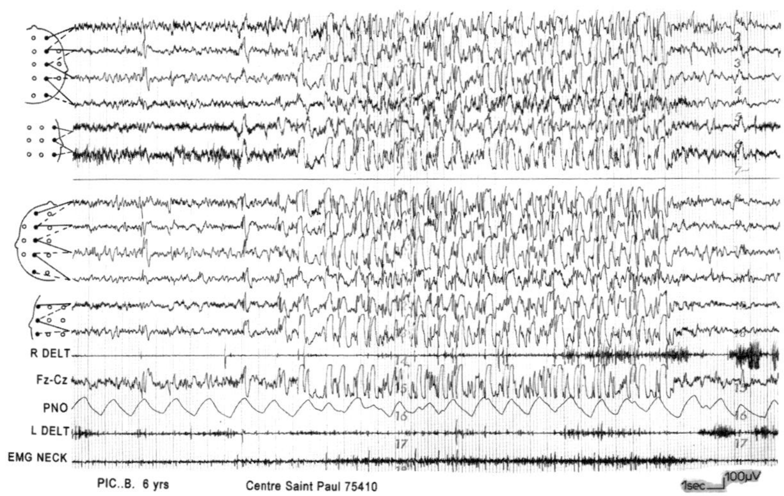

Figure 10

Atypical absence in a 6-year-old girl. Discharge of irregular, high voltage, diffuse SW accompanied by arhythmic, slight myoclonic jerks, visible on the left deltoid and the neck EMG, and a breathing change.

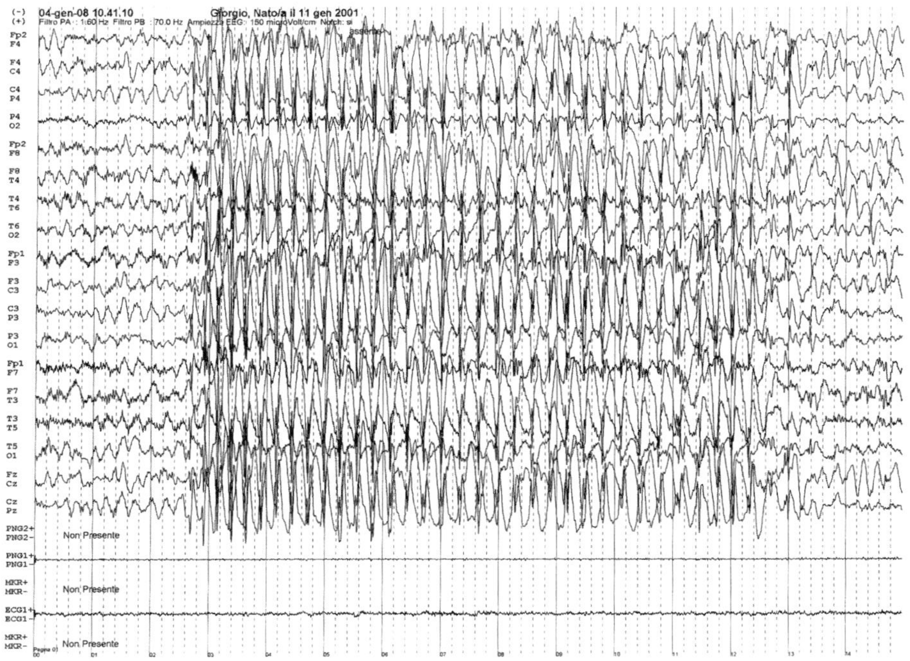

Figure 11

Another type of absence in an 8-year-old boy. Discharge of regular, high voltage, generalized SW at 3 Hz, very similar to the discharge observed in the absences of chilhood absence epilepsy.

in temporal or occipital region. In the literature, the reported focal seizures are CPS with the same characteristics we described above (Ohki *et al.*,1997; Gaily *et al.*, 2013; Specchio *et al.*, 2014). While CPS are reported by most authors, SPS are mentioned only by some (Giovanardi-Rossi *et al.*, 1991; Yakoub *et al.*, 1992; Wang *et al.*, 1996; Sarisjulis *et al.*, 2000; Caraballo & Fejerman, 2006).

Triggering factors

One of the main symptoms that characterize DS patients is their extremely low epileptic threshold to external as well as internal stimuli, especially observed in the small children. The following sections will examine the main factors associated with seizure precipitation.

Temperature variations

"Body temperature variations sensitivity" is a definition more appropriate than "fever sensitivity" because the temperature level that can trigger a seizure is often below the level admitted to define fever (≥ 37°8 Celsius). This increase of temperature is not necessarily accompanied by an infection. Temperature sensitivity is also expressed when the child takes a hot bath, as first described by the Japanese authors since whole body immersion in hot water (39° to 42° for 5-10 minutes) is a common habit in Japan (Ogino *et al.*, 1985). By recording the video-EEG of seven children with DS in hot water immersion and monitoring their temperature continuously, Awaya *et al.* (1989) demonstrated the crucial role of the increasing tempe-

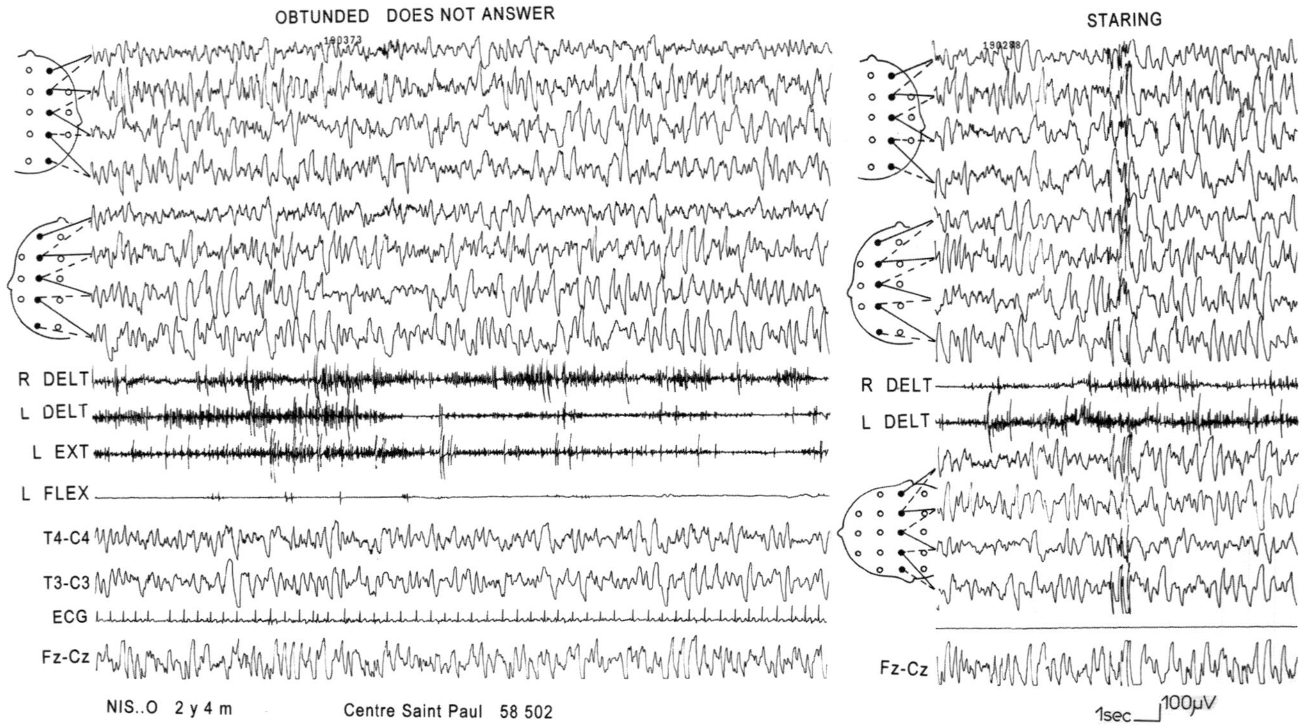

Figure 12

An obtundation status in a 2-year-4-month-old boy.
On the left: **the EEG shows slow waves intermixed with very rare small spikes. Impairment of consciousness and erratic, fragmentary myoclonias associated with a slight tonic component.**
On the right: **during this status occurrence of a SW discharge accompanied by a staring.**

rature unrelated to infection or physical exercise. A more recent study in Taiwan came to similar conclusions (Lee *et al.*, 2015). In European countries precipitation by hot bath is rare (Ragona *et al.*, 2010). External temperature can also represent an aggravating factor and some patients have more seizures in the summer and in hot areas.

Susceptibility to infections is obvious: infections of the upper respiratory tracts are repeated and pneumonia can be severe. Although immunological studies did not show abnormalities that could explain this susceptibility (Nieto *et al.*, 2000a; Oguni *et al.*, 2001, 2005), in our opinion, the chronic use of benzodiazepines may favor respiratory infections via increased secretions.

Photosensitivity and pattern sensitivity

Photosensitivity encompasses a pathological response to intermittent photic stimulation (IPS), or bright environmental light, a wide range of stimuli or images producing high contrast (television, patterns), eye closure (fixation-off sensitivity). These stimuli can provoke eyelid myoclonia, atypical absences, usually with myoclonia, and clonic seizures, with or without focal onset. Pattern sensitivity is not always easy to detect in young children. Different sorts of patterns present in the environment can be effective, including geometrical designs or dotted lines on the walls, clothes, window screens, letters and designs in books for children and so on. It is difficult to properly

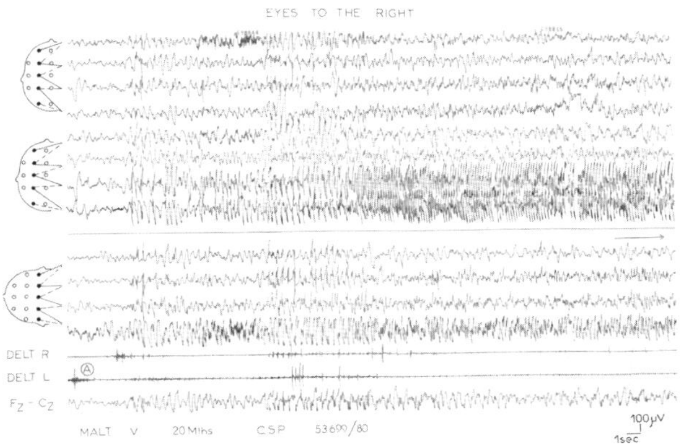

Figure 13 **A 1-year-8-month-old girl. Onset of a focal seizure, occurring on awakening, in the left mid- and posterior areas characterized by fast spikes and waves then by very rapid spikes. Clinically: right deviation of the eyes, loss of contact, arrhythmic myoclonias (of the two deltoids).**

analyze photosensitivity as it may vary over time. A discrepancy between the laboratory EEG and the everyday clinical photosensitivity can be observed, partly due to the use of various photic stimulators of which some are less effective (Specchio *et al.*, 2011; Verbeek *et al.*, 2017). However, photosensitivity has constantly been reported as a main feature (Dravet, 1978; Dravet *et al.*, 1982; Dalla Bernardina *et al.*, 1982). In our 1992 series of 60 patients (Dravet *et al.*, 1992), EEG photosensitivity was observed at least once in the course of the disease in 55% of patients, beginning between three months and five years six months and sometimes disappearing in adolescence. Self-stimulation by eye closure or pattern fixation was observed in 10/60 patients. Eye closure may provoke episodes of "eye fluttering" consisting of subtle eyelid myoclonia and rolling up of eyeballs, with decreased responsiveness.

In one series (Oguni *et al.*, 2001), 6/39 patients had numerous daily attacks (more than 100-200/day) which became very frequent under bright conditions, while they were remarkably reduced in the dark. They were mainly myoclonic seizures and atypical absences with eyelid myoclonia and retropulsion of the head. They became continuous immediately after exposure to bright illumination, easily culminated into GTCS. Takahashi *et al.* (1999) showed that patients with DS have a paroxysmal response which, unlike that in idiopathic generalized epilepsy, is dependent on the quantity of light rather than wavelength. Patients with constant light sensitivity appears to represent the most resistant, especially when children discover self-stimulation (Dalla Bernardina *et al.*, 1987; Fontana *et al.*, 2004). Recently, Verbeek *et al.* (2017) confirmed the high frequency of photosensitivity, which they consider as a marker of the overall severity of the disorder. There is no evidence that AEDs can reduce photosensitivity in DS.

Other stimuli

Among the other precipitating stimuli observed, the most important are physical exercise, excitation and emotions (Verbeek *et al.*, 2015).

Interictal EEG

– EEG background activity remains normal or slightly abnormal in about 50% of patients. In the remaining, background activity becomes slower and poorly organized but is heavily influenced by the time when the EEG is performed with respect to seizures, and can also be influenced by pharmacological treatments. The peculiar theta activity in frontocentral areas observed at onset in some patients appears in most cases and persists throughout follow-up (Ohki *et al.*, 1997; Bureau & Dalla Bernardina, 2011). In some patients there are no epileptiform abnormalities. When present, they are focal or multifocal, frontocentral or centrotemporal and vertex or occipital spikes, SW and polySW, associated with generalized abnormalities *(Figure 8)*. There is no relation between the site of the interictal abnormalities and the site of the seizure origin. Eye closure elicits subclinical or clinical discharges of spikes and SW in 25% of the cases. A strong photosensitivity persists in a large proportion of cases with or without associated clinical events. In other cases there is a fluctuation of the photosensitivity.

– Sleep EEG is usually well organized with physiological patterns, except when several seizures occur during the night. The paroxysmal, generalized as well as localized activities are enhanced or appear. Sometimes the focal abnormalities become continuous or subcontinuous during slow sleep over the frontal regions and decrease during REM sleep *(Figure 14)* as also described by Nabbout *et al.* (2008).

Neurological signs

At the very onset infants appear to have normal developmental skills. Neurological signs progressively appear, simultaneously with the psychomotor delay, but not in all patients.

Hypotonia is the most precocious sign, detectable around one year of age (Dalla Bernardina *et al.*, 1982).

Ataxia appears when the patients start to walk, usually at the normal age (12-18 months). Initially, it seems to be only a delayed walking, but gait remains unbalanced, with enlarged basis and poorly coordinated movements. Ataxia was reported in 83% of our first 42 cases (Dravet *et al.*, 1985), and confirmed by other authors (Dalla

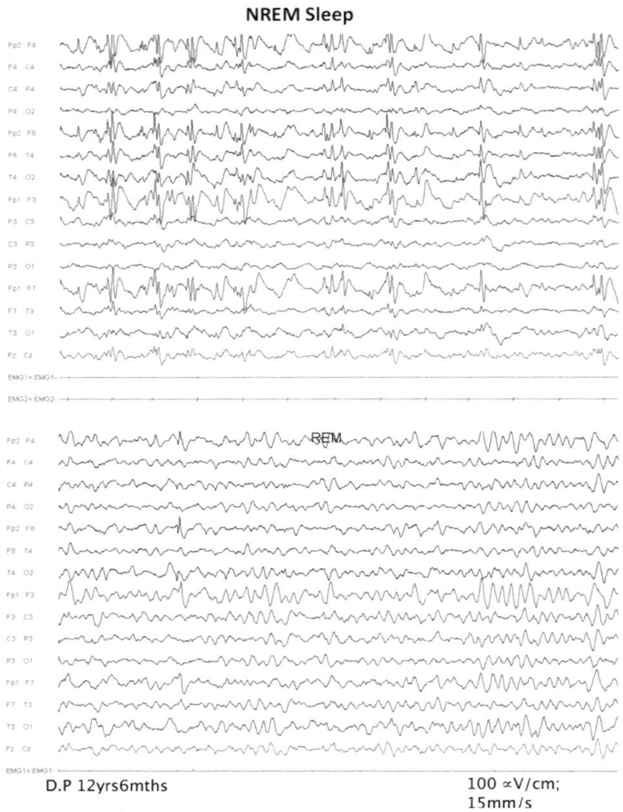

Figure 14 **A sleep EEG recording in a 12-year-6-month-old girl.**
Top: NREM sleep: subcontinuous spikes, polyspikes and SW over the frontal areas.
Bottom: during REM sleep, disappearance of the SW discharges, and existence of diffuse slow waves of higher voltage on the left hemisphere. Note a right fronto-temporal isolated spike.
EMG1+EMG1: right deltoid; EMG2+EMG2: left deltoid.

Bernardina *et al.*, 1982; Oguni *et al.*, 2005; Korff *et al.*, 2007; Ragona *et al.*, 2010; Villeneuve *et al.*, 2014). Ataxia may appear during childhood, often after SE or worsening of seizures. Conversely, in other patients, it tends to attenuate with age.

Pyramidal signs were found in 50% of our initial patients (Dravet *et al.*, 1985), in 80% of those of Dalla Bernadina *et al.* (1982), in 17/21 patients by Villeneuve *et al.* (2014). They consist of increased deep tendon reflexes, prominent at the lower limbs, with Babinski sign. Often the children walk on tip-toes. These signs tend to increase in periods with repeated convulsive seizures, and to decrease when interictal intervals become longer.

Interictal multifocal myoclonic jerks are frequently observed, appearing between age one and five years, at the same time as myoclonic seizures. They are also observed in patients who do not experience myoclonic seizures. They involve either the limbs, with distal predominance, or facial muscles. They are more frequent in the periods of seizure exacerbation, particularly, in older children upon awakening after nocturnal convulsive seizures. Their frequency is variable in the different series, from 30% to 100%. Interictal jerks can be difficult to single out unless polygraphic EEG recordings are performed while the child is involved in fine motor activities such as drinking, piling up cubes, or holding a spoon.

Autonomic symptoms other than the body temperature (Skluzacek *et al.*, 2011) include cold, red or bluish colored extremities, poor sweating, episodes of tachycardia without identifiable cause. In two recent surveys involving caregiver members of DS associations these symptoms do not appear as significant (Villas *et al.*, 2016; Knupp *et al.*, 2017).

Cognitive and motor development

Cognitive and behavioral development

Developmental delay becomes progressively evident from the second year on. Language starts at a normal age, with lallation and babble in the first year, but it progresses very slowly and many patients do not reach the stage of formulating elementary sentences.

The first neuropsychological study was conducted on 20 patients aged from 11 months to 16 years, 10 of them followed up over three years (Cassé-Perrot *et al.*, 2001; Wolff *et al.*, 2006). None of the patients was genetically tested. Cognitive and behavioral difficulties were always present, but of varying degrees *(Figure 15)*. Neuropsychological deficits concerned all skills, motor, linguistic and visual abilities being strikingly affected. Behavior was marked by hyperactivity, psychotic type of relationships and, sometimes, autistic traits. The appearance of neuropsychological disorders appeared to be related to the severity of the epilepsy in the first 2 years of life. Subsequent studies reported similar results (Dalla Bernardina *et al.*, 1987; Giovanardi-Rossi *et al.*, 1991; Yakoub *et al.*, 1992; Wang *et al.*, 1996; Caraballo

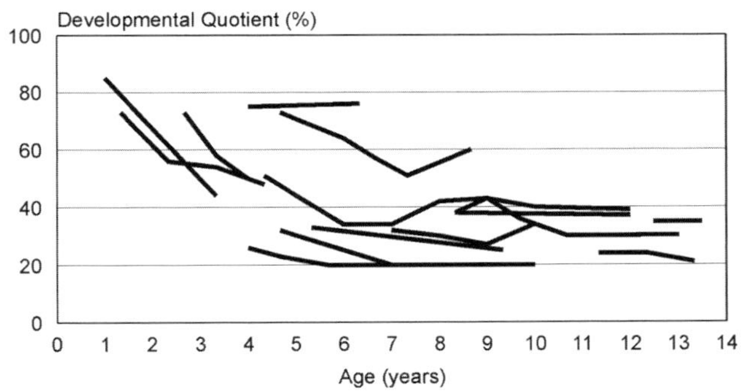

Figure 15 **Evolution of developmental quotient according to age (from Wolff *et al.*, 2006).**

& Fejerman, 2006; Oguni *et al.*, 2001). The more severely impaired functions include attention, visuo-motor abilities, eye-hand coordination, expressive language, verbal planning, auditory working memory, deficit in executive functions, fine motor skills (Cassé-Perrot *et al.*, 2001; Villeneuve *et al.*, 2014). Recently, Turner *et al.* (2017) reported a detailed analysis of the speech motor component they considered as typical for DS.

Studies of the modalities of the cognitive decline (Chieffo *et al.*, 2011a, b; Battaglia *et al.*, 2013, 2016; Ricci *et al.*, 2015; Chieffo *et al.*, 2016) reveal early appearance of visuo-constructive deficit in the first year of life when the development seems normal and the visuo-perceptual assessments results spared, this asymmetry persisting in the following years. Language impairment is also asymmetric with comprehension relatively preserved as regard expression. The possible contribution of a dorsal stream visual processing vulnerability and that of the cerebellum in determining the cognitive decline in DS is suggested (Ricci *et al.*, 2015). Numerous other studies were performed. Some authors emphasize the role of the mutation (Riva *et al.*, 2009; Korff, 2015) supported by experimental studies demonstrating the role of channelopathy on the cognitive decline in mice (Bender *et al.*, 2012, 2016; Han *et al.*, 2012). Conversely, the role of epilepsy is underlined by other authors who favor either the high number of convulsive seizures and SE during the first years or the presence of myoclonic and atypical absence seizures (Passamonti *et al.*, 2015; Ragona *et al.*, 2011; Olivieri *et al.*, 2016). It is difficult to disentangle the two factors and there is rather a consensus about the influence of both (Brunklaus *et al.*, 2012; Nabbout *et al.*, 2013; Ragona *et al.*, 2011; Gataullina & Dulac, 2016; Battaglia *et al.*, 2013, 2016). The recent experimental study in DS mice by Salgueiro-Pereira *et al.* (2019) well demonstrate this double influence: i) the role of the mutation per se does not seem to predominate in the cognitive phenotype; ii) the convulsive seizures have an effect on the phenotype; iii) but an interaction between the seizures and the mutation is necessary and the convulsive seizures without mutation cannot induce a severe phenotype.

Behavioral evolution is characterized by hyperactivity, recalcitrant behavior and stubbornness observed from the second year of life. Children do not acquire autonomy in the daily life. They become provocative, with poor impulse control, absence of danger sense. They have restricted interests and stereotyped activities (puzzles, cartoons), poor relationship with their pairs. Eye contact is fleeting and communication poor (Cassé-Perrot *et al.*, 2001, Villas *et al.*, 2017). Autistic traits are frequent but sociability is better than communication, as confirmed by the Vineland test results and only few children are actually autistic (Villeneuve *et al.*, 2014). However, in adolescents with mild cognitive impairment, poor comprehension and verbal communication deteriorate their social relationship with their pairs and contribute to their isolation, rarely aggressiveness. In the old reports the cognitive decline usually was severe, whereas in the recent series patients may have only mild or moderate deficits (Olivieri *et al.*, 2016).

Motor development

Patients have an *unbalanced gait* and a *poor movement coordination*, partly linked to hypotonia. *Interictal myoclonia and tremor* make the fine movements clumsy, hampering normal daily activities. *Skeletal anomalies* progressively appear during late childhood and adolescence, leading to a "crouch gait" posture, extensively described by Rodda *et al.* (2012). Gitiaux *et al.* (2016) reported a definite motor neuropathy in 7/12 patients presenting with gait disturbance and carrying an *SCN1A* mutation.

Neuroimaging and neuropathology

A main question in DS is whether seizure induced brain damage occurs. Examples have been reported of families in which amongst multiple individuals carrying *SCN1A* gene mutations, those having experienced a limited number of seizures have normal cognition while those with intractable seizures are cognitively impaired (Suls *et al.*, 2010; Guerrini *et al.*, 2011). Ataxic gait, or motor awkwardness and hyperactivity, and a jerky movement pattern are also reported in many of the children who have suffered severe seizures. Since the genetic abnormality does not appear sufficient to cause the impairment *per se*, it is plausible that other factors, possibly seizure related structural changes might contribute to producing cognitive impairment. There are only a few available data on morphologic or functional neuroimaging as well as neuropathology in DS and is therefore difficult to argue to what extent differences in cognitive and motor impairment have a structural anatomic counterpart (Guerrini *et al.*, 2011).

No gross abnormalities were detected on early brain CT or MRI studies, although signs of mild or moderate, diffuse, cerebral or cerebellar atrophy, increased white matter signal were occasionally reported (Dalla Bernardina *et al.*, 1982; Dravet *et al.*, 1992). In a few patients, neuroimaging was normal at the onset but brain atrophy appeared during follow-up (Dravet *et al.*, 2005a, b). Only three studies, all retrospective, have systematically investigated MRI findings (Siegler *et al.*, 2005; Striano *et al.*, 2007a; Catarino *et al.*, 2011). Siegler *et al.* (2005) studied a series of patients in whom no mutation analysis of the *SCN1A* gene had been performed. These authors found MRI changes consistent with hippocampal sclerosis (HS) in 10 out of 14 children with a clinical diagnosis of DS, aged 1.2 to 16 years (mean: 7.2). In six, who had been reported to have normal earlier MRI scans, HS had become obvious on a repeat scan. None of the 10 patients exhibited the clinical features of mesial temporal lobe epilepsy. Cerebral or cerebellar atrophy were observed in 6 out of 14 adult patients; one also exhibiting imaging evidence of hippocampal sclerosis (Jansen *et al.*, 2006).

Striano *et al.* (2007a) reviewed the MRI data of 58 patients (35 with a *SCN1A* mutation) in whom the last scan had been performed at 1.5-T after the age of 4 years. A detailed study of the hippocampal regions was available in all. Thirteen patients (22.4%) had MRI findings that were considered as abnormal; three patients had enlarged ventricles; one had unilateral HS and one had focal cortical dysplasia. Duration of epilepsy and age at seizure onset did not correlate with the presence of MRI abnormalities. There was no correlation between abnormal MRIs and the frequency of episodes of status epilepticus having occurred within the first four years of life. Abnormal findings were more frequently observed in patients without *SCN1A* mutations (39.1% *vs.* 11.4%, $p = 0.02$). Absence of mutations in specific gene makes the latter subgroup likely to be etiologically heterogeneous, however. In the series of adult patients reviewed by Catarino *et al.* (2011), 18 had brain MRI scan. Most frequently, brain imaging was normal, or showed non-specific findings, including cerebral and cerebellar atrophy, or cerebellar atrophy alone. One patient with *SCN1A* mutation had unilateral hippocampal sclerosis on MRI performed at 22 years of age.

A SPECT study (Nieto *et al.*, 1995) showed areas of hypoperfusion in 8 out of 10 patients; the finding was limited to one hemisphere in five patients and was bilateral in the remaining three. Areas of hypoperfusion did not clearly correlate with EEG findings.

The first available neuropathological study in DS was carried on a 19-month-old boy who had died unexpectedly (Renier & Renkawek, 1990). The most striking features included microdysgenesis of the cerebellum and the cerebral cortex and threefold spinal cord channels with surrounding ectopic tissue. The hippocampus and brainstem were normal. An additional autopsy case was reported in a 7-year-old girl who had died of hemorrhagic shock precipitated by an influenza infection (Hayashi *et al.*, 2004). Reported findings included edema and ischemic changes, related to the hemorrhagic shock, as well as fused gyri fused and heterotopic neurons in the adjacent white matter in the frontal and parietal cortex. The hippocampus harbored mild gliosis in the endplate (CA4), and calcified foci were present in the globus pallidus. Myelinated fibers were reduced in the spinal pyramidal tracts. The origin of these subtle structural changes, which in neither of the 2 patients were visible by imaging, remains unclear. Furthermore, it is not known whether a *SCN1A* mutation was present in these two patients.

Le Gal *et al.* (2010) found multifocal micronodular dysplasia of the left temporal cortex and bilateral endfolium gliosis on a neuropathological study of the whole brain of a child with DS and a SCN1A abnormality. In an extensive post mortem neuropathological study of three adult cases, no histological signature of the condition was identified; there was no evidence of cerebral neurodegeneration (Catarino *et al.*, 2011). In particular no significant alteration was found in the distribution and morphology of inhibitory interneuronal subsets in cortex, cerebellum, brainstem or hippocampus in adult DS, compared to that observed in the post-mortem controls with no known neurological disease, even with quantitative analysis. Routine histological stains detected cerebellar atrophy with Purkinje cell loss and gliosis in all adult post-mortem cases. However, as the authors pointed out, cerebellar atrophy was a frequent finding but did not differ, either in pattern or distribution, to that previously described in patients with chronic epilepsy without DS (Crooks *et al.*, 2000). A striking feature was the conspicuous preservation of neurons and interneurons despite decades of poorly controlled seizures.

Chipaux *et al.* (2010) reported unusual anoxo-ischemic-like MRI lesions in three patients with *SCN1A* mutations and DS who following refractory status epilepticus had experienced persistent, severe cognitive and motor deterioration. These MRI abnormalities could not be explained by hemodynamic failure but no plausible causative mechanism could be identified.

Sakakibara *et al.* (2009) reported a 2-year-old girl who had experienced repeated episodes of febrile status epilepticus and myoclonus, and a nonsense *SCN1A* mutation, developing persistent right hemiclonic seizures and left unilateral cortical laminar necrosis followed by progressive cerebral atrophy at age 15 months. The clinical and neuroradiological picture was consistent with the HH syndrome. This observation confirms the potential, though exceedingly rare, risk in children with DS to develop structural changes that can, in turn worsen the epileptic encephalopathy.

Ohmori *et al.* (2008) reported a patient with typical Rasmussen encephalitis in whom a *SCN1A-R1575C* mutation (carried by the unaffected father) was fortuitously identified.

Barba *et al.* (2014) described six patients with DS exhibiting different malformations of cortical development. Sequencing analysis of the *SCN1A* gene detected two missenses, two truncating, and two splice-site mutations. Brain MRI revealed bilateral periventricular nodular heterotopia (PNH) in two patients and focal cortical dysplasia (FCD) in three, and disclosed no macroscopic abnormality in one whose brain, however neuropathologically studied after SUDEP, revealed multifocal micronodular dysplasia in the left temporal lobe. Two patients with FCD underwent epilepsy surgery. Neuropathology revealed FCD type IA and type IIA. Their seizure outcome was unfavorable. All four patients with FCD exhibited multiple seizure types, which always included complex partial seizures, the area of onset of which co-localized with the region of structural abnormality. This study supports a causative role for *SCN1A* mutations in some patients with MCD. This hypothesis is substantiated by subsequent observations of MCD associated with other ion channel disorders, namely *SCN3A* mutations (Miyatake *et al.*, 2018; Smith *et al.*, 2018).

Genetics

The breakthrough for identifying the underlying cause of DS was made by the discovery of voltage-gated sodium-channel gene α1subunit (*SCN1A*) mutations causing generalized epilepsy with FS plus (GEFS+) (Scheffer & Berkovic, 1997; Wallace *et al.*, 2001). Singh *et al.* (2001) subsequently identified patients with DS among GEFS+ family members, and proposed the GEFS+ spectrum, with FS being the most benign phenotype and DS the most severe. Claes *et al.* (2001) identified *de novo SCN1A* mutations in all seven probands with DS they studied. Estimates of the proportion of DS cases carrying *SCN1A* variants have progressively increased (Madia *et al.*, 2006; Mulley *et al.*, 2006; Wang *et al.*, 2008; Nakayama *et al.*, 2010) now reaching up to more than 90. Under ascertainment of *SCN1A* mutations due to human errors or technical limitations (Djémié *et al.*, 2016) in uncovering alternative pathogenic molecular mechanisms, such as genomic rearrangements (Marini *et al;* 2009) or poison exons (Carvill *et al.*, 2018) have contributed to convince clinicians and researchers that DS may be caused by more than one gene. This opinion has been further amplified by description of other genetic disorders, such as *PCDH19-* or *CHD2*-related epilepsy, whose phenotypes included fragments of the Dravet phenotypic spectrum, and by the suboptimal characterization of phenotypes associated with mutations in *SCN1B, HCN1, KCN2A, GABRA1, GABRG2, KCNA2* and *STXBP1*, whose clinical characteristics only share some DS features.

The number of reported DS-associated *SCN1A* variants is now higher than 1 200 (Meng *et al.*, 2015), with more than 90% being *de novo* mutations. The proportion of DS patients with truncation variants has been reported to be between 50 and 60%.

Although genotype phenotype correlations have been largely examined, no consensus has been reached (Nabbout *et al.*, 2003; Ohmori *et al.*, 2003; Fujiwara *et al.*, 2003; Ceulemans *et al.*, 2004; Fukuma *et al.*, 2004; Oguni *et al.*, 2005). In the most recent studies including a large number of *SCN1A* mutation-positive patients, truncation variants were associated with the severe phenotype, particularly with earlier onset of prolonged seizures, the combination of myoclonic and absence seizures, and rapid cognitive decline, and missense variants involving the voltage sensor and ion-pore loop regions critically related to the channel functions were more likely to cause the severe phenotype (Zuberi *et al.*, 2011; Meng *et al.*, 2015; Ishii *et al.*, 2017). On the other hand, a prospective cohort analysis of individuals with *SCN1A* variants, which ultimately resulted in the development of DS, GEFS+, or other types of mild seizure disorders, demonstrated that age at seizure onset allowed the outcomes of DS to be predicted more accurately than mutation types (truncating vs. missense variants), the correlation of which with specific phenotypes was found to be too weak for use in clinical practice (Cetica *et al.*, 2017).

Intrafamilial clinical variability in individuals sharing the same *SCN1A* genotype have been reported in several familial cases, *i.e.* a proband with the SMEI core phenotype, siblings with the SMEI borderline phenotype, or a parent with FS or even no symptoms (Nabbout *et al.*, 2003; Fujiwara *et al.*, 2003; Kimura *et al.*, 2005; Morimoto *et al.*, 2006; Suls *et al.*, 2010; Guerrini *et al.*, 2010). These reports suggest that other modifying factors, such as genes or environmental influences, and also somatic or germline mosaicisms might play a role (Kimura *et al.*, 2005; Gennaro *et al.*, 2006; Morimoto *et al.*, 2006). In a large cohort of DS patients, germline mosaicisms were detected in 7% of parent pairs (Depienne *et al.*, 2010). *De novo SCN1A* mutations largely arise from the paternally derived chromosome, and may occur at any time from the premorula stage of the embryo (causing disease in the subject) to adulthood (with mutations in the germ-line cells of parents causing disease in the offspring) (Heron *et al.*, 2010; Vadlamudi *et al.*, 2010). Modifying genes, including *SCN9A*, *CACNA1A*, and *POLG*, have been suggested to affect disease severity or the combination of absence seizures in patients with *SCN1A* variants (Singh *et al.*, 2009; Gaily *et al.*, 2013; Ohmori *et al.*, 2013). In addition, mosaicisms in *de novo SCN1A* pathogenic variants accounting for 7.5% of DS patients may modify the phenotype severity (de Lange *et al.*, 2018).

Further studies to investigate the molecular and cellular bases of epileptogenicity in DS have been performed using *SCN1A* knockout and knock-in mouse models (Yu *et al.*, 2006; Ogiwara *et al.*, 2007). They reproduced the characteristic temperature- and age-dependent seizures and EEG manifestations of DS (Oakley *et al.*, 2009). In these mouse models, a decrease in the Na current was detected in GABAergic interneurons rather than in pyramidal neurons, indicating that a dysfunction in inhibitory neurons plays a major role in seizure generation. The α type I sodium channel (Nav1.1) protein is predominantly expressed in the axons and somata of inhibitory interneurons and negligible in pyramidal cells (Ogiwara *et al.*, 2007). In heterozygous mutations, there is a 50% reduction in sodium current density in interneurons, without changes in the kinetics of the channels. Thus, the pathogenesis of DS is primarily attributed to a dysfunction in inhibitory interneurons caused by haploinsufficiency. In these mouse models, cognitive and behavioral alterations were detected in the 8th and 10th postnatal weeks when epileptic seizures decreased, indicating that the SCN1A mutation itself causes not only epilepsy, but also neurobehavioral impairment (Ito *et al.*, 2013). Furthermore, impaired GABAergic interneurons in the cerebellum, forebrain, and hypothalamus may cause ataxia, sleep impairment, and thermodysregulation (Kalume *et al.*, 2007, 2015; Gataullina & Dulac, 2017).

Genetic diagnosis is important as it influences management (Brunklaus *et al.*, 2013; Hirose *et al.*, 2013).

Differential diagnosis

An early diagnostic of DS is essential for the management. In the first year of life four main differential diagnoses should be considered, including *febrile seizures*, *epilepsy of infancy with migrating focal seizures*, *other focal epilepsies*, and *female limited epilepsy due to protocadherin 19 mutations*.

Febrile seizures. As the first clonic seizures in DS are often associated with fever, distinction from FS is particularly relevant. In DS: i) onset is early, before 1 year of age; ii) seizures are often clonic and unilateral; iii/ seizures may be prolonged and repeated, even when treated; iiii) body temperature is not necessarily high. After two seizures, having appeared with mild temperature elevation (around 37°5 Celsius), of which at least one prolonged (> 5 minutes) or evolving into status, if the infant is otherwise healthy, DS should be suspected and treatment prescribed, in order to prevent other prolonged seizures and status episodes. The occurrence of additional convulsive seizures, with or without fever, and in spite of treatment, reinforces this suspicion. At this stage, genetic testing should be proposed. The findings presented by Hattori *et al.* (2008), are in keeping with our own observations. These authors compared the clinical characteristics of two groups of infants who presented with FS before age one. Subsequently, one group was diagnosed as DS (46 patients) and a second group had a different diagnosis (50 patients). Age at onset of FS $\leq$ 7 months, a total number of seizures $\geq$ 5, and prolonged seizures lasting > 10 minutes were significant risk factors for DS. Other predictive factors were hemiconvulsions, partial seizures, myoclonic seizures, and hot water-induced seizures.

Epilepsy of infancy with migrating focal seizures. Seizure onset is before the 6th month, sometimes in the first month. Seizures are focal motor, with variable topography. Ictal EEG shows sustained rhythmic theta activity changing localization during the same episode. Seizures are nearly continuous and intractable by conventional AEDs. Severe developmental delay quickly appears. Neuroimaging does not detect brain lesion (Coppola *et al.*, 1995). Mutations in *KCNT1* are the most frequent cause but the *TBC1D24*, *SCN8A*, *SLC12A5*, *SCN2A* genes, and sometimes the *SCN1A* gene, have also been involved (Kearney, 2016).

Early cryptogenic focal epilepsy may also start with FS, rapidly associated with focal seizures. Distinction can be uneasy when the first seizure in DS is focal with or without secondary generalization. In some patients, idiopathic focal epilepsy may be suspected at onset, even Panayiotopoulos syndrome (Hino-Fukuyo *et al.*, 2009). Occurrence of alternating hemiclonic seizures and motor seizures affecting different parts of the body is a strong argument against focal epilepsy (Sarisjulis *et al.*, 2000). However, rare patients with seemingly focal epilepsy share clinical features with DS and also carry SCN1A mutations (Okumura *et al.*, 2007). These cases raise the problem of the limits of the DS.

Female limited epilepsy due to protocadherin 19 mutations. An almost similar semiology with slight variations is observed in girls without *SCN1A* mutation but carrying mutations of the X-linked protocadherin 19 (PCDH19) gene. After initial descriptions (Scheffer *et al.*, 2008; Depienne *et al.*, 2009; Marini *et al.*, 2010), it became progressively clear that this syndrome is distinct from DS. The main elements of diagnosis being: onset at 6-36 months, predominance of focal seizures in clusters, seizures with affective symptoms, rare photosensitivity, seizure remission occurring in childhood (Higurashi *et al.*, 2013; Lotte *et al.*, 2016; Trivisano *et al.*, 2017). EEG features, however, may resemble to those of DS (Trivisano *et al.*, 2018).

Other conditions should also be considered. Some patients with DS belong to families in which other members manifest either FS or another type of epilepsy, in the context of *genetic epilepsy with febrile seizures + (GEFS+)*. (Scheffer *et al.*, 1997; Singh *et al.*, 1999; Yue-Hua Zhang *et al.*, 2017, Camfield *et al.* in this book). Sometimes, an early diagnosis of either GEFS+ or DS is not possible. Other epilepsies should be easily excluded because they have different characteristics, including: *myoclonic epilepsy of infancy* (Guerrini *et al.* in this book); *progressive myoclonus epilepsy*, particularly late infantile neuronal ceroid-lipofuscinosis (Michelucci *et al.*, in this book, Nordli *et al.*, in this book); *epilepsy with myoclonic-atonic seizures (Doose syndrome)* (Guerrini *et al.*, in this book); *Lennox-Gastaut syndrome (LGS)* (Crespel *et al.*, in this book). Some patients affected by DS may present with tonic seizures during the course of the disease (*Figure 15*), but the other characteristics of these patients did not correspond to LGS. Recently epilepsies of genetic origin are reported as Dravet-like syndromes because they present some similarities with DS but should be distinguished from DS (Steel *et al.*, 2017).

Treatment and management

Epilepsy

In spite of recent progresses, treatment of DS remains symptomatic and aim at reducing the number and severity of seizures. Pharmacological treatment is the main basis, although ketogenic diet is increasingly used, whereas surgical treatment of epilepsy is contra-indicated with the exception of palliative procedures. The therapeutic strategy of DS is now relatively well established, at least in Europe and in North America (Aras *et al.*, 2015; Wirrell *et al.*, 2017).

Valproate (VPA) and *benzodiazepines (BZDs)* are largely used as first line AEDs although no controlled studies are available.

Stiripentol (STP) is the only drug approved by the European Medicines Agency (EMA) for the treatment of DS and has been recently recognized as an orphan drug for DS by the US Food and Drug Administration (FDA). It is also approved in New Zeeland, UK and Japan. Its efficacy was demonstrated in two multicenter randomized, double-blind, placebo-controlled add-on trials (Chiron *et al.*, 2000; Guerrini *et al.*, 2002). The long-term efficacy and safety of *STP* were reported in another study (Than *et al.*, 2002). In Japan, Inoue *et al.* in two open-label studies (2009, 2015) obtained results comparable to those of the two European studies. Although in both controlled trials, efficacy of *STP* was demonstrated in association with *VPA* and *CLB*, a direct antiepileptic effect of *STP* is likely (Fisher, 2009, 2011a,b;Wirrell *et al.*, 2013). *STP* has demonstrated its usefulness in decreasing the frequency and duration of convulsive seizures and the number of episodes of SE, and maintained its efficacy over the years (Wirrell *et al.*,2013; De Liso *et al.*, 2017; Myers *et al.*, 2018). Efficacy on the other seizure types, including photosensitive seizures, has not been evaluated yet. As interactions between *STP* and clobazam (*CLB*) are constant through its inhibitory action on the cytochrome P450 isoenzymes (Chiron *et al.*, 2000) it is necessary to adapt doses of the two to avoid their side-effects. Drowsiness, loss of appetite and loss of weight are the main side-effects and they may disappear when the doses of the co-medication are decreased.

Several open-label studies have been conducted on *topiramate (TPM)* and have shown that this medication can prompt a relatively good control of convulsive and focal seizures (Nieto-Barrera *et al.*, 2000a; Coppola *et al.*, 2002; Villeneuve *et al.*, 2002; Grosso *et al.*, 2005; Kroll-Selger *et al.*, 2006) with seizure reduction of ≥ 50% in 50 to 85% of patients, of whom 16 to 18% were seizure-free for 11 to 13 months. Slow titration facilitated better tolerance, but side-effects were observed in approximately 15% of patients, consisting mainly of anorexia and weight loss, but also behavior disturbances, emotional and language regression, risk of dehydration and, more rarely, kidney stones.

Bromides (Br) are used mainly in Germany and in Japan, with interesting results against convulsive seizures and SE (Oguni *et al.*, 1994; Tanabe *et al.*, 2008; Lotte *et al.*, 2012). In Japan, *zonisamide (ZNS)* is considered as one of the best drugs for DS (Kanazawa & Shirane, 1999; Tanabe *et al.*, 2008; Shi *et al.*, 2016). In Europe some patients were treated with a variable efficacy (Kelemen *et al.*, 2011). Only one multicentric, open-label trial evaluated *levetiracetam (LEV)* efficacy (Striano *et al.*, 2007b). The rate of responders was 64.3% of patients for GTCS, 39.2% for GTCS and myoclonic seizures, 44% for absence seizures. Side-effects caused arrest of the trial in 18% (irritability, cutaneous rash, worsening of myoclonic seizures, thrombocytopenia). These results were not confirmed by Chhun *et al.* (2011). *Ethosuximide (ESM) and piracetam (PIR)* are useful for patients suffering from countless myoclonic seizures. *BZDs* other than *CLB* can be used. *Phenobarbital (PB)* is not recommended in infants and children but may be helpful in adolescents and adults, not in association with *STP*. *Corticosteroids*, used in cycles of treatment can be useful in patients with repeated convulsive and myoclonic SE.

Two new drugs are on the point to be introduced in the market, *cannabidiol* and *fenfluramine* after their efficacy was demonstrated in controlled trials.

The pharmaceutical grade plant-derived cannabidiol is a non-psychoactive component of the cannabis plant. Controlled trials have demonstrated its efficacy in strongly reducing the number of seizures in DS (Devinski *et al.*, 2017, 2018, 2019). It has been designated as orphan drug for the treatment of DS by the FDA and the EMA. Its efficacy in patients who do not take clobazam comedication remains unclear, however, because CLB and CBD are both metabolized in the cytochrome P450 (CYP) pathway, and clobazam and norclobazam levels are greatly increased by cannabidiol comedication, due to drug-drug interactions (Geffrey *et al.*, 2015). Antiseizure action might therefore be in part consequent to increased levels of clobazam metabolites.

Fenfluramine is a serotonin receptor agonist which has been used as antiobesity in adults in the years 1980-1997, often in association with other drugs. It was withdrawn from the market after it was suggested that high doses could contribute to valvular heart disease and pulmonary hypertension. As it also has antiepileptic properties at low doses, it continued to be used for clinical antiepileptic purposes in Belgium. These studies have highlighted its efficacy in DS patients (Ceulemans *et al.*, 2012, 2016; Schoonjans *et al.*, 2017; de Witte & Lagae, 2017). No clinical or echographic sign of cardiac valve disease have been observed during the long-term treatment in these studies. They were followed by experiments on a new animal model, the zebrafish (Zhang *et al.*, 2015) that confirmed the clinical results and allowed to study its serotonergic activity. A large international trial is ongoing. *Fenfluramine* obtained orphan drug designations by FDA and EMA for the treatment of DS.

AEDs to be avoided

Carbamazepine (CBZ) and *lamotrigine (LTG)*, have been shown to have an aggravating effect in most patients with DS. For *CBZ*, seizure aggravation was reported by at least three authors (Horn *et al.*, 1986; Wakai *et al.*, 1996b; Wang *et al.*, 1996). An aggravating effect of *LTG* was demonstrated by Guerrini *et al.* (1998) in 17 of 21 patients (80%). Worsening appeared clearly within 3 months in most patients but occasionally had an insidious course, also enhanced by the slow titration of the drug. These findings were confirmed by Wallace (1998). *Lacosamide (LCM)*, a different blocker of voltage-gated sodium channels, might also aggravate seizures in DS. The aggravating effects of *phenytoin (PHT)* were reported anecdotally. *Vigabatrin (VGB)* should also be avoided, especially in children, due to its potential for worsening myoclonic seizures. AED induced seizure worsening does not appear in all patients and might also be influenced by age. In some older patients taking polytherapy including *PHT*, *CBZ* or *LTG*, attempts at withdrawing them were followed by aggravation of epilepsy (Dalic *et al.*, 2015).

Alternative treatments

Ketogenic diet (KD). The KD is based on the biology of starvation, where fat metabolism becomes a major energy source, replacing glucose and other carbohydrates. The KD is high in fat content and low in proteins and carbohydrates. One consensus about the modalities of the diet was reached by a panel of experts and recently updated (Kossoff *et al.*, 2018). Some metabolic disorders, including disorders of fatty acid transport, oxidation and some mitochondrial cytopathies, must be ruled out in the children who are candidates to this diet. The KD requires a good comprehension of the regimen by the parents, and a close collaboration between family, doctors and dieticians. The KD has been shown to benefit children with DS by several retrospective studies (Dressler *et al.*, 2015; Caraballo, 2011; Nabbout *et al.*, 2011). The KD treatment lasted from nine months to at least two years. The reduction in seizure frequency varied from ≥ 50% to ≥ 75%, up to seizure freedom in some patients. Favorable predicting factors were a short duration of epilepsy before starting the diet and the presence of GTCS. A recent prospective study (Yan *et al.*, 2018) evaluated the efficacy and tolerability of the KD on generalized convulsions and SE in 20 Chinese patients. Seventeen were responders at six months with six being seizure-free, two with 90-99% reduction, nine with 50-89% reduction. The KD also improved cognition. KD was considered as a second line therapy in the American consensus (Wirell *et al.*, 2017). Studies of *vagus nerve stimulation (VNS)* for DS are scarce. Dibué-Adjeia (2017) reported a meta-analysis of the results obtained in 68 patients by 13 authors. On the whole 52.9% of patients experienced a 50%-reduction of seizures and the average seizure reduction, assessed in only 28 patients, was 50.8%. Seven out of 13 studies reported additional benefits of *VNS*; however, this could not be assessed systematically. A study employing a social media survey via the Dravet Syndrome Foundation support group (Ali *et al.*, 2017) concludes that *VNS* therapy provides a "significant albeit limited improvement in seizures". The low rate of responders represents a consistent bias in this study. These data contrast with the moderate consensus of the American panel (Wirrell *et al.*, 2017) who considers the place of *VNS* only after failure of both first- and second-line treatments including KD. Three patients with DS submitted to *deep brain stimulation* were reported in the literature (Chabardes *et al.*, 2002; Andrade *et al.*, 2010). No conclusion may be drawn from these few cases.

Future perspectives. Several experimental researches on the pathophysiologic mechanisms of the disease are ongoing in order to find a curative treatment (Mingorance A, 2017). Different procedures are studied: i)selective Nav1.1 activation by venom peptide Hm1a which restores the function of inhibitory interneurons from DS mice without affecting the firing of excitatory neurons (Richards *et al.*, 2018); ii) upregulation of haploinsufficient gene expression in the brain by targeting a long noncoding RNA, using oligonucleotide-based compounds, by administration in the brain of Dravet knock-in mouse model and a non-human primate (Hsiao, 2016); iii) selective NaV1.6 inhibition by a highly selective atypical sodium channel blocker in a mouse model (Anderson *et al.*, 2017); iv) use of Nav1.1 activators (Frederiksen *et al.*, 2017). Other programs attempt to develop vectors to deliver a supplementary copy of *SCN1A* to the brain of the patients.

One clinical trial of Ataluren is ongoing in the US. Ataluren is a translational read-through drug approved in Europe for Duchenne muscular dystrophy. In presence of a nonsense *SCN1A* gene mutation it could enable the cell to move past this defect and complete a functional protein. The use of patient induced pluripotent stem cells (Isom, 2017) and studies on the role of inflammation in the epileptogenesis (French *et al.*, 2017) are other ways of research for better treatments.

The *Figure 16* shows the algorithm we propose for the practical modalities of the treatment.

After the first/second seizure considering DS as a possible diagnosis is reasonable when there is one of the following conditions: i) if two additional seizures, especially if lateralized alternatively, occur after a short interval (days, weeks) without a temperature spike; ii) if one seizure has either evolved to SE or has proven to be resistant to rectal DZ injection; iii) if workup for symptomatic seizures is negative; iv) if other seizure types (focal, myoclonic) appear; v) if spontaneous or light-induced epileptic EEG abnormalities appear, even if convulsive seizures are not frequently repeated at the onset. At this point treatment should be initiated. In most patients, complete control is never reached and subsequent changes in AEDs are necessary, using substitution rather than addition in order to avoid a heavy polytherapy.

KD could be offered early in the course of the disease when the first AEDs are ineffective or poorly tolerated, even in the first year; and at any age when SE are frequently repeated.

Fever. Obviously, body temperature should be monitored regularly. Oral or rectal antipyretic medications should be used without exceeding the recommended doses and with hepatic enzymes monitoring to avoid the risk of reversible hepatic injury favored by interactions with VPA (Nicolai *et al.*, 2008). Prevention of body temperature increase is recommended, by avoiding hot environmental conditions and maintaining a good hydration.

Photo and pattern-sensitivities, variably associated with self-stimulation, are extremely drug-resistant. Watching television requires precautions that are not always sufficient. Outside, wearing sunglasses is recommended but is not sufficient. Takahashi & Tsukahara (1992) showed that photosensitivity in epilepsy could be controlled by blue sunglasses that have an inhibitory effect of short wavelengths and possibly a luminance diminution. Therefore, it is strongly recommended to prescribe this type of lens to patients having photosensitivity and light environmental sensitivity. *Pattern-sensitivity* is only attenuated by these lenses in some patients. Glasses masking one eye are efficacious but they cannot be worn continuously.

Other triggering factors should be avoided: physical exertion, strongly emotional situations and other individual factors.

Seizures and status epilepticus

Clonic and tonic clonic seizures do not require an acute treatment when brief and isolated. One simple protective measure against ictal respiratory failure during sleep is to take any large pillow, fluffy animal and soft toy out the bed. When seizures last more than 5 minutes (potential SE), or when they recur at short intervals it is preferable to interrupt them to reduce the risk of SE. Rectal BZP is reliable for infants and young children, but is difficult to apply in adolescents and adults. Buccal or nasal midazolam (MDZ) has been demonstrated to provide the identical, even better, results (Mc Mullan *et al.*, 2010). No specific guidelines were established for the treatment of *status epilepticus in DS* and the protocols for SE in children are reliable, based on the use of intravenous BZDs (mainly MDZ, LZP, CZP), PHT and fosphenytoin, VPA, barbiturates, more rarely anaesthetic and propofol. LEV was added to this armamentarium (Abend *et al.*, 2010) but further studies are needed to evaluate its usefulness, (Lawton *et al.*, 2018). Attention must be drawn to avoiding accumulation of high doses of AEDs which can induce respiratory depression and metabolic and hemodynamic failure, especially for barbiturates (Chipaux *et al.*, 2010). In Japan, barbiturates are considered to be the most effective against SE (Tanabe *et al.*, 2008). However, barbiturates should be used cautiously, only in the hospital, with plasma levels monitoring. In DS, fever, respiratory infections, vaccinations, and treatment changes are the most frequent causes of SE. When fever is high, in a very young patient and there is no rapid return of consciousness after seizures stop, an acute encephalopathy must be suspected and MRI performed searching to rule out brain edema.

Other seizure types. When atypical absences, myoclonic seizures and focal seizures are frequently repeated, oral/rectal/nasal BZD may be used on occasion. If these seizures evolve into status, acute treatment should be applied to avoid GTCS. *To summarize*, complete seizure control is generally not achievable with current therapies, and the goals of treatment are to balance reduction of seizure burden with adverse effects of therapies that have deleterious effect on behavior and learning. Every family should be provided with a plan for home rescue therapy with precise timing and dosing of the drugs to be applied before hospital admission (Camfield *et al.*, 2016).

Other problems

Compulsory vaccinations

A relationship between vaccination and initial seizures in DS has been reported since the first descriptions. Berkovic *et al.* in 2006 retrospectively analyzed 14 patients with alleged "vaccine encephalopathy" in whom the first seizure happened within 72 hours of

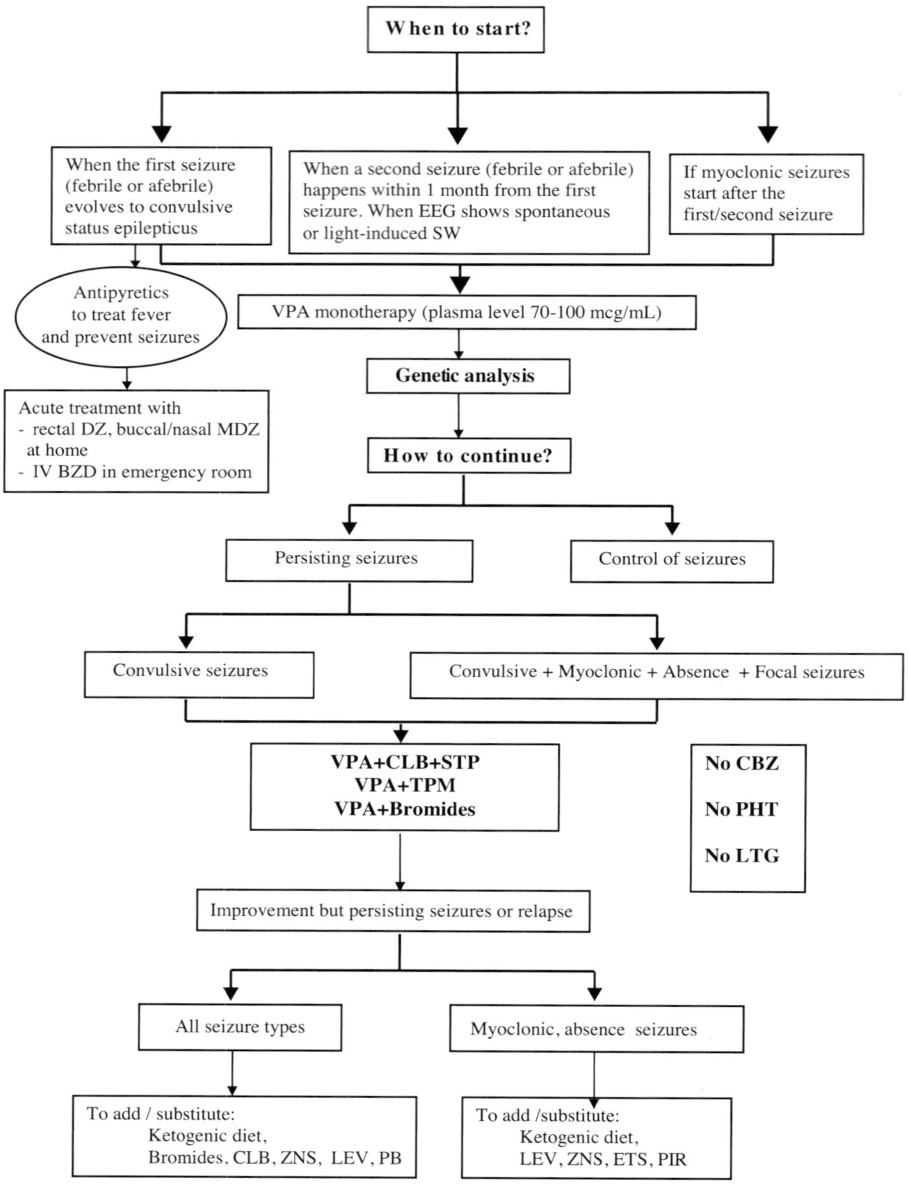

Figure 16

Treatment algorithm.

vaccination. A specific epilepsy syndrome was diagnosed in all cases: DS in 12, 11 carrying an *SCN1A* mutation, LGS in two, without *SCN1A* mutation. This pivotal study allowed to assess that vaccination may trigger epileptic seizures in infants who are prone to have them but is not the cause of epilepsy. Tro-Baumann *et al.* (2011) showed that in one third of 70 patients having seizures following vaccination the seizure was not associated with fever. Pruna *et al.* (2013) advised prophylaxis with antipyretics and BZD for a short time before and after vaccination. In the Netherlands, Verbeek *et al.* (2017) analyzed a cohort (2009-2013) of 77 DS children with (21%) and without (79%) vaccination-associated seizure (VAS) onset. They found: i) no difference in the subsequent course of the disease between the two groups; ii) a younger age at the onset in the VAS group; iii) a lower risk of subsequent VAS for acellular pertussis (9%) and nonpertussis (8%) than whole-cell pertussis (37%); iv) an increased incidence rate ratio of seizures of 2.3 within the risk period of 5 to 12 days following MMR vaccination. The reason for this seizure-triggering effect of the vaccination even without fever is unknown. To our knowledge only one study addressed this question in the literature (Auvin *et al.*, 2018). The authors found that in DS vaccine responsiveness is biased toward a proinflammatory profile with a M1 phenotype of monocytes. This finding is in keeping with the increasing number of studies highlighting the probable role of inflammation in epilepsy. In spite of its possible triggering role in a subset of patients, vaccination must be performed because infectious diseases can be serious and also provoke seizures and neurological complications, as demonstrated by Tanabe *et al.* (2004). There are no true preventative measures but we recommend not to inject one vaccine when the child is ill or febrile, to give antipyretics before and after vaccination, associated with additional BZDs for one week, and if possible to perform the vaccination in hospital.

Cognitive impairment and behavioral disorders

As soon as the diagnosis of DS is confirmed, it is advised to regularly assess the development of infants and children in order to help them and their families when the first difficulties arise. Appropriate educative and rehabilitative methods (psychomotricity, speech therapy, ergotherapy) are helpful. When possible, integration in school, or in classes for children with special needs, is important for socialization. Most adolescent and adult patients need to attend specialized institutions whereas few of them can benefit from sheltered working structures. Management of behavioral disturbances is uneasy and psychological support by a specialized team should be offered. Pharmacological treatment is not appropriate except in case of psychiatric episodes, which are infrequent. Conversely, physicians should be aware of the possible exacerbation of pathological behaviors by some AEDs (LEV, ZNS, TPM, BZD...).

Motor impairment

It can be attenuated by early physiotherapy and psychomotricity. *Kyphoscoliosis* and lower limb deformities should be detected as soon as possible and managed with an orthopedist, keeping in mind there is no definite treatment and results of surgery are variable. This problem is particularly worrying in adolescent patients.

Feeding difficulties and sleep disorders

Feeding difficulties and failure to thrive are frequent and can require a nutritionist counselling. Gastrostomy should be used only exceptionally.

Sleep disorders are difficult to manage. When they are induced by the seizure time-schedule, adaptation of the AEDs administration time should be considered. In other cases, prescription of melatonin or sleep-inducers is helpful. Several special monitoring devices exist but no system is infallible (Wirrell *et al.*, 2017). Many parents know the risk of SUDEP and use one as an alternative to sleep with their child (Villas *et al.*, 2017).

Long-term outcome

Available knowledge indicates that DS has an overall unfavorable outcome. All patients had persistent seizures and were cognitively impaired, often severely. Only one publication has reported one patient who had a normal cognitive outcome in adolescence in spite of a typical DS due to a truncating *SCN1A* mutation (Buoni *et al.*, 2006).

Several authors have published series of patients followed up to adolescence but we could only find one study specifically concerning the evolution in adolescence (Olivieri *et al.*, 2016). In 20 patients (aged 10 to 20 years, median 14 years) cognitive outcome was heterogeneous with mild, moderate, and severe intellectual disability (ID) in one third each. Regression was not observed. Epilepsy improved in eight patients (two seizure-free) while remained severe in the remaining 12. Epilepsy severity was correlated with ID, with some exceptions.

Pulling together various series (Jansen *et al.*, 2006; the Marseille series, published in Dravet *et al.*, 2009 and Genton *et al.*, 2011; Akiyama *et al.*, 2010; Martin *et al.*, 2010; Catarino *et al.*, 2011; Rilstone *et al.*, 2012; Fasano *et al.*, 2014; Takayama *et al.*, 2014; Berkvens *et al.*, 2015) we identified 195 patients followed-up to adulthood, aged from 18 to 66 years, 109 with complete forms, 150 genetically tested, 124 carrying a *SCN1A* mutation (82.6%) whose characteristics can be summarized as follows. *The convulsive seizures* persist. In all series their frequency progressively decreased, up to one per year in some patients but remained monthly or weekly in most. Periods of worsening during adolescence and early adulthood could occur. However, in four studies 14 patients were seizure-free for at least one year and up to 22 years, nine with incomplete DS form. For Rilstone *et al.* (2012) seizure control was observed in most patients after the second decade of life, independently of the type of *SCN1A* mutation, or the presence or number of convulsive SE in infancy and childhood. Convulsive seizures occur mainly during night sleep and can be repeated in clusters during the same night, with or without fever, and be preceded by myoclonic jerks. *Convulsive SE* was no longer observed after the age of ten in two studies (Akiyama *et al.*, 2010; Takayama *et al.*, 2014) but it still occurred after the age of 20 in two (Genton *et al.*, 2011; Catarino *et al.*, 2011). Focal, myoclonic, and atypical absence seizures tended to disappear, but they were still observed in some series. Obtundation status were rare, reported only in two series. Fever and infections kept acting as triggering factors but low-grade fever lost in part its precipitating power.

All authors have reported a tendency of clinical photo-pattern sensitivity to disappear in adolescence and adulthood.

EEG. Background activity fluctuates, depending on the number and severity of seizures. It can be predominantly slow (Catarino *et al.*, 2011) but remain normal with an alpha rhythm in a subset of patients (Dravet *et al.*, 2009; Akiyama *et al.*, 2010; Takayama *et al.*, 2014). Interictal EEG abnormalities can disappear completely or become sporadic, often appearing only during sleep, as focal and multifocal spikes, SW and sharp waves, rarely associated with generalized SW. One study (Takayama *et al.*, 2014) highlighted the positive correlation between the clinical and the EEG outcome in a small series, with five seizure-free patients having alpha rhythm and no epileptic discharges. Photosensitivity was progressively less apparent but persisted in some cases. Bureau & Dalla Bernardina (2011) reported photosensitivity, with or without clinical correlates, in 12% of patients older than 18 years. In our series, cyclic organization of the sleep remained normal in 70% of the patients in whom it was assessed. *Neurologic signs* were not systematically described in the literature and were variable. Few patients presented with permanent hemiplegia acquired during a severe SE in childhood. Ataxia and tremor were regularly reported, and were still present in more than one third of adults. Pyramidal signs, cerebellar signs and dysarthria were less frequent. Interictal myoclonus was reported by only one study in 12/24 patients (Genton *et al.*, 2011) but it is possible they were associated with tremor in the other studies. Six authors (Jansen *et al.*, 2006; Genton *et al.*, 2011; Akiyama *et al.*, 2010; Martin *et al.*, 2010; Catarino *et al.*, 2011; Fasano *et al.*, 2012) reported the appearance of an extrapyramidal symptomatology either limited to rigidity and bradykinesia, or realizing a parkinsonism. The latter has been described in two Canadian studies (Fasano *et al.*, 2012; Aljaafari *et al.*, 2017) in 14 adult patients presenting also "crouch gait" and ID, and they were absent in LGS patients. In another small series of five patients (Martin *et al.*, 2010) the neurologic symptomatology is more detailed: midface hypomimia, action and position tremor of high frequency, dysarthrophonia, thin voice, disturbed eye movements. Only three studies (Catarino *et al.*, 2011; Fasano *et al.*, 2012; Rilstone *et al.*, 2012) reported the "crouch gait" in part of the patients and this posture has been probably underestimated. This posture already starting in adolescence (Rodda *et al.*, 2012) worsens in adulthood, strongly hampering walking, and may lead to wheelchair-bounding. However, Rilstone *et al.* (2012) observed "crouch-gait" in only 5/10 patients of whom 4 aged 30-47 years. In our series of 24 adult patients the six patients with "crouch gait" were also older than 30 years (unpublished data). Catarino *et al.* (2011) reported dysphagia in five patients after the fourth decade of life, causing respiratory infections and leading to percutaneous endoscopic gastrostomy. On the whole, a number of patients experienced deterioration of their motor abilities in adulthood and lost their ability to independently walk. Akiyama *et al.* (2010) found that patients with the most severe motor handicap also had severe mental impairment. Catarino *et al.* (2011) considered there was a continuous neurological deterioration throughout life in all their patients, who were diagnosed very late, mainly after 20 years.

Cognitive, behavioral and social outcome

In most patients there is no further cognitive decline after the first years of life but they tend not to progress or to progress slowly. Therefore, the gap between their acquired skills and the expected skills for chronological age increases and their cognitive level as expressed by IQ scores lowers. Consequently, a child who appeared to be slightly cognitively impaired at pre-school age, could exhibit severe impairment in adolescence and adulthood. One characteristic feature is the extreme slowness in movement, comprehension, thinking and verbal expression. Approximately, when this data is present in the literature (around 130 patients) one finds only one patient with a cognitive level in the normal low range, six with mild ID, 29 with moderate ID and 94 with a severe/profound ID. In two studies in the same center (Akiyama *et al.*,2010; Takayama *et al.*, 2014) the lowest ID degree was significantly correlated with the presence of an alpha rhythm on the last EEG ($p = 0.0085$), patients with incomplete DS tended to have milder ID compared to those with typical DS ($p = 0.0283$), and higher GTCS frequency correlated with more severe ID.

Language impairment is prominent, of variable degree but not detailed in most studies. Sometimes, a simple conversation is possible but language remains poor and dysarthric, with verbal stereotypies and echolalia. Some patients are non verbal, just producing isolated syllables, words and inarticulate sounds or shouting. Usually these patients are rather calm, passive, perseverating in repetitive activities. Nevertheless behavioral problems and autistic features may emerge such as obsessive attitudes, bouts of aggressiveness, nocturnal agitation. In one cohort they were observed in most patients during follow-up (Catarino *et al.*, 2011). In our series six patients of 24 had an autistic or psychotic personality disorder (Genton *et al.*, 2011). Acute psychiatric episodes seem to be rare (Gobbi *et al.*, 2008), but Martin & Kümmerle (2015) reported hallucinations in 10 among 41 patients. Recently Berkvens *et al.* (2015) published a thorough study of autism and behavior of the 13 patients in the same center. They conclude that "*adults with DS exhibit many autistic-like features, though these may be ID-related rather than DS-related, but behavioral problems which are reported in children with DS, are not frequently seen. Thus, the overall behavior of patients with DS seems to become milder in adulthood.*" In general, adult patients with DS did not have aggressive behavior compromising their social integration, but their motor disability, difficulty to communicate, tendency to perseveration and refusal behaviour made them socially isolated. The vast majority of the reported patients were either completely or partially dependent for their daily activities. Many lived in specialized centers, some attended an occupational day center, others attended a sheltered workshop, whereas others could not have any activity. Seven patients were independent and lived in their own apartment, with or without assistance (Jansen *et al.*, 2006; Genton *et al.*, 2011; Takayama *et al.*, 2014). As acknowledged by Takayama *et al.* (2014) such a very unfavorable outcome was observed in patients who had been diagnosed a long time ago, often very late, who did not receive an adequate treatment and were followed in structures specialized for refractoy epilepsies. A small subset of patients experienced less severe disability, as reported by Jansen *et al.* (2006). In our recent child or adolescent patients, seizure frequency and duration are reduced and episodes of SE are better controlled by applying more efficacious drugs. Our study on adolescents (Olivieri *et al.*, 2016) showed less severe epilepsy and ID in one third of them who could have a less severe outcome in adulthood.

Mortality

DS is associated with a mortality rate amongst the highest in the epilepsy population and death may occur at any age, but more frequently during childhoood. The main causes of death are sudden unexpected death in epilepsy (SUDEP) and SE. Several surveys were performed with different methods and have provided variable data concerning the rate of the deaths (from 5.75% to 10%) and their causes. In the published adult series when mortality is noted SUDEP is the main cause of death. The most recent data come from a cohort of 100 consecutive patients with DS, 87 carrying *SCN1A* mutations (Cooper *et al.*, 2016). Seventeen patients died, at a median age of seven years. The most common cause was SUDEP (59%) mainly in childhood, between 2 and 20 years. Four patients (23.5%) died due to SE between 13 months and 11 years, due to preceding viral infection, and evolving to hypoxic encephalopathy and multi-organ failure. Two patients died by drowning and one by asphyxia. The Dravet-specific mortality rate was 15.84/1,000-person-years. The Dravet-specific SUDEP rate was 9.32/1,000-person-years. The authors precise that the Dravet-specific SUDEP rate is the only documented syndrome-specific SUDEP rate. They calculated the probability of survival without SUDEP is 96% at 3 years of FU and 91% at 10 years of FU. The probability of survival without death from Non-SUDEP causes is 97% at 3 years of FU and 94% at 10 years of FU. A review of 177 cases published from 1989 to 2015 (Shmuely *et al.*, 2016) reported similar results.

Circumstances of SUDEP were those generally reported in other epilepsies. Most often it occurred during sleep, in children without recent aggravation and regularly treated, usually by polytherapy. Numerous studies are ongoing in order to elucidate the mechanisms of SUDEP and the role of an ictal-postictal cardio-respiratory dysfunction. Abnormal heart rate variability has been demonstrated in patients with DS (Delogu *et al.*, 2011) and is hypothesized to predispose to autonomic dysfunction and SUDEP. One study (Baysal-Kirac *et al.*, 2012) underlined the possible role of an increased resting heart rate. Other, mainly experimental, studies address the role of the genetic alterations, the *SCN1A* gene being present in the brain and in the heart. Goldman *et al.* (2016) in an extensive review highlighted the complexity of the genetic mechanisms and the need for large collaborative researches. Although evidence-based preventive measures are not available, simple precautions can decrease the risk: frequent monitoring of the child when asleep, avoidance of the prone position, use of smoother-pillows in order to try and minimize the consequences of respiratory obstruction and depression.It is also recommended to perform a cardiac Holter to all children with DS.

The other frequent cause of death in young patients is an "acute encephalopathy after SE". In this condion the child presents with a febrile convulsive status due to an infection, not responding to treatment, followed by a prolonged coma. MRI shows cerebral edema in the acute phase, then lesions in the cortex, subcortical white matter and often in the central nuclei. Either the child dies or he survives with massive neurological and cognitive regression. That has been observed mainly in Japan (Okumura *et al.*, 2012) and also in other countries (Chipaux *et al.*, 2010; Do TTH *et al.*, 2016; Myers *et al.*, 2017; Tian *et al.*, 2018). The etiology of this peculiar sequence is unknown, (Gataullina & Dulac, 2017; Dravet, 2018). The most at risk patients are those aged under 6 years, with an early onset (< 6 months), a severe phenotype and repetitive SE.

Conclusion

Severe myoclonic epilepsy of infancy was first described as an epileptic syndrome of unknown origin which affected the young children. Later on, due to the incredible increase in the knowledge in all the fields of the medical sciences, this syndrome has been recognized as a genetic disease in which epilepsy is associated to cognitive, behavioral, and motor impairment. It is due to loss-of-function mutations of *SCN1A*, the gene encoding a subunit of the voltage-gated sodium channel Nav1.1, which cause reduced GABAergic inhibition leading to seizures. Different degrees of epilepsy severity and cognitive deficit characterize the phenotype but their correlation with the genotype remains a challenge. Clinical and experimental researches tend to demonstrate that genetic background and epilepsy are both at stake in causing cognitive impairment. It is therefore important to treat epilepsy with the right drugs and to stimulate the research to find a treatment targeted against the consequences of the mutations and applicable to the patients as soon as possible after seizure onset. Understanding why SUDEP is particularly frequent in these patients is another challenge for clinicians and researchers. Clinicians face the difficult task to inform the parents about this risk which increases the burden they have to cope with. Over time, families have created associations which may support them in the various aspects of everyday life. Collaboration between doctors and family associations also helps medical research and should be encouraged.

REFERENCES ▶

Abend NS, Gutierrez-Colina AM, Dlugos DJ (2010): Medical treatment of pediatric status epilepticus. *Semin Pediatr Neurol* 17: 169–175.

Aicardi J (1994): *Epilepsy in Children*, 2nd ed. New York: Raven Press.

Akiyama M, Kobayashi K, Yoshinaga H, Ohtsuka Y (2010): A long-term follow-up study of Dravet syndrome up to adulthood. *Epilepsia* 51: 1043–1052.

Ali R, Elsayed M, Kaur M, Air E, Mahmood N, Constantinou J, Schwalb J (2017): Use of social media to assess the effectiveness of vagal nerve stimulation in Dravet syndrome: A caregiver's perspective. *J Neurol Sci* 375: 146–149.

Aljaafari D, Fasano A, Nascimento FA, Lang AE, Andrade DM (2017): Adult motor phenotype differentiates Dravet syndrome from Lennox-Gastaut syndrome and links *SCN1A* to early onset parkinsonian features. *Epilepsia* 58: e44–e48.

Anderson LL, Hawkins NA, Thompson CH, Kearney JA, George AL Jr (2017): Unexpected Efficacy of a Novel Sodium Channel Modulator in Dravet Syndrome. *Sci Rep* 10: 1682.

Andrade DM, Hamani C, Lozano AM, Wennberg RA (2010): Dravet syndrome and deep brain stimulation: Seizure control after 10 years of treatment. *Epilepsia* 51: 1314–1316.

Aras LM, Isla J, Mingorance-Lemeur A (2015): The European patient with Dravet syndrome: Results from a parent-reported survey on antiepileptic drug use in the European population with Dravet syndrome. *Epilepsy Behav* 44: 104–109.

Auvin S, Jeljeli M, Desnous B, Soussi-Yanicostas N, Dournaud P, Sterker G (2018): Altered vaccine-induced immunity in children with Dravet syndrome. *Epilepsia* 59: e45–e50.

Awaya Y, Satoh F, Miyamoto M, Hayashi K, Inaba R, Fukuyama Y (1989): Change of rectal temperature in infants and children during and after hot water immersion. *Clin Therm (Tokyo)* 9: 76–82.

Barba C, Parrini E, Roland Coras R, *et al.* (2014): Co-occurring malformations of cortical development and SCN1A gene mutations. *Epilepsia* 55: 1–11.

Battaglia D, Chieffo D, Siracusano R, *et al.* (2013): Cognitive decline in Dravet syndrome: Is there a cerebellar role? *Epilepsy Res* 106: 211–221.

Battaglia D, Ricci D, Chieffo D, Guzzetta F (2016): Outlining a core neuropsychological phenotype for Dravet syndrome. *Epilepsy Res* 120: 91–97.

Bayat A, Hjalgrim H, Moller RS (2015): The incidence of SCN1A-related Dravet syndrome in Denmark is 1:22,000: A population-based study from 2004 to 2009. *Epilepsia* 56: e36–e39.

Baysal-Kirac L, Güven Serbest N, Erdi Şahin E, *et al.* (2012): Analysis of heart rate variability and risk factors for SUDEP in patients with drug-resistant epilepsy. *Epilepsy Behav* 71: 60–64.

Bender AC, Morse RP, Scott RC, Holmes GL, Lenck-Santini PP (2012): SCN1A mutations in Dravet syndrome: Impact of interneuron dysfunction on neural networks and cognitive outcome. *Epilepsy Behav* 23: 177–186.

Bender AC, Luikart BW, Lenck-Santini PP, *et al.* (2016): Cognitive Deficits Associated with Nav1.1 Alterations: Involvement of Neuronal Firing Dynamics and Oscillations. *PLOS ONE*.

Berg AT, Berkovic SF, Brodie MJ, *et al.* (2010): Revised terminology and concepts of the organization of seizures and epilepsies: Report of the ILAE commission on classification and terminology, 2005-2009. *Epilepsia* 51: 676– 685.

Berkovic SF, Harkin L, McMahon JM, *et al.* (2006): *De novo* mutations of the sodium channel gene SCN1A in alleged vaccine encephalopathy: A retrospective study. *Lancet Neurol* 5: 488–492.

Berkvens JJL, Veugen I, Veendrick-Meekes MJBM, *et al.* (2015): Autism and behavior in adult patients with Dravet syndrome (DS) *Epilepsy Behav* 47: 11–16.

Brunklaus A, Ellis R, Reavey E, Forbes GH, Zuberi SM (2012): Prognostic, clinical and demographic features in SCN1A mutation-positive Dravet syndrome. *Brain* 135: 2329–2336.

Brunklaus A, Dorris L, Ellis R, *et al.* (2013): The clinical utility of an SCN1A genetic diagnosis in infantile-onset epilepsy. *Dev Med Child Neurol* 55: 154–161.

Buoni S, Orrico A, Galli L, *et al.* (2006): SCN1A (2528delG) novel truncating mutation with benign outcome of severe myoclonic epilepsy in infancy. *Neurology* 66: 606–607.

Bureau M, Dalla Bernardina B (2011): Electroencephalographic characteristics of Dravet Syndrome. *Epilepsia* 52 (Suppl. 2): 13–23.

Camfield PR, Camfield CS, McNamara NA, Shellhaas RA, Marini C, Scheffer IE (2019): Febrile seizures and Genetic Epilepsy with Febrile Seizures Plus (GEFS+): *in this book*.

Camfield P, Camfield C, Nolan K (2016): Helping families cope with the severe stress of Dravet Syndrome. *Can J Neurol Sci* 43 (Suppl. 3): S9–S12.

Caraballo RH (2011): Non-pharmacologic treatments of Dravet syndrome: Focus on the ketogenic diet. *Epilepsia* 52 (Suppl. 2): 79–82.

Caraballo R, Cersosimo R, Galicchio S, Fejerman N (1997): Epilepsias en el primer año de vida. *Rev Neurol (Barcelone)* 25: 1521–1524.

Caraballo RH, Fejerman N (2006): Dravet syndrome: A study of 53 patients. *Epilepsy Res* 70 (Suppl. 1): S231–S238.

Carvill GL, Engel KL, Ramamurthy A, *et al.* (2018): Aberrant Inclusion of a Poison Exon Causes Dravet Syndrome and Related SCN1A-Associated Genetic Epilepsies. *Am J Hum Genet* 103: 1022–1029.

Cassé-Perrot C, Wolff M, Dravet C (2001): Neuropsychological aspects of severe myoclonic epilepsy in infancy. In: Jambaqué I, Lassonde M, Dulac O (eds) *The Neuropsychology of Childhood Epilepsy*, pp.131–140. New York: Plenum Press/Kluwer Academic.

Catarino CB, Liu JY, Liagkouras I, *et al.* (2011): Dravet syndrome as epileptic encephalopathy: Evidence from long-term course and neuropathology. *Brain* 134 (Pt 10): 2982–3010.

Cetica V, Chiari S, Mei D, *et al.* (2017): Clinical and genetic factors predicting Dravet syndrome in infants with SCN1A mutations. *Neurology* 88: 1037–1044.

Ceulemans BP, Claes LR, Lagae LG (2004): Clinical correlations of mutations in the SCN1A gene: From febrile seizures to severe myoclonic epilepsy in infancy. *Pediatr Neurol* 30: 236–243.

Ceulemans B, Boel M, Leyssens K, *et al.* (2012): Successful use of fenfluramine as an add-on treatment for Dravet syndrome. *Epilepsia* 53: 1131–1139.

Ceulemans B, Schoonjans A-S, Marchau F, Paelinck BP, Lagae L (2016): Five-year extended follow-up status of 10 patients with Dravet syndrome treated with fenfluramine. *Epilepsia* 57: e129–e134.

Chabardes S, Kahane P, Minotti L, Koudsie A, Hirsch E, Benabid AL (2002): Deep brain stimulation in epilepsy with particular reference to the subthalamic nucleus. *Epileptic Disord* 4 (Suppl. 3): 83–93.

Chieffo D, Ricci D, Baranello G, *et al.* (2011a): Early development in Dravet syndrome; visual function impairment precedes cognitive decline. *Epilepsy Res* 93: 73–79.

Chieffo D, Battaglia D, Lettori D, *et al.* (2011b): Neuropsychological development in children with Dravet syndrome. *Epilepsy Res* 95: 86–93.

Chieffo D, Battaglia D, Lucibello S, *et al.* (2016): Disorders of early language development in Dravet syndrome. *Epilepsy Behav* 54: 30–33.

Chipaux M, Villeneuve N, Sabouraud P, *et al.* (2010): Unusual consequences of status epilepticus in Dravet syndrome. *Seizure* 19: 190–194.

Chiron C, Marchand MC, Tran A, *et al.* (2000): Stiripentol in severe myoclonic epilepsy in infancy: A randomized placebo- controlled syndrome dedicated trial. STICLO study group. *Lancet* 11, 356: 1638–1642.

Chhun S, Troude P, Villeneuve N, *et al.* (2011): A prospective open-labeled trial with levetiracetam in pediatric epilepsy syndromes: Continuous spikes and waves during sleep is definitely a target. *Seizure* 20: 320–325.

Claes L, Del-Favero J, Ceulemans B, Lagae L, Van Broeckhoven C, De Jonghe P (2001): *De novo* mutations in the sodium channel gene SCN1A cause severe myoclonic epilepsy in infancy. *Am J Hum Genet* 68: 1327–1332.

Commission on Classification and Terminology of the International League Against Epilepsy (1989): Proposal for revised classification of epilepsies and epileptic syndromes. *Epilepsia* 30: 289–299.

Cooper MS, Mcintosh A, Crompton DE, *et al.* (2016): Mortality in Dravet syndrome. *Epilepsy Res* 128: 43–47.

Coppola G, Plouin P, Chiron C, Robain O, Dulac O (1995): Migrating Partial Seizures in Infancy: A Malignant Disorder with Developmental Arrest. *Epilepsia* 36: 1017–1024.

Coppola G, Capovilla G, Montagnini A, *et al.* (2002): Topiramate as add-on drug in severe myoclonic epilepsy in infancy: An Italian multicenter open trial. *Epilepsy Res* 49: 45–48.

Crooks R, Mitchell T, Thom M (2000): Patterns of cerebellar atrophy in patients with chronic epilepsy: a quantitative neuropathological study. *Epilepsy Res* 41: 63–73.

Dalic L, Mullen SA, Roulet PerezE, Scheffer E (2015): Lamotrigine can be beneficial in patients with Dravet syndrome. *Dev Med Child Neurol* 57: 200–202.

Dalla Bernardina B, Capovilla G, Gattoni MB, Colamaria V, Bondavalli S, Bureau M (1982): Épilepsie myoclonique grave de la première année. *Rev EEG Neurophysiol* 12: 21–25.

Dalla Bernardina B, Colamaria V, Capovilla G, Bondavalli S (1983): Nosological classification of epilepsies in the first three years of life. In: Nistico G, Di Perri R, Meinardi H (eds) *Epilepsy: an Update on Research and Therapy*, pp. 165–183. New York: Alan Liss.

Dalla Bernardina B, Capovilla G, Chiamenti C, Trevisan E, Colamaria V, Fontana E (1987): Cryptogenic myoclonic epilepsies of infancy and early childhood: Nosological and prognostic approach. In: Wolf P, Dam M, Janz D, Dreifuss FE (eds) *Advances in Epileptology*, pp. 175–180. New York: Raven Press.

de Lange IM, Koudijs MJ, van't Slot R, *et al.* (2018): Mosaicism of *de novo* pathogenic SCN1A variants in epilepsy is a frequent phenomenon that correlates with variable phenotypes. *Epilepsia* 59: 690–703.

De Liso P, Chemaly N, Laschet J, *et al.* (2017): Patients with Dravet syndrome in the era of stiripentol: A French cohort cross-sectional study. *Epilepsy Res* 125: 42–46.

Delogu AB, Spinelli A, Battaglia D, *et al.* (2011): Electrical and autonomic cardiac function in patients affected by Dravet syndrome. *Epilepsia* 52 (Suppl. 2): 55–58.

Depienne C, Bouteiller D, Keren B, *et al.* (2009): Sporadic infantile epileptic encephalopathy caused by mutations in PCDH19 resembles Dravet syndrome but mainly affects females. *PloS Genet* 5: e1000381.

Depienne C, Trouillard O, Gourfinkel-An I, *et al.* (2010): Mechanisms for variable expressivity of inherited SCN1A mutations causing Dravet syndrome. *J Med Genet* 47: 404–410.

Devinski O, Cross JH, Laux L, *et al.* (2017): Trial of Cannabidiol for Drug-Resistant Seizures in the Dravet Syndrome. *N Engl J Med* 37: 2011-2020. doi:10.1056/NEJMoa1611618

Devinski O, Patel AD, Thiele EA, *et al.* (2018): Randomized, dose-ranging safety trial of cannabidiol in Dravet syndrome. *Neurology* 90: e1204–e1211.

Devinsky O, Nabbout R, Miller I, Laux L, Zolnowska M, Wright S, Roberts C (2019): Long term cannabidiol treatment in patients with Dravet syndrome: An open label extension trial. *Epilepsia* 60: 294–302.

de Witte P, Lagae L (2017): Serotonergic modulation as a pharmacological modality in the treatment of Dravet syndrome. *Brain* 140: 1–2.

Dibué-Adjeia M, Fischer I, Steiger HJ, Kamp MA (2017): Efficacy of adjunctive vagus nerve stimulation in patients with Dravet syndrome: A meta-analysis of 68 patients. *Seizure* 50: 147–152.

Djémié T, Weckhuysen S, von Spiczak S, *et al.* (2016): Pitfalls in genetic testing: the story of missed SCN1A mutations. *Mol Genet Genomic Med* 4: 457–464.

Do TTH, Huynh TTK, Van Le TK (2016): Acute encephalopathy in Dravet syndrome: Case reports and literature review. *Neurology Asia* 21: 181–185.

Dravet C (1978): Les épilepsies graves de l'enfant. *Vie Med* 8: 543–548.

Dravet C (2018): Acute encephalopathy after febrile status epilepticus: an underdiagnosed, misunderstood complication of Dravet syndrome. *Dev Med Child Neurol* 60: 534.

Dravet C, Roger J, Bureau M, Dalla Bernardina B (1982): Myoclonic epilepsies in childhood. In: Akimoto H, *et al.* (eds) *Advances in Epileptology, the XIIIth EIS*, pp. 135–140. New York: Raven Press.

Dravet C, Bureau M, Roger J (1985): Severe myoclonic epilepsy in infancy. In: Roger J, Dravet C, Bureau M, Dreifuss FE, Wolf P (eds) *Epileptic Syndromes inInfancy, Childhood and Adolescence*, pp. 58–67. London: John Libbey.

Dravet C, Bureau M, Guerrini R, Giraud N, Roger J (1992): Severe myoclonic epilepsy in infants. In: Roger J, Bureau M, Dravet C, Dreifuss FE, Perret A, Wolf P (eds) *Epileptic Syndromes in Infancy, Childhood and Adolescence*, 2nd ed, pp. 75–88. London: John Libbey.

Dravet C, Bureau M, Oguni H, Fukuyama Y, Cokar O (2005a): Severe myoclonic epilepsy in infancy (Dravet Syndrome). In: Roger J, Bureau M, Dravet C, Genton P, Tassinari CA, Wolf P (eds) *Epileptic Syndromes in Infancy, Childhood and Adolescence*, 4th ed, pp. 89–113. Paris: John Libbey Eurotext.

Dravet C, Bureau M, Oguni H, Fukuyama Y, Cokar O (2005b): Severe myoclonic epilepsy in infancy: Dravet syndrome. In: Delgado-Escueta AV, Guerrini R, Medina MT, Genton P, Bureau M, Dravet C (eds) *Advances in Neurology*, Vol. 95, pp. 71–102. Philadelphia: Lippincott Williams & Wilkins.

Dravet C, Daquin G, Battaglia D (2009): Severe myoclonic epilepsy in infancy (Dravet syndrome). In: Nikanorova M, Genton P, Sabers A (eds), *Long-Term Evolution of Epileptic Encephalopathies*, pp. 29–38. Paris: John Libbey Eurotext.

Dressler A, Trimmel-Schwahofer P, Reithofer E, *et al.* (2015): Efficacy and tolerability of the ketogenic diet in Dravet syndrome – Comparison with various standard antiepileptic drug regimen. *Epilepsy Res* 109: 81–89.

Dulac O, Arthuis M (1982): L'épilepsie myoclonique sévère de l'enfant. In: *Journées parisiennes de pédiatrie*, pp. 259–268. Paris: Flammarion.

Durá-Travé T, Yoldi-Petri ME, Gallinas-Victoriano F (2007): Epilepsy in children in Navarre, Spain: Epileptic seizure types and epileptic syndromes. *J Child Neurol* 22: 823–828.

Engel J Jr (2001): A proposed diagnostic scheme for people with epileptic seizures and with epilepsy. Report of the ILAE Task Force on Classification and Terminology. *Epilepsia* 42: 796–803.

Fasano A, Borlot F, Lang AE, Andrade DM (2014): Antecollis and Levodopa-Responsive Parkinsonism Are Late Features of Dravet Syndrome. *Neurology* 82: 2250–2251.

Fisher JL (2009): The anticonvulsant stiripentol acts directly on the GABAA receptor as a positive allosteric modulator. *Neuropharmacology* 56: 190–197.

Fisher JL (2011a): Interactions between modulators of the GABAA receptor: Stiripentol and benzodiazepines. *Eur J Pharmacol* 2: 160–165.

Fisher JL (2011b): The effects of stiripentol on GABAA receptors. *Epilepsia* 52 (Suppl 2): 76–78.

Fisher RS, Cross JH, French JA, *et al.* (2017): Operational classification of seizure types by the International League Against Epilepsy: Position Paper of the ILAE Commission for Classification and Terminology. *Epilepsia* 5: 522–530.

Fontana E, Dalla Bernardina B, Sgrò V, *et al.* (2004): Epilessia mioclonica severa (EMS) e/o sindrome di Dravet: Studio elettroclinico longitudinale di 53 soggetti. *Boll Lega It Epil* 125/126: 337–340.

Frederiksen K, Lu D, Yang J, Jensen HS, *et al.* (2017): A small molecule activator of Na_v 1.1 channels increases fast-spiking interneuron excitability and GABAergic transmission in vitro and has anti-convulsive effects in vivo. *Eur J Neurosci* 46: 1887–1896.

French J, Koepp M, Naegelin Y, *et al.* (2017): Clinical studies and anti-inflammatory mechanisms of treatments. *Epilepsia*. 58 (Suppl. 3): 69-82.

Fujiwara T, Nakamura H, Watanabe M, *et al.* (1990): Clinicoelectrographic concordance between monozygotic twins with severe myoclonic epilepsy in infancy. *Epilepsia* 31: 281–286.

Fujiwara T, Watanabe M, Takahashi Y, *et al.* (1992): Long-term course of childhood epilepsy with intractable Grand Mal seizures. *Jpn J Psychiatr Neurol* 46: 29.

Fujiwara T, Sugawara T, Mazaki-Miyazaki E, *et al.* (2003): Mutations of sodium channel alpha subunit type 1 (SCN1A) in intractable childhood epilepsies with frequent generalized tonic-clonic seizures. *Brain* 126: 531–546.

Fukuma G, Oguni H, Shirasaka Y, *et al.* (2004): Mutations of neuronal voltage-gated Na+ channel alpha 1 subunit gene *SCN1A* in core severe myoclonic epilepsy in infancy (SMEI) and in borderline SMEI (SMEB). *Epilepsia* 45: 140–148.

Gaily E, Anttonen A K, Valanne L, *et al.* (2013): Dravet syndrome: new potential genetic modifiers, imaging abnormalities, and ictal findings. *Epilepsia* 54: 1577–1585.

Gastaut H, Broughton R, Tassinari CA (1974): Unilateral epileptic seizures. In: Vinken PJ, Bruyn GW (eds) *Handbook of Clinical Neurology: The Epilepsies*, Vol. XV, pp. 235–245. Amsterdam/New-York: Elsevier.

Gataullina S, Dulac O (2017): From genotype to phenotype in Dravet disease. *Seizure* 44: 58–64.

Geffrey AL, Pollack SF, Bruno PL, Thiele EA (2015): Drug-drug interaction between clobazam and cannabidiol in children with refractory epilepsy. *Epilepsia* 56: 1246–1251.

Gennaro E, Santorelli FM, Bertini E, *et al.* (2006): Somatic and germline mosaïcisms in severe myoclonic epilepsy in infancy. *Biochem Biophysl Res Commun* 341: 489–493.

Genton P, Velizarova R, Dravet C (2011): Dravet syndrome: The long-term outcome. *Epilepsia* 52 (Suppl. 2): 44–49.

Giovanardi-Rossi PR, Santucci M, Gobbi G, *et al.* (1991): Long-term follow-up of severe myoclonic epilepsy in infancy. In: Fukuyama Y,

Kamoshita S, Ohtsuka C, Susuki Y (eds) *Modern Perspectives of Child Neurology*, pp. 205–213. Tokyo: Asahi Daily News.

Gitiaux C, Chemaly N, Quijano-Roy S, *et al.* (2016): Motor neuropathy contributes to crouching in patients with Dravet syndrome. *Neurology* 87: 277–281.

Gobbi G, Giovannini S, Boni A, Visconti P, Beghi M, Cornaggia CM (2008): Catatonic psychosis related to forced normalization in a girl with Dravet's syndrome. *Epileptic Disord* 10: 125–129.

Goldman A, Behr ER, Semsarian C, Bagnall RD, Sisodiya S, Cooper PN (2016): Sudden unexpected death in epilepsy genetics: Molecular diagnostics and prevention. *Epilepsia* 57 (Suppl. 1): 17–25.

Grosso S, Galimberti D, Farnetani MA, *et al.* (2005): Efficacy and safety of topiramate in infants according to epilepsy syndromes. *Seizure* 14: 183–189.

Guerrini R, Dravet C, Genton P, *et al.* (1998): Lamotrigine and seizure aggravation in severe myoclonic epilepsy. *Epilepsia* 39: 508–512.

Guerrini, R, Tonnelier, S, D'Athis, P, *et al.* (2002): Stiripentol in severe myoclonic epilepsy in infancy (SMEI): A placebo-controlled trial. *Epilepsia* 43 (Suppl. 9): S155.

Guerrini R, Bonanni P, Parmeggiani L, Hallett H, Oguni H (2005): Pathophysiology of myoclonic epilepsies. In: Delgado-Escueta AV, Guerrini R, Medina MT, Genton P, Bureau M, Dravet C (eds) *Advances in Neurology, Myoclonic Epilepsies*, vol. 95, pp. 23–46. Philadelphia: Lippincott Wilkins & Wilkins.

Guerrini R, Cellini E, Mei D, *et al.* (2010): Variable epilepsy phenotypes associated with a familial intragenic deletion of the SCN1A gene. *Epilepsia* 51: 2474–2477.

Guerrini R, Striano P, Catarino C, Sisodiya SM (2011): Neuroimaging and neuropathology of Dravet syndrome. *Epilepsia* 52 (Suppl. 2): 30–34.

Han S, Taiz C, Westenbroek RE, *et al.* (2012): Autistic behavior in *Scn1a+/–* mice and rescue by enhanced GABAergic transmission. *Nature* 489 (7416): 385–390.

Hattori J, Ouchida M, Ono J, *et al.* (2008): A screening test for the prediction of Dravet syndrome before one year of age. *Epilepsia* 49: 626–633.

Hayashi M, Sugai K, Kurihara E, Tamagawa K (2004): An autopsy case of severe myoclonic epilepsy in infancy, who died of acute encephalopathy associated with influenza infection. *Epilepsia* 45 (Suppl. 8): 65.

Heron SE, Scheffer IE, Iona X, *et al.* (2010): *De novo* SCN1A mutations in Dravet syndrome and related epileptic encephalopathies are largely of paternal origin. *J Med Genet* 47: 137–141.

Higurashi N, Nakamura M, Sugai M, *et al.* (2013): PCDH19-related female-limited epilepsy: Further details regarding early clinical features and therapeutic efficacy. *Epilepsy Res* 106: 191–199.

Hino-Fukuyo N, Haginoya K, Togashi N, *et al.* (2009): Ictal vomiting as an initial symptom of Severe myoclonic epilepsy in infancy: A case report. *J Child Neurol* 24: 228.

Hirose S, Scheffer IE, Marini C, *et al.* (2013): SCN1A testing for epilepsy: application in clinical practice. *Epilepsia* 54: 946–952.

Hsiao J, Yuan TY, Tsai MS, *et al.* (2016): Upregulation of haploinsufficient gene expression in the brain by targeting a long non-coding RNA improves seizure phenotype in a model of Dravet syndrome. *E Bio Medicine* 9: 257–277.

Horn CS, Ater SB, Hurst DL (1986): Carbamazepine-exacerbated epilepsy in children and adolescents. *Pediatr Neurol* 2: 340–345.

Hurst DL (1990): Epidemiology of severe myoclonic epilepsy in infancy. *Epilepsia* 31: 397–400.

Inoue Y, Ohtsuka Y, Oguni H, *et al.* (2009): Stiripentol open study in Japanese patients with Dravet syndrome. *Epilepsia* 50: 2362–2368.

Inoue Y, Ohtsuka Y, STP-1 Study Group (2015): Long-term safety and efficacy of stiripentol for the treatment of Dravet syndrome: A multicenter, open-label study in Japan. *Epilepsy Res* 113: 90–97.

Jansen FE, Sadleir LG, Harkin LA, *et al.* (2006): Severe myoclonic epilepsy in infancy (Dravet syndrome): Recognition and diagnosis in adults. *Neurology* 67: 224–226.

Ishii A, Watkins JC, Chen D, Hirose S, Hammer MF (2017): Clinical implications of SCN1A missense and truncation variants in a large Japanese cohort with Dravet syndrome. *Epilepsia* 58: 282–290.

Isom LL (2017): Opposing Phenotypes in Dravet Syndrome Patient-Derived Induced Pluripotent Stem Cell Neurons: Can Everyone Be Right? *Epilepsy Curr.* 17: 244–247.

Ito S, Ogiwara I, Yamada K, *et al.* (2013): Mouse with Nav1.1 haploinsufficiency, a model for Dravet syndrome, exhibits lowered sociability and learning impairment. *Neurobiol Dis* 49: 29–40.

Kalume F, Yu FH, Westenbroek R., Scheuer T, Catterall WA (2007): Reduced sodium current in Purkinje neurons from Nav1.1 mutant mice: implications for ataxia in severe myoclonic epilepsy in infancy. *J Neurosci* 27: 11065–11074.

Kalume F, Oakley JC, Westenbroek RE, *et al.* (2015): Sleep impairment and reduced interneuron excitability in a mouse model of Dravet Syndrome. *Neurobiol Dis* 77: 141–154.

Kaminska A, Dulac O (2001): Genetic predisposition to severe myoclonic epilepsy in infancy. *Epilepsia* 42: 204–209.

Kanazawa O (1992): Medically intractable generalized tonic-clonic or clonic seizures in infancy. *J Epil* 5: 143–148.

Kanazawa O, Shirane S (1999): Can early zonizamide medication improve the prognosis in the core and peripheral types of severe myoclonic epilepsy in infants? *Brain Dev* 21: 503.

Kearney JA (2016): Locus Heterogeneity in Epilepsy of Infancy with Migrating Focal Seizures. *Epilepsy Currents* 16 (1): 43–45.

Kelemen A, Rásonyl G, Neuwirth M, *et al.* (2011): Our clinical experience with zonisamide in resistant generalized epilepsy syndromes. *Ideggyogy Sz* 64 (5-6): 187–192.

Kimura K, Sugawara T, Mazaki-Miyazaki E, *et al.* (2005): A missense mutation in SCN1A in brothers with severe myoclonic epilepsy in infancy (SMEI) inherited from a father with febrile seizures. *Brain Dev* 27: 424–430.

Knupp K, Knupp G, Scarbro S, *et al.* (2017): Parental Perception of Comorbidities in Children With Dravet Syndrome. *Pediatric Neurology* 76: 60–65.

Kossoff EH, Zupec-Kania BA, Auvin S, *et al.* (2018): Optimal clinical management of children receiving dietary therapies for epilepsy: Updated recommendations of the International Ketogenic Diet Study Group, The Charlie Foundation, Matthew's Friends, and the Practice Committee of the Child Neurology Society. *Epilepsia Open* 3 (2): 175–192.

Korff K, Laux L, Kelley K, Goldstein J, Koh S, Nordli D Jr (2007): Dravet Syndrome (Severe Myoclonic Epilepsy in Infancy): A Retrospective Study of 16 Patients. *J Child Neurol* 22: 185–195.

Korff CM, Brunklaus AM, Zuberi SM (2015): Epileptic activity is a surrogate for an underlying etiology and stopping the activity has a limited impact on developmental outcome. *Epilepsia* 56: 1477–1481.

Kroll-Seger J, Portilla P, Dulac O, *et al.* (2006): Topiramate in the treatment of highly refractory patients with Dravet syndrome. *Neuropediatrics* 37: 325–329.

Lambarri San Martin I, Garaizar Axpe C, Zuazo Zamalloa E, *et al.* (1997): Epilepsia polimorfa de la infancia: revision de 12 casos. *Anal Esp Pediatr* 46: 571–575.

Lawton B, Davis T, Goldstein H, Tagg A (2018): An update in the initial management of paediatric status epilepticus. *Curr Opin Pediatr* (3): 359–363.

Lee HF, Chi CS, Tsai CR, Chen CH, Wang CC (2015): Electroencephalographic features of patients with SCN1A-positive Dravet syndrome. *Brain Dev* 37: 599–611.

Le Gal F, Korff CM, Monso-Hinard C, *et al.* (2010): A case of SUDEP in a patient with Dravet syndrome with SCN1A mutation. *Epilepsia* 51: 191–198.

Losito E, Kuchenbuch M, Chemaly N, *et al.* (2017): Age-related "Sleep/nocturnal" tonic and tonic clonic seizure clusters are underdiagnosed in patients with Dravet Syndrome. *Epilepsy Behav* 74: 33–40.

Lotte J, Haberlandt E, Neubauer B, Staudt M, Kluger GJ (2012): Bromide in patients with SCN1A-mutations manifesting as Dravet syndrome. *Neuropediatrics* 43: 17–21.

Lotte J, Bast T, Borusiak P, *et al.* (2016): Effectiveness of antiepileptic therapy in patients with PCDH19 mutations. *Seizure* 35: 106–110.

Madia F, Gennaro E, Cecconi M, *et al.* (2003): No evidence of GABRG2 mutations in severe myoclonic epilepsy of infancy. *Epilepsy Res* 53: 196–200.

Madia F, Striano P, Gennaro E, *et al.* (2006): Cryptic chromosome deletions involving SCN1A in severe myoclonic epilepsy in infancy. *Neurology* 67: 1230–1235.

Marini C, Scheffer IE, Nabbout R, *et al.* (2009): SCN1A duplications and deletions detected in Dravet syndrome: Implications for molecular diagnosis. *Epilepsia* 50: 1670–1678.

Marini C, Mei D, Parmeggiani L, *et al.* (2010): Protocadherin 19 mutations in girls with infantile-onset epilepsy. *Neurology* 75: 646–653.

Martin P, Rautenstrauß B, Abicht A J. Fahrbach J, Koster S (2010): Severe Myoclonic Epilepsy in Infancy – Adult Phenotype with Bradykinesia, Hypomimia, and Perseverative Behavior: Report of Five Cases. *Mol Syndromol* 1: 231–238.

Martin JP, Kümmerle A (2015): Hallucinations and delusions are frequently reported in individuals with Dravet syndrome. *Epilepsy Behav* 52: 222–224.

McMullan J, Sasson C, Pancioli A, Silbergleit R (2010): Midazolam *versus* diazepam for the treatment of status epilepticus in children and young adults: a meta-analysis. *Acad Emerg Med* 17: 575–582.

Meng H, Xu HQ, Yu L, *et al.* (2015): The SCN1A mutation database: updating information and analysis of the relationships among genotype, functional alteration, and phenotype. *Hum Mutat* 36 (6): 573–580.

Mingorance A (2017): *Dravet syndrome pipeline and opportunities review. Dracaena Report.* Dracaena Consulting.

Miyatake S, Kato M, Sawaishi Y, *et al.* (2018): Recurrent SCN3A p.Ile875Thr variant in patients with polymicrogyria. *Ann Neurol* 84: 159–161.

Morimoto M, Mazaki E, Nishimura A, *et al.* (2006): SCN1A mutation mosaïcism in a family with severe myoclonic epilepsy in infancy. *Epilepsia* 47: 1732–1736.

Mulley JC, Nelson P, Guerrero S, *et al.* (2006): A new molecular mechanism for severe myoclonic epilepsy in infancy: Exonic deletions in SCN1A. *Neurology* 67: 1094–1095.

Myers KA, Scheffer IE (2017): Myoclonic Absence Seizures in Dravet Syndrome. *Pediatr Neurol* 2017: 1–3

Myers KA, McMahon JM, Mandelstam SA, *et al.* (2017): Fatal Cerebral Edema With Status Epilepticus in Children With Dravet Syndrome: Report of 5 Cases. *Pediatrics* 39 (4): e2 0161933.

Myers KA, Lightfoot P, Patil SG, Cross JH, Scheffer IE (2018): Stiripentol efficacy and safety in Dravet syndrome: A 12-year observational study. *Dev Med Child Neurol* 60: 574–578.

Nabbout R, Gennaro E, Dalla Bernardina B, *et al.* (2003): Spectrum of SCN1A mutations in severe myoclonic epilepsy in infancy. *Neurology* 60: 1961–1967.

Nabbout R, Desguerre I, Sabbagh S, *et al.* (2008): An unexpected EEG course in Dravet syndrome. *Epilepsy Res* 81: 90–95.

Nabbout R, Copioli C, Chipaux M, *et al.* (2011): Ketogenic diet also benefits Dravet syndrome patients receiving stiripentol: A prospective pilot study. *Epilepsia* 52: 54–57.

Nabbout R, Chemaly N, Chipaux M. *et al.* (2013): Encephalopathy in children with Dravet syndrome is not a pure consequence of epilepsy. *Orphanet Journal of Rare Diseases* 8: 176.

Nakayama T, Ogiwara I, Ito K, *et al.* (2010): Deletions of SCN1A 5' genomic region with promoter activity in Dravet syndrome. *Hum Mutat* 31: 820–829.

Nicolai J, Gunning B, Leroy PL, Ceulemans B, Vies JSH (2008): Acute hepatic injury in four children with Dravet syndrome: Valproic acid, topiramate or acetaminophen? *Seizure* 17: 92–97.

Nieto M, Márquez E, Candau R, Rufo L, Ruiz del Portal (1995): Tomografia per emission de foton unico (SPECT) en la epilepsia mioclonica severa de la infancia (EMS). *Rev Neurol (Barc)* 23: 1193–1198.

Nieto M, Roldan S, Sanchez B, Candau R, Rodriguez R (2000a): Estudio immunológico en pacientes con epilepsia mioclónica severa en la infancia. *Rev Neurol (Spanish)* 30: 1–15.

Nieto-Barrera M, Candau R, Nieto-Jimenez M, Correa A, del Portal LR (2000a): Topiramate in the treatment of severe myoclonic epilepsy in infancy. *Seizure* 8: 590–594.

Nieto-Barrera M, Lillo MM, Rodriguez-Collado C, Candau R, Correa A (2000b): Severe myoclonic epilepsy in childhood. Epidemiologic analytical study. *Rev Neurol (Spanish)* 30: 620–624.

Oakley JC, Kalume F, Yu FH, Scheuer T, Catterall WA (2009): Temperature-and age-dependent seizures in a mouse model of severe myoclonic epilepsy in infancy. *Proc Natl Acad Sci USA* 106: 3994–3999.

Ogihara M, Hoshika A, Matsuno T, *et al.* (1994): EEG and polygraphical study of vibratory generalized tonic-clonic seizures (vibratory GTCS). *J Jpn Epil Soc* 12: 264-271.

Ogino T (1986): Severe myoclonic epilepsy in infancy – a clinical and electroencephalographic study. *J Jpn Epil Soc* 4: 114–126.

Ogino T, Ohtsuka Y, Mimaki N, *et al.* (1985): Severe myoclonic epilepsy in infancy. *Folia Psychiatr Neurol Japonica* 39: 357–358.

Ogino T, Ohtsuka Y, Yamatogi Y, Oka E, Ohtahara S (1989): The epileptic syndrome sharing common characteristics during early childhood with severe myoclonic epilepsy in infancy. *Jpn J Psychiatry Neurol* 43: 479–481.

Ogiwara I, Miyamoto H, Morita N, *et al.* (2007): Na(v)1.1 localizes to axons of parvalbumin-positive inhibitory interneurons: A circuit basis for epileptic seizures in mice carrying an Scn1a gene mutation. *J Neurosci* 27: 5903–5914.

Oguni H, Kitami H, Oguni M, *et al.* (1994): Treatment of severe myoclonic epilepsy in infants with bromide and its borderline variant. *Epilepsia* 35: 1140–1145.

Oguni H, Hayashi K, Awaya Y, Fukuyama Y, Osawa M (2001): Severe myoclonic epilepsy in infants – a review based on the Tokyo Women's medical university series of 84 cases. *Brain Dev* 23: 736–748.

Oguni H, Hayashi K, Osawa M, *et al.* (2005): Severe myoclonic epilepsy in infants. Typical and borderline groups in relation to SCN1A mutations. In: Delgado-Escueta V, Guerrini R, Medina MT, Genton P, Bureau M, Dravet C (eds) *Advances in Neurology, Myoclonic Epilepsies*, vol. 95, pp. 103–111. Philadelphia: Lippincott Williams & Wilkins.

Ohki T, Watanabe K, Negoro K, *et al.* (1997): Severe myoclonic epilepsy in infancy: Evolution of seizures. *Seizure* 6: 219–224.

Ohmori I, Ohtsuka Y, Murakami N, Asano T, Hattori J, Oka E (2001): Analysis of ictal EEG in severe myoclonic epilepsy in infancy. *Epilepsia* 42 (Suppl. 6): 54.

Ohmori I, Ohtsuka Y, Ouchida M, *et al.* (2003): Is phenotype difference in severe myoclonic epilepsy in infancy related to SCN1A mutations? *Brain Dev* 27: 488–493.

Ohmori I, Ouchida M, Kobayashi K, *et al.*(2008): Rasmussen encephalitis associated with SCN1A mutation. *Epilepsia* 49: 521–526.

Ohmori I, Ouchida M, Kobayashi K, *et al.* (2013): CACNA1A variants may modify the epileptic phenotype of Dravet syndrome. *Neurobiol Dis* 50: 209-217.

Okumura A, Kurahashi H, Hirose S, *et al.* (2007): Focal epilepsy resulting from a *de novo SCN1A* mutation. *Neuropediatrics* 38: 253–256.

Okumura A, Uematsu M, Imataka G, *et al.* (2012): Acute encephalopathy in children with Dravet syndrome. *Epilepsia* 53: 79-86.

Olivieri G, Battaglia D, Chieffo D, *et al.* (2016): Cognitive-behavioral profiles in teenagers with Dravet syndrome. *Brain Dev* 38: 554-562.

Passamonti C, Petrelli C, Mei D, *et al.* (2015): A novel inherited SCN1A mutation associated with different neuropsychological phenotypes: Is there a common core deficit? *Epilepsy Behav* 43: 89-92.

Pruna D, Balestri P, Zamponi N, *et al.* (2013): Epilepsy and vaccinations: Italian guidelines. *Epilepsia* 54 (Suppl. 7): 13-22.

Ragona F, Brazzo D, De Giorgi I, *et al.* (2010): Dravet syndrome: Early clinical manifestations and cognitive outcome in 37 Italian patients. *Brain Dev* 32: 71-77.

Ragona F, Granata T, Dalla Bernardina B, *et al.* (2011): Cognitive development in Dravet syndrome: A retrospective, multicenter study of 26 patients. *Epilepsia* 52: 386-392.

Renier WO, Renkawek K (1990): Clinical and neuropathologic findings in a case of severe myoclonic epilepsy in infancy. *Epilepsia* 31: 287–291.

Ricci D, Chieffo D, Battaglia D, *et al.* (2015): A prospective longitudinal study on visuo-cognitive development in Dravet syndrome: Is there a "dorsal stream vulnerability"? *Epilepsy Res* 109: 57–64.

Richards KL, Milligan CJ, Richardson RJ, *et al.* (2018): Selective NaV1.1 activation rescues Dravet syndrome mice from seizures and premature death. *Proc Natl Acad Sci USA* 115: E8077–E8085.

Rilstone JJ, Coelho FM, Minassian BA, Andrade DM (2012): Dravet syndrome: Seizure control and gait in adults with different SCN1A mutations. *Epilepsia* 53: 1421–1428.

Riva D, Vago C, Pantaleoni C, Bulgheroni S, Mantegazza M, Franceschetti S (2009): Progressive neurocognitive decline in two children with Dravet syndrome, *de novo SCN1A* truncations and different epileptic phenotypes. *Am J Med Genet A* 149A: 2339–2345.

Rodda JM, Scheffer IE, McMahon JM, Berkovic SF,Graham HK (2012): Progressive Gait Deterioration in Adolescents With Dravet Syndrome. *Arch Neurol* 69: 873–878.

Rosander C, Hallböök T (2015): Dravet syndrome in Sweden: A population-based study. *Dev Med Child Neurol* 57: 628–633.

Sakauchi M, Oguni H, Kato I, *et al.* (2011a): Mortality in Dravet syndrome: Search for risk factors in Japanese patients. *Epilepsia* 52 (Suppl. 2): 50–54.

Sakauchi M, Oguni H, Kato I, *et al.* (2011b): Retrospective multi-institutional study of the prevalence of early death in Dravet syndrome. *Epilepsia* 52: 1144–1149.

Sakakibara T, Nakagawa E, Saito Y, *et al.* (2009): Hemiconvulsion hemiplegia syndrome in a patient with severe myoclonic epilepsy in infancy. *Epilepsia* 50: 2158–2162.

Salgueiro-Pereira AR, Duprat F, Pousinha PA, *et al.* (2019): A two-hit story: Seizures and genetic mutation interaction sets phenotype severity in SCN1A epilepsies. *Neurobiol Dis* 125: 31–44.

Sarisjulis N, Gamboni B, Plouin P, Kaminska A, Dulac O (2000): Diagnosing idiopathic/cryptogenic epilepsy syndromes in infancy. *Arch Dis Child* 82: 226–230.

Sato T, Ota M, Matsuo M, Tasaki H, Miyazaki S (1995): Recurrent reversible rhabdomyolisis associated with hyperthermia and status epilepticus. *Acta Paediatr* 84: 1083–1085.

Scheffer IE, Berkovic SF (1997): Generalized epilepsy with febrile seizures plus: A genetic disorder with heterogeneous clinical phenotypes. *Brain* 120: 479–490.

Scheffer IE, Turner SJ, Dibbens LM, *et al.* (2008): Epilepsy and mental retardation limited to females: an under-recognized disorder. *Brain* 131: 918–927.

Scheffer IE, French J, Hirsch E, *et al.* (2017): Classification of the epilepsies: New concepts for discussion and debate – Special report of the ILAE Classification Task Force of the Commission for Classification and Terminology. *Epilepsia Open* 1 (1): 37–44.

Shmuely S, Sisodiya SM, Gunning WB, Sander JW, Thijs RD (2016): Mortality in Dravet syndrome: A review. *Epilepsy Behav* 64: 69–74.

Schoonjans AS, De Keersmaecker S, Van Bouwel B, Ceulemans B (2017): More daytime sleepiness and worse quality of sleep in patients with Dravet Syndrome compared to other epilepsy patients. *Eur J Paediatr Neurol* 23: 61–69.

Shi XY, Tomonoh Y, Wang WZ *et al.* (2016): Efficacy of antiepileptic drugs for the treatment of Dravet syndrome with different genotypes. *Brain Dev* 38: 40–46.

Siegler Z, Barsi P, NeuwirthM, *et al.* (2005): Hippocampal sclerosis in severe myoclonic epilepsy in infancy: A retrospective MRI study. *Epilepsia* 46: 704–708.

Singh R, Scheffer IE, Crossland K, Berkovic SF (1999): Generalized Epilepsy with Febrile Seizures Plus: A Common Childhood-onset Genetic Epilepsy Syndrome. *Ann Neurol* 45: 75–81.

Singh R, Andermann E, Whitehouse WP, *et al.* (2001): Severe myoclonic epilepsy in infancy: Extended spectrum of GEFS+? *Epilepsia* 42: 837–844.

Singh NA, Pappas C, Dahle EJ, *et al.* (2009): A role of SCN9A in human epilepsies, as a cause of febrile seizures and as a potential modifier of Dravet syndrome. *PLoS Genet* 5: e1000649.

Skluzacek JV, Watts KP, Parsy O, *et al.* (2011): Dravet syndrome and parent associations: The IDEA League experience with comorbid conditions, mortality, management, adaptation, and grief. *Epilepsia* 52 (Suppl. 2): 95–101.

Smith RS, Kenny CJ, Ganesh V, *et al.* (2018): Sodium Channel SCN3A ($Na_V1.3$) Regulation of Human Cerebral Cortical Folding and Oral Motor Development. *Neuron* 99: 905–913.

Specchio N, Kasteleijn-Nost-Trenité DGA, Piccioli M, *et al.* (2011): Diagnosing photosensitive epilepsy: Fancy new *versus* old fashioned techniques in patients with different epileptic syndromes. *Brain Dev* 33: 294–300.

Specchio N, Pontrelli G, Serino D, *et al.* (2014): Occipital seizures induced by Intermittent Photic Stimulation in Dravet syndrome. *Seizure* 23: 309–313.

Steel D, Symonds JD, Zuberi SM, Brunklaus A (2017): Dravet syndrome and its mimics: Beyond SCN1A. *Epilepsia* 58: 1807–1816.

Striano P, Mancardi MM, Biancheri R, *et al.* (2007a): Brain MRI findings in severe myoclonic epilepsy in infancy and genotype-phenotype correlations. *Epilepsia* 48: 1092–1096.

Striano P, Coppola G, Pezella M, *et al.* (2007b): An open-label trial of levetiracetam in severe myoclonic epilepsy in infancy. *Neurology* 69: 922–925.

Sugama M, Oguni H, Fukuyama Y (1987): Clinical and electroencephalographic study of severe myoclonic epilepsy in infancy (Dravet). *Jpn J Psychiat Neurol* 41: 463–465.

Suls A, Velizarova R, Yordanova I, *et al.* (2010): Four generations of epilepsy caused by an inherited microdeletion of the SCN1A gene. *Neurology* 75: 72–76.

Takahashi T, Tsukahara Y (1992): Usefulness of blue sunglasses in photosensitive epilepsy. *Epilepsia* 33: 517–521.

Takahashi Y, Fujiwara T, Yagi K, Seino M (1999): Photosensitive epilepsies and pathophysiologic mechanisms of the photoparoxysmal response. *Neurology* 53: 926–932.

Takayama R, Fujiwara T, Shigematsu H, *et al.* (2014): Long-term course of Dravet syndrome: A study from an epilepsy center in Japan. *Epilepsia* 55: 528–538.

Tanabe T, Awaya Y, Matsuishi T, *et al.* (2004): Survey of vaccination and viral infections for children with severe myoclonic epilepsy in infancy. *No To Hattatsu* 36: 318–323.

Tanabe T, Awaya Y, Matsuishi T, *et al.* (2008): Management of and prophylaxis against status epilepticus in children with severe myoclonic epilepsy in infancy (SMEI; Dravet syndrome): A nation-wide questionnaire survey in Japan. *Brain Dev* 30: 629–635.

Than TN, Chiron C, Dellatolas G, *et al.* (2002): Long-term efficacy and tolerance of stiripentol in severe myoclonic epilepsy in infancy (Dravet's syndrome). *Arch Pediatr* 9: 1120–1127.

Tian X, Ye J, Zeng Q, *et al.* (2018): The clinical outcome and neuroimaging of acute encephalopathy after status epilepticus in Dravet syndrome. *Dev Med Child Neurol* 60: 566–573.

Trivisano M, Pietrafusa N, di Ciommo V, *et al.* (2016): PCDH19-related epilepsy and Dravet Syndrome: Face-off between two early-onset epilepsies with fever sensitivity. *Epilepsy Res* 125: 32–36.

Trivisano M, Pietrafusa N, Terracciano A, *et al.* (2018): Defining the electroclinical phenotype and outcome of PCDH19-related epilepsy: A multicenter study. *Epilepsia* 59: 2260–2271.

Tro-Baumann B, von Spiczak S, Lotte J, *et al.* (2011): A retrospective study of the relation between vaccination and occurrence of seizures in Dravet syndrome. *Epilepsia* 52: 175–178.

Tsuda Y, Oguni H, Sakauchia M, Osawa M (2013): An electroclinical study of absence seizures in Dravet syndrome. *Epilepsy Res* 103: 88–96.

Turner SJ, Brown A, Arpone M, Anderson V, Morgan AT, Scheffer IE (2017): Dysarthria and broader motor speech deficits in Dravet syndrome. *Neurology* 88: 743–749.

Vadlamudi L, Dibbens LM, Lawrence KM, *et al.* (2010): Timing of *de novo* mutagenesis – a twin study of sodium-channel mutations. *N Engl J Med* 363: 1335–1340.

Verbeek NE, Wassenaar M, van Campen JS, *et al.* (2015): Seizure precipitants in Dravet syndrome: What events and activities are specifically provocative compared with other epilepsies? *Epilepsy Behav* 47: 39–44.

Verbeek N, Kasteleijn-Nolst T, Wassenaar M, *et al.* (2017): Photosensitivity in Dravet syndrome is under-recognized and related to prognosis. *Clin Neurophysiol* 128 (2): 323–330.

Villas N, Meskis MA, Goodliffe S (2017): Dravet syndrome: Characteristics, comorbidities, and caregiver concerns. *Epilepsy Behav* 74: 81–86.

Villeneuve N, Portilla P, Ferrari AR, *et al.* (2002): Topiramate (TPM) in severe myoclonic epilepsy in infancy (SMEI): Study of 27 patients. *Epilepsia* 43 (Suppl. 8): 155.

Villeneuve N, Laguitton V, Viellard M, *et al.* (2014): Cognitive and adaptive evaluation of 21 consecutive patients with Dravet syndrome. *Epilepsy Behav* 31: 143–148.

Wakai S, Ikehata M, Nihira H, *et al.* (1996a): "Obtundation status (Dravet)" caused by complex partial status epilepticus in a patient with severe myoclonic epilepsy in infancy. *Epilepsia* 37: 1020–1022.

Wakai S, Ito N, Sueoka H, *et al.* (1996b): Severe myoclonic epilepsy in infancy and carbamazepine. *Eur J Pediatr* 155: 724.

Wallace SJ (1998): Myoclonus and epilepsy in childhood: A review of treatment with valproate, ethosuximide, lamotrigine and zonizamide. *Epilepsy Res* 29: 147–154.

Wallace RH, Scheffer IE, Barnett S, *et al.* (2001): Neuronal sodium-channel alpha1-subunit mutations in generalized epilepsy with febrile seizures plus. *Am J Hum Genet* 68: 859–865.

Wang PJ, Fan PC, Lee WT, Young C, Huang CC, Shen YZ (1996): Severe myoclonic epilepsy in infancy: evolution of electroencephalographic and clinical features. *Acta Paed Sin* 37: 428–432.

Wang JW, Kurahashi H, Ishii A, *et al.* (2008): Microchromosomal deletions involving SCN1A and adjacent genes in severe myoclonic epilepsy in infancy. *Epilepsia* 49: 1528–1534.

Wirrell EC, Laux L, Franz DN, *et al.* (2013): Stiripentol in Dravet syndrome: Results of a retrospective U.S. study. *Epilepsia* 54: 1595–1604.

Wirrell EC, Laux L, Donner E, *et al.* (2017): Optimizing the Diagnosis and Management of Dravet Syndrome: Recommendations From a North American Consensus Panel. *Pediatr Neurol.* 68: 18–34.e3.

Wolff M, Cassé-Perrot C, Dravet C (2006): Severe myoclonic epilepsy of infants (Dravet syndrome): Natural history and neuropsychological findings. *Epilepsia* 47 (Suppl. 2): 45–48.

Wu YW, Sullivan J, McDaniel SS, Meisler MH, Walsh EM, Li SX, Kuzniewicz MW (2015): Incidence of Dravet Syndrome in a US Population. *Pediatrics* 136: e1310–e1315.

Yakoub LM, Dulac O, Jambaqué I, Plouin P (1992): Early diagnosis of severe myoclonic epilepsy in infancy. *Brain Dev* 14: 299–303.

Yan N, Xin-Hua W, Lin-Mei Z, *et al.* (2018): Prospective study of the efficacy of a ketogenic diet in 20 patients with Dravet syndrome. *Seizure* 60: 144–148.

Yasuda S, Watanabe M, Fujiwara T, Yagi K, Seino M (1989): A peculiar state observed in 4 patients with severe myoclonic epilepsy in infancy. *Jpn J Psychiatr Neurol* 43: 533–535.

Yu FH, Mantegazza M, Westenbroek RE, *et al.* (2006): Reduced sodium current in GABAergic interneurons in a mouse model of severe myoclonic epilepsy in infancy. *Nat Neurosci* 9: 1142–1149.

Zhang YH, Burgess R, Malone JP, *et al.* (2017): Genetic epilepsy with febrile seizures plus: Refining the spectrum. *Neurology* 89: 1210–1219.

Zhang Y, Kecskés A, Copmans D, *et al.* (2015): Pharmacological characterization of an antisense knockdown zebrafish model of Dravet syndrome: inhibition of epileptic seizures by the serotonin agonist fenfluramine. *PLoS ONE.* 10: e0125898.

Zuberi SM, Brunklaus A, Birch R, Reavey E, Duncan J, Forbes GH (2011): Genotype-phenotype associations in SCN1A-related epilepsies. *Neurology* 76: 594–600.

WITH VIDEO SUPPLEMENTS

CHAPTER 11

MYOCLONIC EPILEPSIES IN INFANCY AND EARLY CHILDHOOD

Renzo Guerrini[1], Francesco Mari[1], Stéphane Auvin[2] and Charlotte Dravet[3]

[1] Pediatric Neurology Unit and Laboratories, Children's Hospital A. Meyer-University of Florence, Italy
[2] Pediatric Neurology Department, Robert-Debré Children Hospital, University of Paris, France
[3] Centre Saint-Paul, Henri-Gastaut Hospital, Marseille, France; Infantile Neuropsychiatric Unit, Fondazione Policlinico Universitario A. Gemelli, IRCCS, Università Cattolica del Sacro Cuore, Roma, Italy

Introduction

General characteristics of myoclonic epilepsies

The term "myoclonic epilepsies" has traditionally been used to designate a large and heterogeneous group of epilepsies characterized by repeated and brief jerks often causing multiple falls, severe course, resistance to antiepileptic drugs, and frequent association with cognitive impairment (Aicardi & Levy Gomes, 1991; Guerrini *et al.*, 2002a). However, ictal manifestations causing the patient to fall to the ground are not always myoclonic in nature and not all "myoclonic" epilepsies are associated to a complicated outcome. Although myoclonic attacks are the only type of seizure in some patients with myoclonic epilepsy, other seizure types are often observed. Generalized tonic-clonic seizures are frequent (Erba & Browne, 1983; Aicardi &Levi Gomes, 1991) but generalized clonic, atypical absences and especially atonic seizures are also observed (Dalla Bernardina *et al.*, 1987; Dravet *et al.*, 2005). Association with tonic seizures is uncommon in myoclonic epilepsies but isolated tonic attacks during sleep are sometimes observed in children with myoclonic astatic epilepsy (Guerrini *et al.*, 2002a; Oguni *et al.*, 2001). Considering the group heterogeneity and variable prognostic outlook, it is therefore not surprising that considerable confusion has dominated attempts to classify myoclonic epilepsies. The fact that a category of myoclonic epilepsies exists is in itself questionable as it carries the risk of overemphasizing one seizure type – which can even be a marginal feature – among multiple, at times complex, clinical manifestations.

Definition of epileptic myoclonus

The term myoclonus is used to describe involuntary muscle jerks, usually involving antagonist muscles (Patel & Jankovic, 1988; Caviness & Brown, 2004). Myoclonus can be classified according to its physiology in epileptic and non-epileptic. Epileptic myoclonus can be comprehensively defined as an elementary electroclinical manifestation of epilepsy involving descending neurons, whose spatial (spread) or temporal (self-sustained repetition) amplification can trigger overt epileptic activity (Guerrini *et al.*, 2002a). According to its distribution, myoclonus is classified as focal, multifocal or generalized (Hallett, 1985). The neurophysiological characteristics of epileptic myoclonus are: i) duration of the myoclonic electromyographic (EMG) burst ranging between 10 and 100 msec; ii) synchronous EMG bursts or silent periods on antagonist muscles; and iii) presence of an EEG correlate detectable by routine surface EEG or burst-locked EEG averaging (Hallet, 1985, Guerrini *et al.*, 2002a; Shibasaki & Hallett, 2005).

Clinical and EEG features common to the myoclonic seizures

Myoclonic seizures (MS) can produce only slight head nodding and/or abduction of the arms or even the patient to fall when the lower limbs are also involved or when the atonic phenomenon immediately following the jerk is prominent (Erba & Browne, 1983; Tassinari *et al.*, 1992). MS are of short duration and may have a saccadic character, with a repetition rate of 2–3 Hz. They most commonly affect axial muscles, but may also involve the external ocular, the eyelids or the facial, especially perioral, muscles in a significant proportion of patients. Most MS occur spontaneously, usually on awakening, as in juvenile myoclonic epilepsy (JME) or during drowsiness, as in myoclonic epilepsy in infancy. In some patients, jerks may be precipitated by photic stimulation in the EEG laboratory or induced by environmental photic stimuli. Tapping or sudden acoustic stimuli may also cause generalized myoclonic jerks of epileptic origin (Ricci *et al.*, 1995). MS are usually isolated events but, at times, they supervene in prolonged series and may even progress to myoclonic status (Doose, 1992a; Dravet *et al.*, 2005).

The EMG recording of a myoclonic seizure is a biphasic or polyphasic EMG potential of 20 to 150-msec. Ictal EEG shows generalized bursts of polyspikes/poly-spike and wave discharges. Interictal EEG may be normal or show slow background activity, depending on the epilepsy syndrome and the etiology *(Figure 1)*. Interictal bursts of irregular poly-spike and wave complexes of short duration (less than 3 seconds) also occur spontaneously or are induced by intermittent photic stimulation (IPS). During NREM sleep, there is often an increase in the frequency of discharges that generally feature multiple spikes and waves (Aicardi & Levy Gomes, 1991; Dravet *et al.*, 2005).

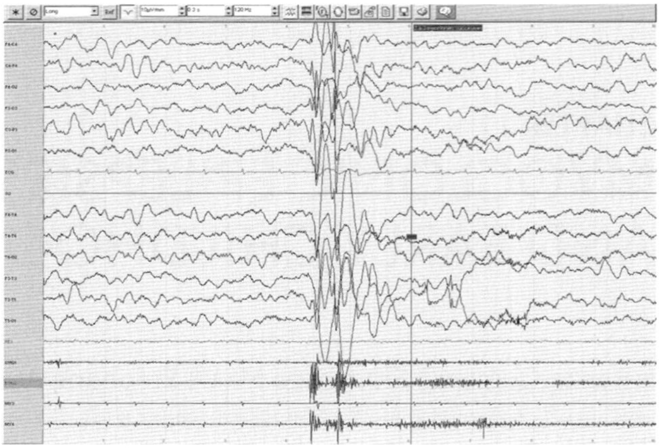

Figure 1 **Ictal polygraphic EEG recording showing spike–wave discharges with two successive myoclonic jerks of the deltoid muscles (EMG 1 right and 2 left) (10sec/page).**

Differential diagnosis of myoclonic seizures

The recognition and classification of seizures described, as a "sudden and brief jerk" is not always easy. Misdiagnosis is possible if not frequent. When the description of the ictal manifestations is combined with EEG, EMG, and video monitoring, three main types of seizures are recognized:

i) During atonic seizures, caused by the loss of muscle tone, the patient falls to the ground, suddenly or slumping in a rhythmic, step by step fashion, mimicking myoclonic seizures (Erba & Browne, 1983). However, if the atonic phenomenon involves only the muscles of the neck, it causes just a brief head nodding. Atonic seizures are accompanied by loss of consciousness: the patient is unaware of falling, although the drop is followed by immediate recovery. On EEG recordings, atonic seizures are associated with various patterns (Rubboli *et al.*, 1997): slow spike and waves (Gastaut *et al.*, 1974), 3-Hz spike and waves (Aicardi & Levy Gomes, 1991), polyspike and waves *(Figure 1)*, or fast recruiting rhythms (Fariello *et al.*, 1979; Chayasirisobhon & Rodin, 1981). The EMG channels show suppression of muscle activity (Gastaut *et al.*, 1974; Rubboli *et al.*, 1997);

ii) Tonic seizures involve the tonic contraction of certain muscle groups, without progression to a clonic phase (Gastaut & Broughton, 1972; Erba & Browne, 1983). They may cause the patient to fall to the ground when the lower limbs are forcibly flexed or the patient is thrown out of balance. During a tonic seizure the EMG shows an interferential muscle discharge similar to that of a voluntary contraction. The EEG may show flattening of background activity, very fast activity (20 Hz) increasing in amplitude, or a 10-Hz rhythmic high amplitude activity similar to the "epileptic recruiting rhythm" (Gastaut *et al.*, 1963; Fariello *et al.*, 1979; Brenner & Atkinson, 1982);

iii) Spasms, symmetrical or asymmetrical, are similar to brief tonic seizures and are an important cause of sudden falls (Egli *et al.*, 1985). They generally occur in clusters. The EEG-EMG recordings of spasms are diagnostic, showing a brief (0.5–3 sec), diamond-shaped EMG burst, which is accompanied by a high amplitude, diffuse slow wave with superimposed fast rhythms. Sometimes it is difficult to distinguish epileptic spasms from epileptic myoclonus and careful polygraphic recording analysis is required.

Etiology of myoclonic epilepsies

Genetic factors play an important role, as indicated by the frequency of a history of epilepsy in family members and, especially, by the numerous association of epilepsies with MS and genetic alterations, from single gene mutations to chromosomal abnormalities. Mutations in the SCN1A gene are reported in almost all patients with Dravet syndrome (DS), former called severe myoclonic epilepsy in infancy (SMEI) – while mutations in the *SCN1B, SCN2A, HCN1, STXBP1, CHD2, KCNA2, GLUT1* genes have been described in patients with a myoclonic astatic epilepsy (MAE) phenotype and in patients with DS-like phenotypes (Wallace *et al.*, 1998; Claes *et al.*, 2001; Marini *et al.*, 2011, Steel *et al.*, 2017; Mullen *et al.*, 2011).

Reports of myoclonic epilepsies that are symptomatic of an acquired, fixed brain lesion are rather uncommon and are most often the result of perinatal hypoxic-ischemic encephalopathy. Patients with brain damage start having MS between a few months of age and the 3rd year of age (Elia *et al.*, 1998; Guerrini *et al.*, 2002a; Dalla Bernardina *et al.*, 2002). Other seizure types usually co-occur. In this chapter, we focus on the previously called idiopathic myoclonic epilepsies in infancy and early childhood (Guerrini *et al.*, 2012), in particular, the myoclonic epilepsy in infancy (MEI, previously defined as benign myoclonic epilepsy of infancy, BMEI) and the epilepsy with myoclonic atonic seizures (MAE, also defined as epilepsy with myoclonic-astatic seizures).

Myoclonic epilepsy in infancy (otherwise known as benign myoclonic epilepsy in infancy)

Historical note and nomenclature

MEI was initially identified through a description of seven infants (Dravet & Bureau, 1981) and called BMEI. It was defined as being characterized by brief and generalized MS without other seizure types (except rare simple febrile seizures, FS), in the first three years of life in cognitively normal infants. In these children MS were easily controlled by a simple treatment and remitted during childhood. Psychomotor development remained normal. The existence of a distinct early and benign myoclonic epileptic syndrome was previously proposed in three infants in a study of early onset epilepsies (Dalla Bernardina *et al.*, 1978) but without known follow up. BMEI was classified among the generalized idiopathic epilepsy syndromes in the 1989 International classification (Commission on Classification and Terminology of the ILAE, 1989) and among the epilepsies of unknown etiology in the proposal of the International League Against Epilepsy (ILAE) Task Force (Berg *et al.*, 2010). Several authors have described a reflex form of MS, triggered by noise or touch (Ricci *et al.*, 1995). The benignity of the syndrome has subsequently been questioned, since the term "benign" should be limited to those forms of epilepsy in which the favorable course and outcome can be predicted from the onset and not in retrospect (Engel, 2006). As that is not the case in all patients with early-onset idiopathic myoclonic epilepsy (Zuberi & O'Reagan, 2006), the name was changed to "myoclonic epilepsy in infancy" (Engel, 2006). However, this denomination is too loose and it was therefore proposed to use the name "idiopathic myoclonic epilepsy in infancy" (IMEI) (Dravet & Vigevano, 2007) which was not accepted by the Commission.

Although the reflex forms appear to be more benign than the non-reflex, we consider the whole group as a single syndrome.

Epidemiology

MEI is rare. Jallon & Latour (2005) mentioned that it is usually excluded from epidemiologic surveys because it is difficult to observe and classify. These authors cite rates from 0.2% of newly diagnosed epilepsies in children to 1% of all childhood epilepsies while Durà-Travé *et al.* (2007) estimated it to represent 0.8% of pediatric epilepsies between 1 month and 15 years in a tertiary center. For comparison, Lennox-Gastaut syndrome accounted for 0.5%, Dravet syndrome for 1.4%, West syndrome for 4.1%. Among epilepsies considered according to age at onset, MEI represented 1.3% and 1.7% of those with onset in the first year of life (Caraballo *et al.*, 1997; Sarisjulis *et al.*, 2000), around 2% of those beginning in the first three years of life (Dalla Bernardina *et al.*, 1983), and 0.39% of those beginning in the first six years of life (Ohtsuka *et al.*, 1993).

Genetics

The genetic contribution to MEI is poorly studied and unclear. There are no familial cases described, with the exception of a pair of monozygotic twins (Doose, 2003). However, a family history of FS or epilepsy is reported by several authors: 17.6% (Auvin *et al.*, 2006), 40% (Lin *et al.*, 1998), 50.5% (Dravet & Bureau, 2005), 55% (Rossi *et al.*, 1997, Darra *et al.*, 2006). These results suggest ill defined genetic influences in the pathogenesis of MEI.

Personal history

No significant antecedents are mentioned prior to the onset of the MS. Only two patients (1.9%) had an associated condition: Down's syndrome and hyperinsulinic diabetes (Dravet *et al.*, 2005). FS were reported in 20% of patients (Dravet & Bureau, 2012). They were always simple, usually rare and often occurring before the onset of the MS and before treatment was started. Darra *et al.* (2006) reported one patient who presented two isolated nocturnal orofacial seizures six months before the appearance of MS.

Clinical and EEG manifestations

When gender is mentioned, it appears that boys outnumber girls. The age at onset is usually between 4 months and 3 years. An earlier onset is uncommon. A later onset, between 3 and 5 years, was reported by some authors (Guerrini *et al.*, 1994; Giovanardi-Rossi *et al.*, 1997; Lin *et al.*, 1998 ; Gentile *et al.*, 2010), which suggests that the same type of epilepsy may appear at different ages, but tends to be more frequent within a narrower age range (Guerrini *et al.*, 1994).

Initially, MS are brief, often rare, involving the upper limbs and the head, rarely the lower limbs. In babies, they may be barely noticeable and the parents may find it difficult to determine their exact onset and frequency. They often report "spasms" or "head nodding". Later, their frequency increases up to several times a day. Video-EEG and polygraphic recordings help providing a precise analysis of these seizures. They are massive myoclonic jerks, involving the axis of the body and the limbs, provoking a head drop and an upward-outward movement of the upper limbs, rarely flexion of the lower limbs, sometimes rolling-up of the eyeballs. Their intensity varies from one child to the other and from one attack to the next in the same child. The most severe jerks cause a sudden projection of the objects held in the hands, sometimes a fall. The mildest forms provoke only a brief forward movement of the head, or, even, a simple closure of the eyes. Myoclonic jerks are very brief (1–3 sec) manifested as either isolated events or as pseudo-rhythmically repeated jerks lasting up to several seconds. They occur several times a day at unpredictable times. Unlike infantile spasms, they do not occur in long series and are not favored by awakening, but rather by drowsiness. In approximately 1/5 of the patients reported by Dravet and Bureau (2005) a clinical and EEG photosensitivity was observed. In the patients with reflex MEI, they are triggered by sudden unexpected noise, or touch, or both (Verrotti *et al.*, 2013). The level of awareness is difficult to assess in isolated MS episodes. In our experience, only repeated jerks may entail impaired awareness. Some authors reported absences associated with the myoclonic jerks (Zafeiriou *et al.*, 2003; Caraballo *et al.*, 2013; Belcastro *et al.*, 2015; 2017). Caraballo *et al.* (2011; 2013) considered the longer MS episodes with apparent reduced awareness as a brief type of absence seizure. However, to appreciate the level of awareness in young children is difficult and the myoclonic component remains predominant. Some reports (Ito *et al.*, 2012; Yang *et al.*, 2017) have highlighted the presence of isolated convulsive afebrile seizure episodes preceding or concurring the appearance of MS. No significant clinical and overall prognostic differences were noticed between these patients and the group with isolated MS.

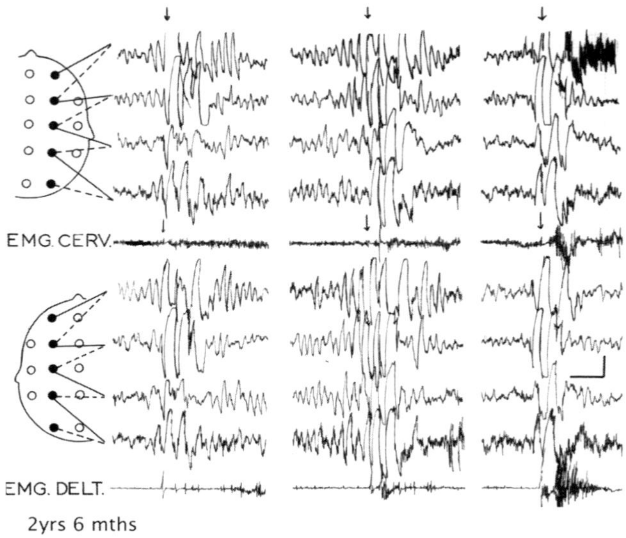

Figure 2 **Three short myoclonic jerks polygraphically recorded in a 2-year-6-month-old boy. Each jerk (arrows) is accompanied by a very high generalized SW discharge. The myoclonia can be followed by an atonia (cervical muscle). In the third manifestation (right) there is also a voluntary movement after the myoclonia. 1 cm = 100 mV.**

We never observed the sudden brief vocalization reported by Lin *et al.* (1998). In reflex MS, jerks can be elicited both in wakefulness and sleep, with a threshold which is lower in stage I and increases gradually during deeper sleep stages (Ricci *et al.*, 1995). As development progresses normally, parents and pediatricians tend not to consider these movements as pathological. Short EEG during wakefulness could be normal in the absence of myoclonic jerks. But the jerks are always associated with generalized fast spike-waves (SW) or polyspike-waves (PSW), lasting as long as the clinical event *(Figures 1 and 2)*. The jerk may be followed by a brief muscular silent period. Darra *et al.* (2006) reported that the mildest seizures, only recognizable as eye blinking, were related to very small spike-waves involving only the fronto-central areas and the vertex. Hirano *et al.* (2009) found predominance in the proximal muscles, a forward flexion and a single occurrence of the jerks.

During drowsiness, there is an enhancement of the myoclonus that usually, but not always, disappears during slow sleep and, sometimes, appears again during arousals (Darra *et al.*, 2006). Myoclonus triggered by tactile and acoustic stimuli has the same characteristics as spontaneous jerks. Ricci *et al.* (1995) noticed that after a reflex myoclonic attack there was a refractory period, lasting 20–30 sec to 1–2 min, during which sudden stimuli did not provoke attacks. IPS can also provoke MS in a minority of patients. The interictal EEG is normal. IPS does not provoke SW without concomitant jerk at onset. Nap sleep recordings show a normal organization of sleep. Generalized SW discharges may occur during REM sleep *(Figure 3)*. No other seizure types are observed in children with MEI in infancy up to age 9 years, even if they are left untreated, except rare FS (Dravet *et al.*, 2005; Capovilla *et al.*, 2007; Gentile *et al.*, 2010). Clinical examination is normal. When brain imaging was performed it was normal.

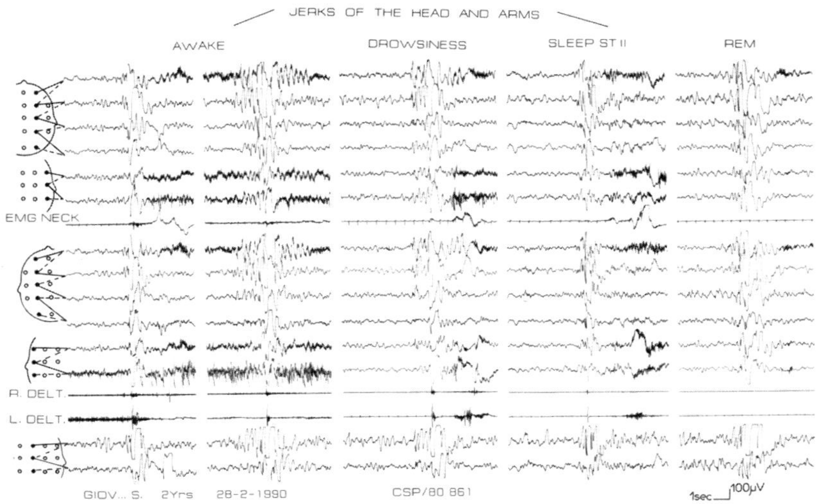

Figure 3

In a 2-year-old girl, before any treatment, several myoclonic jerks are polygraphically recorded when awake, persisting during drowsiness and, attenuated, during sleep stage II. They are accompanied by generalized SW, sometimes preceded by SW localized in the anterior regions. The same type of generalized discharge appears during REM without concomitant clinical event.
R DELT: **right deltoid muscle;** L DELT: **left deltoid muscle.**

Treatment

In 2011 (Guerrini *et al.*, 2012) information about treatment was available for 182 patients (Dravet & Bureau, 2005; Auvin *et al.*, 2006; Darra *et al.*, 2006; Zuberi & O'Regan, 2006; Capovilla *et al.*, 2007; Moutaouakil *et al.*, 2010; Mangano *et al.*, 2011; Gentile *et al.*, 2010; Ong *et al.*, 2011) but not always reported in detail. To summarize, nine patients did not receive any antiepileptic drug (AED) and became seizure-free. Most patients received valproate (VPA) monotherapy from the onset and 82.9% became seizure-free. Other patients received various monotherapies or polytherapies and most became seizure-free after VPA was introduced. Around ten patients were reported as resistant to several antiepileptic drugs (AEDs) and were lost to follow-up. On the whole, in approximately 90% of patients MS disappeared. Literature data suggest that VPA is the first choice in MEI and should be started at high doses with control of the plasma level in case of no answer to avoid a false resistance (Lin *et al.*, 1998, Darra *et al.*, 2006). If MS are not completely controlled by VPA, other options can be chosen: add one benzodiazepine (clobazam (CLB), clonazepam (CNZ)) to VPA, or add ethosuccimide (ETS) to VPA, or substitute VPA by another broad spectrum AED, knowing that lamotrigine (LTG) is not always efficacious. In case of persistent seizures, the diagnosis should be revised. Treatment should be maintained for two years if it is well tolerated. In children with purely reflex seizures some authors suggested that drug treatment can be avoided except in the cases with photosensitive reflex MS (Capovilla *et al.*, 2007). Monitoring cognitive and behavioral development is necessary since it can be impaired, requiring specific help for the child and psychological support to the family.

Long-term outcome and prognosis

In the first, very small, series (Dravet & Bureau, 1981) the outcome seemed to depend on an early diagnosis and treatment. MS were easily controlled by VPA and the child could then develop normally. If left untreated, the patient continued to experience MS, with impaired psychomotor and behavioral development. Currently available information suggests that outcome is less favorable than thirty years ago as underlined by Zuberi & O'Regan(2006). The exact age at follow-up was reported in 2011 for 116 cases. The age range at follow-up was nine months to 30 years *(Figure 4)*. In all these patients but one (Prats Vinas *et al.*, 2002), MS disappeared, lasting less than one year in most, with reflex seizures being more easily controlled. The longest duration of seizures (from four years ten months to nine years four months) was observed only in the first publication, before recognition of the syndrome (Dravet & Bureau, 1981) and in the report by Gentile *et al.* (2010), in patients who were not diagnosed and not treated. In most patients AEDs were withdrawn during childhood. However, the longer the reported follow-up, the higher the number of patients who experienced other seizure types after disappearance of MS. In the review done in 2011, information was available for 162 patients with known outcome after the age of five. Among them, 16% presented other seizures, usually after a free interval after remission of MS. Seventeen patients had isolated GTC or clonic seizures that were either isolated events or easily controlled by a short treatment. Five patients had absence seizures, three of them with marked eyelid myoclonia (Prats-Vinas *et al.*, 2002; Capovilla *et al.*, 2007; Moutaouakil *et al.*, 2010), also well controlled by treatment; two developed JME between 9 and 14 years (Auvin *et al.*, 2006), and one had only photic- induced myoclonic seizures at 14 years (Darra *et al.*, 2006). It is noteworthy that four other patients with JME following MEI were reported in the recent literature (Caraballo *et al.*, 2013, Belcastro *et al.*, 2015). A single patient with the reflex form had a GTCS at 6 years, followed by complex partial seizures, controlled by treatment (Auvin *et al.*, 2006). The EEG data at follow-up reviewed in 2011 were reported for 117 patients, but the ages at recordings were not always indicated. When reported, background activity remained normal and interictal SWs were absent or sporadic. In 34 patients IPS provoked discharges of generalized SW, associated with myoclonic jerks or without clinical correlates. Photosensitivity can appear after MS have disappeared, as reported in some studies (Giovanardi-Rossi *et al.*, 1997; Lin *et al.*, 1998) and can persist on EEG for many years, usually without clinical manifestation. Focal EEG abnormalities were recorded in the EEG in 24 patients, in childhood or in adolescence, usually located in the fronto-central and vertex, sometimes fronto-parieal, fronto-temporal areas, and disappeared during follow-up in most.

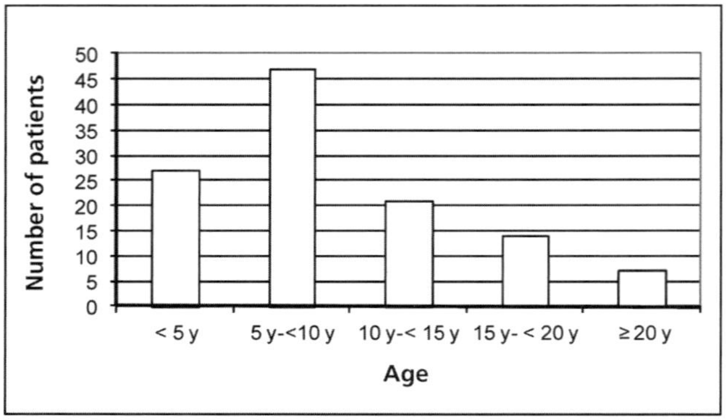

Figure 4 **Age at follow-up in 116 patients.**

Overall, cognitive outcome is not as favorable as initially thought. Although most patients are reported to have normal cognitive skills, follow-up duration was variable *(Figure 4)* and many studies did not mention neuropsychological assessment.

One single study (Mangano *et al.*, 2005) analyzed neuropsychological and behavioral outcome in seven patients, followed up for an average period of 6 years 9 months (range: 4 years 9 months–9 years 2 months). The mean full-scale intelligence quotient of the group as a whole was 74. Five were in the normal limits; one had a mild and one moderate cognitive impairment. All but one also had attention deficit disorder. The authors underlined the young age at onset of the disease in the patients with neuropsychological deficits. Ong *et al.* (2011) reported eight patients of whom only three had normal development (at 3 years 8 months, 6 years 7 months, 8 years). Dyslexia, attention deficit, speech and fine motor delay, and central auditory processing impairment were observed in one patient each.

Among the published cases, 23 patients were followed-up to at least the age of 15 years with a maximum of 28 years. All were seizure-free, including seven who experienced GTCS, absences or photic-induced massive myoclonic jerks after MS remitted. Treatment was known in 8 patients: only two had still VPA due to persistent photosensitivity, while the remaining 6 were without AED since several years. Cognitive outcome was variable *(Table I)*. Fourteen patients (60.9%) had normal abilities, confirmed by psychometric evaluation in five, sometimes with previous learning difficulties. Nine patients (39.1%) had mild to severe cognitive impairment. Except for one

Table I Psychological outcome in 23 patients aged 15 years and more

Authors	Patient Nb	Normal Nb	Abnormal Nb
Guerrini *et al.*, 1994	1	1	
Giovanardi Rossi *et al.*, 1997	2	1	1 moderate MR
Lin *et al.*, 1998	4	3	1 moderate MR
Dravet & Bureau, 2005	3	1	1 severe MR (Down syndrome) 1 severe MR (psychosis)
Prats Vinas *et al.*, 2002	4	2	1 MR 1 MR
Capovilla *et al.*, 2006	1	1	
Darra *et al.*, 2006	2		1 slight MR 1 slight MR
Auvin *et al.*, 2006	6	5	1 severe MR
Total	**23**	**14 (60.8%)**	**9 (39.2%)**

MR: mental retardation.

patient with Down syndrome and one with psychosis, no explanation was found in the remaining patients for this unfavorable outcome. No accurate analysis was performed, but it seems there was no difference in age at onset, response to treatment, EEG abnormalities and appearance of other seizure types between patients with abnormal cognitive outcome and those who remained normal. The role of an onset before two years as a factor of impaired cognitive outcome hypothesized by Mangano *et al.* (2005) is not confirmed by the young age of most patients with reflex MS and a normal development (Verrotti *et al.*, 2013).

MEI with reflex seizures

Dravet and Bureau (2005) compared the patients with and without reflex seizures reported in literature and found no fundamental differences between these two groups, except for the cognitive outcome which is better in the reflex group. Auvin *et al.* (2006) compared their patients with reflex seizures to those with only spontaneous seizures and did not find significant differences in terms of EEG and clinical parameters. However, eight patients out of 13 with reflex seizures were evaluated and all had normal skills, whereas in the group with spontaneous seizures, twelve patients of 21 were evaluated and only nine were normal. Caraballo *et al.* (2003) concluded that reflex MEI may be considered either as an idiopathic stimulo-sensitive syndrome or as a variant of the MEI. Verrotti *et al.* (2013) suggest this syndrome is an early idiopathic generalized epilepsy which should be classified as a distinct nosographic syndrome. At present, as the etiologic substrate of this form of epilepsy remains unknown, this question has no response, but, in practice, it is obvious that the reflex form is the most benign form of MEI.

Differential diagnosis

MS are observed in a wide variety of epilepsies which are frequent in infancy and do not always correspond to a definite syndrome (Dravet, 1990). The differential diagnosis of MS has been discussed in our introduction.

When MS start in the first year of life, the alternative diagnosis that comes in mind is that of cryptogenic infantile spasms (IS) whose interictal and ictal EEG features are radically different. The occurrence of IS is associated with marked behavioral changes, poor communication skills, developmental slowing down and regression.

When both development and the EEG remain normal after several examinations performed while awake and asleep, seizures resembling MS must suggest the diagnosis of benign non epileptic myoclonus described by Lombroso and Fejerman (1977). In these patients, even the ictal EEG is normal (Dravet *et al.*, 1986; Pachatz *et al.*, 1999).

In the first year of life, severe myoclonic epilepsy of infancy (Dravet syndrome) always starts with prolonged and repeated febrile and afebrile convulsive seizures the myoclonic seizures often appearing later and a worse outcome becomes obvious.

If MS are associated with GTCS, an unusual situation, the diagnosis of epilepsy with myoclonic-atonic (previously astatic) seizures must be considered, although the onset of myoclonic astatic seizures in this syndrome is rare before the age of three years (Doose, 1992a). There are two essential differences: i) the first is the clinical aspect of the seizures, which always consist of falls in MAE, while falls are rare in MEI, and which are combined with other types of seizures, particularly status of minor seizures with stupor, which are never observed in MEI (Guerrini *et al.*, 1994); and ii) the EEG features are also different: SW and PSW are more numerous, often grouped in long bursts.

MS seen in progressive myoclonus epilepsy, such as sometimes seen in late infantile ceroid-lipofuscinosis, should not be considered since the general context is clearly different, with rapid developmental decline and specific visual signs, ataxia, fragmentary myoclonus, and grossly abnormal EEG. If MS occur in an infant with language or motor delay, some investigations should be conducted to look for early sign of ceroid lipofuscinosis. This includes EEG with low frequency (0.5 Hz, 1 Hz and 2 Hz) IPS, brain MRI looking for cerebellar atrophy and VEP/ERG.

MS can be observed in other various genetic disorders but they are usually associated with developmental delay, dysmorphic features, other seizure types, or organ deficiency. When the epilepsy satisfies the criteria we have described, we consider the patient to have myoclonic epilepsy in association with a genetic disease, such as Down syndrome or trisomy 12 p (Guerrini *et al.*, 2002b).

Some papers reported patients with mild forms of glucose transporter-1 deficiency (GLUT-1 DS) who exhibited features similar to idiopathic generalized epilepsy (Roullet-Perez *et al.*, 2008) or to MEI (Oguni, 2005; Gaspard *et al.*, 2011). These patients started having MS in the first months of life and their EEG showed generalized SW. However, seizures were pharmacoresistant, and slowing down in development and ataxia became prominent from the second year of life. These reports suggested to look for GLUT-1 DS in those patients with an atypical outcome since this metabolic disorder is easily diagnosed by a lumbar puncture and corrected by the ketogenic diet.

Positive diagnosis

In practice, the diagnosis of IMEI must be restricted to those patients fulfilling the following criteria:
- brief MS, spontaneous or provoked by noise, contact, rarely light;
- starting typically between 4 months and 3 years;
- in a previously normal child, with no evidence of recent cognitive decline;
- no other seizure types except rare, simple FS;
- generalized fast SW and PSW during MS; rare interictal SW when awake;
- SW enhanced by drowsiness and slow sleep, sometimes by IPS;
- normal background; absence of focal discharges;
- good response to VPA monotherapy.

Faced with this typical picture, if treatment is applied without delay, the clinician may predict a good clinical outcome for seizures, while the prognosis is uncertain for cognitive functions and behavior, which could be impaired. The presence of seizures triggered by tactile, auditory or visual stimuli is a factor of good prognosis. In cases with less typical features, particularly in the presence of focal EEG discharges, the diagnosis remains dubious until a long remission is observed (Sarisjulis *et al.*, 2000). When the onset is after age 3 years the diagnostic questions remain the same (Guerrini *et al.*, 1994).

Nosological place

Obviously this syndrome belongs to the group of the generalized genetic (formerly idiopathic generalized – IGE) epilepsies. It seems to be the infantile equivalent of juvenile myoclonic epilepsy. Some data support this hypothesis. The two syndromes have been observed successively in six patients (Auvin *et al.*, 2006; Caraballo *et al.*, 2013; Belcastro *et al.*, 2015) and the mother of another patient suffered from JME (Darra *et al.*, 2006). The patients with later age at onset (Guerrini *et al.*, 1994; Gentile *et al.*, 2010) could be diagnosed as early JME. MEI shares some traits with other probably genetic epilepsies: MAE (Arzimanoglou *et al.*, 1996; Darra *et al.*, 2006, Doose, 1992b; Auvin *et al.*, 2012), childhood absence epilepsy (Mangano *et al.*, 2011), eyelid myoclonia with absence (Prats-Vinas *et al.*, 2002; Moutaouakil *et al.*, 2010), benign centro-temporal epilepsy (Darra *et al.*, 2006). MEI can also be associated with chromosomal aberrations (Guerrini *et al.*,1990). These findings show the complexity of the epilepsies even when they realize a recognizable syndrome.

The term idiopathic myoclonic epilepsy in infancy seemed to be appropriate. However, the ILAE Task Force (Berg *et al.*, 2010) proposed to replace "idiopathic" with "genetic" for those epilepsies which have a presumed genetic basis. According to this approach, MEI should be placed among the epilepsies of unknown etiology although it is likely that genetic factors are involved in this syndrome. In order to take the prognosis into account, the term "self-limited" was suggested by the ILAE Task Force instead of "benign". Thus, the group of MEI with reflex seizures might be designated as self-limited since in some cases MS disappeared without treatment, whereas the other cases might be designated as pharmacosensitive.

Epilepsy with myoclonic-atonic seizures

Nosological aspects

MAE is a childhood non lesional generalized epilepsy with multiple seizure types, including myoclonic -astatic (also called "myoclonic-atonic", Berg *et al.*, 2010), absence, atonic, generalized tonic-clonic, and tonic seizures, and with onset between 7 months and 6 years of age (Commission on Classification and Terminology of the ILAE, 1989). The term myoclonic-astatic epilepsy has been used to designate the primary generalized epilepsies of childhood whose main clinical manifestations include myoclonic and/or astatic seizures (Doose, 1992b). However, major myoclonic attacks and atonic falls attributed to lapses of muscle tone may be impossible to distinguish without adequate polygraphic EEG-EMG recordings. Additional features, which were originally emphasized, include the important role of genetic factors, the idiopathic and generalized nature of the disorder and the accompanying EEG features of biparietal theta activity and prominent generalized spike-wave or polyspike-wave complexes. Doose and coworkers did not propose a "rigidly defined syndrome," but simply identified a large subgroup of epilepsies of idiopathic origin characterized by myoclonic and atonic seizures whose recognized variability was attributed to a multifactorial background (Doose, 1992b). Such defining features, based mainly on etiology, apparently included all forms of idiopathic myoclonic epilepsies, as well as cases that would have subsequently been classified as benign myoclonic epilepsy, severe myoclonic epilepsy as well as other difficult to classify forms. In 1989, the ILAE Classification of epileptic syndromes included "Doose syndrome" among myoclonic epilepsy syndromes (in addition to severe and benign myoclonic epilepsy) based on clinical and EEG characteristics and listed it under the major heading of "cryptogenic and symptomatic epilepsy syndromes". However, this standpoint contrasts with Doose's criteria that were mainly based on a primary or idiopathic etiologic background. Such inconsistencies have contributed to the differences in the way different investigators defined MAE. For example, it is unclear whether falls were considered as a necessary criterion for inclusion in some series (Kaminska *et al.*, 1999; Oguni *et al.*, 2001). In the 2006 Classification amendment (Engel, 2006), MAE was included in the group of IGE and differentiated from other epileptic encephalopathies such as Dravet syndrome and Lennox-Gastaut syndrome. At present MAE should be considered as a generalized genetic epilepsy syndrome.

Long-term prognosis of the patients with MAE has been studied by some authors (Oguni *et al.*, 2002; Kilaru *et al.*, 2007) who have highlighted the almost constant remission of epilepsy within 3.5 years from onset in spite of an uncertain prognosis for cognitive functioning. It is likely that differences in outcome, which are hardly related to clinical course of epilepsy (Guerrini, 2006), reflect instead different etiologic backgrounds.

Etiology and epidemiological data

MAE is a relatively uncommon type of epilepsy; incidence is 1–2.2% of all childhood epilepsy with onset up to age 10 years (Doose, 1992b; Kaminska *et al.*, 1999). There is a male preponderance (Doose,1992b; Kaminska *et al.*, 1999). Genetic factors play an important role as suggested by a family history of epilepsy in 14–32% of affected children (Doose, 1992b; Kaminska *et al.*, 1999). Dominant mutations in the *SLC2A1* gene (GLUT-1) have been demonstrated in some patients with an MAE phenotype (Mullen *et al.*, 2010, 2011). Few patients with MAE were described in the "late-onset" group of patients carrying loss of function mutations in the *SCN2A* gene (Wolff *et al.*, 2017). A few patients with a MAE phenotype have been related to mutations in *GABRB3* (Moller *et al.*, 2017), *SLC6A1* (Carvill *et al.*, 2015; Johannesen *et al.*, 2018), and *SPTAN1* genes (Syrbe *et al.*, 2017).

Clinical and EEG presentation

Onset of seizures is between the age of 7 months and 6 years, with a peak incidence between 2 and 6 years, in previously healthy children (Doose, 1970, 1992b). The characteristic seizures are myoclonic-astatic (or atonic), consisting of brief, massive or axial, symmetrical jerks, involving the neck, shoulders, arms and legs, often resulting in head nodding, abduction of arms and flexion of the legs at the knees. Each jerk is immediately followed by an abrupt loss of muscle tone that contributes causing the drop to the floor (Tassinari *et al.*, 1998). However, falls in MAE can also result from purely myoclonic or atonic seizures (Oguni *et al.*, 1992; Dravet *et al.*, 1997). Violent myoclonus, followed by abrupt fall may result in severe injuries especially of the nose, teeth and face. These episodes last less than 2–3 seconds. The jerks may be isolated or occur in short series at 3 Hz, resulting in saccadic flexion of the head and/or abduction of the arms.

The EEG of myoclonic-atonic seizures shows bursts of spike/polyspike and wave complexes at 2 to 4 Hz *(Figure 5)*. EMG recordings show that the myoclonic potential is usually followed by an EMG silence lasting up to 500 ms. The silent period may also occur without a clear preceding jerk, although it is difficult to exclude a contraction in non-sampled muscles. Neurophysiological study of the myoclonic jerks shows bilateral synchronous EEG discharges and synchronous jerks in muscles from both sides of the body, indicating a primary generalized myoclonus (Bonanni *et al.*, 2002).

Other types of seizures usually occur, including GTCS and atypical absences.

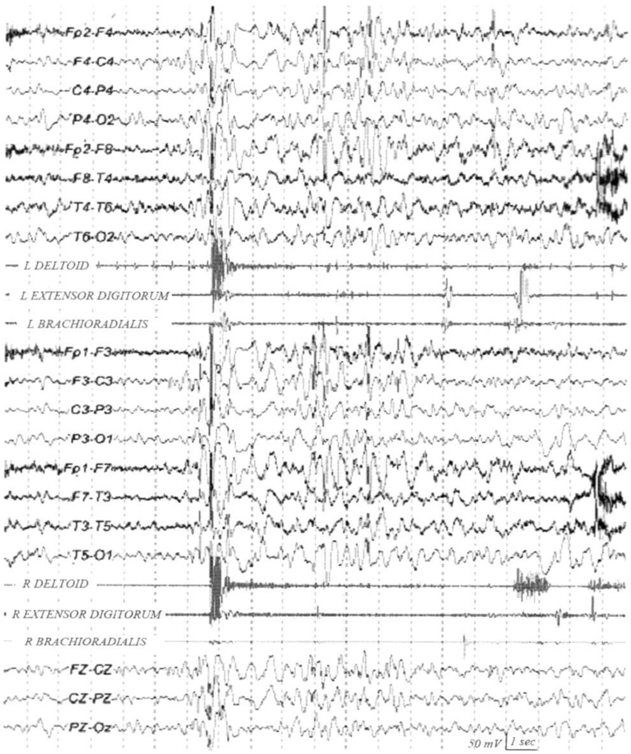

Figure 5 **Ictal EEG-Polygraphic recording in a 3-year 5 month-old boy with myoclonic-astatic (or myoclonic-atonic) epilepsy. A massive myoclonic jerk is correlated with a brief and diffuse spike and wave discharge. Pre-ictal background activity is normal.**

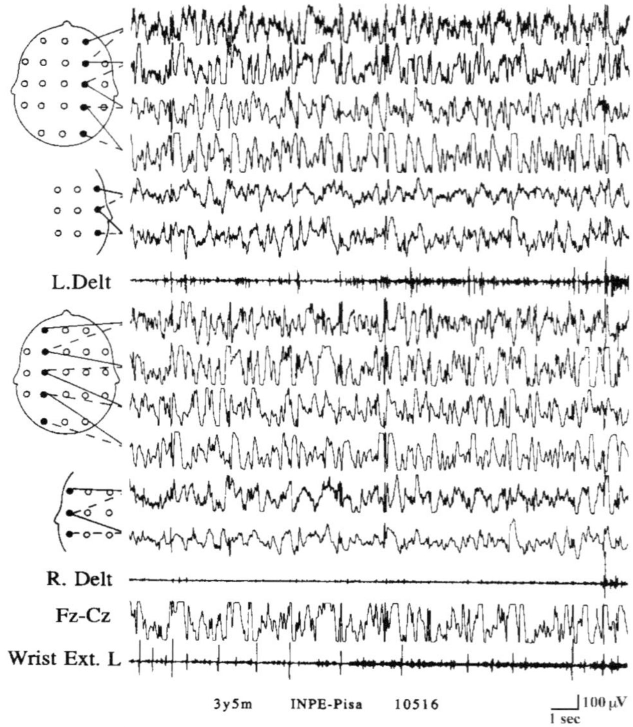

Figure 6 **EEG-Polygraphic recording in a 3-year 5 month-old boy during myoclonic status. The child was vacant, unresponsive, presented increased muscle tone, drooling and tiny, jerky movements on the face and the hands. Note the irregular spike and wave EEG activity and the frequent, multifocal myoclonic jerks.**
Delt.: **deltoids;** Ext.: **extensors;** L.: **left;** m: **months;** R: **right;** y: **years.**

Nonconvulsive status often occurs, manifesting as episodes of stupor, apathy or milder obtundation with drooling, associated with erratic muscle twitching and head nods. Such episodes can begin insidiously and develop progressively. They may last from hours to days or even weeks, often with fluctuations, and have been considered as indicators of a poor prognosis (Kaminska *et al.*, 1999). In our experience, however, this is not necessarily the case. In the EEG, nonconvulsive status is often accompanied by long runs of slow waves or spike-wave complexes *(Figure 6)*.

Tonic seizures, considered to be absent by some authors (Giovanardi Rossi *et al.*, 1997; Oguni *et al.*, 2002), have been found in up to 38% of cases in some series (Kaminska *et al.*, 1999). Their presence is not necessarily associated to an unfavorable outcome. "Vibratory" tonic seizures *(Figure 7)* have also been mentioned by different authors (Kaminska *et al.*, 1999; Oguni *et al.*, 2002).

The interictal EEG of MAE may be normal at onset (Guerrini *et al.*, 2002b). Bursts of 3 Hz spike-waves may occur without apparent clinical manifestations and may be activated by sleep. The most

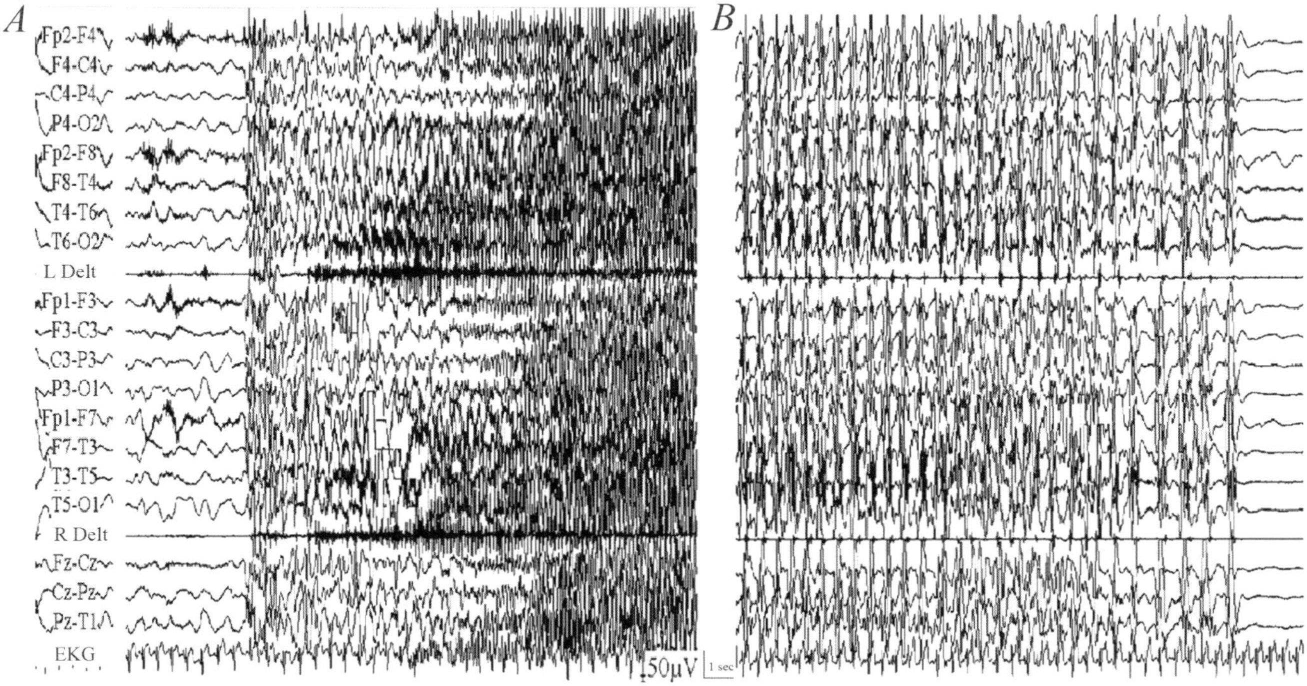

Figure 7

Ictal EEG-Polygraphic recording in a 4-year 9 month-old boy with myoclonic-atonic epilepsy. Vibratory tonic seizure during stormy onset of the syndrome (A, early part), EEG shows abrupt and diffuse recruiting activity correlated with a bilateral and synchronous vibratory contraction. In the later part (B) bilateral and myoclonic jerks are correlated with diffuse spike and wave activity.

suggestive finding is the 4 to 7 Hz theta rhythm with parietal predominance and the occipital 4-Hz rhythm, which is constantly blocked by eye opening (Oguni *et al.*, 2002). Variable lateralization of paroxysmal bursts is possible; however, a consistently localized focus is unusual (Bonanni *et al.*, 2002). A subset of patients is photosensitive.

Course and outcome

The course of MAE is variable and unpredictable. Despite the occurrence of various seizure types, the disorder is often self-limited and seizures abate within three years in 50–89% of patients (Kaminska *et al.*, 1999; Oguni *et al.*, 2002). Cognitive outcome can also be good; up to 58% of patients had normal IQ, while 20% had mild and 22% severe cognitive impairment (Oguni *et al.*, 2002). Some of the children have mild behavioral problems, especially hyperactivity (Kaminska *et al.*, 1999). Other children have a more severe course, with intractable epilepsy. Pathophysiologic factors, which predict the outcome, are poorly understood. The association between a poor mental outcome and the frequent episodes of nonconvulsive status, especially if prolonged, has been emphasized (Doose, 1992b). Young age at onset and presence of focal EEG anomalies have been underlined in a small series of patients (Inoue *et al.*, 2013). Atypical absences, repeated GTCS, and frequent falls have also been variably associated with a less favorable outcome. Nocturnal tonic seizures

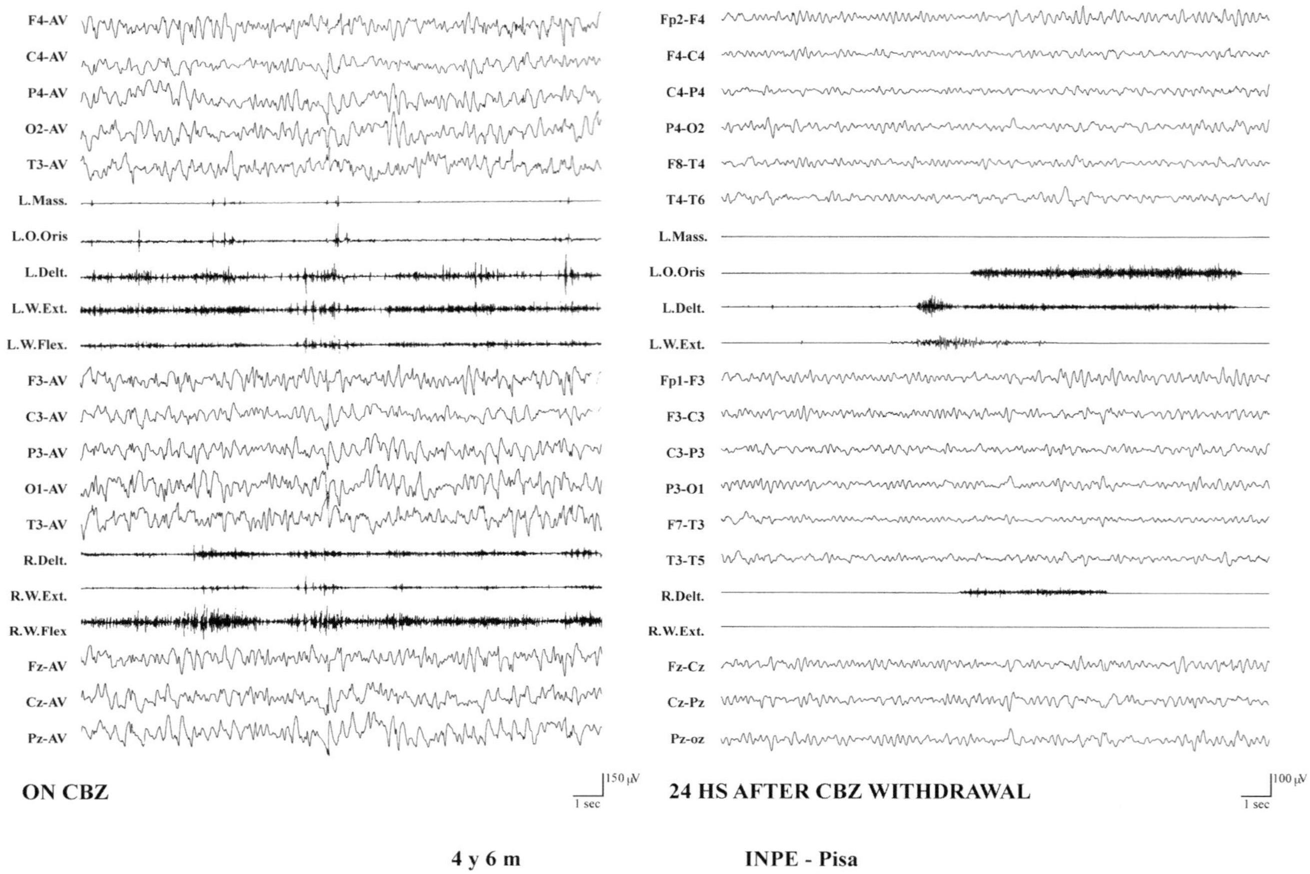

Figure 8

EEG-Polygraphic recording in a 4-year 6 month-old boy. On the left, **recording performed while the child presented with an episode of myoclonic status during carbamazepine (CBZ) treatment. The EEG has an encephalopathic appearance consisting of continuous, high amplitude and rhythmic background activity with superimposed frequent, multifocal discharges. The child is obtunded and presents continuous erratic myoclonic jerks and increased muscle tone.** On the right **– same patient 24 hour after CBZ withdrawal. No clear epileptiform abnormalities are recorded. Backgroung activity is normal. The child was alert at this stage.**

Delt.: **deltoids**; Ext.: **extensors**; Flex.: **flexors**; L.: **left**; Mass.: **masseteris**; m: **months**; O.Oris: **orbicularis oris**; R.: **right**; W.: **wrist**; y: **years.**

have also been considered as a bad prognostic indicator in some, but not in all, series (Kaminska *et al.*, 1999; Guerrini *et al.*, 2002b). In our experience (Guerrini *et al.*, 2002b), about 33% of patients can present with a stormy onset, characterized by either multiple daily generalized seizures (up to 10–12 generalized tonic-clonic or vibratory tonic seizures per day), or episodes of non-convulsive status epilepticus, or multiple daily myoclonic-astatic seizures. This phase, which usually takes place between 1 and 2 months from epilepsy onset, produces great concern and can prompt inappropriate pharmacological treatment, which, in turn, can precipitate seizure worsening and ataxia. However, clinical outcome in these patients is usually rather favorable with interruption of the frequent seizures within a few months and complete seizure freedom in some or persistence of weekly/monthly generalized seizures during sleep or upon awakening. Cognitive outcome is not different from that of patients without stormy onset.

Treatment issues in MAE

Treatment of myoclonic seizures is primarily with VPA, ETS, and the BDZs. Although LTG should be used cautiously in epilepsies with myoclonus, particularly in DS and JME (Guerrini *et al.*, 1998; Panayiotopoulos, 2005), this drug may be useful for treating associated generalized seizures in MAE. Oguni *et al.* found ETS to be most effective with a "good response rate" in 64% of patients (Oguni *et al.*, 2002). A combination of VPA and ETS may be effective and it is worth trying even when either drug alone has failed. CZP may also be very effective but behavioral side effects may limit its use. Other drugs, such as topiramate (TPM), LEV, acetazolamide, methosuximide, and sulthiame, may be effective based on anecdotic reports (Tennison *et al.*, 1991; Mikaeloff *et al.*, 2003). In our experience, patients with stormy onset can respond to low doses of phenobarbital, in order to abate generalized convulsive seizures that usually prove resistant to other medications (Guerrini *et al.*, 2002b). Children who have resistant myoclonic-atonic seizures causing disabling falls pose a serious therapeutic challenge. Uncontrolled trials of steroids or ACTH have been conducted, but have had limited success. Management should include practical measures, such as wearing a helmet, and providing considerable psychosocial support. The ketogenic diet can be effective (Caraballo *et al.*, 2006, Stenger *et al.*, 2017, Wiemer-Kruel *et al.*, 2017). If a mutation on SLC2A1 has been found then the ketogenic diet should be used and maintained even with seizure freedom (Mullen *et al.*, 2010, 2011). Surgery, including callosotomy, is not indicated in the myoclonic epilepsies. Carbamazepine and vigabatrin should be avoided in MAE as they can increase seizure frequency and precipitate myoclonic status *(Figure 8)* (Lortie *et al.*, 1993; Kaminska *et al.*, 1999; Guerrini *et al.*, 2002a).

REFERENCES ▶

Aicardi J, Levy Gomes A (1991): Myoclonic epilepsies in childhood. *Int Pediatr* 6: 195–200.

Arzimanoglou A, Prudent M, Salefranque F (1996): Epilepsie myoclono-astatique et épilepsie myoclonique bénigne du nourrisson dans une même famille: quelques réflexions sur la classification des épilepsies. *Epilepsies* 8: 307–315.

Auvin S, Pandit F, De Bellecize J, *et al.* and the Epilepsy Study Group of the French Pediatric Neurology Society (2006): Benign myoclonic epilepsy in infants: electroclinical features and long-term follow-up of 34 patients. *Epilepsia* 47: 1–7.

Auvin S, Lamblin MD, Cuvellier JC, Vallée L (2012): A patient with myoclonic epilepsy in infancy followed by myoclonic astatic epilepsy. *Seizure* 21: 300–303.

Belcastro V, Giordano L, Pruna D, *et al.* (2015): Do pure absence seizures occur in myoclonic epilepsy of infancy? A case series. *Seizure* 24: 8–11.

Belcastro V, Giordano L, Pruna D, *et al.* (2017): Follow-up study of idiopathic generalized epilepsy with associated absence seizure and myoclonic epilepsy of infancy. *Epilepsy Res* 136: 123–125.

Berg AT, Berkovic SF, Brodie MJ, *et al.* (2010): Revised terminology and concepts for organization of seizures and epilepsies: report of the ILAE Commission on Classification and Terminology, 2005–2009. *Epilepsia* 51: 676–685.

Bonanni P, Parmeggiani L, Guerrini R (2002): Different neurophysiologic patterns of myoclonus characterize Lennox-Gastaut syndrome and myoclonic astatic epilepsy. *Epilepsia* 43: 609–615.

Brenner RP, Atkinson R (1982): Generalized paroxysmal fast activity: electroencephalographic and clinical features. *Ann Neurol* 11: 386–390.

Capovilla G, Beccaria F, Gambardella A, Montagnini A, Avantaggiato P, Seri S (2007): Photosensitive benign myoclonic epilepsy in infancy. *Epilepsia* 48: 96–100.

Caraballo R, Cassar L, Monges S, *et al.* (2003): Reflex myoclonic epilepsy in infancy: a new reflex epilepsy syndrome or a variant ofbenign myoclonic epilepsy in infancy. *Rev Neurol* 2003 36: 429–432.

Caraballo RH, Cersósimo RO, Saks D, Cresta A, Escobal N, Fejerman N (2006): Ketogenic diet in patients with myoclonic astatic epilepsy. *Epil Disord* 8: 151–155.

Caraballo RH, Darra F, Fontana E, Garcia R, Monese E, Dalla Bernardina B (2011): Absence seizures in the first three years of life: an electro- clinical study of 46 cases. *Epilepsia* 52: 393–400.

Caraballo RH, Flesler S, Pasteris MC, *et al.* (2013): Myoclonic epilepsy in infancy: an electroclinical study and long-term follow-up of 38 patients. *Epilepsia* 54: 1605–1612.

Carvill GL, McMahon JM, Schneider A, *et al.* (2015): Mutations in the GABA Transporter SLC6A1 Cause Epilepsy with Myoclonic-Atonic Seizures. *Am J Hum Genet* 96: 808–815.

Caviness JN, Brown P (2004): Myoclonus: current concepts and recent advances. *Lancet Neurol* 3: 598–607.

Chayasirisobhon S, Rodin EA (1981): Atonic-akinetic seizures. *Electr Clin Neurophysiol* 50: 225.

Claes L, Del-Favero J, Ceulemans B, Lagae L, Van Broeckhoven C, De Jonghe P (2001): *De novo* mutations in the sodium-channel gene SCN1A cause severe myoclonic epilepsy of infancy. *Am J Hum Genet* 68: 1327–1332.

Commission on Classification and Terminology of the International League Against Epilepsy (1989): Proposal for revised classification of epilepsies and epileptic syndromes *Epilepsia* 30: 389–399.

Dalla Bernardina B, Plouin P, Lerique A, Beghini G, Trevisan C (1978): Aspects électrocliniques des crises survenant dans les deux premières années de la vie. *Boll Lega It* 22/23: 137–144.

Dalla Bernardina B, Colamaria V, Capovilla G, Bondavalli S (1983): Nosological classification of epilepsies in the first three years of life. In: Nistico G, Di Perri R, Meinardi H (eds) *Epilepsy: an Update on Research and Therapy*, pp. 165–183. NewYork: Alan Liss.

Dalla Bernardina B, Capovilla G, Chiamenti C, Trevisan E, Colamaria V, Fontana E (1987): Cryptogenic myoclonic epilepsies of infancy and early childhood: Nosological and prognostic approach. In: Wolf P, Janz D, Dreifuss FE (eds) *Advances in Epileptology*, pp. 175–179. New York: Raven Press.

Dalla Bernardina B, Fontana E, Darra F (2002): Myoclonic status in non-progressive encephalopathies. In: Roger J, Bureau M, Dravet C, Genton P, Tassinari CA, Wolf P (eds) *Epileptic Syndromes in Infancy, Childhood and Adolescence, 3rd ed*, pp. 137–144. London: John Libbey.

Darra F, Fiorini E, Zoccante L, *et al.* (2006): Benign myoclonic epilepsy in infancy (BMEI): a longitudinal electro-clinical study of 22 cases. *Epilepsia* 47 (Suppl 5): 31–35.

Doose H, Gerken H, Leonhardt R, Volzke E, Volz C (1970): Centrencephalic myoclonic-astatic petit mal. Clinical and genetic investigation. *Neuropediatrie* 2: 59–78.

Doose H (1992a): Myoclonic-astatic epilepsy. *Epilepsy Res* (Suppl) 6: 163–168.

Doose H (1992b): Myoclonic astatic epilepsy of early childhood. In: Roger J, Bureau M, Dravet C, Dreifuss FE, Perret A, Wolf P (eds) *Epileptic Syndromes in Infancy, Childhood and Adolescence, 2nd ed*, pp. 103–114. London, Paris: John Libbey Eurotext.

Doose H (2003): Benign myoclonic epilepsy. In: Doose H (ed) *EEG in Childhood Epilepsy*, p. 133. Montrouge: John Libbey Eurotext.

Dravet C (1990): Les épilepsies myocloniques bénignes du nourrisson. *Epilepsies* 2: 95–101.

Dravet C, Bureau M (1981): L'épilepsie myoclonique bénigne du nourrisson. *Rev EEG Neurophysiol* 11: 438–444.

Dravet C, Giraud N, Bureau M, Roger J, Gobbi G, Dalla Bernardina B (1986): Benign myoclonus of early infancy or benign non-epileptic infantile spasms. *Neuropediatrics* 1986 17: 33–38.

Dravet C, Guerrini R, Bureau M (1997): Epileptic syndromes with drop seizures in children. In: Beaumanoir A, Andermann F, Avanzini G, Mira L (eds) *Falls in Epileptic and Non-Epileptic Seizures during Childhood*, pp. 95–111. London: John Libbey & Company Ltd.

Dravet C, Bureau M (2005): Benign myoclonic epilepsy in infancy. In: Roger J, Bureau M, Dravet C, Genton P, Tassinari CA, Wolf P (eds) *Epileptic Syndromes in Infancy, Childhood and Adolescence, 4th ed*, pp. 77–88. London: John Libbey & Co Ltd.

Dravet C, Bureau M, Oguni H, Fukuyama Y, Cokar O (2005): Severe myoclonic epilepsy in infancy (Dravet syndrome). In: Roger J, Bureau M, Dravet C, Genton P, Tassinari CA, Wolf P (eds) *Epileptic Syndromes in Infancy, Childhood and Adolescence, 4th ed*, pp. 81–103. London: John Libbey & Co Ltd.

Dravet C, Bureau M (2012): Idiopathic myoclonic epilepsy in infancy. In: Gilman S (ed) *Medlink Neurology*. San Diego: Medlink Corporation. Available at www.medlink.com. Last updated: February 2012.

Dravet C, Vigevano F (2007): Idiopathic myoclonic epilepsy in infancy. In: Engel J Jr, Pedley TA (eds) *Epilepsy. A comprehensive Textbook, 2nd ed*, pp. 2343–2348. Philadelphia: Wolters Kluwer/Lippincott Williams & Wilkins.

Durá-Travè T, Yoldi-Petri ME, Gallinas-Victoriano F (2007): Epilepsy in children in Navarre, Spain: epileptic seizure types and epileptic syndromes. *J Child Neurol* 22: 823–828.

Egli M, Mothersill I, O'Kane M, O'Kane F (1985): The axial spasm – the predominant type of drop seizure in patients with secondary generalized epilepsy. *Epilepsia* 26: 401–415.

Elia M, Musumeci SA, Ferri R, Cammarata M (1998): Trisomy 12p and epilepsy with myoclonic absences. *Brain Dev* 20: 127–130.

Engel, J (2006): Report of the ILAE Classification Core Group. *Epilepsia* 47: 1558–1568.

Erba G, Browne TR (1983): Atypical absence, myoclonic, atonic, and tonic seizures, and the Lennox-Gastaut syndrome. In: Browne T, Feldman RG (eds) *Epilepsy: Diagnosis and Management*, pp. 75–94. Boston: Little Brown.

Fariello RG, Doro JM, Forster FM (1979): Generalized cortical electrodecremental event. Clinical and neurophysiological observations in patients with dystonic seizures. *Arch Neurol* 36: 285–291.

Gaspard N, Suls A, Vilain C, De Jonghe P, Van Bogaert P (2011): "Benign" myoclonic epilepsy of infancy as the initial presentation of glucose transporter-1 deficiency. *Epil Disord* 13: 300–303.

Gastaut H, Roger J, Ouahchi S, Timsit M, Broughton R (1963): An electroclinical study of generalized epileptic seizures of tonic expression. *Epilepsia* 4: 15–44.

Gastaut H, Broughton R (1972): *Epileptic Seizures*. Springfield: CC Thomas.

Gastaut H, Broughton R, Roger J, Tassinari CA (1974): Generalized convulsive seizures without local onset. In: Vinken P, Bruyn GW (eds) *The Epilepsies. Handbook of Clinical Neurology*, pp. 107–129. Amsterdam: Elsevier.

Gentile V, Brunetto D, Leo I, Bonetti S, Cerrotti A, Franzoni E (2010): Clinical and neuropsychological considerations in a case of unrecognized myoclonic epileptic jerks dramatically controlled by levetiracetam. *Neuropediatrics* 41: 270–272.

Giovanardi Rossi P, Parmeggiani A, Posar A, Santi A, Santucci M (1997): Benign myoclonic epilepsy: long-term follow-up of 11 new cases. *Brain Dev* 19: 473–479.

Guerrini R (2006): Epilepsy in children. *Lancet* 367: 499–524.

Guerrini R, Bureau M, Mattei MG, Battaglia A, Galland MC, Roger J (1990): Trisomy 12p syndrome: a chromosomal disorder associated with generalized 3-Hz spike and wave discharges *Epilepsia* 31: 557–566.

Guerrini R, Dravet C, Gobbi G, Ricci S, Dulac O (1994): Idiopathic generalized epilepsies with myoclonus in infancy and childhood. In: Malafosse A, Genton P, Hirsch E, Marescaux C, Broglin D, Bernasconi R (eds) *Idiopathic Generalized Epilepsies: Clinical, Experimental, and Genetic Aspects*, pp. 267–280. London, Paris: John Libbey Eurotext Ltd.

Guerrini R, Dravet C, Genton P, Belmonte A, Kaminska A, Dulac O (1998): Lamotrigine and seizure aggravation in severe myoclonic epilepsy. *Epilepsia* 39: 508–512.

Guerrini R, Bonanni P, Rothwell J, Hallett M (2002a): Myoclonus and epilepsy. In: Guerrini R, Aicardi J, Andermann F, Hallett M (eds) *Epilepsy and Movement Disorders*, pp. 165–210. Cambridge: Cambridge University Press.

Guerrini R, Parmeggiani L, Kaminska A, Dulac O (2002b): Myoclonic astatic epilepsy. In: Roger J, Bureau M, Dravet C, Genton P, Tassinari CA, Wolf P (eds) *Epileptic Syndromes in Infancy, Childhood and Adolescence, 3rd ed*, pp. 105–112. London-Paris: John Libbey & Co Ltd.

Guerrini R, Mari F, Dravet C (2012): Idiopathic myoclonic epilepsies in infancy and early childhood. In: Bureau M, Genton P, Dravet C, Delgado-Escueta AV, Tassinari CA, Thomas P, Wolf P (eds) *Epileptic Syndromes in Infancy, Childhood and Adolescence, 5th ed*, pp. 157–173. London-Paris: John Libbey & Co Ltd.

Hallett M (1985): Myoclonus: relation to epilepsy. *Epilepsia* 26: S67–S77.

Hirano Y, Oguni H, Funatsuka M, Imai K, Osawa M (2009): Differentiation of myoclonic seizures in epileptic syndromes: a video-polygraphic study of 26 patients. *Epilepsia* 50: 1525–1535.

Inoue T, Ihara Y, Tomonoh Y, Nakamura N, Ninomiya S, Fujita T (2014) Early onset and focal spike discharges as indicators of poor prognosis for myoclonic-astatic epilepsy. *Brain Dev* 36: 613–619.

Ito S, Oguni H, Osawa M. (2012): Benign myoclonic epilepsy in infancy with preceding afebrile generalized tonic-clonic seizures in Japan. *Brain Dev* 34: 829–833.

Jallon P, Latour P (2005): Epidemiology of idiopathic generalized epilepsies. *Epilepsia* 46 (Suppl 9): 10–14.

Johannesen KM, Gardella E, Linnankivi T, *et al.* (2018): Defining the phenotypic spectrum of SLC6A1 mutations. *Epilepsia* 59: 389–402.

Kaminska A, Ickowicz A, Plouin P, Bru MF, Dellatolas G, Dulac O (1999): Delineation of cryptogenic Lennox-Gastaut syndrome and myoclonic astatic epilepsy using multiple correspondence analysis. *Epilepsy Res* 36: 15–29.

Kilaru S, Bergqvist AG (2007): Current treatment of myoclonic astatic epilepsy: clinical experience at the children's hospital of Philadelphia. *Epilepsia* 48: 1703–1707.

Lin YP, Itomi K, Takada H, *et al.* (1998): Benign myoclonic epilepsy in infants: video-EEG features and long-term follow-up. *Neuropediatrics* 29: 268–271.

Lombroso CT, Fejerman N (1977): Benign myoclonus of early infancy. *Ann Neurol* 1: 138–143.

Lortie A, Chiron C, Mumford J, Dulac O (1993): The potential for increasing seizure frequency, relapse, and appearance of new seizure types with vigabatrin. *Neurology* 43: (Suppl 5): 24–27.

Mangano S, Fontana A, Cusumano L (2005): Benign myoclonic epilepsy in infancy: neuropsychological and behavioural outcome. *Brain Dev* 27: 218–223.

Mangano S, Fontana A, Spitaleri C, *et al.* (2011): Benign myoclonic epilepsy in infancy followed by childhood absence epilepsy. *Seizure* 20: 727–730.

Marini C, Scheffer IE, Nabbout R, *et al.* (2011): The genetics of Dravet syndrome. *Epilepsia* 52 (Suppl 2): 24–29.

Mikaeloff Y, de Saint-Martin A, Mancini J, *et al.* (2003): Topiramate: efficacy and tolerability in children according to epilepsy syndromes. *Epilepsy Res* 53: 225–232.

Møller RS, Wuttke TV, Helbig I, Marini C, Johannesen KM, Brilstra EH (2017): Mutations in GABRB3: From febrile seizures to epileptic encephalopathies. *Neurology* 88: 483–492.

Moutaouakil F, El Otmani H, Fadel H, El Moutawakkil B, Slassi I (2010): Benign myoclonic epilepsy of infancy evolving to Jeavons syndrome. *Pediatr Neurol* 43: 213–216.

Mullen SA, Suls A, De Jonghe P, Berkovic SF, Scheffer IE (2010): Absence epilepsies with widely variable onset are a key feature of familial GLUT1 deficiency. *Neurology* 75: 432–440.

Mullen SA, Marini C, Suls A, Mei D, *et al.* (2011): Glucose transporter 1 deficiency as a treatable cause of myoclonic astatic epilepsy. *Arch Neurol* 68: 1152–1155.

Oguni H (2005): Symptomatic epilepsies imitating idiopathic generalized epilepsies. *Epilepsia* 46 (Suppl 9): 84–90.

Oguni H, Fukuyama Y, Imaizumi Y, Uehara T (1992): Video-EEG analysis of drop seizures in myoclonic astatic epilepsy of early childhood (Doose syndrome). *Epilepsia* 33: 805–813.

Oguni H, Fukuyama Y, Tanaka T, *et al.* (2001): Myoclonic-astatic epilepsy of early childhood – clinical and EEG analysis of myoclonic-astatic seizures, and discussions on the nosology of the syndrome. *Brain Dev* 23: 757–764.

Oguni H, Tanaka T, Hayashi K, *et al.* (2002): Treatment and long-term prognosis of myoclonic- astatic epilepsy of early childhood. *Neuropediatrics* 33: 122–132.

Ohtsuka Y, Ohno S, Oka E, Ohtahara S (1993): Classification of epilepsies and epileptic syndromes of childhood according to the 1989 ILAE classification. *J Epilepsy* 6: 272–276.

Ong HT, Lim K, Tay S, Low PS (2011): Neuropsychological outcome following benign myoclonic epilepsy of infancy. Poster sessions. *Epilepsia* 52: 23–263.

Pachatz C, Fusco L, Vigevano F (1999): Benign myoclonus of early infancy. *Epil Disord* 1: 57–61.

Panayiotopoulos CP (2005): *The Epilepsies: Seizures, Syndromes and Management.* Bladon Medical Publishing, Oxfordshire.

Patel V, Jankovic J (1988): Myoclonus. *Curr Neurol* 8: 109–156.

Prats-Vinas, JM, Garaizar C, Ruiz-Espinosa C (2002): Benign myoclonic epilepsy in infants. *Rev Neurol* (Spanish) 34: 201–204.

Ricci S, Cusmai R, Fusco L, Vigevano F (1995): Reflex myoclonic epilepsy: a new age-dependent idiopathic epileptic syndrome related to startle reaction. *Epilepsia* 36: 342–348

Roullet-Perez E, Ballhausen D, Bonafè L, Cronel-Ohayon S, Maeder-Ingvar M (2008): Glut-1 deficiency syndrome masqueranding as idiopathic generalized epilepsy. *Epilepsia* 49: 1955–1958.

Sarisjulis N, Gamboni B, Plouin P, Kaminska A, Dulac O (2000): Diagnosing idiopathic/cryptogenic epilepsy syndromes in infancy. *Arch Dis Child* 82: 226–230.

Shibasaki H, Hallett M (2005): Electrophysiological studies of myoclonus. *Muscle Nerve* 31: 157–174.

Stenger E, Schaeffer M, Cances C, *et al.* (2017): Efficacy of ketogenic diet in resistant myoclono-astatic epilepsy: A French multicenter retrospective study. *Epilepsy Res* 131: 64–69.

Syrbe S, Harms FL, Parrini E, Montomoli M, Mütze U, Helbig KL (2017): Delineating SPTAN1 associated phenotypes: from isolated epilepsy to encephalopathy with progressive brain atrophy. *Brain* 2017; 140: 2322–2336.

Steel D, Symonds JD, Zuberi SM, Brunklaus A (2017): Dravet syndrome and its mimics: Beyond SCN1A. *Epilepsia* 58: 1807–1816.

Tassinari CA, Bureau M, Thomas P (1992): Epilepsy with myoclonic absences. In: Roger J, Bureau M, Dravet Ch, Dreifuss FE, Perret A, Wolf P (eds) *Epileptic Syndromes in Infancy, Childhood and Adolescence, 2nd ed*, pp. 151–60. London: John Libbey Eurotext Ltd.

Tassinari CA, Rubboli G, Shibasaki H (1998): Neurophysiology of positive and negative myoclonus. *Electroencephalogr Clin Neurophysiol* 107: 181–195.

Tennison MB, Greenwood RS, Miles MV (1991): Methsuximide for intractable childhood seizures. *Pediatrics* 87: 186–189.

Verrotti A, Matricardi S, Pavone P, Marino R, Curatolo P. (2015): Reflex myoclonic epilepsy in infancy: a critical review. *Epil Disord* 15: 114–122.

Wallace RH, Wang DW, Singh R, *et al.* (1998): Febrile seizures and generalized epilepsy associated with a mutation in the Na+- channel beta1 subunit gene *SCN1B*. *Nat Genet* 19: 366–370.

Wiemer-Kruel A, Haberlandt E, Hartmann H, Wohlrab G, Bast T (2017): Modified Atkins diet is an effective treatment for children with Doose syndrome *Epilepsia* 58: 657–662.

Wolff M, Johannesen KM, Hedrich UBS, *et al.* (2017): Genetic and phenotypic heterogeneity suggest therapeutic implications in SCN2A-related disorders. *Brain* 140: 1316–1336.

Yang Z, Li H, Xue J, Qian P, Liu X, Zhang Y (2017): Myoclonic epilepsy in infancy with preceding or concurrent afebrile generalized tonic-clonic seizures in Chinese children. *Brain Dev* 39: 828–835.

Zafeiriou D, Vargiami E, Kontopoulos E (2003): Reflex myoclonic epilepsy in infancy: a benign age- dependent idiopathic startle epilepsy. *Epil Disord* 5: 121–122.

Zuberi SM, O'Regan ME (2006): Developmental outcome in benign myoclonic epilepsy in infancy and reflex myoclonic epilepsy in infancy: a literature review and six new cases. *Epilepsy Res* 70 (Suppl 1): 110–115.

Zullini E, Santorum E, Piardi F, Mastella L, Segala R, Dalla Bernardina B (1996): Epilessia mioclonica benigna riflessa del primo anno di vita. *Boll Lega It Epi* 95/96: 517–518.

WITH VIDEO SUPPLEMENTS

CHAPTER 12
LENNOX-GASTAUT SYNDROME

Arielle Crespel[1], Philippe Gélisse[1], Greta Macorig[1], Marina Nikanorova[2], Edoardo Ferlazzo[3] and Pierre Genton[4]

[1] Epilepsy Unit, Montpellier, France
[2] Children Department, Danish Epilepsy Centre, Dianalund, Denmark
[3] Regional Epilepsy Centre, Bianchi-Melacrino-Morelli Hospital, Reggio Calabria, Italy
[4] Centre Saint-Paul, Henri-Gastaut Hospital, Marseille, France

Anne Beaumanoir (Beaumanoir, 1985) and Charlotte Dravet (Beaumanoir & Dravet, 1992) were the first authors of this chapter devoted to the Lennox-Gastaut syndrome in this "Blue Guide" so well-known to all of us. It is a great honor for us to continue in their steps.

Historical background

The Lennox-Gastaut syndrome (LGS) remains one of the most severe childhood epileptic encephalopathies with high seizure frequency, including sudden falls, progressive cognitive impairment and drug resistance. In spite of new therapeutic approaches developed in recent years, the treatment of LGS remains challenging. Cognitive impairment and deterioration of psychomotor skills require complex therapeutic management as well as specialized social and educational support. Moreover, most epileptic encephalopathies with diffuse slow spike-waves were considered until recently to be LGS, leading to overdiagnosis.

In 1770, Tissot first identified young children presenting with severe seizures, myoclonic jerks, falls, loss of consciousness and cognitive impairment. Further similar cases were reported by Herpin (1867), Jackson (cited by Taylor, 1958) and Hunt in 1922 (cited by Gastaut,1982). In 1885, Gowers accurately described tonic seizures. In 1938, the first EEG data were presented by Gibbs, and then in 1939 by Gibbs *et al.* They described a characteristic slow wave pattern at 2 Hz which they called the "Petit Mal variant" as opposed to the typical spike-wave pattern at 3 Hz observed in "Petit Mal". Shortly after participating in the description of the EEG pattern, Lennox described a syndrome in children presenting with mental retardation, three different types of epileptic seizures (myoclonias, absences and falls), and the latter EEG pattern, *i.e.*, diffuse slow spike-waves (Lennox, 1945; Lennox & Davis, 1950).

In 1952, Gibbs & Gibbs described an EEG pattern with tonic seizures generally occurring during sleep which they called "Grand Mal seizures in sleep", but they did not identify this as the main characteristic of the syndrome. In 1964, the term "myokinetic epilepsy" was used by Sorel while the term "akinetic petit mal" was used by Doose (1964) to describe the syndrome.

Charlotte Dravet's medical dissertation (Dravet, 1965) was the basis of a paper published in Epilepsia (Gastaut *et al.*, 1966), with observations of 50 subjects. This led to the complete identification of the LGS: "a very severe variety of childhood epilepsy which is refractory to treatment and characterized by: i) frequent tonic seizures and variant of petit mal absences; ii) pronounced homogeneous mental retardation; iii) interictal EEG records showing pseudo rhythmical (1.5 to 2 Hz) diffuse slow spikes and waves". Gastaut proposed to describe this condition under the name of the epileptologist who first described it in detail as Lennox syndrome. Subsequently, William Lennox's daughter Margaret Buchtal-Lennox suggested that the syndrome be called the Lennox-Gastaut syndrome in honour of her father's first description later confirmed and completed by the Marseille school.

It took nearly three more decades to fully identify the LGS. Beaumanoir's definition in the first edition of the "Blue Guide" published in 1985 was subsequently approved by the International Classification of Epilepsies and Epileptic Syndromes in 1989. The LGS has been and continues to be the subject of numerous articles, revisions, and monographs that have been published since its identification by the Marseille school (Gastaut, 1982; Beaumanoir *et al.*, 1968; Beaumanoir,

1981, 1982, 1985; Niedermeyer, 1969; Janz 1969, 1972; Karbowski *et al.*, 1970; Chevrie & Aicardi, 1972; Aicardi, 1973; Ohtahara *et al.*, 1976, 1995; Markand, 1977, 2003; Blume, 1987; Boniver *et al.*, 1987; Niedermeyer & Degen, 1988; Aicardi & Levy-Gomes, 1988; Roger *et al.*, 1989; Blatter-Arifi, 1991; Dulac & NGuyen, 1993; Dravet, 1996; Hirt, 1996; Oguni *et al.*, 1996; Yagi, 1996; Wheless & Constantinou, 1997; Rantala & Putkonen, 1999; Genton *et al.*, 2000, 2009; Beaumanoir & Blume, 2005; Genton & Dravet, 2007; Morita & Glauser, 2008, Arzimanoglou *et al.*, 2009).

Definition

In the 2017 International League Against Epilepsy (ILAE) classification of epilepsies, LGS is classified in the new group of combined generalised and focal epilepsies, because patients have both generalised and focal seizures. The term epileptic encephalopathy applies to LGS, since the epileptic activity itself contributes to severe cognitive and behavioural impairment. (Scheffer *et al.*, 2017). LGS is characterized by a triad of symptoms as defined by Anne Beaumanoir (1985) and approved in 1989 (Commission, 1989).

The typical LGS is indeed described according to the following symptomatic triad: i) epileptic seizures: axial tonic, atonic and atypical absence; ii) EEG abnormalities: bursts of diffuse slow spike-waves (Petit Mal variant) during wakefulness and bursts of fast rhythmic waves and slow polyspikes and above all generalized fast rhythms at about 10 Hz during sleep; and iii) a slowing of intellectual growth and associated personality disorders.

Although the clinical presentation, EEG patterns and characteristic course of this syndrome are all typical, the aetiological spectrum is broad (due to lesional, congenital or acquired, metabolic, or other causes). LGS is currently thought to be either symptomatic or cryptogenic.

Epidemiology

Despite the large number of studies in the literature, few of them respect the inclusion criteria as defined in 1989. Instead, criteria are often limited to a typical seizure and/or the presence of diffuse slow spike-waves on EEG recordings. Although it is known to be essential in order to establish the diagnosis of LGS, a sleep EEG is often not included in the criteria. As a result, the prevalence and incidence of the LGS cannot be estimated accurately. In the literature, LGS is estimated at 1.5 to 10% of childhood epilepsies (Beilmann *et al.*, 1999: 1%; Kramer *et al.*, 1998: 1.5%; Eriksson & Koivikko, 1997: 2%; Beaumanoir, 1982: 2 to 3%; Camfield & Camfield, 2007: 2.5%; Rantala & Putkonen, 1999: 2.8%; Cavazzuti, 1980: 3.2%; Trevathan *et al.*, 1997: 4%; Janz, 1972: 5%; Sidenvall *et al.*, 1996: 5.8%; Bourrous *et al.*, 2010: 6%; Genton & Dravet 2007: 6.6%; Steffenburg *et al.*, 1998; 7%; Alving, 1979: 10%; Gastaut *et al.*, 1973: 10%). As mentioned by Beaumanoir & Blume (2005), prevalence estimates decrease sharply to 1 to 3% when proper criteria are met. In 1988, when Gastaut and Zifkin reexamined the data from an earlier study by Gastaut *et al.* (1973) in which a 10% prevalence had been found, the prevalence of LGS dropped to 4%.

Annual incidence was estimated to be 2.1/100,000 by Heiskala (1997) and 1.93/100,000 by Rantala & Putkonen (1999), but a loose definition of LGS was used. If subjects with non-specific generalized epilepsy or myoclonic-astatic epilepsy with normal development had not been classified as LGS, the incidence would have been approximately 1.2/100,000 in the Heiskala study (1997).

In a specialized reference centre with strict inclusion criteria including sleep EEG, the frequency was 3.7% overall and 6.6% in children under 10 years (Genton *et al.*, 2000). Male predominance as high as fivefold has been described in several studies (Loubier, 1974; Markand, 1977; Oguni *et al.*, 1996; Trevathan *et al.*, 1997; Beilman *et al.*, 1999; Herranz *et al.*, 2010). LGS occurs in children with a previous West syndrome in 39% (Trevathan *et al.*, 1997), in 40% (Rantala & Putkanen 1999), and in 65% of cases (Camfield & Camfield, 2007). A family history of epilepsy has been found in 2.5% of cases (Chevrie & Aicardi, 1972). Familial cases of LGS have been observed in subjects with mutations causing cortical malformations (Guerrini, 2005; Parrini *et al.*, 2009; Lawrence *et al.*, 2010). In 2001, Nokelainen *et al.* described two brothers with a syndrome similar to LGS presenting with mental retardation, facial dysmorphia, macrocephalia, cerebral atrophy, and fetal exposure to alcohol. Thus, except with populations in specialized centres, LGS is a rare syndrome when defined accurately, accounting for 1 to 3% of childhood epilepsies. According to Genton *et al.* (2009), the incidence of LGS in a reference centre is approximately the same as for Dravet syndrome and myoclonic-astatic epilepsy (MAE).

Physiopathology

LGS physiopathology remains unclear. The difficulty lies in the comprehension of how this syndrome, which sometimes occurs following earlier encephalopathy, and whose etiologies vary, can exhibit a typical pattern of clinical signs and EEG abnormalities. As yet, there is no animal model for this particular electroclinical entity. It is likely that LGS physiopathology shares traits with the physiopathology of generalized epilepsies and existing animal models for absences epilepsy, generalized tonic-clonic seizures, and tonic seizures.

The following characteristics should be taken into account:

1. The physiopathology of an epileptic seizure as defined by the ILAE (Fisher *et al.*, 2005), which highlights "the transitory occurrence of signs and symptoms due to excessive activity or abnormal synchrony of neurons".

2. Secondary bilateral synchrony as defined by Tükel & Jasper (1952), in which an internal frontal lesion induces diffuse spike-waves such as those observed in generalized epilepsies. The action of the internal frontal lesion was thought to occur *via* a centrencephalic system.

3. The existence of a centrencephalic system, enabling pathways between the two hemispheres *via* subcortical projections toward the cortex (Penfield & Jasper, 1954).

4. Variations of the excitatory and inhibitory systems including the reticular formation, the thalamus, and the caudate nucleus correspond to the different generalized seizures. This hypothesis was put forward by Gastaut & Broughton (1972). Tonic seizures and fast EEG rhythms are induced by the recruiting action of the thalamus whereas the slow elements are induced by its inhibitory system. Absences can be induced by stimulating the iterative action of the two systems at the same time. Atonic seizures are induced by the preponderant action, first of the inhibitory system, and then of the activatory system. Generalized tonic-clonic seizures can be induced by stimulating the thalamus, the medullary reticular formation, and the reticulo-spinal medullary sympathetic efferences.

In animal models of absence epilepsies, thalamo-cortical loop oscillations have been demonstrated to induce EEG abnormalities and absences (Gloor *et al.*, 1977; Avoli & Gloor, 1981, 1982; Pellegrini *et al.*, 1979). The oscillations may originate in the thalamus or in the cortex (Mereen *et al.*, 2002), or they may be caused by thalamo-cortical loop dysfunction (Blume, 2001). Both the thalamus and the corpus callosum can have a synchronizing effect (Vergnes & Marescaux, 1994). Spikes can be induced by the thalamus (Avanzini *et al.*, 1989) through the T-type Ca++ channels (Coulter *et al.*, 1989; Kely *et al.*, 1990) for which ethosuximide and valproate have a selective inhibiting action. Slow spike-waves observed in LGS may indicate a higher excitability than in the case of other generalized epilepsies.

In the rodent, tonic seizures observed in audiogenic reflex models originate in the brainstem (Buchhalter, 1993). However, deep brain recordings in patients with LGS have demonstrated frontal cortex activity (Fisher & Niedermeyer, 1987). Bursts of fast rhythms, which are an EEG characteristic of LGS, appear to be due to cortical neuronal activity. These neurons, which can produce very fast oscillations, have a high capacity to induce seizures (Blume, 2001; Timofeev & Steriade, 2004).

In models of generalized tonic-clonic seizures (GTCS), the entire brain is involved (Blume, 2006). The motor component stems from the cortex (Marcus *et al.*, 1968). The flexion-extension components may stem from action in the medullar system (Blume, 2006). Substantia nigra may have a modulating and anticonvulsive effect (Gale, 1985; Velisek *et al.*, 2002). The tonic and clonic components may involve the brainstem as well as the mesencephalon (Browning, 1985; Burnham, 1985). Myoclonias and GTCS can be induced with stimulation of the mesencephalon (Kreindler *et al.*, 1958). Studies in quail-chick chimeras have demonstrated that transfer of the entire brain was required in order to observe all the components of the seizure (Teillet *et al.*, 1991; Guy *et al.*, 1993).

Physiopathology of LGS thus appears to involve the entire brain, which may explain the diversity of etiologies in this syndrome. LGS can be conceptualized as a "secondary network epilepsy", in which epileptic activity is amplified through cerebral networks. Cortical lesions, if present, interact with these networks to produce network instability (Archer *et al.*, 2014a). This hypothesis is supported by different functional neuroimaging studies, which confirm the involvement of diffuse zones of association cortex in the epileptogenesis of the disease (Archer *et al.*, 2014b; Pillay *et al.*, 2013). Deep brain structure involvement could be a pathway to adjuvant therapeutic approaches such as deep brain stimulation.

Clinical presentation

Onset

LGS usually begins before the age of 8 years, with a peak between 3 and 5 years. Onset after the age of 10 years is rare, and usually occurs in particular clinical settings, such as Down syndrome (Ferlazzo *et al.*, 2009). Although symptoms can appear *de novo* in a normally developing child, without any apparent cause, LGS generally develops in children with a variety of prenatal, perinatal, and postnatal conditions. In cryptogenic LGS, onset is usually later than in symptomatic LGS. LGS can evolve from West syndrome or from unspecified epilepsies, or may represent the first seizure disorder. Approximately one-third of patients with symptomatic LGS have a history of spasms occurring in infancy and early childhood (Gastaut *et al.*, 1966; Trevathan *et al.*, 1997). When LGS follows a previous West syndrome, infantile spasms may be replaced by tonic seizures without a free interval, or after a period during which both EEG recordings and psychomotor development improve. When LGS is a continuation of other forms of epilepsies, the diagnosis is marked by the onset of falls, behavioural abnormalities and cognitive decline.

Fully developed Lennox-Gastaut syndrome

Different seizure types occur in LGS, including tonic seizures, atypical absences, GTCS, myoclonic as well as focal seizures.

Tonic seizures

Tonic seizures represent the most distinctive and most common seizure type in LGS and their presence is a requisite for diagnosis, although they are not specific to this condition. At onset, tonic seizures may be absent or very brief, and therefore they may not be recognized by parents, especially if occurring during sleep. The full clinical picture is usually expressed several months later with the appearance of atypical absences or other seizure types, as well as cognitive decline, which may develop rapidly or insidiously after the first seizure. Thus, the diagnosis of LGS may not be easy at the very beginning. In young children, LGS usually begins with drop attacks, followed by other seizure types. In the school-age group, behavioral disturbances may be the heralding signs, along with drop attacks, soon followed by frequent seizures, episodes of status epilepticus, progressive cognitive decline, personality disturbances, and chronic psychosis (Roger *et al.*, 1989).

Tonic seizures are usually short. Consciousness is frequently but not always impaired. Depending on the extent and groups of muscles involved, tonic seizures may be limited to head and trunk flexion (occasionally preceded by cries), with apnoea, mouth opening, upward rolling of the eyes (axial tonic seizures), or associated with elevation, abduction and semiflexion of the upper limbs and elevation of the shoulders (axorhizomelic tonic seizures). If most muscles are involved, including the distal parts of limbs, extension or triple flexion of the lower limbs may be observed (global tonic seizures). Tonic seizures may have hemicorporeal predominance at times. If the patient is standing, he may fall either forward or backward (Gastaut *et al.*, 1966). Autonomic signs such as apnoea, facial flushing, acceleration of heart, dilation of pupils and loss of urine may occur. Tonic seizures may manifest only with upward rolling of the eyes, hypopnoea or apnoea, associated or not with other minor motor phenomena such as head flexion and slight elevation of the shoulders, especially if they occur during sleep. Such subtle tonic seizures are usually revealed only by video-polygraphic recording including EEG, electromyography and pneumography. Frequent arousals provoked by tonic seizures may lead to diurnal drowsiness. Gestural or ambulatory automatisms may follow the tonic phase, and they may last from several minutes to several hours (tonic-automatic seizures) (Oller Daurella, 1970); such seizures occur more often in patients with later onset, and in older patients. When tonic seizures last more than 10 seconds, they can culminate in a tremor that affects the whole body ("tonic-vibratory" seizures) (Dravet & Roger, 1988). The tremor is characterized by a series of rapid low amplitude jerks affecting the entire body, and they should not be confused with the clonic phase of a GTCS. Such seizures occur more typically towards the end of the night.

Tonic seizures can be isolated or serial, day and night. In the most severe patients, they can be repeated during sleep and occur up to 40–50 times or more during one night. Often there is a series on awakening or on falling asleep. In the series, they are of various intensities from the beginning to the end of the series, as infantile spasms, and may be first subclinical before evolving to clinical. Tonic seizures may also be precipitated by stimuli such as noise, contact, or movement (Roger *et al.*, 1989), especially in patients with Down syndrome (Ferlazzo *et al.*, 2009).

Atypical absences

Atypical absences are the second characteristic seizure type of LGS, and can be observed in approximately two-thirds of patients. In contrast to typical absences, which present sudden onset and offset with a short duration (usually 5–30 seconds), atypical absences have a gradual onset and offset, and duration is usually longer. During atypical absences, there is "clouding" rather than complete loss of consciousness, so that patients can continue their activity to a certain extent (Gastaut *et al.*, 1966). For these reasons, diagnosis of atypical absences may be difficult based solely on clinical grounds; quantification of atypical absences is impossible without continuous EEG monitoring. Perioral and eyelid myoclonias may occur, as well as drooling and gradual head drop. As in tonic seizures, atypical absences may also be precipitated by stimuli such as noise, contact, or movement (Roger *et al.*, 1989), especially in patients with Down syndrome (Ferlazzo *et al.*, 2009).

Atonic, myoclonic-atonic, and myoclonic seizures

Their diagnosis is usually difficult, based only on the patient's history or clinical observation, so a polygraphic study is often necessary. Most authors group these seizures with falls under the name of akinetic or astatic seizures or drop attacks. Seizures are characterized by sudden fall either of the head only or of the whole body (Roger *et al.*, 1989). Attacks are usually short (~ 1 second) and loss of contact is very brief, except in case of head concussion.

Other seizures

They may occur in the LGS (*e.g.*, generalized tonic-clonic, generalized clonic, and focal seizures). Such seizures do not play a prominent part in diagnosis, and are associated with the more typical seizure types outlined above. Reflex seizures may be seen in some cases, like seizures provoked by eating (Lee *et al.*, 2001) or in Down syndrome patients, in whom a "startle" reaction may trigger tonic seizures or atypical absences (Ferlazzo *et al.*, 2009). Psychogenic, non-epileptic seizures may also occur, coexisting with the other seizures.

Clinical variants

The prominent occurrence of myoclonic jerks led to the individualization of a "myoclonic" variant of the LGS, which may represent as much as 18% of the cases (Aicardi & Chevrie, 1972): most of these cases were reported as cryptogenic, less severe, and a part would probably be diagnosed nowadays as myoclonic-astatic epilepsy (Doose, 1992). Late-onset LGS has been studied by several authors (Oller Daurella, 1973; Bauer *et al.*, 1983; Roger *et al.*, 1987). These LGS can follow idiopathic generalized epilepsy, focal epilepsy, or appear initially as the typical cryptogenic syndrome. The age of onset is usually between 10 and 20 years but in some cases was between 20 and 30 years. Patients with Down syndrome will usually initiate LGS between the ages of 8 and 12 years (Ferlazzo *et al.*, 2009).

Status epilepticus

Most patients (about 90%) with LGS have one or more episodes of status epilepticus (Dulac & N'Guyen, 1993). A variety of forms of status epilepticus may occur, representing a continuum from absence status, consisting of an insidious confused state lasting for up to several days or weeks and periodically interrupted by recurrent brief tonic seizures, to pure tonic status epilepticus. The latter is observed more often in adolescents or adults than in children. Status usually mixes several seizure types in the LGS.

– *Absence status* may be difficult to recognize, particularly in children with severe mental retardation. During absence status, the EEG becomes almost hypsarrhythmic and may represent a temporary worsening of the usual interictal symptomatology. These episodes of status are heralded by the appearance or worsening of cognitive deficit or behavioural disorders. Aggravation of the neurological state occurs insidiously. In some patients, oral expression may be hindered by hypertonia of the buccal and neck muscles with a velopalatal maximum (Beaumanoir *et al.*, 1968). Return to the previous state occurs gradually. Absence status is usually resistant to drug therapy, and tends to be recurrent. No permanent sequelae are observed in most cases, although a high status frequency has been related to poor cognitive outcome.

– *Tonic status* is usually characterized by tonic seizures occurring subcontinuously during waking and sleep. At times, tonic seizures are intermingled with GTCS. At the onset of the status, consciousness is preserved between tonic seizures, and patients are able to speak, eat and walk. A gradual clouding of consciousness sets in afterwards, along with swallowing difficulties and respiratory congestion. Life-threatening autonomic dysfunction (respiratory failure, hyperthermia, tachycardia) may occur in rare cases. This status has been reported to be occasionally elicited by intravenous administration of benzodiazepines (Tassinari *et al.*, 1972) in patients who were already in atypical absence status with numerous spike-wave discharges in their EEG.

– *Atonic status* is less common and appears as an inability to maintain the upright position due to recurrent seizures or serial head drops when the patient is sitting, without interictal clouding of consciousness.

Neurologic and neuropsychiatric symptomatology

Interictal neurologic symptoms are not specific to the LGS but they are determined by the location and extent of the underlying pathology. Hence, the neurologic examination may be normal in subjects without preexisting brain pathology. Motor signs occur in 59% of cases, but cerebellar signs or gait ataxia may be difficult to differentiate from effects of antiepileptic drugs (Markand, 1977). Recurrent injuries, lack of physical exercise, or natural evolution of the disease may also lead to impaired gait stability.

Progressive behavioural disorders may be linked to the polymorphism of EEG abnormalities. In the past, abnormalities were sometimes linked to side-effects of drugs (phenytoin, barbiturates) but have become far less frequent with recent medications. Cognitive decline is progressive as well, and an age-related pattern can be observed (Blume, 1978). The decline begins with stagnation and then a slowing of psychomotor skills, after which a deterioration of abilities sets in. Several other features can be seen, including instability, mood disorders, impaired expression and ideation, and difficulty acquiring new skills. Psychiatric symptoms may also appear, including aggressiveness, irritability, isolation, personality disorders, and loss of social contact, all of which may lead to "disintegrative psychosis" (Viani, 1991). Severe mental retardation, associated with autistic traits, is often observed in patients with a pre-existing encephalopathy or symptomatic LGS (Kieffer-Renaux *et al.*, 1997). Mental retardation is not as severe in children with cryptogenic LGS whose development was normal prior to onset, but they do develop behavioural and personality disorders.

Etiology

Although LGS is phenotypically a homogenous syndrome with a well-defined clinical pattern and typical EEG characteristics, there is a diversity of etiologies including various structural causes as well as infectious, tumoral, traumatic, malformational, immunologic, metabolic, toxic, genetic, or chromosomal causes. Some authors described idiopathic cases (Boniver *et al.*, 1987; Ohtahara *et al.*, 1988) before the category of cryptogenic was introduced in the international classification (1989). Their series may have included patients with myoclonic astatic epilepsy, which can be sometimes difficult to distinguish from LGS. But most of the patients should be classified now as cryptogenic – or the etiology as "unknown" – when no etiological factors were found and they were normal before the epilepsy onset.

Several common etiologies of LGS have been described. LGS is observed with ante-, peri- or postnatal sequelae of anoxo-ischemia, cerebrovascular accidents and cerebromeningeal infections. LGS is also caused by malformations of cortical development, including hemimegalencephaly and band heterotopia (Palmini *et al.*, 1991; Ricci *et al.*, 1992; Soucek *et al.*, 1992). These malformations can be genetic or not, as in lissencephaly or pachygyria resulting from mutations in the doublecortin gene (DCX) (Guerrini, 2005; Lawrence *et al.*, 2010), bilateral perisylvian polymicrogyrias and polygyrias resulting from a mutation in Xq28, recessive autosomic transmission or 22q11.2 deletion (Guerrini, 2005), or else bilateral frontoparietal polymicrogyrias resulting from a mutation of the *GPR56* gene which encodes for a G protein (Parrini *et al.*, 2009). LGS is also found in subjects with chromosomal disorders. Several cases of LGS have been reported with 15q11-q13 inversion-duplication (Battaglia *et al.*, 1997; Kobayashi & Yoshino, 1999; Orrico *et al.*, 2009; Rocha *et al.*, 2012), Rett syndrome (Olmos Garcia de Alba *et al.*, 1987), Leigh's disease (Matsuishi *et al.*, 1985), or juvenile ceroid-lipofuscinosis (Lagenstein *et al.*, 1978). Down syndrome is frequently associated with late onset LGS and reflex seizures (Guerrini *et al.*, 1993; Ferlazzo *et al.*, 2009). In tuberous sclerosis, the LGS can occur with or without previous infantile spasms (Ohtsuka *et al.*, 1998). Exome studies or case reports of patients with LGS without a history of infantile spasms have shown the role of other genes mutations such as *GABRB3, ALG13, SCN8A, STXBP1, DNM1, FOXG1, CHD2* (Allen *et al.*, 2013; Terrone *et al.*, 2014; Lund *et al.*, 2014). A heteroplasmic variant in the mithocondrial *MT-ND1* gene, resulting in a reduced stability of the protein, was demonstrated in a patient with a LGS evolving from a West syndrome (Delmiro *et al.*, 2013). LGS can also occur after concussion, or tumoral, infectious, or vascular lesions.

Findings also suggest immunologic etiologies with some evidence in subjects with LGS presenting with an abnormally frequent expression of the HLA-B7 antigen (Smeraldi *et al.*, 1975), or with an abnormally frequent expression of the DR5 antigen and a decreased expression of the DR4 antigen (van Engelen *et al.*, 1994). In 2005, Kondo *et al.* reported the occurrence of LGS following acute disseminated encephalomyelitis in a girl with an immune deficiency syndrome. Toxic causes of LGS have been suggested in the case of treatment for acute lymphoblastic leukemia with intravenous and intrathecal methotrexate prior to radiotherapy (Mitsufugi *et al.*, 1996). Several cases of LGS have also been reported with neurocysticercosis (Frochtengarten & Scarante, 1973; Agapejev *et al.*, 2000), with Sturge-Weber disease (Bosten & Reznick, 1967, cited by Roger & Gambarelli-Dubois, 1988), or with hypothalamic hamartoma (Andermann & Berkovic, 1988).

No cases of LGS have been described in the literature in GEFS+ families. LGS is not an epileptic encephalopathy caused by a mutation of the *SCN1A* gene. Nevertheless, Selmer *et al.* (2009) have described a mutation of the *SCN1A* gene in one subject in a series of 22 LGS subjects. In a study of 14 subjects with post-vaccinal epileptic encephalopathy, it is to be noted that Berkovic *et al.* (2006) found no mutation of the *SCN1A* gene in the two LGS subjects, but found the mutation in a subject presenting with a clinical pattern evocative of Dravet syndrome.

Pathology

In 1988, Roger & Garambelli-Dubois reviewed 30 cases of LGS studied after autopsy and 8 cases of cortical biopsy. All the subjects died of status epilepticus or anoxia. Lesions were found in most cases (malformations of cortical development, heterotopias, phacomatosis, microcephalia, multiple malformations). Cerebellar lesions were observed in 20 cases, 4 of which were isolated lesions. Neuronal necrosis was observed in 23 cases, with several cases of selective neuronal necrosis. In the biopsies, the authors found neuronal loss with mild diffuse reactive gliosis, and a rarefaction of cortical dendrites and their synaptic contacts. In the literature, cortical biopsy was performed on two other subjects thought to have had idiopathic LGS (Renier, 1988). In both cases, a rarefaction of cortical dendrites was observed on the fifth layer of pyramidal cells.

EEG

Wake and sleep EEG are characteristic in LGS subjects. Typical sleep EEG is one of the three characteristics used to diagnose LGS. Sleep recordings are therefore of utmost importance, and should be performed routinely with the 10–20 international system and associated with electromyography (EMG), pneumography, and an electrocardiogram. Systematic video recording is important to link EEG with clinical events which may at times be discrete. Prolonged video monitoring helps provide sufficient periods of sleep.

Interictal EEG

Interictal EEG often shows slow and poorly organized background activity *(Figure 1)* which is observed either frequently or only during phases of exacerbation *(Figure 2)*. It varies with age and etiology. It can also be normal, particularly in older patients. Bursts of diffuse slow spike- or polyspike-wave activity at 2–2.5 Hz are recorded (Blume, 1988) *(Figure 2)*. Predominance is generally anterior and more rarely posterior (Markand, 1977). The spike-waves can be isolated, in bursts or in discharges leading to atypical absences. Classically bilateral and synchronous, the discharges can be asymmetric,

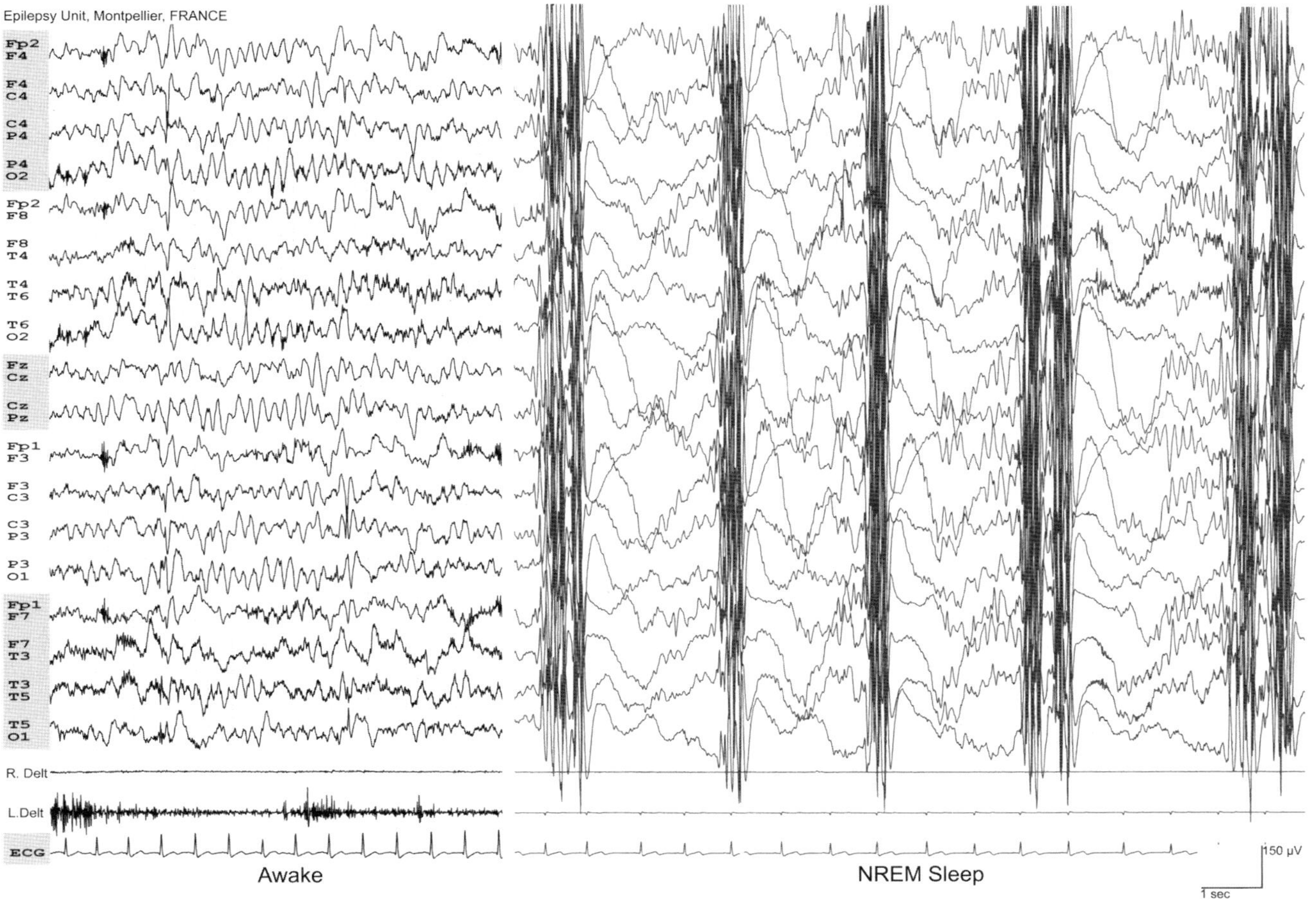

Figure 1

8-year-old boy with cryptogenic Lennox-Gastaut syndrome. On the left, slow background activity with diffuse slow waves with superimposed spike-waves. On the right (NREM sleep), generalized polyspikes followed by flattening.

or they can vary during the EEG recording. Amplitude and frequency vary in the same subject. Discharges are activated by drowsiness and NREM sleep *(Figure 3)*. Although hyperpnoea is often without effect, it can sometimes lead to an increased frequency of spike-waves and occurrence of an atypical absence. No photosensitivity has been observed (Markand, 1977). Focal abnormalities mostly occur in symptomatic LGS but can also be found in cryptogenic cases. Triphasic waves or anterior slow delta waves can also be present (Blume, 1988).

Diagnosis of LGS should not rest on the presence of diffuse slow spike-waves alone. The full-night sleep EEG is characterised by: i) increase and change of diffuse slow spike-waves during NREM sleep; ii) increase of fast rhythms with or without subtle seizures or tonic

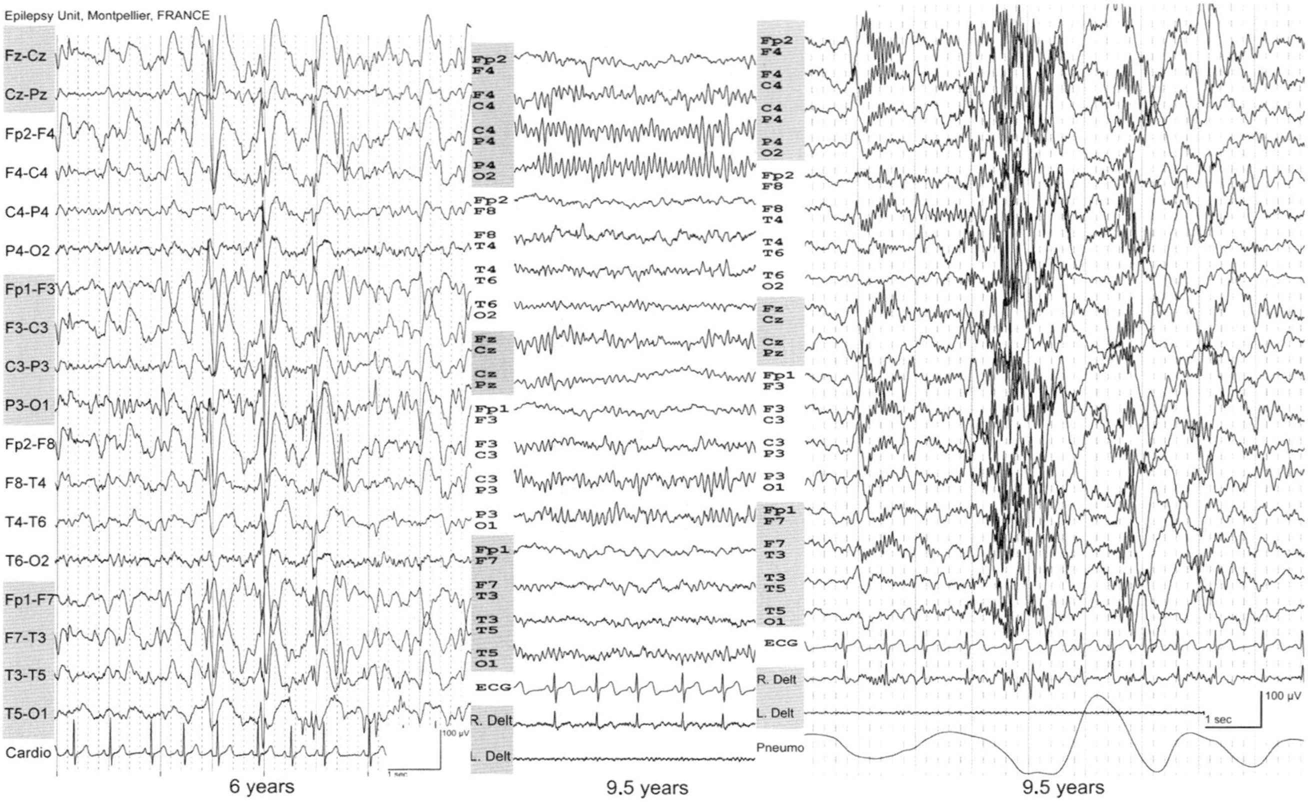

Figure 2

Left: **girl seen at age 6 years. The child is awake. Slow background activity with a series of slow spike-waves with anterior predominance. Epilepsy remained very active until age 9, when, under antiepileptic polytherapy and vagus nerve stimulation, the parents noted that daytime as well as nocturnal seizures had ceased.** Middle: **recording at age 9.5 years, normal background activity.** Right: **same recording: generalized discharges of fast rhythms during NREM sleep. After the discharge, increased amplitude of breathing.**

seizure; iii) reduction of interictal changes and seizures during REM sleep; iv) total disappearance of interictal changes only seen in patients with well-controlled seizures (Baldy-Moulinier *et al.*, 1988). Diffuse discharges of fast rhythms at 10 c/s during NREM sleep lasting from 0.5 to several seconds are the most characteristic EEG element in LGS *(Figure 4)*. Diffuse polyspikes and polyspike-waves with persistence of diffuse slow spike-waves can also be observed during sleep.

In sleep, intercritical abnormalities which become more rhythmic and synchronous occur at increased frequency, and these abnormalities are more generalized than in waking *(Figure 1)*. Subtle tonic seizures may occur with subclinical fast rhythms and only a slight change in breathing and/or muscle activity *(Figure 2)*. Physiological transients are rare or absent because of the frequency of abnormalities and the fragmented sleep pattern. During REM sleep, the abnormalities

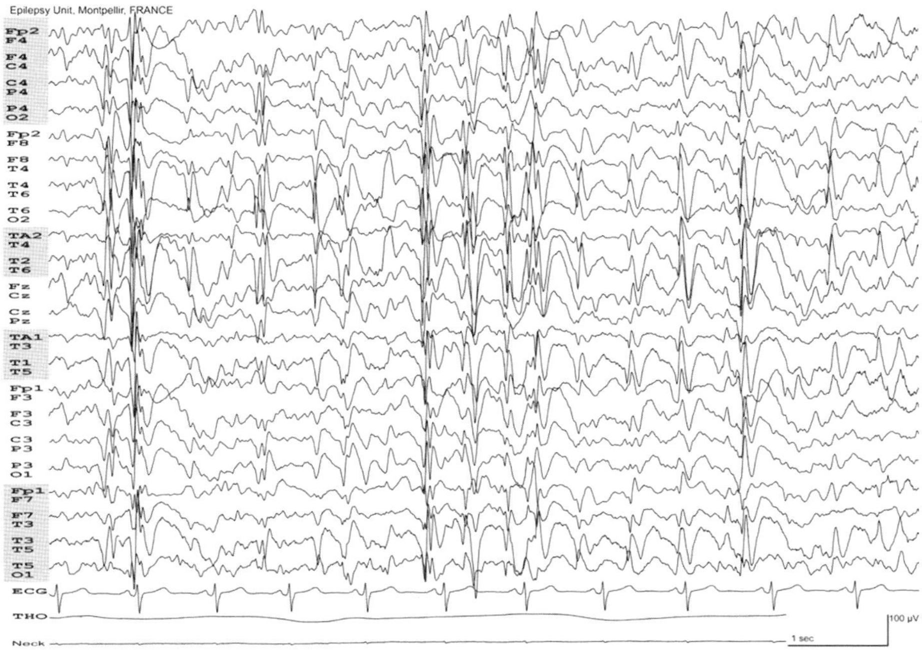

Figure 3 26-year-old woman with a cryptogenic Lennox-Gastaut syndrome. Supplementary anterior/inferior temporal electrodes (TA1, T1, TA2, T2). Stage 2 NREM sleep; the EEG shows diffuse slow spike-waves.

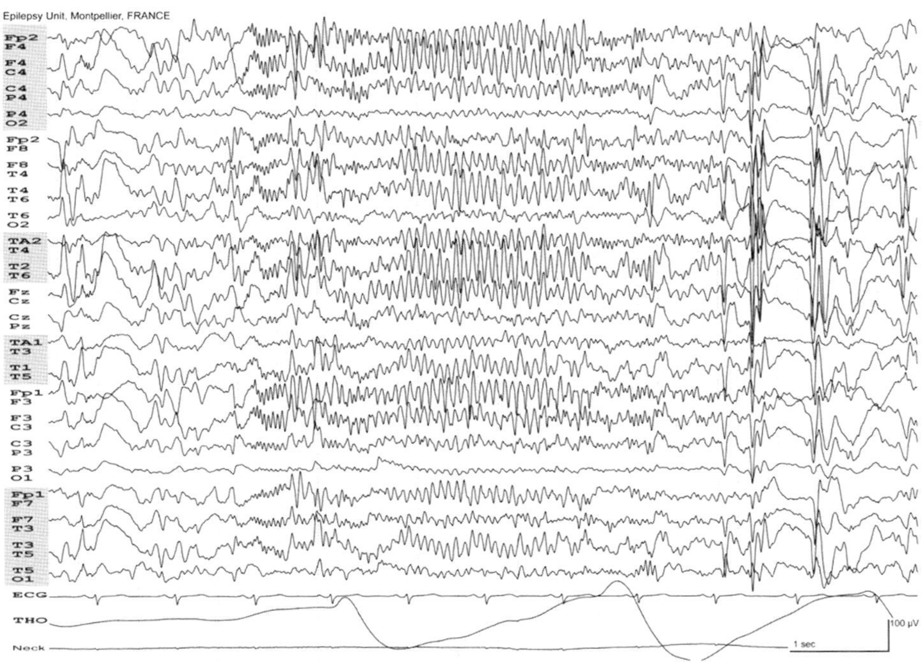

Figure 4 Same patient as in *Figure 3*. Recording during NREM sleep. Polymorphic changes including prominent fast rhythms with slightly higher amplitude over the right hemisphere.

predominate anteriorly, fast rhythms, polyspikes and polyspike-waves are less frequent and less typical, and may be associated with focal or multifocal changes.

Depending on the etiologies, further clinical and EEG characteristics can be described. For instance, focal abnormalities can be observed more frequently in LGS subjects with a focal lesion, and diffuse, fast rhythms can be seen in LGS subjects with malformations of cortical development.

Ictal EEG

Atypical absences

Long lasting (more than 20 seconds) diffuse slow spike-wave (2–2.5 Hz) discharges can be present on the EEG *(Figure 5)*. They are irregular, predominate anteriorly, and are sometimes asymmetric. Spike-wave morphology can vary during the absence *(Figure 6)*. Drowsiness can be an activating factor of atypical absences. Spike-waves discharges at more than 3.5 Hz can also be seen, and fast abnormalities can be intermingled with slow diffuse changes.

Tonic seizures

Tonic seizures can sometimes be observed in waking EEG, but they occur more often during NREM sleep. When they are subclinical or subtle, they may be evidenced only by EEG. Bilateral discharges of rapid rhythms (10–20 Hz) with anterior predominance lasting 5 to 15 seconds are typical of these seizures. The discharges of fast rhythms occur after a slow complex *(Figure 7)* or a diffuse flattening. Amplitude may be maximal at onset *(Figure 8)* or it may increase gradually *(Figure 9)*. Offset is sudden, and several diffuse ample delta waves can be observed. Sometimes the tonic seizure is fragmented with slow components or flattening which intermix with the discharge of fast rhythms. Muscle contraction and apnoea are followed by deep breathing *(Figure 10)* which resumes at the offset of the seizure without prolonged post-critical distress.

In tonic seizures with automatisms, the discharges of fast rhythms are followed by diffuse slow spike-waves or high-voltage slow-waves of long duration (Beaumanoir & Blume, 2005). In tonic vibratory seizures, a long-lasting discharge of fast rhythms is followed by generalized spike-waves (clonic phase) clinically associated with jerks and sometimes followed by diffuse slow waves.

Atonic seizures

Atonic seizures are associated with polyspike-waves and generalized spike-waves with resumption of muscle tone clinically corresponding to slow wave components. A discharge of fast rhythms preceding generalized spike-waves may also be recorded. Bradycardia or apnoea are sometimes observed.

Myoclonic-atonic seizures

Generalized discharges of slow spike-waves or polyspike-waves are associated with myoclonic-atonic seizures. Myoclonia is associated with spike and atonia is associated with slow waves.

Myoclonias

Myoclonias may occur in LGS. They are associated with bilateral symmetric spike-waves preceding one or more slow waves. Bonanni *et al.* (2002) demonstrated that myoclonias in LGS are frontal at onset, leading to secondary bilateral synchrony with a 20 ms interhemispheric latency period.

Miscellaneous seizures

When generalized tonic-clonic seizures occur in LGS, the seizures exhibit the typical EEG characteristics of this type of seizure.

Status epilepticus

Stuporous states are associated with mixed irregular, diffuse or anterior slow spike-waves or polyspikes-waves, usually at a lower frequency than at baseline (Morita & Glauser, 2008). The EEG reveals fast activity intermixed with discharges of slow spike-waves during tonic status epilepticus.

Evolution with age

At onset, a transitory period can be observed in young children, after which the more typical EEG patterns appear gradually (spasms/brief tonic seizures/diffuse slow spike-waves).

In adolescence and adulthood, evolution continues to be gradual, with decreasing frequency of diffuse slow spike-waves at later stages (Blume, 1988). Rhythms in the background activity tend to improve, and the wake EEG becomes normal or almost normal in some cases (Ferlazzo *et al.*, 2010). However, seizures may persist even though they are the only remaining pathological abnormality in the waking EEG.

In a long-term follow-up study of 89 subjects with LGS, Ohtsuka *et al.* (1991) demonstrated the gradual disappearance of diffuse slow spike-waves and the occurrence of focal epileptic discharges, especially multifocal spikes, after 1–2 decades following onset of LGS. Hughes & Patil (2002) followed the evolution of the diffuse slow spike-wave EEG pattern in 64 subjects with LGS. They found that the average age at onset of slow spike-wave patterns was 8.2 years and the average pattern duration was 8.6 years. After the age of 16 years, the interictal EEG in 95% of patients did not exhibit diffuse slow spike-wave patterns, and EEG changes comprised slowing of the background activity and focal discharges. In the study of Ferlazzo *et al.* (2010), slowing of the EEG background activity was observed in 21 out of 27 patients at the early stages of LGS, while the EEG was

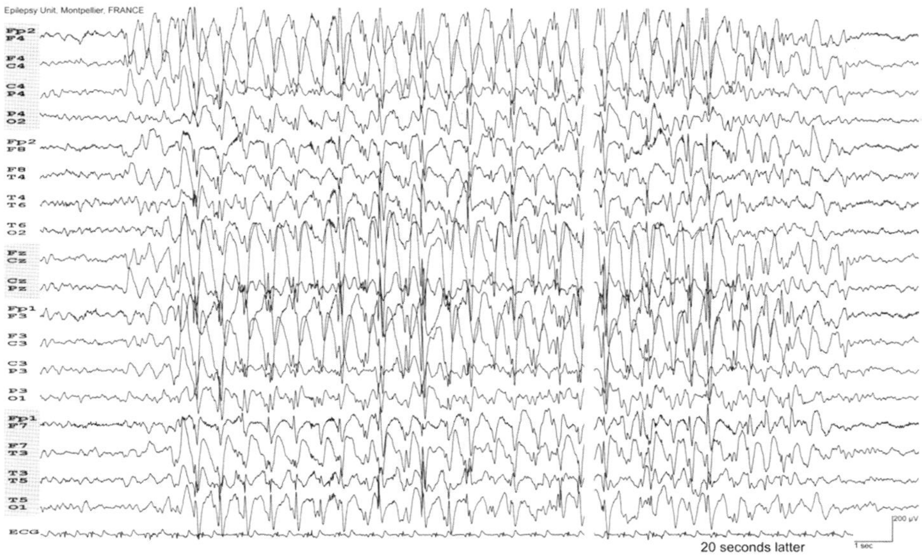

Figure 5 Same patient as in *Figure 1* (8-year-old boy). Atypical absence. The child is awake, the EEG shows slow spike-waves predominating anteriorly.

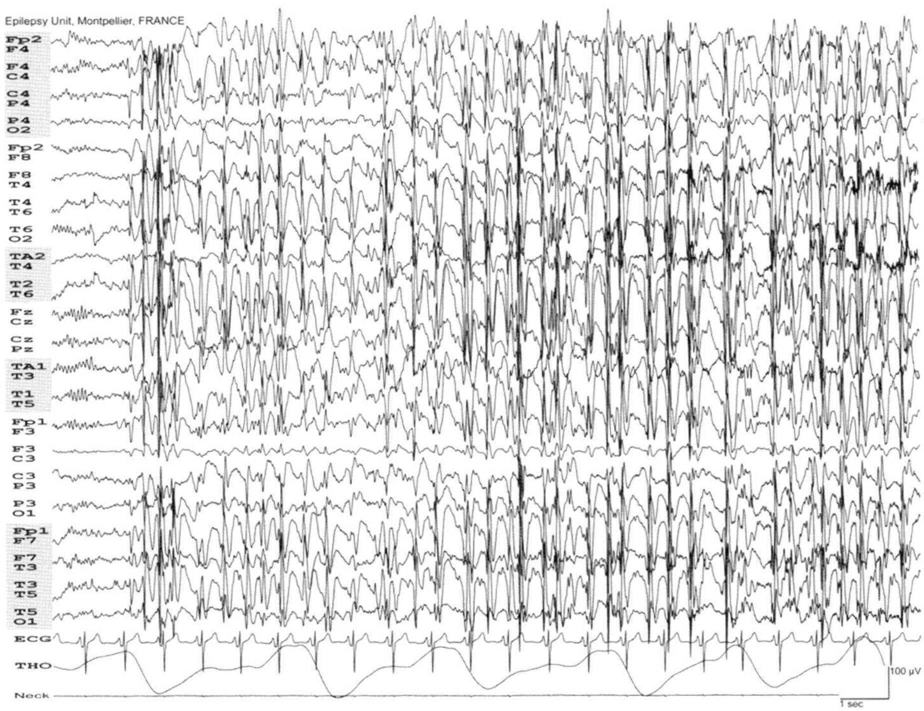

Figure 6 Same patient as in *Figures 3 and 4* (26-year-old woman). Atypical absence. Note the variable morphology and amplitude of the spike-waves.

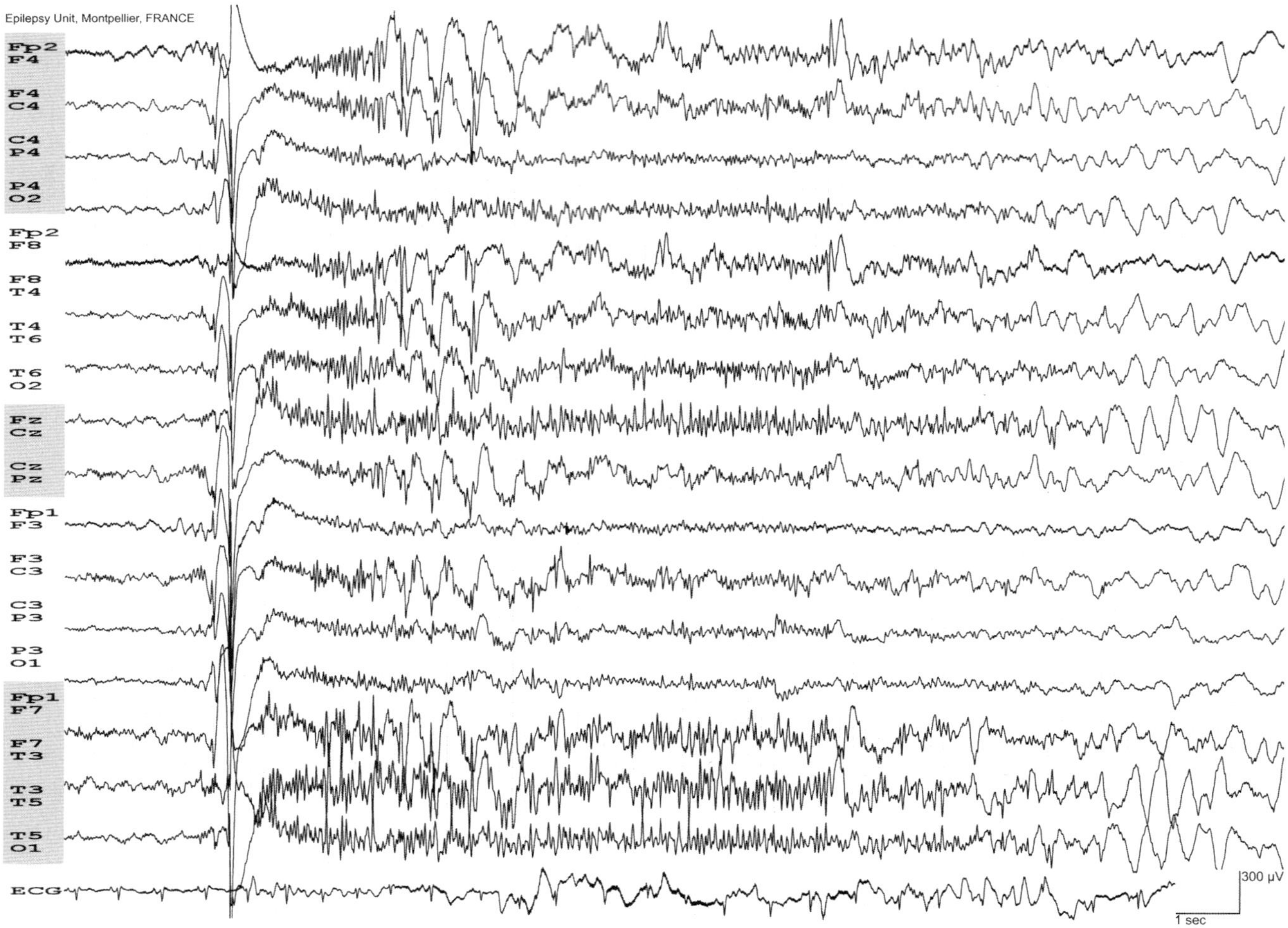

Figure 7

Same patient as in *Figures 1 and 5*. Tonic seizure with an initially high-amplitude complex, followed by low-voltage activity with fast rhythms of increasing amplitude. The discharge ends with slow delta waves.

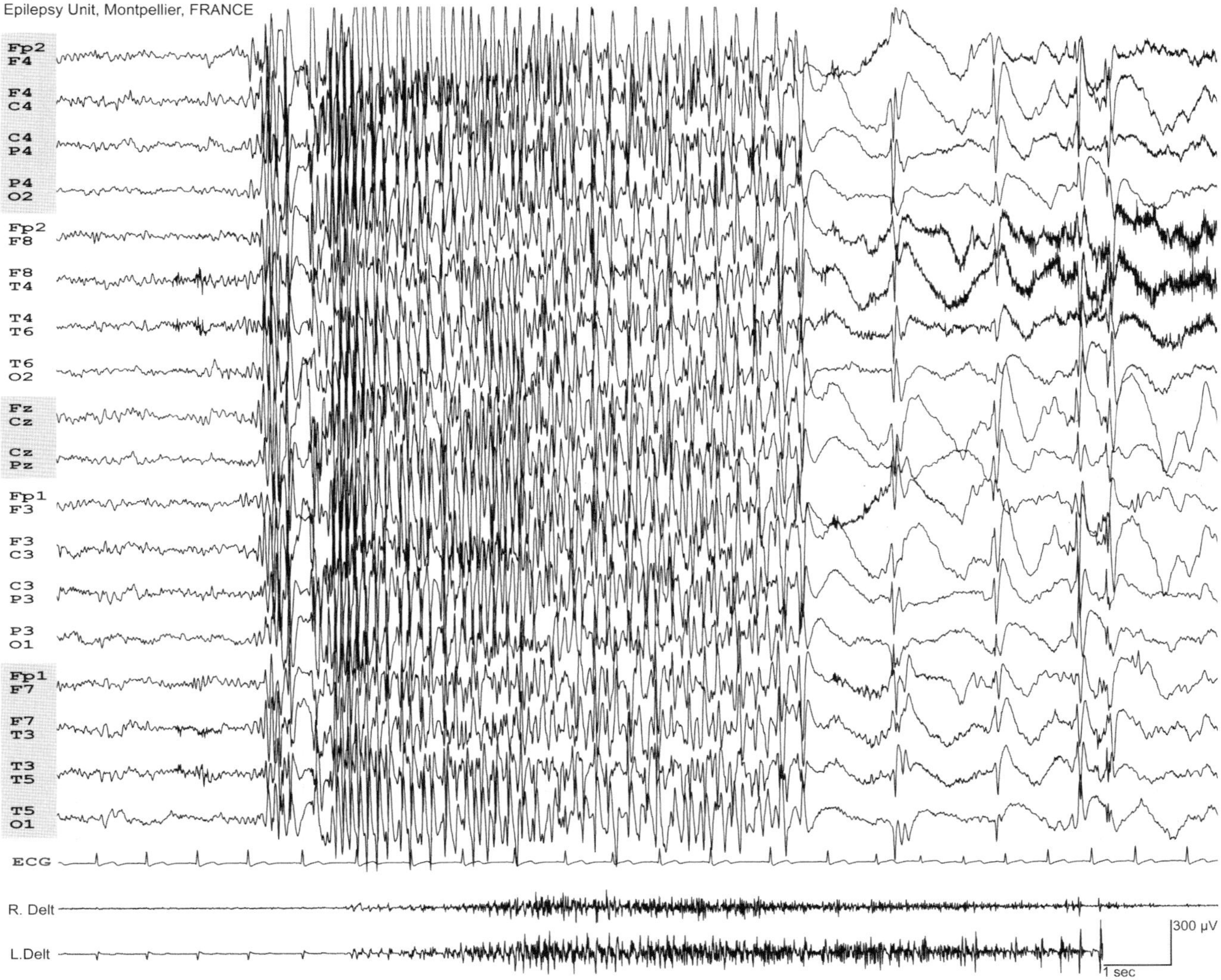

Figure 8

Same patient as in *Figures 1, 5 and 7* but seen later at age 13 years. The recording includes polygraphic EMG of deltoid muscles. Tonic seizure with fast discharge that has maximal amplitude from the start on, and becomes fragmented with intermixed low voltage activity. The tonic muscular contraction is shown by the EMG leads. The onset is delayed, with progressive increase in amplitude and a relative decrease during the low-voltage EEG periods.

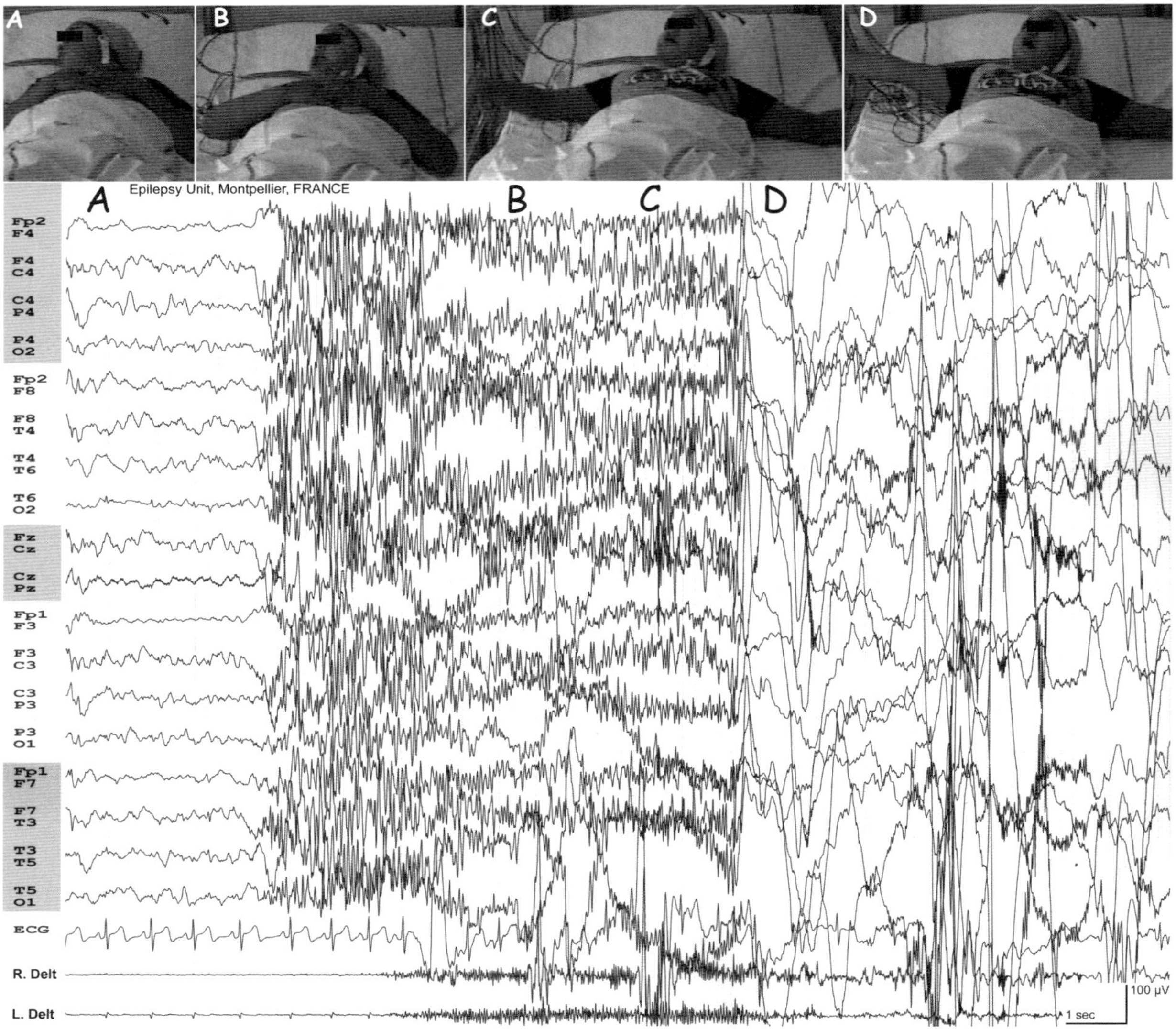

Figure 9

Same patient as in *Figure 2* seen at age 9.5 years. The child is in NREM sleep (A). A tonic seizure with fast discharge occurs. Note the contraction shown by the EMG leads, beginning 2 seconds after seizure onset. The patient opens her eyes and raises her arms (B). She opens her mouth and extends her arms (C, D). The tonic contraction decreases on the EMG leads when the EEG activity becomes depressed.

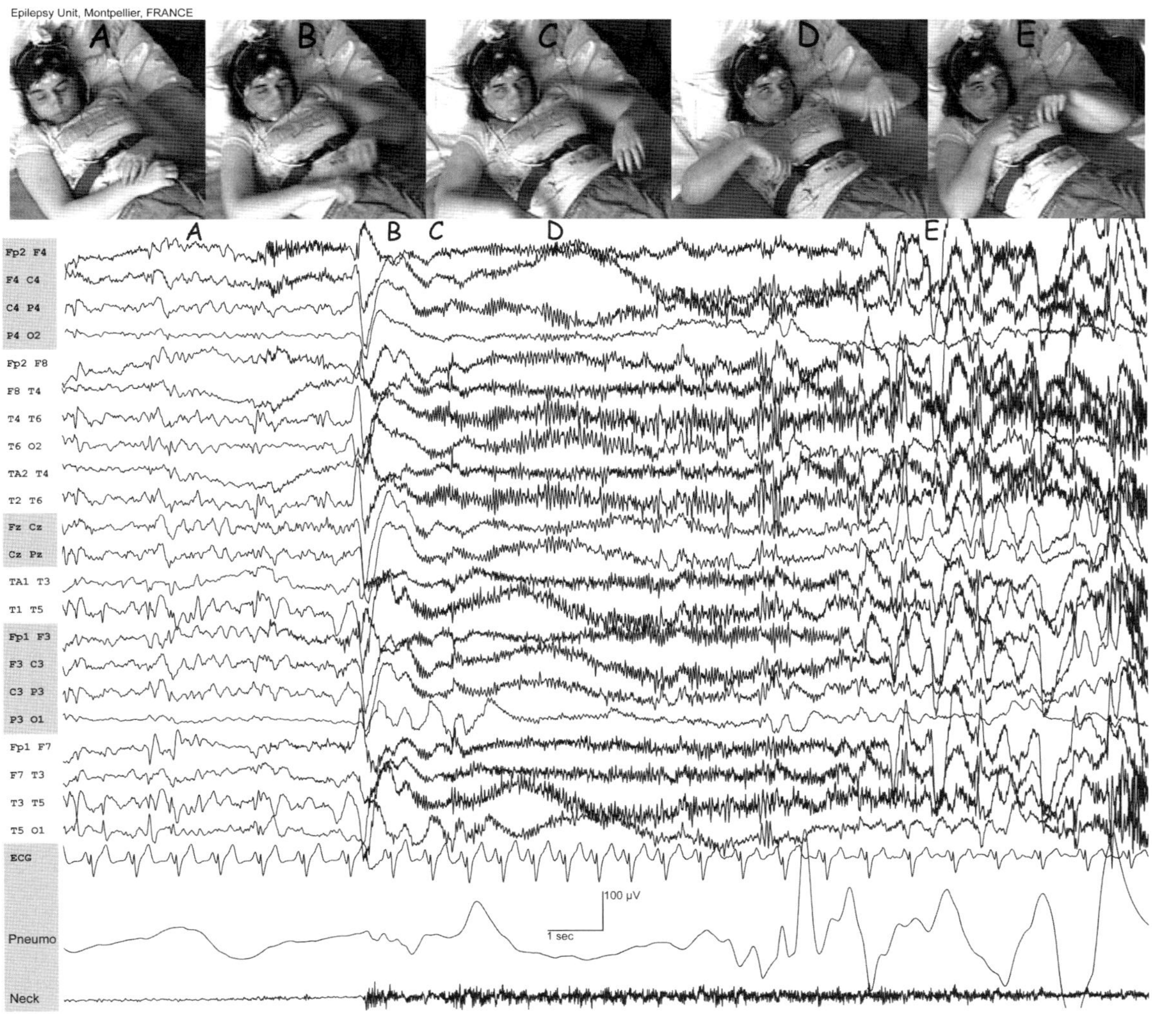

Figure 10

Same patient as in *Figures 3, 4 and 6*. The patient is in NREM sleep (A). There are bilateral interictal changes on posterior temporal regions, predominating on T5. Tonic seizure: there is a large diphasic complex followed by low voltage activity, then fast activity lasting 10 seconds, followed by slow waves. Hypopnea with acceleration of breathing at the end of the tonic discharge. On the EMG lead, there is a tonic contration associated with the high-amplitude slow complex. The patient bends her head, raises her arms (B). There is upward deviation of eyeballs (C, D). The arms are semi-flexed (E).

normal in 12 and slow in 15 patients at the last follow-up observation. Diffuse slow spike-waves were present in 22 out of 27 patients at LGS onset, whereas at the end of the follow-up period, they persisted only in 7 patients. However, the typically sleep-related changes are always present in LGS, with typical fast discharges, so that sleep EEG is required to establish a diagnosis of LGS in adults.

Morphological and functional imaging

All imaging studies have clearly demonstrated the heterogeneity of LGS. In their series of 42 subjects evaluated with the first available CT scan, Gastaut & Gastaut (1976) reported absence of abnormalities, diffuse subcortical cortical atrophies, porencephalic lesions, parieto-occipital tumor, tuberous sclerosis, leucoblastic infiltration, calcification, and several undetermined focal lesions. Etiologies undiagnosed at the time, in particular malformations of cortical development, have been visualized with MRI. In their series of 47 subjects, Goldsmith *et al.* (2000) reported ante- and perinatal lesions, malformations of cortical development, infectious sequelae, and abnormalities linked with genetic causes. In 1993, Velasco *et al.* reported the presence of a mesencephalic hypersignal in T2 in 7 subjects presenting with non-symptomatic LGS without other abnormalities. Siniatchkin *et al.* (2011) demonstrated the activation of the brainstem and the centro-median anterior part of the thalamic nuclei with FMRI during EEG discharges in 11 LGS subjects. This activation did not occur in the control group of 9 epileptic children. HMPAO/SPECT findings in fMRI in three LGS subjects exhibited multiple hypoperfusion zones (Heiskala & Launes, 1993). PET findings in LGS are normal or there can be evidence of hypometabolism not always associated with MRI abnormalities (Theodore *et al.*, 1987; Chugani *et al.*, 1987). Hypometabolism can be temporal (Gur *et al.*, 1982), involve the inferior frontal gyrus and the posterior part of the superior temporal gyrus (Iinuma *et al.*, 1987), or it can be temporal and frontal (Miyauchi *et al.*, 1988). Ferrie *et al.* (1996) reported cortical hypometabolism in LGS following West syndrome while hypometabolism was not observed in *de novo* LGS.

Differential diagnosis

Not all encephalopathies presenting with falls and/or diffuse slow spike-waves are LGS. Indeed, diffuse slow spike-waves can be observed in other generalized epilepsies which are symptomatic, cryptogenic, or even idiopathic in borderline cases or during worsening due to inadequate medication. It is important to distinguish LGS from other specific epileptic encephalopathies, focal epilepsies followed by tonic seizures, and/or EEG with secondary bisynchrony. Although some encephalopathies may be evocative of LGS at certain periods of their evolution, the clinical triad of LGS is not observed, and the typical clinical pattern of other specific encephalopathies should be used to distinguish them from LGS.

– *Epilepsy with myoclonic-atonic seizures (Doose syndrome)* was often misdiagnosed as LGS in the past, and still remains one of the most difficult differential diagnoses (Doose, 1992). Although evolution can be similar to LGS, several characteristics are more evocative of Doose syndrome, including the existence of a family history of idiopathic epilepsy, early onset, appearance of fast spike-waves on the EEG, absence of focal EEG changes, occurrence of myoclonias, myoclonic-astatic and generalized tonic-clonic seizures, and absence of focal seizures (Kaminska *et al.*, 1999).

– *Epilepsy with myoclonic absences* is characterized by typical absences associated with axial hypertonia and rhythmic myoclonias at 3 Hz (Genton & Bureau, 2006). However, subjects with a severe form and a pejorative evolution may present with the LGS clinical pattern.

– *Idiopathic generalized epilepsies modified by iatrogenic factors:* narrow-spectrum anti-epileptic drugs (most commonly vigabatrin, tiagabine, gabapentine, carbamazepine, oxcarbazepine and phenytoin) can lead to electroclinical aggravation of idiopathic generalized epilepsies, and in particular absence epilepsies (Perucca *et al.*, 1998). Worsening is associated with modification of electroclinical features which may evoke an epileptic encephalopathy with atypical absences, and/or negative myoclonias with falls. In 2006, Thomas *et al.* also demonstrated absence status and mixed status epilepticus with absences and myoclonias in this context. However, aggravation is not associated with onset of tonic seizures or intellectual decline. Moreover, all of the typical LGS electric characteristics are not observed, and the background activity is preserved in wake and sleep EEG with preservation of the physiological sleep transients.

– *Idiopathic generalized epilepsies with sleep-related fast activities:* some idiopathic generalized epilepsies exhibit "intermediate", atypical EEG characteristics, such as diffuse slow spike-waves, generalized polyspikes and fast rhythms during sleep, and are refractory to medication. Due to these abnormalities, the epilepsy is said to be "intermediate" between an idiopathic and a symptomatic/cryptogenic generalized epilepsy such as LGS; transitional forms of absence epilepsy have been described in children with polyspikes and fast rhythms during sleep (Lugaresi *et al.*, 1973; Guye *et al.*, 2001). Some children with absence epilepsy at onset develop generalized tonic-clonic seizures with falls in adolescence. Tonic seizures and myoclonias are absent, or they are not predominant features. There is no cognitive decline at onset or during evolution. EEG sleep recordings exhibit diffuse slow spike-waves, generalized polyspike-waves and fast rhythms. However, these epilepsies do not constitute a specific entity.

– *Dravet syndrome* constitutes a precise diagnostic entity. Patients sometimes present with atypical absences, but tonic seizures are not frequent (Nabbout *et al.*, 2008). EEG characteristics also differ from LGS. Moreover, a *SCN1A* mutation is found in a large majority of cases, and is not found in the LGS, with a single exception (Selmer *et al.*, 2009).

– *Angelman syndrome* differs from LGS in its clinical presentation as well as its typical dysmorphia, although in some very rare instances patients may exhibit an epilepsy that is close to LGS. Subjects usually do not have tonic seizures or falls. Recordings are characteristic with long discharges of slow spike-waves in awake EEG, often associated with fast-bursting cortical myoclonus often reported as tremor (Guerrini *et al.*, 1996).

– *Late infantile ceroid-lipofuscinosis (Jansky-Bielschowsky)* can be mistaken for LGS at onset (Genton *et al.*, 2005). Indeed, onset generally occurs between ages 1 and 4 years and regression of psychomotor skills is observed. The infant presents with generalized tonic-clonic seizures associated with myoclonias and atypical absences followed by neurological signs and progressive blindness. Background EEG activity is modified with slowing. The EEG abnormalities include slow waves and spikes, spike-waves and polyspike-waves. Characteristic posterior polyphasic spikes occur with low-frequency ILS.

– *The encephalopathy with electrical status epilepticus during sleep* (syndrome of continuous spike-waves during slow sleep), first described by Patry *et al.* (1971), is age-dependent and is associated with remission at puberty and was often misdiagnosed as LGS. In primary school-age children, the main characteristics at onset are behavioural difficulties, cognitive decline, and sometimes absences and falls, but no tonic seizures. EEG recordings show bursts of diffuse spike-waves during waking, which become continuous during sleep and last during more than 80% of NREM sleep. Contrary to LGS, no fast rhythms during sleep can be observed.

– *Atypical benign partial epilepsy* (Aicardi & Chevrie, 1982) or pseudo-Lennox syndrome in the German-speaking area (Hahn *et al.*, 2001) is an idiopathic focal epilepsy of childhood with transient or longlasting aggravation, associated with atypical absences, negative myoclonus, and falls. Subjects also present with clinical aggravation on recordings with diffuse slow spike-waves, and increased frequency of centro-temporal spike-waves during sleep similar to continuous spike-waves during slow sleep over short periods. There are no tonic seizures. Such aggravation can occur spontaneously or be activated by antiepileptic medication. Subjects recover at puberty.

– *Secondary bilateral synchrony and transitory LGS:* in children with symptomatic focal epilepsy, abnormal EEG characteristics can be observed such as symmetric diffuse slow spike-waves with anterior predominance, which correspond to secondary bilateral synchrony. The notion of secondary bilateral synchrony was described in 1952 by Tükel & Jasper. They observed that internal frontal lesions caused diffuse spike-waves similar to those observed with generalized epilepsies. Age of onset is later in children with focal epilepsy and secondary bilateral synchrony than in LGS. Other differences observed are focal abnormalities during neurological examination, milder cognitive decline, fewer seizures with predominance of focal seizures rather than tonic seizures (Gastaut & Zifkin, 1988). The typical characteristics of secondary bilateral synchrony are fully expressed several months or years after onset. Periods of "generalization" of the focal epilepsy can sometimes be iatrogenic due to inadequate administration of antiepileptic drugs or drug overloading. These children, who usually exhibit frontal lobe epilepsy, present with transitory LGS, with appearance of atypical absences, seizures associated with falls, and tonic seizures (Beaumanoir, 1982).

Outcome and prognosis

In most cases, LGS has a chronic course and constitutes a lifelong disease. More than 80% of patients continue to have seizures in adulthood and only a few of them are able to live independently. Transitory LGS has been described, most likely corresponding to a mild variant of the syndrome (Beaumanoir, 1982; Roger *et al.*, 1989). Longitudinal studies evaluating the long-term outcome of LGS patients have demonstrated that in general it is unfavourable (Gastaut *et al.*, 1973; Ohtahara *et al.*, 1976; Beaumanoir, 1982; Roger *et al.*, 1987, 1989; Ohtsuka *et al.*, 1990; Oguni *et al.*, 1996; Yagi, 1996). Seizure frequency tends to decrease after puberty, but 2/3 of patients still have daily or weekly seizures (Ohtsuka *et al.*, 1990). The factors consistent with an unfavourable long-term prognosis include a previous history of West syndrome, age of onset before 3 years, high seizure frequency, long periods of exacerbation, frequent episodes of status epilepticus, constantly slow background activity and multifocal localized abnormalities on the EEG, overtreatment in chronic cases, and numerous iatrogenic complications (Roger *et al.*, 1989; Genton & Dravet, 2007). Complete seizure remission in LGS is exceptional and varies in different series from 0 to 6.7% (Gastaut *et al.*, 1973; Beaumanoir *et al.*, 1988; Camfield & Camfield, 2007). The prerequisites for seizure-free recovery are cryptogenic etiology, short duration of full-blown LGS symptomatology, swift therapeutic response and vigorous treatment from the onset (Genton & Dravet, 2007). The mortality rate in LGS is estimated at around 5–17% (Gastaut *et al.*, 1973; Loubier, 1974). Deaths are usually related to accidents or episodes of status epilepticus.

Several longitudinal studies have shown that 33 to 67% of patients maintain a complete LGS profile in adulthood, whereas about 55% lose the typical LGS features and evolve to non-specific generalized epilepsy, severe multifocal epilepsy with independent spike foci or other focal epilepsies (Roger *et al.*, 1987; Ohtsuka *et al.*, 1990; Blatter-Arifi *et al.*, 1991; Oguni *et al.*, 1996). The slow spike-wave complexes usually disappear at this stage and are replaced by multiple independent focal discharges and diffuse slowing (Ohtsuka *et al.*, 1990; Hughes & Patil, 2002). Roger *et al.* (1987) reported a seizure evolution in 53% of patients with a transition in 16% of patients to severe unifocal epilepsy with frontal lobe dysfunction and in 20% to epilepsy with rare partial seizures. Oguni *et al.* (1996) found that maintaining the complete LGS profile in adulthood was more characteristic for cryptogenic cases, whereas the evolution to other epilepsy syndromes was more frequently observed in patients with symptomatic LGS. In the Yagi series (1996), only 33% of patients retained full-blown LGS symptomatology at adult age. However, no significant differences in seizure outcome was found between cryptogenic and symptomatic cases by Goldsmith *et al.* in 2000.

The age-dependent seizure evolution in LGS has been shown in several series (Holmes, 1988; Roger *et al.*, 1989; Ohtsuka *et al.*, 1990; Oguni *et al.*, 1996; Dravet, 1999, Vignoli *et al.*, 2017). The most prominent finding was the persistence of tonic seizures with time and their tendency to become more prolonged. Atonic falls were also retained in most of the adult patients with LGS, while atypical absences may subside. Ferlazzo *et al.* (2010) evaluated the electroclinical features of 27 adult patients with LGS followed for an average period of 35 years. They showed that tonic seizures were dominant throughout the evolution in all patients *(Table I)*. At onset, tonic seizures occurred with equal frequency during wakefulness and sleep, whereas at the end of the follow-up period tonic seizures were still present in all patients during sleep but only in less than 50% of patients (11/27) during wakefulness. The frequency of absences, atonic and myoclonic seizures decreased with time, while generalized tonic-clonic and focal seizures remained almost unchanged. Status epilepticus occurred in 15 patients at the early stages of the disease, whereas it was experienced by none of the patients at the last follow-up. There was no significant difference between cryptogenic and symptomatic cases of LGS in terms of seizure evolution, seizure frequency and response to treatment (Ohtsuka *et al.*, 1990; Oguni *et al.*, 1996; Yagi, 1996; Ferlazzo *et al.*, 2010; Vignoli *et al.*, 2017).

The neuropsychological outcome of LGS is poor. Although there might be some improvement in terms of seizure frequency and EEG findings, most patients (85–92%) have a progressive intellectual decline.

Progressive mental deterioration is determined by many factors, amongst which are the following: the development of epileptic encephalopathy due to a chronic course of epilepsy with high seizure frequency, recurrent episodes of status epilepticus, especially detrimental if they occur at early age, the cumulative neurotoxic effect of antiepileptic drugs and lack of social stimulation (Tassinari & Ambrosetto, 1988; Ohtsuka *et al.*, 1990; Oguni *et al.*, 1996). Ohtsuka *et al.* (1990) found a correlation between seizure evolution and mental outcome. Persisting LGS features were associated with low IQ scores, while in seizure-free patients the IQ scores were higher, with one third of patients having IQ scores between 25 and 75. In adults, the course of LGS is characterized by periods of regression associated with a deterioration of mental functions and behaviour. Mental functions are characterized by slow expression and ideation, decreased reaction time and speech latency.

Extrapyramidal and cerebellar neurological symptoms and signs are common and lead to progressive gait disturbances, dysphagia, drooling, and dysarthria (Ohtsuka *et al.*, 1990; Trevathan *et al.*, 1997). The appearance of "frontal" deficits and psychiatric symptoms is not uncommon (Roger *et al.*, 1987; Beaumanoir *et al.*, 1988; Goldsmith *et al.*, 2000; Genton & Dravet, 2007). Aggressiveness, stereotypes and loss of ability to control behaviour are typical patterns and suggest frontal lobe involvement. Numerous iatrogenic complications may contribute to the neurological and behavioural impairment.

Many patients are chronically treated with multiple antiepileptic drugs including benzodiazepines, and often in combination with neuroleptics which may impair cognitive function by fatiguing the patient. Apathy can be a result of social isolation and also interfere with mental processes. In a study by Hoffmann-Riem *et al.* (2000), on 101 patients with LGS who were followed for an average period of 16 years, 24% had evolved to a severe encephalopathy with language disability, and in almost half of the patients, motor skills were significantly impaired. In the Ferlazzo *et al.* series (2010) at the end of a 35-year follow-up period, 26 out of 27 patients had moderate or severe cognitive impairment, and 14 exhibited behavioral disturbances, mostly hyperactivity and aggressiveness. Fifteen patients were institutionalized, 11 lived withtheir family, and only one patient, with mild mental retardation and rare tonic seizures during sleep, was married and had a child. Few adult LGS patients are able to live independently. The majority of the patients become institutionalized eventually. Some patients, in particular those who were normal before the disease onset, can manage partial or sheltered employment. Among 102 patients followed up by Yagi (1996) for 16 years, 12 worked normally, 36 had part time work and 54 were under home or institutional care.

The recent study of Vignoli *et al.* (2017) showed that 3 patients of the cohort presented paroxysmal nonepileptic seizures (PNES), which have been recorded with video-EEG/home videos. Adjustments in the environment such as education of the caregivers and improvement of day care centers, improved the psychogenic features of these patients.

Treatment

The LGS is one of the most pharmacoresistant epileptic syndromes, and patient management remains very difficult. Different treatments are currently used, including conventional and unconventional drug therapies, as well as non-pharmacological therapies such as the ketogenic diet, vagus nerve stimulation, callosotomy, or deep brain stimulation. Social and psychological support is of course necessary.

Antiepileptic treatments: rational polytherapy

It is currently acknowledged that antiepileptic drug polytherapy is the most appropriate treatment due to the severity of this type of epilepsy and to the wide range of seizure types with varying reactions to the different molecules. Several controlled drug trials have been carried out for LGS: felbamate in 1993 (The Felbamate Study Group in Lennox-Gastaut Syndrome), lamotrigine in 1997 (Motte *et al.*, 1997), topiramate in 1999 (Sachdeo *et al.*, 1999), rufinamide (Glauser *et al.*, 2008), clobazam (Conry *et al.*, 2009), and the effectiveness of these molecules has been demonstrated. Non-masked trials have been carried out on benzodiazepines (Vassella *et al.*, 1973; Hosain *et al.*, 2003), zonisamide (Ohtahara, 2006; You *et al.*, 2008), levetiracetam (de los Reyes *et al.*, 2004), vigabatrin (Dulac *et al.*, 1991; Feucht & Brantner-Inthaler, 1994), rufinamide (Kluger *et al.*, 2009; Coppola *et al.*, 2010), topiramate (Glauser *et al.*, 2000; Guerreiro *et al.*, 1999; Coppola *et al.*, 2002), lamotrigine (Timmings & Richens, 1992; Donaldson *et al.*, 1997; Chen *et al.*, 2006), also demonstrating the effectiveness of these molecules. However, none of these drugs brings seizure freedom.

Valproate (VPA) used to be considered the first-line treatment for LGS (Covanis *et al.*, 1982), and its combination with lamotrigine (LTG) is particularly beneficial for LGS patients (Bisulli *et al.*, 2001; Thomé-Souza *et al.*, 2003; Huber *et al.*, 2007; Velizarova *et al.*, 2011), so that the VPA + LTG cotherapy can nowadays be considered the actual first-line pharmacological treatment in LGS. Valproate (or VPA + LTG) may also be combined with topiramate or clobazam (Schmidt & Bourgeois, 2000), or with one or two of the following medications: felbamate, levetiracetam, rufinamide, topiramate, or zonisamide (Ferrie & Patel, 2009). Two anticonvulsants have a special status as "orphan drugs" in the LGS: felbamate (FBM) and rufinamide (RUF). Hence, a relative consensus has been reached concerning a therapy combining several broad-spectrum antiepileptic drugs, starting with the VPA + LTG combination, as using if necessary FBM or RUF, or one of many other options.

In the recent study of Auvin *et al.* (2017) perampanel as adjunctive therapy showed to be efficacious and generally well tolerated in 13 children and adolescents with the LGS. After a mean follow-up of 10.8 months, 9/13 patients (69.2%) were responders (≥ 50% reduction in total seizure frequency); 4/13 patients (30.8%) discontinued perampanel due to lack of efficacy (2/13 patients) and seizure aggravation (2/13 patients). For 7/13 patients (53.8%) an improvement of cognitive functions and/or behavior was reported. With perampanel, similar results were found in an adult Lennox Gastaut population. In this study forty-five of the seventy patients were responders (63% of population) with a decrease of seizure frequency ≥ 50% (Crespel *et al.*, submitted 2019).

Potential exacerbation with antiepileptic drugs

It has long been demonstrated that intravenous injections of benzodiazepine can induce or worsen tonic status epilepticus: nitrazepam (Martin, 1970), nitrazepam or clonazepam (Tassinari *et al.*, 1972), diazepam (Prior *et al.*, 1972). Gabapentin can also worsen seizures in LGS (Vossler, 1996). Cuzzola *et al.* (2010) observed paradoxical aggravation in 3 consecutive LGS subjects at onset of treatment with lacosamide, a finding confirmed by Andrade-Machado *et al.* (2015), who nevertheless found that some patients (3 out of 19) experienced improvement, particularly in GTCS and in focal seizures, while Miskin *et al.* (2016) found improvement in 7 out of 8 patients, with no case of aggravation.

Management during periods of exacerbation

During periods of exacerbation due to natural evolution of the syndrome or an intercurring event, treatment of non-convulsive status epilepticus or an increased incidence of seizures should be non-aggressive and limited to avoid overtreatment. Indeed, transitory exacerbation can often be controlled by maintaining or increasing the patient's usual drug therapy, or with adjuvant use of benzodiazepines. In more severe cases, IV injections of benzodiazepines can be administered, provided that the patient is closely monitored to avoid aggravation of tonic seizures (Garcia de Alba *et al.*, 1987). Effectiveness of propofol has also been reported in absence status (Crouteau *et al.*, 1998). In cases of severe aggravation, the authors of several studies have recommended steroids (Brett, 1988; Nair & Snead, 2008), but their administration should remain exceptional due to the risk of side effects, dependence; barbiturate-induced coma may be used (Riikonen *et al.*, 1987; Saukkonen, 1987). Status epilepticus with generalized tonic-clonic seizures or refractory tonic seizures can be treated with IV phenytoin or fosphenytoin.

Non-conventional drug therapies

Because LGS remains a very serious syndrome, many trials with non-conventional drug therapies have been carried out, with mostly anecdotal evidence (overview, Genton *et al.*, 2009). The most commonly tested therapies are: bromide salts, TRH (thyreotropin releasing hormone) and its analogues, allopurinol, vitamin B6 (pyridoxine), tryptophane, carnitine, immunoglobulins, ACTH and corticosteroids, and general anesthesia with barbiturates.

– *Cannabidiol (CBD)* has some evidence of efficacy and an adequate safety profile as adjunctive therapy in children and young adults with treatement-resistant epilepsies (Stockings *et al.*, 2018). An open-label uncontrolled trial (Devinsky *et al.*, 2016) including 30 LGS patients treated with CBD, showed a median reduction of 36.8% of motor seizures over a period of 12 weeks, with a prominent efficacy in atonic (- 68.8%) and tonic seizures (-44%). In the recent randomized, double-blind, placebo-controlled phase 3 trial (Thiele *et al.*, 2018) 171 LGS patients received 20 mg/kg oral CBD daily (86 patients) or placebo (85 patients). The median reduction in monthly drop seizure frequency was 43.9% in the CBD group and 21.8% in the placebo group, with an estimated median difference between the two groups of -17.21. Adverse events occurred in 86% of patients of the CBD group and 69% of patients in the placebo group and the most common adverse events were diarrhea, somnolence, pyrexia, decreased appetite and vomiting.

– *The ketogenic diet* has been recommended by several authors for children with severe epilepsy, amongst which LGS. Freeman *et al.* (2009) have studied the effectiveness of the ketogenic diet *vs.* an inactivated ketogenic diet with glucose intake in a series of 20 LGS subjects. Seizure frequency decreased significantly and rapidly in the ketogenic diet group. A literature review of 18 studies that included outcome data specifically for patients with LGS found that 47% of children experienced > 50% of seizure frequency reduction after 3–36 months of ketogenic diet (Lemmon *et al.*, 2012). This diet can be proposed in young LGS patients during periods of aggravation, but implementation is more difficult in adults. The ketogenic diet has been found to be effective in particular when combined with valproate (Lyczkowski *et al.*, 2005).

Surgical treatment

Vagus nerve stimulation

The effect of vagus nerve stimulation (VNS) has been studied in subjects with refractory epilepsies, including some cases of LGS (Hornig *et al.*, 1997; Lundgren *et al.*, 1998; Ben-Menachem *et al.*, 1999; Shahwan *et al.*, 2009; Müller *et al.*, 2010; Cersosimo *et al.*, 2010). The effectiveness of VNS was demonstrated, with more than 50% responders in the LGS group. However, the results in several other trials were less favourable for LGS compared to the other epilepsies (Labar, 2004; Buoni *et al.*, 2004; Casazza *et al.*, 2006; Rychlicki *et al.*, 2006; Colicchio *et al.*, 2010). In studies with LGS subjects only (Hosain *et al.*, 2000; Frost *et al.*, 2001; Kostov *et al.*, 2009), patient response was favourable with decreased seizure frequency ranging from 50 to 60%. In 2001, Frost *et al.* observed an 88% decrease in fall frequency and an 81% decrease in atypical absences, and in 2009, Kostov *et al.* observed an 80% decrease in atonic seizures, and a 73% decrease in tonic seizures. An evidence-based guideline published by the American Academy of Neurology (AAN) included a pooled analysis of 4 studies with a total of 113 LGS patients treated with VNS and demonstrated a responder rate of 55% (Morris *et al.*, 2013). On the basis of this evidence, the AAN recommended that VNS may be considered as a treatment option for patients with LGS with a level of evidence C. The results were less favourable in several other studies (Majoie *et al.*, 2001; Aldenkamp *et al.*, 2002; Majoie *et al.*, 2005) with approximately 20% responders and better results with atypical absences. VNS can also improve cognitive skills, alertness, behaviour, and sometimes intellectual abilities and mood control in LGS (Frost *et al.*, 2001; Majoie *et al.*, 2001, 2005). Improved cognitive skills were observed regardless of seizure control. When assessed, quality of life is improved as well (Lundgren *et al.*, 1998; Frost *et al.*, 2001; Aldenkamp *et al.*, 2002). The few side effects observed in the studies were transitory (cough, modified voice, dyspnea, neck stiffness). The cost of VNS (ca 9,500 euros) is compensated within 2.3 years (Boon *et al.*, 1999; Majoie *et al.*, 2001). In a comparative study of callosotomy *vs.* VNS in LGS subjects, You *et al.* (2008) found no statistically significant difference between the two methods (63.7% responders with callosotomy *vs.* 70% with VNS). No statistically significant difference was reported for side effects, although morbidity appeared to be lower with VNS.

Corpus callosotomy

The technique of corpus callosotomy was described by Van Wagenen & Herren in 1940. It has mainly been used as a surgical therapy for LGS (Williamson, 1985). The more complete the resection is, the higher the risk of complications, in particular neuropsychological (Gazzaniga *et al.*, 1975; Ledoux *et al.*, 1977; Sass *et al.*, 1988; Smith *et al.*, 2001). Callosotomy has been discussed in a large number of publications for severe epilepsy, including LGS (Blume, 1984; Spencer *et al.*, 1987; Andermann & Berkovic, 1988; Engel *et al.*, 1993; Rougier *et al.*, 1997; Kwan *et al.*, 2000; Roberts & Siegel, 2001; Smith *et al.*, 2001; Gates & de Paola, 2004; Cukiert *et al.*, 2006; Roberts, 2008; Tanriverdi *et al.*, 2009). Clinical improvement was observed in 50 to 90% of subjects with a more than 50% decrease in seizure frequency. Callosotomy is particularly effective in reducing falls during atonic and tonic seizures as well as generalized tonic-clonic seizures, especially with posterior resection (Cendes *et al.*, 1993; Spencer *et al.*,

1987; Roberts *et al.*, 1995; Rougier *et al.*, 1997; Kwan *et al.*, 2000, 2001; Maehara & Shimizu, 2001; Cukiert *et al.*, 2006; Turanli *et al.*, 2006; Tanriverdi *et al.*, 2009; Cukiert *et al.*, 2013). Callosotomy is more effective when performed at an early stage (Rougier *et al.*, 1998) and during childhood (Maehara & Shimizu, 2001). Callosotomy is thus currently considered as a palliative treatment in case of failure to respond to drug therapies and VNS, whose efficacy is comparable to callosotomy with lower morbidity rates (Fandino-Franky *et al.*, 2000; Karceski, 2001; Nei *et al.*, 2006; You *et al.*, 2008).

Deep brain stimulation

In the early 2000s, five LGS subjects underwent deep brain stimulation of the centromedian nucleus of the thalamus with favourable results (Velasco *et al.*, 2000, 2001a, 2001b). Thirteen other LGS subjects have undergone deep brain stimulation since (Velasco *et al.*, 2006). Seizure frequency decreased by more than 80% in 8 subjects. Decreased seizure frequency is correlated with improved quality of life. Two patients were seizure-free at the 60- and 93-month follow-up visits. Ictal and interictal EEG abnormalities decreased in all, with normalization in two of them. Cukiert *et al.* (2009) reported observations of four subjects with generalized epilepsy who had undergone callosotomy prior to deep brain stimulation of the centromedian nucleus of the thalamus. Seizure frequency decreased by 65 to 95%. EEG abnormalities were also less frequent (25 to 95%).

Resective epilepsy surgery

Some authors reported successful treatment of a localized lesion in patients with LGS (Dravet, 2008). This situation remains exceptional and most of the time the diagnostic criteria for LGS are not well defined. Wyllie *et al.* (2007) and Gupta *et al.* (2007) published good results of surgery in children with generalized EEG findings and focal lesions, mainly a cortical dysplasia. Lee *et al.* (2010) identified 27 subjects with LGS. Preoperative MRI showed focal cortical dysplasia (18 cases), encephalomalacia (4 cases), unilateral infarction (1 case). Four were classified nonlesional. Ten patients had multilobar resection, 11 had single lobar resection and 6 had a functionnal hemisphrotomy. At a mean of 33.1 months postoperative follow-up, in patients with single lobar resection, 45.5% had no seizure and 9.1% had infrequent seizures. The nonlesional patients had frontal resection. Two became seizure-free but the other two did not have any change. In patients with multilobar resection, 60% had no seizure and 20% had infrequent seizures. In patients with hemispherotomy, 83.3% had no seizure and 16.7% had infrequent seizures. After surgery, an increase in developmental quotient was observed in 14 patients who had no seizure and in two who had infrequent seizures. The authors propose that resective surgery could be considered for children with LGS. In fact, these cases probably correspond to a focal epilepsy with a secondary bilateral synchrony (see differential diagnosis). In these patients a surgical issue can be proposed when MRI, ictal video-EEG and functional neuroimaging show accurate focal onset of seizures.

Other aspects of patient management

Measures should be taken to avoid physical trauma due to seizures and falls (helmets, wheelchair). The living environment should also be adapted to limit the risk of accidents. Education should be provided to the family and caregivers so that they can recognize a phase of exacerbation and adopt the proper attitude by administering the appropriate treatment at onset. At-home management can limit hospitalizations which may be harmful for fragile patients. Treatment should be provided for associated disorders and copathologies. Behavioural and psychiatric disorders associated with LGS should be managed appropriately. In clinical practice, only a very slight worsening of seizures can be observed with classical neuroleptics or other psychotropic substances at moderate dosages, so that there is no reason to deprive patients who could benefit from such medications (Kanner, 2008; Holzhausen *et al.*, 2007).

Conclusion

Lennox-Gastaut syndrome can be considered as a true epileptic syndrome, the archetype of the epileptic encephalopathy, with fairly homogenous clinical presentation and prognosis, and multiple etiologies. It has a chronic course, and in approximately 50% of patients, it evolves in adulthood into non-specific generalized or multifocal epilepsy. It remains a therapeutic challenge, with many treatment options, of which few are highly efficacious. It also remains a challenge to our understanding of physiopathological mechanisms of seizures and of associated disorders characteristic of epileptic encephalopathies. There is ample room for major progress.

REFERENCES ▶

Agapejev S, Padula NA, Morales NM, Lima M (2000): Neurocysticercosis and Lennox-Gastaut syndrome: case report. *Arq Neuropsiquiatr* 58: 538–547.

Aicardi J (1973): The problem of the Lennox syndrome. *Dev Med Child Neurol* 15: 77–80.

Aicardi J, Chevrie JJ (1982): Atypical benign partial epilepsy in childhood. *Dev Med Child Neurol* 24: 281–292.

Aicardi J, Levy-Gomes A (1988): The Lennox Gastaut syndrome: clinical and electroencephalographic features In: Niedermeyer E, Degen R (eds) *The Lennox Gastaut Syndrome*, pp. 25–46. New York: Alan R Liss, Inc.

Aldenkamp AP, Majoie HJ, Berfelo MW, *et al.* (2002): Long-term effects of 24-month treatment with vagus nerve stimulation on behaviour in children with Lennox-Gastaut syndrome. *Epilepsy Behav* 3: 475–479.

Allen AS, Berkovic SF, Cossette P, *et al.* (2013): pi4KConsortium; Epilepsy Phenome/Genome Project. *De novo* mutations in epileptic encephalopathies. *Nature* 501(7466): 217–221.

Alving J (1979): Classification of the epilepsies. An investigation of 402 children. *Acta Neurol Scand* 60: 157–163.

Andermann F, Berkovic S (1988): Secondary generalized epilepsy in patients with hypothalamic hamartoma, precocious puberty and laughing attacks: a study of five patients. In: Niedermeyer E, Degen R (eds) *The Lennox Gastaut Syndrome*, pp. 433–446. New York: Alan R Liss Inc.

Andrade-Machado R, Luque-Navarro-de Los Reyes J, Benjumea-Cuartas V *et al.* (2015): Efficacy and tolerability of add-on Lacosamide treatment in adults with Lennox-Gastaut syndrome: An observational study. *Seizure* 33: 81–87.

Archer JS, Warren AE, Jackson JD, Abbott DF (2014a): Conceptualizing Lennox-Gastaut syndrome as a secondary network epilepsy. *Front Neurol* 5: 225.

Archer AS, Warren AE, Stagnitti MR, Masterton RA, Abbott DF, Jackson GD (2014b): Lennox-Gastaut syndrome and phenotype: secondary network epilepsy. *Epilepsia* 55: 1245–1254.

Arzimanoglou A, French J, Blume WT, *et al.* (2009): Lennox-Gastaut syndrome: a consensus approach on diagnosis, assessment, management, and trial methodology. *Lancet Neurol* 8: 82–93.

Auvin S, Dozieres B, Ilea A, Delanoë C (2017): Use of perampanel in children and adolescents with Lennox-Gastaut Syndrome. *Epilepsy Behav* 74: 59–63.

Avanzini G, de Curtis M, Panzica F, Spreafico R (1989): Intrinsic properties of nucleus reticularis thalami neurones of th rat studied *in vitro*. *J Physiol* 416: 111–122.

AvoliM, Gloor P (1982): Interaction of cortex and thalamus in spike and wave discharges of feline generalized penicillin epilepsy. *Exp Neurol* 76: 196–217.

Avoli M, Goor P (1981): The effects of transients functional depression of the thalamus on spindles and on synchronous epileptic discharges of feline generalized penicillin epilepsy. *Epilepsia* 22: 443–452.

Baldy-Moulinier M, Touchon J, Billiard M, Carriere A, Besset A. Nocturnal sleep studies in the Lennox-Gastaut syndrome. In: Niedermeyer E, Degen R (eds) *The Lennox-Gastaut Syndrome*, pp. 243–260. New York: Alan R Liss Inc.

Battaglia A, Gurrieri F, Bertini E, *et al.* (1997): The inv dup(15) syndrome: a clinically recognizable syndrome with altered behavior, mental retardation, and epilepsy. *Neurology* 48: 1081–1086.

Bauer G, Aichner F, Saltuari L (1983): Epilepsies with diffuse slow spikes and waves of late onset. *Eur Neurol* 22: 344–350.

Beaumanoir A (1981): Les limites du syndrome de Lennox-Gastaut. *Rev EEG Neurophysiol* 11: 468–473.

Beaumanoir A (1982): The Lennox-Gastaut syndrome: a personal study. In: Broughton RJ (ed) *Henri Gastaut and the Marseilles School's Contribution to the Neurosciences*, pp. 85–99. Amsterdam: Elsevier Biomedical Press.

Beaumanoir A (1985): The Lennox-Gastaut syndrome. In: Roger J, Dravet C, Bureau M, Dreifuss FE, Wolf P (eds) *Epileptic Syndromes in Infancy, Childhood and Adolescence*, pp. 89–100. London: John Libbey.

Beaumanoir A, Blume WT (2005): The Lennox-Gastaut syndrome. In: Roger J, Bureau M, Dravet C, Genton P, Tassinari CA, Wolf P (eds) *Epileptic Syndromes in Infancy, Childhood and Adolescence* (4th ed) pp. 125–148. London: John Libbey.

Beaumanoir A, Dravet C (1992): The Lennox-Gastaut syndrome. In: Roger J, Bureau M, Dravet C, Deifuss FE, Perret A, Wolf P (eds) *Epileptic Syndromes in Infancy, Childhood and Adolescence* (2nd ed) pp. 115–132. London: John Libbey.

Beaumanoir A, Foletti G, Magistris M, Volanschi D (1988): Status epilepticus in the Lennox-Gastaut syndrome. In: Niedermeyer E, Degen R (eds) *The Lennox-Gastaut Syndrome*, pp. 283–299.New York: AR Liss.

Beaumanoir A, Martin F, Panagopoulos M, Mundler F (1968): Le syndrome de Lennox. *Schweiz Arch Neurl Neurochr Psychiat* 102: 31–62.

Beilmann A, Napa A, Sööt A, Talvik I, Talvik T (1999): Prevalence of childhood epilepsy in Estonia. *Epilepsia* 40: 1011–1019.

Ben-Menachem E, Hellström K, Waldton C, Augustinsson LE (1999): Evaluation of refractory epilepsy treated with vagus nerve stimulation for up to 5 years. *Neurology* 52: 1265–1267.

Berkovic SF, Harkin L, McMahon JM, *et al.* (2006): *De-novo* mutations of the sodium channel gene SCN1A in alleged vaccine encephalopathy: a retrospective study. *Lancet Neurol* 5: 488–492.

Bisulli F, Baruzzi A, Rosati A, *et al.* (2001): Efficacy of lamotrigine add-on therapy in severe partial epilepsy in adults with drop seizures and secondary bilateral synchrony on EEG. *Epileptic Disord* 3: 151–156.

Blatter-Arifi V (1991): Long term follow-up with Lennox-Gastaut syndrome. Epileptological aspects, psychomotor development and social adaptation. *Shweiz Rund sch Med Praxis* 36: 909–918.

Blume WT (1978): Clinical and electroencephalographic correlates of the multiple independant spike foci pattern in children. *Ann Neurol* 4: 541–547.

Blume WT (1984): Corpus callosum section for seizure control: rationale and review of experimental and clinical data. *Cleve Clin Q* 51: 319–332.

Blume WT (1987): Lennox-Gastaut syndrome. In: Luders HO, Lesser RP (eds) *Epilepsy: Electroclinical Syndrome*, pp. 73–92. Berlin, Heidelberg: Springer Verlag.

Blume WT (1988): The EEG features of the Lennox-Gastaut syndrome. In: Niedermeyer E, Degen R (eds) *The Lennox-Gastaut Syndrome*, pp. 159–176. New York: Allan R Liss Inc.

Blume WT (2001): Pathogenesis of Lennox-Gastaut syndrome: considerations and hypothesis. *Epileptic Disord* 3: 183–196.

Blume WT (2006): Systems and network in tonic seizures and epilepsies in humans. In: Hirsch E, Andermann F, Chauvel P, Engel J, Lopes da Silva F, Luders H (eds) *Generalized Seizures: from Clinical Phenomenology to Underlying Systems and Networks*, pp. 53–67. Paris: John Libbey Eurotext.

Bonanni P, Parmeggiani L, Guerrini R (2002): Different neurophysiologic patterns of myoclonus characterize Lennox-Gastaut syndrome and myoclonic astatic epilepsy. *Epilepsia* 43: 609–615.

Boniver C, Dravet C, Bureau M, Roger J (1987): Idiopathic Lennox-Gastaut syndrome. In: Wolf P, Dam M, Janz D, Dreifuss FE (eds) *Advances in Epileptology*, vol. 16, pp. 195–200. New York: Raven Press.

Boon P, Vonck K, D'Have M, O'Connor S, Vandekerckhove T, De RJ (1999): Cost-benefit of vagus nerve stimulation for refractory epilepsy. *Acta Neurol Belg* 99: 275–280.

Bourrous M, Elibrahimi I, Draiss G, Safini F, Amine M, Bouskraoui M (2010): Characteristics of the children with epilepsy followed in the Marrakech University Hospital. *Rev Neurol (Paris)* 166: 921–926.

Brett EM (1988): The Lennox-Gastaut syndrome: therapeutic aspects. In: Niedermeyer E, Degen R (eds) *The Lennox-Gastaut Syndrome*, pp. 329–339. New York: Allan R Liss Inc.

Browning RA (1985): Role of the brain-stem reticular formation in tonic-clonic seizures: lesion and pharmalogical studies. *Fed Proc* 44: 2425–2431.

Buchhalter JR (1993): Animals models of inherited epilepsy. *Epilepsia* 34 (Suppl 3): 31–41.

Buoni S, Mariottini A, Pieri S, *et al.* (2004): Vagus nerve stimulation for drug-resistant epilepsy in children and young adults. *Brain Dev* 26: 158–163.

Burnham WM (1985): Core mechanisms in generalized convulsions. *Fed Proc* 44: 2442–2445.

Camfield P, Camfield C (2007): Long-term prognosis for symptomatic (secondarily) generalized epilepsies: a population-based study. *Epilepsia* 48: 1128–1132.

Casazza M, Avanzini G, Ferroli P, Villani F, Broggi G (2006): Vagal nerve stimulation: relationship between outcome and electroclinical seizure pattern. *Seizure* 15: 198–207.

Cavazzuti GB (1980): Epidemiology of different types of epilepsy in school age children of Modena, Italy. *Epilepsia* 21: 57–62.

Cendes F, Ragazzo PC, da Costa V, Martins LF (1993): Corpus callosotomy in treatment of medically resistant epilepsy: preliminary results in a pediatric population. *Epilepsia* 34: 910–917.

Cersosimo RO, Bartuluchi M, De Los Santos C, Bonvehi I, Pomata H, Caraballo RH (2010): Vagus nerve stimulation: effectiveness and tolerability in patients with epileptic encephalopathies. *Childs Nerv Syst* 27: 787–792.

Chen SJ, Chang KP, Wong TT, Kwan SY, Hsu ML, Wang CC (2006): Lamotrigine adjunctive therapy in children with refractory epilepsy: a medical center study. *Acta Paediatr Taiwan* 47: 123–126.

Chevrie JJ, Aicardi J (1972): Childhood encephalopathy with slow spike wave. A statistical study of 80 cases. *Epilepsia* 13: 259–271.

Chugani HT, Mazziotta JC, Engel J, Phelps ME (1987): The Lennox Gastaut syndrome. Metabolic subtypes determined by 2deoxy 2 (18 F) fluoroglucose positron emission tomography. *Ann Neurol* 21: 4–13.

Colicchio G, Policicchio D, Barbati G, *et al.* (2010): Vagal nerve stimulation for drug-resistant epilepsies in different age, aetiology and duration. *Childs Nerv Syst* 26: 811–819.

Commission on Classification and Terminology of the International League Against Epilepsy (1989): Proposal for revised classification of epilepsies and epileptic syndromes. *Epilepsia* 50: 389–399.

Conry JA, Ng YT, Paolicchi JM, *et al.* (2009): Clobazam in the treatment of Lennox-Gastaut syndrome. *Epilepsia* 50: 1158–1166.

Coppola G, Caliendo G, Veggiotti P, *et al.* (2002): Topiramate as add-on drug in children, adolescents and young adults with Lennox-Gastaut syndrome: an Italian multicentric study. *Epilepsy Res* 51: 147–153.

Coppola G, Grosso S, Franzoni E, *et al.* (2010): Rufinamide in children and adults with Lennox-Gastaut syndrome: First Italian multicenter experience. *Seizure* 19: 587–591.

Coulter DA, Huguenard JR, Prince DA (1989): Characterization of ethosuximide reduction of low-threshold calcium current in thalamic neurons. *Ann Neurol* 25: 582–593.

Covanis A, Gupta AK, Jeavons PM (1982): Sodium valproate: monotherapy and polytherapy. *Epilepsia* 23: 693–720.

Crespel A, Gélisse P, Tang NPL, Macorig G, Genton P (submitted 2019): Open trial of perampanel in 70 adult patients with Lennox-Gastaut syndrome.

Crouteau D, Shevell M, Rosenblatt B, Dilenge ME, Andermann F (1998): Treatment of absence status in the Lennox-Gastaut syndrome with propofol. *Neurology* 51: 315–316.

Cukiert A, Burattini JA, Mariani PP, *et al.* (2006): Extended, one-stage callosal section for treatment of refractory secondarily generalized epilepsy in patients with Lennox-Gastaut and Lennox-like syndromes. *Epilepsia* 47: 371–374.

Cukiert A, Burattini JA, Cukiert CM, *et al.* (2009): Centro-median stimulation yields additional seizure frequency and attention improvement in patients previously submitted to callosotomy. *Seizure* 18: 588–592.

Cukiert A, Cukiert CM, Burattini JA, *et al.* (2013): Long-term outcome after callosotomy or vagus nerve stimulation in consecutive prospective cohorts of children with Lennox-Gastaut or Lennox-like syndrome and non-specific MRI findings. *Seizure* 22: 396–400.

Cuzzola A, Ferlazzo E, Italiano D, Calabro RS, Bramanti P, Genton P (2010): Does lacosamide aggravate Lennox-Gastaut syndrome? Report on three consecutive cases. *Epilepsy Behav* 19: 650–651.

De Los Reyes EC, Sharp GB, Williams JP, *et al.* (2004): Levetira-cetam in the treatment of Lennox-Gastaut syndrome. *Pediatr Neurol* 30: 254–256.

Delmiro A, Rivera H, García-Silva MT, *et al.* (2013): Whole-exome sequencing identifies a variant of the mitochondrial MT-ND1 gene associated with epileptic encephalopathy: west syndrome evolving to Lennox-Gastaut syndrome. *Hum Mutat* 34: 1623–1627.

Devinsky O, Marsh E, Friedman D, *et al.* (2016): Cannabidiol in patients with treatment-resistant epilepsy: an open-label interventional trial. *Lancet Neurol* 15: 270–278.

Donaldson JA, Glauser TA, Olberding LS (1997): Lamotrigine adjunctive therapy in childhood epileptic encephalopathy (the Lennox-Gastaut syndrome). *Epilepsia* 38: 68–73.

Doose H (1964): Das akinetische Petit Mal. *Arch Psychiatr Nervenk* 205: 625–654.

Doose H (1992): Myoclono-astatic epilepsy. In: Roger J, Bureau M, Dravet C, Deifuss FE, Perret A, Wolf P (eds) *Epileptic Syndromes in Infancy, Childhood and Adolescence* (2nd ed), pp. 103–114. London: John Libbey Eurotext.

Dravet C (1965): *Encéphalopathie épileptique de l'enfant avec pointe-onde lente diffuse*. Thèse, Marseille.

Dravet C (1996): Le syndrome de Lennox-Gastaut et ses frontières. *Epilepsies* 8: 73–88.

Dravet C (1999): The Lennox-Gastaut syndrome from baby to adolescent. In: Nehlig A, Motte J, Moshé SL, Plouin P (eds) *Childhood Epilepsies and Brain Development*, pp. 103–112. London: John Libbey & Co Ltd.

Dravet C (2008): The Lennox-Gastaut syndrome: a surgically remediable epilepsy? In: Luders HO (eds) *Textbook of Epilepsy Surgery*, pp. 384–393. London: Informa Healthcare.

Dravet C, Roger J (1988): The Lennox Gastaut syndrome: historical aspects from 1966 to 1987. In: Niedermeyer E, Degen R (eds) *The Lennox-Gastaut Syndrome*, pp. 9–23. NewYork: Allan R Liss Inc.

Dulac O, N'Guyen T (1993): The Lennox Gastaut syndrome. *Epilepsia* 34 (Suppl 7): 7–17.

Dulac O, Chiron C, Luna D, *et al.* (1991): Vigabatrin in childhood epilepsy. *J Child Neurol* (Suppl 2): 30–37.

Engel J Jr, Van Ness PC, Rasmussen TB, Ojemann LM (1993): Outcome with respect to epileptic seizures. In: Engel J Jr (ed) *Surgical Treatment of the Epilepsies*, pp. 509–521. New York: Raven Press.

Eriksson KJ, Koivikko MJ (1997): Prevalence, classification, and severity of epilepsy and epileptic syndromes in children. *Epilepsia* 38: 1275–1282.

Fandino-Franky J, Torres M, Narino D, Fandino J (2000): Corpus callosotomy in Colombia and some reflections on care and research among the poor in developing countries. *Epilepsia* 41 (Suppl 4): 22–27.

Ferlazzo E, Adjien CK, Guerrini R, *et al.* (2009): Lennox-Gastaut syndrome with late-onset and prominent reflex seizures in trisomy 21 patients. *Epilepsia* 50: 1587–1595.

Ferlazzo E, Nikanorova M, Italiano D, *et al.* (2010): Lennox-Gastaut syndrome in adulthood: clinical and EEG features. *Epilepsy Res* 89: 271–277.

Ferrie CD, Maisey M, Cox T, *et al.* (1996): Focal abnormalities detected by 18FDG PET in epileptic encephalopathies. *Arch Dis Child* 75: 102–107.

Ferrie CD, Patel A (2009): Treatment of Lennox-Gastaut syndrome (LGS). *EurJ Paediatr Neurol* 13: 493–504.

Feucht M, Brantner-Inthaler S (1994): Gamma-vinyl-GABA (vigabatrin) in the therapy of Lennox-Gastaut syndrome: An open study. *Epilepsia* 35: 993–998.

Fisher RS, Niedermeyer E (1987): Depth EEG studies in the Lennox Gastaut syndrome. *Clin Electroencephalogr* 18: 191–200.

Fisher RS, van Emde Boas W, Blume W, *et al.* (2005): Epileptic seizures and epilepsy: definitions proposed by the International League Against Epilepsy (ILAE) and the International Bureau for Epilepsy (IBE). *Epilepsia* 46: 470–472.

Freeman JM, Vining EP, Pillas DJ, Pyzik PL, Casey JC, Kelly LM (1998): The efficacy of the ketogenic diet: a prospective evaluation of intervention in 150 children. *Pediatrics* 102: 1358–1363.

Freeman JM, Vining EP, Kossoff EH, Pyzik PL, Ye X, Goodman SN (2009): A blinded, crossover study of the efficacy of the ketogenic diet. *Epilepsia* 50: 322–325.

Frochtengarten ML, Scarante O (1973): West's syndrome developing into Lennox-Gastaut syndrome in a patient with cerebral cysticercosis. *Arq Neuropsiquiatr* 31: 319–325.

Frost M, Gates J, Helmers SL, *et al.* (2001): Vagus nerve stimulation in children with refractory seizures associated with Lennox-Gastaut syndrome. *Epilepsia* 42: 1148–1152.

Gale K (1985): Mechanisms of seizure control mediated by gamma aminobutyric acid: role of the substantia nigra. *Fed Proc* 44: 2414–2424.

Garcia de Alba GO, Malagon Valdez J, Franco Delgadillo J, Ramos Peek J (1987): Status epilepticus within the Lennox-Gastaut syndrome: clinical characteristics and management. *Clin Electroencephalogr* 18: 89–92.

Gastaut H (1982): The Lennox-Gastaut syndrome: Comments on the syndrome's terminology and nosological position amongst secondary generalized epilepsies of childhood. In: Broughton R (ed) *Henri Gastaut and the Marseilles School's Contribtion to the Neurosciences*, pp. 71–84. Amsterdam: Elsevier Biomedical Press.

Gastaut H, Broughton R (1972): *Epileptic Seizures*. Springfield: Ch C Thomas.

Gastaut H, Gastaut JL (1976): Computerized transverse axial tomography in epilepsy. *Epilepsia* 17: 325–336.

Gastaut H, Zifkin B J (1988): Secondary bilateral synchony and Lennox-Gastaut syndrome. In: Niedermeyer E, Degen R (eds) *The Lennox-Gastaut Syndrome*, pp. 221–242. NewYork: Allan R Liss Inc.

Gastaut H, Roger J, Soulayrol R, *et al.* (1966): Childhood epileptic encephalopathy with diffuse slow spike-waves (otherwise known as "petit mal variant") or Lennox syndrome. *Epilepsia* 7: 139–179.

Gastaut H, Dravet C, Loubier D, *et al.* (1973): Évolution clinique et pronostic du syndrome de Lennox-Gastaut. In: Lugaresi E, Pazzaglia P, Tassinari CA (eds) *Evolution and Prognosis of Epilepsies*, pp. 133–154. Bologna: Aulo Gaggi.

Gates JR, de Paola L (2004): Corpus callosum section for epilepsy. In: Shorvon S, Perucca E, Fish D and Dodson E (eds) *The Treatment of Epilepsy* (2nd ed), pp. 798–811. Oxford: Blackwell Publishing.

Gazzaniga MS, Risse GL, Springer SP, Clark DE, Wilson DH (1975): Psychologic and neurologic consequences of partial and complete cerebral commissurotomy. *Neurology* 25: 10–15.

Genton P, Bureau M (2006): Epilepsy with myoclonic absences. *CNS Drugs* 20(11): 911–916.

Genton P, Dravet C (2007): Lennox-Gastaut syndrome. In: Engel J, Pedley TA, Aicardi J, Moshé S (eds) *Epilepsy: A Comprehensive Textbook*, 2nd ed., pp. 2417–2427. Philadelphia: Lippincott Williams & Wilkins.

Genton P, Gélisse P, Crespel A (2009): *Le syndrome de Lennox-Gastaut*. Paris: John Libbey Eurotext.

Genton P, Guerrini R, Dravet C (2000): The Lennox-Gastaut syndrome. In: Pierre J, Vinken PJ, Bruyn GW (eds) *Handbook of Clinical Neurology*. Vol. 73, revised series 23, pp. 211–222. Amsterdam: Elsevier.

Genton P, Malafosse A, Moulard B, *et al.* (2005): Progressive myoclonus epilepsies. In: Roger J, Bureau M, Dravet C, Genton P, Tassinari CA, Wolf P (eds) *Epileptic Syndromes in Infancy, Childhood and Adolescence* (4th ed.), pp. 441–465. Paris: John Libbey Eurotext.

Gibbs FA (1938): The electroencephalogram in epileptic seizures. *Tabul Biol* 16: 128.

Gibbs FA, Gibbs EL (1952): *Atlas of Electroencephalography*, vol. 1, pp. 31–54. Adison-Wesley: Reading Mass.

Gibbs FA, Gibbs EL, Lennox WG (1939): The influence of the blood sugar level on the wave and spike formation in Petit Mal epilepsy. *Arch Neurol Psychiat* 41: 111–116.

Glauser TA, Levisohn PM, Ritter F, Sachdeo RC (2000): Topiramate in Lennox-Gastaut syndrome: open-label treatment of patients completing a randomized controlled trial. Topiramate YL Study Group. *Epilepsia* 41 (Suppl 1): 86–90.

Glauser TA, Kluger G, Sachdeo R, Krauss G, Perdomo C, Arroyo S (2008): Rufinamide for generalized seizures associated with Lennox-Gastaut syndrome. *Neurology* 71: 1950–1958.

Gloor P, Quesney LF, Zumstein H (1977): Pathophysiology of generalized penicillin epilepsy in the cat: the role of cortical and subcortical structures. II. Topical application of penicillin to the cerebral cortex and the subcortical structures. *Electroencephalogr Clin Neurophysiol* 43: 79–94.

Goldsmith IL, Zupanc ML, Buchhalter JR (2000): Long-term outcome in 74 patients with Lennox-Gastaut syndrome: effects of incorporating MRI head imaging in defining the cryptogenic subgroup. *Epilepsia* 41: 395–399.

Gowers WR (1885): *Epilepsy and Other Convulsive Disorders. Their Causes, Symptoms and Treatment.* London: Wood.

Guerreiro MM, Manreza ML, Scotoni AE, *et al.* (1999): A pilot study of topiramate in children with Lennox-Gastaut syndrome. *Arq Neuropsiquiatr* 57: 167–175.

Guerrini R (2005): Genetic malformations of the cerebral cortex and epilepsy. *Epilepsia* 46 (Suppl 1): 32–37.

Guerrini R, Dravet C, Ferrari AR, *et al.* (1993): The evolution of epilepsy in the most common genetic forms with mental retardation (Down's syndrome and the fragile X syndrome). *Pediatr Med Chir* 15 (Suppl 1): 19–22.

Gupta A, Chirla A, Wyllie E, Lachhwani DK, Kotagal P, Bingaman WE (2007): Pediatric epilepsy surgery in focal lesions and generalized electroencephalogram abnormalities. *Pediatr Neurol* 37: 8–15.

Gur RC, Sussman NM, Alavi A, *et al.* (1982): Positron emission tomography in two cases of childhood epileptic encephalopathy (Lennox-Gastaut syndrome) *Neurology* 32: 1191–1194.

Guy NTM, Batini C, Naquet R, Teillet MA (1993): Avian photogenic epilepsy and embryogenic chimeras: neuronal activity of the adult prosencephalon and mesencephalon. *Exp Brain Res* 93: 196–204.

Guye M, Bartolomei F, Gastaut JL, Chauvel P, Dravet C (2001): Absence epilepsy with fast rhythmic discharges during sleep: an intermediary form of generalized epilepsy? *Epilepsia* 42: 351–356.

Hahn A, Pistohl J, Neubauer BA, Stephani U (2001): Atypical "benign" partial epilepsy or pseudo-Lennox syndrome. Part I: symptomatology and long-term prognosis. *Neuropediatrics* 32: 1–8.

Heiskala H (1997): Community-based study of Lennox Gastaut syndrome. *Epilepsia* 38: 526–531.

Heiskala H, Launes J, Pihko H, Nikkinen P, Santavuori P (1993): Brain perfusion SPECT in children with frequent fits. *Brain Dev* 15: 214–218.

Herpin T (1867): *Des accès incomplets d'épilepsie*. Paris: Baillère.

Herranz JL, Casas-Fernândez C, Campistol J, *et al.* (2010): Lennox-Gastaut syndrome in Spain: a descriptive retrospective epidemiological study. *Rev Neurol* 50: 711–717.

Hirt HR (1996): Nosology of Lennox-Gastaut syndrome. *Nervenarzt* 67: 109–122.

Hoffmann-Riem M, DienerW, BenningerC, *et al.* (2000): Nonconvulsive status epilepticus-a possible cause of mental retardation in patients with Lennox-Gastaut syndrome. *Neuropediatrics* 31: 169–174.

Holmes GL (1988): Myoclonic, tonic and atonic seizures in children. *J Epilepsy* 1: 173–195.

Holzhausen SP, Guerreiro MM, Baccin CE, Montenegro MA (2007): Use of risperidone in children with epilepsy. *Epilepsy Behav* 10: 412–416.

Hornig GW, Murphy JV, Schallert G, Tilton C (1997): Left vagus nerve stimulation in children with refractory epilepsy: an update. *South Med J* 90: 484–488.

Hosain S, Nikalov B, Harden C, *et al.* (2000): Vagus nerve stimulation treatment for Lennox-Gastaut syndrome. J *Child Neurol* 15: 509–512.

Hosain SA, Green NS, Solomon GE, Chutorian A (2003): Nitrazepam for the treatment of Lennox-Gastaut syndrome. *Pediatr Neurol* 28: 16–19.

Huber B, Hauser I, Horstmann V, *et al.* (2007): Long-term course of epilepsy in a large cohort of intellectually disabled patients. *Seizure* 16: 35–42.

Hughes JR, Patil VK (2002): Long-term electro-clinical changes in the Lennox-Gastaut syndrome before, during and after the slow spike-wave pattern. *Clin Electroencephalogr* 33: 1–7.

Iinuma K, Yanai K, Yanagisawa T, *et al.* (1987): Cerebral glucose metabolism in five patients with Lennox-Gastaut syndrome. *Pediatr Neurol* 3: 12–18.

Janz D (1969): *Die Epilepsien.* Stuttgart: Georg Thieme.

Janz D (1972): Lennox syndrom (akinetisches Petit Mal myoclonisch-astatisches Petit Mal). Epilepsie mit langsamer Spike-Wave Variante. In: *Psychiatric Gegenwart. Forschung und Praxis*, 2nd ed, vol. 2, pp. 585–587. Berlin: Springer.

Kaminska A, Ickowicz A, Plouin P, Bru MF, Dellatolas G, Dulac O (1999): Delineation of cryptogenic Lennox Gastaut syndrome and myoclonic astatic epilepsy using multiple correspondence analysis. *Epilepsy Res* 36: 15–29.

Kanner AM (2008): The use of psychotropic drugs in epilepsy: what every neurologist should know. *Semin Neurol* 28: 379–388.

Karbowski K, Vasella F, Schneider J (1970): Electroencephalographic aspects of Lennox syndrome. *Eur Neurol* 4: 301–311.

Karceski S (2001): Vagus nerve stimulation and Lennox-Gastaut syndrome: a review of the literature and data from the VNS patient registry. *CNS Spectr* 6: 766–770.

Kelly KM, Gross RA, Macdonald RM (1990): Valproic acid selectively reduces the low-threshold (T) calcifum current in rat nodose neurons. *Neurosci Lett* 116: 233–238.

Kieffer-Renaux V, Jambaqué I, Kaminska A, Dulac O (1997): Evolution neuropsychologique des enfants avec syndromes de Lennox-Gastaut et de Doose. *ANAE* 42: 84–88.

Kluger G, PellockJM, Perucca E, Wheless JW (2009): Lennox-Gastaut syndrome: a consensus approach on diagnosis, assessment, management, and trial methodology. *Lancet Neurol* 8: 82–93.

Kobayashi Y, Yoshino A (1999): Acaseof invdup (15) mosaic with mental retardation and symptomatic generalized epilepsy. No *To Shinkei* 51: 259–262.

Kondo M, Fukao T, Teramoto T, *et al.* (2005): A common variable immunodeficient patient who developed acute disseminated encephalomyelitis followed by the Lennox-Gastaut syndrome. *Pediatr Allergy Immunol* 16: 357–360.

Kostov K, Kostov H, Taubell E (2009): Long-term vagus nerve stimulation in the treatment of Lennox-Gastaut syndrome. *Epilepsy Behav* 16: 321–324.

Kramer U, Nevo Y, Neufeld MY, Fatal A, Leitner Y, Harel S (1998): Epidemiology of epilepsy in childhood: a cohort of 440 consecutive patients. *Pediatr Neurol* 18: 46–50.

Kreindler A, Zuckermann E, Steriade M, Chiminion D (1958): Electroclinical features of convulsions induced by stimulation of the brain stem. *J Neurophysiol* 2: 430–436.

Kwan SY, Wong TT, Chang KP, *et al.* (2000): Seizure outcome after corpus callosotomy: the Taiwan experience. *Childs Nerv Syst* 16: 87–92.

Kwan SY, Wong TT, Chang KP, Yang TF, Lee YC, Guo WY, Su MS (2001): Seizure outcomes after anterior callosotomy in patients with posterior-dominant and with anterior-dominant epileptiform discharges. *Childs Nerv Syst* 17: 71–75.

Labar D (2004): Vagus nerve stimulation for 1 year in 269 patients on unchanged antiepileptic drugs. *Seizure* 13: 392–398.

Lagenstein I, Sternowsky HJ, Koepp P, Leiber U (1978): Myoclonic-astatic seizures (Lennox syndrome) in the course of juvenile neuronal ceroid-lipofuscinosis. *Klin Padiatr* 190: 507–511.

Lawrence KM, Mei D, Newton MR, Leventer RJ, Guerrini R, Berkovic SF (2010): Familial Lennox-Gastaut syndrome in male siblings with a novel DCX mutation and anterior pachygyria. *Epilepsia* 51: 1902–1905.

Ledoux JE, Risse GL, Springer SP, Wilson DH, Gazzaniga MS (1977): Cognition and commissurotomy. *Brain* 100: 87–104.

Lee IH, Kwan SY, Su MS (2001): Eating seizures in Lennox-Gastaut syndrome. *Eur Neurol* 45: 123–125.

Lee YJ, Kang HC, Lee JS, *et al.* (2010): Resective pediatric epilepsy surgery in Lennox-Gastaut syndrome. *Pediatrics* 125: e58–66.

Lemmon ME, Terao NN, Ng YT, Reisig W, Rubenstein JE, Kossoff EH (2012): Efficacy of the ketogenic diet in Lennox-Gastaut syndrome: a retrospective review of one institution's experience and summary of the literature. *Dev Med Child Neurol* 54: 464–468.

Lennox WG (1945): The petit mal epilepsies. Their treatment with tridione. *JAMA* 129: 1069–1074.

Lennox WG, Davis JP (1950): Clinical correlates of the fast and the slow spikes-waves electroencephalogram. *Pediatrics* 5: 626–644.

Linuma K, Yanai K, Yanagisawa T, *et al.* (1987): Cerebral glucose metabolism in five patients with Lennox-Gastaut syndrome. *Pediat Neurol* 3: 12–18.

Loubier D (1974): *Le syndrome de Lennox-Gastaut: modalités évolutives.* Marseille. Thesis.

Lugaresi E, Pazzaglia P, Franck L, *et al.* (1973): Evolution and prognosis of primary generalized epilepsy of the petit mal absence type. In: Lugaresi E, Pazzaglia P, Tassinari CA (eds) *Evolution and Prognosis of Epilepsy*, pp. 2–22. Bologna: Aulo Gaggi.

Lund C, Brodtkorb E, Øye AM, Røsby O, Selmer KK (2014): CHD2 mutations in Lennox-Gastaut syndrome. *Epilepsy Behav* 33: 18–21.

Lundgren J, Amark P, Blennow G, Strömblad LG, Wallstedt L (1998): Vagus nerve stimulation in 16 children with refractory epilepsy. *Epilepsia* 39: 809–813.

Lyczkowski DA, Pfeifer HH, Ghosh S, Thiele EA (2005): Safety and tolerability of the ketogenic diet in pediatric epilepsy: effects of valproate combination therapy. *Epilepsia* 46: 1533–1538.

Maehara T, Shimizu H (2001): Surgical outcome of corpus callosotomy in patients with drop attacks. *Epilepsia* 42: 67–71.

Majoie HJ, Berfelo MW, Aldenkamp AP, *et al.* (2005): Vagus nerve stimulation in patient with catastrophic childhood epilepsy, a 2-year follow-up study. *Seizure* 14: 10–18.

Majoie HJ, Berfelo MW, Aldenkamp AP, Evers SM, Kessels AG, Renier WO (2001): Vagus nerve stimulation in children with therapy-resistant epilepsy diagnosed as Lennox-Gastaut syndrome: clinical results, neuropsychological effects, and cost-effectiveness. *J Clin Neurophysiol* 18: 419–428.

Marcus EM Watson CW, Simon SA (1968): An experimental model of some varieties of petit mal epilepsies. Electrical-behavioral correlations of acute bilateral epileptogenic foci in cerebral cortex. *Epilepsia* 9: 233–248.

Markand ON (1977): Slow spike-wave activity in EEG and associated clinical features: often called "Lennox" or "Lennox-Gastaut" syndrome. *Neurology* 27: 746–757.

Markand ON (2003): The Lennox Gastaut syndrome (chilhood epileptic encephalopathy). *J Clin Neurophysiol* 20: 426–441.

Martin D (1970): Intravenous nitrazepam (Mogadon) in the treatment of epilepsy. *Neuropediatrie* 2: 27–37.

Matsuishi T, Yoshino M, Tokunaga O, Katafuchi Y, Yamashita F (1985): Subacute necrotizing encephalomyelopathy (Leigh disease): report of a case with Lennox-Gastaut syndrome. *Brain Dev 7:* 500–504.

Mereen HK, Pijn JP, Van Luijtelaar EL, Coenen AM, Lopes da Silva FH (2002): Cortical focus drives widespread corticothalamic networks during spontaneous absence seizures in rats. *J Neurosci* 22: 1480–1495.

Miskin C, Khurana DS, Valencia I, *et al.* (2016):Efficacy and Tolerability of Lacosamide in the Treatment of Children With Refractory Generalized Epilepsy. *J Child Neurol* 31: 925–928.

Mitsufuji N, Ikuta H, Yoshioka H, Sawada T (1996): Lennox-Gastaut syndrome associated with leukoencephalopathy. *Pediatr Neurol* 15: 63–65.

Miyauchi T, Nomura Y, Ohno S, Kishimoto H, Matsushita M (1988): Positron emission tomography in three case of Lennox-Gastaut syndrome. *Jp J Psychiatry Neurol* 42: 795–804.

Morita DA, GlauserTA (2008): Lennox-Gastaut syndrome. In: PellockJM, Bourgeois BFD, Dodson WE (eds) *Pediatric Epilepsy*, 3rd ed., pp. 307–322. New York: Demos.

Morris GL III, Gloss D, Buchhalter J, Mack KJ, Nickels K, Harden C (2013): Evidence-based guideline update: vagus nerve stimulation for the treatment of epilepsy: report of the Guideline Development Subcommittee of the American Academy of Neurology. *Neurology* 81: 1453–1459.

Motte J, Trevathan E, Arvidsson JF, Barrera MN, Mullens EL, Manasco P (1997): Lamotrigine for generalized seizures associated with the Lennox-Gastaut syndrome. Lamictal Lennox-Gastaut Study Group. *N Engl J Med* 337: 1807–1812.

Müller K, Fabo D, Entz L, *et al.* (2010): Outcome of vagus nerve stimulation for epilepsy in Budapest. *Epilepsia* 51 (Suppl 3): 98–101.

Nabbout R, Desguerre I, Sabbagh S, *et al.* (2008): An unexpected EEG course in Dravet syndrome. *Epilepsy Res* 81: 90–95.

Nair RR, Snead OC III (2008): ACTH and steroids. In: Pollock JM, Bourgeois BFD, Dodson WE, Nordli DR, Sankar R (eds) *Pediatric Epilepsy. Diagnosis and Therapy*, 3rd ed., pp. 543–546. New York: Demos.

Nei M, O'Connor M, Liporace J, Sperling MR (2006): Refractory generalized seizures: response to corpus callosotomy and vagal nerve stimulation. *Epilepsia* 47: 1115–1122.

Niedermeyer E (1969): The Lennox-Gastaut syndrome, a severe type of childhood epilepsy. *Dtsch Z Nervenheilk* 195: 263–282.

Niedermeyer E, Degen R (1988): *The Lennox-Gastaut Syndrome*. New York: Allan R. Liss.

Nokelainen P, Heiskala H, Raininko R, *et al.* (2001): Two brothers with macrocephaly, progressive cerebral atrophy and abnormal white matter, severe mental retardation, and Lennox-Gastaut spectrum type epilepsy: an inherited encephalopathy of childhood? *AmJ Med Genet* 103: 198–206.

Oguni H, Hayashi K, Osawa M (1996): Long term prognosis of Lennox-Gastaut syndrome. *Epilepsia* 37 (Suppl 3): 44–47.

Ohtahara S (2006): Zonisamide in the management of epilepsy-Japanese experience. *Epilepsy Res* 68 (Suppl 2): 25–33.

Ohtahara S, Yamamoshi Y, Ohtsuka Y (1976): Prognosis of the Lennox-Gastaut syndrome. *Folia Psychiatr Neurol Jpn* 30: 275–287.

Ohtahara S, Ohtsuka Y, Yoschinaga H, *et al.* (1988): Lennox-Gastaut syndrome: etiological considerations. In: Niedermeyer E, Degen R (eds) *The Lennox-Gastaut Syndrome*, pp. 47–63. New York: Allan R Liss Inc.

Ohtahara S, Ohtsuka Y, Kobayashi K (1995): Lennox-Gastaut syndrome: a new vista. *Psychiatr Clin Neurosc* 49: S179-S183.

Ohtsuka Y, Amato R, Mizukawa M, Ohtahara S (1990): Long-term prognosis of the Lennox-Gastaut syndrome. *Japan J Psych Neurol* 44: 257–264.

Ohtsuka Y, Amano R, Mizukawa M, Maniwa S, Ohtahara S (1991): Long term prognosis of the Lennox-Gastaut syndrome: considerations in its evolutional changes. In: Fukuyama Y, Kamoshita S, Ohtsuka C, Suzuki Y (eds) *Modern Perspectives of Child Neurology*, pp. 215–222. Tokyo: The Japanese Society of Child Neurology.

Ohtsuka Y, Ohmori I, Oka E (1998): Long-term follow-up of childhood epilepsy associated with tuberous sclerosis. *Epilepsia* 39: 1158–1163.

Oller Daurella L (1970): Un type spécial de crises observées dans le syndrome de Lennox-Gastaut d'apparition tardive. *Rev Neurol (Paris)* 122: 459–462.

Oller Daurella L (1973): Évolution et pronostic du syndrome de Lennox-Gastaut. In: Lugaresi E, Pazzaglia P, Tassinari C (eds) *Evolution and Prognosis of Epilepsies*, pp. 155–164. Bologna: Auto Gaggi.

Olmos Garcia de Alba G, Gamboa Marrufo JD, Rengifo Ramos O, *et al.* (1987): Rett's syndrome with Lennox-Gastaut pattern. *Clin Electroencephalogr* 18: 187–190.

Orrico A, Zollino M, Galli L, Buoni S, Marangi G, Sorrentino V (2009): Late-onset Lennox-Gastaut syndrome in a patient with 15q11.2-q13.1 duplication. *Am J Med Genet* 149: 1033–1035.

Palmini A, Andermann F, Aicardi J, *et al.* (1991): Diffuse cortical dysplasia, or the "double cortex" syndrome: the clinical and epileptic spectrum in 10 patients. *Neurology* 41: 1656–1662.

Parrini E, Ferrari AR, Dorn T, Walsh CA, Guerrini R (2009): Bilateral frontoparietal polymicrogyria, Lennox-Gastaut syndrome, and GPR56 gene mutations. *Epilepsia* 50: 1344–1353.

Patry G, Lyagoubi S, Tassinari CA (1971): Subclinical electrical status epilepticus induced by sleep. An electroencephalographical study of six cases. *Arch Neurol* 24: 242–252.

Pellegrini A, Musgrave J, Gloor P (1979): Role of imput of subcortical origin in the genesis of bilaterally synchonous epileptic discharge ob feline generalized penicillin epilepsy. *Exp Neurol* 64: 155–173.

Penfield W, Jasper H (1954): *Epilepsy and the Functional Anatomy of the Human Brain*. London: J & A Churchill.

Perucca E, Gram L, Avanzini G, Dulac O (1998): Antiepileptic drugs as a cause of worsening seizures. *Epilepsia* 39: 5–17.

Pillay N, Archer JS, Badawy RA, Flanagan DF, Berkovic SF, Jackson G (2013): Networks underlying paroxusmal fast activity and slow spike and wave in Lennox-Gastaut syndrome. *Neurology* 81: 665–673.

Prior PD, Maclaine GN, Scott DF, Laurance BM (1972): Tonic status epilepticus precipitated by intravenous diazepam in a child with Petit Mal Status. *Epilepsia* 13: 467–472.

Rantala H, Putkonen T (1999): Occurrence, outcome, and prognostic factors of infantile spasm and Lennox-Gastaut. *Epilepsia* 40: 286–289.

Renier WO (1988): Neuromorphological and biochemical analysis of a brain biopsy in a second case of idiopathic Lennox-Gastaut syndrome. In: Niedermeyer E, Degen R (eds) *The Lennox-Gastaut Syndrome*, pp. 427–432. New York: Allan R Liss Inc.

Ricci S, Cusmai R, Fariello G, Fusco L, Vigevano F (1992): Double cortex. A neuronal migration anomaly as a possible cause of Lennox-Gastaut syndrome. *Arch Neurol* 49: 61–64.

Riikonen R, Santavuori P, Mertoja O, Sainio K, Neuvonen PJ, Tokola RA (1987): *Effect of short barbiturate anesthesia on infantile spasms*. Paper presented at the EFCNS meeting in Helsinki.

Roberts DW (2008): Corpus callosotomy. In: Engel J, Pedley TA (eds) *Epilepsy. A Comprehensive Textbook*, 2nd ed., pp. 1907–1913. Philadelphia: Lippincott-Raven New York.

Roberts DW, Siegel AM (2001): Corpus callosotomy. In: Luders HO, Comair YG (eds) *Epilepsy Surgery*, 2nd ed., pp. 747–756. Philadelphia: Lippincott Williams & Wilkins.

Roberts DW, Reeves AG, Nordgren RE (1995): The role of posterior callosotomy in patients with suboptimal response to anterior callosotomy. In: Reeves AG, Roberts DW (eds) *Epilepsy and the Corpus Callosum*, 2nd ed., pp. 183–190. New York: Plenum Press.

Rocha J, Guerra C, Oliveira R, Dória S, Rego R, Rosas MJ (2012): Late onset Lennox-Gastaut syndrome as a phenotype of 15q11.1q13.3 duplication. *Epileptic Disord* 14: 159–162.

Roger J, Gambarelli-Dubois D (1988): Neuropathological studies of the Lennox-Gastaut syndrome In: Niedermeyer E, Degen R (eds) *The Lennox-Gastaut Syndrome*, pp. 73–93. New York: Allan R Liss Inc.

Roger J, Remy C, Bureau M, *et al.* (1987): Le syndrome de Lennox-Gastaut de l'adulte. *Rev Neurol (Paris)* 143: 401–405.

Roger J, Bureau M, Dravet C (1989): The Lennox-Gastaut syndrome. *Clev ClinJ Med* 56 (Suppl 2): 172–177.

Rougier A, Claverie B, Pedespan JM, Marchal C, Loiseau P (1997): Callosotomy for intractable epilepsy: Overall outcome. *J Neurosurg Sci* 41: 51–57.

Rougier A, Pedespan JM, Marchal C, Loiseau P (1998): Indications et résultats des callosotomies chez l'enfant. In: Bureau M, Kahane P, Munari C (eds) *Epilepsies partielles graves pharmaco-résistantes de l'enfant: stratégies diagnostiques et traitements chirurgicaux*, pp. 236–240. Paris: John Libbey Eurotext.

Rychlicki F, Zamponi N, Trignani R, Ricciuti RA, Iacoangeli M, Scerrati M (2006): Vagus nerve stimulation: clinical experience in drug-resistant pediatric epileptic patients. *Seizure* 15: 483–490.

Sachdeo RC, Glauser TA, Ritter F, Reife R, Lim P, Pledger G (1999): A double-blind, randomized trial of topiramate in Lennox-Gastaut syndrome. Topiramate YL Study Group. *Neurology* 52: 1882–1887.

Sass KJ, Spencer DD, Spencer SS, Novelly RA, Williamson PD, Mattson RH (1998): Corpus callosotomy for epilepsy. II. Neurologic and neuropsychological outcome. *Neurology* 38: 24–28.

Saukkonen AL (1987): *Clinical experience in barbiturate anesthesia in the treatment of intractable epilepsy.* Paper presented on the EFCN meeting in Helsinki.

Scheffer IE, Berkovic S, Capovilla G, *et al.* (2017): ILAE Classification of the epilepsies: position paper of the ILAE commission for classification and terminology. *Epilepsia* 58: 512–521.

Schmidt D, Bourgeois B (2000): A risk-benefit assessment of therapies for Lennox-Gastaut syndrome. *Drug Saf* 22: 467–477.

Selmer KK, Lund C, Brandal K, Undlien DE, Brodtkorb E (2009): *SCN1A* mutation screening in adult patients with Lennox-Gastaut syndrome features. *Epilepsy Behav* 16: 555–557.

Shahwan A, Bailey C, Maxiner W, Simon Harvey A (2009): Vagus nerve stimulation for refractory epilepsy in children: More to VNS than seizure frequency reduction. *Epilepsia* 50: 1220–1228.

Sidenvall R, Forsgren L, Forsgren L, Heijbel J (1996): Prevalence and characteristics of epilepsy in children in northern Sweden. *Seizure* 5: 139–146.

Siniatchkin M, Coropceanu D, Moeller F, Boor R, Stephani U (2011): EEG-fMRI reveals activation of brainstem and thalamus in patients with Lennox-Gastaut syndrome. *Epilepsia* 28: 1528–1567.

Smeraldi E, Sorza-Smeraldi R, Cazzullo CL, Guareschi-Cazzullo A, Fabio G, Canger R (1975): Immunogenetics of Lennox-Gastaut syndrome: Frequency of HLA antigens and halotypes in patients and first degrees relative. *Epilepsia* 16: 699–704.

Smith MC, Byrne R, Kanner AM (2001): Corpus callosotomy and multiple subpial transection. In: Elaine W (ed) *The Treatment of Epilepsy*, 3rd ed., pp. 1175–1184. Philadelphia: Lippincott Williams & Wilkins.

Sorel L (1964): L'épilepsie myokinétique grave de la première enfance avec pointe-ondes lentes (petit mal variant) et son traitement. *RevNeurol (Paris)* 110: 215–233.

Soucek D, Birbamer G, Luef G, Felber S, Kristmann E, Bauer G (1992): Laminar heterotopic grey matter (double cortex) in a patient with late onset Lennox-Gastaut syndrome. *Wien Klin Wochenschr* 104: 607–608.

Spencer SS, Gates JR, Reeves AG, *et al.* (1987): Corpus callosum section for uncontrolled epilepsy. In: Engel J Jr (ed) *Surgical Treatment of the Epilepsies*, pp. 425–444. New York: Raven Press.

Steffenburg U, Hedström A, Lindroth A, Wirklund LM, Hagberg G, Kyllerman M (1998): Intractable epilepsy in a population-based series of mentally retarded children. *Epilepsia* 39: 767–775.

Stockings E, Zagic D, Campbell G, *et al.* (2018): Evidence for cannabis and cannabinoids for epilepsy: a systematic review of controlled and observational evidence. *J Neurol Neurosurg Psychiatry* [Epub ahead of print].

Tanriverdi T, Olivier A, Poulin N, Andermann F, Dubeau F (2009): Long-term seizure outcome after corpus callosotomy: a retrospective analysis of 95 patients. *J Neurosurg* 110: 332–342.

Tassinari CA, Ambrosetto G (1988): Tonic seizures in the Lennox-Gastaut syndrome: semiology and differential diagnosis. In: Niedermeyer E, Degen R (eds). *The Lennox-Gastaut Syndrome*, pp. 109–124. New York: Allan R Liss Inc.

Tassinari CA, Dravet C, Roger J, Cano JP, Gastaut H (1972): Tonic status epilepticus precipitated by intravenous benzodiazepine in five patients with Lennox-Gastaut syndrome. *Epilepsia* 13: 421–435.

Taylor J (1958): *Selected Writings of John Hughlings Jackson*, Vol. I and II. New York: Basic Book Inc.

Teillet MA, Naquet R, Le Gal La Salle G, Merat P, Schuler B, Le Douarin NM (1991): Transfer of genetic epilepsy by ebryonic brain grafts in the chicken. *Proc Natl Acad Sci* 88: 6966–6970.

Terrone G, Bienvenu T, Germanaud D, *et al.* (2014): A case of Lennox-Gastaut syndrome in a patient with FOXG1-related disorder. *Epilepsia* 55(11): e116–e119.

The Felbamate Study Group in Lennox Gastaut syndrome (1993): Efficacy of felbamate in childhood epileptic encephalopathy (Lennox-Gastaut syndrome). *N EnglJ Med* 328: 29–33.

Theodore WH, Rose D, Patronas N, *et al.* (1987): Cerebral glucose metabolism in the Lennox-Gastaut syndrome. *Ann Neurol* 21: 14–21.

Thiele EA, Marsh ED, French JA, *et al.*; GWPCARE4 Study Group (2018): Cannabidiol in patients with seizures associated with Lennox-Gastaut syndrome (GWPCARE4): a randomised, double-blind, placebo-controlled phase 3 trial. *Lancet* 391(10125): 1085–1096.

Thomas P, Valton L, Genton P (2006): Absence and myoclonic status epilepticus precipitated by antiepileptic drugs in idiopathic generalized epilepsy. *Brain* 129: 1281–1292.

Thomé-Souza S, Freitas A, Fiore LA, Valente KD (2003): Lamotrigine and valproate: efficacy of co-administration in a pediatric population. *Pediatr Neurol* 28: 360–364.

Timmings PL, Richens A (1992): Lamotrigine as add-on drug in the management of Lennox-Gastaut syndrome. *Eur Neurol* 32: 305–307.

Timofeev I, Steriade M (2004): Neocortical seizures: initiation, development and cessation. *Neuroscience* 123: 299–336.

Tissot SA (1770): *Traité de l'épilepsie, faisant le Tome troisième du Traité des nerfs et de leurs maladies.* Lausanne: Antoine Chapuis.

Trevathan E, Murphy CC, Yeargin-Allsopp M (1997): Prevalence and descriptive epidemiology of Lennox-Gastaut syndrome among Atlanta children. *Epilepsia* 38: 1283–1288.

Tukel K, Jasper H (1952): The electroencephalogram in parasagittal lesions. *Electroencephal Clin Neurophysiol* 4: 481–494.

Turanli G, Yalnizoglu D, Genç-Açikgöz D, Akalan N, Topçu M (2006): Outcome and long term follow-up after corpus callosotomy in childhood onset intractable epilepsy. *Childs Nerv Syst* 22: 1322–1327.

Van Engelen B, Renier WO, Weemaes CM, *et al.* (1994): High-dose intravenous immunoglobulin treatment in cryptogenic West and Lennox-Gastaut syndrome; an add-on study. *Eur J Pediatr* 153: 762–769.

Van Wagenen WP, Herren RY (1940): Surgical division of commissural pathways in the corpus callosum: relation to spread of an epileptic attack. *Arch Neurol Psychiatry* 44: 740–759.

Vassella F, Pavlincova E, Schneider HJ, *et al.* (1973): Treatment of infantile spasms and Lennox-Gastaut syndrome with clonazepam (Rivotril). *Epilepsia* 14: 165–175.

Velasco AL, Boleaga B, Santos N, Velasco F, Velasco M (1993): Electroencephalographic and magnetic resonance correlations in children with intractable seizures of Lennox-Gastaut syndrome and *Epilepsia partialis continua*. *Epilepsia* 34: 262–270.

Vignoli A, Oggioni G, De Maria G, Peron A, Savini MN, Zambrelli E, Chiesa V, La Briola F, Turner K, Canevini MP (2017): Lennox-Gastaut syndrome in adulthood: Long-term clinical follow-up of 38 patients and analysis of their recorded seizures. *Epilepsy Behav* 77: 73–78.

Velasco AL, Velasco F, Jimenez F, *et al.* (2006): Neuromodulation of the centromedian thalamic nuclei in the treatment of generalized seizures and the improvement of the quality of life in patients with Lennox-Gastaut syndrome. *Epilepsia* 47: 1203–1212.

Velasco F, Velasco M, Jimenez F, *et al.* (2000): Predictors in the treatment of difficult-to-control seizures by electrical stimulation of the centromedian thalamic nucleus. *Neurosurgery* 47: 295–304.

Velasco F, Velasco M, Jimenez F, Velasco AL, Marquez I (2001a): Stimulation of the central median thalamic nucleus for epilepsy. *Stereotact Funct Neurosurg* 77: 228–232.

Velasco M, Velasco F, Velasco AL (2001b): Centromedian-thalamic and hippocampal electrical stimulation for the control of intractable epileptic seizures. *J Clin Neurophysiol* 18: 495–513.

Velizarova R, Gélisse P, Pageaux GP, Genton P, Crespel A (2011): Valproate treatment after liver transplant in a patient with Lennox-Gastaut syndrome. *Seizure* 20: 500–501.

Velisek L, Veliskovâ J, Moshé SL (2002): Electrical stimulation of substantia nigra pars reticulata is anticonvulsant in adult and young male rats. *Exp Neurol* 173: 145–152.

Vergnes M, Marescaux C (1994): Pathophysiological mechanisms underlying genetic absence epilepsy in rats. In: Malafosse A, Genton P, HirschE, Marescaux C,Broglin D, Bernasconi R (eds) *Idiopathic Generalized Epilepsies: Clinical, Experimental and Genetic Aspects*, pp. 151–168. London: John Libbey.

Viani F (1991): Le syndrome de Lennox-Gastaut. Problèmes actuels et perspectives de recherche. *Epilepsies* 3: 179–190.

Vossler DG (1996): Exacerbation of seizures in Lennox-Gastaut syndrome by gabapentin. *Neurology* 46: 852–853.

Wheless JW, Constantinou JEC (1997): Lennox-Gastaut syndrome. *Pediatr Neurol* 17: 203–211.

Williamson PD (1985): Corpus callosum section for intractable epilepsy: criteria for patient selection. In: Reeves AG (ed) *Epilepsy and the Corpus Callosum*, pp. 243–257. New York: Plenum Press.

Wyllie E, Lachhwani DK, Gupta A, *et al.* (2007): Successful surgery for epilepsy due to early brain lesions despite generalized EEG findings. *Neurology* 69: 389–397.

Yagi K (1996): Evolution of Lennox-Gastaut syndrome: a long-term longitudinal study. *Epilepsia* 37 (Suppl 3): 48–51.

You SJ, Kang HC, Ko TS, *et al.* (2008): Comparison of corpus callosotomy and vagus nerve stimulation in children with Lennox-Gastaut syndrome. *Brain* 30: 195–199.

WITH VIDEO SUPPLEMENTS

CHAPTER 13

SELF-LIMITED FOCAL EPILEPSIES IN CHILDHOOD

Veysi Demirbilek[1], Michelle Bureau[2], Özlem Çokar[3] and Chrysostomos P. Panayiotopoulos[4]

[1] Department of Neurology, Cerrahpasa Faculty of Medicine, Istanbul University-Cerrahpasa, Istanbul, Turkey
[2] Centre Saint-Paul, Henri-Gastaut Hospital, Marseille, France
[3] Department of Neurology, Haseki Research and Training Hospital, Health Sciences University, Istanbul, Turkey
[4] Clinical Neurophysiology Dpt, St Thomas'NHS Foundation Trust, London, United Kingdom

Introduction

Self-limited focal epilepsies in childhood, formerly considered as idiopathic focal epilepsies (Pal *et al.*, 2016), affect 25% of children with non-febrile seizures and constitute a significant part of the everyday practice of paediatricians, neurologists and electroencephalographers. They comprise three identifiable electroclinical syndromes recognized by the International League against Epilepsy (ILAE): Rolandic epilepsy, Panayiotopoulos syndrome (PS), a common autonomic epilepsy, which is currently more readily diagnosed and the idiopathic childhood occipital epilepsy of Gastaut (ICOE-G) including the idiopathic photosensitive occipital lobe epilepsy, a less common form with uncertain prognosis. There are also reports of children with benign syndromes of focal seizures with predominantly affective symptoms, and claims have been made for other clinical phenotypes associated with specific interictal EEG foci, such as frontal, midline or parietal, with or without giant somatosensory evoked spikes. Neurological and mental states and brain imaging are normal, though because of their high prevalence any type of benign childhood focal seizures may incidentally occur in children with neurocognitive deficits or abnormal brain scans. The most useful diagnostic test is the EEG. All these conditions may be linked together in a broad, age-related and age-limited, benign childhood seizure susceptibility syndrome (BCSSS) which may be genetically determined (Panayiotopoulos, 1993, 2010). Considering a number of diagnostic, pathogenetic and management uncertainties, BCSSS may need proper multidisciplinary re-assessment in an evidence-based manner.

Classification and nomenclature

The currently valid 1989 ILAE classification recognized three "age-related and localization–related (focal, local, partial) epilepsies and syndromes" (Commission, 1989): i) benign childhood epilepsy with centro-temporal spikes (BCECTS); ii) childhood epilepsy with occipital paroxysms; iii) primary reading epilepsy.

The 2010 ILAE report lists three syndromes of idiopathic focal epilepsies in childhood (Berg *et al.*, 2010): i) benign childhood epilepsy with centro-temporal spikes (BCECTS) (rating score 3); ii) Panayiotopoulos syndrome (rating score 3); and iii) late-onset childhood occipital epilepsy (Gastaut type) (rating score 2) that we prefer to call idiopathic childhood occipital epilepsy of Gastaut (ICOE-G).

The rating score in parenthesis reflects on the certainty with which the ILAE Core Group believed that each syndrome represents a unique diagnostic entity on a range of 1–3 (with 3 being the most clearly and reproducibly defined) (Engel, 2006).

BCECTS and Rolandic epilepsy are used synonymously, although we would prefer the latter because: i) the term "Rolandic epilepsy" has long been established and is better known than BCECTS among paediatricians; ii) most "centro-temporal spikes" (CTSs) are Rolandic spikes; they are rarely located in the temporal electrodes; iii) the word "temporal" is misleading because children with this form of epilepsy do not have symptoms from the temporal lobes, BCECTS may occur without CTSs and conversely CTSs may occur in children without seizures or other clinical phenotypes of BCSSS; iv) similar clinical features may appear in patients with spikes in locations other than at centro-temporal sites.

Benign childhood epilepsy with occipital paroxysms has undergone significant terminological and classification changes because: i) occipital paroxysms may not occur in a significant proportion of patients; hence the new term "occipital epilepsy" has replaced "occipital paroxysms"; ii) the recognition of Panayiotopoulos syndrome as a common idiopathic epilepsy in childhood that is multifocal rather than occipital and clearly different than the ICOE-G; hence only the eponymic nomenclature is now used by the ILAE Commission (Berg *et al.*, 2010). The previous descriptive nomenclature of "early-onset benign childhood occipital epilepsy (Panayiotopoulos type)" has been abandoned (Berg *et al.*, 2010).

A problem in the classification is the new proposal to abandon the terms benign and idiopathic (Berg *et al.*, 2010) which may be unjustifiable and many experts disagree (Vigevano *et al.*, 2009; Wolf, 2010; Ferrie, 2010c). The possible existence of cognitive and language impairment and behavioral disturbances led to the replacement of the terms "idiopathic" or "benign" by "self-limited" in the recent ILAE classification (Scheffer *et al.*, 2017).

Among self-limited focal epilepsies in childhood, RE and PS are age-limited and at least a third of patients have only a single seizure. They should be classified among "Conditions with epileptic seizures that are traditionally not diagnosed as a form of epilepsy *per se*" like benign neonatal seizures and febrile seizures.

Rolandic epilepsy (self-limited epilepsy with centro-temporal spikes)

Rolandic epilepsy is the best known and the most common self-limited focal epilepsy of childhood formerly called "idiopathic or benign childhood epilepsy with centro-temporal spikes" (Beaussart & Faou, 1978; Loiseau *et al.*, 1988; Bouma *et al.*, 1997; Beaussart *et al.*, 1999; Panayiotopoulos, 1999a; Dalla Bernardina *et al.*, 2005; Wirrell *et al.*, 2006; Fejerman *et al.*, 2007; Panayiotopoulos *et al.*, 2008).

Demographic data

The age of onset ranges from 1 to 14 years with 75% starting between 7–10 years. There is a 1.5 male predominance, prevalence is around 15% in children aged 1–15 years with non-febrile seizures and incidence is 10–20/100,000 of children aged 0–15 years (Heijbel *et al.*, 1975; Cavazzuti, 1980; Sidenvall *et al.*, 1996; Astradsson *et al.*, 1998; Berg *et al.*, 1999; Larsson & Eeg-Olofsson, 2006).

Clinical manifestations

The cardinal features of Rolandic seizures are infrequent, often single, focal seizures consisting of: i) unilateral facial sensorimotor symptoms (30% of patients); ii) oropharyngolaryngeal manifestations (53% of patients); iii) speech arrest (40% of patients); iv) hypersalivation (30% of patients) (Beaussart, 1972; Lerman & Kivity, 1975; Bouma *et al.*, 1997; Panayiotopoulos, 1999a; Dalla Bernardina *et al.*, 2005; Wirrell *et al.*, 2006; Fejerman, 2010).

Ictal manifestations indicative of temporal lobe involvement do not occur in Rolandic epilepsy, and the term "centro-temporal" refers only to the spike topography and it is partly a misnomer (see EEG section below).

Hemifacial sensorimotor seizures are often entirely localized in the lower lip or spread to the ipsilateral hand. Motor manifestations are sudden, continuous or bursts of clonic contractions, usually lasting from a few seconds to a minute. Concurrent ipsilateral tonic deviation of the mouth is also common. Hemifacial sensory symptoms consist of unilateral numbness mainly in the corner of the mouth.

Hemifacial seizures are often associated with an inability to speak and hypersalivation: "The left side of my mouth felt numb and started jerking and pulling to the left, and I could not speak to say what was happening to me."

Sensorimotor ictal signs localized to one leg have been reported in some rare instances (Panayiotopoulos *et al.*, 2008; Fusco *et al.*, 2010).

Negative myoclonus can be observed in some cases, as an interruption of tonic muscular activity; the polygraphic EEG/EMG recording will in such instance show that it is time locked to the contralateral spike without evidence of a preceding myoclonus (Watemberg *et al.*, 2009).

Oropharyngolaryngeal ictal manifestations are unilateral sensorimotor symptoms inside the mouth. Numbness, and more commonly paraesthesias (tingling, prickling, freezing), are usually diffuse on one side or, exceptionally, may be highly localised even to one tooth. Motor oropharyngolaryngeal symptoms produce strange sounds, such as death rattle, gargling, grunting and guttural sounds, and combinations: "In his sleep, he was making guttural noises, with his mouth pulled to the right, as if he was chewing his tongue." "We heard her making strange noises like roaring and found her unresponsive, head raised from the pillow, eyes wide open, rivers of saliva coming out of her mouth, rigid."

Arrest of speech is a form of anarthria. The child is unable to utter a single intelligible word and attempts to communicate with gestures. "My mouth opened and I could not speak. I wanted to say I cannot speak. At the same time, it was as if somebody was strangling me."

Hypersalivation, a prominent autonomic manifestation, is often associated with hemifacial seizures, oropharyngolaryngeal symptoms and speech arrest. Hypersalivation is not just frothing: "Suddenly my mouth is full of saliva, it runs out like a river and I cannot speak."

Ictal syncope may occur, probably as a concurrent symptom of Panayiotopoulos syndrome: "She lies there, unconscious with no movements, no convulsions, like a wax work, no life."

Consciousness and recollection are fully retained in more than half (58%) of Rolandic seizures. "I felt that air was forced into my mouth, I could not speak and I could not close my mouth. I could understand well everything said to me. Other times I feel that there is food in my mouth and there is also a lot of salivation. I cannot speak."

In the remainder (42%), consciousness becomes impaired during the ictal progress and in one third there is no recollection of ictal events.

Progression to hemiconvulsions or generalized tonic-clonic seizures (GTCS) occurs in around half of children and hemiconvulsions may be followed by postictal Todd's hemiparesis (Panayiotopoulos, 1999a).

Duration and circadian distribution: Rolandic seizures are usually brief, lasting for 1–3 min. Three-quarters of seizures occur during non-rapid eye movement (NREM) sleep, mainly at sleep onset or just before awakening.

Status epilepticus: Although rare, focal motor status or hemiconvulsive status epilepticus is more likely to occur than secondarily generalised convulsive status epilepticus, which is exceptional (Deonna *et al.*, 1986; Wirrell *et al.*, 1995; Panayiotopoulos, 1999a). Opercular status epilepticus usually occurs in children with atypical evolution (Colamaria *et al.*, 1991; Deonna *et al.*, 1993; Fejerman *et al.*, 2000) or may be induced by carbamazepine or lamotrigine (Caraballo *et al.*, 1989; Parmeggiani *et al.*, 2004). This state lasts for hours to months and consists of ongoing unilateral or bilateral contractions of the mouth, tongue or eyelids, positive or negative subtle perioral or other myoclonus, dysarthria, speech arrest, difficulties in swallowing, buccofacial apraxia and hypersalivation. These are often associated with continuous spikes and waves on an EEG during NREM sleep.

Other seizure types: Despite prominent hypersalivation, focal seizures with primarily autonomic manifestations (autonomic seizures) are not considered part of the core clinical syndrome of Rolandic epilepsy. However, some children may present with independent autonomic seizures or seizures with mixed Rolandic-autonomic manifestations including emesis (see below in the relations between Rolandic epilepsy and PS).

Primarily GTCS are considered part of Rolandic epilepsy by the ILAE (Engel, 2006) and their occurrence cannot be excluded. However, from the published ictal recordings (Watanabe, 1996; Panayiotopoulos, 1999a; Wirrell *et al.*, 2006) and the electroclinically unequivocal focal nature of Rolandic epilepsy, it can be inferred that at least the majority of the GTCS follow Rolandic activation, and are therefore secondarily GTCS. Short lived initial focal symptoms may pass unnoticed in daytime GTCS and are bound to be missed in nocturnal GTCS.

Atypical forms: Rolandic epilepsy may present with atypical manifestations such early age at onset, developmental delay or learning difficulties at inclusion, other seizure types, atypical EEG abnormalities (Datta & Sinclair 2007; Kramer, 2008; Fejerman, 2009; Callenbach *et al.*, 2010).

Diagnostic procedures

Apart from the EEG, all the tests are normal. Brain imaging is not needed for typical cases, although 15% of patients with Rolandic seizures may have abnormal findings because of static or other brain diseases unrelated to the pathophysiology of Rolandic epilepsy (Santanelli *et al.*, 1989; Gélisse *et al.*, 2003; Lundberg *et al.*, 2003).

The presence of brain lesions has no influence on the prognosis of Rolandic seizures (Gélisse *et al.*, 2003).

Electroencephalography

By definition, CTSs are the hallmark of benign childhood epilepsy with CTSs *(Figures 1 and 2)*. However, although called centrotemporal, these spikes are mainly localised in the C3 and C4 (high central) or C5 and C6 (low central) supra-sylvian and not temporal electrodes (Legarda *et al.*, 1994; Panayiotopoulos, 1999a). CTSs are often bilateral and typically activated by drowsiness and NREM sleep, but not by overbreathing (Smith & Kellaway, 1964; Blom & Brorson, 1966; Clemens & Majoros, 1987). CTSs amplify during stages I-IV of sleep by a factor of two to five times without disturbing sleep organization. Somatosensory stimulation is common form of activation of CTSs (10–20%) (De Marco & Tassinari, 1981; Panayiotopoulos, 1999a; Fonseca & Tedrus, 2000; Kubota *et al.*, 2000; Langill & Wong, 2003) and evokes extreme (giant) somatosensory evoked spikes (GSES) *(Figure 2)*, which correspond to mid- or long-latency somatosensory evoked potentials (Manganotti *et al.*, 1998). GSES, like spontaneous CTSs, occur in children with or without seizures and disappear with age. They may be detected in EEGs with or without spontaneous CTSs or other functional spikes of childhood.

In serial EEGs of the same child, CTSs may occur right or left, infrequently or frequently, and appear small or giant, alone or with spikes in other locations. Rarely, children with Rolandic epilepsy may have normal EEG or CTSs may appear only during NREM sleep (3–35%) (Panayiotopoulos, 1999a). The incidence of extra-Rolandic spikes in Rolandic epilepsy is not precisely known but may be significant when these are sought (Drury & Beydoun, 1991).

Dipole EEG (Gregory & Wong, 1992; Tsai & Hung, 1998; Jung *et al.*, 2003), magnetoencephalography (MEG) (Minami *et al.*, 1996; Huiskamp *et al.*, 2004; Pataraia *et al.*, 2008) and functional MRI (Boor

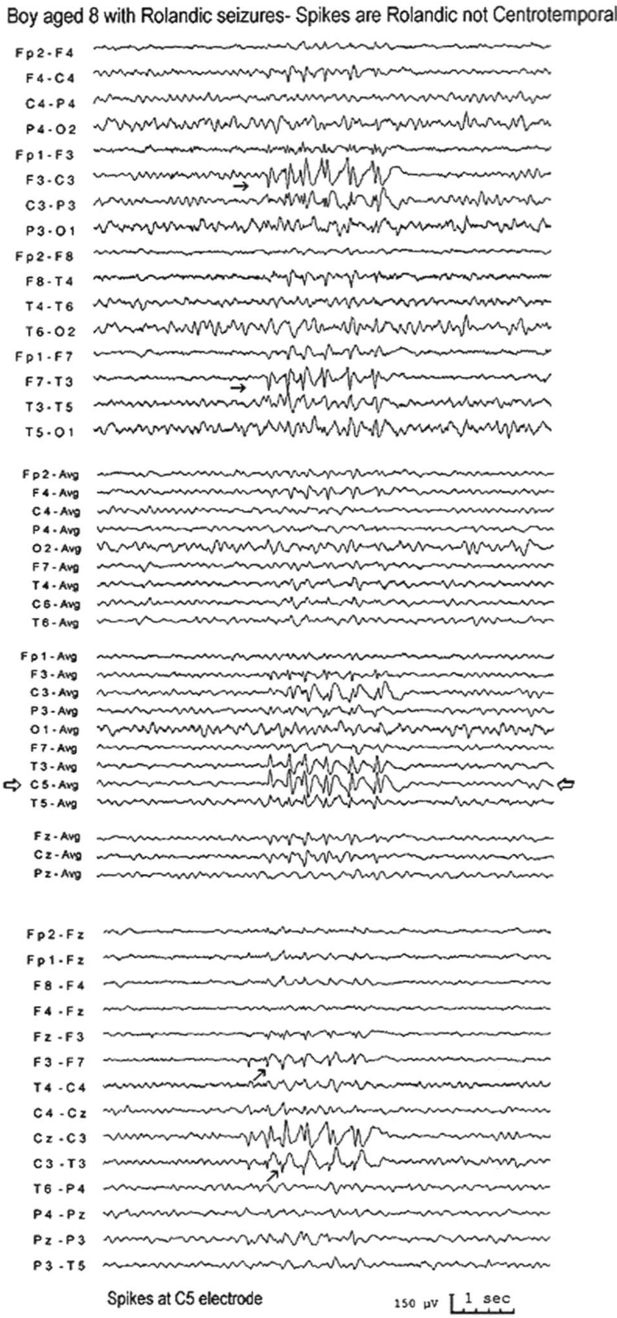

Figure 1 **Centro-temporal spikes are mainly Rolandic not temporal spikes.** Top, middle and bottom: **The same EEG sample is shown in 3 different montages. This is from an 8-year-old boy referred for an EEG because of "recent GTCS and a 2-year history of unilateral facial spasms. Previously, the EEG and CT brain scan were normal. No medication. Focal seizures with secondarily generalized convulsions?" The EEG showed frequent clusters of repetitive centrotemporal spikes on the left. Because the spikes appeared to be of higher amplitude in the temporal electrode (T3) (black arrows), the technologist rightly applied additional electrodes at C5 and C6 (Rolandic localization). This showed that the spike is of higher amplitude in the left Rolandic region (C5) (open arrows). Another EEG 16 months later, showed a few small spikes in the right frontal and central midline electrodes. From Panayiotopoulos (2010) with permission.**

et al., 2007) studies have demonstrated that the main negative spike component of CTS is usually modelled by a single and stable tangential dipole source with the negative pole maximum in the central region and the positive pole maximum in the frontal region.

Typical 3 Hz spike-wave discharges and absence seizures are rare (Beydoun *et al.*, 1992; Gélisse *et al.*, 1999; Panayiotopoulos, 1999a; Verrotti *et al.*, 2017a, 2017b) though a high incidence of them has been reported (Beaumanoir *et al.*, 1974). Brief generalised 4–5 Hz waves with small spikes may be common. Diffuse, often asymmetrical spike-wave discharges, occurring mostly with sleepiness are found in about 25% of cases (Gélisse *et al.*, 1999).

CTSs are diagnostic markers of Rolandic epilepsy only in a suggestive clinical presentation. Their frequency, location and persistence do not determine the clinical manifestations, severity and frequency of seizures or the prognosis. It is well established that CTSs are not specific to Rolandic epilepsy (Kellaway, 1980; Panayiotopoulos, 1999a) as they: i) occur in 2–3% of normal school-aged children, of whom less than 10% develop Rolandic seizures (Gibbs & Gibbs, 1967; Petersen & Eeg-Olofsson, 1971; Cavazzuti *et al.*, 1980; Okubo *et al.*, 1994); ii) are common among relatives of children with Rolandic epilepsy (Bray & Wiser, 1965; Bali *et al.*, 2007); iii) may occur in a variety of organic brain diseases with or without seizures, such as cerebral tumours, Rett syndrome, fragile X syndrome and focal cortical dysplasia (Kellaway, 1980; Panayiotopoulos, 1999a); iv) may incidentally be found in non-epileptic children with various symptoms, such as headache, speech, and behavioural and learning difficulties (Gibbs & Gibbs, 1967).

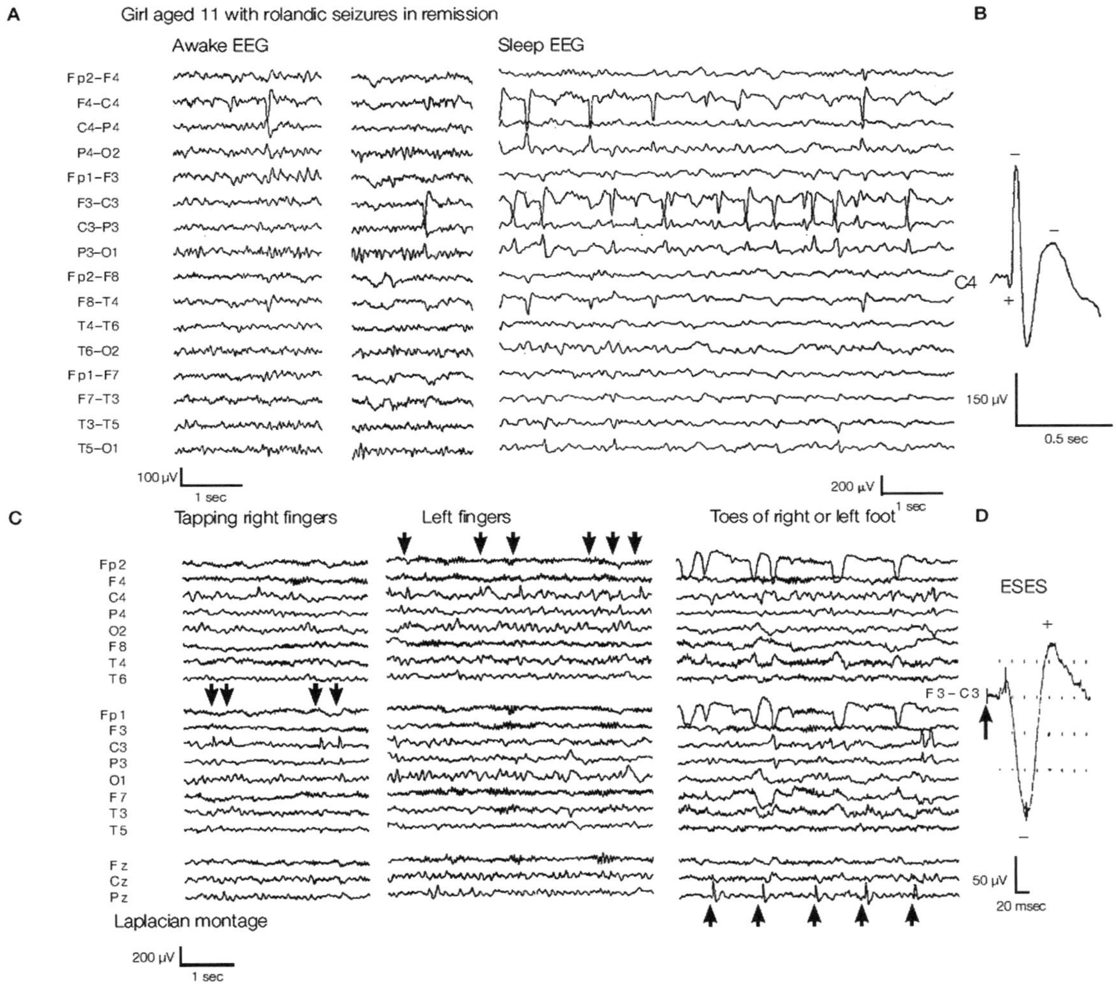

Figure 2

Samples from a video-EEG of an 11-year-old girl with Rolandic seizures who has been in remission since the age of 8 years. (A) High-amplitude CTSs (in fact, these are central spikes) occur independently on the right and left, and are markedly exaggerated during natural sleep. (B) Typical morphology and polarity of CTSs in laplacian montage. (C) GSES, which are evoked by tapping fingers or toes. Note that their location corresponds to the location of the activating stimulus (black arrows). (D) GSES from another patient, which was evoked by electrical stimulation of the right thumb (onset at redarrow). Peak latency of the somatosensory evoked spike is 58 ms. From Panayiotopoulos (2010) with permission.

Ictal EEG: There have been around 50 reported ictal EEGs of Rolandic seizures showing an initial paucity of spontaneous CTSs before the onset of the ictal discharge, which appears in the Rolandic regions contralateral to the clinical manifestations and consists of slow waves intermixed with spikes (Dalla Bernardina & Tassinari 1975; Panayiotopoulos, 1999a; Wirrell *et al.*, 2006; Fejerman *et al.*, 2007) *(Figure 3)*. GTCS, when occurred, were preceded by focal clinical and EEG features (Watanabe, 1996; Panayiotopoulos, 1999a; Wirrell *et al.*, 2006).

In a study of 34 seizures recorded in 30 patients, 4 different ictal EEG patterns (A-D) were identified (Capovilla *et al.*, 2011). The most frequent (pattern A) was characterized by low voltage activity of fast rhythmic spikes, increasing in amplitude and decreasing in frequency, and occurred in 14 children. Pattern B (6 patients) was constituted by a discharge of spikes intermixed with sharp waves increasing in frequency and amplitude. Pattern C (7 children) consisted of monomorphic theta which progressively formed a discharge increasing in amplitude and decreasing in frequency. Pattern D (5 children) was characterized by an initial focal depression of the electrical activity, followed by one of the three above described patterns. In 21 out of 28 children, the initial ictal pattern, altered from one pattern to another one. No clinical or EEG feature was predictive of a specific ictal pattern (Capovilla *et al.*, 2011).

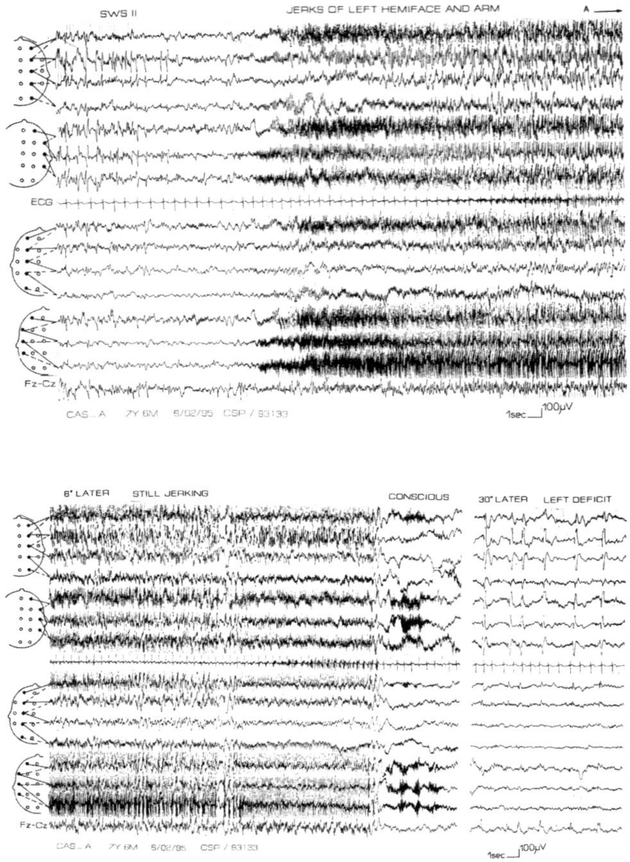

Figure 3 **EEG plates with a seizure in Rolandic epilepsy. A 7 years and 6 months old untreated boy with a history of typical Rolandic seizures during sleep.** Top: **onset of seizure, in NREM sleep stage 2; note the suppression of interictal Rolandic spikes preceding the onset of fast activity over the right Rolandic leads.** Bottom: **continuation of the seizure. Note the abrupt offset with immediate return to baseline waking EEG. Right Rolandic spikes recurred after 30 seconds. The long term evolution was fine.**

Aetiology

Rolandic epilepsy is genetically determined but the genetic factors and the full phenotype spectrum of this epilepsy syndrome are both complex (Vadlamudi *et al.*, 2004, 2006; Pal *et al.*, 2007; Kugler *et al.*, 2008; Strug *et al.*, 2009; Vears *et al.*, 2012). In studying the genetics of Rolandic epilepsy, the three main phenotypes within family members of Rolandic epilepsy patients, namely speech sound disorder/dyslexia, the EEG centro-temporal spikes and Rolandic seizures are usually addressed. Patients with Rolandic epilepsy are 2.5 times more likely than the general population to have a speech sound disorder and 5.8 times more likely to have dyslexia. These same speech sound disorder and dyslexia also appear in family members of Rolandic epilepsy patients even though these same family members have no epilepsy (Clark *et al.*, 2007). Siblings or parents of patients with Rolandic epilepsy may rarely have the same type of seizures or other phenotypes of BCSSS such as PS. Reported occurrence of febrile seizures range from 10–20% (Kajitani *et al.*, 1992).

The EEG CTS has been addressed as an integral and central component of the epilepsy syndrome. Proof that the EEG CTS is a highly penetrant autosomal dominant trait was obtained in family studies of the EEG CTS. Thirty siblings of 23 probands with clinical Rolandic epilepsy underwent sleep deprived EEG (Bali *et al.*, 2007). Eleven of 23 recordings demonstrated CTSs, yielding a corrected segregation ratio of 0.48 (95% CI: 0.27–0.69). The segregation ratio of CTSs in families of Rolandic epilepsy is therefore an autosomal dominant trait and recessive and X-linked inheritance can be rejected (Bali *et al.*, 2007; Pal *et al.*, 2007). These results on the autosomal dominant inheritance of the EEG CTS is consistent with the results of Bray & Wiser (1965).

The advances of Pal and associates (2010) have genetically associated the EEG CTS with SNPs in ELP4 introns using both family based analysis and case control analysis (Strug *et al.*, 2009). Genome wide linkage analysis of the EEG CTS was then conducted by Pal *et al.* (2010) in 38 families from New York, ascertained through a Rolandic epilepsy proband. Strong evidence for linkage to chromosome 11p13 was obtained with maximum two-point LOD score of 4.01 and multipoint LOD score of 4.30. Pal *et al.* then tested for genetic association of the EEG CTS with SNPs distributed across genes in the chromosomes 11p13 region in 68 Rolandic epilepsy cases and 187 controls. Significant association with SNPs in ELP4 introns 9,6 and 5 was obtained with significant ratios 1.80–2.04 at these markers. Joint analysis with a replication dataset from Canada confirmed the association with maximum likelihood ratio for association at intron 9 at 589:1. Speech dyspraxia and the EEG CTS share genetic linkage to chromosome 11p13. When the phenotype of Rolandic epilepsy families are broadened from CTS to CTS plus speech sound disorder, multipoint LOD score rose to 7.5 at D11S914.4. However, dyslexia in Rolandic epilepsy does not share linkage to the same site emphasizing the complexity of the genetics in Rolandic epilepsy (Pal *et al.*, 2010).

Pal *et al.* speculate that ELP4 might partially abrogate Elongator function as a scaffold protein involved in transcriptional elongation of nuclear and cytoplasmic proteins, regulating migration of multiple cell types, specifically to the centro-temporal speech/vocal tract functions and neuronal circuits. These results could explain the premorbid speech sound disorder that presents in the first two years of life preceding the median age at onset for the Rolandic seizures.

Clearly, there are more undefined epilepsy genes other than *ELP4*, that underlie Rolandic epilepsy as the syndrome has been linked to two other chromosome loci, namely 15q14 (Neubauer *et al.*, 1998) and 16p12–11.2 (Guerrini *et al.*, 1999). Kugler *et al.* (2008) reported a three generation family with 11 of 22 affected with a variant form of Rolandic epilepsy, speech impairment, oromotor apraxia, and cognitive deficit. Linkage analysis excluded loci at 11p,15q, 16p12 and Xq22 suggesting genetic heterogeneity for the Rolandic epilepsy syndrome. In addition, mutations in *SRPX2* (*sushi-repeat containing protein X-linked 2*) in two families with mental retardation, severe language dysfunction, orofacial dyspraxia and Rolandic seizures have been reported (Roll *et al.*, 2006). Rare mutations in *KCNQ2* and *KCNQ3* were identified in a small number of patients with RE (Neubauer *et al.*, 2008).

Mutations in other genes are shown to be risk factors for RE. Mutations in *GRIN2A*, a gene on chromosome 16p13 that encodes a subunit of the glutamate N-methyl-D-aspartate receptor, have been identified in patients with RE, also seen in Landau-Kleffner syndrome (LKS) and epileptic encephalopathy with continuous spike and wave during sleep (CSWS) (Lemke *et al.*, 2013, Carvill *et al.*, 2013, Lesca *et al.*, 2013). A linguistic phenotype expressed as speech dyspraxia as well as dysarthria, with poor articulation and disturbances in prosody is described (Turner *et al.*, 2015). One study found an increased risk of RE with mutations of the neuronal splicing regulators genes-involved in the homeostatic control of neuronal excitability-RBFOX1 and RBFOX3 (Lal *et al.*, 2013). However, mutations in *RFBOX* have also been reported in other neurologic disorders, including generalized epilepsy. Another genetic risk factor for typical and atypical RE including atypical benign partial epilepsy (ABPE), LKS and CSWS is 16p11.2 duplication (Reinthaler *et al.*, 2014).

Recently Reinthaler *et al.* (2015) reported that mutations of the *GABRG2* gene may increase the risk for RE. In the other study, *ZDHHC9* mutations are associated with susceptibility to focal seizure and EEG futures sharing characteristics with RE (Baker *et al.*, 2015). Panjwani *et al.* (2016) found that a microRNA-328 binding site in PAX6 is disrupted in 7% of RE patients and strongly associated with CTS on electroencephalogram.

In conclusion, recent studies have yielded genetic and phenotypic heterogeneties; supporting polygenic and complex inheritance pattern.

Pathophysiology

As indicated by the distribution of centro-temporal spikes, the epileptogenic zone in Rolandic epilepsy involves neuronal networks within the Rolandic cortex surrounding the central fissure bilaterally. This is congruent with the seizure symptomatology (symptomatogenic zone) and in agreement with those described by Penfield & Rasmussen (1957) during electrical stimulation of the lower part of the precentral and postcentral gyrus in man.

The speech arrest is due to anarthia attributed to loss of the power and coordination of the musculature responsible for the articulation of words. There is no impairment of the cortical language networks. Hypersalivation most probably relates to the involvement of the superior bank of the sylvian fissure (Luders *et al.*, 1987), but defining ictal symptomatogenesis by plotting the simple topographic coordinates of an ictal discharge can hardly explain the high prevalence of hypersalivation in benign Rolandic epilepsy compared to its exceptional occurrence in adults with symptomatic foci of similar topography. Nor can it explain the opercular status epilepticus, with the hours-long speech arrest, drooling and bilateral regional twitching that is associated with diffuse or bilateral Rolandic spike wave activity, but does not propagate in a conventional way and does not involve other systems like for instance the motor strip or the language function. Therefore, at variance with the symptomatic adult focal epilepsies of comparable but more discretely localized topography, Rolandic epilepsy reflects an age related maturational instability of the lower Rolandic (somatosensory) cortex that represents the face and the oropharynx bilaterally (Koutroumanidis, 2007).

Evolution and prognosis

The prognosis for Rolandic seizures is invariably excellent, with probably less than 2% risk of developing absence seizures and less often GTCS in adult life (Beaumanoir *et al.*, 1974; Lerman & Kivity, 1975; Blom & Heijbel, 1982; Loiseau *et al.*, 1983; Panayiotopoulos, 1999a; Datta & Sinclair, 2007; Panayiotopoulos *et al.*, 2008; Caraballo *et al.*, 2008b; Callenbach *et al.*, 2010). Remission usually occurs within 2–4 years from onset and before the age of 16 years. The total number of seizures is low, the majority of patients having fewer than 10 seizures; 10–20% have just a single seizure. About 10–20% may have frequent seizures, but these also remit with age.

Rarely (< 1%) Rolandic epilepsy may evolve to more severe syndromes with linguistic, behavioural and neuropsychological deficits, such as Landau-Kleffner syndrome, atypical focal epilepsy of childhood or epilepsy with CSWS and negative myoclonus (Dalla Bernardina *et al.*, 1978, 1989; Caraballo *et al.*, 1989; Fejerman *et al.*, 2000). However, many of these cases may be epileptic encephalopathies and not genuine Rolandic epilepsy.

Shared susceptibility between Rolandic epilepsy and migraine has been suggested (Clarke *et al.*, 2009).

Cognitive functions/Language impairment/Comorbities

Children with Rolandic seizures may develop usually mild and reversible linguistic, cognitive and behavioural abnormalities during the active phase of the disease (Giordani *et al.*, 2006; Nicolai *et al.*, 2006; Riva *et al.*, 2007; Kossoff *et al.*, 2007; Perkins *et al.*, 2008; Kavros *et al.*, 2008; Danielsson & Petermann, 2009; Tedrus *et al.*, 2009; Goldberg-Stern *et al.*, 2010, Kirby *et al.*, 2017). These may be worse in children with onset of seizures before 8 years of age. Detailed neuropsychological studies have shown deficits in many subdomains, including attention (Kavros *et al.*, 2008), verbal and visual memory (Danielsson & Petermann, 2009, Verrotti *et al.*, 2014a), fine motor skills (Vannest *et al.*, 2016; Kirby *et al.*, 2017) processing speed (Ebus *et al.*, 2012, Vannest *et al.*, 2016), visuo-spatial and visuo-motor skills, (Pinton *et al.*, 2006), and executive functions (Filippini *et al.*, 2016). In studies investigating standardized language and verbal memory outcomes, the performance of patients with RE was poorer than age-matched healthy controls (Piccinelli *et al.*, 2008; Goldberg-Stern *et al.*, 2010). Other studies have documented lower performance among patients with RE on visuospatial tasks and nonverbal memory (Vintan *et al.*, 2012; Ebus *et al.*, 2012). In one of the largest studies, children with RE performed more poorly than controls on verbal fluency, speeded naming, and instruction comprehension tasks, with earlier age of onset associated with lower language scores (Jurkeviciene *et al.*, 2012). A meta-analysis of 23 studies on language and literacy skills shows the most prominent impairments are in single word reading, receptive and expressive language, and phonologic processing in children with RE (Smith *et al.*, 2015). Language difficulties at the word, sentence, and discourse levels (Overvliet *et al.*, 2013), reading and comprehension difficulties have been found (Currie *et al.*, 2017).

Behavioural disorders have also been observed in children with RE (Kim *et al.*, 2014). In a larger study of 43 patients, aggressive behaviour, social and attention problems and anxiety/depression have been documented and these showed correlation with sleep problems (Samaitiene *et al.*, 2013). Attention and inhibition problems have also been reported (Verrotti *et al.*, 2013). Recently, higher incidence of ADHD was reported (Kim *et al.*, 2014). These are associated with a high frequency of learning disorders (10 to 40%) and academic issues (Piccinelli *et al.*, 2008; Smith *et al.*, 2015).

The children with early-onset epileptic seizures have lower scores in language tests; especially in verbal fluency and comprehension. The language difficulties were more pronounced in older children. Both in the active and remission phase of the disease; specific language disorders have been reported (Monjauze *et al.*, 2011). In another study, the intensity of cognitive deficits showed correlation with the abundance of nocturnal epileptiform discharges (Overvliet *et al.*, 2010). In addition, NREM sleep interictal epileptiform discharges are shown to have negative impact on declarative memory (Verrotti *et al.*, 2014a). However, another study did not show negative cognitive effect of abundant epileptiform activity in RE with aggressive treatment (Nissenkorn *et al.*, 2017). There are some studies with no significant difference in memory, language, or executive functions between adolescents and young adults who had recovered from RE, when compared to controls. The development, social adaptation and occupations of adults with a previous history of Rolandic seizures were found normal (Blom & Heijbel, 1982; Loiseau *et al.*, 1983). A recent study of neuropsychological functioning in unmedicated children with newly diagnosed RE found only small, nonsignificant differences in language and cognitive skills compared with healthy control subjects at the early course of their epilepsy disorder (Vannest *et al.*, 2016).

It is unclear if the cognitive or linguistic disabilities of children with RE are related to the disease itself or the centro-temporal spike activities in EEG or antiepileptic drugs.

Functional neuroimaging

Functional MRI (fMRI) or simultaneous EEG-fMRI studies of RE have shown regional functional abnormalities involving central, temporal and frontal regions related to epileptogenesis (Masterton *et al.*, 2013) or anterior language impairment (Besseling *et al.*, 2013a, Datta *et al.*, 2013). The involved regions have been proposed as the components of sensorimotor network (Besseling *et al.*, 2013b). On the other hand, in previous studies, using quantitative structural magnetic resonance imaging have shown widespread morphological changes in RE (Overvliet *et al.*, 2013; Pardoe *et al.*, 2013). Pardoe *et al.* 2013 found that grey matter volume and cortical thickness were increased in the frontal gyri, insula and parietal regions, and these regions were involved in both language and attention networks. Studies using diffusion tensor imaging have revealed altered integrity of white matter tracts associated with cognitive impairments (Ciumas *et al.*, 2014; Kim SE *et al.*,2014; Besseling *et al.*, 2013c; Xiao *et al.*, 2014). It was reported that abnormal cognition and behaviour were related to the changes of structural and functional neuroanatomy in patients with RE.

Management

Children with Rolandic seizures may not need AEDs, particularly if the seizures are infrequent, mild or nocturnal, or the onset is close to the natural age of remission of this age-limited disorder (Panayiotopoulos *et al.*, 2008). Patients with either frequent seizures and secondarily GTCSs or comorbid conditions may need medication (Al Twajri & Shevell, 2002). Some AEDs may significantly reduce GTCSs without reduction of focal seizures (Peters *et al.*, 2001).

Some children might experience learning difficulties, aggravation and new types of seizures when receiving either carbamazepine or lamotrigine. "Within days after re-introduction of carbamazepine, she suffered nearly continuous, brief atonic attacks of head and arm drop and also absences" (case 17.3 in Panayiotopoulos) (Panayiotopoulos, 1999a).

Childen with Rolandic seizures having difficulties in academic and social life need guidance during follow-up. It is important to point out that only comprehensive neuropsychometric assesment can unravel the cognitive, linguistic, attention and behavioural disorders. Parental education and psychological support is also the most important aspect of management (Valeta, 2005; 2011). For details see the section on "Idiopathic focal seizures in childhood".

Panayiotopoulos syndrome

Panayiotopoulos syndrome (PS) is a common childhood-related idiopathic benign susceptibility to autonomic seizures and autonomic status epilepticus (Panayiotopoulos 2002; 2007). The syndrome has been confirmed in over 700 children with an impressive uniformity in Asia, Canada, Europe, Japan, North and South America and in all races through independent studies (Ferrie *et al.*, 1997; Oguni *et al.*, 1999; Caraballo *et al.*, 2000, 2007; Lada *et al.*, 2003; Covanis, 2006; Ferrie *et al.*, 2006; Koutroumanidis, 2007; Dura-Trave *et al.*, 2008; Ohtsu *et al.*, 2008; Michael *et al.*, 2010; Specchio *et al.*, 2010a; Gonzalez-Duarte *et al.*, 2011; Degerliyurt *et al.*, 2014).

Demographic data

Onset is from age 1 to 14 years with 76% starting between 3–6 years. Both sexes are probably equally affected, though a female preponderance was found in some studies (Lada *et al.*, 2003; Dura-Trave *et al.*, 2008; Specchio *et al.*, 2010a). Children of all races are affected. Prevalence of PS may be high though this syndrome is practically absent in designed controlled epidemiological studies, which is understandable as this syndrome was only recently formally recognized, its features imitate many other conditions and often it manifests with a single seizure only. In the original cohort of Panayiotopoulos (1988), prevalence was around 13% in children aged 3–6 years with one or more non-febrile seizures, and 6% in the age group 1–15 years. These figures may be higher if children who are currently considered to have atypical clinical presentation are included in the syndrome (Panayiotopoulos, 2002; Covanis, 2006). PS is the most common specific cause of non- febrile status epilepticus in childhood (Okanishi *et al.*, 2008).

Clinical manifestations

Autonomic seizures and autonomic status epilepticus are the cardinal manifestations of PS. Seizures comprise an unusual constellation of autonomic, mainly emetic, symptoms, behavioural changes, unilateral deviation of the eyes and other more conventional ictal manifestations. Consciousness and speech, as a rule, are preserved at seizure onset but commonly become impaired in the progression of the attacks. The seizure commonly starts with autonomic manifestations (81%), which are mainly emetic (74–82%). In a typical presentation, the child is initially fully conscious, able to speak and understand, complains "I feel sick", looks pale and vomits.

Ictus emeticus in PS

The full emetic triad (nausea, retching, vomiting) culminates in vomiting in 74–82% of seizures in PS, in others, only nausea or retching occur and in a quarter, emesis may not be apparent. Emesis is usually the first apparent ictal symptom, but may also occur long after the onset of other manifestations.

Typically, nausea is the first complaint of a child who suffers a seizure (while awake or waking from sleep) prior to vomiting and other ictal manifestations. This initial stage does not suggest an epileptic seizure, the child simply complains of feeling sick and being unwell, and looks pale. The patient may be quiet or agitated, vacant or restless but fully conscious and able to understand and answer questions. Ictus emeticus at this stage is no different from any other disease that causes emesis just a child who feels sick or wants to be sick.

When vomiting occurs, it commonly starts 1–5 min after the onset of nausea, while the child is still conscious and otherwise well. Less often, vomiting may occur later during other more conventional seizure symptoms. See also "Ictal EEG recordings".

The intensity and duration of vomiting varies considerably from mild to often severe and repetitive. Usually, the child vomits 3–5 times; however, some children repeatedly vomit for hours leading to dehydration, while others may vomit only once.

Other autonomic manifestations

Autonomic manifestations other than ictus emeticus may occur prior, concurrently or appear later in the course of the ictus. These include pallor and less often flushing or cyanosis, mydriasis and less often miosis, cardiorespiratory and thermoregulatory alterations, coughing, incontinence of urine and/or faeces, modifications of intestinal motility, lacrimation and diaphoresis. Tachycardia is often the first ictal manifestation in ictal EEG recordings. Hypersalivation (probably a concurrent Rolandic symptom) may occur. Headache and more often other cephalic auras occur particularly at onset.

Pallor is one of the commonest ictal manifestations. It mainly occurs at onset, usually with emetic symptoms. Exceptionally, pallor may be among the first symptoms without apparent emesis.

Cyanosis is less common than pallor. It principally occurs during the evolution of the seizures, often while the child is unresponsive. Redness of the face with or without fever may be a prominent and lengthy symptom in some children.

Incontinence of urine and faeces occur when consciousness is impaired prior to, or without, convulsions: "became unresponsive and incontinent of urine" is a common association. These symptoms do not occur at onset.

Mydriasis is sometimes so prominent that witnesses may report it spontaneously: "pupils were as big as the eyes". Mydriasis occurs concurrently with other marked autonomic manifestations. Dilated pupils may or not be reactive to light.

Miosis is rare and occurs with other severe autonomic manifestations while the child is unresponsive.

Hypersalivation is also rare in PS (6%), in contrast to its common occurrence in Rolandic seizures. Combined speech arrest and hypersalivation, as in Rolandic epilepsy, is even rarer.

Cephalic auras, though rare, are of interest, because they are considered to be autonomic manifestations and because of the diagnostic confusion they may cause with migraine if not properly evaluated. Cephalic auras commonly occur with other autonomic symptoms, mainly nausea, at seizure onset. Occasionally, the child may also complain of "headache" but whether the complaint of "headache" is a true perception of pain, discomfort or some odd sensation in the head is uncertain.

Coughing may occur as an initial ictal symptom either with or without ictus emeticus. It is described as "strange coughing" or "cough as if about to vomit".

Thermoregulatory changes: raised temperature may be subjectively or objectively documented during the seizure or immediately postictally. Whether this is a coincidental finding, a precipitating factor or an ictal abnormality is uncertain. It could be any of these. However, pyrexia recorded immediately after seizure onset is probably an ictal autonomic manifestation.

Abnormalities of intestinal motility: diarrhoea (3%) is occasionally reported during the progression of seizures.

Breathing and cardiac irregularities are rarely reported, but may be much more common in their mild forms. Breathing changes prior to convulsions include descriptions of "heavy, irregular, abnormal breathing" or "brief cessation of breathing for a few seconds". Tachycardia is a consistent finding, often at the onset, of ictal EEG. Priapism that is consistent with parasympathetic autonomic manifestations has also been reported (Brabec *et al.*, 2013).

Cardiorespiratory arrest is rare, probably occurring in 1 per 200 individuals with PS, but it is potentially life threatening without immediate medical intervention (Ferrie *et al.*, 2007, Dirani *et al.*, 2015, Yalcın & Toydemir, 2017). Ictal cardiopulmonary arrest, at disease onset, has been reported in children with PS (Verrotti *et al.*, 2005; Mujawar *et al.*, 2011).

Syncopal-like manifestations (ictal syncope or syncope-like epileptic seizures) occur in at least one-fifth of seizures (Panayiotopoulos, 2002; Ferrie *et al.*, 2006; Covanis, 2006; Ferrie *et al.*, 2007; Caraballo *et al.*, 2007; Gonzalez-Duarte *et al.*, 2011; Koutroumanidis *et al.*, 2012). The child becomes "completely unresponsive and flaccid like a rag doll" which may precede, be concurrent with other seizure symptoms or be the sole manifestation of a seizure (Oguni *et al.*, 1999; Panayiotopoulos, 2002). They may occur while the patient is standing, sitting, lying down or asleep and last from 1–2 minutes to half an hour or more.

This seizure type of the developing brain is not featured in any ILAE classification. "Ictal syncope" or "syncope-like epileptic seizures" is descriptive term to express this state, because "unresponsiveness with loss of postural tone" are the defining clinical symptoms of syncope (Panayiotopoulos, 2002, 2004; Ferrie *et al.*, 2007; Koutroumanidis *et al.*, 2012).

Ictal behavioural changes

Ictal behavioural changes usually consist of restlessness, agitation, terror or quietness, which appear at the onset of seizures, often concurrently with emetic or other autonomic manifestations. These symptoms are often similar to those occurring in "Benign childhood epilepsy with affective symptoms".

Ictal non-autonomic symptoms

Pure autonomic seizures and pure autonomic status epilepticus appear to occur in 10% of patients. They commence and terminate solely with autonomic symptoms. In all other seizures, autonomic manifestations are followed or occasionally start with conventional seizure symptoms. The child gradually or suddenly becomes confused and unresponsive.

Unilateral deviation of the eyes with, or rarely without, ictal vomiting is a common ictal manifestation (60–83%), which seldom occurs at onset. The eyes shift to the extreme of one side and the head may also turn ipsilaterally. This pursuit-like deviation of the eyes may be brief (for minutes) or prolonged (for hours). It may be continuous or less often intermittent, with eyes returning to the midline and shifting again towards the same side. The eyelids remain open, but may be half open or open wide and, at this stage, consciousness is often, but not invariably, impaired. Deviation of the eyes may occur without vomiting in 10–20% of patients and, in some children, the eyes may be open wide and remain in the midline before other convulsions occur.

Other non-autonomic ictal symptoms include Rolandic symptoms such as speech arrest (8%), hemifacial spasms (6%) and oropharyngolaryngeal movements (3%). Ictal visual symptoms (6%), such as visual hallucinations, illusions or blindness, usually occur after more typical seizure symptoms of PS have started. Unilateral drooping of the mouth, mild myoclonic jerks, eyelid fluttering or eyelid jerks, ictal nystagmus or automatisms occur less than 3% each. The seizures may end with hemiconvulsions often with jacksonian marching (19–30%) or generalized convulsions (21–36%).

Impairment of consciousness

Though initially fully conscious, the child gradually or suddenly becomes confused and unresponsive. Impairment of consciousness may be mild or moderate, with the child retaining some ability to respond to verbal commands, but often talking out of context. Complete unresponsiveness is probably exceptional at the beginning of the seizure. In diurnal seizures observed from onset, cloudiness of consciousness usually starts after the appearance of autonomic and behavioural symptoms, becoming progressively worse until complete unresponsiveness is reached. Good awareness may be preserved throughout the ictus in around 6% of seizures.

Seizures without autonomic manifestations

The same child may have seizures with marked autonomic manifestations and seizures during which autonomic manifestations may be inconspicuous or absent. Seizures without autonomic manifestations are rare (7%).

The clinical seizure manifestations are roughly the same irrespective of EEG localizations though there may be slightly less autonomic and slightly more focal motor features at onset in children without occipital spikes.

Duration of seizures and autonomic status epilepticus

The seizures are usually lengthy of over 6 minutes and almost half of them last for more than 30 minutes to many hours, thus constituting autonomic status epilepticus (Panayiotopoulos, 2002; Ferrie *et al.*, 2007). Lengthy seizures are equally common in sleep and wakefulness. Even after the most severe seizures and autonomic status epilepticus, the patient is normal after a few hours' sleep. There is no record of residual neurological abnormalities. Hemiconvulsive or convulsive status epilepticus (CSE) is rare (4%) however one study demonstrates that CSE can occur at the onset of PS, although it is not associated with a poor prognosis (Verrotti *et al.*, 2014b).

Circadian distribution and precipitating factors

Two-thirds of seizures start in sleep. There are no apparent precipitating factors other than sleep. Fixation off sensitivity is an EEG phenomenon, which may not be clinically important. Many seizures have been witnessed as occurring whilst the child is travelling in a car, boat or aeroplane. There are two explanations for this: i) the seizures are more likely to be witnessed during travelling, or ii), children are more vulnerable because travelling also precipitates sleep and motion sickness which is particularly common in children.

Furthermore, fever may be a precipitant of autonomic seizures in PS (Cordelli *et al.*, 2012).

Intra-individual seizure variability

The same child may have brief and lengthy seizures, diurnal and nocturnal, with marked, inconspicuous, or even without apparent autonomic changes. Even cardinal symptoms (such as vomiting or eye deviation) may be present in one but be absent in another seizure. Seizures without conspicuous autonomic manifestations are rare (7%) and occur in patients who also have additional autonomic seizures

(Panayiotopoulos, 2002). Ictal video EEG recordings have documented that autonomic symptoms and signs may vary between seizures of the same child (Koutroumanidis *et al.*, 2005). There is no correlation between ictal semiology and topography of interictal spikes.

Atypical clinical presentations of Panayiotopoulos syndrome

The previous descriptions refer to relatively typical cases. However, as in any other disease including Rolandic epilepsy, atypical presentations are expected particularly in children who may have a combined predisposition, genetic or otherwise, to a number of age-related diseases such as cyclic vomiting syndrome, abdominal migraine or other common disorders such as migraines or other forms of epilepsies. Atypical presentations may also result from combined clinical manifestations of the clinical phenotypes of benign childhood seizure susceptibility syndrome with Rolandic, Gastaut, Panayiotopoulos and affective features or occipital photosensitivity. Examples of atypical cases have been detailed by Panayiotopoulos (2002) and include children with seizures manifesting with only lengthy "episodes of suddenly falling asleep or collapse without convulsions", prolonged episodes of behavioural changes, cephalic sensations or autonomic disturbances other than emesis, alone or usually in combination.

The term "atypical cases" of PS is often used in the literature for children who have frequent, but otherwise typical seizures of PS and whose EEG are typical (Ferrie & Livingston, 2010). Their ultimate prognosis, in terms of eventual seizure remission, is the same as that of "typical cases". In statistical terms when considering seizure frequency, they lie within the "expected distribution" but relatively distant from the median. Other "atypical cases" include children with PS with atypical evolution as in Rolandic epilepsy (Caraballo *et al.*, 2001; Fejerman, 2009).

Diagnostic procedures

By definition neurological and mental states and high resolution MRI are normal in PS. However, as in Rolandic epilepsy, static brain abnormalities unrelated to the pathogenetic process of PS may occur by chance (Yalcin *et al.*, 2009; Specchio *et al.*, 2010a). The most useful laboratory test is the EEG *(Figures 4 to 8)*.

The most important determinant of the neurodiagnostic procedures is the state of the child at the time of first medical attendance.

(a) *The child has a typical brief or lengthy seizure of PS, but has fully recovered before arriving at the accident and emergency department or being seen by a physician*. A child with the distinctive clinical features of PS, particularly ictus emeticus and lengthy seizures, may not need any investigations other than EEG. However, because approximately 10–20% of children with similar seizures may have brain pathology, an MRI may be indicated in the non-acute state. In young children the risks of giving a general anaesthetic need to be considered.

(b) *The child with a typical lengthy seizure of PS has partially recovered, though is still in a postictal stage, tired, mildly confused and drowsy on arrival at the accident and emergency department or when seen by a physician*. The child should be kept under medical supervision until full recovery, which is the rule in PS after a few hours of sleep. Then guidelines are the same as in (a).

(c) *The child is brought to the accident and emergency department or is seen by a physician while ictal symptoms continue*. This is the most difficult and challenging situation. Symptoms may dramatically accumulate in succession, and demand rigorous and experienced evaluation and management. A history of a previous similar seizure is reassuring and may help to avoid unnecessary investigations.

Electroencephalography

Interictal EEG

Interictal EEG shows great variability in functional focal spikes at various electrode locations as illustrated in *Figures 4 to 8* (Panayiotopoulos, 1988, 2002, 2010; Oguni *et al.*, 1999, 2001; Ohtsu *et al.*, 2003; Lada *et al.*, 2003; Covanis *et al.*, 2003; Sanders *et al.*, 2004; Caraballo *et al.*, 2007; Ohtsu *et al.*, 2008; Yalcin *et al.*, 2009; Kokkinos *et al.*, 2010; Specchio *et al.*, 2010a). All brain regions are involved, though posterior areas predominate *(Figure 6)*. In about 90% of cases, the EEG reveals functional, mainly multifocal, high amplitude sharp-slow wave complexes *(Figures 4 to 8)*. Spikes may appear anywhere. They are often independent, and occur at various posterior locations and, less often anterior locations, in the same or the contralateral hemisphere, and may appear as cloned-like, repetitive, multifocal spike-wave complexes. In order of prevalence, the complexes occur in occipital, frontal and centro-temporal regions. Right and left regions are equally involved *(Figure 6)*. Midline spikes occur in 17% of cases.

Spikes are usually of high amplitude and morphologically similar to centro-temporal spikes. Small and even inconspicuous spikes may appear in the same or a previous EEG of children with giant spikes. Though rare, positive spikes or other unusual EEG spike configurations may occur (Panayiotopoulos, 2002).

Two-thirds of patients (68%) have at least one EEG with occipital paroxysms or, more commonly, occipital spikes, which are often (64%) concurrent with extra-occipital spikes in at least one EEG. The other third (32%) never show occipital spikes *(Figure 5)*. Instead, they have extra-occipital spikes (21%) only, a consistently normal EEG

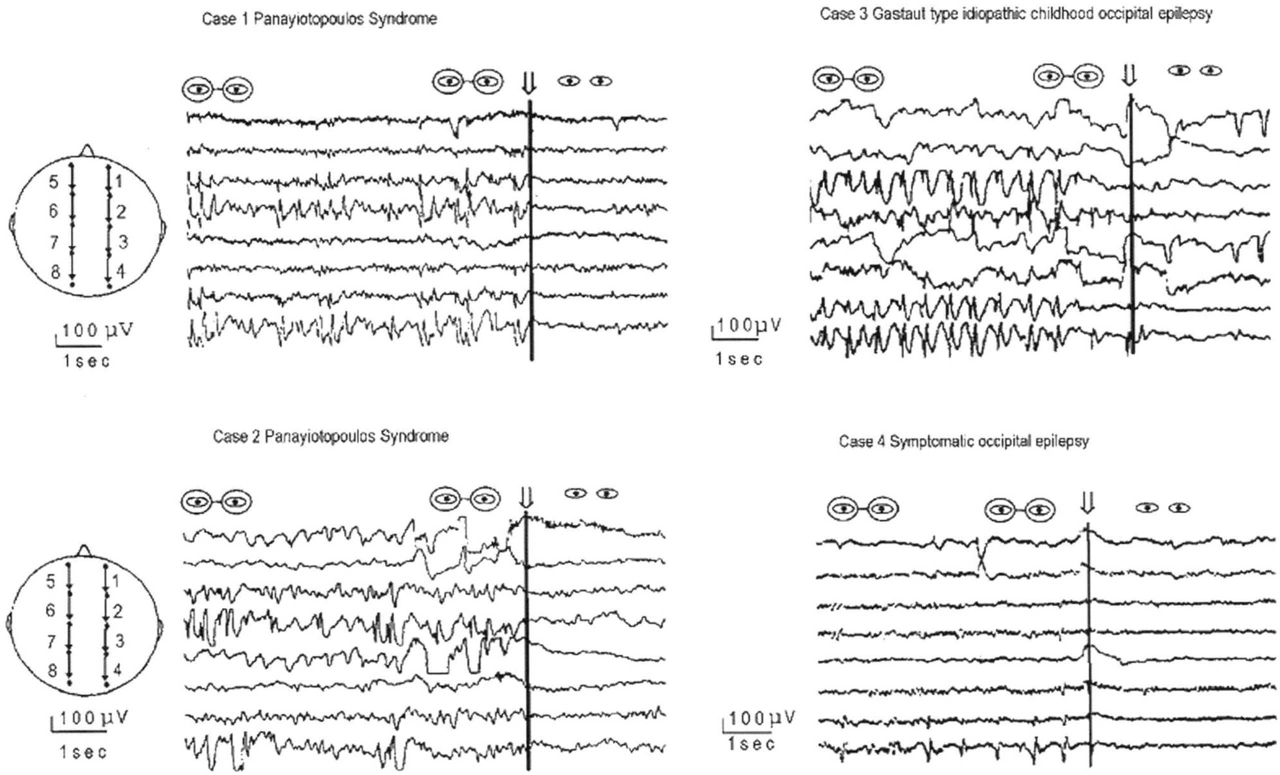

Figure 4

Occipital paroxysms with fixation-off sensitivity as first reported by Panayiotopoulos (1981). Despite similar EEG features, these four patients had different clinical manifestations showing that this EEG phenomenon was not a specific abnormality. Cases 1 and 2 suffered from Panayiotopoulos syndrome, case 3 reported in 1980 had idiopathic childhood occipital epilepsy as described later by Gastaut (1982) and case 4 had symptomatic occipital epilepsy. In routine EEG high amplitude, continuous occipital sharp and slow wave complexes (occipital paroxysms) occurred immediately after closing of the eyes, lasting as long as the eyes were closed. The EEG normalized immediately after opening of the eyes and as long as the eyes were open though some break through occipital spikes could occur. It was documented that the activation of the occipital paroxysms was due to the elimination of central vision and fixation (left of the vertical bar, symbol of eyes with glasses) and inhibition by fixation (right of the vertical bar, symbol of eyes without glasses). Note, that the occipital paroxysms are similar in Panayiotopoulos syndrome and ICEO-G which contrast with the strictly localized occipital spikes of the symptomatic occipital epilepsy for which fixation-off sensitivity was not tested. Modified from Panayiotopoulos (1981) with permission.

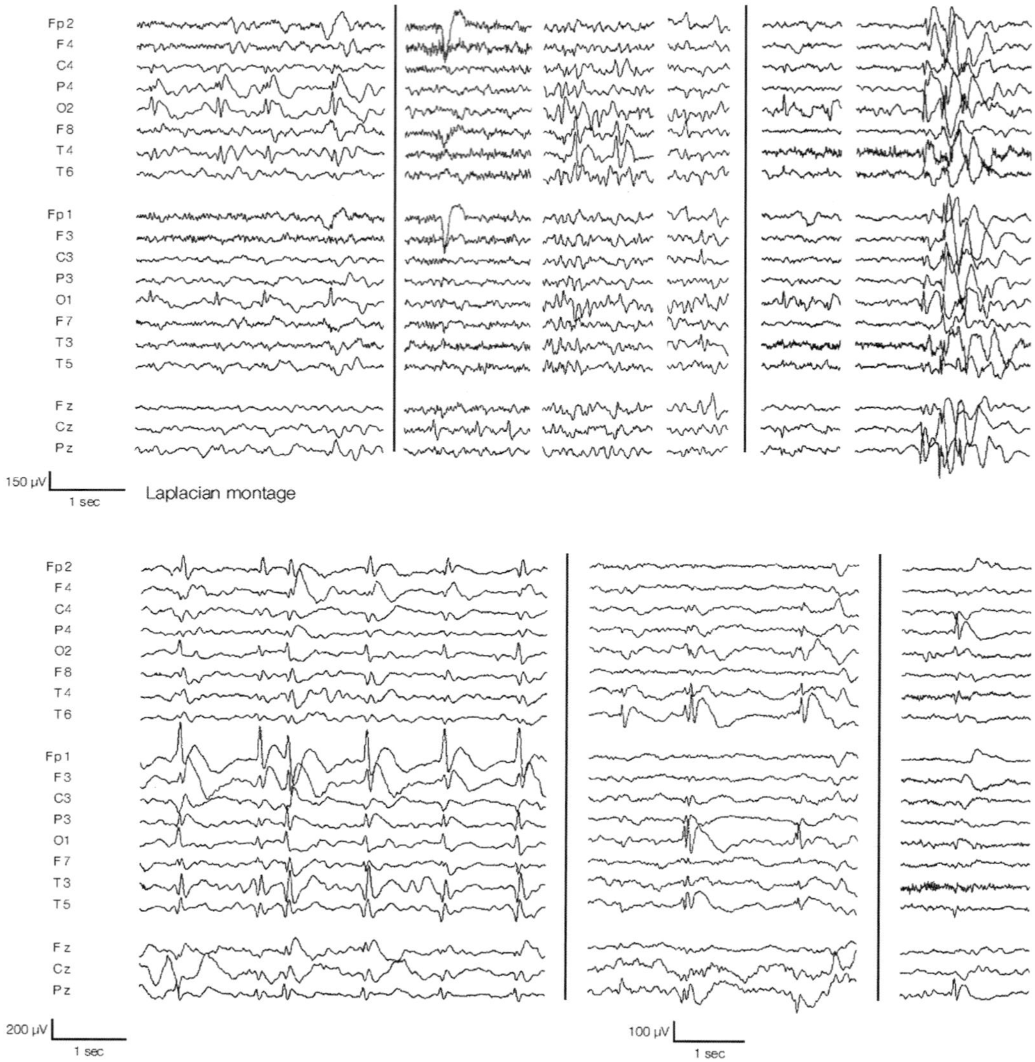

Figure 5

Samples from EEGs of 6 children with typical clinical manifestations of PS. Spikes may occur in all electrode locations, and they are usually of high amplitude and frequent or repetitive (clone-like repetitive multifocal spike-wave complexes), although they may also be small and sparse. Brief generalized discharges of small spikes and slow waves may be present. From Panayiotopoulos (2002) with permission.

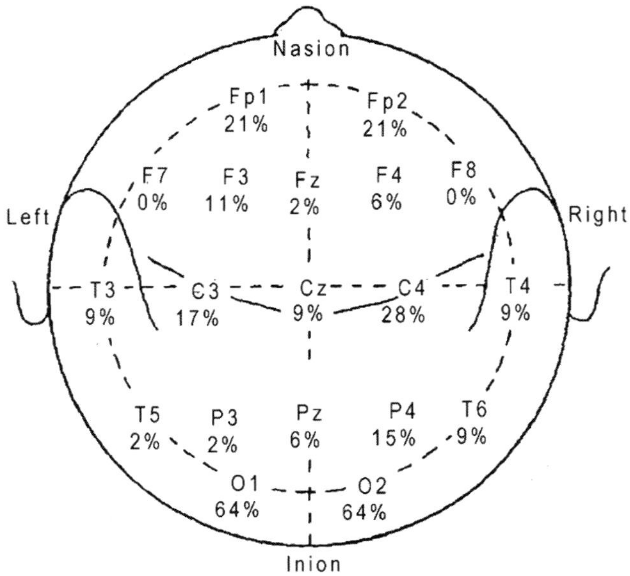

Figure 6 **Prevalence of spike localization as estimated from the analysis of EEG of 47 patients with PS. All but the anterior temporal regions are involved. Note that frontal spikes are second more frequent after the occipital, followed by central spikes. Right and left occipital and frontal regions are equally involved. Midline spikes occurred in 17%. From Panayiotopoulos (2002) with permission.**

(9%) or brief generalized discharges only (2%). An EEG with multifocal spikes in more than two, and often many, brain locations occurs in one-third of patients, single spike foci are rare (9%).

Cloned-like, repetitive, multifocal spike-wave complexes may be characteristic features when they occur (19%). These are repetitive spike or sharp and slow wave complexes that appear concurrently in different brain locations of one or both hemispheres *(Figure 5)*. There may be just two discrete foci unilaterally or contralaterally, but the complexes are usually multifocal and often give the impression of generalized discharges or secondary bilateral synchrony. They are stereotypically and identically repetitive in the same and often subsequent EEGs from the same patient, which is the reason that the name "cloned-like" was coined. On routine surface EEG recordings, they appear synchronous but usually one spike focus precedes (leads) the others by a few milliseconds. Also the leading spike-focus commonly occurs alone without spikes in other locations which may be anterior or posterior, medial or lateral (Leal *et al.*, 2008; Yoshinaga *et al.*, 2009; Kokkinos *et al.*, 2010). Cloned-like repetitive multifocal spike-wave complexes can occur without the primary leading spike and can be so abundant that they dominate the EEG and obscure its background, which is otherwise normal. On other occasions, they are scarce and appear in a well-organized EEG with normal background. Longitudinal EEG studies indicate that the cloned-like repetitive multifocal spike wave complexes are frequently shifting location, multiplying and propagating diffusely with age, rather than persistently localizing in the occipital regions (Ueno *et al.*, 2001; Kokkinos *et al.*, 2010). At times, the occipital EEG spikes appeared initially and then shifted to the fronto-polar regions or appeared synchronously with them. In this fronto-polar-occipital EEG pattern occipital spikes constantly lead to fronto-polar spikes, resulting in secondary occipito-frontopolar synchrony (Ueno *et al.*, 2001). Thus, the variable localizations of EEG foci seen in PS may merely depend on the timing of initial EEG recording of the patients. Cloned-like repetitive multifocal spike-wave complexes have never been studied or reported before in idiopathic epilepsies. On the contrary, multifocal repetitive spikes are usually considered as indicative of a bad prognosis and of symptomatic epilepsies (Yamatogi & Ohtahara, 2003). Cloned-like, repetitive, multifocal spike-wave complexes do not determine the prognosis, because they occur equally in children with single or multiple seizures.

Brief generalized discharges of slow waves intermixed with small spikes may occur either alone (4%) or more often with focal spikes (15%). Diffuse discharges at onset as the sole EEG manifestation, which lasted throghout the course of the typical cases of PS has been reported (Caraballo *et al.*, 2015).

The EEG spikes may be stimulus sensitive, occipital paroxysms are commonly (47%) activated by the elimination of central vision and fixation, while centro-temporal spikes may be elicited by somatosensory stimuli *(Figures 2 and 4)*. Occipital photosensitivity in EEG is an exceptional finding in PS.

Functional spikes in whatever location are accentuated by NREM sleep *(Figure 7)*. If a routine EEG is normal, a sleep EEG should be performed. There is no particular relationship between the likelyhood of an abnormal EEG and the interval since the last seizure. EEGs recorded a short or long time after a seizure are equally likely to manifest with functional spikes, which may occur only once in serial routine and sleep EEGs.

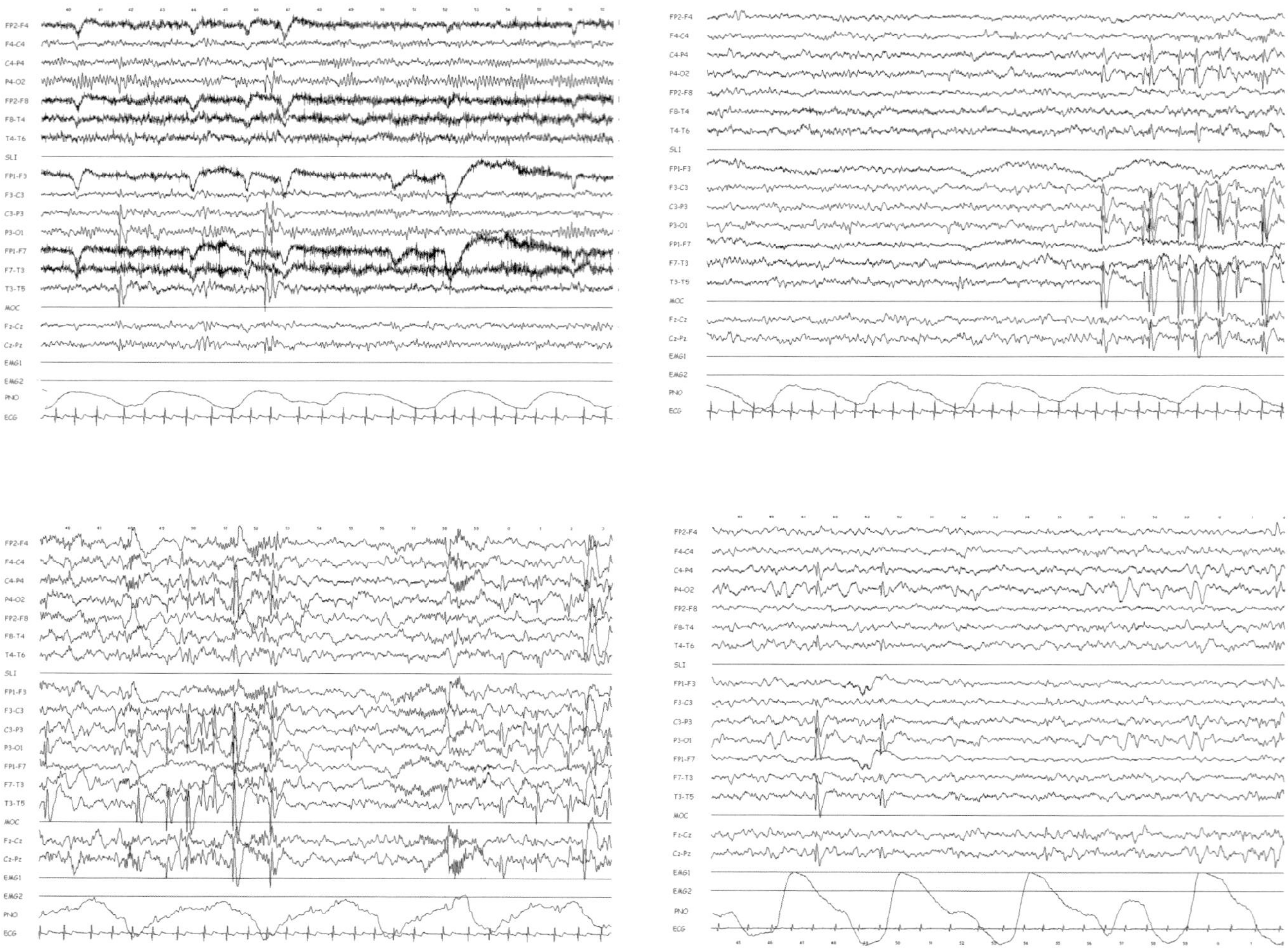

Figure 7

Interictal EEG of a 5-year-old girl with Panayiotopoulos syndrome. Top, left: **waking EEG showing left occipital sharp waves.** Top, right: **at somnolence, increase in density and voltage of the spikes with increased diffusion to the right.** Bottom, left: **EEG changes remain active in stage 2 NREM sleep.** Bottom, right: **during REM sleep, the spikes have reduced amplitude and diffusion.**
Callibration: 15 mm/s, 100 μv.

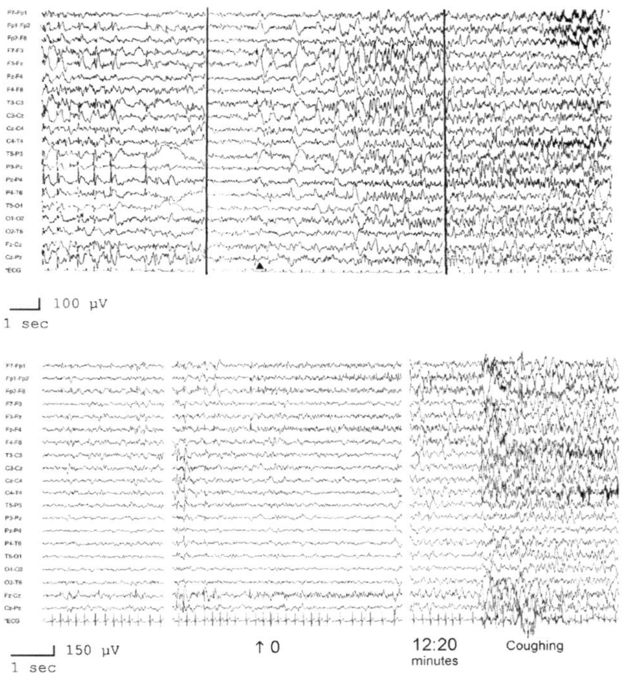

Figure 8 **Ictal EEG of autonomic status epilepticus of non-occipital onset in two children with PS.** Top: **This child had an EEG with interictal cloned-like repetitive multifocal spike-wave complexes that were mainly bi-frontal, left more than right, midline and occipital. Clinically, while asleep, "he suddenly got up with both eyes open, vomited several times and then showed a prolonged atonic state with cyanosis and irregular respiration for 3 minutes". The first EEG change consisted of periodic slow waves from the left fronto-temporal region (F3) for 3 seconds followed by rhythmic generalized discharge of mainly monomorphic rhythmic slow waves intermixed with spikes. ECG showed significant tachycardia during the ictus (see ECG trace). Modified from Oguni *et al.* (1999) with the permission of the editor of *Epilepsia*.**

Bottom: **From video EEG of a 4-year-old boy with autonomic status epilepticus recorded from onset to termination. High amplitude spikes and slow waves are recorded from the bifrontal regions prior to the onset of the electrical discharge, which is also purely bifrontal (arrow). First clinical symptoms with three or four coughs and marked tachycardia appeared 13 min after the onset of the electrical discharge, when this had become bilaterally diffuse. Subsequent clinical symptoms were tachycardia, ictus emeticus (without vomiting) and impairment of consciousness. No other ictal manifestations occurred until termination of the seizure with intravenous lorazepam 70 min after onset.**

Modified from Koutroumanidis *et al.* (2005) with permission of the editor of *Epilepsy & Behaviour*.

The background EEG is usually normal, but diffuse or localized slow wave abnormalities may also occur in at least one EEG in 20% of cases, particularly postictally.

EEG abnormalities, particularly functional spikes, may persist for many years after clinical remission; they disappear when the patient reaches the mid-teens. Conversely, spikes may appear only once in one of a series of EEGs or the EEG may be consistently normal (Specchio *et al.*, 2010b).

Frequency, location and persistence of functional spikes do not determine clinical manifestations, duration, severity and frequency of seizures, or prognosis.

Ictal EEG

Typical autonomic seizures and autonomic status epilepticus of PS have been documented by ictal EEG (Vigevano & Ricci, 1993; Beaumanoir, 1993b; Oguni *et al.*, 1999; Vigevano *et al.*, 2000; Oguni *et al.*, 2001; Demirbilek & Dervent, 2004; Parisi *et al.*, 2005; Koutroumanidis *et al.*, 2005; Battaglia *et al.*, 2007; Iannetti *et al.*, 2009; Specchio *et al.*, 2010) in 20 patients, all during sleep *(Figure 8)*, as reviewed by Specchio *et al.* (2010b). Recorded ictal onsets of typical autonomic seizures start in the posterior (9 cases), frontal (8 cases) regions or diffusely (1 case). Ictal electrical discharge may last long, sometimes 10 minutes or longer, before the first apparent clinical manifestation. There are no significant differences in the clinical manifestations of seizures irrespective of their origin of onset. The first clinical manifestation is usually opening of the eyes. The eyes just open as if the child awakes from sleep. There are no any other abnormal seizure symptoms of tonic or clonic movements of the eyeballs and the eyelids. At this stage, usually the child responds, often correctly, to simple questions. On other occasions, the first clinical symptoms consist of tachycardia or coughing just before eyes opening. Ictal vomiting and other autonomic manifestations as well as deviation of the eyes did not appear to relate to any specific region of EEG activation.

A report of a seizure recorded during tilt-testing documented small increase in blood pressure, significant tachycardia and pronounced increase of norepinephrine, epilenephrin and vasopressin (Gonzalez-Duarte *et al.*, 2011; Koutroumanidis, 2011).

Figure 8 shows ictal EEG of autonomic status epilepticus captured from onset which was non-occipital. Overt ictal clinical manifestations may start minutes after the onset of the electrical seizure discharge.

Magnetoencephalography (MEG)

Thirteen patients with adequate clinical and EEG follow-up documenting PS were investigated with advanced MEG technology combined with MRI (Kanazawa *et al.*, 2005). Equivalent current dipoles (ECD) clustered preferentially in cortical locations along the parietal-occipital, the calcarine or the Rolandic sulci. ECDs along the parietal-occipital sulcus were more often superior (affecting entirely the parietal cortex) than inferior. The ECD clustering was unilateral or bilateral, monofocal or multifocal. Despite the high prevalence of frontal spikes in surface EEG, no frontal ECDs were detected with MEG.

To investigate correlations between developmental brain maturation and spike origin in PS, Saito *et al.* (2008) evaluated age-related or duration-related MEG spike localization in 25 patients with PS. Patients with frontal spikes were significantly older than patients with spikes on Rolandic, parieto-occipital, or calcarine sulci. Both calcarine and parieto-occipital localizations were seen at around the same age. Follow-up MEG demonstrated shifting localization or disappearance of MEG spikes.

Aetiology

PS, like Rolandic epilepsy, is probably genetically determined although conventional genetic influences may be less important than other mechanisms. Usually, no family history of similar seizures exists, though siblings and twins with PS or PS and Rolandic epilepsy have been reported (Ferrie *et al.*, 1997; Caraballo *et al.*, 2000, 2007; Lada *et al.*, 2003; Covanis *et al.*, 2003; Taylor *et al.*, 2008; Specchio *et al.*, 2010a). Families with 3 affected siblings with PS have been reported (Kuzniecky & Rosenblatt, 1987; Gonzalez-Duarte *et al.*, 2011).

There is a high prevalence of febrile seizures ranging from 16% (Ferrie *et al.*, 1997), 26% (Caraballo *et al.*, 2000), 30% (Vigevano & Ricci, 1993) to 45% (Oguni *et al.*, 1999) of children with PS.

SCN1A mutations have been reported in a child (Grosso *et al.*, 2007) and two siblings (Livingston *et al.*, 2009) with relatively early onset of seizures, prolonged time over which many seizures have occurred and strong association with febrile precipitants even after the age of 5 years. However, no such mutations were found in another couple of siblings (personal communication with J. Livingston), homozygous twins (Martin del Valle, 2010) with typical PS and no febrile seizure precipitants as well as 10 patients with PS and febrile seizures (Cordelli *et al.*, 2012). These data indicate that SCN1A mutations when found contribute to a more severe clinical phenotype of PS.

Alteration in *CACNA1H* may have contributed to seizure susceptibility in a Finnish family with a complex seizure phenotype of febrile seizures, childhood absence epilepsy and PS (Siren *et al.*, 2010).

Pathophysiology

In PS, the neuroanatomical and neurophysiological underpinnings of autonomic manifestations are unknown. Any hypothesis of the pathophysiology of PS should explain significant pieces of evidence that converge from clinical, EEG and magnetoencephalographic studies (Panayiotopoulos *et al.*, 2008).

First, autonomic seizures and autonomic status epilepticus with the symptomatology and sequence as in PS, appear to be specific for childhood (Panayiotopoulos, 2004; Ferrie *et al.*, 2007). For example, in adults ictal vomiting occurs scarcely, and as a rule when consciousness is impaired following other focal mainly temporal lobe symptoms, and is attributed to non-dominant mesial temporal lobe involvement (Kramer *et al.*, 1988; Schauble *et al.*, 2002; Koutroumanidis, 2003). In contrast, ictal vomiting in children is common, usually occurs when consciousness is intact without preceding focal cortical symptoms, and probably has no localizing or lateralizing value (see ictal EEG). A possible explanation for this discrepancy may relate to the fact that children are constitutionally more vulnerable to emetic disturbances as exemplified by the "cyclic vomiting syndrome", a non-seizure disorder of unknown aetiology that is also specific to childhood (Li *et al.*, 1999) and associated with autonomic dysfunction (Chelimsky & Chelimsky, 2007). Thus, the preferential involvement of emetic and other autonomic manifestations in PS may be attributed to a maturation-related susceptibility of the central autonomic network (Panayiotopoulos, 2002, 2004). Emesis in PS has been attributed to ictal increase of vasopressin (Gonzalez-Duarte *et al.*, 2011).

Second, the epileptogenic zone in PS is wide and bilateral with multifocal pockets in cortical areas surrounding major fissures such as central, sylvian and mainly calcarine (Kanazawa *et al.*, 2005; Yoshinaga *et al.*, 2006; Saitoh *et al.*, 2007, 2008).

Third, ictal autonomic symptomatology appears to pertain to any epileptogenic cortical onset zone, be this occipital, fronto-temporal or frontal, and usually precede other focal cortical semiology (see the section on ictal EEG). It is likely, that central autonomic networks have a lower threshold to epileptogenic activation than those producing focal cortical semiology (occipital, frontal, central, parietal and probably exceptionally temporal). Irrespective of the localization of their onset, ictal discharges may activate the lower-threshold autonomic centres (and therefore produce autonomic manifestations) before other cortical regions of relatively higher threshold that generate focal cortical symptoms (sensory, motor, visual or other). Seizures remain purely autonomic if ictal neuronal activation of non-autonomic cortical areas fails to reach threshold; otherwise they consist of autonomic and localization-related cortical symptoms and signs that may only rarely occur from onset. This hypothesis may explain why similar autonomic manifestations may appear from anterior or posterior, right or left brain onsets. As seizures primarily involve a particular system (the autonomic), PS may be considered as an electroclinical example of a "system epilepsy" (Koutroumanidis, 2007).

To explain the paradoxical discrepancy between the prolonged and ample-looking ictal discharges that have invariably featured in all published ictal recordings and the also consistent lack of conspicuous cortical (motor or sensory) manifestations for several minutes into the seizure, one may also hypothesize a suboptimal "strength" of the ictal electrical activity. Despite their scalp EEG phenomenology discharges presumably fail to transform into dynamic cortico-cortical propagation and generate conventional cortical symptoms according to their distribution over the cerebrum (being though still capable of activating a more hyperexcitable central autonomic system network).

Syncopal-like attacks are difficult to explain. They may be a distinct seizure-type symptom similar to atonic seizures, but on some occasions they may be due to cardiac asystole (ictal syncope) generated by the seizure discharge.

Differential diagnosis

Despite sound clinical and EEG manifestations, PS escaped recognition for a number of reasons (Ferrie & Livingston, 2010) and mainly because emetic and other autonomic manifestations were often erroneously considered as symptoms of other non-epileptic diseases.

Differentiation from encephalitis, migraine, gastroenteritis and other non-epileptic disorders

The main problem in PS is to recognize emetic and other autonomic manifestations as seizure events, and not to dismiss them or erroneously consider them as unrelated to the ictus and as a feature of encephalitis, migraine, syncope or gastroenteritis. Otherwise, the result is avoidable morbidity, erroneous treatments and costly hospital admissions.

When vomiting is associated with a deteriorating level of consciousness, followed by convulsions, encephalitis or other acute cerebral insults are the prevailing diagnoses in the acute stage. If the child is seen after complete recovery, atypical migraine, gastroenteritis, motion sickness or a first seizure are likely diagnoses. Similarly, ictal syncope has only recently been recognized as an important clinical manifestation of PS and may be misdiagnosed as cardiogenic syncope, pseudoseizure or a more severe encephalopathic state.

Differentiating Panayiotopoulos syndrome from other epileptic disorders is easy

(a) Symptomatic autonomic seizures: One tenth of autonomic seizures and autonomic status epilepticus with a similar presentation to PS are due to heterogeneous cerebral pathology, such as focal or diffuse brain lesions of diverse aetiology. These autonomic seizures are also restricted to childhood. In these symptomatic cases, there is often abnormal neurological or mental symptomatology, abnormal brain imaging, and background EEG abnormalities. Also, patients commonly have additional types of seizures without autonomic symptoms that continue in adult life. Management and treatment is similar to any other form of focal lesional epilepsy.

(b) Childhood occipital epilepsy of Gastaut has entirely different clinical manifestations, despite common interictal EEG features when occipital paroxysms occur in PS *(Table I)*. There is undue emphasis on whether PS manifests with visual hallucinations, which is the prominent seizure type in COE-G. This makes no difference. Even if visual hallucinations were the starting ictal symptom in all patients and for all seizures, there are more significant and striking differences between them. Visual symptoms in PS, when present, occur with other typical clinical, mainly autonomic, vomiting and behavioural manifestations. They are not the predominant seizure symptom. They are never the sole symptom of a seizure and do not occur alone. Usually, they develop after the seizure has started. Their presence signifies spreading of the discharge to the occipital regions of the brain. Exceptionally (in 1% of cases), visual symptoms occur at onset suggesting an occipital origin for the epileptic discharge in these patients.

Furthermore, ictal EEG, when performed is also markedly different as shown in *Figures 8 and 9*.

Table I Differential diagnosis of Panayiotopoulos syndrome *vs.* COE-G

	Panayiotopoulos syndrome	COE-G
Prevalence amongst self-limited focal seizures of childhood	20–30%	1–10%
Mean age at onset	5 year	8 years
Seizure characteristics		
Duration for seconds to 1 minute	None	As a rule
Duration of more than 3 minutes to hours	As a rule	Exceptional
Total number of seizures 1–15	Exclusively	Exceptional
High, sometimes daily, seizure frequency	None	As a rule
Nocturnal	Two thirds	Less than one third
Visual hallucinations	Rare	As a rule
Deviation of the eyes	Frequent	Frequent
Autonomic disturbances (pallor, sweating)	Frequent	Exceptional
Ictal vomiting	Frequent	Exceptional
Ictal behavioural disturbances	Frequent	Exceptional
Blindness	Exceptional	Frequent
Impairment of consciousness	Frequent	Rare
Ictal headache	Rare	Rare
Postictal headache	Exceptional	Frequent
Prognosis		
Remission within 1–2 years from first seizure	As a rule	Exceptional
Seizures after the age of 15 years	Exceptional	Frequent
Ictal EEG	Slow activity with spikes of variable localization	Fast occipital spikes

(c) Rolandic seizures have different clinical manifestations. Emesis, when it occurs, is a concomitant symptom of PS even in children with centro-temporal spikes only (Covanis *et al.*, 2003). Conversely, in some cases of PS, there are concurrent Rolandic symptoms such as hypersalivation.

(d) Photosensitive occipital seizures may have similar symptoms of autonomic disturbances and ictal vomiting but these are usually preceded by elementary visual hallucinations triggered by photic stimuli (Guerrini *et al.*, 1995; Panayiotopoulos, 2005, 2010).

(e) Cases of PS with seizures occurring when the child is febrile may be diagnosed as febrile seizures.

Interpretation of the EEG may also have similar pitfalls. Multiple independent spike foci that occur in at least one EEG of a third of children with PS are considered as features of intractable epilepsies and often occur in the transitional state between hypsarrhythmia and generalized slow wave discharges (see review in Panayiotopoulos, 2005). Cloned-like repetitive multifocal spike-wave complexes are one of the most fascinating EEG aspects of PS. An EEG demonstrating

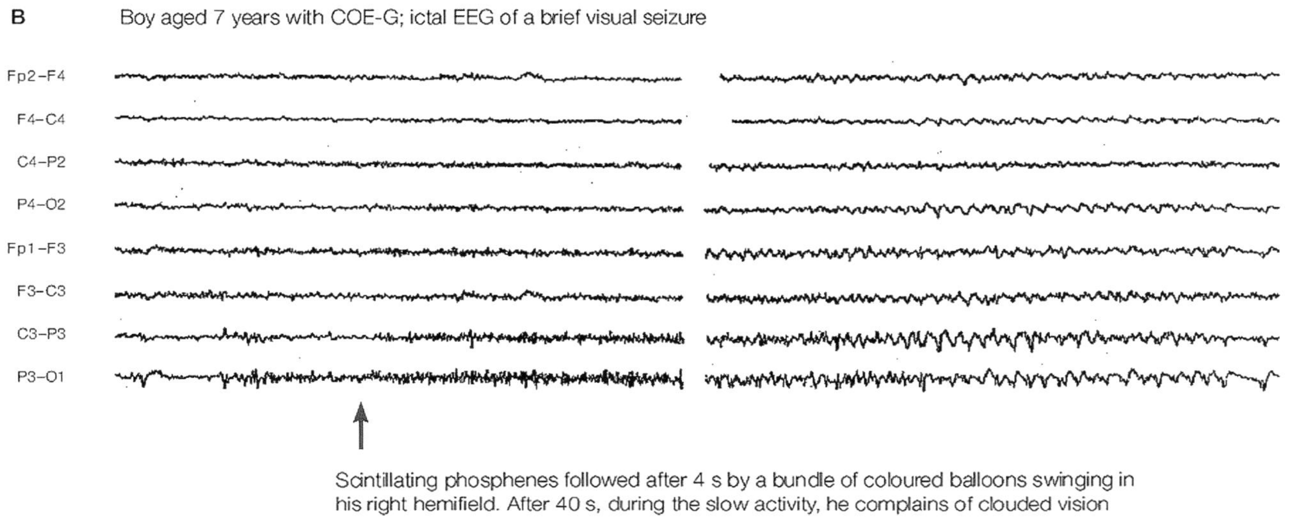

Figure 9

Ictal EEG during a visual seizure in a boy with COE-G. The seizure starts in the left occipital region with fast spikes associated with visual symptoms. This spreads, 4 s later, to the parietal regions and the child sees a bundle of coloured balloons swinging in his right hemifield.This lasted for 40 s and was followed by slow waves that progressively became slower and diffused over the whole brain. At this stage, he complained of clouded vision. This boy was normal physically and intellectually, and also had a normal CT brain scan. At the age of 3 years, he had a nocturnal, left hemiconvulsion. His first EEG showed occipital paroxysms with fixation-off sensitivity. From the age of 4 years, he had started having frequent, brief, visual seizures (simple, coloured, visual hallucinations) provoked by sudden darkness. Modified with permission from Beaumanoir (1993b).

multifocal spikes may be indispensable in the diagnosis of patients with PS if clinical information is inadequate or emetic manifestations are inconspicuous.

Improving diagnosis of Panayiotopoulos syndrome

PS, autonomic seizures and autonomic status epilepticus are still significantly underdiagnosed and often misdiagnosed as encephalitis, atypical migraine, gastroenteritis, motion sickness or first febrile or afebrile seizure. By increasing awareness, diagnosis is expected to improve (Covanis & Panayiotopoulos, 2008). The contribution of EEG technologists is crucial (Sanders *et al.*, 2004). In a prospective study, at the end of 3 years 228 consecutive children aged 1 to 14 years had one or more afebrile epileptic seizures. Fourteen patients (6.1%) had PS diagnosed mainly on clinical grounds. This did not include 11 additional patients with probable PS, either with atypical clinical and EEG features or inadequate information. Of the 14 children with typical PS, only 3 were appropriately diagnosed on referral. Alarmingly, 9 patients were suspected of suffering from encephalitis, a diagnosis that demanded further invasive procedures such as lumbar puncture, erroneous treatment, and costly hospital admissions. For most of the patients, the correct diagnosis and management was prompted by the EEG technologist who obtained the appropriate history through a simple questionnaire while preparing the patient for an EEG (Sanders *et al.*, 2004).

Retrospective analysis and audits of the last 200 children with definite or probable seizures seen or admitted in paediatric departments is recommended for the detection of PS. It is expected that at least 12 of them have autonomic seizures or autonomic status epilepticus with ictal vomiting, 11 of PS and 1 of symptomatic epilepsy (Covanis & Panayitopoulos, 2008). These should follow a dual approach, which is based i) on clinical evidence (ictal autonomic manifestations of which ictus emeticus is more apparent); and ii) EEG evidence (multifocal spikes of which occipital are more prominent).

Prognosis

PS is remarkably benign in terms of its evolution (Panayiotopoulos, 1988, 2002; Oguni *et al.*, 1999; Lada *et al.*, 2003; Ohtsu *et al.*, 2003; Covanis *et al.*, 2003; Caraballo *et al.*, 2007; Specchio *et al.*, 2010a). However, autonomic seizures are of concern in the rare context of cardiorespiratory arrest, though all five reported patients with cardiorespiratory arrest had complete recovery either spontaneously or through cardiopulmonary resuscitations (Panayiotopoulos, 2002; Verrotti *et al.*, 2005; Ferrie *et al.*, 2006; 2007; Mujawar *et al.*, 2011).

The majority of patients with PS have a single or less than 5 seizures until remission. Only one quarter have multiple and sometimes very frequent and prolonged seizures that may be resistant to treatment. Furthermore, the active seizure period is usually very brief with remission commonly occurring within 1–2 years from onset though longer periods of more than 7 years have been reported (Caraballo *et al.*, 2000). Cumulative probability of recurrence was 57.6%, 45.6%, 35.1%, and 11.7% at 6, 12, 24, and 36 months, respectively, after the first seizure (Specchio *et al.*, 2010a). In patients with PS preexisting mild neurobehavioral disorders, seizures tend to be pharmacoresistant and frequent despite final remission by 12 years of age (Oguni *et al.*, 2001; Hirano *et al.*, 2009).

Subtle neuropsychological deficits in some children during the active phase (Germano *et al.*, 2005) may be syndrome-related symptoms in PS, but may also reflect effects of AED (most of the children were on AEDs including phenobarbital and vigabatrin) and/or other contributing factors. In a review of 7 studies on neuropsychological assessments in patients with PS, the overall conclusions were that children with PS have normal IQ, some minor statistically significant differences were found in arithmetic, comprehension picture arrangement, attention and memory (Specchio *et al.*, 2010a). In one of the most complete investigation of visual and visuoperceptual function in 28 children with PS, such abnormalities were mild and uncommon (De Rose *et al.*, 2010). Mild learning difficulties, behavioural problems, visual-perceptive attention abnormalities, visual processing and visual memory problem have also reported (Pérez-Villena *et al.*, 2012; Bedoin *et al.*, 2012; Lopes *et al.*, 2014; Hodges *et al.*, 2016). Prognosis of cognitive function is good even for patients with atypical evolutions (Caraballo *et al.*, 2007).

The risk of epilepsy in adult life appears to be no higher than in the general population (Panayiotopoulos, 2002; Ferrie *et al.*, 2006; Caraballo *et al.*, 2007). However, a fifth of patients develop Rolandic and less often occipital or other seizures but these are also age-related and remit (Panayiotopoulos, 2002). Atypical evolution of PS with absences and drop attacks similar to those described in Rolandic epilepsy is rare probably less than 3% (Caraballo *et al.*, 2001, 2007; Ferrie *et al.*, 2002; Kikumoto *et al.*, 2006).

Management

In the absence of official guidelines regarding neurodiagnostic procedures and management of PS, these may be reasonably assumed by appropriate modifications of the current recommendations regarding febrile seizures (American Academy of Pediatrics, 1999). In the acute stage control of the seizures is para- mount. Half of them are relatively brief and self-limited. The other half, or autonomic status epilepticus, demand appropriate and vigorous evaluation and treatment (see the section "Management of self-limited focal epilepsies in childhood"). The risk of giving multiple drugs that may cause respiratory depression and hypotension should be addressed. Early, parental treatment with oral midazolam is usually effective.

Prophylactic treatment with antiepileptic medication is not recommended even for patients with lengthy seizures or more than 2 recurrences. There is no increased risk of subsequent epilepsy or neurological deficit. Prophylactic treatment may be desired if a child has multiple recurrences or in the unlikely event of parental insistence. Though there is no evidence of superiority amongst monotherapy with various drugs most authors prefer carbamazepine or valproate. Of new AEDs levetiracetam has been used successfully in cases pharmacoresistant to valproate (Garcia & Rubio, 2005).

The traumatizing, sometimes long-lasting effect on parents, even of febrile seizures, is worse for autonomic seizures that may last for many hours compounded by physicians' uncertainty regarding diagnosis, management and prognosis (Valeta, 2005). Supportive family management includes education about PS, psychological support and specific instructions about emergency procedures for possible subsequent seizures (Valeta, 2005; 2010).

Childhood occipital epilepsy of Gastaut (COE-G)

COE-G is a form of self-limited childhood epilepsy manifesting purely with occipital seizures formerly called "benign occipital epilepsy" or "idiopathic childhood occipital epilepsy of Gastaut" (Gastaut, 1981, 1982a, 1982b; Beaumanoir, 1983; Gastaut & Zifkin, 1987;

Gastaut *et al.*, 1992; Ferrie *et al.*, 1997; Panayiotopoulos, 1999a, 1999b; Kivity *et al.*, 2000; Covanis *et al.*, 2005; Gobbi *et al.*, 2008; Caraballo *et al.*, 2008a, 2009).

Demographic data

COE-G is rare (Gastaut *et al.*, 1992) with a reported prevalence of 0.3% of children with newly diagnosed non-febrile seizures (Berg *et al.*, 1999) and 2–7% of those with self-limited focal seizures of childhood (Berg *et al.*, 1999; Panayiotopoulos, 1999a; Kivity *et al.*, 2000; Caraballo *et al.*, 2008a; Gaggero *et al.*, 2014). Peak age at onset is 8–9 years with a reported range from 15 months to 19 years (Gastaut & Zifkin, 1987; Panayiotopoulos, 1999a; Caraballo *et al.*, 2008a). Boys and girls are equally affected.

Clinical manifestations

Seizures are occipital and primarily manifest with elementary visual hallucinations, blindness or both (Gastaut, 1982a; Gastaut & Zifkin, 1987; Gastaut *et al.*, 1992; Panayiotopoulos, 1999a, 1999b; Gobbi *et al.*, 2008; Caraballo *et al.*, 2008a, 2009). They are usually frequent, brief and diurnal.

Visual ictal symptoms

Elementary visual hallucinations are the most common and most characteristic ictal symptom of COE-G. They are frequently the first and often the only seizure symptom. They develop rapidly within seconds and consist mainly of small multicoloured circular patterns that often appear in the periphery of a visual field, becoming larger and multiplying during the course of the seizure, frequently moving towards the other side: "I see millions of small, very bright, mainly blue and green coloured, circular spots of light, which appear on the left side and sometimes move to the right."

Ictal blindness is probably the second commoner symptom after visual hallucinations. It is sudden, usually total and it is frequently the first and often the only seizure symptom in patients who may also have other visual seizures without blindness: "Everything went suddenly black, I could not see and I had to ask other swimmers to show me the direction to the beach."

Impairment of visual awareness is consistently reported by some patients before the appearance of visual hallucinations.

Complex visual hallucinations such as faces and figures and visual illusions such as micropsia, palinopsia and metamorphopsia occur in less than 10% of patients and mainly after the appearance of other visual symptoms (Gastaut & Zifkin, 1987).

Non-visual ictal occipital lobe symptoms

Non-visual occipital symptoms usually appear after the elementary visual hallucinations and these in order of prevalence are deviation of the eyes, eyelid fluttering or repetitive eye closures and sensory hallucinations of ocular movements (Gastaut, 1982a; Gastaut & Zifkin, 1987; Panayiotopoulos, 1999a, 1999b; Gobbi *et al.*, 2008; Caraballo *et al.*, 2008a).

Deviation of the eyes, often associated with ipsilateral turning of the head, is the most common (in about 70% of cases) non-visual ictal symptom. It usually starts after the commencement of visual hallucinations and may be mild, but more often it is forceful tonic and may progress to hemiconvulsions and GTCS. Some children may have seizures of eye deviation from the start without visual hallucinations and it is likely that these cases have a better prognosis (Beaumanoir, 1983; Ferrie *et al.*, 1997). Other ocular manifestations may include unidirectional ocular clonic seizures (oculo-clonic seizures) that are rare, and eyelid fluttering or repetitive eye closures that occur in about 10% of patients, usually at a later stage when consciousness is impaired. They signal an impending secondary GTCS.

Ictal headache, or mainly orbital pain, is a common ictal symptom, and in a small number of patients it may start before the first visual or other ictal occipital symptoms.

Consciousness is intact during the visual symptoms (simple focal seizures), but may be disturbed or lost in the course of the seizure, usually before or at the time of eye deviation or convulsions.

Syncopal-like attacks are rare (Panayiotopoulos, 2002).

A single case, a 7-year-old girl who presented with acute onset elemental visual hallucination and complex partial status epilepticus, followed by ictal respiratory arrest necessitating endotracheal intubation and mechanical ventilation has been reported (Funata *et al.*, 2018).

Extra-occipital seizure progression

Elementary visual hallucinations or other ictal symptoms may progress to complex focal seizures (14%), hemiconvulsions (43%) or GTCS (13%) (Gastaut & Zifkin, 1987). Complex focal seizures of temporal lobe symptomatology are extremely rare and may indicate a symptomatic cause (Panayiotopoulos, 1999b). Ictal vomiting may occur with progression to the non-dominant temporal lobe (Guerrini *et al.*, 1995).

Postictal headache

Postictal headache, mainly diffuse, but also severe, unilateral, pulsating and indistinguishable from migraine headache, occurs in half the patients, in 10% of whom it may be associated with nausea and vomiting (Gastaut & Zifkin, 1987; Panayiotopoulos, 1999a,

1999b; Caraballo *et al.*, 2008a). This occurs immediately, or 5 to 10 minutes after the end of the visual hallucinations. The duration and severity of the headache appears to be proportional to the duration and severity of the preceding seizure although it may also occur after brief simple visual seizures.

Seizure stereotype

For any patient, in every seizure the elementary visual hallucinations have a fingerprint with a stereotypic appearance regarding morphology, colours, location, movement and other characteristics. Most of patients also know at what stage of their ictal manifestations a secondarily GTCS may occur.

Duration and circadian distribution

Visual seizures are usually brief, lasting from a few seconds to 1–3minutes if they occur alone without other occipital or extra-occipital spreading (Gastaut, 1982a; Gastaut & Zifkin, 1987; Panayiotopoulos, 1999a, 1999b; Covanis *et al.*, 2005; Gobbi *et al.*, 2008; Caraballo *et al.*, 2008a). However, a few patients with brief visual seizures may later develop lengthy visual seizures lasting for 10–20 minutes.

Visual seizures are predominantly diurnal and occur at any time of the day but some patients may also have infrequent seizures in sleep or on awakening.

Frequency of seizures

If untreated, the majority of patients experience frequent brief visual seizures ranging from several every day to one per week or month. However, propagation to other seizure manifestations, such as focal or generalized convulsions, is much less frequent occurring once per month, year or even rarer.

Precipitating factors and self-limited photosensitive occipital epilepsy

This is a matter of inclusion criteria. Gastaut considers photosensitivity as part of COE-G (Gastaut, 1982a; Gastaut & Zifkin, 1987) while the ILAE Task Force recognizes "*idiopathic photosensitive occipital lobe epilepsy*" as a syndrome of reflex epilepsy with age-related onset (Engel, 2001, 2006; Berg *et al.*, 2010). Reflex occipital seizures induced by television, video games, and intermittent photic stimulation (IPS) manifest with similar semiology as the spontaneous visual seizures (Aso *et al.*, 1987; Michelucci & Tassinari, 1993; Guerrini *et al.*, 1995, 1998; Yalcin *et al.*, 2000; Panayiotopoulos, 2007). Deviation of the eyes, epigastric discomfort and vomiting, headache, and generalized convulsions may follow. Prognosis is uncertain. Some children may have only 1 or 2 seizures, but others may not remit. Interictal EEG shows spontaneous and photically induced occipital spikes. Centro-temporal spikes may coexist. Ictal EEG documented the occipital origin and the spreading of the discharges to the temporal regions (Guerrini *et al.*, 1995, 1998). There remain no other significant precipitating factors in COE-G if photosensitive patients are excluded. Despite fixation off sensitivity (FOS) in EEG, only a few patients report seizure precipitation by going from bright light to darkness or by darkness itself (Beaumanoir *et al.*, 1989).

Aetiology

There is an increased family history of epilepsies (21–37%) or migraine (9–16%) (Gastaut & Zifkin, 1987; Caraballo *et al.*, 2008a) but familial COE-G appears to be rare (Nagendran *et al.*, 1990; Grosso *et al.*, 2008; Taylor *et al.*, 2008). Monozygotic twin pairs did not show a higher concordance rate than dizygotic twin pairs suggesting that COE-G may not be a purely genetic disorder and that non-conventional genetic influences or environmental factors may play a major role (Taylor *et al.*, 2008).

Pathophysiology

The seizures are purely of occipital lobe origin. The epileptogenic zone involves wide and bilateral networks within the occipital lobes and this localization is congruent with the symptomatogenic zone. Elementary visual hallucinations originate from the visual cortex, complex visual hallucinations from the junction of the occipital with the parietal and temporal lobes, formed visual illusions from the lateral occipital-posterior temporal junction and tonic deviation of the eyes from the medial occipital cortex, above or below the calcarine sulcus. Ictal blindness may reflect bi-occipital seizure spreading but this may not explain its sudden onset, without any other preceding manifestations. From the EEG standpoint, the occipital paroxysms are usually bilateral and synchronous because they are activated in both occipital regions by the elimination of fixation and central vision (FOS) (Panayiotopoulos, 1981) and not by thalamo-cortical activation proposed by Gastaut & Zifkin (1987).

The mechanisms for postictal headache are unknown. It is likely that the occipital seizure discharge triggers a genuine migraine headache through trigeminovascular or brainstem mechanisms (Panayiotopoulos, 1999b, 1999c).

Diagnostic procedures

By definition, all tests other than the EEG are normal. However, high-resolution MRI is mandatory, because symptomatic occipital epilepsy present with the same clinical-EEG manifestations (Adcock & Panayiotopoulos, 2012). Early age of seizure onset and an abnormal neurological examination were significant predictors of abnormal MR imaging in children with epilepsy with occipital features (Schrader *et al.*, 2011).

Electroencephalography

The interictal EEG shows occipital paroxysms (Gastaut, 1982a; Gastaut & Zifkin, 1987), often demonstrating FOS (Panayiotopoulos, 1981) *(Figure 10)*. Because terminology is often unclear and FOS is not always tested, the prevalence of classical occipital paroxysms with FOS is uncertain and ranges from 100% (Gastaut & Zifkin, 1987), 88% (Caraballo *et al.*, 2008a) to 19% (Panayiotopoulos, 1999a) or even less (Tsiptsios *et al.*, 2010). However, it should also be emphasized that FOS is not specific for any syndrome, and may also occur in patients without childhood occipital epilepsy of Gastaut and adults (Fattouch *et al.*, 2013; Karkare *et al.*, 2018). Occipital paroxysms may also be suppressed during various neuro-psychologic conditions that required attention and different mental processes (Rots *et al.*, 2012).

Some patients may have only random occipital spikes, whereas others may have occipital spikes only in sleep EEG and some may have a consistently normal EEG (Panayiotopoulos, 1999b; Tsiptsios *et al.*, 2010). Centro-temporal, frontal and GSES occur together with occipital spikes in around 16–20% of patients (Herranz Tanarro *et al.*, 1984; Gastaut & Zifkin, 1987; Wakamoto *et al.*, 2011). IPS consistently elicits occipital spikes and/or generalized discharges in photosensitive patients.

As it happens with the Rolandic spikes, occipital spikes are not pathognomonic of any particular syndrome, because they also occur in a variety of organic brain diseases with or without seizures, in children with congenital or early onset visual and ocular deficits, and even in 0.5–1.2% of normal preschool age children (Gibbs & Gibbs, 1952, 1967; Kellaway, 1980).

They are common in young children with a peak age at first discovery of 4–5 years, and "tend to disappear in adult life, and the subsidence of the EEG abnormality is usually accompanied by a cessation of seizures" (Gibbs & Gibbs, 1952, 1967).

Ictal EEG: There are many reported ictal EEGs (Gastaut, 1982a; Gastaut & Zifkin, 1987; Aso *et al.*, 1987; De Romanis *et al.*, 1988, 1991; Beaumanoir, 1993a, 1993b; Thomas *et al.*, 2003). Seizure onset is preceded by the disappearance of occipital paroxysms, and is characterized by the sudden appearance of an occipital discharge that consists of fast rhythms, fast spikes or both and is of much lower amplitude than the occipital paroxysms *(Figure 9)*. Elementary visual hallucinations relate to the initially fast spike activity and complex visual hallucinations may occur when the ictal discharge is slower. In oculo-clonic seizures, spikes and spike-wave complexes are slower, and a localised ictal fast spike rhythm may occur before deviation of the eyes. Ictal EEG during blindness is characterized by pseudo-periodic slow waves and spikes, which differ from those seen in ictal visual hallucinations. There are usually no postictal abnormalities.

Differential diagnosis

The differential diagnosis of COE-G is mainly from symptomatic occipital epilepsy, migraine with aura, acephalgic and basilar migraine where misdiagnosis is very high (Panayiotopoulos, 1999a, 1999b, 2006; Belcastro *et al.*, 2011).

Patients with symptomatic occipital epilepsy may often have identical symptoms as COE-G with normal neuro-ophthalmological examination and routine brain imaging. Thus, high-resolution MRI is required to detect subtle lesions (Kuzniecky *et al.*, 1997). Occipital seizures of mitochondrial disorders, Lafora disease and coeliac disease should be considered (Panayiotopoulos, 1999a; Taylor *et al.*, 2003).

The differential diagnosis of COE-G from migraine is usually easy if all clinical elements are properly assessed and synthesised *(Table II)*. Contrary to visual seizures, the visual aura of migraine develops slowly within minutes, lasts long for 10–20 minutes and consists of mainly achromatic and linear patterns (Panayiotopoulos, 1994; Russell & Olesen, 1996; Schott, 2007). Illustration of the visual symptoms of the attacks by the patient is a powerful tool in differential diagnosis and to inform objective analysis *(Figure 11)*. Orbital pain in the ictal phase of visual hallucinations is typical of occipital seizures and does not occur in migraine. However, post-attack headache is common and similar for both occipital epilepsy and migraine. Basilar migraine attacks also develop slowly within minutes, last for 30 to 60 minutes and consist of mainly bilateral impairment of vision associated with, or followed by, neurological symptoms such as vertigo, tinnitus, ataxia, bilateral weakness and dysaesthesiae which do not occur in occipital lobe epilepsy (Panayiotopoulos, 1999c).

Mistaking visual seizures as migraine attacks may be common in publications referring to controversial diagnostic terms such as "migralepsy" and "basilar migraine with occipital paroxysms". Critical reviews of such reported cases indicate that these are likely to be genuine occipital seizures imitating migraine (Panayiotopoulos, 1999c).

Despite some overlapping features, COE-G is distinctive from PS *(Table I)* and the differences have been statistically validated (Panayiotopoulos, 1999a). As a rule of thumb seizure onset is primarily with visual symptoms in COE-G and with autonomic manifestations in PS.

Prognosis

The prognosis of COE-G is not as predictable as that of Rolandic epilepsy and Panayiotopoulos syndrome. The main reason is that the boundaries of this syndrome are still undefined, because symptomatic and generalized epilepsies have been included by Gastaut (Gastaut, 1982a; Gastaut & Zifkin, 1987) in what, by definition,

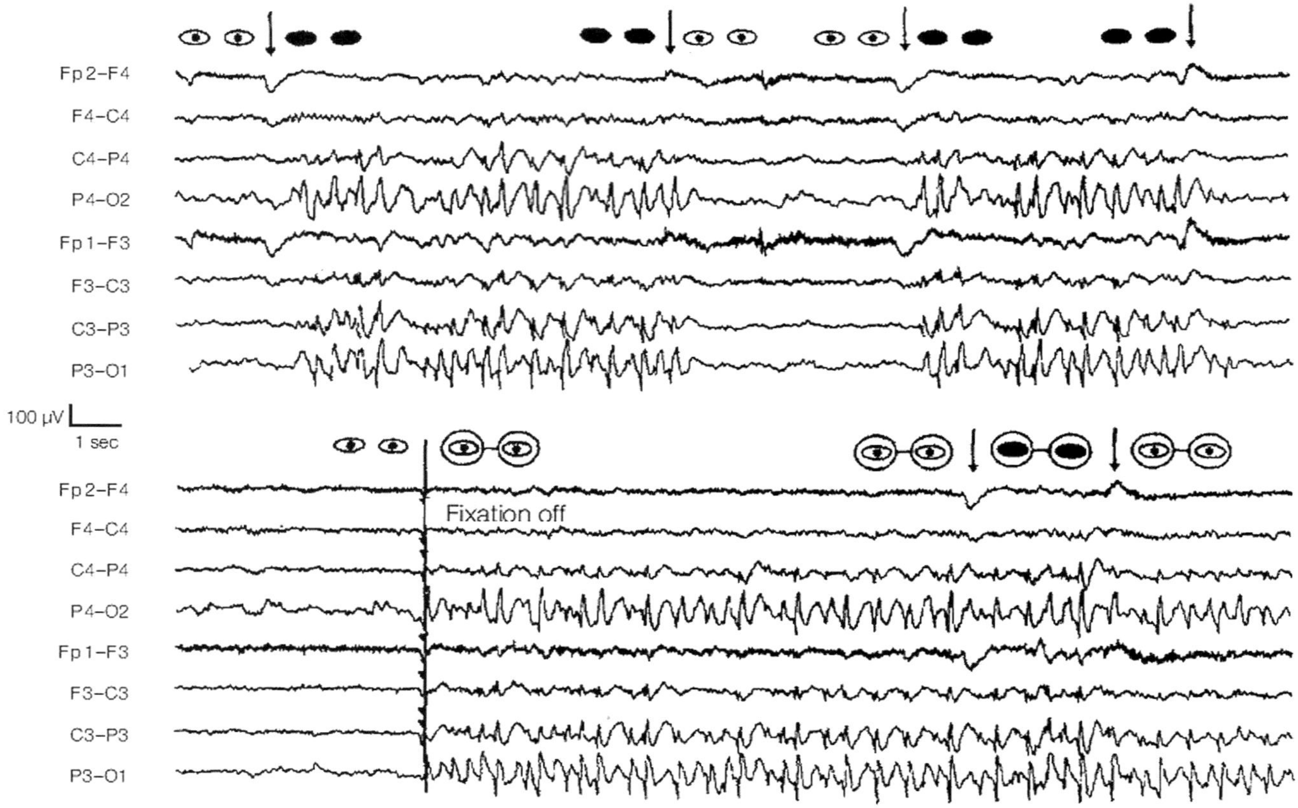

Figure 10

Case 26 of COE-G in Panayiotopoulos (1999a). Occipital paroxysms occur as long as fixation and central vision are eliminated by any means (eyes closed, darkness + 10 spherical lenses, Ganzfeld stimulation). Under these conditions, eye opening cannot inhibit the spikes. Symbols of the eyes open or closed without glasses denote that the recording was made with the lights on and whenever fixation was possible. Symbols of the eyes open or closed with glasses denote that the recording was made when fixation and central vision were eliminated by any of the above means.

is an idiopathic condition with focal occipital seizures. Nevertheless, available data indicate that remission occurs in 50–60% of patients within 2–4 years after onset (Gastaut & Zifkin, 1987; Panayiotopoulos, 1999b; Fejerman *et al.*, 2007; Caraballo *et al.*, 2008a). Seizures show a dramatically good response to carbamazepine in more than 90% of patients. However, 40–50% of patients may continue having visual seizures and infrequent secondarily GTCS. Rarely, atypical evolutions to epilepsy with CSWS and cognitive deterioration have been reported (Tenembaum *et al.*, 1997). Also, rarely children with COE-G may manifest with typical absence seizures, which appear before or after the onset of occipital seizures (Wakamoto *et al.*, 2011; Caraballo *et al.*, 2005). The possibility of subtle cognitive deficits should be considered in some patients. Neuropsychological evaluation of patients with COE-G indicate lower scores for attention,

Table II **Main clinical differences between occipital seizures of COE-G and migraine with visual aura (from Caraballo *et al.* [2009] with permission)**

	COE-G	Migraine
Daily occurrence	Common	Rare
Rapid development of visual symptoms (in seconds)	As a rule	Probably none
Brief duration (1–3 minutes)	Frequent	Rare
Long duration (> 10 minutes)	Rare	As a rule
Mainly colored and circular visual hallucinations	As a rule	Rare
Mainly achromatic or black and white linear visual hallucinations	Rare	As a rule
Tonic deviation of eyes, repetitive eyelid blinking and other oculoclonic phenomena	As a rule	None
Progression to impairment of consciousness	Common	Very rare (unless when basilar migraine is involved)

memory, and intellectual functioning, poor scholastic achievement and behavioral impairment, as well as for specific deficits in the visuo-perceptual or visuospatial domain (Gulgonen *et al.*, 2000; Chilosi *et al.*, 2006 ; Gagliano *et al.*, 2007 ; Brancati *et al.*, 2012; Shu *et al.*, 2013 ; Ferrari-Marinho *et al.*, 2013).

Management

In contrast to other phenotypes of self-limited focal epilepsy of childhood, patients with COE-G often suffer from frequent seizures and therefore prophylactic treatment, mainly with carbamazepine, is likely to be mandatory. Secondarily GTCS are probably unavoidable without medication.

A slow reduction in the dose of medication 2 or 3 years after the last visual or other minor or major seizure should be advised, but if visual seizures reappear, treatment should be restored.

Benign childhood seizure susceptibility syndrome: a unified concept of self-limited (idiopathic benign) focal seizures in childhood

Self-limited focal epilepsies in childhood are probably a group of syndromes of one nosological continuum of benign childhood seizure susceptibility syndrome (BCSSS) (Panayiotopoulos, 1993, 2002; Panayiotopoulos *et al.*, 2008; Ferrie, 2010a). They share common clinical and EEG characteristics. Seizures are infrequent, usually nocturnal and remit within 1–3 years of onset. Brief or prolonged seizures, even focal status epilepticus, may be the only clinical event in the patient's lifetime. Ictal autonomic manifestations, such as hypersalivation, emesis, headache and ictal syncope, which are unusual in other epileptic syndromes or in adults, are frequent and may occasionally appear in isolation. The clinical and EEG characteristics of one syndrome may evolve into another or a child may simultaneously develop features of another form of self-limited childhood focal seizures. Affected siblings may have the same or another type of self-limited childhood focal seizures.

Febrile seizures are common. Neurological and intellectual states are normal, but some children may experience mild and reversible neuropsychological problems during the active stage of the disorder. Brain imaging is normal. There are usually severe EEG abnormalities of spikes, which commonly are disproportionate to the frequency of seizures. EEG spikes are regional (bilateral and multifocal) rather than strictly focal, and there is a significant overlap of interictal topographies. Epileptogenic foci, irrespective of their location, manifest as abundant, high-amplitude, sharp-slow wave complexes which occur mainly in clusters. They are often bilateral, independent or synchronous, frequently combined with foci from other cortical areas or brief generalized discharges, and are exaggerated in sleep stages I-IV. A normal EEG is rare and should prompt a sleep EEG study. Similar EEG features, which resolve with age, are found in normal school-age children (*Table III*) and 1% of children who have had an EEG for reasons other than seizures.

There is no justification for suggesting that all these syndromes differ merely because an "epileptogenic" focus is a little anterior or posterior, or lateral or medial to the centro-temporal regions. A unified concept of self-limited childhood focal seizures is also suggested by the frequency of more than one type of self-limited childhood focal

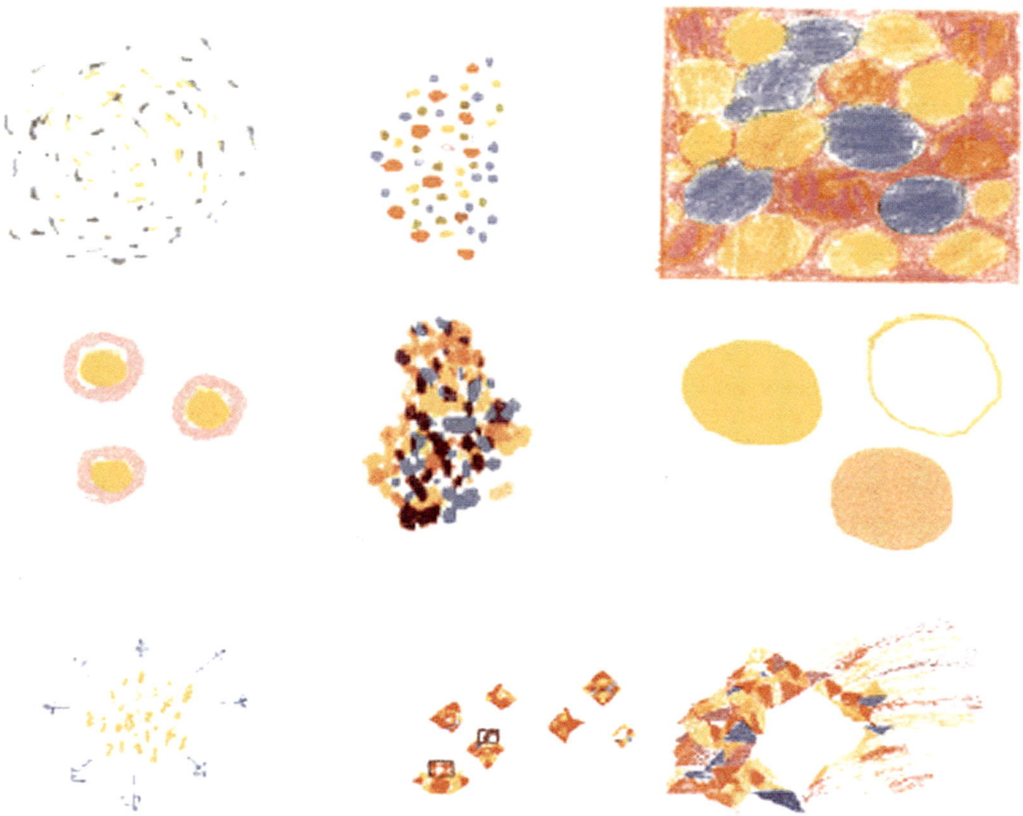

Figure 11

Elementary visual hallucinations as perceived and drawn by patients with COE-G. From Panayiotopoulos (1999a).

Table III EEG functional spikes in normal children (% median and range) (modified from Panayiotopoulos [1999a])

Age (years)	Centrotemporal spikes	Occipital spikes	Frontal spikes	Generalized discharges
5–12	2.25 (0.7–3.5)	0.15 (0.0–0.4)	0.10 (0.1–0.6)	1.00 (0.1–1.1)
1–5	0.40 (0.3–0.4)	0.90 (0.8–1)	0.05 (0–0.1)	0.20 (0.1–0.3)

seizures in an affected child, siblings or both. The relevant ictal semeiologies and EEG findings suggest that each one of these forms reflects constitutional hyperexcitability of a particular functional brain area or system: the lower Rolandic (somatosensory) cortex that represents the face and the oropharynx bilaterally in Rolandic epilepsy, the occipital areas (cortical visual system) in COE-G and of the central autonomic network bilaterally and diffusely in PS (Koutroumanidis, 2007). In all probability, all these conditions are linked together by a common, genetically determined, mild and reversible, functional derangement of the maturational process of the brain (Panayiotopoulos, 1993, 2002; Panayiotopoulos *et al.*, 2008). This derangement is often clinically silent and presents in more than 90% with EEG sharp and slow waves that are age related. The remaining minority have infrequent focal seizures with symptoms that are localization and age related and dependent. A few of these children, with or without seizures, could also possibly have minor and fully reversible neuropsychological symptoms that are rarely clinically overt and can be detected only by formal neuropsychological testing. Finally, there may be a very small number of patients (< 1%) in whom this derangement of brain maturation may be further derailed to a more aggressive condition with seizures, neuropsychological manifestations and EEG abnormalities of various combinations and various degrees of severity, such as atypical benign focal epilepsy of childhood, Landau-Kleffner syndrome and epilepsy with continuous spike-and-slow-wave during sleep (Panayiotopoulos, 1999a; Caraballo *et al.*, 2011).

This concept of BCSSS is in agreement with previously expressed views of "functional epilepsies of maturation" (Sorel & Rucquoy-Ponsar, 1969), "multifactorial pathogenesis of epilepsies with benign focal epileptiform sharp waves" (Doose *et al.*, 1997, 2002), "selective rates of maturation of the different cortical areas" (Luders *et al.*, 1987) and more recently of possible "neurobiological relationships" between BCSSS and IGE (Taylor *et al.*, 2003).

BCSSS, febrile and other self-limited (idiopathic) focal seizures in neonates and infants

One of the most interesting aspects of self-limited childhood seizures is their striking age-related sequence that appears to reflect enhanced epileptogenicity of the developing brain, as a whole and also of its functional systems, in different stages of maturation. Benign neonatal and infantile seizures, Rolandic epilepsy, PS, COE-G and other clinical phenotypes of BCSSS are specific to early life and do not occur in adults. This is also the case with most febrile seizures whose different genetic influences may explain their high prevalence amongst patients with BCSSS and other more severe types of epilepsy, including the febrile plus phenotypes and genotypes (Harkin *et al.*, 2007; Scheffer *et al.*, 2007). It appears that there are three main periods of age-related childhood susceptibility to benign seizures: Febrile, mainly generalized, convulsions first appear in early childhood at a peak age of around 18–22 months. Rolandic epilepsy and COE-G manifest with purely focal seizures and occur in late childhood age. PS presents with mainly autonomic seizures and covers the intermediate early childhood period with peak at 4 or 5 years *(Figure 12)*. The neonatal and early infantile periods are not immune to focal seizure susceptibility either, as indicated by the benign neonatal seizures of the first few days of life (Plouin & Anderson, 2005) and the benign infantile focal seizures of Watanabe-Vigevano syndrome (Vigevano *et al.*, 2008). This point is exemplified by reports of children with neonatal seizures who later developed Rolandic epilepsy (Maihara *et al.*, 1999) or PS (Lada *et al.*, 2003; Panayiotopoulos, 2005).

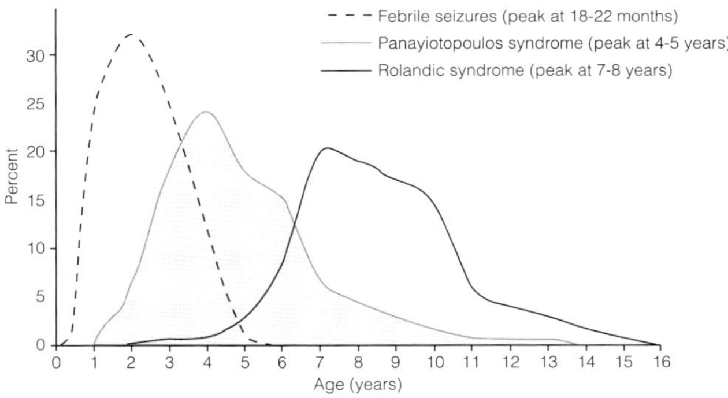

Figure 12 **Diagramatic age-related presentation of febrile seizures, Panayiotopoulos syndrome and Rolandic epilepsy. Reproduced with permission from Panayiotopoulos (2002).**

BCSSS and idiopathic generalized epilepsies

The majority of BCSSS if properly diagnosed do not have any clinical or EEG resemblance to idiopathic generalized epilepsies though others may disagree (Taylor *et al.*, 2003). Overlap of BCSSS with IGE is limited (see above). However, a possible link, the type and extent of which should be explored further with clinical and genetic studies may be suggested by: i) the occurrence of EEG generalized discharges in BCSSS (though these are often markedly different from the classical generalized spike or polyspike discharges of

IGE); ii) an undetermined but probably small proportion of patients with any type of BCSSS that may also suffer typical generalized convulsive or absence seizures either during the active phase of BCSSS or more often at a later stage (Caraballo *et al.*, 2004); iii) an undetermined but probably small proportion of patients with syndromes of IGE including childhood absence epilepsy that may also have EEG focal spikes only or together with any type of seizures of BCSSS (Beaumanoir *et al.*, 1974; Taylor *et al.*, 2003; Caraballo *et al.*, 2008b)

Other phenotypes of BCSSS

There are reports of children suffering from benign childhood focal seizures with clinical-EEG manifestations that cannot be classified as Rolandic epilepsy, PS or COE-G. They may represent rare, atypical or overlapping presentations of BCSSS.

Benign childhood seizures with affective symptoms

Benign childhood epilepsy with affective symptoms, reported in approximately 50 patients (Nascimento *et al.*, 2017), is a clinical phenotype of BCSSS with features common in both PS (behavioural and autonomic symptoms) and Rolandic epilepsy (speech arrest and hypersalivation) (Dalla Bernardina *et al.*, 1992, 2007; Capovilla & Beccaria, 2010; Nascimento *et al.*, 2017). Onset is between 2 and 9 years of age and both sexes are equally affected.

Seizures manifest with terror and screaming, autonomic disturbances (pallor, sweating, abdominal pain, hypersalivation), chewing and other automatisms, speech arrest and mild impairment of consciousness.

"This terror was expressed by the child starting to scream, to yell or to call his mother; he clung to her or to anyone nearby or went to a corner of the room hiding his face in his hands. His terrorized expression was sometimes associated with either chewing or swallowing movements, distressed laughter, arrest of speech with glottal noises, moans and salivation, or some kind of autonomic manifestation, such as pallor, sweating or abdominal pain, that the child expressed by bringing his hands onto his abdomen and saying 'It hurts me, it hurts me'. These phenomena were associated with changes in awareness (loss of contact) that did not amount to complete unconsciousness" (Dalla Bernardina *et al.*, 1992).

These are usually brief for 1–2 minutes, frequent occurring several times a day in wakefulness or sleep. A fifth of patients have febrile seizures and some may also have infrequent Rolandic seizures. Generalized seizures do not occur.

The interictal EEG shows high-amplitude fronto-temporal and parieto-temporal spikes that are exaggerated by sleep. Ictal EEG discharges are mainly localized in the fronto-temporal, centro-temporal or parietal regions and are stereotypical for each patient.

The response to treatment is excellent and remission occurs within 1–2 years from onset. Behavioural problems may be prominent during the active stage of the disease, but subside later with seizure remittance.

Benign childhood epilepsy with parietal spikes and frequent extreme somatosensory-evoked spikes (Giant somatosensory evoked spikes)

Benign childhood epilepsy with parietal spikes and frequent GSES (De Marco & Tassinari, 1981; Dalla Bernardina *et al.*, 1991; Tassinari & De Marco, 1992; Fonseca & Tedrus, 2000) has been proposed as another phenotype of BCSSS. The defining features are EEG spikes in the parietal regions, which are often elicited by tactile stimulation *(Figure 2)*. However, GSES are not specific for any syndrome because they also occur in 10–20% of children with Rolandic seizures (Fonseca & Tedrus, 2000), in a few patients with PS (Panayiotopoulos, 1999a, 2002) and in children with no seizures (Negrin & De Marco, 1977).

Versive seizures of the head and body, often without impairment of consciousness, are mainly diurnal and infrequent. Frequent seizures and focal status epilepticus are exceptional.

Remission usually occurs within one year from seizure onset, but EEG abnormalities may persist for longer.

Benign childhood focal seizures associated with frontal or midline spikes

Benign childhood focal seizures associated with frontal (Beaumanoir & Nahory, 1983; Martin-Santidrian *et al.*, 1998; Panayiotopoulos, 1999a) or midline spikes (Bagdorf & Lee, 1993; Panayiotopoulos, 1999a) have been described and long follow-up reports have confirmed a benign course, although no systematic studies have been published. However, EEG spike foci specificity is questionable, as EEG spike foci of various locations (including frontal and midline) are also seen in Rolandic epilepsy and more commonly in PS, and midline spikes are more common in children than in adults (Kutluay *et al.*, 2001; Sanders *et al.*, 2002).

"Benign infantile focal epilepsy with midline spikes during sleep" has been described as a new syndrome of BCSSS (Bureau *et al.*, 2002; Capovilla *et al.*, 2006; Flesler *et al.*, 2010). Age at onset is in the first 3 years of life and both sexes are equally affected. Seizures consist mainly of staring, motion arrest, cyanosis, loss of consciousness and stiffening of the arms. Clonic convulsions and automatisms are rare.

Seizures are brief from 1 to 5 minutes, mainly diurnal and are generally infrequent from one to three per year. There is a strong family history of undefined types of epileptic seizures with benign epilepsies prevailing.

Interictal EEG abnormalities are seen mainly in NREM sleep and consist of small, mostly singular, midline and Rolandic spikes. The prognosis is excellent, with remission of seizures, normal development and normalization of the EEG before the age of 4 years.

Differential diagnosis between syndromes of BCSSS

The differential diagnosis between the main phenotypes of BCSSS is easy in their typical presentations. Problems may arise in children with clinical symptoms that fall into two (or more) phenotypes or from overemphasizing on EEG localization. As in any other medical condition, a single symptom is of limited syndromic significance. The differential diagnosis requires that symptoms are meaningfully synthesized in regard to quality and quantity, chronological sequence, consistency, relation to other seizure manifestations, the circumstances of their appearance and the overall clustering of clinical-EEG manifestations.

Rolandic epilepsy *vs.* Panayiotopoulos syndrome

Their differential diagnosis is usually easy. However, there are some cases with overlapping features:

(a) One tenth of children with PS often have typical and lengthy autonomic seizures with concurrent Rolandic features such as speech arrest, hemifacial convulsions, hypersalivation and OPS but these appear after the onset of autonomic symptoms and emesis (Ferrie *et al.*, 1997; Oguni *et al.*, 1999; Kivity *et al.*, 2000; Panayiotopoulos, 2002; Lada *et al.*, 2003; Caraballo *et al.*, 2007; Specchio *et al.*, 2010b;Yoshinaga *et al.*, 2015). Conversely, these ictal symptoms occur at onset and usually without autonomic symptoms in Rolandic epilepsy.

(b) One tenth of children with PS develop pure Rolandic seizures, either in parallel with autonomic seizures, or at a later age prior to final remission (Oguni *et al.*, 1999; Panayiotopoulos, 2002; Lada *et al.*, 2003; Caraballo *et al.*, 2004, 2007; Specchio *et al.*, 2010a; Yoshinaga *et al.*, 2015).

(c) The topography of interictal spikes may overlap. Covanis *et al.*, (2003) studied 24 otherwise normal children with focal non-febrile seizures who had emetic manifestations in at least one seizure and CTS in at least one EEG; 21 (83%) had ictal semiology typical of PS but 5 also had concurrent Rolandic symptoms and 4 later developed pure Rolandic seizures. The other 4 children (17%) had typical Rolandic seizures with concurrent ictus emeticus. Ohtsu *et al.* (2007) found that in early-onset Rolandic epilepsy vomiting usually happened in the middle of the ictus, seizures, neurocognitive and behavioral abnormalities were more frequent while focal status epilepticus and prolonged seizures were less common than in PS.

(d) Of siblings one may have Rolandic seizures and another PS and there is a high prevalence of febrile seizures in both (Ferrie *et al.*, 1997; Oguni *et al.*, 1999; Panayiotopoulos, 2002; Caraballo *et al.*, 2007).

Self-limited childhood occipital epilepsy of Gastaut *vs.* Panayiotopoulos syndrome

The differentiation here is more straightforward *(Table I)*. The seizures of COE-G are purely occipital and as such start and often end only with occipital lobe symptomatology. Further, seizures are mainly brief, frequent and diurnal. Rarely, seizures may be longer and also occur in sleep but these are also fundamentally different to the Rolandic epilepsy or the autonomic seizures and autonomic status epilepticus of PS.

Exceptionally ictal vomiting may occur in COE-G but this follows the appearance of visual symptomatology as it happens with reflex photosensitive occipital seizures (Guerrini *et al.*, 1995, 1998) and the same patient usually has frequent brief occipital seizures. Conversely, visual symptoms in PS, when present, are not the sole manifestation of a seizure, stereotypical and only exceptionally (1%) are reported at seizure onset (Ferrie *et al.*, 1997; Yalcin *et al.*, 1997; Panayiotopoulos, 2002; Caraballo *et al.*, 2007). From the EEG standpoint, occipital paroxysms or occipital spikes which characterize COE-G are also common in PS but these often occur with extra-occipital spikes and with shifting locations in sequential EEG. Further, ictal EEG is markedly different in these syndromes.

Reported difficulties in the differential diagnosis of COE-G and PS may arise when assessing them on individual symptoms and features without considering quality, chronological sequence from onset, stereotypical appearance or not that may be common even amongst different disorders including migraine with aura (visual hallucinations, lengthy durations, vomiting and headache) *(Table I)*.

Further, the commonly quoted argument that PS is not essentially different from COE-G considering that "the younger the children are, the less likely they are to describe visual symptoms" (Andermann & Zifkin, 1998) is not tenable: i) more than two thirds of children with

PS are older than 4 years and therefore able to describe their visual experiences; ii) there is no difference in seizure presentation between younger and older children with PS.

A few patients with either PS or Rolandic epilepsy may later develop purely occipital seizures as of COE-G (Guerrini *et al.*, 1997; Parmeggiani & Guerrini, 1999; Panayiotopoulos, 2002). These cases are easy to diagnose and indicate the intimate links of these disorders within the framework of BCSSS.

Management of self-limited focal epilepsies in childhood

Short- and long-term treatment strategies of self-limited focal epilepsies in childhood are largely empirical and need re-evaluation (Panayiotopoulos *et al.*, 2008; Ferrie, 2010b).

Acute management

Control of the seizure is paramount. Long-lasting seizures (> 10 minutes) or status epilepticus (> 30 minutes to hours) is a feature in two-thirds of children (70%) with PS. This is a genuine paediatric emergency that demands appropriate and vigorous diagnosis and treatment as for status epilepticus. Early, usually parental administration of appropriate drugs and mainly buccal midazolam is more effective than late emergency treatment. Aggressive treatment (particularly when intravenous lorazepam or diazepam are used) should be avoided because of the risk of iatrogenic complications, including cardiorespiratory arrest (Ferrie *et al.*, 2007; Lacroix *et al.*, 2011).

Continuous antiepileptic treatment

Continuous antiepileptic medication is not usually recommended. Although effective AED may prevent the occurrence of additional seizures, potential adverse effects may not commensurate with the benefit. Decisions on management must take into account the following:

(a) Most children have excellent prognosis: 10–30% may have only a single seizure and 60–70% may have less than 10 in total. However, 10–20% of children may have frequent seizures, which are sometimes resistant to treatment.

(b) Remission of benign childhood focal seizures is expected in all patients by the age of 15–16 years at the latest.

(c) There is no evidence that the long-term prognosis is worse in untreated children (Ambrosetto & Tassinari, 1990), although they may not be protected against seizure recurrences and particularly GTCS Peters *et al.*, 2001).

(d) Some children become frightened, even by simple focal seizures, and some parents are unable to cope with the possibility of another fit despite firm reassurances.

(e) Persistence and frequency of EEG functional spikes do not predict clinical severity, frequency or degree of liability to seizures.

(f) In contrast to the other phenotypes of the BCSSS, patients with COE-G often suffer from frequent seizures and therefore prophylactic AED treatment may be mandatory. Secondarily GTCS are probably unavoidable without medication.

Continuous prophylaxis consists of daily monotherapy using any AED that has proven efficacy in focal seizures and minimal adverse effects in children. The 2006 ILAE treatment guidelines found that "no AED had level A or level B efficacy and effectiveness evidence as initial monotherapy" in Rolandic epilepsy (Glauser *et al.*, 2006). Of older AED most authorities prefer carbamazepine in USA (Wheless *et al.*, 2005) and valproic acid in Europe (Wheless *et al.*, 2007) though these may have equivalent efficacy with all others (phenobarbital, valproic acid, phenytoin, clonazepam) (Ferrie *et al.*, 1997; Bouma *et al.*, 2002); carbamazepine may exaggerate seizures in a minority of children with BCSSS including PS (Kikumoto *et al.*, 2006) and valproate is associated with significant adverse effects. Sulthiame has been revived as an excellent drug for the treatment of Rolandic epilepsy with EEG normalisation (Bast *et al.*, 2003; Ben Zeev *et al.*, 2004) but this may be associated with cognitive abnormalities (Wirrell *et al.*, 2008). Recommended newer AEDs include levetiracetam (Verrotti *et al.*, 2007; Kossoff *et al.*, 2007), gabapentin (Bourgeois, 2000) and lamotrigine (Wheless *et al.*, 2005). Lamotrigine on rare occasions may cause seizure exacerbation and cognitive deterioration (Cerminara *et al.*, 2004). "Kepprarage" is a well-known adverse effect of levetiracetam (Keppra®) in around 10% of children.

Stopping medication

Strategies of withdrawing medication differ among experts, although all agree that there is no need to continue medication 1–3 years after the last seizure and certainly not after age 14 when most self-limited childhood focal seizures remit, or age 16, when they are practically non-existent. Withdrawal of AED medications should be very slow, reducing the dose in monthly steps until complete discontinuation. This is because it is expected that any possible seizure recurrence during the process of very slow drug withdrawal would manifest with mild, brief and simple focal seizures with no secondarily GTCSs. In the case of phenobarbital and benzodiazepines, slow withdrawal of medication is mandatory to avoid risking withdrawal seizures.

Parental needs and support

Despite their excellent prognosis, self-limited childhood focal seizures usually have a dramatic impact to parents as documented in long-term studies by Valeta (2005; 2007; 2011). The most dominant points of parental anxiety and concerns refer to their uncertainty of the nature, the cause and the impact of the events on their child's development as well as the lack of appropriate information (Valeta, 2005; 2010; 2011). There is a need for supportive family management, education and specific instructions about emergency procedures for possible subsequent seizures. Education about BCSSS is the cornerstone of the optimal management. Parents should be given general information about self-limited childhood focal seizures and, in particular PS, in which seizures may have dramatic features and last for many hours; the situation is frequently compounded by physicians' uncertainty over diagnosis, management and prognosis (Valeta, 2010). Parents who have watched their child during a seizure may need specific psychological support to overcome anxiety and panic that may result in overprotection and interfere in turn with parent-child separation and independence (Valeta, 2007).

REFERENCES ▶

Adcock JE, Panayiotopoulos CP (2012): Occipital lobe seizures and epilepsies. *J Clin Neurophysiol* 29: 397–407.

Al Twajri WA, Shevell MI (2002): Atypical benign epilepsy of childhood with Rolandic spikes: features of a subset requiring more than one medication for seizure control. *J Child Neurol* 17: 901–904.

Ambrosetto G, Tassinari CA (1990): Antiepileptic drug treatment of benign childhood epilepsy with Rolandic spikes: is it necessary? *Epilepsia* 31: 802–805.

American Academy of Pediatrics. Committee on Quality Improvement, Subcommittee on Febrile Seizures (1999): Practice parameter: long-term treatment of the child with simple febrile seizures. *Pediatrics* 103: 1307–1309.

Andermann F, Zifkin B (1998): The benign occipital epilepsies of childhood: an overview of the idiopathic syndromes and of the relationship to migraine. *Epilepsia* 39 (Suppl 4): S9-S23.

Aso K, Watanabe K, Negoro T, *et al.* (1987): Visual seizures in children. *Epilepsy Res* 1: 246–253.

Astradsson A, Olafsson E, Ludvigsson P, Bjorgvinsson H, Hauser WA (1998): Rolandic epilepsy: an incidence study in Iceland. *Epilepsia* 39: 884–886.

Bagdorf R, Lee SI (1993): Midline spikes: is it another benign EEG pattern of childhood? *Epilepsia* 34: 271–274.

Baker K, Astle DE, Scerif G, *et al.* (2015): Epilepsy, cognitive deficits and neuroanatomy in males with ZDHHC9 mutations. *Ann Clin Tran Neurol* 2: 559–569.

Bali B, Kull LL, Strug LJ, *et al.* (2007): Autosomal dominant inheritance of centrotemporal sharp waves in Rolandic epilepsy families. *Epilepsia* 48: 2266–2272.

Bast T, Volp A, Wolf C, Rating D (2003): The influence of sulthiame on EEG in children with benign childhood epilepsy with centrotemporal spikes (BECTS). *Epilepsia* 44: 215–220.

Battaglia D, Martinelli D, Perrino F, *et al.* (2007): Ictal video-EEG and atypical evolution in a child with Panayiotopoulos syndrome. *Boll Lega It Epil* 136/137: 51–54.

Beaumanoir A (1983): Infantile epilepsy with occipital focus and good prognosis. *Eur Neurol* 22: 43–52.

Beaumanoir A (1993a): An EEG contribution to the study of migraine and of the association between migraine and epilepsy in childhood. In: Andermann F, Beaumanoir A, Mira L, Roger J, Tassinari CA (eds) *Occipital Seizures and Epilepsy in Children*, pp. 101–110. London: John Libbey & Company Ltd.

Beaumanoir A (1993b): Semiology of occipital seizures in infants and children. In: Andermann F, Beaumanoir A, Mira L, Roger J, Tassinari CA (eds) *Occipital Seizures and Epilepsy in Children*, pp. 71–86. London: John Libbey & Company Ltd.

Beaumanoir A, Ballis T, Varfis G, Ansari K (1974): Benign epilepsy of childhood with Rolandic spikes. A clinical, electroencephalographic and telencephalographic study. *Epilepsia* 15: 301–315.

Beaumanoir A, Capizzi G, Nahory A, Yousfi Y (1989): Scotogenic seizures. In: Beaumanoir A, Gastaut H, Roger J (eds) *Reflex Seizures and Reflex Epilepsies*, pp. 219–223. Geneva: Medecine and Hygiene.

Beaumanoir A, Nahory A (1983): Benign partial epilepsies: 11 cases of frontal partial epilepsy with favorable prognosis. *Rev Electroencephal Neurophysiol Clin* 13: 207–211.

Beaussart M (1972): Benign epilepsy of children with Rolandic (centrotemporal) paroxysmal foci. A clinical entity. Study of 221 cases. *Epilepsia* 13: 795–911.

Beaussart M, de Faou R (1978): Evolution of epilepsy with Rolandic paroxysmal foci: a study of 324 cases. *Epilepsia* 19: 337–342.

Beaussart M, Loiseau P, Roger H. (1999): The discovery of "benign Rolandic epilepsy". In: Berkovic SF, Genton P, Hirsch E, Picard F (eds) *Genetics of Focal Epilepsies*, pp. 3–6. London: John Libbey & Company.

Bedoin N, Ciumas C, Lopez C, Redsand G, Herbillon V, Laurent A, *et al.* (2012): Disengagement and inhibition of visual-spatial attention are differently impaired in children with rolandic epilepsy and Panayiotopoulos syndrome. *Epilepsy Behav* 25: 81–91.

Belcastro V, Striano P, Kasteleijn-Nolst Trenite DG, Villa MP, Parisi P (2011): Migralepsy, hemicrania epileptica, postictal headache and "ictal epileptic headache": a proposal for terminology and classification revision. *J Headache Pain* 12: 289–294.

Ben Zeev B, Watemberg N, Lerman P, Barash I, Brand N, Lerman-Sagie T (2004): Sulthiame in childhood epilepsy. *Pediatr Int* 46: 521–524.

Berg AT, Shinnar S, Levy SR, Testa FM (1999): Newly diagnosed epilepsy in children: presentation at diagnosis. *Epilepsia* 40: 445–452.

Berg AT, Berkovic SF, Brodie MJ, *et al.* (2010): Revised terminology and concepts for organization of seizures and epilepsies: Report of the ILAE Commission on Classification and Terminology, 2005–2009. *Epilepsia* 51: 676–685.

Besseling RM, Jansen JF, Overvliet GM, *et al.* (2013a): Reduced functional integration of the sensorimotor and language network in rolandic epilepsy. *Neuroimage Clin* 2: 239–246.

Besseling RM, Overvliet GM, Jansen JF, van der Kruijs SJ, Vles JSH, Ebus SC *et al.* (2013b): Aberrant functional connectivity between motor and language networks in rolandic epilepsy. *Epilepsy Res* 107: 253–262.

Besseling RM, Jansen JF, Overvliet GM, *et al.* (2013c): Reduced structural connectivity between sensorimotor and language areas in rolandic epilepsy. *PLoS ONE*, vol. 8, no. 12, Article ID e83568.

Beydoun A, Garofalo EA, Drury I (1992): Generalized spike-waves, multiple loci, and clinical course in children with EEG features of benign epilepsy of childhood with centrotemporal spikes. *Epilepsia* 33: 1091–1096.

Blom S, Brorson LO (1966): Central spikes or sharp waves (Rolandic spikes) in children's EEG and their clinical significance. *Acta Paediatr Scand* 55: 385–393.

Blom S, Heijbel J (1982): Benign epilepsy of children with centrotemporal EEG foci: a follow-up study in adulthood of patients initially studied as children. *Epilepsia* 23: 629–632.

Boatman DF, Trescher WH, Smith C, *et al.* (2008): Cortical auditory dysfunction in benign Rolandic epilepsy. *Epilepsia* 49: 1018–1026.

Boor R, Jacobs J, Hinzmann A, *et al.* (2007): Combined spike-related functional MRI and multiple source analysis in the non-invasive spike localization of benign Rolandic epilepsy. *Clin Neurophysiol* 118: 901–909.

Bouma PA, Bovenkerk AC, Westendorp RG, Brouwer OF (1997): The course of benign partial epilepsy of childhood with centrotemporal spikes: a meta-analysis. *Neurology* 48: 430–437.

Bouma PA, Peters AC, Brouwer OF (2002): Long term course of childhood epilepsy following relapse after antiepileptic drug withdrawal. *J Neurol Neurosurg Psychiatry* 72: 507–510.

Bourgeois BF (2000): Drug treatment of benign focal epilepsies of childhood. *Epilepsia* 41: 1057–1058.

Brabec J, Chaudhary S, Ng YT (2013): Ictal priapism as an autonomic manifestation of Panayiotopoulos syndrome. *J Child Neurol* 28: 1686–1688.

Brancati C, Barba C, Metitieri T, Melani F, Pellacani S, Viggiano MP (2012): Impaired object identification in idiopathic childhood occipital epilepsy. *Epilepsia* 53: 686–694.

Bray PF, Wiser WC (1965): Hereditary characteristics of familial temporal-central focal epilepsy. *Pediatrics* 36: 207–221.

Bulgheroni S, Franceschetti S, Vago C, *et al.* (2008): Verbal dichotic listening performance and its relationship with EEG features in benign childhood epilepsy with centrotemporal spikes. *Epilepsy Res* 79: 31–38.

Bureau M, Cokar O, Maton B, Genton P, Dravet C (2002): Sleep-related, low voltage Rolandic and vertex spikes: an EEG marker of benignity in infancy-onset focal epilepsies. *Epileptic Disord* 4: 15–22.

Callenbach PM, Bouma PA, Geerts AT, *et al.* (2010): Long term outcome of benign childhood epilepsy with centrotemporal spikes: Dutch Study of Epilepsy in Childhood. *Seizure* 19: 501–506.

Capovilla G, Beccaria F (2010): Other phenotypes of benign childhood seizure susceptibility syndrome. In: Panayiotopoulos CP (ed) *Atlas of Epilepsies*, pp. 977–982. London: Springer.

Capovilla G, Beccaria F, Montagnini A (2006): "Benign focal epilepsy in infancy with vertex spikes and waves during sleep". Delineation of the syndrome and recalling as "benign infantile focal epilepsy with midline spikes and waves during sleep" (BIMSE). *Brain Dev* 28: 85–91.

Capovilla G, Beccaria F, Bianchi A, *et al.* (2011): Ictal EEG patterns in epilepsy with centro-temporal spikes. *Brain Dev* 33(4): 301–309.

Caraballo R, Fontana E, Michelizza B, *et al.* (1989): Carbamazepina, "assenze atipiche", "crisi atoniche", "crisi ato- niche" e stato di PO continua del sonno. *Boll Lega It Epil* 66/67: 379–381.

Caraballo R, Cersósimo R, Fejerman N (1998): Idiopathic partial epilepsies with Rolandic and occipital spikes appearing in the same children. *J Epilepsy* 11: 261–264.

Caraballo R, Cersosimo R, Medina C, Fejerman N (2000): Panayiotopoulos-type benign childhood occipital epilepsy: a prospective study. *Neurology* 55: 1096–1100.

Caraballo RH, Astorino F, Cersosimo R, Soprano AM, Fejerman N (2001): Atypical evolution in childhood epilepsy with occipital paroxysms (Panayiotopoulos type). *Epileptic Disord* 3: 157–162.

Caraballo RH, Sologuestua A, Granana N, *et al.* (2004): Idiopathic occipital and absence epilepsies appearing in the same children. *Pediatr Neurol* 30: 24–28.

Caraballo RH, Cersosimo RO, Fejerman N (2005): Late-onset, "Gastaut type", childhood occipital epilepsy: an unusual evolution. *Epileptic Disord* 7: 341–346.

Caraballo R, Cersosimo R, Fejerman N (2007): Panayiotopoulos syndrome: a prospective study of 192 patients. *Epilepsia* 48: 1054–1061.

Caraballo RH, Cersosimo RO, Fejerman N (2008a): Childhood occipital epilepsy of Gastaut: A study of 33 patients. *Epilepsia* 49: 288–297.

Caraballo RH, Fontana E, Darra F, *et al.* (2008b): Childhood absence epilepsy and electroencephalographic focal abnormalities with or without clinical manifestations. *Seizure* 17: 617–624.

Caraballo R, Koutroumanidis M, Panayiotopoulos CP, Fejerman N (2009): Idiopathic childhood occipital epilepsy of Gastaut: a review and differentiation from migraine and other epilepsies. *J Child Neurol* 24: 1536–1542.

Caraballo RH, Aldao MR, Cachia P (2011): Benign childhood seizure susceptibility syndrome: three case reports. *Epileptic Disord* 13: 133–139.

Caraballo R, Pasteris MC, Portuondo E, Fortini PS (2015): Panayiotopoulos syndrome and diffuse paroxysms as the first EEG manifestation at clinical onset: a study of nine patients. *Epileptic Disord* 17: 143–149.

Carvill GL, Regan BM, Yendle SC, *et al.* (2013): *GRIN2A* mutations cause epilepsy-aphasia spectrum disorders. *Nat. Genet* 45: 1073–1076.

Cavazzuti GB (1980): Epidemiology of different types of epilepsy in school age children of Modena, Italy. *Epilepsia* 21: 57–62.

Cavazzuti GB, Cappella L, Nalin A (1980): Longitudinal study of epileptiform EEG patterns in normal children. *Epilepsia* 21: 43–55.

Cerminara C, Montanaro ML, Curatolo P, Seri S (2004): Lamotrigine-induced seizure aggravation and negative myoclonus in idiopathic Rolandic epilepsy. *Neurology* 63: 373–375.

Chelimsky TC, Chelimsky GG (2007): Autonomic abnormalities in cyclic vomiting syndrome. *J Pediatr Gastroenterol Nutr* 44: 326–330.

Chilosi AM, Brovedani P, Moscatelli M, Bonani P, Guerrini R (2006): Neuropsychological findings in idiopathic occipital lobe epilepsies. *Epilepsia* 47 (Suppl) 2: 76–78.

Ciumas C, Saignavongs M, Ilski F, *et al.* (2014): White matter development in children with benign childhood epilepsy with centro-temporal spikes. *Brain* 137: 1095–1106.

Clarke T, Baskurt Z, Strug LJ, Pal DK (2009): Evidence of shared genetic risk factors for migraine and Rolandic epilepsy. *Epilepsia* 50: 2428–2433.

Clarke T, Strug LJ, Murphy PL, *et al.* (2007): High risk of reading disability and speech sound disorder in Rolandic epilepsy families: case control study. *Epilepsia* 48: 2258–2265.

Clemens B, Majoros E (1987): Sleep studies in benign epilepsy of childhood with Rolandic spikes. II. Analysis of discharge frequency and its relation to sleep dynamics. *Epilepsia* 28: 24–27.

Colamaria V, Sgro V, Caraballo R, *et al.* (1991): Status epilepticus in benign Rolandic epilepsy manifesting as anterior operculum syndrome. *Epilepsia* 32: 329–334.

Commission on Classification and Terminology of the International League Against Epilepsy (1989): Proposal for revised classification of epilepsies and epileptic syndromes. *Epilepsia* 30: 389–399.

Cordelli DM, Aldrovandi A, Gentile V, *et al.* (2012): Fever as a seizure precipitant factor in Panayiotopoulos syndrome: a clinical and genetic study. *Seizure* 21: 141–143.

Covanis A (2006): Panayiotopoulos syndrome: a benign childhood autonomic epilepsy frequently imitating encephalitis, syncope, migraine, sleep disorder, or gastroenteritis. *Pediatrics* 118: e1237-e1243.

Covanis A, Ferrie CD, Koutroumanidis M, Oguni H, Panayiotopoulos CP (2005): Panayiotopoulos syndrome and Gastaut type idiopathic childhood occipital epilepsy. In: Roger J, Bureau M, Dravet C, Genton P, Tassinari CA, Wolf P (eds) *Epileptic Syndromes in Infancy, Childhood and Adolescence*, 4th ed, pp. 227–253. Paris: John Libbey Eurotext.

Covanis A, Lada C, Skiadas K (2003): Children with Rolandic spikes and ictus emeticus: Rolandic epilepsy or Panayiotopoulos syndrome? *Epileptic Disord* 5: 139–143.

Covanis A, Panayiotopoulos CP (2008): Improving the diagnostic yield in Panayiotopoulos syndrome. *Eur J Neurol* 15: 317–319.

Currie NK, Lew AR, Palmer TM, Basu H, de Goede C, Iyer A, Cain K (2018): Reading comprehension difficulties in children with rolandic epilepsy. *Dev Med Child Neurol* 60: 275–282.

Dalla Bernardina B, Tassinari CA (1975): EEG of a nocturnal seizure in a patient with "benign epilepsy of childhood with Rolandic spikes". *Epilepsia* 16: 497–501.

Dalla Bernardina B, Tassinari CA, Dravet C, Bureau M, Beghini G, Roger J (1978): Épilepsie partielle bénigne et état de électroencéphalique pendant le sommeil. *Rev EEG Neurophysiol* 8: 350–353.

Dalla Bernardina B, Fontana E, Michelizza B, Colamaria V, Capovilla G, Tassinari CA (1989): Partial epilepsies of childhood, bilateral synchronization continuous spike-waves during slow sleep. In: Manelis J, Bental E, Loeber JN, Dreifuss FE (eds) *Advances in Epileptology*, pp. 295–302. New York: Raven Press.

Dalla Bernardina B, Sgrò V, Caraballo R, *et al.* (1991) Sleep and benign partial epilepsies of childhood: EEG and evoked potentials study. *Epilepsy Res* (Suppl): 83–96.

Dalla Bernardina B, Colamaria V, Chiamenti C, Capovilla G, Trevisan E, Tassinari CA (1992): Benign partial epilepsy with affective symptoms ("benign psychomotor epilepsy"). In: Roger J, Bureau M, Dravet C, Dreifuss FE, Perret A, Wolf P (eds) *Epileptic Syndromes in Infancy, Childhood and Adolescence*, 2nd ed, pp. 219–223. London: John Libbey & Company Ltd.

Dalla Bernardina B, Sgro M, Fejerman N (2005): Epilepsy with centrotemporal spikes and related syndromes. In: Roger J, Bureau M, Dravet C, Genton P, Tassinari CA, Wolf P (eds) *Epileptic Syndromes in Infancy, Childhood and Adolescence*, 4th ed, pp. 203–225. Paris: John Libbey Eurotext.

Dalla Bernardina B, Fontana E, Darra F (2007): Are there other types of benign focal epilepsies in childhood? In: Fejerman N, Caraballo RH (eds) *Benign Focal Epilepsies in Infancy, Childhood and Adolescence*, pp. 169–178. Paris: John Libbey Eurotext.

Danielsson J, Petermann F (2009): Cognitive deficits in children with benign Rolandic epilepsy of childhood or Rolandic discharges: A study of children between 4 and 7 years of age with and without seizures compared with healthy controls. *Epilepsy Behav* 16: 646–651.

Datta A, Sinclair DB (2007): Benign epilepsy of childhood with Rolandic spikes: typical and atypical variants. *Pediatr Neurol* 36: 141–145.

Datta AN, Oser N, Bauder F, *et al.* (2013): Cognitive impairment and cortical reorganization in children with benign epilepsy with centrotemporal spikes. *Epilepsia* 54: 487–494.

De Marco P, Tassinari CA (1981): Extreme somatosensory evoked potential (ESEP): an EEG sign forecasting the possible occurrence of seizures in children. *Epilepsia* 22: 569–575.

De Romanis F, Feliciani M, Cerbo R (1988): Migraine and other clinical syndromes in children affected by EEG occipital spike-wave complexes. *Function Neurol* 3: 187–203.

De Romanis F, Buzzi MG, Cerbo R, Feliciani M, Assenza S, Agnoli A (1991): Migraine and epilepsy with infantile onset and electroencephalographic findings of occipital spike-wave complexes. *Headache* 31: 378–383.

De Rose P, Perrino F, Lettori D, *et al.* (2010): Visual and visuoperceptual function in children with Panayiotopoulos syndrome. *Epilepsia* 51: 1205–1211.

Degerliyurt A, Teber S, Bektaş O, Senkon G (2014). Panayiotopoulos syndrome: a case series from Turkey. *Epilepsy Behav* 36: 24–32.

Demirbilek V, Dervent A (2004): Panayiotopoulos syndrome: video-EEG illustration of a typical seizure. *Epileptic Disord* 6: 121–124.

Deonna T, Ziegler AL, Despland PA, van Melle G (1986): Partial epilepsy in neurologically normal children: clinical syndromes and prognosis. *Epilepsia* 27: 241–247.

Deonna TW, Roulet E, Fontan D, Marcoz JP (1993): Speech and oromotor deficits of epileptic origin in benign partial epilepsy of childhood with Rolandic spikes (BPERS): Relationship to the acquired aphasia-epilepsy syndrome. *NeuroPediatrics* 24: 83–87.

Dirani M, Yamak W, Beydoun A (2015): Panayiotopoulos syndrome presenting with respiratory arrest: A case report and literature review. *Epilepsy Behav: Case Reports* 3: 12–14.

Doose H, Brigger-Heuer B, Neubauer B (1997): Children with focal sharp waves: clinical and genetic aspects. *Epilepsia* 38: 788–796.

Doose H, Petersen B, Neubauer BA (2002): Occipital sharp waves in idiopathic partial epilepsies-clinical and genetic aspects. *Epilepsy Res* 48: 121–130.

Drury I, Beydoun A (1991): Benign partial epilepsy of childhood with monomorphic sharp waves in centrotemporal and other locations. *Epilepsia* 32: 662–667.

Dura-Trave T, Yoldi-Petri ME, Gallinas-Victoriano F (2008): Panayiotopoulos syndrome: epidemiological and clinical characteristics and outcome. *Eur J Neurol* 15: 336–341.

Ebus S, Arends J, Hendriksen J, *et al.* (2012): Cognitive effects of interictal epileptiform discharges in children. *Eur J Paediatr Neurol* 16: 697–706.

Engel J Jr (2001): A proposed diagnostic scheme for people with epileptic seizures and with epilepsy: Report of the ILAE Task Force on Classification and Terminology. *Epilepsia* 42: 796–803.

Engel J Jr (2006): Report of the ILAE classification core group. *Epilepsia* 47: 1558–1568.

Fattouch J, Casciato S, Lapenta L, *et al.* (2013): The spectrum of epileptic syndromes with fixation off sensitivity persisting in adult life. *Epilepsia* 54 (Suppl 7): 59–65.

Fejerman N (2009): Atypical Rolandic epilepsy. *Epilepsia* 50 (Suppl 7): 9–12.

Fejerman N (2010): Benign childhood epilepsy with centrotemporal spikes. In: Panayiotopoulos CP (ed) *Atlas of Epilepsies*, pp. 957–964. London: Springer.

Fejerman N, Caraballo RH (2007): *Benign Focal Epilepsies in Infancy, Childhood and Adolescence*. Paris: John Libbey Eurotext.

Fejerman N, Caraballo R, Tenembaum SN (2000): Atypical evolutions of benign localization-related epilepsies in children: are they predictable? *Epilepsia* 41: 380–390.

Ferrari-Marinho T, Macedo EF, Costa Neves RS, *et al.*, (2013): Gastaut type idiopathic childhood occipital epilepsy. *Epileptic Disord* 15: 80–83.

Ferrie CD (2010a): Benign childhood seizure susceptibility syndrome. In: Panayiotopoulos CP (ed) *Atlas of Epilepsies*, pp. 983–987. London: Springer.

Ferrie CD (2010b): Managemenet of the benign focal epilepsies of childhood. In: Panayiotopoulos CP (ed) *Atlas of Epilepsies*, pp. 995–1000. London: Springer.

Ferrie CD (2010c): Terminology and organization of seizures and epilepsies: radical changes not justified by new evidence. *Epilepsia* 51: 713–714.

Ferrie CD, Livingston JH (2010): Panayiotopoulos syndrome: learning lessons from atypical cases. *Epileptic Disord* 12: 92–94.

Ferrie CD, Beaumanoir A, Guerrini R, *et al.* (1997): Early-onset benign occipital seizure susceptibility syndrome. *Epilepsia* 38: 285–293.

Ferrie CD, Koutroumanidis M, Rowlinson S, Sanders S, Panayiotopoulos CP (2002): Atypical evolution of Panayiotopoulos syndrome: a case report. *Epileptic Disord* 4: 35–42.

Ferrie C, Caraballo R, Covanis A, *et al.* (2006): Panayiotopoulos syndrome: a consensus view. *Dev Med Child Neurol* 48: 236–240.

Ferrie CD, Caraballo R, Covanis A, *et al.* (2007): Autonomic status epilepticus in Panayiotopoulos syndrome and other childhood and adult epilepsies: a consensus view. *Epilepsia* 48: 1165–1172.

Filippini M, Ardu E, Stefanelli S, Boni A, Gobbi G, Benso F (2016): Neuropsychological profile in new-onset benign epilepsy with centrotemporal spikes (BECTS): focusing on executive functions. *Epilepsy Behav* 54: 71–79.

Flesler S, Saler D, Cersosimo R, Caraballo RH (2010): Benign infantile focal epilepsy with midline spikes and waves during sleep: a new epileptic syndrome or a variant of benign focal epilepsy? *Epileptic Disord* 12: 205–211.

Fonseca LC, Tedrus GM (2000): Somatosensory evoked spikes and epileptic seizures: a study of 385 cases. *Clin Electroencephalogr* 31: 71–75.

Funata K, Shike T, Takenouchi T, Yamashita Y, Takao Takahashi T (2018): Respiratory arrest at the onset of idiopathic childhood occipital epilepsy of Gastaut. *Brain Dev* 40: 74–76.

Fusco L, Trivisano M, Specchio N, Vigevano F (2010): Rolandic epilepsy: an uncommon presentation with leg motor seizures. *Epilepsia* 51: 2488–2491.

Gaggero R, Pistorio A, Pignatelli S, *et al.* (2014): Early classification of childhood focal idiopathic epilepsies: is it possible at the first seizure? *Eur J Paediatr Neurol* 18: 376–380.

Gagliano A, Ferlazzo E, Germano E, *et al.* (2007): Neuropsychological deficits in monozygotic twins with childhood epilepsy with occipital paroxysms. *J Clin Exp Neuropsychol* 29: 488–495.

Garcia C, Rubio G (2005): Efficacy of levetiracetam in the treatment of Panayiotopoulos syndrome. *Epilepsy Res* 85: 318–320.

Gastaut H (1981): Benign epilepsy with occipital spike waves in children. *Bull Mem Acad Roy Med Belg* 136: 540–555.

Gastaut H (1982a): A new type of epilepsy: benign partial epilepsy of childhood with occipital spike-waves. *Clin Electroencephal* 13: 13–22.

Gastaut H (1982b): The benign epilepsy in childhood with occipital spike wave complexes. *EEG-EMG Z Elektroenzephalograph Elektromyograph Verwandte Geb* 13: 3–8.

Gastaut H, Zifkin BG. (1987): Benign epilepsy of childhood with occipital spike and wave complexes. In: Andermann F, Lugaresi E (eds) *Migraine and Epilepsy*, pp. 47–81. Boston: Butterworths.

Gastaut H, Roger J, Bureau M. (1992): Benign epilepsy of childhood with occipital paroxysms. Update. In: Roger J, Bureau M, Dravet C, Dreifuss FE, Perret A, Wolf P (eds) *Epileptic Syndromes in Infancy, Childhood and Adolescence*, 2nd ed, pp. 201–217. London: John Libbey & Company Ltd.

Gélisse P, Corda D, Raybaud C, Dravet C, Bureau M, Genton P (2003): Abnormal neuroimaging in patients with benign epilepsy with centrotemporal spikes. *Epilepsia* 44: 372–378.

Gélisse P, Genton P, Bureau M, Dravet C, Guerrini R, Viallat D, Roger J (1999): Are there generalized spike waves and typical absences in benign Rolandic epilepsy? *Brain Dev* 21: 390–396.

Germano E, Gagliano A, Magazu A, Sferro C, Calarese T, Mannarino E, Calamoneri F (2005): Benign childhood epilepsy with occipital paroxysms: Neuropsychological findings. *Epilepsy Res* 64: 137–150.

Gibbs FA, Gibbs EL (1952): *Atlas of Electroencephalography*, vol. 2. Epilepsy. Reading, Massachusetts: Addison-Wesley.

Gibbs FA, Gibbs EL (1967): *Medical Electroencephalography*. Reading, Massachusetts: Addison-Wesley Publishing Company.

Giordani B, Caveney AF, Laughrin D, *et al.* (2006): Cognition and behavior in children with benign epilepsy with centrotemporal spikes (BECTS): *Epilepsy Res* 70: 89–94.

Glauser T, Ben-Menachem E, Bourgeois B, *et al.* (2006): ILAE treatment guidelines: evidence-based analysis of antiepileptic drug efficacy and effectiveness as initial monotherapy for epileptic seizures and syndromes. *Epilepsia* 47: 1094–1120.

Gobbi G, Guerrini R, Grosso S. (2008): Late onset childhood occipital epilepsy (Gastaut type): In: Engel J Jr, Pedley TA (eds) *Epilepsy, A Comprehensive Textbook*, pp. 2387–2395. Philadelphia: Lippincott Williams & Wilkins.

Gonzales-Duarte A, Norcliffe-Kaufmann L, Martinez J, *et al.* (2011): Cardiovascular and neuroendocrine features of Panayiotopoulos syndrome. *Epilepsy Behav* 21: 296–300.

Goldberg-Stern H, Gonen OM, Sadeh M, Kivity S, Shuper A, Inbar D (2010): Neuropsychological aspects of benign childhood epilepsy with centrotemporal spikes. *Seizure* 19: 12–16.

Gregory DL, Wong PK (1992): Clinical relevance of a dipole field in Rolandic spikes. *Epilepsia* 33: 36–44.

Grosso S, Orrico A, Galli L, Di BR, Sorrentino V, Balestri P (2007): SCN1A mutation associated with atypical Panayiotopoulos syndrome. *Neurology* 69: 609–611.

Grosso S, Vivarelli R, Gobbi G, Bartolo RD, Berardi R, Balestri P (2008): Late-onset childhood occipital epilepsy (Gastaut type): A family study. *Eur J Paediatr Neurol* 12: 421–426.

Guerrini R, Bonanni P, Nardocci N, *et al.* (1999): Autosomal recessive Rolandic epilepsy with paroxysmal exercise-induced dystonia and writer's cramp: delination of the syndrome and gene mapping to chromosome 16p12–11.2. *Ann Neurol* 45: 344–352.

Guerrini R, Bonanni P, Parmeggiani L, Belmonte A (1997): Adolescent onset of idiopathic photosensitive occipital epilepsy after remission of benign Rolandic epilepsy. *Epilepsia* 38: 777–781.

Guerrini R, Bonanni P, Parmeggiani L, *et al.* (1998): Induction of partial seizures by visual stimulation. Clinical and electroencephalographic features and evoked potential studies. *Adv Neurol* 75: 159–178.

Guerrini R, Dravet C, Genton P, *et al.* (1995): Idiopathic photosensitive occipital lobe epilepsy. *Epilepsia* 36: 883–891.

Gulgonen S, Demirbilek V, Korkmaz B, Dervent A, Townes BD (2000): Neuropsychological functions in idiopathic occipital lobe epilepsy. *Epilepsia* 41: 405–411.

Harkin LA, McMahon JM, Iona X, *et al.* (2007): The spectrum of SCN1A-related infantile epileptic encephalopathies. *Brain* 130: 843–852.

Heijbel J, Blom S, Bergfors PG (1975): Benign epilepsy of children with centrotemporal EEG foci. A study of incidence rate in outpatient care. *Epilepsia* 16: 657–664.

Herranz Tanarro FJ, Saenz Lope E, Cristobal Sassot S (1984): La pointe-onde occipitale avec et sans épilepsie bénigne chez l'enfant. *Rev Electroencephalograph Neurophysiol Clin* 14: 1–7.

Hirano Y, Oguni H, Funatsuka M, Imai K, Osawa M (2009): Neurobehavioral abnormalities may correlate with increased seizure burden in children with Panayiotopoulos syndrome. *Pediatr Neurol* 40: 443–448.

Hodges SL, Gabriel MT, Perry MS (2016): Neuropsychological findings associated with Panayiotopoulos syndrome in three children. *Epilepsy Behav* 54: 158–162.

Huiskamp G, Van der MW, Van Huffelen A, Van Nieuwenhuizen O (2004): High resolution spatio-temporal EEG-MEG analysis of Rolandic spikes. *J Clin Neurophysiol* 21: 84–95.

Iannetti P, Spalice A, Rocchi V, Verrotti A (2009): Diffuse onset of ictal electroencephalography in a typical case of Panayiotopoulos syndrome and review of the literature. *J Child Neurol* 24: 472–476.

Jung KY, Kim JM, Kim DW (2003): Patterns of interictal spike propagation across the central sulcus in benign Rolandic epilepsy. *Clin Electroencephalogr* 34: 153–157.

Jurkeviciene G, Endziniene M, Laukiene I, *et al.* (2012): Association of language dysfunction and age of onset of benign epilepsy with centrotemporal spikes in children. *Eur J Paediatr Neurol* 16: 653–661.

Kajitani T, Kimura T, Sumita M, Kaneko M (1992): Relationship between benign epilepsy of children with centro-temporal EEG foci and febrile convulsions. *Brain Dev* 14: 230–234.

Kanazawa O, Tohyama J, Akasaka N, Kamimura T (2005): A magnetoencephalographic study of patients with Panayiotopoulos syndrome. *Epilepsia* 46: 1106–1113.

Karkare KD, Menon RN, Radhakrishnan A, Cherian A, Thomas SV (2018): Electroclinical characteristics and syndromic associations of "eye-condition" related visual sensitive epilepsies – A cross-sectional study. *Seizure* 58: 62–71.

Kavros PM, Clarke T, Strug LJ, Halperin JM, Dorta NJ, Pal DK (2008): Attention impairment in Rolandic epilepsy: Systematic review. *Epilepsia* 40: 1570–1580.

Kellaway P (1980): The incidence, significance and natural history of spike foci in children. In: Henry CE (ed) *Current Clinical Neurophysiology. Update on EEG and Evoked Potentials*, pp. 151–175. New York: Elsevier.

Kikumoto K, Yoshinaga H, Oka M, Ito M, Endoh F, Akiyama T, Ohtsuka Y (2006): EEG and seizure exacerbation induced by carbamazepine in Panayiotopoulos syndrome. *Epileptic Disord* 8: 53–56.

Kim EH, Yum MS, Kim HW, Ko TS (2014): Attention-deficit/hyperactivity disorder and attention impairment in children with benign childhood epilepsy with centrotemporal spikes. *Epilepsy Behav* 37: 54–58.

Kim SE, Lee JH, Chung HK, Lim SM, Lee HW (2014): Alterations in white matter microstructures and cognitive dysfunctions in benign childhood epilepsy with centrotemporal spikes. *Eur J Neurol* 21: 708- 717.

Kirby A, Williams N, Koelewijn L, *et al.* (2017): Benign childhood epilepsy with centrotemporal spikes (BECTS) and developmental coordination disorder. *Epilepsy Behav* 72: 122–126.

Kivity S, Ephraim T, Weitz R, Tamir A (2000): Childhood epilepsy with occipital paroxysms: Clinical variants in 134 patients. *Epilepsia* 41: 1522–1533.

Kokkinos V, Koutroumanidis M, Tsatsou K, Koupparis A, Tsiptsios D, Panayiotopoulos CP (2010): Multifocal spatiotemporal distribution of interictal spikes in Panayiotopoulos syndrome. *Clin Neurophysiol* 121: 859–869.

Kossoff EH, Los JG, Boatman DF (2007): A pilot study transitioning children on to levetiracetam monotherapy to improve language dysfunction associated with benign Rolandic epilepsy. *Epilepsy Behav* 11: 514–517.

Koutroumanidis M (2003): Ictal vomiting in association with left temporal lobe seizures in a left hemisphere language-dominant patient. *Epilepsia* 44: 1259.

Koutroumanidis M (2007): Panayiotopoulos syndrome: an important electroclinical example of benign childhood system epilepsy. *Epilepsia* 48: 1044–1053.

Koutroumanidis M (2011): Cardiovascular and neuroendocrine features of Panayiotopoulos syndrome. *Epilepsy Behav* 21: 217–218.

Koutroumanidis M, Rowlinson S, Sanders S (2005): Recurrent autonomic status epilepticus in Panayiotopoulos syndrome: Video/EEG studies. *Epilepsy Behav* 7: 543–547.

Koutroumanidis M, Ferrie CD, Valeta T, Sanders S, Michael M, Panayiotopoulos CP (2012): Syncope-like epileptic seizures in Panayiotopoulos syndrome. *Neurology* 79: 463–467.

Kramer U (2008): Atypical presentations of benign childhood epilepsy with centrotemporal spikes: a review. *J Child Neurol* 23: 785–790.

Kramer RE, Luders H, Goldstick LP, Dinner DS, Morris HH, Lesser RP, Wyllie E (1988): Ictus emeticus: an electroclinical analysis. *Neurology* 38: 1048–1052.

Kubota M, Takeshita K, Sakakihara Y, Yanagisawa M (2000): Magnetoencephalographic study of giant somatosensory evoked responses in patients with Rolandic epilepsy. *J Child Neurol* 15: 370–379.

Kugler SL, Bali B, Lieberman P, *et al.* (2008): An autosomal dominant genetically heterogenous variant of Rolandic epilepsy and speech disorder. *Epilepsia* 49: 1086–1090.

Kutluay E, Passaro EA, Gomez-Hassan D, Beydoun A (2001): Seizure semiology and neuroimaging findings in patients with midline spikes. *Epilepsia* 42: 1563–1568.

Kuzniecky R, Gilliam F, Morawetz R, Faught E, Palmer C, Black L (1997): Occipital lobe developmental malformations and epilepsy: clinical spectrum, treatment, and outcome. *Epilepsia* 38: 175–181.

Kuzniecky R, Rosenblatt B (1987): Benign occipital epilepsy: a family study. *Epilepsia* 28: 346–350.

Lacroix L, Fluss J, Gervais A, Korff CM (2011): Benzodiazepines in the acute management of seizures with autonomic manifestations: anticipate complications! *Epilepsia* 52: e156–e159.

Lada C, Skiadas K, Theodorou V, Covanis A (2003): A study of 43 patients with Panayiotopoulos syndrome: A common and benign childhood seizure suceptibility. *Epilepsia* 44: 81–88.

Lal D, Reinthaler EM, Altmuller J, *et al.* (2013): RBFOX1 and RBFOX3 mutations in Rolandic epilepsy. PLoS One, 8, e73323.

Langill L, Wong PK (2003): Tactile-evoked Rolandic discharges: a benign finding? *Epilepsia* 44: 221–227.

Larsson K, Eeg-Olofsson O (2006): A population based study of epilepsy in children from a Swedish county. *Eur J Paediatr Neurol* 10: 107–113.

Leal AJ, Ferreira JC, Dias AI, Calado E (2008): Origin of frontal lobe spikes in the early onset benign occipital lobe epilepsy (Panayiotopoulos syndrome). *Clin Neurophysiol* 119: 1985–1991.

Legarda S, Jayakar P, Duchowny M, Alvarez L, Resnick T (1994): Benign Rolandic epilepsy: high central and low central subgroups. *Epilepsia* 35: 1125–1129.

Lemke JR, Lal D, Reinthaler EM, *et al.* (2013): Mutations in GRIN2A cause idiopathic focal epilepsy with Rolandic spikes. *Nat Genet* 45: 1067–1072.

Lerman P, Kivity S (1975): Benign focal epilepsy of childhood. A follow-up study of 100 recovered patients. *Arch Neurol* 32: 261–264.

Lesca G, Rudolf G, Bruneau N, *et al.* (2013): GRIN2A mutations in acquired epileptic aphasia and related childhood focal epilepsies and encephalopathies with speech and language dysfunction. *Nat Genet* 45: 1061–1066.

Li BU, Issenman RM, Sarna SK (1999): Consensus statement-2nd International Scientific Symposium on CVS. The Faculty of the 2nd International Scientific Symposium on Cyclic Vomiting Syndrome. *Dig Dis Sci* 44: 9S-11S.

Livingston JH, Cross JH, McLellan A, Birch R, Zuberi SM (2009): A novel inherited mutation in the voltage sensor region of SCN1A is associated with Panayiotopoulos syndrome in siblings and generalized epilepsy with febrile seizures plus. *J Child Neurol* 24: 503–508.

Loiseau P, Pestre M, Dartigues JF, Commenges D, Barberger-Gateau C, Cohadon S (1983): Long-term prognosis in two forms of childhood epilepsy: typical absence seizures and epilepsy with Rolandic (centrotemporal) EEG foci. *Ann Neurol* 13: 642–648.

Loiseau P, Duche B, Cordova S, Dartigues JF, Cohadon S (1988): Prognosis of benign childhood epilepsy with centrotemporal spikes: a follow-up study of 168 patients. *Epilepsia* 29: 229–235.

Lopes R, Simões MR, Leal AJR (2014): Neuropsychological abnormalities in children with the Panayiotopoulos syndrome point to parietal lobe dysfunction. *Epilepsy Behav* 31: 50–55.

Luders HO, Lesser RP, Dinner DS, Morris III HH (1987): Benign focal epilepsy of childhood. In: Luders H, Lesser RP (eds) *Epilepsy. Electroclinical Syndromes*, pp. 303–346. Berlin Heidelberg: Springer-Verlag.

Lundberg S, Weis J, Eeg-Olofsson O, Raininko R (2003): Hippocampal region asymmetry assessed by 1H-MRS in Rolandic epilepsy. *Epilepsia* 44: 205–210.

Maihara T, Tsuji M, Higuchi Y, Hattori H (1999): Benign familial neonatal convulsions followed by benign epilepsy with centrotemporal spikes in two siblings. *Epilepsia* 40: 110–113.

Manganotti P, Miniussi C, Santorum E, Tinazzi M, Bonato C, Marzi CA, *et al.* (1998): Influence of somatosensory input on paroxysmal activity in benign Rolandic epilepsy with "extreme somatosensory evoked potentials". *Brain* 121: 647–658.

Masterton RA, Jackson GD, Abbott DF (2013): Mapping brain activity using event-related independent components analysis (eICA): specific advantage for EEG-fMRI. *NeuroImage* 70: 164–174.

Monjauze C, Broadbent H, Boyd SG, Neville BGR, Baldeweg T (2011): Language deficits and altered hemispheric lateralization in young people in remission from BECTS. *Epilepsia* 52: 79–83.

Martin del Valle F, Diaz NA, Ares MG, Sanz Santaeufemia FJ, Del Rosal RT, Gonzalez-Valcarcel Sanchez-Puelles FJ (2010): Panayiotopoulos syndrome: Probable genetic origin, but not in SCN1A. *Eur J Paediatr Neurol* 15: 155–157.

Martin-Santidrian MA, Garaizar C, Prats-Vinas JM (1998): Frontal lobe epilepsy in infancy: is there a benign partial frontal lobe epilepsy? *Rev Neurol* 26: 919–923.

Michael M, Tsatsou K, Ferrie CD (2010): Panayiotopoulos syndrome: an important childhood autonomic epilepsy to be differentiated from occipital epilepsy and acute non-epileptic disorders. *Brain Dev* 32: 4–9.

Michelucci R, Tassinari CA (1993): Television-induced occipital seizures. In: Andermann F, Beaumanoir A, Mira L, Roger J, Tassinari CA (eds) *Occipital Seizures and Epilepsies in Children*, pp. 141–144. London: John Libbey & Company Ltd.

Minami T, Gondo K, Yamamoto T, Yanai S, Tasaki K, Ueda K (1996): Magnetoencephalographic analysis of Rolandic discharges in benign childhood epilepsy. *Ann Neurol* 39: 326–334.

Mujawar QM, Sen S, Ali MD, Balakrishnan P, Patil S (2011): Panayiotopoulos syndrome presenting with status epilepticus and cardiorespiratory arrest: a case report. *Pediatr Emerg Care* 27: 754–757.

Nagendran K, Prior PF, Rossiter MA (1990): Benign occipital epilepsy of childhood: a family study. *J R Soc Med* 83: 804–805.

Nascimento FA, Sotero de Menezes MA,Simão CA, Takeshita BT,Blattes da Rocha SM, Kowacs PA (2017): The semiology of benign focal epilepsy with affective symptoms. *Epileptic Disord* 19: 202–206.

Negrin P, De Marco P (1977): Parietal focal spikes evoked by tactile somatotopic stimulation in sixty non-epileptic children: the nocturnal sleep and clinical and EEG evolution. *Electroencephalogr Clin Neurophysiol* 43: 312–316.

Neubauer BA, Fiedler B, Himmelein B, *et al.* (1998): Centrotemporal spikes in families with Rolandic epilepsy: linkage to chromosome 15q14. *Neurology* 51: 1608–1612.

Neubauer BA, Waldegger S, Heinzinger J, *et al.* (2008): KCNQ2 and KCNQ3 mutations contribute to different idiopathic epilepsy syndromes. *Neurology* 71: 177–183.

Nicolai J, Aldenkamp AP, Arends J, Weber JW, Vles JS (2006): Cognitive and behavioral effects of nocturnal epileptiform discharges in children with benign childhood epilepsy with centrotemporal spikes. *Epilepsy Behav* 8: 56–70.

Nissenkorn A, Pappo A, Feldmann Y, *et al.* (2017): Influence of epileptic activity during sleep on cognitive performance in benign childhood epilepsy with centrotemporal spikes. *Eur J Paediatr Neurol* 21: 858–863.

Oguni H, Hayashi K, Imai K, Hirano Y, Mutoh A, Osawa M (1999): Study on the early-onset variant of benign childhood epilepsy with occipital paroxysms otherwise described as early-onset benign occipital seizure susceptibility syndrome. *Epilepsia* 40: 1020–1030.

Oguni H, Hayashi K, Funatsuka M, Osawa M (2001): Study on early-onset benign occipital seizure susceptibility syndrome. *Pediatr Neurol* 25: 312–318.

Ohtsu M, Oguni H, Hayashi K, Funatsuka M, Imai K, Osawa M (2003): EEG in children with early-onset benign occipital seizure susceptibility syndrome: Panayiotopoulos syndrome. *Epilepsia* 44: 435–442.

Ohtsu M, Oguni H, Imai K, Funatsuka M, Osawa M (2008): Early-onset form of benign childhood epilepsy with centro-temporal EEG foci – a different nosological perspective from panayiotopoulos syndrome. *Neuropediatrics* 39: 14–19.

Okanishi T, Maegaki Y, Ohno K, Togari H (2008): Underlying neurologic disorders and recurrence rates of status epilepticus in childhood. *Brain Dev* 30: 624–628.

Okubo Y, Matsuura M, Asai T, *et al.* (1994): Epileptiform EEG discharges in healthy children: prevalence, emotional and behavioral correlates, and genetic influences. *Epilepsia* 35: 832–841.

Overvliet GM, Besseling RMH, van der Kruijs SJM, *et al.* (2013): Clinical evaluation of language fundamentals in Rolandic epilepsy, an assessment with CELF-4. *Eur J Paediatr Neurol* 17: 390–396.

Pal DK, Li W, Clarke T, Lieberman P, Strug LJ (2010): Pleiotropic effects of the 11p13 locus on developmental verbal dyspraxia and EEG centrotemporal sharp waves. *Genes Brain Behav* 9: 1004–1012.

Pal DK, Strug LJ, Clarke T, Murphy PL (2007): Major genetic loci for reading disability in Rolandic epilepsy families. *Epilepsia* 48: 376.

Pal DK, Ferrie C, Addis L, *et al.* (2016): Idiopathic focal epilepsies: the "lost tribe". *Epileptic Disord* 18: 252–288.

Panayiotopoulos CP (1981): Inhibitory effect of central vision on occipital lobe seizures. *Neurology* 31: 1330–1333.

Panayiotopoulos CP (1988): Vomiting as an ictal manifestation of epileptic seizures and syndromes. *J Neurol Neurosurg Psychiatr* 51: 1448–1451.

Panayiotopoulos CP (1993): Benign childhood partial epilepsies: benign childhood seizure susceptibility syndromes. *J Neurol Neurosurg Psychiatry* 56: 2–5.

Panayiotopoulos CP (1994): Elementary visual hallucinations in migraine and epilepsy. *J Neurol Neurosurg Psychiatr* 57: 1371–1374.

Panayiotopoulos CP (1999a): *Benign Childhood Partial Seizures and Related Epileptic Syndromes*. London: John Libbey & Company Ltd.

Panayiotopoulos CP (1999b): Elementary visual hallucinations, blindness, and headache in idiopathic occipital epilepsy: differentiation from migraine. *J Neurol Neurosurg Psychiatry* 66: 536–540.

Panayiotopoulos CP (1999c): Visual phenomena and headache in occipital epilepsy: a review, a systematic study and differentiation from migraine. *Epileptic Disord* 1: 205–216.

Panayiotopoulos CP (2002): *Panayiotopoulos Syndrome: a Common and Benign Childhood Epileptic Syndrome*. London: John Libbey & Company.

Panayiotopoulos CP (2004): Autonomic seizures and autonomic status epilepticus peculiar to childhood: diagnosis and management. *Epilepsy Behav* 5: 286–295.

Panayiotopoulos CP (2005): Idiopathic photosensitive occipital lobe epilepsy. In: Panayiotopoulos CP (ed) *The Epilepsies: Seizures, Syndromes and Management*, pp. 469–474. Oxford: Bladon Medical Publishing.

Panayiotopoulos CP (2006): "Migralepsy" and the significance of differentiating occipital seizures from migraine. *Epilepsia* 47: 806–808.

Panayiotopoulos CP (2007): The birth and evolution of the concept of Panayiotopoulos syndrome. *Epilepsia* 48: 1041–1043.

Panayiotopoulos CP (2010): *A Clinical Guide to Epileptic Syndromes and their Treatment* (revised 2nd ed). London: Springer.

Panayiotopoulos CP, Michael M, Sanders S, Valeta T, Koutroumanidis M (2008): Benign childhood focal epilepsies: assessment of established and newly recognized syndromes. *Brain* 131: 2264–2286.

Panjwani N, Wilson MD, Addis L, *et al.* (2016): A microRNA binding site in PAX6 is associated with centrotemporal spikes of rolandic epilepsy. *Ann Clin Trans Neurol* 3: 512–522.

Pardoe HR, Berg AT, Archer JS, Fulbright RK, Jackson GD (2013): A neurodevelopmental basis for BECTS: evidence from structural MRI. *Epilepsy Res* 105: 133–139.

Parisi P, Ferri R, Pagani J, Cecili M, Montemitro E, Villa MP (2005): Ictal video-polysomnography and EEG spectral analysis in a child with severe Panayiotopoulos syndrome. *Epileptic Disord* 7: 333–339.

Parisi P, Matricardi S, Tozzi E, Sechi E, Martini C, Verrotti A (2012): Benign epilepsy of childhood with centro-temporal spikes (BECTS) versus migraine: a neuropsychological assessment. *Childs Nerv Syst* 28: 2129–2135.

Parmeggiani L, Guerrini R (1999): Idiopathic partial epilepsy: electroclinical demonstration of a prolonged *Seizure* with sequential Rolandic and occipital involvement. Seizure spread due to regional susceptibility? *Epileptic Disord* 1: 35–40.

Parmeggiani L, Seri S, Bonanni P, Guerrini R (2004): Electrophysiological characterization of spontaneous and carbamazepine-induced epileptic negative myoclonus in benign childhood epilepsy with centro-temporal spikes. *Clin Neurophysiol* 115: 50–58.

Pataraia E, Feucht M, Lindinger G, ull-Watschinger S, Baumgartner C (2008): Combined electroencephalography and magnetoencephalography of interictal spikes in benign Rolandic epilepsy of childhood. *Clin Neurophysiol* 119: 635–641.

Penfield W, Rasmussen T (1957): *The Cerebral Cortex of Man: A Clinical Study of Localisation of Function*. New York: The Macmillan Company.

Pérez-Villena A, López-Marín L, García-Peñas JJ, *et al.* (2012): Benign childhood epilepsies: academic difficulties and behavioural disorders. *Rev Neurol* 54: 17–23.

Perkins FF Jr, Breier J, McManis MH, *et al.* (2008): Benign Rolandic epilepsy-perhaps not so benign: use of magnetic source imaging as a predictor of outcome. *J Child Neurol* 23: 389–393.

Peters JM, Camfield CS, Camfield PR (2001): Population study of benign Rolandic epilepsy: Is treatment needed? *Neurology* 57: 537–539.

Petersen I, Eeg-Olofsson O (1971): The development of the electroencephalogram in normal children from the age of 1 through 15 years. Non-paroxysmal activity. *Neuropadiatrie* 2: 247–304.

Piccinelli P, Borgatti R, Aldini A, *et al.* (2008): Academic performance in children with Rolandic epilepsy. *Dev Med Child Neurol* 50: 353–356.

Pinton F, Ducot B, Motte J, *et al.* (2006): Cognitive functions in children with benign childhood epilepsy with centrotemporal spikes (BECTS). *Epileptic Disord* 8: 11–23.

Plouin P, Anderson VE (2005): Benign familial and non-familial neonatal seizures. In: Roger J, Bureau M, Dravet C, Genton P, Tassinari CA, Wolf P (eds) *Epileptic Syndromes in Infancy, Childhood and Adolescence*, 4th ed, pp. 3–15. Paris: John Libbey Eurotext.

Reinthaler EM, Lal D, Lebon S, *et al.* (2014): 16p11.2 600 kb Duplications confer risk for typical and atypical Rolandic epilepsy. *Hum Mol Genet* 23 (22): 6069–6080.

Reinthaler EM, Dejanovic B, Lal D, *et al.* (2015): Rare variants in gamma-aminobutyric acid type A receptor genes in rolandic epilepsy and related syndromes. *Ann Neurol* 77: 972–986.

Riva D, Vago C, Franceschetti S, *et al.* (2007): Intellectual and language findings and their relationship to EEG characteristics in benign childhood epilepsy with centro- temporal spikes. *Epilepsy Behav* 10: 278–285.

Roll P, Rudolf G, Pereira S, *et al.* (2006): SRPX2 mutations in disorders of language cortex and cognition. *Hum Mol Genet* 15: 1195–1207.

Rots ML, De Vos CC, Smeets-Schouten JS, Portier R, van Putten MJAM (2012): Suppressors of interictal discharges in idiopathic childhood occipital epilepsy of Gastaut. *Epilepsy Behav* 25: 189–191.

Russell MB, Olesen J (1996): A nosographic analysis of the migraine aura in a general population. *Brain* 119: 355–361.

Saito N, Kanazawa O, Tohyama J, *et al.* (2008): Brain maturation-related spike localization in Panayiotopoulos syndrome: magnetoencephalographic study. *Pediatr Neurol* 38: 104–110.

Saito N, Kanazawa O, Toyama J, Akasaka N, Kamimura T (2007): Magnetoencephalographic findings of Panayiotopoulos syndrome with frontal epileptic discharges. *Pediatr Neurol* 36: 190–194.

Samaitiene R, Norkuniene J, Tumiene B, Grikiniene J (2013): Sleep and behavioral problems in Rolandic epilepsy. *Pediatr Neurol* 48: 115–122.

Sanders S, Rowlinson S, Koutroumanidis M, Ferrie CD, Panayiotopoulos CP (2002): Midline spikes in children and clinical correlations. *Epilepsia* 43: 1436–1439.

Sanders S, Rowlinson S, Manidakis I, Ferrie CD, Koutroumanidis M (2004): The contribution of the EEG technologists in the diagnosis of Panayiotopoulos syndrome (susceptibility to early onset benign childhood autonomic seizures. *Seizure* 13: 565–573.

Santanelli P, Bureau M, Magaudda A, Gobbi G, Roger J (1989): Benign partial epilepsy with centrotemporal (or Rolandic) spikes and brain lesion. *Epilepsia* 30: 182–188.

Schauble B, Britton JW, Mullan BP, Watson J, Sharbrough FW, Marsh WR (2002): Ictal vomiting in association with left temporal lobe seizures in a left hemisphere language-dominant patient. *Epilepsia* 43: 1432–1435.

Scheffer IE, Harkin LA, Grinton BE, *et al.* (2007): Temporal lobe epilepsy and GEFS+ phenotypes associated with SCN1B mutations. *Brain* 130: 100–109.

Scheffer IE, Berkovic S, Capovilla G, *et al.* (2017): ILAE classification of the epilepsies: Position paper of the ILAE Commission for Classification and Terminology. *Epilepsia* 58: 512–521.

Schott GD (2007): Exploring the visual hallucinations of migraine aura: the tacit contribution of illustration. *Brain* 130: 1690–1703.

Schrader D, Shukla R, Gatrill R, Farrell K, Connolly M (2011): Epilepsy with occipital features in children: factors predicting seizure outcome and neuroimaging abnormalities. *Eur J Pediatr Neurol* 15: 15–20.

Shu XM, Zhang GP, Yang BZ, Li J (2013): The Characterization of Childhood Occipital Epilepsy of Gastaut: A Study of Seven Patients. *Cell Biochem Biophys* 67: 991–995.

Sidenvall R, Forsgren L, Heijbel J (1996): Prevalence and characteristics of epilepsy in children in northern Sweden. *Seizure* 5: 139–146.

Smith JMB, Kellaway P (1964): Central (Rolandic) foci in children: an analysis of 200 cases. *Electroencephalogr Clin Neurophysiol* 17: 460–461.

Smith AB, Bajojo O, Pal DK (2015): A meta-analysis of literacy and language in children with Rolandic epilepsy. *Dev Med Child Neurol* 57: 1019–1026.

Sorel L, Rucquoy-Ponsar M (1969): L'épilepsie fonctionnelle de maturation. Apport des montages verticaux en EEG dans le diagnostic de cette forme d'épilepsie. *Rev Neurol* 121: 289–297.

Specchio N, Trivisano M, Balestri M, *et al.* (2010a): Panayiotopoulos syndrome: a clinical, EEG and neuropsychological study of 93 consecutive patients. *Epilepsia* 51: 2098–2107.

Specchio N, Trivisano M, Claps D, Battaglia D, Fusco L, Vigevano F (2010b): Documentation of autonomic seizures and autonomic status epilepticus with ictal EEG in Panayiotopoulos syndrome. *Epilepsy Behav* 19: 383–393.

Strug LJ, Clarke T, Chiang T, *et al.* (2009): Centrotemporal sharp wave EEG trait in Rolandic epilepsy maps to Elongator Protein Complex 4 (ELP4). *Eur J Hum Genet* 17: 1171–1181.

Strug LJ, Addis L, Chiang T, *et al.* (2012): The genetics of reading disability in an often excluded sample: novel loci suggested for reading disability in rolandic epilepsy. *PLoS One* 7: e40696.

Tassinari CA, De Marco P (1992): Benign partial epilepsy with extreme somato-sensory evoked potentials. In: Roger J, Bureau M, Dravet C, Dreifuss FE, Wolf P, Perret A (eds) *Epileptic Syndromes in Infancy, Childhood and Adolescence*, 2nd ed, pp. 225–229. London: John Libbey & Company.

Taylor I, Berkovic SF, Kivity S, Scheffer IE (2008): Benign occipital epilepsies of childhood: clinical features and genetics. *Brain* 131: 2287–2294.

Taylor I, Scheffer IE, Berkovic SF (2003): Occipital epilepsies: identification of specific and newly recognized syndromes. *Brain* 126: 753–769.

Tedrus GM, Fonseca LC, Melo EM, Ximenes VL (2009): Educational problems related to quantitative EEG changes in benign childhood epilepsy with centrotemporal spikes. *Epilepsy Behav* 15: 486–490.

Tenembaum S, Deonna T, Fejerman N, Medina C, Ingvar-Maeder M, Gubser-Mercati D (1997): Continuous spike-waves and dementia in childhood epilepsy with occipital paroxysms. *J Epilepsy* 10: 139–145.

Thomas P, Arzimanoglou A, Aicardi J (2003): Benign idiopathic occipital epilepsy: report of a case of the late (Gastaut) type. *Epileptic Disord* 5: 57–59.

Tsai ML, Hung KL (1998): Topographic mapping and clinical analysis of benign childhood epilepsy with centrotemporal spikes. *Brain Dev* 20: 27–32.

Tsiptsios D, Kokkinos V, Sanders S, *et al.* (2010): Electroencephalographic manifestations and their prognostic significance in idiopathic childhood occipital epilepsy of Gastaut. *Epilepsia* 51 (Suppl 4): 156.

Turner SJ, Mayes AK, Verhoeven A, Mandelstam SA, Morgan AT, Scheffer IE (2015): GRIN2A: an aptly named gene for speech dysfunction. *Neurology* 84: 586–593.

Ueno M, Oguni H, Yasuda K, Osawa M (2001): Neurophysiological study of secondary synchronous occipito-frontopolar spikes in childhood. *Clin Neurophysiol* 112: 2106–2112.

Vadlamudi L, Harvey AS, Connellan MM, *et al.* (2004): Is benign Rolandic epilepsy genetically determined? *Ann Neurol* 56: 129–132.

Vadlamudi L, Kjeldsen MJ, Corey LA, *et al.* (2006): Analyzing the etiology of benign Rolandic epilepsy: a multicenter twin collaboration. *Epilepsia* 47: 550–555.

Valeta T (2005): Parental attitude, reaction and education in benign childhood focal seizures. In: Panayiotopoulos CP (ed) *The Epilepsies: Seizures, Syndromes and Management*, pp. 258–261. Oxford: Bladon Medical Publishing.

Valeta T (2007): Impact of newly identified epileptic seizures in patients and family. In: Panayiotopoulos CP (ed) *Newly Identified Epileptic Seizures: Diagnosis, Procedures and Management*, vol. 3, pp. 138–144. Oxford: Medicinae.

Valeta T (2010): Psychosocial impact of epilepsy in children and family. In: Panayiotopoulos CP (ed) *Atlas of Epilepsies*, pp. 1371–1373. London: Springer.

Valeta T (2011): Parental reactions and needs in benign childhood focal seizures. *Epilepsia* 52 (Suppl 6): 122–123.

Vannest J, Tenney JR, Altaye M, *et al.* (2016): Impact of frequency and lateralization of interictal discharges on neuropsychological and fine motor status in children with benign epilepsy with centrotemporal spikes. *Epilepsia* 57: 161–167.

Vears DF, Tsai MH, Sadleir LG, *et al.* (2012): Clinical genetic studies in benign childhood epilepsy with centrotemporal spikes. *Epilepsia* 53: 319–324.

Verrotti A, Coppola G, Manco R, *et al.* (2007): Levetiracetam monotherapy for children and adolescents with benign Rolandic seizures. *Seizure* 16: 271–275.

Verrotti A, Salladini C, Trotta D, di Corcia G, Chiarelli F (2005): Ictal cardiorespiratory arrest in Panayiotopoulos syndrome. *Neurology* 64: 1816–1817.

Verrotti A, Matricardi S, Di Giacomo DL, Rapino D, Chiarelli F, Coppola G (2013): Neuropsychological impairment in children with rolandic epilepsy and in their siblings. *Epilepsy Behav* 28: 108–112.

Verrotti A, Filippini M, Matricardi S, Agostinelli MF, Guiseppe G (2014a): Memory impairement and benign epilepsy with centrotemporal spike (BECTS): A growing suspicion. *Brain and Cognition* 84: 123–131.

Verrotti A, Sebastiani M, Giordano L, Striano P, Belcastro V, Franzoni E (2014b): Panayiotopoulos syndrome with convulsive status epilepticus at the onset: a long-term study. *Seizure* 2: 728–731.

Verrotti A, D'Alonzo R, Rinaldi VE, Casciato S, D'Aniello A, Di Gennaro G (2017a): Childhood absence epilepsy and benign epilepsy with centrotemporal spikes: a narrative review analysis. *World J Pediatr* 13: 106–111.

Verrotti A, Casciato S, Spalice A, *et al.* (2017b): Coexistence of childhood absence epilepsy and benign epilepsy with centrotemporal spikes: A case series. *Eur J Paediatr Neurol* 21: 570–575.

Vintan MA, Palade S, Cristea A, Benga I, Muresanu DF (2012): A neuropsychological assessment, using computerized battery tests (CANTAB), in children with benign rolandic epilepsy before AED therapy. *J Med Life* 5: 114–119.

Vigevano F, Capovilla G, Genton P, Gobbi G, Hirsch E, Specchio N (2009): Revisiting the concept of "benign" (April 18–20, 2008, Monreale, Italy). *Epilepsia* 50: 1648–1649.

Vigevano F, Lispi ML, Ricci S (2000): Early onset benign occipital susceptibility syndrome: video-EEG documentation of an illustrative case. *Clin Neurophysiol* 111 (Suppl 2): S81-S86.

Vigevano F, Ricci S (1993): Benign occipital epilepsy of childhood with prolonged seizures and autonomic symptoms. In: Andermann F, Beaumanoir A, Mira L, Roger J, Tassinari CA (eds) *Occipital Seizures and Epilepsies in Children*, pp. 133–140. London: John Libbey & Company Ltd.

Vigevano F, Specchio N, Caraballo R, Watanabe K. (2008): Benign familial and nonfamilial seizures. In: Engel J Jr and Pedley TA (eds) *Epilepsy, A Comprehensive Textbook*, pp. 2313–2321. Philadelphia: Lippincott Williams & Wilkins.

Wakamoto H, Nagao H, Fukuda M, *et al.* (2011): Idiopathic Childhood Occipital Epilepsy of Gastaut: Report of 12 Patients. *Pediatr Neurol* 44: 183–186.

Watanabe K (1996): Benign partial epilepsies. In: Wallace S (ed) *Epilepsy in Children*, pp. 293–313. London: Chapman & Hall.

Watemberg N, Leitner Y, Fattal-Valevski A, Kramer U (2009): Epileptic negative myoclonus as the presenting seizure type in Rolandic epilepsy. *Pediatr Neurol* 41: 59–64.

Wheless JW, Clarke DF, Arzimanoglou A, Carpenter D (2007): Treatment of pediatric epilepsy: European expert opinion, 2007. *Epileptic Disord* 9: 353–412.

Wheless JW, Clarke DF, Carpenter D (2005): Treatment of pediatric epilepsy: expert opinion, 2005. *J Child Neurol* 20 (Suppl 1): S1-S56.

Wirrell E, Camfield CS, Camfield PR (2006): Idiopathic and benign partial epilepsies of childhood. In: Wyllie E, Gupta A, Lachhwani D (eds) *The Treatment of Epilepsy*, 4th ed, pp. 373–389. Philadelphia: Lippincott Williams & Wilkins.

Wirrell E, Sherman EM, Vanmastrigt R, Hamiwka L (2008): Deterioration in cognitive function in children with benign epilepsy of childhood with central temporal spikes treated with sulthiame. *J Child Neurol* 23: 14–21.

Wirrell EC, Camfield PR, Gordon KE, Dooley JM, Camfield CS (1995): Benign Rolandic epilepsy: atypical features are very common. *J Child Neurol* 10: 455–458.

Wolf P (2010): Much ado about nothing? *Epilepsia* 51: 717–718.

Xiao F, Chen Q, Yu X, *et al.* (2014): Hemispheric lateralization of microstructural white matter abnormalities in children with active benign childhood epilepsy with centrotemporal spikes (BECTS): a preliminary DTI study. *Journal of the Neurological Sciences* 336: 171–179.

Yalcin AD, Kaymaz A, Forta H (1997): Childhood occipital epilepsy: Seizure manifestations and electroencephalographic features. *Brain Dev* 19: 408–413.

Yalcin AD, Kaymaz A, Forta H (2000): Reflex occipital lobe epilepsy. *Seizure* 9: 436–441.

Yalcin AD, Toydemir HE, Celebi LG, Forta H (2009): Panayiotopoulos syndrome with coincidental brain lesions. *Epileptic Disord* 11: 270–276.

Yalcin AD, Toydemir HE (2017): Panayiotopoulos syndrome with a special emphasis of ictal semiologic features. *Epilepy Research* 131: 37–43.

Yamatogi Y, Ohtahara S (2003): Severe epilepsy with multiple independent spike foci. *J Clin Neurophysiol* 20: 442–448.

Yoshinaga H, Kobayashi K, Ohtsuka Y (2009): Characteristics of the synchronous occipital and frontopolar spike phenomenon in Panayiotopoulos syndrome. *Brain Dev* 32: 603–608.

Yoshinaga H, Koutroumanidis M, Kobayashi K, *et al.* (2006): EEG dipole characteristics in Panayiotopoulos syndrome. *Epilepsia* 47: 781–787.

Yoshinaga H, Kobayashi K, Shibata T, Inoue T, Oka M, Akiyama T (2015): Manifestation of both emetic seizures and sylvian seizures in the same patients with benign partial epilepsy. *Brain Dev* 37: 13–17.

WITH VIDEO SUPPLEMENTS

CHAPTER 14

ENCEPHALOPATHY RELATED TO STATUS EPILEPTICUS DURING SLOW SLEEP (ESES) INCLUDING LANDAU-KLEFFNER SYNDROME

Carlo Alberto Tassinari[1], Gaetano Cantalupo[2,3], Bernardo Dalla Bernardina[3], Francesca Darra[3], Michelle Bureau[4], Chiara Cirelli[5], Giulio Tononi[5] and Guido Rubboli[6,7]

[1] University of Bologna, Bologna, Italy; Neuroscience Department, University of Parma, Parma, Italy
[2] Child Neuropsychiatry Unit, University of Parma, Parma, Italy
[3] Child Neuropsychiatry Unit, University of Verona, Verona, Italy
[4] Centre Saint-Paul, Henri-Gastaut Hospital, Marseille, France
[5] Center for Sleep and Consciousness, University of Wisconsin – Madison School of Medicine, Department of Psychiatry, Madison, USA
[6] Danish Epilepsy Center, Filadelfia, Dianalund, Denmark
[7] University of Copenhagen, Copenhagen, Denmark

Introduction

The first description of subclinical electrical status epilepticus induced by sleep in children dates back to 1971, when Patry, Lyagoubi and Tassinari described in six children a peculiar EEG pattern occurring almost continuously during sleep, characterized by apparently "subclinical" spike-and-waves, for a variable length of time (months to years). Five of the six children were mentally retarded, and two of them had failed to acquire speech (Patry *et al.*, 1971). Tassinari *et al.* (1977) introduced the term *"Encephalopathy related to electrical status epilepticus during slow sleep"* and "suggested that the condition of a protracted (years) SES (status epilepticus during sleep) can be the factor leading to severe mental deterioration and psychic disturbances". A quarter of century later, this concept of "epileptic encephalopathy" was recognized by the ILAE (Engel, 2001).

The term "continuous spikes and waves during slow sleep (CSWS)" is for us a simplistic and inexact synonym of SES (see "Electroencephalography" paragraph). Kellerman (1978) first documented that patients with acquired epileptic aphasia or Landau-Kleffner syndrome (LKS) had an extreme activation of spike-and-wave discharges during slow sleep consistent with SES – as described by Patry *et al.* (1971); and actually LKS is now considered a clinical variant or a subtype of ESES (see among others De Negri, 1997; Galanopoulou *et al.*, 2000; Halâsz *et al.*, 2005; Van Bogaert *et al.*, 2006; Nickels & Wirrel, 2008; Rudolf *et al.*, 2009; Garcia-Penas, 2010; Overvliet *et al.*, 2010; Caraballo *et al.*, 2014) as we already proposed (Tassinari *et al.*, 1992; Tassinari, 1995).

ESES syndrome is typically characterized by: i) *epilepsy:* focal and apparently generalized seizures (unilateral or bilateral clonic seizures, tonic-clonic seizures, absences), partial motor seizures, complex partial seizures or epileptic falls; ii) *encephalopathy:* neurological deterioration, involving cognitive, behavioural and/or motor domains; III) *typical EEG findings:* status epilepticus during sleep (SES), defined as the appearance at sleep onset of a pattern of diffuse spike-and-waves (with different degrees of symmetry or even unilateral or focal) occurring in up to 85% of slow sleep and persisting for months or years (see below the quantification of the paroxysmal activity).

In general, ESES syndrome is considered to be rare. Morikawa *et al.* (1989) reported 31 cases out of a population of 12,854 patients, corresponding approximately to 0.5% of all childhood epilepsies examined in their centre. Thirty-one cases have been observed at the Centre Saint-Paul of Marseille between 1968 and 1992 (Bureau, 1995a). Seventy-one new cases, showing a 3:2 male preponderance were reported at the meeting on ESES syndrome and related disorders held in Venice in 1993 (Bureau, 1995b). For Kramer *et al.* (1998), in a cohort of 440 consecutive pediatric patients with at least two seizures, ESES accounted for 0.2% of all cases. As in Galanopoulou *et al.'s* comprehensive review (2000), including the cases presented at the Venice symposium (Beaumanoir *et al.*, 1995), and other descriptions in the literature (see Yan Liu & Wong, 2000; Nickels & Wirrell, 2008), several hundred cases have been described so far all over the world: ESES is no more a Marseille specialty "like the bouillabaisse" (Tassinari, 1995). Loddenkemper *et al.* (2009) found that in a population of 415 pediatric patients undergoing video-EEG evaluation and epilepsy surgery at Cleveland Clinic, 8 (1.9%) had ESES. In a review of 1,497 overnight video-EEG monitoring studies performed over a 5-year interval, Van Hirtum-Das *et al.* (2006) found 102 records that showed "significant sleep activation" of spike-and-waves. Clinical information was available for 90 of these children, 20% of whom met criteria for LKS. Teixeira *et al.* (2009) reported, in their series of 40 patients with polymicrogyria, that 6 children (15%) presented with continuous epileptiform abnormalities over a focal area on wakefulness, which became bilateral and synchronous during sleep; the observation of this electrical status was correlated with the worsening of school performance. A relatively large-scale retrospective study including 196 patients with benign childhood epilepsy with centro-temporal spikes (BCECTS) suggested that an "atypical" evolution into ESES or LKS is more common than previously reported, accounting for a total of 6.6% of patients (4.6 and 2 respectively) and representing the 65% of all "atypical" presentations of BCECTS (Tovia *et al.*, 2011). On the other hand, patients with a previous diagnosis of idiopathic partial epilepsy account for about one-third of the ESES cases (Saltik *et al.*, 2005; Kramer *et al.*, 2009).

Anatomo-electro-clinical features

Predisposing factors: personal antecedents and genetics

Personal antecedents are found in about one-third of cases, such as congenital or early-acquired brain lesions, *i.e.*, pre- or perinatal insults, hydrocephalus, malformations of cortical development; accordingly clinical features preceding ESES onset can include fixed encephalopathy, mental retardation, congenital hemiparesis, or spastic diplegia. In the Centre Saint-Paul, in a series of 20 cases, reviewed by Bureau (1999), neuroimaging was abnormal in more than 60% of cases. MRI was abnormal in 10 out of 14 patients; in four of them it showed perisylvian polymicrogyria (one case), left temporal focal dysplasia (one case), and extensive fronto-parietal polymicrogyria (two cases). According to Galanopoulou *et al.* (2000), personal antecedents and neuroradiological abnormalities range from 30 to 61%. Polymicrogyria, particularly perisylvian, has been reported in up to 81% of ESES (Guerrini *et al.*, 1998; Caraballo *et al.*, 2013). Of particular interest for their pathophysiological implication are two – possibly related – factors: i) an impressive 30% of patients presents with shunted hydrocephalus (Veggiotti *et al.*, 1999; Caraballo *et al.*, 2008); and ii) early thalamic lesions are strongly associated with sleep-enhanced epileptiform discharges (Guzzetta *et al.*, 2005; Tas *et al.*, 2009; Sanchez Fernandez *et al.*, 2012a; Quigg & Noachtar, 2012; Losito *et al.*, 2015). Furthermore, SES has been observed, as a rare unfavourable evolution, in children with idiopathic partial epilepsies, either epilepsy with centro-temporal spikes (Dalla Bernardina *et al.*, 1978, 1982, 1989) or Panayiotopoulos type occipital childhood epilepsy (Dalla Bernardina *et al.*, 1991; Lerman & Kivity, 1991; Panayiotopoulos, 1999).

Genetic factors are particularly difficult to define; a vague family history of epilepsy has been mentioned in about 15% of cases; however, there is one report in monozygotic twins (Blennow & Ors, quoted in Beaumanoir *et al.*, 1995, pp. 185–186), another familial aggregate has been reported by Praline *et al.* (2006), and, interestingly, two families have been described, characterized by coexistent BECTS and cryptogenic epilepsy with ESES in first-degree relatives (De Tiège *et al.*, 2006), suggesting a possible genetic basis for the syndrome. Supporting this idea, Rudolf *et al.* (2009) pointed out that mutations in *SRPX2* gene are found in an X-linked form of Rolandic epilepsy with speech dyspraxia (Roll *et al.*, 2006) as well as in bilateral perisylvian polymicrogyria, a brain developmental abnormality associated with both ESES (Guerrini *et al.*, 1998; Teixeira *et al.*, 2007) and LKS (Huppke *et al.*, 2005); furthermore, they suggested a possible overlap between brain malformations and idiopathic focal epilepsy of childhood, based on the association between "Rolandic EEG trait" and variants of the *ELP4* (Strug *et al.*, 2009), a gene involved in cell motility and migration (Rudolf *et al.*, 2009). Extending this concept, we can hypothesize that some "benign" form of childhood focal epilepsy maybe not idiopathic *sensu stricto*, but due to a subtle – undetectable with current imaging techniques – developmental abnormality.

ESES can also appear in different genetic diseases, in fact about one-fifth of the girls with genetically confirmed Rett syndrome who started having seizures between 1 and 5 years of age developed SES (Nissenkorn *et al.*, 2010). Furthermore, in a series of children with epilepsy and mitochondrial respiratory chain defects, two out of the 32 patients with Complex I deficiency were classified as LKS while no SES was described in the 11 subjects with defect in Complex IV (Lee *et al.*, 2008). Besides, the increasing accuracy of genetic analysis allowed researchers to find a growing number of chromosomal micro-rearrangements that might play a role in about 10% of "cryptogenic"

ESES (Mefford *et al.*, 2011; Kevelam *et al.*, 2012). These Copy-Number Variations (CNVs) include partial duplications of chromosome X (Giorda *et al.*, 2009; Broli *et al.*, 2011), chromosome 1 (Mefford *et al.*, 2011) or chromosome 9 (Nakayama *et al.*, 2012); micro-deletions of 16p13 (Reutlinger *et al.*, 2010), 4p16 (Mefford *et al.*, 2011), 15q13 (Kevelan *et al.*, 2012), 8p (Nakayama *et al.*, 2012), 8q (Verhoeven *et al.*, 2011), or partial trisomy 13/21 (Atkins & Nikanorova, 2011); however, the pathogenic role of such CNVs is largely undefined, and further studies on larger numbers of patients are needed (Kevelan *et al.*, 2012), in concert with more accurate analysis of the functions of the involved genes.

Studies based on the combination of different genetic investigations have led to the identification of genetic mutations in the *GRIN2A* gene in various childhood epileptic disorders with "acquired" language deficits with variable degree of severity, encompassed in the epilepsy-aphasia spectrum, including also ESES (Lesca *et al.*, 2013; Lemke *et al.*, 2013; Carvill *et al.*, 2013). However, whether several evidences demonstrate a role of *GRIN2A* mutations in these disorders, how the various genetic and genomic events concurring with *GRIN2A* mutations participate in the remarkable phenotypic variability observed in these patients remains to be elucidated. Several genetic and genomic defects have been identified also in the *CNKSR2* gene in patients with clinical features reminiscent to the epilepsy-aphasia spectrum, encompassing ESES (Lesca *et al.*, 2012; Vaags *et al.*, 2014; Damiano *et al.*, 2017).

A recent systematic review has provided on overview of all genetic etiologies which have been reported to be associated with ESES spectrum. The conclusion was that *SCN2A, KCNQ2, KCNB1, KCNA2* and *GRIN2A* contributed to the etiology of many patients with ESES. Since the common underlying functions of these genes is to encode important channels in brain neurons, channelopathies seems to play a major role in pathogenesis of ESES and conditions comprised in the epilepsy aphasia spectrum (Kessi *et al.*, 2018).

Epilepsy

Seizures can occur before the recognition of SES. Age of onset of seizures can vary from 2 to 12 years, with a peak around 4–5 years. The first seizures are frequently nocturnal and of unilateral type in almost half of the cases, sometimes presenting in the form of unilateral status. Less commonly absences, focal seizures, and "secondary generalized" tonic-clonic seizures have also been reported as onset seizure types during wakefulness. In the majority of cases, seizures are present during SES, but in some cases there is no history of clinical seizures at all. Interestingly, Morrell (1995) reported, in his series of patients with LKS, the occurrence of subtle seizures, often missed by the family. Semeiology and frequency of seizures are variable. We proposed three groups, based on seizure patterns:

– Group 1: patients with motor seizures, rare and nocturnal throughout their evolution.

– Group 2: patients with unilateral partial motor seizures or "secondarily generalized" tonic-clonic seizures mainly occurring during sleep, who also had, during wakefulness, absences (similar to typical absences of childhood absence epilepsy) at the onset, when SES was detected.

– Group 3: patients with rare nocturnal seizures in whom atypical absences, frequently with atonic or tonic components leading to sudden falls, developed during the ESES, after a variable period of evolution. Negative myoclonus (Rubboli & Tassinari, 2006) is frequent during wakefulness, contributing to the development of motor impairment (Dalla Bernardina *et al.*, 1989; Tassinari *et al.*, 1995, 1998).

Other seizure types, usually partial motor seizures (Morikawa *et al.*, 1989), auditory seizures (Morrell, 1995), and falls heralded the appearance of ESES in 23% of cases (Bureau, 1995b).

Seizure types and seizure frequency generally increase during SES. However, in 7% of patients seizures are rare and occur only during sleep; in 50% they occur several times a week, with "atypical" daily absences and partial motor seizures. In 43%, the absences occur with daily frequency, associated with falls, absence status and motor seizures. Interestingly, sleep studies failed to demonstrate the occurrence of "tonic seizures" (Billard *et al.*, 1982; Dulac *et al.*, 1983).

Bureau's data on follow-up of patients, based on the original Marseille cohort, specified that seizures disappeared whether epilepsy had been severe or not (Bureau, 1999). Mean duration of epilepsy was about 12 years in our series, ranging from 4 years and 4 months up to 14 years and 11 months. In 31%, the disappearance of seizures was simultaneous with the end of SES. In 44%, seizures disappeared before the end of SES, whereas in 25% they persisted after the end of SES, becoming rare and consisting of absences without falls, generalized clonic or tonic-clonic seizures. The overall outcome of epilepsy can be considered as good also in patients with organic pathology, including neuronal migration disorders (Guerrini *et al.*, 1998).

Encephalopathy

Neurological deterioration occurs, by definition, in all cases of ESES syndrome, usually being coincidental with the detection of SES and representing one of the crucial signs of the syndrome. This encephalopathy is represented most frequently by a combination of disturbances in one or more domains, including language, cognition, behavior, and motor abilities.

Language impairment
"Syndrome of acquired aphasia with convulsive disorder in children" or Landau-Kleffner syndrome

Van Bogaert & Paquier (2009) organized a symposium where William Landau and Frank Kleffner presented a video depicting one of their first aphasic girl while being tested in 1957 *(Figure 1A)*, and another one in which, fifty years later *(Figure 1B)*, the same patient reported on her experience with a fluent speech; in *Figure 1C*, the mother is discussing about the illness period of her daughter with William Landau.

By convention the "acquired epileptic aphasia" – referred to as Landau-Kleffner syndrome (LKS) – is not related to brain organic lesions and occurs in previously normal children who have already developed age-appropriate speech. However, there are reports of "clinically defined" LKS in patients with congenital or acquired brain lesion (Solomon *et al.*, 1993; Hirsch *et al.*, 1995; Galanopoulou *et al.*, 2000; Huppke *et al.*, 2005).

The disorder makes its appearance between 2 and 8 years of age with a peak between 5 and 7 years. LKS manifests in only 5% of the cases after 9 years and never after the age of 12 (Bureau, 1995b). The first symptom is epilepsy in 50% of cases and neuropsychological disorders in the remaining cases. The onset of aphasia is usually subacute, progressive with spontaneous fluctuations; the type of aphasia typically is a verbal auditory agnosia (Rapin *et al.*, 1977; Deonna & Roulet, 1995). Verbal auditory agnosia implies the failure to give a semantic significance to the different sounds. Common first symptoms are inability to understand spoken words followed by inarticulation and a decreased amount of speech. Spontaneous speech is rapidly reduced: children can show perseverations, paraphasias, phonological errors; they tend to use verbal stereotypes – a sort of telegraphic style with a jargon. *"Ultimately, the child may become completely mute and fails to respond even to non-verbal sounds such as the telephone ringing or door knocking, etc."* (Morrell, 1995). Kaga (1999) suggested a *"sequential language disorder beginning with sensory aphasia followed by auditory agnosia and finally word deafness"*. The final indifferent attitude of these children towards acoustic messages can lead to a misdiagnosis of acquired deafness or autism (Humphrey *et al.*, 1975; Kale *et al.*, 1995).

Aphasia often shows a waxing and waning course characterized by remissions and exacerbations usually, but not necessarily, related to quantitative variations of paroxysmal activity during sleep (Deonna *et al.*, 1977; Rapin *et al.*, 1977; Mantovani & Landau, 1980; Landau & Kleffner, 1957; Toso, 1981; Hirsch *et al.*, 1990). The recurrence of aphasia or its worsening can occur even many years after the initial episode (Dugas *et al.*, 1995). The duration of the disease is extremely variable. Spontaneous remissions have been reported within weeks or months after onset (Landau & Kleffner, 1957; Deonna *et al.*, 1977; Mantovani & Landau, 1980; Deonna, 1991; Deonna & Roulet, 1995). However, if symptoms persist unchanged for more than a year, spontaneous recovery is rare (Morrell, 1995). After a variable time, aphasia stabilizes and usually improves before adulthood (Deonna *et al.*, 1989; Hubert-Franc, 1990). Dugas *et al.* (1995) analyzed the long-term outcome of 55 cases with a minimum follow-up of 7 years: 47.5% presented no oral expression or unintelligible or significantly reduced oral language; 34.5% had persistence of oral or written language difficulties which did not prevent normal life; 18% did not show language abnormalities. However, the long-term deterioration of intellectual functioning is uncommon even when a severe aphasia persists in adulthood (Mantovani & Landau 1980; Deonna *et al.*, 1989; Dugas *et al.*, 1995).

Other language deficits

Other language dysfunctions associated with ESES may consist of expressive aphasia as well as difficulties predominant in lexical and grammar judgment, with relatively spared oral comprehension (Debiais *et al.*, 2007); this profile, influenced by selection bias (exclusion of patients classified as LKS), is consistent with a previously reported predominance of frontal dysexecutive syndrome in ESES (Roulet-Perez *et al.*, 1993; Veggiotti *et al.*, 2001). Nevertheless, at least in some patients, these permanent language disturbances cannot be explained by a more global cognitive deficit and are likely related to SES (Seegmüller *et al.*, 2012).

Other neuropsychological disturbances

During SES, there is the occurrence or a further decrease in performance, a marked impairment of IQ, deterioration of language, temporo-spatial disorientation, behavioural changes, reduced attention span, hyperactivity, aggressiveness, impaired social interaction and communication (Tassinari *et al.*, 1985, 1992b). Data presented at the Venice Colloquium (Beaumanoir *et al.*, 1995; Mira *et al.*, 1995) showed that SES is associated with a disruption of all cognitive functions, with sometimes a greater impairment of logical-structural intelligence and of infrastructural intelligence, possibly in relation to a previously different intellectual organization. The pattern of these disturbances may vary from patient to patient, or in the same patient during the evolution, presumably depending on the localization of the paroxysmal discharges: predominant over one or both temporal regions in severe deterioration of language (Patry *et al.*, 1971; Kellerman, 1978; Billard *et al.*, 1982; Tassinari *et al.*, 1982, 1985; De Marco, 1988; Badinand Hubert *et al.*, 1995), or involving the frontal regions when mental and behavioural deterioration occur, evoking a frontal lobe syndrome (Billard *et al.*, 1982; Roulet Perez *et al.*, 1993).

Cases with very selective neuropsychological deficits, related to a focal ESES (Kuki *et al.*, 2014) can be easily misdiagnosed or overlooked. A proper diagnosis demands a careful and appropriate

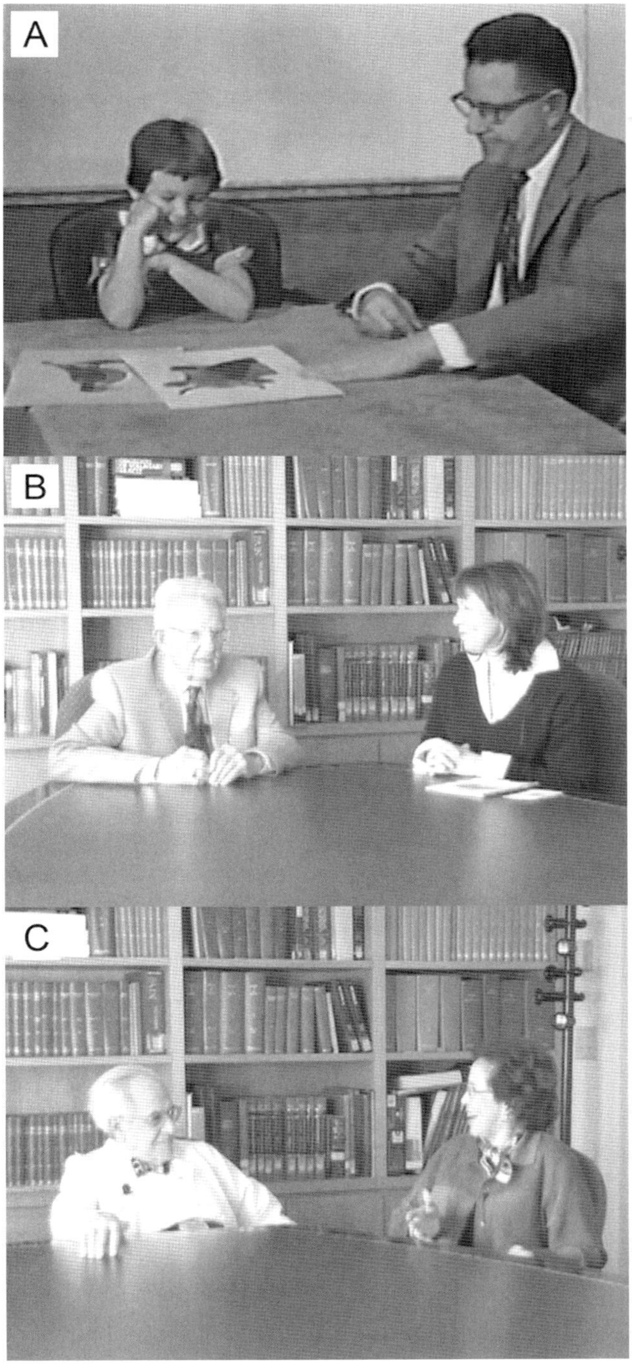

Figure 1 **One of the first children with a diagnosis of "syndrome of acquired aphasia with convulsive disorder", Jill, at age 6 years (1961), while being tested (A), and in 2006 (53 years old) interviewed by Frank Kleffner (B). William Landau in 2006 discussing about the illness period with Jill's mother (C).**

neuropsychological evaluation, eventually with test tailored for the specific cognitive deficit and complemented with adequate neurophysiological and neuroimaging investigations (Tassinari *et al.*, 2015).

Long-term outcome studies (Seegmüller *et al.*, 2012) confirmed previous observations (Praline *et al.*, 2006; Debiais *et al.*, 2007) indicating that a sharp distinction between patients with predominant language impairment and those with global cognitive regression cannot always be made. Variability in the long-term neurocognitive outcome has been hypothesized to depend on treatment response, disease duration and etiology (Pera *et al.*, 2013). In addition, cognitive deterioration is not the only consequence of ESES; in fact a pattern of slowing or stagnation of development, associated with behavioral problemes persisting beyond epilepsy resolution has been reported (De Giorgis *et al.*, 2017).

Behavioural disturbances

Hyperactivity, sometimes associated with attention deficits, has been reported in about half of the cases; disturbances of personality with psychotic characteristics have been described (Dugas *et al.*, 1982; Gordon, 1990; Zivi *et al.*, 1990), as well as a global cognitive regression and impairment of affective development, with aggressiveness and outbursts of rage (White & Sreenivasan, 1987; Roulet-Perez *et al.*, 1991). These disturbances can show different degrees of severity and are possibly related to increasing difficulties in communication (Humphrey *et al.*, 1975).

Motor impairment

Dystonia, dyspraxia and ataxia (Dalla Bernardina *et al.*, 1989; Neville & Boyd 1995; Neville *et al.*, 1998) or unilateral deficit, with possible relation to negative myoclonus, are the most disabling motor disturbances. Ansink *et al.* (1989) have described the association with a mild form of apraxia. Transitory motor dysfunctions have also been described on awakening (Veggiotti *et al.*, 2005). A peculiar type of motor impairment is probably represented by the acquired epileptiform opercular syndrome, a condition characterized by oro-facio-lingual dysfunction with dysarthria, weakness of facial and tongue muscles, Rolandic seizures and atypical absences (Colamaria *et al.*, 1991; Prats *et al.*, 1992; Shafrir& Prensky, 1995; Pascual-Castroviejo *et al.*, 1999).

Neurophysiology

Waking EEG

EEG during wakefulness shows usually focal, or multifocal, slow spikes with frequent associated diffuse slow spikes and waves. In a proportion of cases, the EEG can show similarities to what one observes in "idiopathic" focal ("Rolandic", frontal or, less frequently, parieto-occipital) epilepsies or syndromes. In other cases, a clear background asymmetry, the presence of fast spikes, or other features can evoke the presence of organic pathologies (*e.g.*, disorders of neuronal migration).

During SES, the interictal EEG abnormalities during wakefulness are similar to those before SES, but are usually more marked (Beaumanoir, 1995a, 1995b); diffuse bursts of 2–3 Hz spike-and-wave discharges, with or without clinical manifestations can occur *(Figure 2)*.

Sleep EEG

The characteristic feature of this disorder occurs during non-rapid-eye-movement (NREM) sleep. As soon as the patients fall asleep, continuous bilateral and diffuse slow spike-and-waves appear, mainly at 1.5–2.5 Hz, persisting through all the slow sleep stages *(Figures 2 to 4)*. This pattern is generally found between the ages of 4 and 14 years and it seems to develop 1 or 2 years after the appearance of seizures. According to Patry *et al.* (1971), a spike-and-wave index ranging from 85 to 100%, calculated during all night sleep EEG recordings was considered an essential feature for the diagnosis.

However, years later, and with several hundred additional reported cases, one should admit that this criterion was useful to identify only the "tip of the iceberg". Unilateral or more or less focal (frontal, centrotemporal, etc.), subcontinuous paroxysmal discharges during slow sleep have been described in different patients, in relation to various factors (aetiology, topography of the spikes, evolution; etc.) with shifting from unilateral *(Figure 5)* to diffuse paroxysmal activity in the same patient (Michelucci *et al.*, 1987; Giovanardi Rossi *et al.*, 1999).

A spike-and-wave index under 85% has been used for the diagnosis of ESES syndrome (Calvet, 1978; Billard *et al.*, 1982; Yasuhara *et al.*, 1991); such cases have a less regression in their performance scores, as compared to patients with higher sleep related spike-and-wave index (Beaumanoir, 1995b).

Morphology and distribution of the paroxysms during slow wave sleep can be relevant as well. During REM sleep, paroxysmal activity becomes fragmented, less continuous, whereas focal discharges may become more evident (Genton *et al.*, 1992). Discharges organized as a subclinical seizure are observed, as documented in *Figure 6*.

A recent study in ESES with different etiologies failed to demonstrate in the follow-up a correlation between the spike-and-wave index and maximum amplitude of the ESES pattern (anterior *versus* posterior) with seizure control and reduction of SWI (Gencpinar *et al.*, 2016).

Auditory evoked potentials

The auditory system has been explored mostly in presence of receptive language impairment. Audiometric tests are normal (Rapin *et al.*, 1977; Kale *et al.*, 1995; Stroink *et al.*, 1997). Auditory evoked potentials gave normal responses in the cases studied by Nakano *et al.* (1989) and Shu-Xian *et al.* (1989), but Isnard *et al.* (1995) found alterations in central components of early and middle latency auditory evoked potentials. Seri *et al.* (1998) demonstrated, in a group of six children with LKS, that spikes in temporal regions could produce a reduction in amplitude and an increment in latency of the N1 auditory evoked responses. These results were consistent with a dysfunction of the central auditory pathways and with a deficit in the activation of auditory cortical areas. Paetau *et al.* (1999) described alterations of the auditory evoked magnetic fields in five children with LKS. The neural generators of the auditory evoked magnetic fields coincided with the sources of the spontaneous spikes, both located along the sylvian fissure, and suggested a participation of sound-responsive neurons in the non-primary auditory cortex, within the middle and posterior sylvian region, in the genesis of epileptic activity.

EEG after the end of SES

In the group of 25 patients (Bureau *et al.*, 1990) EEG was normal during wakefulness and sleep in eight cases, with normalization being progressive and occurring with a mean of 3 months after the end of SES. Repeated awake and sleep EEG recordings show that the normalization may continue for an average of 15 years, after the end of SES. In five cases, it was normal during wakefulness while showing focal abnormalities during sleep. In 12 cases, however, focal abnormalities existed during awake and sleep recordings. In none of the patients diffuse abnormalities were recorded. In all cases, the cyclic organization of sleep was normal. All stages of sleep were present at a normal percentage, with normal sleep patterns in all.

Quantitative and qualitative EEG parameters

The description of the EEG pattern of ESES has been based almost exclusively on the abundance of epileptic abnormalities, while other quantitative and qualitative measures have been usually neglected. In fact, since the earliest descriptions, the amount of epileptic discharges, expressed as percentage of the total duration of slow sleep occupied by spike-and-waves, was referred as spike-index (Patry *et al.*, 1971). In the following years different threshold values were considered, ranging from > 85% (Tassinari *et al.*, 2000) to 25% (Van Hirtum-Das, 2006), and, more significantly, the methods to

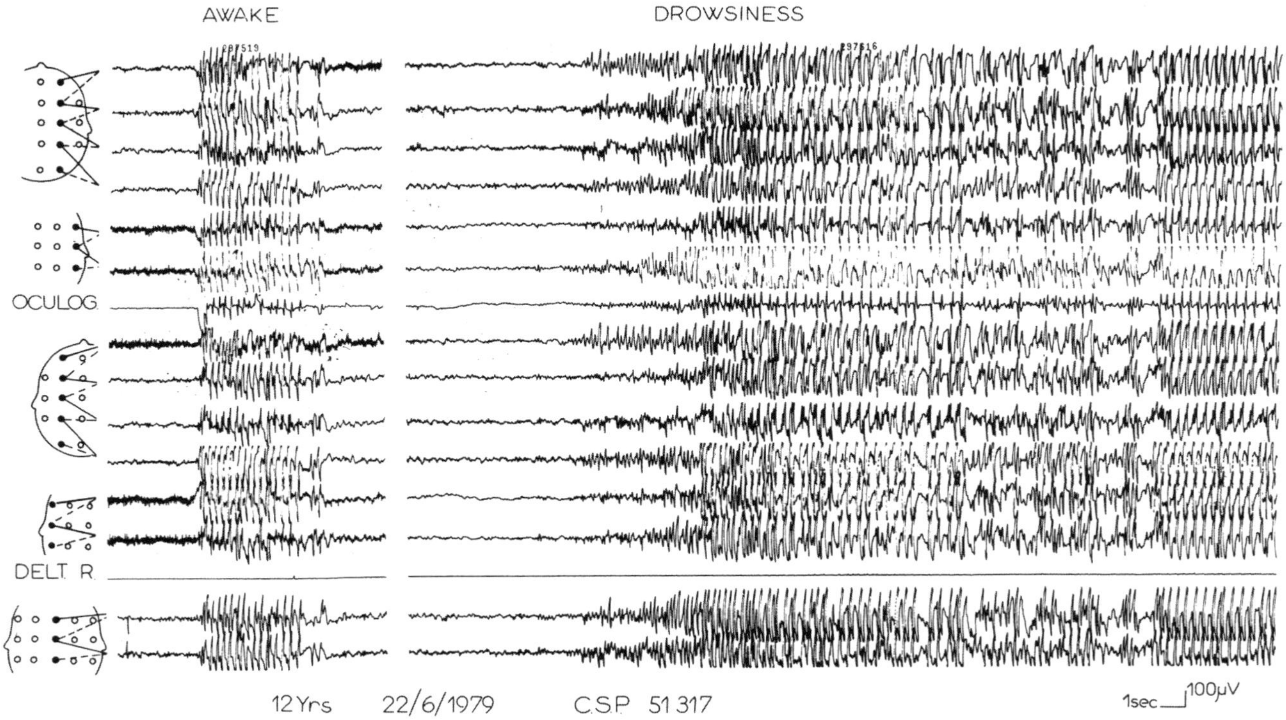

Figure 2

Awake and sleep EEG recording in a 12-year-old-boy. Left: awake EEG: subclinical burst of diffuse SW around 3 Hz/sec. Right: drowsiness showing the onset of SES.

determine the spike-index vary considerably across different studies, considering the percentage of either the whole-night NREM sleep, or at least 15 minutes slow wave sleep, or a nap, or the total duration of each cycle of slow wave sleep, or percentage of seconds with more than 1 spike-wave complex during the first and last sleep cycles (for a detailed review see Scheltens-de Boer, 2009). Apart from spike-index cut-off used as inclusion criteria, several authors developed grading scales to quantify evolution of EEG, in order to assess the efficacy of treatment (*i.e.*, Aeby *et al.*, 2005); however, differences between studies forbid comparisons. Furthermore, a single spike-index value for each recording cannot illustrate the temporal evolution of the SES across the night that, even if never quantified in detail, has been variably described as continuous, but also as subcontinuous, or fragmented, or periodic (according or not with sleep stages, cycle ordinal or maybe CAP phases). This latter consideration on discontinuity of SES led us to consider the CSWS acronym proposed by the ILAE Task Force on Classification and Terminology as inadequate to describe the full spectrum of EEG pattern encountered in ESES. To better describe this pattern, Scheltens-de Boer (2009) proposed to express spike-index as mean, range and most encountered value. Quantification of epileptiform activity in EEG has mainly been done by visual inspection of the recorded EEG; semi-automated methods have been proposed (Larsson *et al.*, 2009; Nonclerq *et al.*, 2009; Peltola *et al.*, 2012) giving the possibility to extract information on the time-course of spike-index value or when the spike wave index is of limited value (Peltola *et al.*, 2014). Topographic

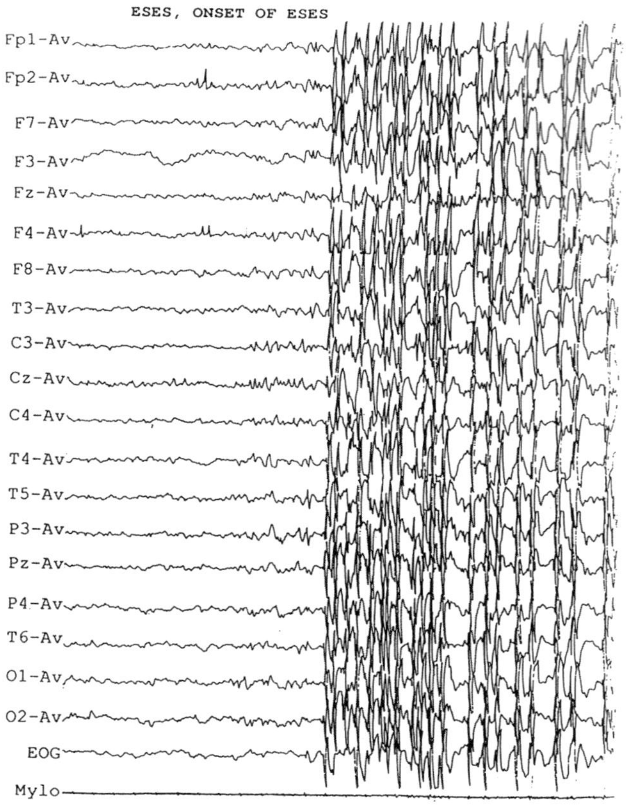

Figure 3 **Diffuse onset of SES in a patient with wakefulness multifocal abnormalities (right frontal and left temporo-parietal foci are evident). Horizontal scale: 1 sec; vertical scale: 100 mV.**

distribution of epileptiform activity mostly is described as secondary bilateral synchronized (Kobayashi *et al.*, 1994, Morrell *et al.*, 1995), nevertheless, different grades of hemispheric lateralization are reported (hemi-SES or asymmetric SES) as well as bitemporal, focal and multifocal distributions. Few studies analyze quantitatively these topographic features. In the clinical variant of ESES with acquired aphasia (or LKS), EEG (Morrell *et al.*, 1995) or MEG (Paetau *et al.*, 1999; Paetau, 2009) studies were performed in order to localize the "pace-maker" abnormalities for surgical purposes. Even this fast

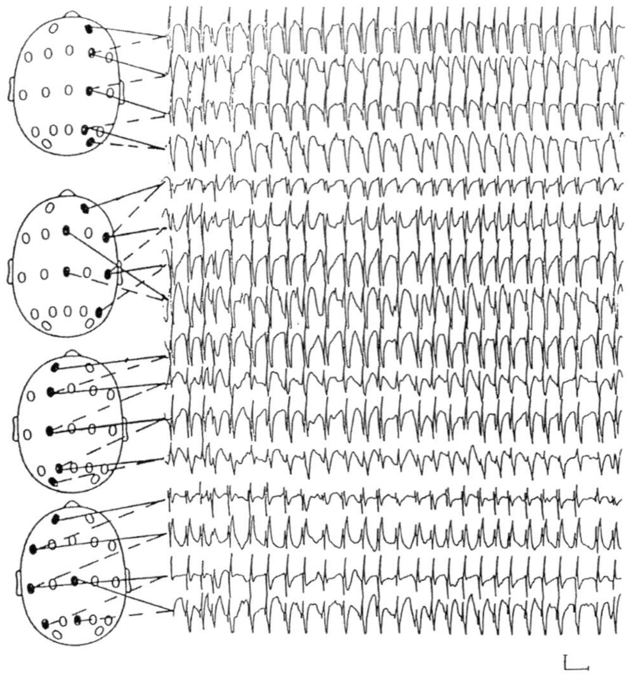

Figure 4 **Continuous, diffuse SW activities during NREM sleep in a 4-year-old-boy with ESES syndrome. Horizontal scale: 1 sec; vertical scale: 100 mV.**

propagation of the epileptiform activity between different brain areas, usually considered a qualitative parameter (*i.e.*, presence or absence of secondary bilateral synchrony – SBS), has been analyzed quantitatively (Larsson *et al.*, 2010; Martin Miguel *et al.*, 2011). Furthermore, it has to be considered that the amplitude of epileptiform activity has been measured only rarely (Tassinari *et al.*, 2000; Veggiotti *et al.*, 2001), whereas morphology only almost incidentally has been described, and probably the reciprocal influence between sleep and epileptic discharges would be different according to these variables. In particular, topography seems to be important also for the clinical features of the encephalopathy. In fact, it is already known that, during wakefulness, the interictal focal spike activity itself can be associated with a transient disruption of the specific function mediated by the cortical area involved, *i.e.*, visual (Shewmon & Erwin,

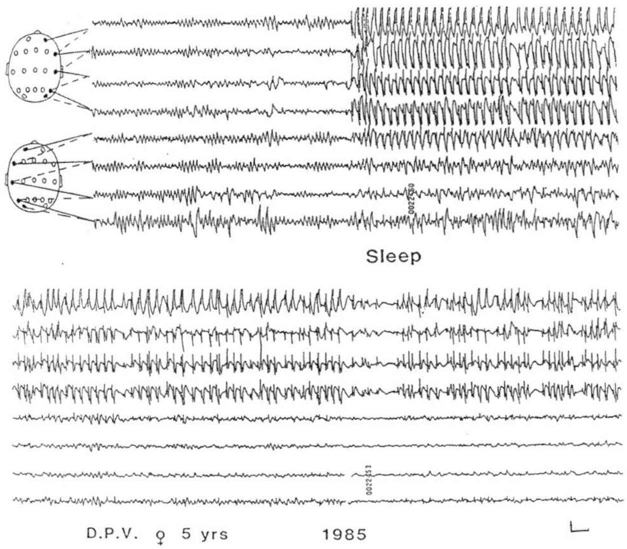

Figure 5 **Asymmetrical, continuous 2–2.5 Hz/sec SW discharge appeared at sleep onset on the right hemisphere and persisted during slow wave sleep stages. During wakefulness, sporadic left side sharp waves were evident. The patient was submitted twice to surgical shunt procedure for hydrocephalus at the age of 40 days and 2 years; neurological examination was normal; mild subcortical atrophy, predominent on the right side was demonstrated by brain CTscan. Horizontal scale: 1 sec; vertical scale: 100 mV.**

1988a, 1988b, 1989) or auditory (Seri *et al.*, 1998). It led to the relevant concept of short-term "transitory cognitive impairment" (Aarts *et al.*, 1984; Binnie, 1993) in the domain subserved by the cortical neuronal network involved by paroxysmal activity. Also the chronic cognitive dysfunctions have been demonstrated to selectively correlate with accurate location of interictal focal abnormalities in children with idiopathic partial epilepsy (Wolff *et al.*, 2005). Similarly, visuo-spatial deficits have been documented during occipito-temporal SES (Eriksson *et al.*, 2003) while a frontal dysexecutive syndrome was reported in association with SES predominance on anterior leads (Roulet-Perez *et al.*, 1991; Veggiotti *et al.*, 2001).

Treatment

Therapeutic options must intend not only to reduce *epileptic seizures* but above all to "treat" – *i.e.*, obtaining the disappearance of the SES responsible for the *encephalopathy*. Benzodiazepines, sodium valproate, ethosuximide, carbamazepine and phenytoin are the drugs most commonly used to treat the seizures, as well as newer antiepileptic drugs (AEDs), based on seizure type, comorbidities and side-effect profile. As already mentioned, although the response may only be partial, the long-term seizure outcome is favorable. Taking into account the relationship between the occurrence of SES and the neuropsychological deterioration, a rapid aggressive therapy of SES is mandatory, with accurate follow-up by means of i) repeated sleep-EEG recordings (at least monthly), in order to verify the suppression of SES; and ii) concomitant evaluation of the neuropsychological status. Treatment options include a variety of antiepileptic medications, immunosuppressant/immunomodulatory treatments or surgical approach (Kellerman, 1978; Billard *et al.*, 1982; Morikawa *et al.*, 1985; Yan Liu & Wong, 2000; Tsuru *et al.*, 2000; Peltola *et al.*, 2010).

All classical types of AEDs have been used. While improvements have been reported with some drugs, such as valproate, ethosuximide or benzodiazepines (Marescaux *et al.*, 1990; Sanchez Fernandez *et al.*, 2013), other AEDs, such as phenytoin, carbamazepine, oxcarbazepine and phenobarbital have been proved either ineffective or even worsening the clinical and EEG picture (Snead & Hosey, 1985; Lerman, 1986; Caraballo *et al.*, 1989; Pavlidis *et al.*, 2015). Moreover, these latter drugs can induce or unleash the appearance of ESES in otherwise benign conditions (Dalla Bernardina *et al.*, 2005), in which discontinuation of these AEDs results in a prompt recovery. Intravenous benzodiazepine can be rapidly and dramatically effective in suppressing the EEG abnormalities during slow sleep *(Figure 7)* and in improving verbal communication, but this result is transitory and brief (Ravnik, 1985). Chronic oral treatment with clobazam (Larrieu *et al.*, 1986; Vega *et al.*, 2018), lorazepam (Boel & Casaer, 1989) and clonazepam (Yasuhara *et al.*, 1991), associated with other AEDs (usually sodium valproate and ethosuximide) seems to have more durable efficacy. Also treatment with short cycles of high-dose DZP (one to 3 weeks) can lead to transient remission (De Negri *et al.*, 1995), but the cycle should be repeated after each relapse, occurring generally within 18 months (Inutsuka *et al.*, 2006; Kramer *et al.*, 2009), although more recent studies lack of long-term follow-up (Sanchez Fernandez *et al.*, 2012b). Similarly, a tolerance/habituation phenomenon – after initial efficacy – has been reported for sulthiame (Wirrell *et al.*, 2006) and aceta-zolamide (Pisani *et al.*, 1999), albeit longstanding effects have been reported in some cases (Fejerman *et al.*, 2012; Fine *et al.*, 2015). The efficacy of some AEDs, especially

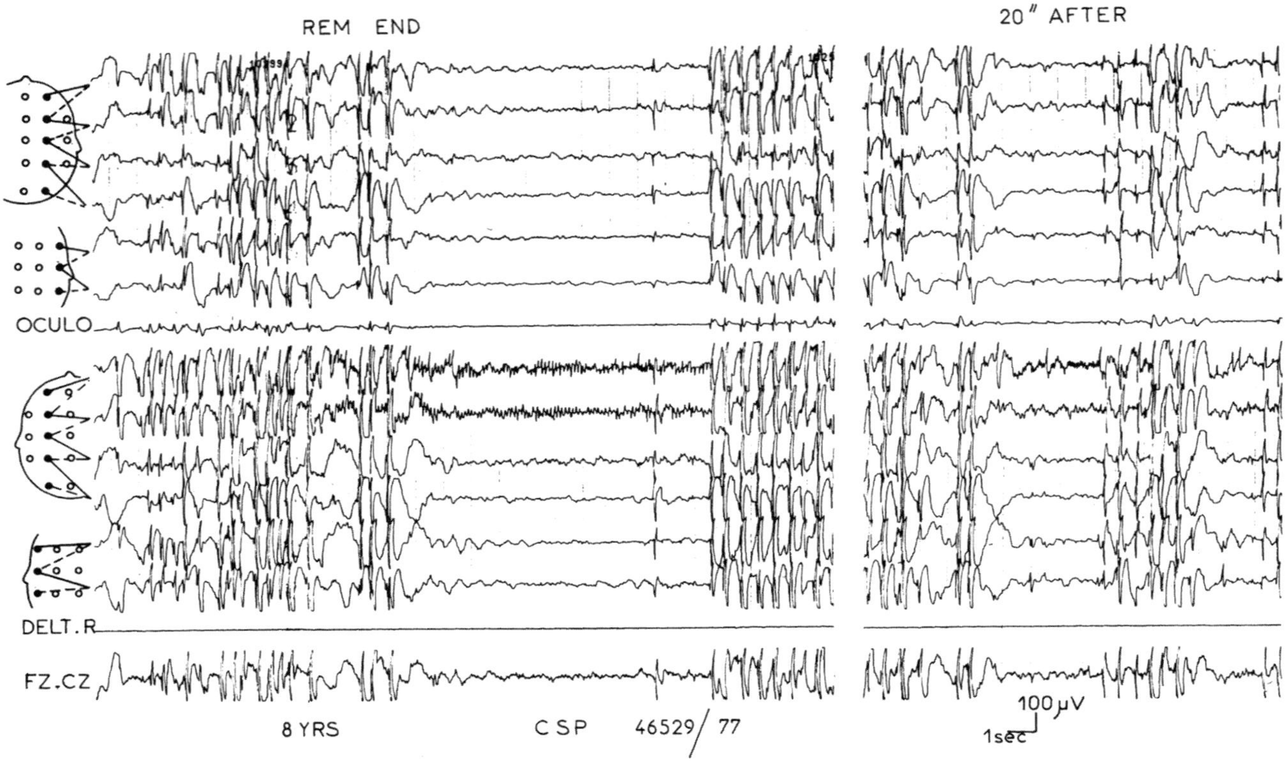

Figure 6

Left: at the end of REM stage, when the diffuse SW reappear, occurrence of a subclinical ictal discharge in the left fronto-central area. Right: after 20 sec another shorter ictal discharge.

levetiracetam, has been suggested in the treatment of ESES (Hoppen *et al.*, 2003; Capovilla *et al.*, 2004; Aeby *et al.*, 2005; Chhun *et al.*, 2011; Larsson *et al.*, 2012); moreover, in a prospective study on 20 patients, levetiracetam, as an add-on treatment, has been suggested as an effective and lasting treatment for children with ESES resulting from symptomatic epilepsy, in whom the paroxysmal activity displayed a regional location without SBS (Atkins & Nikanorova, 2011). Furthermore, levetiracetam's efficacy can be tested acutely by means of intravenous formulation, obtaining a prompt EEG improvement (Cesaroni *et al.*, 2009). The particular effectiveness of this new drug might be related at least partially to its anti-inflammatory effects (Stieten *et al.*, 2011). Finally, recent reports in children with ESES have suggested that lacosamide, topiramate and amantadine might be also effective (Grosso *et al.*, 2014; Vrielynck *et al.*, 2017; Wilson *et al.*, 2018), however, due to the limited size of the patients cohorts, these findings need to be replicated.

Although polytherapy with the smallest number of drugs has been reported to improve the clinical picture (Van Lierde, 1995), at present an association therapy seems to be the most effective treatment in clinical practice. This polytherapy is mainly achieved after a rather strict sequential association of valproate, ethosuximide, levetiracetam and benzodiazepines (Dalla Bernardina *et al.*, 1989; Inutsuka *et al.*, 2006; Veggiotti *et al.*, 2011). We agree with this "energic approach"

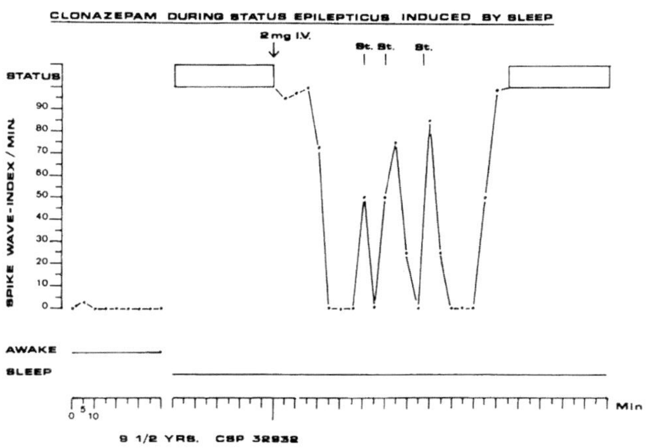

Figure 7 **9 years 6 months old girl with ESES. Diagram showing the interruption (for about 85 min) of the SW discharges of SES following administration of clonazepam, 2 mg e.v. Arousing stimuli (St) evoked SW activity, whose number and duration increases at time from the benzodiazepine injection elapses.**

as we must consider ESES an emergency, so we cannot wait more than few weeks of persisting SES before considering it drug-resistant and taking into account all further therapeutic options.

In drug-resistant cases, steroid treatment has been proposed by several authors (McKinney & McGreal, 1974; Lerman & Lerman-Sagie, 1989; Marescaux *et al.*, 1990; Lerman *et al.*, 1991; Raha *et al.*, 2012) adopting different regimens, including intravenous, oral prednisone, pulse methylprednisolone, or ACTH injections, followed or not by oral prednisone, subsequently slowly tapered. Buzatu *et al.* (2009) and van Munckhof *et al.* (2018) provided two large series of patients (n = 44 and n = 43, respectively) addressing the efficacy of corticosteroids in ESES. Buzatu *et al.* (2009) accordingly to their literature review on previously reported series, found a response rate of about 77%. Van Munckhof *et al.* (2018) evaluated various treatments regimens and concluded that steroids were the most effective treatment in improving cognitive function, as shown in a previous meta-analysis (van Munckhof *et al.*, 2015), in comparison with non-steroid treatments. However, major concern with the use of steroids, aside from side-effects, is the SES relapse after discontinuation or during tapering, suggesting that a prolonged trial should be done (Buzatu *et al.*, 2009; Veggiotti *et al.*, 2011), with careful electroclinical follow up. No clear results can be extrapolated from the few studies on vagus nerve stimulation (Park *et al.*, 2003; Veggiotti *et al.*, 2012) while transcranial direct current stimulation (TDCS) has been demonstrated to be ineffective (Varga *et al.*, 2011).

There are also some reports of successful use of intravenous immunoglobulins: however, after the first 3 patients described (Lagae *et al.*, 1998; Fayad *et al.*, 1997; Mikati *et al.*, 1998), none of the 9 additional cases prospectively treated by Mikati *et al.* responded (Mikati & Saab, 2000; Mikati & Shamseddine, 2005); 4 out of 15 showed a positive response in two retrospective series (Kramer *et al.*, 2009; Arts *et al.*, 2009). Moreover, a recent study in a limited cohort of ESES patients has shown that immunomodulating treatments with intravenous immunoglobulin or steroids significantly reduced interleukin IL-6 levels and this reduction was associated with improvement of the EEG and of the neurocognitive status. These findings have been interpreted as suggesting that IL-6 might correlate with disease activity and efficacy of immunomodulalting treatment (van den Munckhof *et al.*, 2016).

Limited evidence is available in favour of ketogenic diet; however, Bergqvist *et al.* (1999) have reported an enduring improvement in language, behavior, and seizures in 3 children with drug-resistant LKS, and two out of five patients were successfully treated by Nikanorova *et al.* (2009).

In the subgroup of patients with ESES, in which a focal perinatal damage, or a focal malformation of cortical development can be documented, surgery can be an effective strategy both for control of seizures and avoidance of detrimental effects of SES. In fact, Loddenkemper *et al.* (2009) demonstrated that 8 patients with drug-resistant epilepsy with unilateral congenital or early-acquired brain lesions underwent hemispherectomy or focal resection, and experienced good seizure outcome and additional developmental benefits. Functional hemispherectomy has been successfully employed also in a patient with an early brain injury involving thalamus associated with refractory partial seizures and ESES (Battaglia *et al.*, 2009). A Finnish study further reported on the utility of hemispherectomy and focal resection, adding interesting evidence on neurological, cognitive and behavioural improvements also after callosotomy (Peltola *et al.*, 2010). Finally, improvement of neurocognitive status, cessation of seizures and resolution of ESES have been described in 9 children with a unilateral lesion who underwent hemispherotomy (Jeong *et al.*, 2017).

Resective surgery, by means of left temporal lobectomy, has been performed also in two cases without brain lesion, resulting in a transitory improvement of aphasia (Cole *et al.*, 1988; Nass *et al.*, 1999).

In pharmacoresistant ESES patients without brain lesions, the technique of multiple subpial transection (MST) was proposed by Morrell *et al.* (1989). MST selectively interrupts the intracortical horizontal fibres, preserving the vertical columnar organization, therefore preventing the synchronization through horizontal linkages necessary for the epileptic discharge to occur, whilst not altering the normal physiological transactions mediated by the vertically oriented cortical columns. MST represents an alternative choice also in lesional ESES in whom resective surgery is not indicated (Spencer *et al.*, 2002; Cross & Neville, 2009). Over the years, a growing evidence of progressive and long-lasting improvement of the language function after MST performed in the region of focal epileptic discharges, as defined by ECoG recordings *(Figure 8)*, has been provided (Morrell *et al.*, 1995; Grote *et al.*, 1999; Spencer *et al.*, 2002); since only a small number of selected patients have been treated by means of MST data on efficacy are still controversial (Cross & Neville, 2009).

Physiopathogenic considerations

Two main issues are relevant to physiopathology of ESES: i) the mechanism generating SES; and ii) the mechanism responsible for the encephalopathy with neuropsychological disturbances.

The mechanism generating SES

Besides the seminal works of Morrell (1985, 1995) and Morrell *et al.* (1995) *(Figure 9)*, several neurophysiological data support the hypothesis that SES is the result of a secondary bilateral synchrony (SBS). These include: i) the main seizure type, usually focal; ii) focal EEG activity during both wakefulness and REM sleep; iii) interhemispheric peak latencies and phase reversal of spikes on unilateral regions (Morikawa *et al.*, 1989, 1995); iv) coherence and phase analyses (Kobayashi *et al.*, 1990); v) intracranial EEG recordings (Cole *et al.*, 1988; Solomon *et al.*, 1993) and vi) EEG spectrum studies (Nakano *et al.*, 1989). It has also been observed that metabolic abnormalities revealed by means of functional imaging such as PET (Maquet *et al.*, 1990; Hirsch *et al.*, 1995), SPECT (Mouridsen *et al.*, 1993; Harbord *et al.*, 1999), and fMRI studies (De Tiège *et al.*, 2009; Siniatchkin *et al.*, 2010) seem to indicate either a dysfunction predominant over the temporal areas (mainly in patients with language disturbances), or diffuse abnormalities, distant from the EEG focus (De Tiège *et al.*, 2009).

Paroxysmal activity is greatly increased by slow sleep in different conditions, such as the Lennox-Gastaut syndrome, BECTS and, above all, ESES. Accordingly, it was considered that "the underlying cellular mechanism generating spike-and-waves are similar regardless of etiology and in spite of the clinical varieties of epileptic seizures" (Amzica & Steriade, 2002). A clinical fundamental comment is that activation of paroxysmal activities during sleep is an age-dependent condition. According to experimental work of Steriade's school (Steriade *et al.*, 1993; Steriade & Amzica, 1994, Steriade & Contreras, 1998) during natural sleep, slow oscillation of < 1 Hz occur both in cats and humans (Acherman & Borbely, 1997).

The physiological excitatory component of the slow oscillation arising from neocortex could, in epileptic conditions, become "the seed" of increased synchrony within cortical network, leading to paroxysmal epileptic discharges evident in the EEG.

A secondary role of the thalamo-cortical network in the recruitment and progression of the paroxysmal activity has been documented experimentally (Neckelmann *et al.*, 1998; Amzica & Steriade, 2002) leading to an avalanche process. This could also be one of the mechanism in maintaining the SES. Reports of patients with early thalamic injury (Monteiro *et al.*, 2001; Guzzetta *et al.*, 2005; Kelemen *et al.*, 2006), reduced thalamic volume (Sanchez Fernandez *et al.*, 2017), thalamic abnormalities at PET scanning (Agarwal *et al.*, 2016) and ESES are also in favor of this mechanism, and should be carefully looked for.

Role of sleep in cognitive development and interference by sleep-related epileptiform EEG activities

Overall trends in the literature confirm a causal relationship between SES and the encephalopathy in humans. Experimental evidence has shown that some cognitive and motor performances can improve after sleep (Smith, 1995; Mednick *et al.*, 2002; Stickgold *et al.*, 2000; Walker *et al.*, 2002; Fenn *et al.*, 2003). A role of sleep in neuroplastic remodelling of neural networks mediating cognitive performances and behavior, particularly in children, is supported by a growing body of experimental data, demonstrating, for instance, the crucial role of sleep in learning and memory consolidation (Stick-gold *et al.*, 2002; Benington & Frank, 2003; Walker & Stickgold, 2004), whereas, sleep deprivation has an opposite, deleterious effect on these processes (Peigneux *et al.*, 2001). Finally, several experimental evidences have demonstrated the important role played by slow wave sleep in normal cortical plasticity during developmental critical periods, thus lending support to hypothesis that postulate a disruptive effect of sleep-related electrographic seizures on cortical maps and cortical development (Issa, 2014).

EEG activity for most of normal sleep is characterized by slow wave activity (SWA), that corresponds at a cellular level, to slow oscillations of membrane potentials of cortical neurons (Steriade, 2000). The

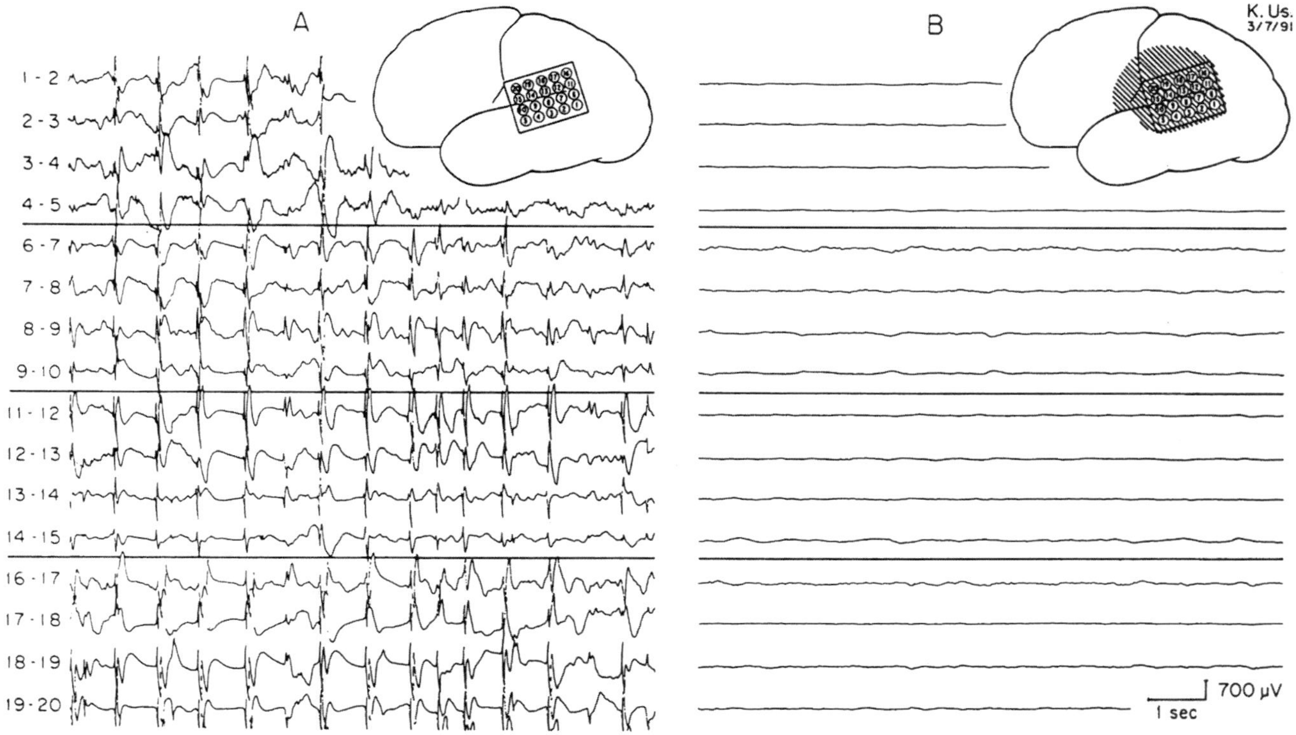

Figure 8

Electrocorticographic recording showing: (A) widespread distribution of the spike activity in the perisylvian cortex; (B) complete disappearance of spikes immediately following multiple subpial transect ions of the planum temporale and peri sylvian cortex (indicated by the slanted lines). Reproduced from Morrell (1995) with kind permission.

amount of EEG SWA is homeostatically regulated, showing an increment during wakefulness and returning to baseline during sleep (Borbely & Achermann, 2000). Slow wave sleep (SWS) has always been associated with the restorative functions of sleep, but what these functions might be remains unclear. A hypothesis – the synaptic homeostasis hypothesis (Tononi & Cirelli, 2006) – suggests that a consequence of staying awake is a progressive increase in synaptic strength in many brain circuits, since the awake brain learns and adapts to an ever-changing environment mostly through synaptic potentiation. A progressive increase in synaptic strength is unsustainable, because stronger synapses consume more energy, occupy more space (they are more numerous and/or larger) and saturate the ability to learn. Thus, sleep may serve an essential function by promoting a homeostatic reduction in synaptic strength. According to this hypothesis (detailed in *Figure 10*), the larger the wake-related synaptic potentiation, the larger the slow waves at the beginning of SWS. Moreover, these slow waves are instrumental to produce synaptic renormalization. Sudies in flies, zebrafish, mice, rats and humans, using multiple anatomical, molecular and electrophysiological approaches, have provided evidence in support of synaptic

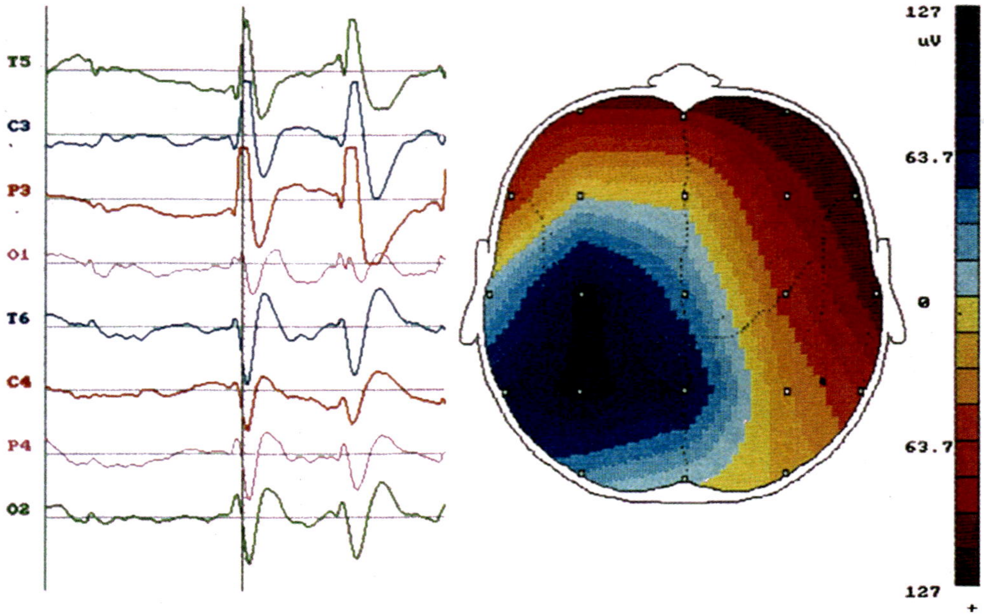

Figure 9 Computerized topographic mapping of the spike component of the SW complexe at the onset of SES illustrated in *Figure 3* shows that the leading activity appears at the P3 electrode, to spread then diffusely to both hemispheres.

homeostasis. For instance, after ruling out effects of time of day and stress, it was shown that in many brain areas synapses are larger/more numerous (Gilestro *et al.*, 2009), contain more synaptic proteins and AMPA receptors (Vyazovskiy *et al.*, 2008), and generate stronger excitatory currents (Liu *et al.*, 2010) after wake than after sleep. Moreover, there is evidence that synaptic renormalization is tied to the beneficial effects of sleep on brain function and performance, for instance after motor learning (Huber *et al.*, 2004; Landsness *et al.*, 2009).

In particular, it has been demonstrated that a learning task involving a specific brain region may influence sleep homeostasis (Huber *et al.*, 2004): in fact, a local change of EEG SWA (*i.e.*, a local increment of SWA) during sleep after a learning task can be observed in correspondence of the cortical regions involved in the performance of that task. This local increment of SWA results in a significant improvement in the task performance after sleep. The opposite effect has been reported in subjects with prolonged immobilization of an arm in whom a local decrement of EEG SWA during sleep occurred in the corresponding arm cortical area (Huber *et al.*, 2006). These data have led to hypothesize that the electrophysiological marker of sleep homeostasis, SWA, can be selectively modulated in circumscribed cortical areas, suggesting therefore a local regulation of sleep (Huber *et al.* 2004). In addition, a local SWA increment following a learning task suggests the direct or indirect involvement of local plastic changes in learning processes. These data, therefore, may demonstrate a correlation between local SWA homeostasis during sleep and learning/cognitive performance related to the cortical areas where SWA homeostasis was modulated.

Considering these data, it can be postulated that prolonged focal epileptic activity during sleep (as it occurs in ESES) interferes with local SWA at the site of the epileptic focus, impairing the neural processes and, possibly, the local plastic changes associated with learning and other cognitive functions (Tassinari & Rubboli, 2006; Rubboli *et al.*, 2018). In this respect, ESES might represent a model of the clinical effects of a localized disruption of EEG activity during sleep caused by long-lasting sleep-related focal epileptic activity, adding further evidences on the crucial role of sleep in neuroplasticity mechanisms underlying higher cognitive functions (Tassinari *et al.*, 2009). The plausibility of this hypothesis has been demonstrated by Bölsterli *et al.* (2011). These authors, in a retrospective case control study, analyzed the time course of the slope of EEG slow waves in nine patients with ESES. It was shown that the slope of slow waves is an even more sensitive measure of cortical synaptic strength than SWA (references in Vyazovskiy *et al.*, 2009). It was found that, as expected, control subjects showed a decrease of the slope of slow waves from the first to the last hour of sleep, which parallels the decline in SWA in the course of sleep. ESES patients, by contrast, showed no significant change in slope across the night, and this effect was more

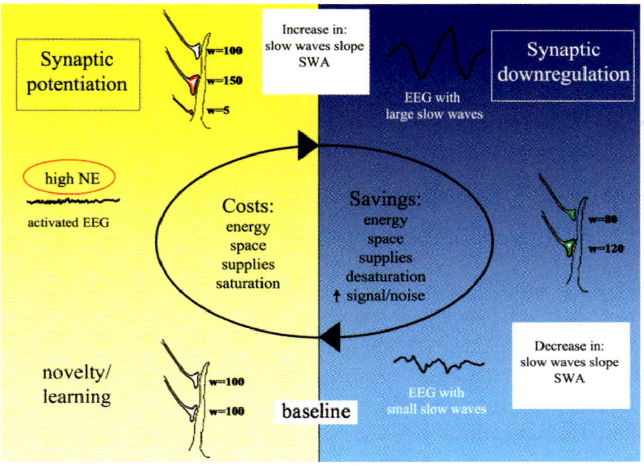

Figure 10 The synaptic homeostasis hypothesis of sleep. During wake (yellow background), we interact with an ever-changing environment and acquire information about it. The EEG is activated, and the neuro-modulatory milieu (*e.g.*, high levels of norepinephrine, NE) favors the storage of information, which occurs largely through long-term potentiation (increase in synaptic strength). This potentiation occurs when the firing of a presynaptic neuron is followed by the depolarization or firing of a postsynaptic neuron, and the neuro-modulatory milieu signals the occurrence of salient events (in the figure strengthened synapses are in red, with their strength given by a number). Due to the net increase in synaptic strength, wake plasticity has a cost in terms of energy and space requirements, and progressively saturates our capacity to learn. When we sleep (blue background), we become virtually disconnected from the environment. Changes in the neuro-modulatory milieu trigger slow oscillations in membrane potential, comprising depolarized and hyperpolarized phases, which affect every neuron in the cerebral cortex, and which are reflected in the EEG as slow waves and in EEG power spectra as slow wave activity (SWA, the EEG power in the 0.5–4.5 Hz range during NREM sleep, is a measure of the number and amplitude of sleep slow waves). The changed neuro-modulatory milieu (*e.g.*, low NE) ensures that synaptic activity is not followed by synaptic potentiation, which makes adaptive sense given that synaptic activity during sleep is not driven by interactions with the environment. Because average synaptic strength at the end of wake is high, neurons undergoing sleep slow oscillations are highly synchronized. As a result, the EEG of early sleep shows slow waves of high amplitude. The slow waves, however, are not just an epiphenomenon of the increased synaptic strength, but have a role to play. The repeated sequences of depolarization-hyperpolarization cause the downregulation of the synapses impinging on each neuron, which means that they decrease in strength (the assumption is that most, if not all synapses do so, perhaps proportionally; green color in the figure). The reduced synaptic strength reduces the amplitude and synchronization of the slow oscillations in membrane potential, which is reflected in a reduced SWA in the sleep EEG, and thus smaller slow waves. Because of the dampening of the slow waves, synaptic renormalization is progressively reduced, making the process self-limiting when synaptic strength reaches an appropriate baseline level. Thus, when we wake up, neural circuits do preserve a trace of the previous experiences, but are kept efficient at a renormalized level of synaptic strength, and the cycle can begin again.

pronounced in the hemisphere with more spike-wave activity. In addition, it was shown that the impairment of the slope decrease was more pronounced at the site of the epileptic focus, with a positive correlation with the spike wave index (Bolsterli *et al.*, 2014). Finally, a recent study by Bolsterli *et al.* (2017) in a limited cohort children with idiopathic ESES has reported a correlation between the neuropsychological and behavioural outcome and the degree of impairment of the slope of the sleep slow waves during active ESES. Children who completely recovered cognitively and behaviourally after ESES showed a partial preservation of the overnight decline of the slope of sleep slow waves during ESES active phase, at variance with those children who continued to have cognitive deficits and behavioral disorders after ESES resolution who completely lack the physiological decline of the slope of sleep slow waves during active ESES. Other studies showed that in healthy children the recall of learned word pairs increased after a night of sleep, whereas the opposite, *i.e.* a decrease of word recall, was observed in children with ESES (Urbain *et al.*, 2011), suggesting that impairment of sleep homeostasis may be responsible for the lack of memory consolidation. Additional data have shown that homeostatic regulation of sleep SWA undergoes maturational changes across adolescence (Campbell *et al.*, 2011) that parallel the anatomical markers of cortical maturation and synaptic pruning (Buchmann *et al.*, 2010). In addition, the observation that younger patients have spike focus more posteriorly than older children has suggested that the posterior-anterior trajectory of maximal spike-waves that has been observed in ESES children at different ages parallels a similar maturational-related trajectory of the maximal expression of sleep slow waves. This has led to the hypothesis that the epileptic activity in sleep tends to occur where there is an age-related higher susceptibility to synchronization (Bolsterli Heinze *et al.*, 2017).

An interesting finding is the observation of spike-related high-frequency oscillations (HFO) in ESES (Kobayashi *et al.*, 2010) that might suggest a role of HFO in synaptic strengthening of pathological cortico-thalamic network associated with secondary bisynchronous spikes of ESES (Siniatchkin *et al.*, 2010), as suggested by the tendency to an increase in SWA slope across the night (Bösterli *et al.*, 2011). Based on these findings, it can be postulated that pathological conditions interfering with sleep-related synaptic downscaling are predicted to be harmful, particularly during the critical time-window of childhood and pre-adolescence (Cantalupo *et al.*, 2011; Rubboli *et al.*, 2018). Moreover, this approach introduces a new methodological perspective in the field of electroclinical correlations, opening a new way for the analysis and understanding of the ESES syndrome, and providing a new background to evaluate the relevance of paroxysmal activities during sleep, not only for ESES but for a large population of children with significant activation of focal paroxysmal activity during sleep.

The "Penelope syndrome" (an eponym conveying the encephalopathy mechanism)

One of the most intriguing issues of ESES is the relationship between SES and the pattern of neuropsychological and/or motor derangement. Based on the recent data, quoted above, on the role of sleep in the normal cognitive and psychomotor development and functionality, we hypothesize that prolonged, focal epileptic activity, occurring almost exclusively during sleep (as in ESES) interferes with local slow wave activity at the site of the epileptic focus, leading to neuropsychological impairment and behavioural disorders, possibly by altering cortical plasticity processes necessary for normal cognitive development, therefore adding further evidences on the crucial role of sleep in neuroplasticity mechanisms underlying higher cognitive functions (Tassinari & Rubboli, 2006; Rubboli *et al.*, 2018). Indeed, it seems appropriated to label ESES as "Penelope syndrome" (Tassinari *et al.*, 2009), in which the diurnal "spinning" to make up a thread (a neuronal network) is erased by the SES, *i.e.*, "spiking" during sleep.

REFERENCES ▶

Aarts JHP, Binnie CD, Smit AM, Wilkins AJ (1984): Selective cognitive impairment during focal and generalized epileptiform EEG activity. *Brain* 107: 293–308.

Achermann P, Borbély AA (1997): Low-frequency (< 1 Hz) oscillations in the human sleep electroencephalogram. *Neuroscience* 81: 213–222.

Aeby A, Poznanski N, Verheulpen D, Wetzburger C, Van Bogaert P (2005): Levetiracetam efficacy in epileptic syndromes with continuous spikes and waves during slow sleep: experience in 12 cases. *Epilepsia* 46: 1937–1942.

Agarwal R, Kumar A, Tiwari VN, Chugani H (2016): Thalamic abnormalities in children with continuous spike-wave during slow-wave sleep: An F-18-fluorodeoxyglucose positron emission tomography perspective. *Epilepsia* 57: 263–271.

Amzica F, SteriadeM (2002): Cellular mechanisms underlying seizure activity during sleep. In: Bazil C, Malow B, Sammaritano M (eds) *Sleep and Epilepsy: the Clinical Spectrum*, pp. 109–126. Amsterdam: Elsevier.

Ansink BJ, Sarphatie H, Van Dongen HR (1989): The Landau-Kleffner syndrome: case report and theoretical consideration. *Neuropediatrics* 20: 170–172.

Arts WF, Aarsen FK, Scheltens-de Boer M, Catsman-Berrevoets CE (2009): Landau-Kleffner syndrome and CSWS syndrome: treatment with intravenous immunoglobulins. *Epilepsia* 50 (Suppl 7): 55–58.

Atkins M, Nikanorova M (2011): A prospective study of levetiracetam efficacy in epileptic syndromes with continuous spikes-waves during slow sleep. *Seizure* 20: 635–639.

Badinand Hubert N, Bastuji H, De Bellescize J, Cortinovis P, Kocher L, Rousselle C, Revol M (1995): Three unpublished new cases of continuous spikes and waves during slow sleep. In: Beaumanoir A, Bureau M, Deonna T, Mira L, Tassinari CA (eds) *Continuous Spikes and Waves During Slow Sleep. Electrical Status Epilepticus During Slow Sleep*, pp. 186–187. London: John Libbey.

Battaglia D, Veggiotti P, Lettori D, *et al.* (2009): Functional hemispherectomy in children with epilepsy and CSWS due to unilateral early brain injury including thalamus: sudden recovery of CSWS. *Epilepsy Res* 87: 290–298.

Beaumanoir A (1995a): About continuous or subcontinuous spike-wave activity during wakefulness: electroclinical correlations. In: Beaumanoir A, Bureau M, Deonna T, Mira L, Tassinari CA (eds) *Continuous Spikes and Waves during Slow Sleep. Electrical Status Epilepticus during Slow Sleep*, pp. 115–118. London: John Libbey.

Beaumanoir A (1995b): EEG data. In: Beaumanoir A, Bureau M, Deonna T, Mira L, Tassinari CA (eds) *Continuous Spikes and Waves during Slow Sleep. Electrical Status Epilepticus during Slow Sleep*, pp. 217–223, London: John Libbey.

Beaumanoir A. Bureau M, Deonna T, Mira L, Tassinari CA (1995): *Continuous Spikes and Waves during Slow Sleep. Electrical Status Epilepticus during Slow Sleep*. London: John Libbey.

Benington JH, Frank MG (2003): Cellular and molecular connections between sleep and synaptic plasticity. *Prog Neurobiol* 69: 71–101.

Bergqvist AGC, Brooks-Kayal AR (1997): Ketogenic diet in the treatment of acquired epileptic aphasia. *Ann Neurol* 42: 504.

Billard C, Autret A, Laffont F, Lucas B, Degiovanni E (1982): Electrical status epilepticus during sleep in children: a reappraisal from eight new cases. In: Sterman MB, Shouse MN, Passouant P (eds) *Sleep and Epilepsy*, pp. 481–491. London and New York: Academic Press.

Binnie CD (1993): Significance and management of transitory cognitive impairment due to subclinical EEG discharges in children. *Brain Dev* 15: 23–30.

Boel M, Casaer P (1989): Continuous spikes and waves during slow sleep: a 30 month follow up study of neuropsychological recovery and EEG finding. *Neuropediatrics* 20: 176–180.

Bölsterli BK, Schmitt B, Bast T, Critelli H, Heinzle J, Jenni OG, Huber R (2011): Impaired slow wave sleep downscaling in encephalopathy with status epilepticus during sleep (ESES). *Clin Neurophysiol* 122: 1779–1787.

Bölsterli Heinzle BK, Fattinger S, Kurth S, *et al.* (2014): Spike wave location and density disturb sleep slow waves in patients with CSWS (continuous spike waves during sleep). *Epilepsia* 55: 584–591.

Bölsterli Heinzle BK, Bast T, Critelli H, Huber R, Schmitt B (2017): Age-Dependency of Location of Epileptic Foci in "Continuous Spike-and-Waves during Sleep": A Parallel to the Posterior-Anterior Trajectory of Slow Wave Activity. *Neuropediatrics* 48: 36–41.

Bölsterli BK, Gardella E, Pavlidis E, *et al.* (2017): Remission of encephalopathy with status epilepticus (ESES) during sleep renormalizes regulation of slow wave sleep. *Epilepsia* 58: 1892–1901.

Borbély AA, Achermann P (2000): Sleep homeostasis and models of sleep regulation. In: Kryger M, Roth T, Dement W (eds) *Principles and Practice of Sleep Medicine*, pp. 377–390. Philadelphia: W.B. Saunders.

Broli M, Bisulli F, Mastrangelo M, *et al.* (2011): Definition of the neurological phenotype associated with dup (X) (p11.22-p11.23). *Epileptic Disord* 13: 240–251.

Buchmann A, Ringli M, Kurth S, Schaerer M, Geiger A, Jenni OG, Huber R (2011): EEG sleep slow-wave activity as a mirror of cortical maturation. *Cereb Cortex* 21(3): 607–615.

Bureau M (1995a): Continuous spikes and waves during slow sleep (ESES): definition of the syndrome. In: Beaumanoir A, Bureau M, Deonna T, Mira L, Tassinari CA (eds) *Continuous Spikes and Waves during Slow Sleep. Electrical Status Epilepticus during Slow Sleep*, pp. 17–26. London: John Libbey.

Bureau M (1995b): Outstanding cases of ESES and LKS: analysis of the data sheets provided by the participants. In: Beaumanoir A, Bureau M, Deonna T, Mira L, Tassinari CA (eds), *Continuous Spikes and Waves during Slow Sleep. Electrical Status Epilepticus during Slow Sleep*, pp. 213–216. London: John Libbey.

Bureau M (1999): Electro-clinical aspects and evolution of the syndrome of epilepsy with continuous spikes and waves during slow sleep (CSWS). *Epilepsi (Turkey)* 3: 102–110.

Bureau M, Cordova S, Dravet C, Roger J, Tassinari CA (1990): Épilepsie avec pointe-ondes continues pendant le sommeil lent (POCS): évolution à moyen et long terme (à propos de 15 cas). *Epilepsies* 2: 6–94.

Buzatu M, Bulteau C, Altuzarra C, Dulac O, Van Bogaert P (2009): Corticosteroids as treatment of epileptic syndromes with continuous spikes-waves during slow-waves sleep. *Epilepsia* 50 (Suppl 7): 68–72.

Calvet U (1978): *Épilepsies nocturnes de l'enfant: épilepsies bénignes.* Toulouse: Medicine thesis.

Campbell IG, Darchia N, Higgins LM, Dykan IV, Davis NM, de Bie E, Feinberg I (2011): Adolescent changes in homeostatic regulation of EEG activity in the delta and theta frequency bands during NREM sleep. *Sleep* 34: 83–91.

Cantalupo G, Rubboli G, Tassinari CA (2011): Night-time unravelling of the brain web: Impaired synaptic downscaling in ESES – The Penelope syndrome. *Clin Neurophysiol* 122: 1691–1692.

Capovilla G, Beccaria F, Cagdas S, Montagnini A, Segala R, Paganelli D (2004): Efficacy of levetiracetam in pharmacoresistant continuous spikes and waves during slow sleep. *Acta Neurol Scand* 110: 144–147.

Caraballo R, Fontana E, Michelizza B, *et al.* (1989): Carbamazepina, "assenze atipiche", crisi "ato-niche" e stato di PO continua del sonno (POCS). *Boll Lega It Epil* 66–67: 379–381.

Caraballo RH, Bongiorni L, Cersosimo R, Semprino M, Espeche A, Fejerman N (2008): Epileptic encephalopathy with continuous spikes and waves during sleep in children with shunted hydrocephalus: a study of nine cases. *Epilepsia* 49: 1520–1527.

Caraballo RH, Cejas N, Chamorro N, Kaltenmeier MC, Fortini S, Soprano AM (2014): Landau-Kleffner syndrome: a study of 29 patients. *Seizure* 23: 98–104.

Caraballo RH, Cersósimo RO, Fortini PS, *et al.* (2013): Congenital hemiparesis, unilateral polymicrogyria and epilepsy with or without status epilepticus during sleep: a study of 66 patients with long-term follow-up. *Epileptic Disord* 15: 417–427.

Carvill GL, Regan BM, Yendle SC, *et al.* (2013): GRIN2A mutations cause epilepsy-aphasia spectrum disorders. *Nat Genet* 45: 1073–1076.

Cesaroni E, Zamponi N, Cappanera S, Cardinali C (2009): The Landau-Kleffner syndrome responsive to levetiracetam i.v. *Epilepsia* 50 (Suppl 4): 235.

Chhun S, Troude P, Villeneuve N, *et al.* (2011): A prospective open-labeled trial with levetiracetam in pediatric epilepsy syndromes: continuous spikes and waves during sleep is definitely a target. *Seizure* 20: 320–325.

Colamaria V, Sgro V, Simeone R, *et al.* (1991): Status epilepticus in benign Rolandic epilepsy manifesting as anterior operculum syndrome. *Epilepsia* 32: 329–334.

Cole AJ, Andermann F, Taylor L, *et al.* (1988): The Landau-Kleffner syndrome of acquired epileptic aphasia. Unusual clinical outcome, surgical experience and absence of encephalitis. *Neurology* 38: 31–38.

Cross JH, Neville BG (2009): The surgical treatment of Landau-Kleffner syndrome. *Epilepsia* 50 (Suppl 7): 63–67.

Dalla Bernardina B, Dravet C, Bureau M, Beghini G, Roger J (1978): Épilepsie partielle bénigne et état de mal électroencéphalographique pendant le sommeil. *Rev EEG Neurophysiol Clin* 8: 350–353.

Dalla Bernardina B, Bondavalli S, Colamaria V (1982): Benign epilepsy of childhood with Rolandic spikes during sleep. In: Sterman MB, Shouse MN, Passouant P (eds) *Sleep and Epilepsy*, pp. 495–506. London and New York: Academic Press.

Dalla Bemardina B, Fontana E, Michelizza B, Colamaria V, Capovilla G, Tassinari CA (1989): Partial epilepsies of childhood, bilateral synchronization, continuous spike-waves during slow sleep. In: Manelis S, Bental E, Loeber JN, Dreifuss FE (eds) *Advances in Epileptology*, pp. 295–302. New York: Raven Press.

Dalla Bernardina B, Sgro V, Caraballo R, *et al.* (1991): Sleep and benign partial epilepsies of childhood: EEG and evoked potentials study. *Epilepsy Res* 2 (Suppl): 83–96.

Dalla Bernardina B, Sgro V, Fejerman N (2005): Epilepsy with centro-temporal spikes and related syndromes. In: Roger J, Bureau M, Dravet C, *et al.* (eds) *Epileptic Syndromes in Infancy, Childhood and Adolescence*, 4th ed., pp. 203–226. Paris: John Libbey Eurotext.

Damiano JA, Burgess R, Kivity S, *et al.* (2017): Frequency of CNKSR2 mutation in the X-linked epilepsy-aphasia spectrum. *Epilepsia* 58: e40–43.

De Giorgis V, Filippini M, Macasaet JA, Masnada S, Veggiotti P (2017): Neurobehavioral consequences of continuous spike and waves during slow sleep (CSWS) in a pediatric population: A pattern of developmental hindrance. *Epilepsy Behav* 74: 1–9.

De Marco P (1988): Electrical status epilepticus during slow sleep: one case with sensory aphasia. *Clin Electroencephalogr* 19: 111–113.

De Negri M, Baglietto M, Battaglia F, Gaggero R, Pessagno A, Recanati L (1995): Treatment of electrical status epilepticus by short diazepam (DZP) cycles after DZP rectal bolus test. *Brain Dev* 17: 330–333.

De Negri M (1997): Electrical status epilepticus during sleep (ESES). Different clinical syndromes: towards a unifying view? *Brain Dev* 19: 447–451.

De Tiège X, Goldman S, Verheulpen D, Aeby A, Poznanski N, Van Bogaert P (2006): Coexistence of idiopathic Rolandic epilepsy and CSWS in two families. *Epilepsia* 47: 1723–1727.

De Tiège X, Goldman S, Van Bogaert P (2009): Insights into the pathophysiology of psychomotor regression in CSWS syndromes from FDG-PET and EEG-fMRI. *Epilepsia* 50 (Suppl 7): 47–50.

Debiais S, Tuller L, Barthez MA, Monjauze C, Khomsi A, Praline J, *et al.* (2007): Epilepsy and language development: the continuous spike-waves during slow sleep syndrome. *Epilepsia* 48: 1104–1110.

Deonna T (1991): Acquired epileptiform aphasia in children (Landau-Kleffner syndrome). *J Clin Neurophysiol* 8: 288–298.

Deonna T, Beaumanoir A, Gaillard A, Assal G (1977): Acquired aphasia in childhood with seizure disorder: a heterogeneous syndrome. *Neuropadiatrie* 8: 263–273.

Deonna T, Peter CL, Ziegler A (1989): Adult follow-up of the acquired aphasia epilepsy syndrome in childhood: report of seven cases. *Neuropediatrics* 20: 132–138.

Deonna T, Roulet E (1995): Acquired epileptic aphasia (AEA): definition of the syndrome and current problems. In: Beaumanoir A, Bureau M, Deonna T, Mira M, Tassinari CA (eds) *Continuous Spikes and Waves during Slow Sleep. Electrical Status Epilepticus during Slow Sleep*, pp. 37–45. London: John Libbey.

Dugas M, Masson M, Le Heuzey MF, Regnier N (1982): Aphasie acquise de l'enfant avec épilepsie (syndrome de Landau et Kleffner). *Rev Neurol* 138: 755–780.

Dugas M, Gérard CL, Franc S, Lecendreux M (1995): Late onset acquired epileptic aphasia. In: Beaumanoir A, Bureau M, Deonna T, Mira M, Tassinari CA (eds) *Continuous Spikes and Waves during Slow Sleep. Electrical Status Epilepticus during Slow Sleep*, pp. 143–147. London: John Libbey.

Dulac O, Billard C, Arthuis M (1983): Aspects électrocliniques et évolutifs de l'épilepsie dans le syndrome aphasie-épilepsie. *Arch Franc Pediatr* 40: 299–308.

Engel J Jr (2001): A proposed diagnostic scheme for people with epileptic seizures and with epilepsy: Report of the ILAE task force on classification and terminology. *Epilepsia* 42: 796–803.

Eriksson K, Kylliainen A, Hirvonen K, Nieminen P, Koivikko M (2003): Visual agnosia in a child with non-lesional occipito-temporal CSWS. *Brain Dev* 25: 262–267.

Fayad MN, Choueiri R, Mikati M (1997): Landau-Kleffner syndrome: consistent response to repeated intravenous gamma-globulin doses: a case report. *Epilepsia* 38: 489–494.

Fejerman N, Caraballo RH, Cersosimo R, Ferraro SM, Gallicchio S, Amartino H (2012): Sulthiame add-on therapy in children with focal epilepsies associated with encephalopathy related to electrical status epilepticus during slow sleep (ESES). *Epilepsia* 53: 1156–1161.

Fenn KM, Nusbaum HC, Margoliash D (2003): Consolidation during sleep of perceptual learning of spoken language. *Nature* 425: 614–616.

Fine AL, Wirrell EC, Wong-Kisiel LC, Nickels KC (2015): Acetazolamide for electrical status epilepticus in slow-wave sleep. *Epilepsia* 56: e134–8.

Galanopoulou AS, Bojko A, Lado F. Moshé SL (2000): The spectrum of neuropsychiatric abnormalities associated with electrical status epilepticus in sleep. *Brain Dev* 21: 279–295.

Garcia-Penas JJ (2010): Disfuncion neurocognitiva en el syndrome de estado de mal electrico durante el sueno lento: podemos modificar la evolucion natural del syndrome con un tratamiento farmacologico precoz? *Rev Neurol* 50 (Suppl 3): S37-S47.

Gencpinar P, Dundar NO, Tekgul H (2016): Electrical status epilepticus in sleep (ESES)/continuous spikes and waves during slow sleep (CSWS) syndrome in children: An electroclinical evaluation according to the EEG patterns. *Epilepsy Behav* 61: 107–111.

Genton P, Maton B, Ogihara M, *et al.* (1992): Continuous focal spikes during REM sleep in a case of acquired aphasia (Landau-Kleffner syndrome). *Sleep* 15: 454–460.

Gilestro GF, Tononi G, Cirelli C (2009): Widespread changes in synaptic markers as a function of sleep and wakefulness in Drosophila. *Science* 324: 109–112.

Giorda R, Bonaglia MC, Beri S, *et al.* (2009): Complex segmental duplications mediate a recurrent dup(X)(p11.22-p11.23) associated with mental retardation, speech delay, and EEG anomalies in males and females. *Am J Hum* Genet 85(3): 394–400.

Giovanardi Rossi P, Parmeggiani A, Posar A, Scaduto MC, Chiodo S, Vatti G (1999): Landau-Kleffner syndrome (LKS): long-term follow-up and links with electrical status epilepticus during sleep (ESES). *Brain Dev* 21: 90–98.

Gordon N (1990): Acquired aphasia epilepsia in childhood: the Landau-Kleffner syndrome. *Dev Med Child Neurol* 32: 267–274.

Grosso S, Parisi P, Giordano L, di Bartolo R, Balestri P (2014): Lacosamide efficacy in epileptic syndromes with continuous spike and waves during slow sleep (CSWS). *Epilepsy Res* 108: 1604–1608.

Grote CL, Van Slyke P, Hoeppner LA (1999): Language outcome following multiple subpial transection for Landau-Kleffner syndrome. *Brain* 122: 561–566.

Guerrini R, Genton P, Bureau M, *et al.* (1998): Multilobar polymicrogyria, intractable drop attack seizures and sleep-related electrical status epilepticus. *Neurology* 51: 504–512.

Guzzetta F, Battaglia D, Veredice C, *et al.* (2005): Early thalamic injury associated with epilepsy and continuous spike-wave during slow sleep. *Epilepsia* 46: 889–900.

Halâsz P, Kelemen A, Clemens B, *et al.* (2005): The perisylvian epileptic network. A unifying concept. *Ideggyogy Sz* 58: 21–31.

Harbord MG, Singh R, Morony S (1999): SPECT abnormalities in Landau-Kleffner syndrome. *J Clin Neurosci* 6: 9–15.

Hirsch E, Marescaux C, Maquet P, *et al.* (1990): Landau-Kleffner syndrome: a clinical and EEG study of five cases. *Epilepsia* 31: 756–767.

Hirsch E, Pierre M, Metz-Lutz MN, Motte I, Finck S, Marescaux C (1995): The eponym "Landau-Kleffner syndrome" should not be restricted to childhood-acquired aphasia with epilepsy. In: Beaumanoir A, Bureau M, Deonna T, Mira L, Tassinari CA (eds) *Continuous Spikes and Waves during Slow Sleep. Electrical Status Epilepticus during Slow Sleep*, pp. 57–62. London: John Libbey.

Hoppen T, Sandrieser T, Rister M (2003): Successful treatment of pharmacoresistant continuous spike wave activity during slow sleep with levetiracetam. *Eur J Pediatr* 162: 59–61.

Huber R, Ghilardi MF, Massimini M, Tononi G (2004): Local sleep and learning. *Nature* 430: 78–81.

Huber R, Ghilardi MF, Massimini M, *et al.* (2006): Arm immobilization causes cortical plastic changes and locally decreases sleep slow wave activity. *Nat Neurosci* 9: 1169–1176.

Hubert-Franc S (1990): *Le syndrome de Landau-Kleffner 33 ans après (histoire naturelle, devenir socio-professionnel, évolution des troubles du langage, aspects électroencéphalographiques)*. Paris. Thèse Médecine.

Humphrey IL, Knipstein R, Bumpass ER (1975): Gradually developing aphasia in children. A diagnostic problem. *J Am Acad Child Psychiatr* 14: 625–655.

Huppke P, Kallenberg K, Gärtner J (2005): Perisylvian polymicrogyria in Landau-Kleffner syndrome. *Neurology* 64: 1660.

Inutsuka M, Kobayashi K, Oka M, Hattori J, Ohtsuka Y (2006): Treatment of epilepsy with electrical status epilepticus during slow sleep and its related disorders. *Brain Dev* 28: 281–286.

Isnard I, Fisher C, Bastuji H, Badinand N, de Villard R (1995): Auditory early (BAEP) and middle-latency (MLAEP) evoked potentials in patients with ESES and Landau-Kleffner syndrome. In: Beaumanoir A, Bureau M, Deonna T, Mira L, Tassinari CA (eds) *Continuous Spikes and Waves during Slow Sleep. Electrical Status Epilepticus during Slow Sleep*, pp. 99–103. London: John Libbey.

Issa NP (2014): Neurobiology of continuous spike-wave in slow-wave sleep and Landau-Kleffner syndromes. *Pediatr Neurol* 51: 287–296.

Jeong A, Strahle J, Vellimana AK, Limbrick DD Jr, Smyth MD, Bertrand M (2017): Hemispherotomy in children with electrical status epilepticus of sleep. *J Neurosurg Pediatr* 19: 56–62.

Kaga M (1999): Language disorders in Landau-Kleffner syndrome. *J Child Neurol* 14: 118–122.

Kale U, El-Naggar M, Hawthorne M (1995): Verbal auditory agnosia with focal EEG abnormality: an unusual case of child presenting to an ENT surgeon with "deafness". *J Laryngol Otol* 109: 431–432.

Kelemen A, Barsi P, Gyorsok Z, Sarac J, Szucs A, Halâsz P (2006): Thalamic lesion and epilepsy with generalized seizures, ESES and spike-wave paroxysms-report of three cases. *Seizure* 15: 454–458.

Kellerman K (1978): Recurrent aphasia with subclinical bioelectric status epilepticus during sleep. *Eur J Pediatr* 128: 207–212.

Kessi M, Peng J, Yang L, *et al.* (2018): Genetic etiologies of the electrical status epilepticus during slow wave sleep: systematic review. *BMC Genetics* 19: 40.

Kevelam SH, Jansen FE, Van Binsbergen E, *et al.* (2012): Copy number variations in patients with electrical status epilepticus in sleep. *J Child Neurol* 27: 178–182.

Kobayashi K, Ohtsuka Y, Ohtahara S (1990): Epilepsy and sleep: with special reference to non convulsive status epilepticus with continuous spike-wave discharges during slow-wave sleep. *No-To-Hattasu (Tokyo)* 22: 136–142.

Kobayashi K, Nishibayashi N, Ohtsuka Y, Oka E, Ohtahara S (1994): Epilepsy with electrical status epilepticus during slow sleep and secondary bilateral synchrony. *Epilepsia* 35: 1097–1103.

Kobayashi K, Watanabe Y, Inoue T, Oka M, Yoshinaga H, Ohtsuka Y (2010): Scalp-recorded high-frequency oscillations in childhood sleep-induced electrical status epilepticus. *Epilepsia* 51: 2190–2194.

Kramer U, Nevo M, Neufeld Y, Fatal A, Leitner Y, Harel S (1998): Epidemiology of epilepsy in childhood: a cohort of 440 consecutive patients. *Pediatr Neurol* 18: 46–50.

Kramer U, Sagi L, Goldberg-Stern H, Zelnik N, Nissenkorn A, Ben-Zeev B (2009): Clinical spectrum and medical treatment of children with electrical status epilepticus in sleep (ESES). *Epilepsia* 50: 1517–1524.

Kuki, I., Kawawaki, H., Okazaki, S., Ikeda, H. & Tomiwa, K (2014): Epileptic encephalopathy with continuous spikes and waves in the occipito-temporal region during slow-wave sleep in two patients with acquired Kanji dysgraphia. *Epileptic Disord* 16: 540–45.

Lagae LG, Silberstein J, Gillis PL, Casaer PJ (1998): Successful use of intravenous immunoglobulins in Landau-Kleffner syndrome. *Pediatr Neurol* 19: 399–400.

Landau W, Kleffner FR (1957): Syndrome of acquired aphasia with convulsive disorder in children. *Neurology* 7: 523–530.

Landsness EC, Crupi D, Hulse BK, *et al.* (2009) Sleep-dependent improvement in visuomotor learning: a causal role for slow waves. *Sleep* 32: 1273–1284.

Larrieu JL, Lagueny A, Ferrer X, Jullien J (1986): Épilepsie avec décharges continues au cours du sommeil lent. Guérison sous clobazam. *Rev EEG Neurophysiol Clin* 16: 383–394.

Larsson PG, Wilson J, Eeg-Olofsson O (2009): A new method for quantification and assessment of epileptiform activity in EEG with special reference to focal nocturnal epileptiform activity. *Brain Topogr* 22: 52–59.

Larsson PG, Eeg-Olofsson O, Michel CM, Seeck M, Lantz G (2010): Decrease in propagation of interictal epileptiform activity after introduction of levetiracetam visualized with electric source imaging. *Brain Topogr* 23: 269–278.

Larsson PG, Bakke KA, Bjernses H, *et al.* (2012): The effect of levetiracetam on focal nocturnal epileptiform activity during sleep – a placebo-controlled double-blind crossover study. *Epilepsy Behav* 24: 44–48.

Lee YM, Kang HC, Lee JS, *et al.* (2008): Mitochondrial respiratory chain defects: underlying etiology in various epileptic conditions. *Epilepsia* 49: 685–690.

Lemke JR, Lal D, Reinthaler EM, *et al.* (2013): Mutations in *GRIN2A* cause idiopathic focal epilepsy with rolandic spikes. *Nat Genet* 45: 1067–1072.

Lerman P (1986): Seizures induced or aggravated by anticonvulsants. *Epilepsia* 27: 706–710.

Lerman P, Lerman-Sagie T (1989): Early steroid therapy in Landau-Kleffner syndrome. In: Manelis J, Bental E, Loeber JN, Dreifuss FE (eds) *Advances in Epileptology*, Vol. XVII, pp. 330–332. New York: Raven Press.

Lerman P, Kivity S (1991): The benign partial non-Rolandic epilepsies. *J Clin Neurophysiol* 8: 275–287.

Lerman P, Lerman-Sagie T (1995): The relation of electro-clinical syndromes with continuous spike-waves in waking and sleep to mental retardation. In: Beaumanoir A, Bureau M, Deonna T, Mira L, Tassinari CA (eds) *Continuous Spikes and Waves during Slow Sleep. Electrical Status Epilepticus during Slow Sleep*, pp. 119–122. London: John Libbey.

Lerman P, Lerman-Sagie T, Kivity S (1991): Effect of early corticosteroid therapy for Landau-Kleffner syndrome. *Dev Med Child Neurol* 33: 257–266.

Lesca G, Rudolf G, Labalme A, *et al.* (2012): Epileptic encephalopathies of the Landau-Kleffner and continuous spike and waves during slow-wave sleep types: genomic dissection makes the link with autism. *Epilepsia* 53: 1526–1538.

Lesca G, Rudolf G, Bruneau N, *et al.* (2013): *GRIN2A* mutations in acquired epileptic aphasia and related childhood focal epilepsies and encephalopathies with speech and language dysfunction. *Nat Genet* 45: 1061–1066.

Liu ZW, Faraguna U, Cirelli C, Tononi G, Gao XB (2010): Direct evidence for wake-related increases and sleep-related decreases in synaptic strength in rodent cortex. *J Neurosci* 30: 8671–8675.

Loddenkemper T, Cosmo G, Kotagal P, *et al.* (2009): Epilepsy surgery in children with electrical status epilepticus in sleep. *Neurosurgery* 64: 328–337.

Loddenkemper T, Sanchez Fernandez J, Peters JM (2011): Continuous spike and waves during sleep and electrical status epilepticus in sleep. *J Clin Neurophysiol* 28: 154–164.

Losito E, Battaglia D, Chieffo D, *et al.* (2015): Sleep-potentiated epileptiform activity in early thalamic injuries: Study in a large series (60 cases). *Epilepsy Res* 109: 90–99.

Mantovani JF, Landau WM (1980): Acquired aphasia with convulsive disorder: course and prognosis. *Neurology* 30: 524–529.

Maquet P, Hirsch E, Dive D, Salmon E, Marescaux C, Franck G (1990): Cerebral glucose utilization during sleep in Landau-Kleffner syndrome: a PET study. *Epilepsia* 31: 778–783.

Marescaux C, Hirsh E, Finck S, *et al.* (1990): Landau-Kleffner syndrome. A pharmacologic study of five cases. *Epilepsia* 31: 768–777.

Martin Miguel MdC, Garcia Seoane JJ, (2011): EEG latency analysis for hemispheric lateralisation in Landau-Kleffner syndrome. *Clin Neurophysiol* 122: 244–252.

McKinney W, McGreal DA (1974): An aphasic syndrome in children. *Can MedAssocJ* 110: 636–639.

Mednick SC, Nakayama K, Cantero JL, Atienza M, Levin AA, Pathak N, Stickgold R (2002): The restorative effect of naps on perceptual deterioration. *Nat Neurosci* 5: 677–681.

Mefford HC, Yendle SC, Hsu C, Cook J, Geraghty E, McMahon JM, *et al.* (2011): Rare copy number variants are an important cause of epileptic encephalopathies. *Ann Neurol* 70: 974–985.

Michelucci R, Rubboli G. Plasmati R (1987): Clinical relevance of various EEG features of electrical status epilepticus during slow sleep. *17th Epilepsy International Congress*, 79. Book of Abstracts, Jerusalem.

Mikati MA, Fayad M, Choueri R (1998): IVIG in Landau-Kleffner syndrome. *Pediatr Neurol* 19: 399–400.

Mikati MA, Saab R (2000): Successful use of intravenous immunoglobulin as initial monotherapy in Landau-Kleffner syndrome. *Epilepsia* 41: 860–886.

Mikati MA, Shamseddine AN (2005): Management of Landau-Kleffner syndrome. *Paediatr Drugs 7:* 377–389.

Mira L, BonaO, Van Lierde A (1995): Cognitive assessment of children with ESES syndrome: a critical review of data from 155 cases submitted to the Venice colloquium. In: Beaumanoir A, Bureau M, Deonna T, Mira L, Tassinari CA (eds) *Continuous Spikes and Waves during Slow Sleep. Electrical Status Epilepticus during Slow Sleep*, pp. 229–242. London: John Libbey.

Monteiro JP, Roulet-Perez E, Davidoff V, Deonna T (2001): Primary neonatal thalamic haemorrhage and epilepsy with continuous spike-wave during sleep: a longitudinal follow-up of a possible significant relation. *EurJ Paediatr Neurol* 5: 41–44.

Morikawa T, Seino M, Osawa T, Yagi K (1985): Five children with continuous spike-waves discharges during sleep. In: Roger J, Dravet C, Bureau M, Dreifuss FE, Wolf P (eds) *Epileptic Syndromes in Infancy, Childhood and Adolescence*, pp. 205–212. London: John Libbey.

Morikawa T, Seino M. Watanabe Y, Watanabe M, Yagi K (1989): Clinical relevance of continuous spike-waves during slow wave sleep. In: Manelis S, Bental E, Loeber JN, Dreifuss FE (eds) *Advances in Epileptology*, pp. 359–363. New York: Raven Press.

Morikawa T, Seino M, Watanabe M (1995): Long-term outcome of ESES syndrome. In: Beaumanoir A, Bureau M, Deonna T, Mira L, Tassinari CA (eds) *Continuous Spikes and Waves during Slow Sleep. Electrical Status Epilepticus during Slow Sleep*, pp. 27–36. London: John Libbey.

Morrell F (1985): Secondary epileptogenesis in man. *Arch Neurol* 42: 318–335.

Morrell F (1995): Electrophysiology of ESES in Landau-Kleffner syndrome. In: Beaumanoir A, Bureau M, Deonna T, Mira L, Tassinari CA (eds) *Continuous Spikes and Waves during Slow Sleep. Electrical Status Epilepticus during Slow Sleep*, pp. 77–90. London: John Libbey.

Morrell F, Whisler WW, Bleck TP (1989): Multiple subpial transection: a new approach to the surgical treatment of focal epilepsy. *J Neurosurg* 70: 231–239.

Morrell F, Whisler WW, Smith MC, *et al.* (1995): Landau-Kleffner syndrome. Treatment with subpial intracortical transection. *Brain* 118: 1529–1546.

Mouridsen SE, Videbaek C, Sogaard H, Andersen AR (1993): Regional cerebral blood-flow measured by HMPAO and SPECT in a 5-year-old boy with Landau-Kleffner syndrome. *Neuropediatrics* 24: 47–50.

Nakano S, Okuno T, Mikawa H (1989): Landau-Kleffner syndrome: EEG topographic studies. *Brain Dev* 11: 43–50.

Nakayama T, Nabatame S, Saito Y, *et al.* (2012): 8p deletion and 9p duplication in two children with electrical status epilepticus in sleep syndrome. *Seizure* 21: 295–299.

Nass R, Gross A, Wisoff I, Devinsky O (1999): Outcome of multiple subpial transections for autistic epileptiform regression. *Pediatr Neurol* 21: 464–470.

Neckelmann D, Amzica F Steriade M (1998): Spike-wave complexes and fast components of cortically generated seizures. III. Synchronizing mechanisms. *J Neurophysiol* 80: 1480–1494.

Neville BGR, Boyd SG (1995): Selective epileptic gait disorder. *J Neurol Neurosurg Psychiatry* 58: 371–373.

Neville BGR, Burch V, Cass H, Lees J (1998): Motor disorders in Landau-Kleffner syndrome (LKS). *Epilepsia* 39 (Suppl 6): 123.

Nickels K, Wirrell E (2008): Electrical status epilepticus in sleep. *Semin Pediatr Neurol* 15(2): 50–60.

Nikanorova M, Miranda MJ, Atkins M, Sahlholdt L (2009): Ketogenic diet in the treatment of refractory continuous spikes and waves during slow sleep. *Epilepsia* 50: 1127–1131.

Nissenkorn A, Gak E, Vecsler M, Reznik H, Menascu S, Ben Zeev B (2010): Epilepsy in Rett syndrome-the experience of a National Rett Center. *Epilepsia* 51: 1252–1258.

Nonclercq A, Foulon M, Verheulpen D, *et al.* (2009): Spike detection algorithm automatically adapted to individual patients applied to spike-and-wave percentage quantification. *Neurophysiol Clin* 39: 123–131.

Overvliet GM, Besseling RM, Vles JS, *et al.* (2010): Nocturnal epileptiform EEG discharges, nocturnal epileptic seizures, and language impairments in children: review of the literature. *Epilepsy Behav* 19: 550–558.

Paetau R (2009): Magnetoencephalography Landau-Kleffner syndrome. *Epilepsia* 50 (Suppl 7): 51–54.

Paetau R, Granstrom ML, Blomstedt G, Jousmaki V, Chuchman M, Liukkonen E (1999): Magnetoencephalography in presurgical evaluation of children with the Landau-Kleffner syndrome. *Epilepsia* 40: 326–335.

Panayiotopoulos CP (1999): Severe syndromes of mainly linguistic and neuropsychological deficits, seizures or both and marked EEG abnormalities from the Rolandic and neighbouring regions. In: Panayiotopoulos CP (ed) *Benign Childhood Partial Seizures and Related Epileptic Syndromes*, pp. 337–360. John Libbey: London.

Park YD (2003): The effects of vagus nerve stimulation therapy on patients with intractable seizures and either Landau-Kleffner syndrome or autism. *Epilepsy Behav* 4: 286–290.

Pascual Castroviejo I, Pascual-Pascual S, Pena W, Talavera M (1999): Status epilepticus-induced brain damage and opercular syndrome in childhood. *Dev Med Child Neurol* 41: 420–423.

Patry G, Lyagoubi S, Tassinari CA (1971): Subclinical electrical status epilepticus induced by sleep in children. *Arch Neurol* 24: 242–252.

Pavlidis E, Rubboli G, Nikanorova M, Kölmel MS, Gardella E (2015): Encephalopathy with status epilepticus during sleep (ESES) induced by oxcarbazepine in idiopathic focal epilepsy in childhood. *Funct Neurol* 30: 139–141.

Peltola ME, Liukkonen E, Granström ML, *et al.* (2011): The effect of surgery in encephalopathy with electrical status epilepticus during sleep. *Epilepsia* 52: 602–609.

Peltola ME, Palmu K, Linkkonen E, Gaily E, Vanhatalo S (2012): Semiautomatic quantification of spiking in patients with continuous spike and waves in sleep: Sensitivity to settings and correspondence to visual assessment. *Clin Neurophysiol* 123: 1284–1290.

Peltola ME, Sairanen V, Gaily E, Vanhatalo S (2014): Measuring spike strength in patients with continuous spikes and waves during sleep: comparison of methods for prospective use as a clinical index. *Clin Neurophysiol* 125: 1639–1646.

Pera MC, Brazzo D, Altieri N, Balottin U, Veggiotti P (2013): Long-term evolution of neuropsychological competences in encephalopathy with status epilepticus during sleep: a variable prognosis. *Epilepsia* 54 (Suppl 7): 77–85.

Pisani F, Seri S, Pelliccia A (1999): Landau-Kleffner syndrome and atypical benign partial epilepsy of childhood: the effectiveness of acetazolamide. *Neuropediatrics* 30: 164.

Praline J, Barthez MA, Castelnau P, *et al.* (2006): Atypical language impairment in two siblings: relationship with electrical status epilepticus during slow wave sleep. *J Neurol Sci* 249: 166–171.

Prats JM, Garaizar C, Uterga JM, Urroz MJ (1992): Operculum syndrome in childhood: a rare case of persistent speech disturbance. *Dev Med Child Neurol* 34: 359–364.

Quigg M, Noachtar S (2012): Sleep-potentiated epileptic discharges, language regression and pediatric thalamic lesions. *Neurology* 78: 1708–1709.

Raha S, Shah U, Udani V (2012): Neurocognitive and neurobehavioral disabilities in Epilepsy with Electrical Status Epilepticus in slow sleep (ESES) and related syndromes. *Epilepsy Behav* 25: 381–385.

Rapin I, Mattis S, Rowan AJ, Golden GG (1977): Verbal auditory agnosia in children. *Dev Med Child Neurol* 19: 192–207.

Ravnik I (1985): A case of Landau-Kleffner syndrome: effect of intravenous diazepam. In: Roger J, Dravet C, Bureau M, Dreifuss FE, Wolf P (eds) *Epileptic Syndromes in Infancy, Childhood and Adolescence*, pp. 192–193. London: John Libbey.

Reutlinger C, Helbig I, Gawelczyk B, *et al.* (2010): Deletions in 16p13 including GRIN2A in patients with intellectual disability, various dysmorphic features, and seizure disorders of the Rolandic region. *Epilepsia* 51: 1870–1873.

Roll P, Rudolf G, Pereira S, *et al.* (2006): SRPX2 mutations in disorders of language cortex and cognition. *Hum Mol Genet* 15: 1195–1207.

Roulet-Perez E, Deonna T, Gaillard F, Peter-Favre C, Despland PA (1991): Acquired aphasia, dementia, and behavior disorder with epilepsy and continuous spike and waves during sleep in a child. *Epilepsia* 32: 495–503.

Roulet-Perez E, Davidoff V, Despland PA. Deonna T (1993): Mental and behavioural deterioration of children with epilepsy and ESES: acquired epileptic frontal syndrome. *Dev Med Child Neurol* 35: 661–674.

Rubboli G, Tassinari CA (2006): Negative myoclonus. An overview of its clinical features, pathophysiological mechanisms, and management. *Neurophysiol Clin* 36: 337–343.

Rubboli G, Huber R, Tononi G, Tassinari CA (2018). Encephalopathy related to status epilepticus during sleep (ESES). A link with sleep homeostasis? *Epileptic Dis* [Epub ahead of print].

Rudolf G, Valenti MP, Hirsch E, Szepetowski P (2009): From Rolandic epilepsy to continuous spike-and-waves during sleep and Landau-Kleffner syndromes: insights into possible genetic factors. *Epilepsia* 50 (Suppl 7): 25–28.

Saltik S, Uluduz D, Cokar O, Demirbilek V, Dervent A (2005): A clinical and EEG study on idiopathic partial epilepsies with evolution into ESES spectrum disorders. *Epilepsia* 46: 524–533.

Sanchez Fernandez I, Takeoka M, *et al.* (2012a): Early thalamic lesions in patients with sleep-potentiated epilep-tiform activity. *Neurology* 78: 1721–1727.

Sanchez Fernandez I, Hadjiloizou S, *et al.* (2012b): Short-term response of sleep-potentiated spiking to high-dose diazepam in electric status epilepticus during sleep. *Pediatr Neurol* 46: 312–318.

Sánchez Fernández I, Peters JM, An S, Bergin AM, Takeoka M, Rotenberg A, *et al.* (2013): Long-term response to high-dose diazepam treatment in continuous spikes and waves during sleep. *Pediatr Neurol* 49: 163–170.

Sánchez Fernández I, Peters JM, Akhondi-Asl A, Klehm J, Warfield SK, Loddenkemper T (2017): Reduced thalamic volume in patients with Electrical Status Epilepticus in Sleep. *Epilepsy Res* 130: 74–80.

Scheltens-de Boer M (2009): Guidelines for EEG in encephalopathy related to ESES/CSWS in children. *Epilepsia* 50 (Suppl 7): 13–17.

Seegmüller C, Deonna T, Mayor Dubois C, *et al.* (2012): Long-term outcome after cognitive and behavioral regression in nonlesional epilepsy with continuous spike-waves during slow-wave sleep. *Epilepsia* 53: 1067–1076.

Seri S, Cerquiglini A, Pisani F (1998): Spike-induced interference in auditory sensory processing in Landau-Kleffner syndrome. *Electroencephalogr Clin Neurophysiol* 108: 506–510.

Shafrir Y, Prenski AL (1995): Acquired epileptiform opercular syndrome: a second case report, review of the literature, and comparison to the Landau-Kleffner syndrome. *Epilepsia* 36: 1050–1057.

Shewmon AD, Erwin RJ (1988a): The effect of focal interictal spikes on perception and reaction time. I. General considerations. *Electroencephalogr Clin Neurophysiol* 69: 319–337.

Shewmon AD, Erwin RJ (1988b): The effect of focal interictal spikes on perception and reaction time. II. Neuroanatomic specificity. *Electroencephalogr Clin Neurophysiol* 69: 338–352.

Shewmon DA, Erwin RJ (1989): Transient impairment of visual perception induced by single interictal occipital spikes. *J Clin Exp Neuropsychol* 11: 675–691.

Shu-Xian H, Xi Ru W, Chin L, Shou-Yu H (1989): Landau-Kleffner syndrome with unilateral EEG abnormalities. Two cases from Bejing. *Brain Dev* 11: 420–422.

Siniatchkin M, Groening K, Moehring J, *et al.* (2010): Neuronal networks in children with continuous spikes and waves during slow sleep. *Brain* 133: 2798–2813.

Smith C (1995): Sleep states and memory processes. *Behav Brain Res* 69: 137–145.

Snead OC 3rd, Hosey LC (1985): Exacerbation of seizures in children with carbamazepine. *N Engl J Med* 313: 916–921.

Solomon GE, Carson D, Pavalkis S, Fraser R, Labar D (1993): Intracranial EEG monitoring in Landau-Kleffner syndrome associated with left temporal lobe astrocytoma. *Epilepsia* 34: 557–560.

Spencer SS, Schramm J, Wyler A, *et al.* (2002): Multiple subpial transection for intractable partial epilepsy: an international meta-analysis. *Epilepsia* 43: 141–145.

Steriade M (2000): Corticothalamic resonance, states of vigilance and mentation. *Neuroscience* 101: 243–275.

Steriade M, McCormick DA, Sejnowski TJ (1993): Thalamocortical oscillations in the sleeping and aroused brain. *Science* 262(5134): 679–685.

Steriade M, Amzica F (1994): Dynamic coupling among neocortical neurons during evoked and spontaneous spike-wave seizure activity. *J Neurophysiol* 72: 2051–2069.

Steriade M, Contreras D (1998): Spike-wave complexes and fast components of cortically generated seizures. I. Role of neocortex and thalamus. *J Neurophysiol* 80: 1439–1455.

Stickgold R, James L, Hobson JA (2000): Visual discrimination learning requires sleep after training. *Nat Neurosci* 3: 1237–1238.

Stickgold R, Fosse R, Walker MP (2002): Linking brain and behavior in sleep-dependent learning and memory consolidation. *Proc Natl Acad Sci USA* 99(26): 16519–16521.

Stienen MN, Haghikia A, Dambach H, *et al.* (2011): Anti-inflammatory effects of the anticonvulsant drug levetira-cetam on electrophysiological properties of astroglia are mediated *via* TGFβ1 regulation. *BrJ Pharmacol* 162: 491–507.

Stroink H, Van Dongen HR, Meulstee J, Scheltens-de Boer M, Geesink HH (1997): A special case of "deafness"; Landau-Kleffner syndrome. *Ned Tijdschr Geneeskd* 141: 1623–1625.

Strug LJ, Clarke T, Chiang T, *et al.* (2009): Centrotemporal sharp wave EEG trait in Rolandic epilepsy maps to Elon-gator Protein Complex 4 (ELP4). *EurJ Hum* Genet 17: 1171–1181.

Tas E, Takeoka M, Molino J, *et al.* (2009): Thalamic lesions increase the frequency of spiking during sleep. *Epilepsia* 50 (Suppl 11): 479.

Tassinari CA (1995): The problems of "continuous spikes and waves during slow sleep" or "electrical status epilepticus during slow sleep" today. In: Beaumanoir A, Bureau M, Deonna T, Mira L, Tassinari CA (eds) *Continuous Spikes and Waves during Slow Sleep. Electrical Status Epilepticus during Slow Sleep*, pp. 251–255. London: John Libbey.

Tassinari CA, Dravet C, Roger J (1977): ESES: encephalopathy related to electrical status epilepticus during slow sleep. *Electroencephalogr Clin Neurophysiol* 43: 529–530.

Tassinari CA, Bureau M, Dravet C, Roger J, Daniele-Natale O (1982): Electrical status epilepticus during sleep in children (ESES). In: Sterman MB, Shouse MN, Passouant P (eds) *Sleep and Epilepsy*, pp. 465–479. London and New York: Academic Press.

Tassinari CA, Bureau M, Dravet C, Dalla Bernardina B, Roger J (1985): Epilepsy with continuous spike and waves during slow sleep. In: Roger J, Dravet C, Bureau M, Dreifuss FE, Wolf P (eds) *Epileptic Syndromes in Infancy, Childhood and Adolescence*, pp. 194–204. London: John Libbey.

Tassinari CA, Michelucci R, Forti A, *et al.* (1992a): The electrical status epilepticus syndrome. In: Degen R, Dreifuss FE (eds) *Benign Localized and Generalized Epilepsies of Early Childhood*, pp. 111–115. Amsterdam: Elsevier.

Tassinari CA, Bureau M. Dravet C, Dalla Bernardina B, Roger J (1992b): Epilepsy with continuous spikes and waves during slow sleep – otherwise described as ESES (epilepsy with electrical status epilepticus during slow sleep). In: Roger J, Bureau M, Dravet C, Dreifuss FE, Perret A, Wolf P (eds) *Epileptic Syndromes in Infancy, Childhood and Adolescence*, 2nd ed, pp. 245–256. London: John Libbey.

Tassinari CA, Rubboli G, Parmeggiani L, *et al.* (1995): Epileptic negative myoclonus. In: Fahn S, Hallet M, Lüders HO, Marsden CD, *et al.* (eds) *Negative Motor Phenomena, Advances in Neurology*, vol. 67, pp. 181–197. Philadelphia: Lippincott-Raven.

Tassinari CA, Rubboli G, Shibasaki H (1998): Neurophysiology of positive and negative myoclonus. *Electroencephalogr Clin Neurophysiol* 107: 181–195.

Tassinari CA, Rubboli G, Volpi L, *et al.* (2000): Encephalopathy with electrical status epilepticus during slow sleep or ESES syndrome including the acquired aphasia. *Clin Neurophysiol* 111 (Suppl 2): 94–102.

Tassinari CA, Rubboli G (2006): Cognition and paroxysmal EEG activities: from a single spike to electrical status epilepticus during sleep. *Epilepsia* 47 (Suppl 2): 40–43.

Tassinari CA, Cantalupo G, Rios-Pohl L, Giustina ED, Rubboli G (2009): Encephalopathy with status epilepticus during slow sleep: "the Penelope syndrome". *Epilepsia* 50 (Suppl 7): 4–8.

Tassinari CA, Cantalupo, G, Rubboli G (2015): Focal ESES as a selective focal brain dysfunction: a challenge for clinicians, an opportunity for cognitive neuroscientists. *Epileptic Disord* 17: 1–3.

Teixeira KC, Montenegro MA, Cendes F, Guimarâes CA, Guerreiro CA, Guerreiro MM. (2007): Clinical and electroencephalographic features of patients with polymicrogyria. *J Clin Neurophysiol* 24: 244–251.

Teixeira KCS, Cendes F, Guerreiro CAM, Guerreiro MM (2009): Focal electrical status (FES): a new finding associated with polymicrogyria. *J Clin Neurophysiol* 26: 155–159.

Tononi G, Cirelli C (2006): Sleep function and synaptic homeostasis. *Sleep Med Rev* 10: 49–62.

Toso V, Moschini M, Gagnin G, Antoni D (1981): Aphasie acquise de l'enfant avec épilepsie. Trois observations et revue de la littérature. *Rev Neurol* 137: 425–434.

Tovia E, Goldberg-Stern H, Ben Zeev B, *et al.* (2011): The prevalence of atypical presentations and comorbidities of benign childhood epilepsy with centrotemporal spikes. *Epilepsia* 52: 1483–1488.

Tsuru T, Mori M, Mizuguchi M, Momoi MY (2000): Effects of high-dose intravenous corticosteroid therapy in Landau-Kleffner syndrome. *Pediatr Neurol* 22: 145–147.

Urbain C, Di Vincenzo T, Peigneux P, Van Bogaert P (2011): Is sleep-related consolidation impaired in focal idiopathic epilepsies of childhood? A pilot study. *Epilepsy Behav* 22: 380–384.

Vaags AK, Bowdin S, Smith ML, *et al.* (2014): Absent *CNKSR2* causes seizures and intellectual, attention, and language deficits. *Ann Neurol* 76: 758–764.

Van Bogaert P, Aeby A, De Borchgrave V, *et al.* Groupe de travail des centres francophones de référence de l'epi-lepsie réfractaire (2006): The epileptic syndromes with continuous spikes and waves during slow sleep: definition and management guidelines. *Acta Neurol Belg* 106(2): 52–60.

Van Bogaert P, Paquier PF (2009): Fifty years of Landau-Kleffner syndrome. Proceedings of an international symposium. November 2–4, 2007. Alden-Biesen, Belgium. *Epilepsia* 50 (Suppl 7): 1–82.

van den Munckhof B, van Dee V, Sagi L, *et al.* (2015): Treatment of electrical status epilepticus in sleep: a pooled analysis of 575 cases. *Epilepsia* 56: 1738–1746.

van den Munckhof B, de Vries EE, Braun KP, *et al.* (2016): Serum inflammatory mediators correlate with disease activity in electrical status epilepticus in sleep (ESES) syndrome. *Epilepsia* 57: e45–50.

van den Munckhof B, Alderweireld C, Davelaar S, *et al.* (2018): Treatment of electrical status epilepticus in sleep: Clinical and EEG characteristics and response to 147 treatments in 47 patients. *Eur J Paediatr Neurol* 22: 64–71.

Van Hirtum-Das M, Licht EA, Koh S, Wu JY, Shields WD, Sankar R (2006): Children with ESES: variability in the syndrome. *Epilepsy Res* 70 (Suppl 1): S248-S258.

Van Lierde A (1995): Therapeutic data. In: Beaumanoir A, Bureau M, Deonna T, Mira L, Tassinari CA (eds) *Continuous Spikes and Waves during Slow Sleep. Electrical Status Epilepticus during Slow Sleep*, pp. 225–227, London: John Libbey.

Varga ET, Terney D, Atkins MD, *et al.* (2011): Transcranial direct current stimulation in refractory continuous spikes and waves during slow sleep: a controlled study. *Epilepsy Res* 97: 142–145.

Vega C, Sánchez Fernández I, Peters J, *et al.* (2018): Response to clobazam in continuous spike-wave during sleep. *Dev Med Child Neurol* 60: 283–289.

Veggiotti P, Beccaria F, Guerrini R, Capovilla G, Lanzi G (1999): Continuous spike-and-wave activity during slow-wave sleep: syndrome or EEG pattern? *Epilepsia* 40: 1593–1601.

Veggiotti P, Bova S, Granocchio E, Papalia G, Termine C, Lanzi G (2001): Acquired epileptic frontal syndrome as long-term outcome in two children with CSWS. *Neurophysiol Clin* 31: 387–397.

Veggiotti P, Cardinali S, Granocchio E, *et al.* (2005): Motor impairment on awakening in a patient with an EEG pattern of "unilateral, continuous spikes and waves during slow sleep". *Epileptic Disord* 7: 131–136.

Veggiotti P, Pera MC, Teutonico F, Brazzo D, Balottin U, Tassinari CA (2012): Therapy of encephalopathy with status epilepticus during sleep (ESES-CSWS syndrome): an update. *Epileptic Disord* 14: 1–11.

Verhoeven WM, Egger JI, Feenstra I, de Leeuw N (2011): A *de novo* 3.57 Mb microdeletion in 8q12.3q13.2 in a patient with mild intellectual disability and epilepsy. *EurJ Med Genet* 55: 358–361.

Vrielynck P, Marique P, Ghariani S, *et al.* (2017): Topiramate in childhood epileptic encephalopathy with continuous spike-waves during sleep: A retrospective study of 21 cases. *Eur J Paediatr Neurol* 21: 305–311.

Vyazovskiy VV, Cirelli C, Pfister-Genskow M, Faraguna U, Tononi G (2008): Molecular and electrophysiological evidence for net synaptic potentiation in wake and depression in sleep. *Nat Neurosci* 11: 200–208.

Walker MP, Brakefield T, Morgan A, Hobson JA, Stickgold R (2002): Practice with sleep makes perfect: sleep-dependent motor skill learning. *Neuron* 35: 205–211.

Walker MP, Stickgold R (2004): Sleep-dependent learning and memory consolidation. *Neuron* 44: 121–133.

White H, Sreenivasan V (1987): Epilepsy-aphasia syndrome in children: an unusual presentation to psychiatry. *Can J Psychiatr* 32: 599–601.

Wilson RB, Eliyan Y, Sankar R, Hussain SA (2018): Amantadine: A new treatment for refractory electrical status epilepticus in sleep. *Epilepsy Behav* 84: 74–78.

Wirrell E, Ho AW, Hamiwka L (2006): Sulthiame therapy for continuous spike and wave in slow-wave sleep. *Pediatr Neurol* 35: 204–208.

Wolff M, Weiskopf N, Serra E, Preissl H, Birbaumer N, Kraegeloh-Mann I (2005): Benign partial epilepsy in childhood: selective cognitive deficits are related to the location of focal spikes determined by combined EEG/MEG. *Epilepsia* 46: 1661–1667.

Yan Liu X, Wong V (2000): Spectrum of epileptic syndromes with electrical status epilepticus during sleep in children. *Pediatr Neurol* 22: 371–379.

Yasuhara A, Yoshida H, Hatanaka T, Sugimoto T, Kobashi Y, Dyken E (1991): Epilepsy with continuous spike-waves during slow sleep and its treatment. *Epilepsia* 32: 59–62.

Zivi A, Broussaud C, Daymas S, Hazard J, Sicard C (1990): Syndrome aphasie acquise-épilepsie avec psychose: à propos d'une observation. *Ann Pédiatr* 37: 391–394.

WITH VIDEO SUPPLEMENTS

CHAPTER 15

ABSENCE EPILEPSIES

Marco T. Medina[1], Pierre Genton[2], Michelle Bureau[2], Édouard Hirsch[3], Philippe Gélisse[4], Peter Wolf[5] and Carlo Alberto Tassinari[6]

[1] School of Medical Sciences, National Autonomous University of Honduras, Tegucigalpa, Honduras
[2] Centre Saint-Paul, Henri-Gastaut Hospital, Marseille, France
[3] Strasbourg University Hospital, Strasbourg, France
[4] Epilepsy Unit, Montpellier, France
[5] Epilepsihospitalet, Dianalund, Denmark; Florianopolis, Brazil
[6] University of Bologna, Bologna, Italy

Introduction

Typical absence seizures (TA) have been defined in 1981 (Commission, 1981). Typical absence seizures occur in several forms of genetic (idiopathic) generalized epilepsies (IGE). In the past, considering only a type of seizures and not the syndrome they belong to led to a misunderstanding of their prognostic significance. For this reason, a meta-analysis of the many published papers would be meaningless. Absence epilepsies are a heterogeneous group of genetic or presumed genetic generalized epilepsies with usual onset on childhood or adolescence (Scheffer *et al.*, 2017; Berger *et al.*, 2012). The absence epilepsies represent several epilepsy syndromes, *e.g.* childhood absence epilepsy (CAE), juvenile absence epilepsy (JAE), epilepsy with myoclonic absences EMA), childhood absence epilepsy evolving to juvenile myoclonic epilepsy among others (Tassinari *et al.*, 1992; Medina *et al.*, 2005; Martinez-Juarez *et al.*, 2006; Scheffer *et al.*, 2017). Other epilepsies with absences as the main seizure type have also been reported, like early onset absence epilepsies (EOAEs) (Chaix *et al.*, 2003; Agostinelli *et al.*, 2013), absence status epilepsy (Genton *et al.*, 2008) and the spectrum of absence epilepsies includes also elderly patients, with *"de novo"* absence status epilepsy of late onset (Thomas, 1999).

CAE and JAE were recognized as discrete epileptic syndromes by the International League Against Epilepsy in 1989 and in 2017 (Commission, 1989; Scheffer *et al.*, 2017). Further ILAE classifications included CAE and JAE as IGE syndromes (Engel, 2001) or genetic epilepsy syndromes (Berg *et al.*, 2010; Scheffer *et al.*, 2017). The studies published on absence seizures before 1981 and on absence epilepsies before 1989 have to be read with caution. A monography was dedicated to a detailed review on all aspects of typical absences and related epileptic syndromes (Duncan & Panayiotopoulos, 1995). This chapter updates the comprehensive reviews published in the fifth edition and covers CAE, JAE, EMA and others, less common and less consensual syndromes.

History

Clinical period

According to Temkin (1971) the first description of absences was made by Poupart in 1705. However, Tissot's description (Tissot, 1770) (*Figure 1*) is more familiar to us: *"La jeune malade avait eu fréquemment, dans l'intervalle des grands accès, de petits accès très courts, qui n'étaient marqués que par une perte instantanée de connaissance, qui lui coupait la parole avec un très léger mouvement dans les yeux; souvent, en revenant à elle, elle achevait la phrase au milieu de laquelle elle avait été interrompue; d'autres fois, elle l'avait oubliée."* (In the intervals between major attacks, the young patient had frequently had very short minor attacks which were recognized only by an instantaneous loss of consciousness which stopped her speech, accompanied by a very slight movement in the eyes. Often, on recovery, she completed the sentence which had been interrupted; on other occasions she had forgotten it). This girl was 14 years old. Her "petits accès" had begun at 7 years of age. A few months later she also had had "very intense and very frequent true epileptic attacks" (generalized tonic-clonic seizures – GTCS).

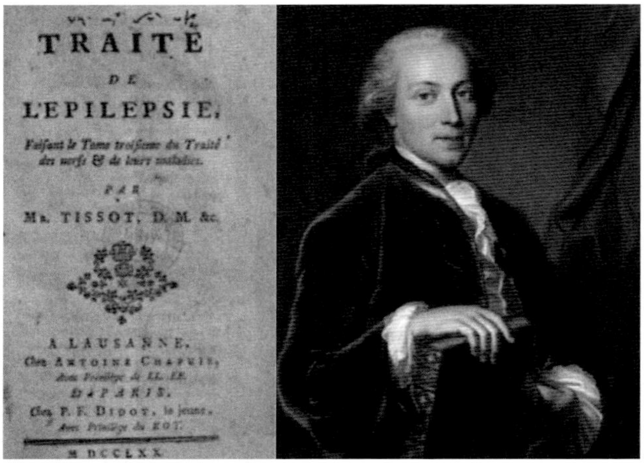

Figure 1 **Samuel Auguste Tissot and the *Traité de l'épilepsie*, published in 1770.**

The contrast between GTCS and seizures without convulsions, and even without fall, "petits accès", has always struck medical attention, hence terms such as "absences" (Calmeil in 1824), "petit mal" (Esquirol in 1838), and "epilepsia mitior" (Reynolds in 1861).

Even if, at the end of the XIXth century, focal seizures with impaired awareness and absences were probably mistaken one for the other, absences were clearly recognized. Gowers gave a most accurate description of the absence seizures "without conspicuous convulsion" (Gowers, 1881). Their epileptic nature was accepted, despite a short moment of doubt at the beginning of the XXth century: *"nicht epileptische Absencen oder kurze narkoleptische Anfälle"* (Friedmann in 1906). This error did not last.

The frequency of absences had also been conspicuous and Sauer coined in 1916 the name "pyknolepsy". Hyperventilation as a test to induce absences was first described by Brain in 1924 (cited by Peterman, 1945). In the same year, Adie (1924) summarized *"pyknolepsy, a form of epilepsy occurring in children with a good prognosis"* as follows: *"A disease with an explosive onset between the age of 4 and 14 years of frequent, short, very slight, monotonous minor epileptiform seizures of uniform severity which recur almost daily for weeks, months or years, are uninfluenced by antiepileptic remedies, do not impede normal mental and psychological development, and ultimately cease spontaneously never to return"*. Doose *et al.* (1965) conducted a study with the purpose of determining whether all cases of "spike-wave-absences" belonged to one syndrome or not. They found that apart from pyknolepsy with a peak age of onset from 4 to 8 years and a female preponderance there were cases of earlier or later onset, and these were in some respects clinically different. Particularly, these authors found a second manifestation peak for absences from age 10 to 12. For these patients there was no sex difference, and the recurrence of absences was infrequent especially when the patient also had grand mal seizures. Thus, the age of onset became the first distinctive feature of this group of cases, which therefore were subsequently referred to as "juvenile absences".

Electroclinical period

Absence were the first seizure types to which a typical EEG pattern became attached. It began in 1935, when Gibbs, Davis and Lennox showed that petit mal absences were associated with a rhythmic 3 cycles per second discharge of regular spike and wave complexes on the EEG (Gibbs *et al.*, 1935). The enthusiasm provoked by this new technique gave rise to some excess: *"There can be no question of the propriety of speaking of a petit mal type of dysrhythmia when it occurs during a clinical petit mal seizure... we believe that it is equally proper to speak of a petit mal type of dysrhythmia when the same pattern appears in a routine record in the absence of clinically obvious seizures, even if the particular patient has no history of petit mal or of epilepsy"* (Gibbs *et al.*, 1943). And: *"The electroencephalographic classification of alternate spikes and waves brings together a triad of seizures having diverse clinical manifestations"* (Lennox, 1945). It was the petit mal triad, with: i) absences; ii) myoclonic seizures; iii) akinetic seizures. This triad was misunderstood and misused. All minor seizures accompanied by bilateral spikes and waves were considered as petit mal, despite Lennox's warning (Lennox & Davis, 1950): *"Minor seizures other than petits have to be called minor epilepsy or given their proper designation, such as myoclonic or atonic members of the petit mal triad"*. The discovery of tridione gave the first anti-absence drug (Lennox, 1945).

Janz & Christian (1957), in their description of what is now called juvenile myoclonic epilepsy (JME), observed that there were patients who had absences of identical appearance as in pyknolepsy, and the same EEG characteristics but occurring much less frequently. Doose *et al.* (1965) conducted a study with the purpose of determining whether all cases of "spike-wave-absences" belonged to one syndrome or not. They found that apart from pyknolepsy with a peak age of onset from 4 to 8 years and a female preponderance, they found a second manifestation peak for absences from ages 10 to 12. For these patients there was no sex difference, recurrence of absences was infrequent and the patient also had GTCS.

Video-EEG analysis allowed a better description of TA (Penry *et al.*, 1975) as well as their syndromic-related characterization (Panayiotopoulos *et al.*, 1989; Panayiotopoulos, 2005). An important progress is due to the operational classification of seizure types by the ILAE (Fisher *et al.*, 2017). Different absence seizures types have been defined: typical absence seizures (TAS), atypical absence, absence with eyelid myoclonia and myoclonic absence (Commission,1981; Fisher *et al.*, 2017; Scheffer *et al.*, 2017). Absence seizures were recently classified as nonmotor generalized onset seizures (Fisher *et al.*, 2017; Scheffer *et al.*, 2017).

In the past decades, two opposite views developed regarding the syndromic classification of IGE with absences. The syndromic approach differentiates the patient population into more relatively homogeneous groups, largely on the basis of clinical and EEG criteria (Hirsch *et al.*, 1994; Panayiotopoulos, 2005; Loiseau & Panayiotopoulos, 2005). In contrast, the neurobiological approach unifies all genetic generalized epilepsies or IGE into one entity (Berkovic *et al.*, 1987; Holmes *et al.*, 1987; Mullen & Berkovic, 2018). At present, CAE, JAE and EMA are classified as a genetic or presumed genetic electro-clinical syndromes (Berg *et al.*, 2010; Scheffer *et al.*, 2017).

Genetics basis and mechanisms of absence epilepsies

Although absence epilepsies are genetically determined, the precise mode of inheritance and the genes involved remain largely unidentified (Crunelli & Leresche, 2002). The genetic character of the typical absence syndromes has been recognized by early authors. A positive family history of epilepsy was found in 15% to 44% of cases with CAE (Lennox & Lennox, 1960; Currier *et al.*, 1963; Bergamini *et al.*, 1965; Hirsch *et al.*, 1994; Sgro *et al.*, 1996).

Lennox and Lennox (1960) reported a genetic contribution to the spike-wave EEGs abnormalities in CAE, supported by 74% concordance for monozygotic twins and 27% concordance for dizygotic twins. Metrakos & Metrakos (1960; 1961a; 1961b) and Tanaka *et al.* (2008) reported that siblings and offspring had i) 50% risk of inheriting the 3-Hz spike-wave trait; ii) 35% risk of expressing the EEG trait in their lifetime, and iii) 12% risk for tonic-clonic seizures and 8% risk for absences.

Ascertainment of family history of epilepsy has to be considered: when keeping only epilepsy in parents and siblings, the frequency decreases from 42.6% to 20.7% (Holowach *et al.*, 1962). In two series, epilepsy in first-degree relatives was found in 17% of CAE (Loiseau *et al.*, 1995a; Callenbach *et al.*, 1998). These seizures are TA and GTCS. In studies on twins, 84% of monozygotic twins had 3-Hz spike-waves, TA developed in 75% of pairs and dizygotic twins 16 times less often (Lennox & Lennox, 1960). An Australian study of epilepsy in twins confirmed that in concordant pairs, twins developed similar syndrome (Berkovic *et al.*, 1994). Bianchi *et al.* (1995) found that in 24 families with a CAE proband there was a high concordance (33.3%) for the same clinical form in first degrees relatives, while febrile seizures (46.7%) and GTCS (30%) were more common in distant relatives. Epilepsy risk in children of patients with CAE would be 6.8% (Beck-Mannagetta *et al.*, 1989).

Currently, various chromosomal loci have been identified in families with absences of childhood onset (not necessarily equated with CAE) (Weber & Lerche, 2008). Linkage to chromosome 1 was found in families with absences starting in childhood and the later development of myoclonic jerks and GTCS, as in JME (Delgado-Escueta *et al.*, 1999). Linkage analysis in five generations of a family in which affected patients had childhood absences and GTCS provided evidence of a locus on chromosome 8q24 (Fong *et al.*, 1998; Delgado-Escueta *et al.*, 1999; Sujimoto *et al.*, 2000). The candidate region for this locus, designated ECA 1, has been refined, but a gene remains to be identified. According to the criteria proposed in this chapter, neither of these groups is CAE. There are also reports implicating chromosome 5q31.1 and 19p13.2 (see for review Crunelli & Leresche, 2002). Furthermore, there is now evidence available to suggest that mutations in genes encoding GABA receptors (Feucht *et al.*, 1999; Wallace *et al.*, 2001; Marini *et al.*, 2003) or brain-expressed voltage-dependent calcium channels (Chen *et al.*, 2003) may underlie CAE. Feucht *et al.* (1999) found a significant association between a polymorphism in GABA-A receptor gamma 3 subunit in chromosome 15q11 in 50 families with CAE. Marini *et al.* (2003) found GABA-A receptor gamma 2 subunit gene mutations on chromosome 5 in a large family with CAE and febrile seizures (including febrile seizures plus and other seizure phenotypes). This gene mutation segregated with febrile seizures and CAE, and also occurred in individuals with the other phenotypes. The clinical and molecular data suggested that the GABA-A receptor subunit mutation alone could account for the febrile seizure phenotype, but an interaction of this gene with another gene or genes was required for the childhood absence phenotype in this family. Linkage analysis for a putative second gene contributing to the childhood absence phenotype suggested possible loci on chromosomes 10, 13, 14 and 15 (Marini *et al.*, 2003). Chen *et al.* (2003) found 68 variations, including 12 missense mutations in the calcium channel CACNA1H gene in CAE patients. The identified missense mutations occurred in the highly conserved residues of the T-type calcium channel gene. However, another study of 33 nuclear families, each with two or more individuals with CAE each provided conclusive evidence that the genes encoding GABA-A and GABA-B receptors, voltage-dependent calcium channels and the ECA1 region on chromosome 8q do not account independently for the childhood absence trait in a majority of the families (Robinson *et al.*, 2002).

Tanaka *et al.* (2008) reported mutations on the GABAA receptor beta 3 subunit gene (GABRB3) in four out 48 probands and families with remitting CAE. They found one heterozygous missense mutation (P1 1S) in exon 1a segregated with four CAE-affected persons in one multiplex, two-generation Mexican family. P1 1S was also found in a singleton from Mexico. Another heterozygous missense mutation (S15F) was present in asingleton from Honduras. An exon 2 heterozygous missense mutation (G32R) was present in two CAE-affected persons and two persons affected with EEG-recorded spike and/or sharp wave in a two-generation Honduran family. All mutations were absent in 630 controls. All the mutations showed hypergycolsylation and reduced GABA currents of the mutated GABRB3 polypetide.

Striano *et al.* (2012) reported nine family members affected mainly by absence epilepsies with variable age at onset (from early childhood to adulthood) and an individual with CAE that evolved into JME with a novel nonsynonymous SLC2A1 mutation (c.694C>T, p.R232C). The SLC2A1 gene encodes the glucose transporter type 1 (GLUT1). Functional analysis revealed a reduced maximum uptake velocity for glucose, whereas the affinity to glucose and the protein expression were not different in wild-type and mutant transporters. SLC2A1 pathogenic variants leading to GLUT1 deficiency is seen in 10% of those with typical absence seizures starting before 4 years of age and around 1% of people with typical Genetic Generalized Epilepsies (Suls *et al.*, 2009; Mullen & Berkovic, 2018).

Concerning JAE, identical twins who both have the syndrome have been reported by Berkovic *et al.* (1994) and by Panayiotopoulos *et al.* (1989). Obeid (1994) reported that in a Saudi-Arabian population consanguineous marriages were found in 47% of the families of patients with JME (Panayiotopoulos & Obeid, 1989), while this was only true for one out of 14 JAE families. In the clinical genetic study of families with IGE (Marini *et al.*, 2004), phenotypic concordance within families of JAE was 10% which was low compared to families of other IGE syndromes. Because 31% of JAE relatives had CAE but only 2.5% had JME, they suggested that CAE and JAE share a close genetic relation, whereas JME might be a more distinct entity. A similar observation was done by Winawer *et al.* (2003).

Sander *et al.* (1997) studied the relation of JAE to glutamate receptor polymorphism. In the investigated family, evidence was found "that allelic variants of [the kainate-selective GluR5 receptor gene] GRIK1 contribute a major genetic determinant to the pathogenesis of JAE-related phenotypes". However, the role of the mGluR5 (group I) in animal models of absences is not well established (Ngomba *et al.*, 2011). But group III mGlu receptors seem to play a crucial role in the physiopathology of absences (Ngomba *et al.*, 2011). This group includes mGlu4, mGlu6, mGlu7 and mGlu8. mGlu4 receptor gene is localized within the EJM1 susceptibility locus for JME at 6p21.3 (Ngomba *et al.*, 2011). mGluR7 receptor is a presynaptic receptor expressed at synapses of the cotico-thalomo-cortical circuitry that generates spike-wave discharges. It negatively regulates neurotransmitter release (glutamate and GABA). Disruption of the mGluR7 complex provoke absences in rats and mice (Bertaso *et al.*, 2008).

There are several reports of mutation of CACNA1A, alpha 1 subunit of the CaV2.1 Ca2+ channel, or CACNB4, beta 4 subunit, with the phenotype of absence seizures with ataxia (Escayg *et al.*,2000; Imbrici *et al.*, 2004), which does not fit in any of the known absence epilepsies. The paper of Escayg *et al.* (2000) comprises an observation of a mutation in a family with an identical locus in CACNB4 as in the lethargic mouse mutant but which resulted in a quite different human phenotype.

Acquired factors

As concordance in monozygotic twins is not 100%, non genetic factors are likely (Berkovic, 1996). Perinatal complications, postnatal head trauma and cerebral inflammatory disease were found in the case histories of 7 to 30% of patients (Weir, 1965; Lugaresi *et al.*, 1973), and only 3.9% in Janz'series (Janz *et al.*, 1994). However, these cerebral aggressions are very common in children and were not risk factors in a population-based case-control study (Rocca *et al.*, 1987). A history of febrile seizures is frequent: 20 to 23% of cases (Rocca *et al.*, 1987; Sgro *et al.*, 1996). More than a risk factor, febrile seizures are probably the first manifestation of an epileptic diathesis (Rocca *et al.*, 1987). This is in accordance with results of studies on the phenotype of families with "febrile seizures plus" related or not to mutations of voltage-dependant sodium channel gene mutations (*SCN1A* or *SCN1B*). In such families, tonic-clonic, tonic and also absence seizures have been reported (Lerche *et al.*, 2001; Audic-Gerard *et al.*, 2003).

A valid animal model of generalized absence seizures should reflect the clinical and pharmacologic characteristics of this disorder. The criteria for animal models of absence seizures are: electroencephalographic findings and behavior analogous to human absence epilepsy; reproductibility, predictability; ability to standardize and quantitate; attenuation or blockage by ethosuximide, trimethadione, valproic acid, and benzodiazepines; appropriate ontogeny; exacerbation by GABA-ergic drugs; blockage by GABAB antagonists; spike-wave discharges that originate in thalamus, cortex, or both; hippocampus silent during seizure activity.

There are two main genetic models of absence seizures in rats: WAG/Rij (Coenen & Van Luijetelaar, 2003) and GAERS (Genetic Absence Epilepsy Rats from Strasbourg) (Danober *et al.*, 1998). Spike-and-wave discharges are initiated in the primary somatosensory cortex and then rapidly propagate to motor cortices and thalamic nuclei (Sarkisova & van Luijtelaar, 2011; Depaulis *et al.*, 2016; Depaulis & Charpier, 2018). The WAG/Rij rats have a susceptibility locus located at 2q33-37. In human, an association analysis at 2q36 showed a candidate susceptibility gene for JAE and/or absence seizures associated with GTCS (Yalçin *et al.*, 2011). According to these authors, the inhibin alpha subunit precursor (INHA) could be a novel gene contributing to the pathogenesis of JAE.

The animal data suggest that three interacting neuropharmacologic forces within the context of the thalamo-cortical circuitry are involved in the pathogenesis of absence seizures:

– Post synaptic events required for the occurrence of generalized absence seizures are glutamate-mediated EPSP followed by GABAA-and GABAB-mediated inhibition that triggers a low-threshold calcium current in Nucleus Reticularis Thalamus neurons.

– The overall setpoint of thalamic and cortical excitability is modulated by means of ascending cholinergic pathways that project to the thalamus and noradrenergic and dopa-minergic neurons projecting to the cortical end of the thalamocortical loop.

– Presynaptic GABAB and GHB receptors may contribute to the regulation of thalamocortical rhythmicity by means of precise control of excitation and inhibition through modulation of GABA and glutamate release within the involved thalamocortical circuitry.

Studies have uncovered the causative genes for absence-like mice models. Tottering and leaner mice have defects in the calcium channel alpha subunit, lethargic mouse in the calcium channel beta4 gene, and stargazer and waggler mice in the calcium channel gamma subunit gene. These mice mutants show some characteristics of absence epilepsy; however, all affected mice show some degree of cerebellar degeneration, which is quite different from human absence epilepsy (Hirose *et al.*, 2000).

Attempts to identify the genetic defects in calcium channel genes that underlie human absence epilepsy have so far failed (Sander *et al.*, 1998). Similar mutations of P/Q-type voltage-gated calcium channel CaV2.1. have been reported in a family with autosomal dominant transmission of absences and episodic ataxia (Imbrici *et al.*, 2003). A genetic study in GAERS suggests a polygenic mode of inheritance of the EEG phenotype with at least three gene loci on chromosome 4, 7, and 8 (Rudolf *et al.*, 2004).

Absence epilepsies clearly have a genetic basis. Initially, an autosomal dominant monogenic mode of inheritance with age-dependent penetrance was described in several families (Tanaka *et al.*, 2008), while polygenic factors had been suggested before (Doose *et al.*, 1973). In fact, one or several genetic abnormalities are responsible for a predisposition and for the EEG trait, but absence epilepsies are likely to be multifactorial and associated to complex inheritance factors (Andermann, 1980; Mullen & Berkovic, 2018).

Pathology, structural and functional brain imaging

Autopsy (Meencke & Janz, 1985; Meencke, 1995) and MRI (Woermann *et al.*, 1998) studies found microdysgenesis and other cerebral structural changes in some patients with CAE which may be inconceivable for this benign, age-dependent and age-limited epileptic syndrome. Meencke (1995) reviewed autopsy findings in CAE and confirmed his previous reports on microdysgenesis (Meencke & Janz, 1985) with the frontal lobe more severely affected. Using quantitative MRI, Woermann *et al.* (1998) found that patients with IGE had epilepsy had significantly larger cortical grey matter volumes than control subjects.

Abnormalities of the regional distribution of cerebral grey and sub-cortical matter were frequent in other patients with IGE but only in one out of 10 patients with CAE. However, all cases of Meenke (1995) had frequent absences from childhood to adulthood and GTCS, which would not conform with a strict diagnosis of the syndrome of CAE. Similar may be the single patient with abnormal MRI of Woermann *et al.* (1998).

Functional imaging with positron emission tomography demonstrates normal cerebral glucose metabolism and benzodiazepine receptor density in absence epilepsies with diffuse hypermetabolism during 3-Hz spike and wave discharges (Ryvlin & Mauguière, 1998; Duncan, 1999). There is no evidence of any interictal overall abnormality of opioid receptors though typical absences have been found to displace 11C-diprenorphine from the association areas of the neocortex. In contrast, binding of 11C-flumazenil to cBZRs has been shown not to be affected by serial absences (Duncan, 1999). fMRI-EEG study of absences seizures in an adult patient with JAE demonstrated bilateral activation of thalamus and widespread deactivation of cortex maximal in frontal regions (Salek-Haddadi *et al.*, 2003). Similar results were reported using fMRI-EEG in 14 patients with 3-Hz generalized discharges (Aghakhani *et al.*, 2004). Substraction interictal-ictal SPECT co-registered to MRI (SISCOM) was used to evaluate cerebral blood flow changes during the ictal and immediate postictal phase in 4 children with CAE (Nehlig *et al.*, 2004). The authors reported a widespread decrease of cerebral blood flow during ictal phase and an increase during post ictal phase. Those studies confirm in human data observed in animal models, which suggest a crucial role of the thalamo-cortical loop and specific metabolic modifications during absence seizures.

Physiopathology of absence seizures

Current thinking about the pathogenesis of absence seizures dates to the landmark experiments of Jasper (Jasper & Droogleever-Fortuyn, 1947). They demonstrated that 3 cycles per sec stimulation of the midline and intralaminar nuclei of the thalamus in cats could produce bilaterally synchronous spike-wave discharges in the cortical EEG of those animals. Over the next 50 years, a debate ensued in the literature as to which was preeminent in controlling synchronous spike-wave discharge that characterized absence seizures: the cortex, the thalamus or both. With the advent of number of animal models of generalized absence seizures, this controversy has been at least partially resolved (Snead *et al.*, 1999). Moreover, the availability of these models has advanced our understanding of the basic mechanisms of absence seizures. The unifying hypothesis coming from animal data and *in vitro* neurophysiological data will be briefly summarized in this chapter.

Childhood absence epilepsy

Definition

In the international classification of epilepsies (Commission, 1989; Scheffer *et al.*, 2017) CAE is a genetic generalized epilepsy or IGE defined as follows: pyknolepsy occurs in children of school age (peak manifestation age 6–7 years), with a strong genetic predisposition in otherwise normal children. It appears more frequently in girls than in boys. It is characterized by very frequent (several to many per day) absences. The EEG reveals bilateral, synchronous symmetrical spike-waves, usually 3-Hz, on a normal background activity. During adolescence, GTCS often develop. Otherwise, absences may remit or, more rarely, persist as the only seizure type.

This brief definition mainly based on retrospective studies was a source of confusion. Thus, many authors make the arbitrary interpretation that CAE is any type of epilepsy with onset of absences in childhood, which is not correct. Therefore, epidemiology, genetics, age at onset, clinical manifestations, other types of seizures, long-term prognosis and treatment do not accurately reflect the syndrome of CAE. A more precise definition of CAE has been proposed by the ILAE Task Force on Classification defining inclusion and exclusion criteria (Loiseau & Panayiotopoulos, 2005). It takes several important diagnostic points into account, such as the degree of impairment of consciousness, the morphology of spike-wave discharges, the place of GTCS and clear exclusion criteria. This proposal (Loiseau & Panayiotopoulos, 2005) considers eyelid myoclonia (which is predominantly myoclonic and less of an absence) and TA consistently provoked by specific stimuli as exclusion criteria. Whether perioral myoclonia or single violent jerks during the ictus of an absence seizure are exclusion criteria may be debatable; however, their presence indicates worse prognosis (Panayiotopoulos 1997; 2005). The same applies for multiple spikes (more than 3 spikes per wave) that also indicate a bad prognosis and co-existent myoclonic jerks or GTCS (Panayiotopoulos *et al.*, 1989; Fong *et al.*, 1998; Fakhoury & Abou-Khalil, 1999).

The following definition may better represent CAE *(Table I)*: CAE is an age-related IGE, which occurs in otherwise normal children, more frequently girls, with a strong genetic predisposition. Age of onset is between 4 and 10 years of age, with a peak at 5–7 years. CAE is the archetypal childhood epileptic syndrome of typical absence seizures. Absences are severe and frequent, tens to hundreds per day. Their duration varies from 4-20 seconds though most of them last around 10 seconds. Clinically, there is abrupt and severe impairment (loss) of consciousness, with cessation of voluntary activity, which is not restored during the ictus. The eyes spontaneously open, overbreathing, speech and other voluntary activity stop within the first 3 seconds from the onset of the discharge. Automatisms are frequent but have no significance in the diagnosis. The eyes stare or move slowly, random eyelid blinking (usually not sustained) may occur.

Persistent eyelid myoclonia, perioral myoclonia, rhythmic massive limb jerking, single or arrhythmic myoclonic jerks of the head, trunk or limbs are probably not compatible with CAE. However, milder myoclonic elements particularly at the onset of the seizure discharge may be a feature of CAE. Generalized tonic-clonic seizures and other types of seizures like myoclonic jerks should not be featured in CAE. Visual (photic) and other sensory precipitation is most likely against a diagnosis of CAE. Mild or no impairment of consciousness is not compatible with CAE.

The EEG has a normal background, with sometimes rhythmic posterior delta activity. Ictal discharges consist of generalized high-amplitude spike and double (maximum occasional three spikes are allowed) spike– and slow-wave complexes. They are rhythmic at around 3–4 Hz (> 2.5 Hz) with a gradual and regular (0.5–1 Hz) slowdown from the initial to the terminal phase of the discharge. The first 1–2 seconds of the onset of the discharge is usually fast and unreliable for these measurements. There are no marked variations in the relation of spike to the slow wave, no fluctuations in the intradischarge frequency and certainly no fragmentations of the ictal discharges. Remission usually occurs before the age of 12 years but infrequent GTCS may develop in adolescence.

Epidemiology

The annual incidence rate of CAE in children < 15 years of age (for obvious reasons, a global, non age-specific incidence rate is meaningless) has been estimated between 6.3/100,000 (Olsson, 1988; Loiseau *et al.*, 1990) and 8.0/100,000 (Blom *et al.*, 1978). Though most cases in these studies were genuine CAE, in Olsson' series for example, 11 of 108 included patients had JME. Due to

Table I **Inclusion and exclusion criteria for CAE (from Loiseau & Panayiotopoulos (2000), with permission of the publisher of *Neurobase*).**

Inclusion criteria for CAE	Exclusion criteria for CAE
– Age at onset between 4 and 10 years and a peak at 5–7 – Normal neurological state and development – Brief (4–20 seconds, exceptionally longer) and frequent (tens per day) absence seizures with abrupt and severe impairment (loss) of consciousness. Automatisms are frequent but have no significance in the diagnosis – EEG ictal discharges of generalized high-amplitude spike and double (maximum occasional three spikes are allowed) spike– and slow-wave complexes. They are rhythmic at around 3-Hz with a gradual and regular slowdown from the initial to the terminal phase of the discharge. Their duration varies from 4–20 seconds	– Other than typical absence seizures such as GTCS, or myoclonic jerks prior to or during the active stage of absences – Eyelid myoclonia, perioral myoclonia, rhythmic massive limb jerking and single or arrhythmic myoclonic jerks of the head, trunk, or limbs – However, mild myoclonic elements of the eyes, eyebrows, and eyelids may be featured particularly in the first 3 seconds of the absence seizure – Mild or no impairment of consciousness during the 3-to 4-Hz discharges – Brief EEG 3-4 Hz spike wave paroxysms of less than 4 seconds, multiple spikes (more than 3) or ictal discharge fragmentations. – Visual (photic) and other sensory precipitation of clinical seizures

recruitment bias, the frequency of CAE among childhood epilepsies has been very differently assessed, ranging from 2.3% to 37.7% of cases. In two prospective community-based studies prevalence of CAE was 10% (Callenbach *et al.*, 1998) and 12.3% (Berg *et al.*, 1999; 2000) for children with epilepsy younger than 16 years of age. CAE is clearly more frequent in girls than in boys. Sixty to 70% of affected children are girls (Lennox & Lennox, 1960; Currier *et al.*, 1963; Hertoft, 1963; Bergamini *et al.*, 1965).

Age at onset is one of the main diagnostic components. Classically, CAE starts between 4–10 years with a peak at 5–7 years (Lennox & Lennox, 1960; Currier *et al.*, 1963; Livingston *et al.*, 1965; Panayiotopoulos, 2005). Lowest and highest age at onset compatible with CAE is uncertain. An earlier onset is a rare possibility (Beaumanoir, 1976; Cavazzuti *et al.*, 1989; Darra *et al.*, 1996). Ten years is usually considered as the upper limit of onset (Bergamini *et al.*, 1965; Loiseau *et al.*, 1995a). Onset after this age may be exceptional (Loiseau *et al.*, 1995a; Panayiotopoulos, 2005). CAE is an epileptic syndrome, and age at onset is not the only diagnostic criterion.

Seizures

TA in CAE are characterized by: short duration; abrupt onset and abrupt termination; severe impairment of consciousness; high frequency. The duration varies from 4-20 seconds, usually around 10 seconds. Duration of less than 4 seconds or more than 30 seconds may be incompatible for CAE (Loiseau & Panayiotopoulos, 2005). Reported mean duration is 8.0 ± 0.2 seconds (Hirsch *et al.*, 1994) and 12.4 ± 2.1 seconds (Panayiotopoulos *et al.*, 1989). In the literature, reported range varies from 2–3 seconds to 1–2 minutes but in most cases this is 5–10 seconds (Penry *et al.*, 1975), 5–30 seconds (Lennox & Lennox, 1960), 9–18 seconds (Panayiotopoulos *et al.*, 1989), and 3–27 seconds (Hirsch *et al.*, 1994). As a rule, the onset of absence seizures is abrupt. "If warning occurs, the diagnosis of petit mal may be questioned" (Lennox & Lennox, 1960). A brief retrograde amnesia (4 to 15 seconds) may occur (Jus & Jus, 1962). The attack ends as abruptly as it has commenced. The patient usually resumes the pre-ictal activity as if nothing had happened. However, it can take a few seconds before returning to a normal behavior: "The occasional patient will 'come to' rather slowly over a period of seconds" (Lennox & Lennox, 1960). The child is usually unaware the attack. A stimulus (call, pain) can interrupt the TA (Lennox & Lennox, 1960).

Severe impairment of consciousness is the essential feature of the absence seizure in CAE, with complete loss of awareness and responsiveness and cessation of on-going activities. The patient stops talking, eating, walking. The child may remain motionless, with vacant eyes, staring or drifting upwards. Mild impairment of consciousness in untreated patients is an exclusion criterion (Loiseau & Panayiotopoulos, 2005). Regarding other associated ictal clinical features, automatisms are common in CAE. In perseverative automatisms, the patient persists in what he is doing, *i.e.*, eating, walking, handling objects. These activities can be correctly done but are often distorted: walking more slowly, pouring water in a full glass. *De novo* automatisms are in the great majority of cases very simple: lip licking, swallowing, face rubbing, scratching, fumbling with clothes. They can be more complex: catching objects, grunting, mumbling, humming or singing but are shorter and less elaborate than in partial seizures. Automatisms occur in more than 60% of attacks (Penry *et al.*, 1975). They are related to the duration of seizures. They were noted in 95% of TA longer than 16 seconds (Penry *et al.*, 1975). Mild tonic or clonic symptoms often occur, particularly in the first second of the absence seizure. However, marked eyelid or perioral or limb and trunk myoclonic jerks particularly if they continue in the course of the absence seizure may be exclusion criteria (Loiseau & Panayiotopoulos, 2005). Atonic falls do not occur (Loiseau, 1992). Pallor is common. Incontinence of urine is exceptional.

Frequency of TA in CAE

Frequent TAs, tens or hundreds per day, is another defining criterion of CAE; hence the synonym term "pyknolepsy". "If attacks do not recur daily, the diagnosis may be questioned" (Lennox & Lennox, 1960). "They begin in driblets, the parents noting short episodes of immobility or eye-rolling but passing it off as day-dream or an emotional display. In time, however, the blackout periods increase in frequency or in duration and cannot be disregarded any longer" *(ibid.)*. At this moment, they range from 10 to 200 per day. The true frequency of TA is difficult to assess without prolonged video-EEG monitoring because the clinical manifestations can be easily missed. Parents' assessment is often an underestimation. These are important factors in assessing the efficacy of therapy (Browne *et al.*, 1983; Panayiotopoulos, 2001, 2005).

Precipitating factors

TA occur spontaneously but they are also influenced by various other factors and mainly hyperventilation. A diagnosis of CAE should be seriously questioned in an untreated child who does not have an attack on hyperventilation (Holowach *et al.*, 1962). In a series from Strasbourg, hyperventilation provoked TA in 100% of patients with CAE (Hirsch *et al.*, 1994). Further, there may be numerous other precipitating or facilitating factors such as: emotional (anger, sorrow, fear, surprise, embarrassment), intellectual (lack of interest, release of attention, mealtime for some children, school-time for others), nycthemeral (evening or awakening), metabolic (hypoglycemia). Whether in certain cases an emotional or conflicting situation such as reading difficulties (Bureau *et al.*, 1968) provokes an absence seizure, TA generally do not occur when a child is busy and stimulated by physical or mental activity, or has a sustained attention. It is worth noting that in a given patient TA are often triggered by the same factor. TA that are consistently elicited by specific stimuli such as flickering light or patterns do not belong to CAE (Hirsch *et al.*, 1994; Loiseau *et al.*, 1995a, 1995b; Panayiotopoulos, 2005; Loiseau & Panayiotopoulos, 2005).

Other types of seizures

Other seizures than TA are not part of CAE. In particular, GTCS or myoclonic jerks preceding TA or concomitant with the stage of active absence seizures do not occur in CAE (Hirsch *et al.*, 1994; Loiseau *et al.*, 1995a, 1995b; Panayiotopoulos, 2005; Loiseau & Panayiotopoulos, 2005). Also, though absence status may occur in 5 to 16% of cases with TA starting before the age of 10 years (Livingston *et al.*, 1965; Dieterich *et al.*, 1985; Wirrell *et al.*, 1996a) this is probably incompatible with CAE (Panayiotopoulos, 2005; Agathonikou *et al.*, 1998).

Electroencephalography

The EEG, preferably video-EEG, is the single-most important diagnostic procedure in diagnosing CAE.

Ideally, all children with absence seizures should have video-EEG recordings in an untreated state. The EEG accompaniment of TA is a bilaterally synchronous and symmetrical discharge of rhythmic 3-Hz spike-and-slow wave complexes (Commission 1989) *(Figures 2 and 3)*. The ictal EEG shows generalized, spike- or double-spike (no more

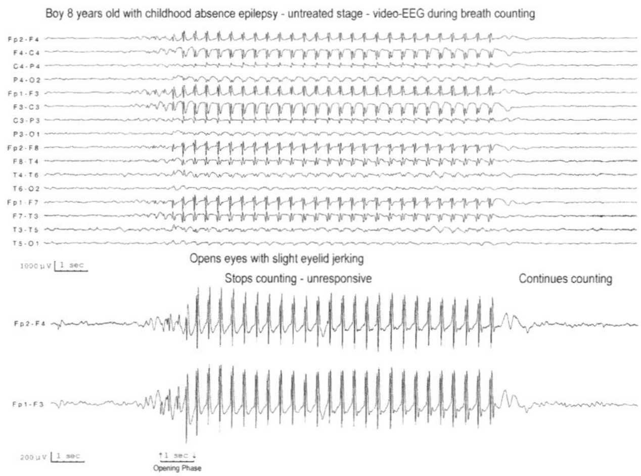

Figure 2 **Ictal EEG of an archetypal TAS of CAE. Note the regular rhythm of the discharge, the constant spike and slow wave relation, the abrupt onset and termination. The opening phase (first one second) is often variable and unreliable.**
This is from video-EEG of an 8 years boy. Suddenly, he stopped counting and opened his eyes within the first 2 seconds from the onset of the discharge. There was an initial brief eyelid flickering followed by eyes and head deviating upwards and to the right. He was totally unresponsive from the onset of the initial to the onset of the terminal phase of the discharge.
This child, despite severe absences, remained undiagnosed for 1 year. In a neuropsychological assessment, several absences were considered as frequent distractions affecting his performance.
The last 2 EEG traces are amplified frontal derivations.

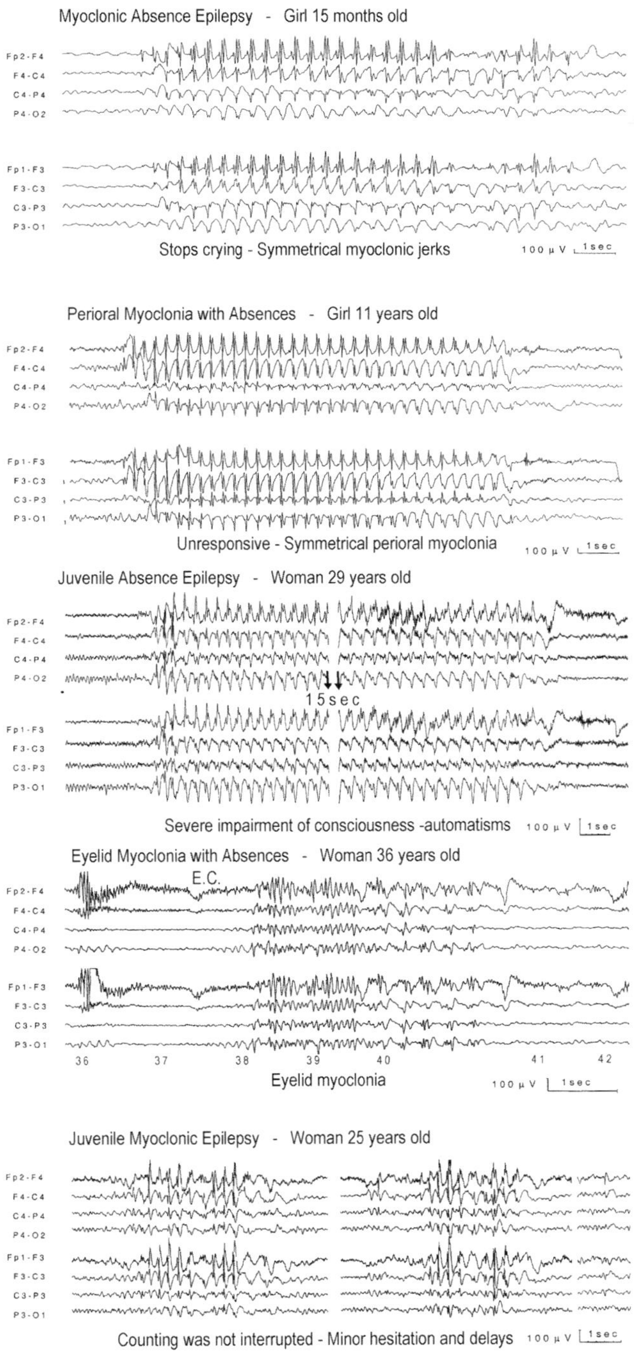

Figure 3 **Samples of video-EEG from patients with several syndromes of IGE manifested with TAS who do not have CAE.**
First from the top. **Typical absence seizure of a girl with symptomatic myoclonic absence epilepsy (birth anoxia), at age 15 months. There were marked, rhythmic and synchronous bilateral myoclonic jerks of limbs and head. Note, the multiple spikes of the discharge.**
She had many of them per day, lasting for 8–10 seconds. Subsequently, she developed frequent, mainly nocturnal GTCS while myoclonic absences continued. These are intractable to any appropriate mediation. At age 8 years she has severe learning difficulties and spastic quadraparesis (video-EEG demonstration can be viewed in Panayiotopoulos, 2000).
Second from the top. **TAS of perioral myoclonia with absences. This is case 1 of Panayiotopoulos *et al.* (1994). Onset of these TAS with profound perioral myoclonia, preceded by GTCS, was at age 3 years. Note that ictal EEG, without video, would not be sufficient to differentiate these from CAE. According to exclusion criteria, GTCS and marked myoclonia during the absence, she does not belong to CAE.**
Third from the top. **TAS of juvenile absence epilepsy of a woman aged 29 years. Note the prolonged and severe absence (around 30 seconds). She started having frequent (tens per day) typical absence seizures with severe impairment of consciousness at age 11 years. At age 14 years she had her first GTCS. Since then long absences of 20–30 seconds continue daily. Also she has 3–5 GTCS every year mainly in the morning, after awakening. These are preceded by clusters of absences. Occasionally, she may have random, infrequent and mild limb myoclonic jerks which started at age 20. Treatment with various appropriate anti-absence drugs was ineffective (video-EEG demonstration can be viewed in Panayiotopoulos, 2000).**
Fourth from the top. **Eyelid myoclonia with mild absence of a 35 years old woman with EMA from early childhood (case 9 of Giannakodimos & Panayiotopoulos, 1996). Note that the discharge is predominated by multiple spikes and it markedly different from others of IGE with typical absence seizures (video-EEG demonstration can be viewed in Panayiotopoulos 2000).**
Bottom. **Typical discharges of 3–4 Hz spike/multiple spike and slow wave discharges of a 25 years old woman with typical juvenile myoclonic epilepsy. Note, the multiple spike components, the brief duration and the fragmentations of the discharges. On video-EEG these were associated with only minor clinical changes during breath counting (a practical and easy procedure that is rarely performed in EEG evaluation of patients with TAS).**

than 3 spikes are allowed) and slow wave complexes at 3 Hz (no less than 2.7 Hz and no more than 4 Hz) at the initial phase of the discharge with gradual and smooth decline in frequency from the initial to the terminal phase *(Figure 3)* The discharge is regular, with well-formed spikes, which retain a constant relation with the slow-waves. The duration is usually around 10–12 seconds, no less than 4 seconds and exceptionally more than 20 seconds *(Figure 2)*. The opening phase of the discharge (1–2 seconds of onset) may be faster, irregular and asynchronous and therefore unreliable for such measurements *(Figure 3)*. Fragmentation of the ictal discharges, *i.e.*, transient discontinuation of the rhythmic spike-wave and multiple spike- and slow-waves discharges are considered as exclusion criteria for CAE (Panayiotopoulos *et al.*, 1989; Hirsch *et al.*, 1994; Loiseau & Panayiotopoulos, 2005). However, in an unpublished study of one of us (P.L.) no difference in evolution and prognosis was found between patients with either regular 3 Hz or irregular generalized SW discharge.

Background EEG is normal (Commission, 1989). However, some patients exhibit a rather particular posterior delta rhythm (Cobb *et al.*, 1961). This usually occurs in long runs of 3 Hz sinusoidal high amplitude activities, either symmetrical or more often asymmetrical in the occipital and occipito-parietal areas. It is blocked by eye-opening and enhanced by hyperventilation. Asymmetrical posterior slow waves, usually with a right predominance, are physiological in children.

Interictal paroxysmal activity, consisting of single or brief discharges of bilateral spike-waves may occur particularly during NREM sleep with important morphologic changes. Transient asymmetries of ictal or interictal spike-wave discharges are frequent mainly in treated patients. Transient focal epileptiform abnormalities such as centro-temporal sharp waves (Beaumanoir *et al.*, 1974; Hedström & Olsson, 1991) or persistent focal abnormalities (Lombroso, 1997) may occur in CAE.

Response to intermittent photic stimulation is not mentioned by the Commission (1989). Clinical photosensitivity is proposed as an exclusion criterion (Hedström & Olsson, 1991; Hirsch *et al.*, 1994; Panayiotopoulos, 2005) but this is not accepted by others (Wolf & Goosses, 1986).

Clinical interictal presentation

By definition of an idiopathic epileptic syndrome, CAE, formerly "pure petit mal", occurs in neurologically and intellectually normal children (Lennox & Lennox, 1960; Currier *et al.*, 1963; Livingston *et al.*, 1965; Beaumanoir, 1976). However, it may also occur in children with an idiopathic mild mental subnormality (they belong to the so-called normal population). Attention disturbances and scholastic difficulties may be frequent. Behavioral abnormalities may be due to TA as well as to parents' attitude and medication.

Evolution and prognostic factors

Most of the available evidence is inconclusive regarding evolution and prognosis of CAE. This is because of markedly different classification criteria in the relevant reports or of too short follow-up periods. Most authors include in CAE any child with absences before the age of 10 years which may not be CAE (see for review Bouma *et al.*, 1996; Panayiotopoulos 2005; Loiseau & Panayiotopoulos, 2005). Retrospective studies in adults may lack accurate initial data. Patients must be followed beyond eighteen or twenty years of age (Loiseau *et al.*, 1983, 1995b; Loiseau & Duché, 1995). The literature and hence the text of the International Classification of epileptic syndromes are likely to be too pessimistic. Our view is that CAE, if properly defined, has an excellent prognosis. However, as to date this optimism is not based on indisputable data, some older studies will be quoted, in spite of their selection bias. The included patients had received anti-absence medication, diones since 1945, then ethosuximide since 1951, and later sodium valproate. At a time when no anti-absence drug existed, Adie (1924) concluded that even if absence seizures in pyknolepsy persisted for a long time, they ultimately ceased, never to return. This is consistent with findings that absences of CAE, even if they may persist several years, they finally disappear with age in more than 90% of cases (Loiseau *et al.*, 1983, 1995a, 1995b). In a Swedish population-based study, a 91% remission rate was found when patients with absence epilepsy had only absences (Hedström & Olsson, 1991).

TA persist for a mean time of 6.6 years (Currier *et al.*, 1963), disappear between age 3–19 years, mean age 10.5 (Hertoft, 1963) or 14 years (Currier *et al.*, 1963). "The tendency for petit mal to cease is present at all ages and not just at puberty. In about a quarter of patients the attacks cease before the age of 15 and by the age of 30 years petit mal had ceased in about three quarters of the patients" (Gibberd, 1966). In this study, with a follow-up of about 5 years, only 3% of patients experienced TA beyond 50 years of age. In another study (Livingston *et al.*, 1965), of the 92 controlled patients, 89 were aged 20 or younger at the time of cessation of absence seizures. Thus, TA persistence is rare, reported to occur in about 6% of patients (Oller-Daurella & Sanchez, 1981). In adults, attacks tend to be infrequent, milder and occur with precipitating factors such as fatigue, sleep deprivation, menstruation (Currier *et al.*, 1963; Gastaut *et al.*, 1986; Panayiotopoulos *et al.*, 1992; Panayiotopoulos, 2005) though in some of them absences may be very severe (Agathonikou *et al.*, 1998; Panayiotopoulos, 1997, 2005). Two favorable prognostic signs are age at onset of TA and medication efficacy. In patients early diagnosed and followed beyond 20 years of age, TA had disappeared in 95 and 90% of cases according to an age at onset of 8 or 10 years (Loiseau *et al.*, 1995a; 1995b). Their cessation soon after prescription of a convenient antiepileptic drug is considered as a favorable sign (Currier *et al.*, 1963; Loiseau *et al.*, 1966).

However, cessation of absence seizures may not mean remission. This again depends on diagnostic inclusion and exclusion criteria. Considering all absences with onset in childhood as CAE, prognosis is uncertain and with great variations (see for review Bouma *et al.*, 1996; Panayiotopoulos, 1997, 2005; Loiseau & Panayiotopoulos, 2005). GTCS may appear and patients may develop JME (Wirrell *et al.*, 1996a; Delgado-Escueta *et al.*, 1999). Medina *et al.* (2005) suggested that CAE evolving to JME belongs under the concept of absence epilepsies for the following reasons: i) it starts with absences with 3-Hz single spike-and-slow wave in childhood; ii) absences are the most common seizure type in affected members; iii) absence are the most common persisting seizure type in probands; iv) like typical CAE the affected persons are most often females and transmission is predominantly maternal; and v) despite treatment with VPA monotherapy or poly-therapy, absences persist lifelong (Martinez-Juarez *et al.*, 2006).

It has been estimated that GTCS occurred in 36–60% of patients with onset of TA in childhood (Currier *et al.*, 1963; Livingston *et al.*, 1965; Charlton & Yahr, 1967; Oller-Daurella & Sanchez, 1981; Loiseau *et al.*, 1983). Most often, GTCS occur 5 to 10 years after onset of TA (Loiseau *et al.*, 1983), *i.e.*, mainly between 8 and 15 years of age (Livingston *et al.*, 1965; Charlton & Yahr, 1967; Dieterich *et al.*, 1985), and sometimes beyond 20 and even 30 years of age (Gastaut *et al.*, 1986). They have been considered as infrequent and easily controlled (Currier *et al.*, 1963; Charlton & Yahr, 1967; Oller-Daurella & Sanchez, 1981; Loiseau *et al.*, 1983). Some authorities proposed to distinguish two groups of patients; in one of them, GTCS begin usually beyond 16 years of age, are rare, and even a unique seizure, and a precipitating factor (sleep deprivation, stress) is constant; in the other group, they usually begin between 8 and 15 years of age and recur without provocative factor other than irregular therapy (Dieterich *et al.*, 1985).

Different trisk factors have been suggested, as follows.

Age at onset of TAS. The later the onset of TAS, the higher the risk for subsequent convulsive seizures (Lennox & Lennox, 1960; Bergamini *et al.*, 1965; Livingston *et al.*, 1965; Charlton & Yahr, 1967; Oller-Daurella & Sanchez, 1981; Loiseau *et al.*, 1983; Guiwer *et al.*, 2004). Loiseau *et al.* (1995a) followed-up beyond the age of 20 years 52 patients with strictly defined CAE. GTCS developed in 16% of those with onset of TA before 9 years of age; this rose to 44% of those with onset of TA between 9 and 10 years.

Absence status, especially when they occur late in the course of epilepsy (Dieterich *et al.*, 1985) but this may not be CAE (Agathonikou *et al.*, 1998; Panayiotopoulos *et al.*; 2001, Guye *et al.*, 2001).

Sex: whether TASs are more frequent in girls, TA + GTCS are more frequent in boys (Oller-Daurella & Sanchez, 1981).

EEG. Usually, clinical/EEG correlation is fair. However, the predictive value of the EEG is not absolute; SW discharges may persist after clinical recovery and conversely GTCS may occur in spite of a normalized EEG (Hedström & Olsson, 1991). When initial tracings show posterior delta rhythms, GTCS rarely occur (Cobb *et al.*, 1961; Oller-Daurella & Sanchez, 1981; Loiseau *et al.*, 1983; Hedström & Olsson, 1991). An abnormal background activity, multiple spikes, focal abnormalities are considered as unfavorable signs, but are likely to correspond to erroneous diagnoses.

Therapy. With an early institution of effective therapy, GTCS occurred in 30% of cases and 68% after incorrect therapy (Bergamini *et al.*, 1965). GTCS manifested in 85% of incorrectly treated patients (Dieterich *et al.*, 1985).

Many other symptoms and clinical signs were examined as predictors of outcome without conclusive result (Wirrell *et al.*, 1996a).

A change of CAE into epilepsy with focal seizures has been reported. It corresponds to erroneous diagnosis: either TA with automatisms (Currier *et al.*, 1963; Sato *et al.*, 1976; Dieterich *et al.*, 1985), or absence epilepsy other than CAE such as in febrile seizures plus (Kobayashi *et al.*, 2004).

When stricter criteria are applied for CAE, GTCS are infrequent and easily controlled by medication. A series of 52 patients older than 20 years at last follow-up was studied (Loiseau *et al.*, 1995a). Inclusion criteria were age at onset (3–10 years) of daily and EEG recorded typical absences as a presenting sign of normal children, with no history of preceding seizures other than febrile convulsions and seen within the first year of onset or treatment. EEG with multiple or irregular spike-waves and/or photosensitivity were exclusion criteria. Absences persisted in 5 (< 10%) and in 2 of them as the only type of seizure. GTCS occurred in 14 patients (26%) but in 11 of them GTCS were isolated or rare. GTCS were more common amongst patients with onset of absences from 9-10 years and without posterior delta rhythms. Control of absences with treatment varied: it was achieved in 12 patients within weeks but in most cases they persisted for years. In another approach, Agathonikou *et al.* (1997) studied 39 adults with IGE and TA starting before 10 years of age. All were older than 18 years (31.5 ± 10.5; range 18–56) and all had EEG recorded TA (15 with video-EEG). Typical absences had onset at 6.2 ± 1.9 years (range 2–9) and still persisted in 28 (71.8%). GTCS occurred in 87.2% (onset 13 ± 7.2 years; range 2–36). Myoclonic jerks occurred in 38.5% (onset 12.6 ± 4.1 years; range 7–18). Women (82%) and photosensitivity (56.4%) markedly predominated. Only one of them fulfilled strict criteria of CAE and was well controlled on medication. Of the others, 8 were classified as eyelid myoclonia with absence, 5 JAE, 4 perioral myoclonia with absence,

3 JME, 3 absences with single myoclonic jerk, 3 predominantly photosensitive IGE with TAS. Twelve patients had unclassified IGE (8 with photosensitivity).

Complete remission

A wide range of remission rates has been given: 78 to 33%. Reasons are as follows: i) patients with absence epilepsies other than CAE were included; ii) patient's age at last clinic visit, with for instance control in 82% of patients when beyond 18 years of age but only 65% in those beyond 20 (Dieterich *et al.*, 1985); iii) follow-up duration, with relapse in 19% of patients who had been seizure-free 2 years or more (Dieterich *et al.*, 1985); and iv) therapy (Oller-Daurella & Sanchez, 1981; Dieterich *et al.*, 1985): with an early and adequate therapy, 70% of patients were controled and only 18% with an incorrect therapy (Bergamini *et al.*, 1965).

Social prognosis

Social adaptation of patients having had CAE would be poor in one third of patients, even when in remission (Hertoft, 1963; Lugaresi *et al.*, 1973; Loiseau *et al.*, 1983; Dieterich *et al.*, 1985; Guiwer *et al.*, 2004). In CAE, TA are very frequent and EEG also shows brief discharges of bilateral spike-waves without apparent clinical impairment. Neuropsychological studies have documented cognitive dysfunctioning (reaction time tasks and sustained attention tests) during these discharges. "The transitory bursts of spike-wave activity represent the tip of an iceberg. Below the surface there may be a more or less continuously active pathophysiological process, which is reflected in impaired performance on tests of attention and in alterations in event-related brain potentials" (Mirsky *et al.*, 1986; 1995). Therefore, long-term sequelae of scholastic difficulties are not surprising. A psychomotor slowing beginning late in follow-up has been found in some patients with TA persisting after the age of 30 to 61 years (Gastaut *et al.*, 1986). It was supposed to be multifactorial in origin.

Juvenile absence epilepsy

According to the ILAE (1989), JAE is an idiopathic generalized epilepsy (IGE) characterized by a genetic predisposition, an average age at onset around puberty, no evidence of neurological or intellectual deficit. Seizures are typical absences in 100% of the patients, longer and less frequent than in CAE, GTCS in 80% and sporadic myoclonic jerks in 20%. More recent proposals have classified JAE as a syndrome of adolescence-adulthood (Berg *et al.*, 2010).

JAE is less frequent than CAE or JME. In large cohorts, it was estimated from 0.2 to 2.4% (Jallon & Latour, 2005). According to Janz (1969), JAE represented 10% of the age-related epilepsies with "petit mal" seizures. Panayiotopoulos (1997) reported a prevalence of 13.3% among adult patients with absences and 10.2% among IGEs. From 14 epilepsy centers in Lombardy including 8,570 patients, 1,494 (17.4%) had various types of IGEs and 160 (2.2%) of these had JAE (Osservatore Regionale per l'Epilessia Lombardy, ILAE 1996). Of 2,841 consecutive newly referred patients first seen between 1986 and 1997 at the Centre Saint-Paul in Marseilles, the group of IGE represented 15.3% of all cases. JME was the most frequent form of IGE (26.7% of IGE; 4.1% of all epilepsies), preceding CAE (23.3% of IGE; 3.6% of all epilepsies); JAE (11% of IG E; 1.7% of all epilepsies); photogenic epilepsy (9.1% of IGE; 1.4% of all epilepsies) and awakening grand mal (6,2% of IGE; 0,96% of all epilepsies) (Genton *et al.*, 2000). Of 1,123 patients seen at least one time over one year (April 2009–2010) in Montpellier, 23 patients with JAE (2% of the active file) and 80 patients with JME (7% of the active file) were identified (Gélisse *et al.*, 2011).

There is a female preponderance in CAE and JME. The sex distribution seems to be equal in JAE. In the material of Janz (1969), there were 62 females (53%) and 54 males (47%). In the investigation of Wolf & Inoue (1984), there were 48 females (45%) and 59 males (55%). However, Trinka *et al.* (2008) reported in a group of 64 patients, 42 (66%) females *vs.* 22 males (34%) and Lu *et al.* (2008) 15 females (60%) and 10 males (40%) in group of 25 patients.

Clinical presentation

According to the 1989 Classification (Commission, 1989), "the absences of JAE are the same as in pyknolepsy, but absences with retropulsive movements are less common. Manifestation occurs around puberty. Seizure frequency is lower than in pyknolepsy, with absences occurring less frequently than every day, mostly sporadically. Association with GTCS is frequent, and GTCS precede the absence manifestations more often than in childhood absence epilepsy, often occurring on awakening. Not infrequently, the patients also have myoclonic seizures."

Age of onset is mostly in the range of 7–17 years with a peak at 10–12 years; TA are relatively rare (spanioleptic) and often longer than in CAE but may happen several times a day. They can occur in clusters during the hour that follows awakening. The same types of TA occur as in CAE, but absences with retropulsive movements are less common. There is a sudden more or less complete suspension of consciousness. Loss of consciousness is less pronounced than in CAE. In one video-based study, expressive speech and overbreathing was less disturbed in JAE than in CAE (Panayiotopoulos *et al.*, 1989). In some seizures, interrupted speech and overbreathing were restored during the absence. Spontaneous eye opening was rare. Some simple automatisms are frequent during the absence especially when the absence lasts more than 10 seconds. Subtle myoclonia of the eyelids are common but marked eyelid or perioral myoclonus, marked myoclonic jerks of the limbs, trunk, head during the absence are incompatible with JAE (Panayiotopoulos, 2010).

One of us (Wolf, 1995, case 1) reported a patient where the onset of JAE was monitored with video-EEGs. This was a 10-year-old girl, and her first seizure manifestation was a GTCS. Her video-EEG presented subclinical generalized irregular spike-wave paroxysms of up to 3 seconds duration and photosensitivity at 20 Hz. She had a second GTCS 3 months later. A new video-EEG investigation revealed, at hyperventilation, three bursts of generalized spike-waves, and tests with acoustic stimuli during these, now demonstrated impaired consciousness along with initial slight eyelid moyclonus.

The majority of patients also have GTCS, and these precede absences more often than in CAE. Most frequently, they belong to the awakening type. Association with myoclonic seizures is more common than in CAE, probably in the order of 15–20%. Praxis-induced seizures have been reported in JAE but are less frequent than in JME. Among 32 subjects with a history of praxis-induced seizures, 21 were diagnosed as having JME, 3 JAE, and 4 unspecified IGE (Wolf & Inoue, 2005).

Absence status seems to be more frequent in JAE than in JME (Agathonikou *et al.*, 1998). The episodes can be spontaneous or precipitated by drug withdrawal or by inappropriate drugs especially carbamazepine. A case in an elderly patient (aged 68 at the last episode) with recurrent absence status was reported recently (Muccioli *et al.*, 2018). In a series of 14 patients with absence status precipitated by antiepileptic drugs, the final diagnosis was JAE in 6, JME in four, epilepsy with grand mal on awakening in two and CAE in 2 (Thomas *et al.*, 2006). All the JAE patients were on carbamazepine and absence status was precipitated by an increase of dose in three. Oxcarbazepine is chemically related to carbamazepine. Paradoxal aggravation was reported in one case with JAE (Gélisse *et al.*, 2004) who developed frequent absences one month after the introduction of the drug and evolved to an absence status. Fatigue, sleep deprivation and abnormal lifestyle play an aggravating role.

Interictal EEG

The interictal EEG shows a normal background and generalized symmetric spike-waves (SW) or polyspike-waves (PSW) with frontal accentuation. These elements are isolated or grouped in brief bursts. The frequency is usually faster than 3 Hz (3.5–4 Hz), the first complex of a group sometimes even faster. SW or PSW are mainly seen during sleep *(Figure 4)* whereas awake EEGs show absence seizures. In some patients, long discharges of generalized spike-waves at 3 Hz are sometimes observed in NREM sleep and can provoke an arousal. As in JME, focal or asymmetrical abnormalities can be observed but tend to shift from one hemisphere to the other during the same recording *(Figure 5)*. The occurrence of fast rhythms during NREM sleep is indicative of drug resistance (see paragraph differential diagnosis).

Temporal intermittent rhythmic delta activity is an EEG pattern observed in 13% of JAE *(Figure 6)* (Gélisse *et al.*, 2011). The frequency is around 3 Hz. This activity is activated by hyperventilation and drowsiness. It decreases in NREM sleep and reappears in REM sleep. This activity could represent a continuum with the posterior delta waves seen in CAE but with an anterior location toward the temporal lobes.

For Wolf and Goosses (1986), photosensitivity is less common than in other IGE: 7.5% in JAE, 18% in CAE and 30.6% in JME, 13% in epilepsy with GTCS on awakening. But this was not confirmed by Lu et al. (2008). In 25 patients (8 males, 15 females), a photoparoxysmal reaction was found in 56% of the cases, higher in males (80%) than in females (40%).

Ictal EEG

Absences are likewise made of spike-wave and polyspike-wave discharges at 3.5-4 Hz that are bilateral, synchronous with anterior predominance *(Figures 7 and 8)*. The preliminary study of Panayiotopoulos *et al.* (1989) indicated that the ictal discharges may be longer in JAE (16.3 ± 7.1 sec) than in CAE (12.4 ± 2.1 sec) and in JME (6.6 ± 4.2 sec). They were more regular than in JME but could show fragmentation unlike in CAE.

Outcome and prognosis

JAE is not considered severe, but the condition is lifelong. The response to therapy is good in spite of the frequent combination with GTCS. Approximately 80% of cases become seizure-free with the traditional drugs such as ethosuximide and valproate, but the rate of relapse after drug discontinuation is probably close to 100% (Healy *et al.*, 2018). Wolf & Inoue (1984) reported in their cross-sectional study of 229 adolescents and adults who had a diagnosis of absences and still were in treatment, that all were seizure free if they had only had absences (n = 21), and 87% if there had not been more than 10 GTCS in addition. If there were more GTCS (which was the case in 123 patients), the response was still very good but 24% were not seizure free. The response was better in JAE (85% seizure free) than in CAE (80%, $p < 0.02$), and combination with myoclonic seizures did not affect the therapy prognosis. In these patients, the absences were mostly treated with ethosuximide, valproate or both – in some cases with methsuximide – and if necessary the doses were increased

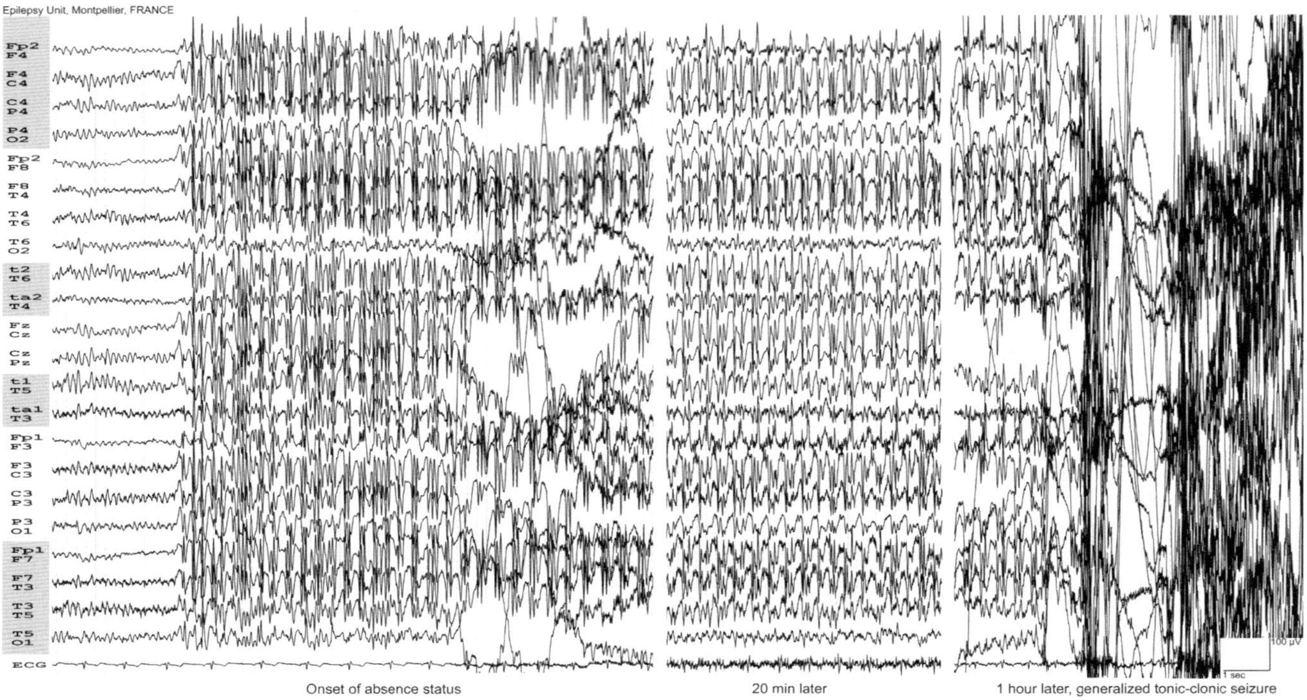

Figure 4

EEG with international 10–20-electrode system with supplementary anterior/inferior temporal electrodes (TA1, T1, TA2, T2). Spontaneous absence status occurring in the morning in a 43-year-old woman. The EEG shows continuous generalized spike-and-wave activity. Mild impairment of the consciousness during the status. It ends with a generalized tonic-clonic seizure.

to the maximum the patients could tolerate. If GTCS were present, these were often treated with a combination. In the follow-up study of Bartolomei *et al.* (1997) which included 53 cases of CAE and 27 cases of JAE, in both groups, absences or GTCS persisted in about 40%. In the study of Trinka *et al.* (2004), 40 (62%) of 64 JAE patients were seizure free for at least 2 years, which was almost similar to the seizure free rate of CAE patients (56%). Siren *et al.* (2002) reported that the 4 patients with intractable JAE had rhythmic, random eyelid blinking in addition to GTCS.

JAE is a well-delineated syndrome of IGE. JAE has found its place as an easily recognizable form of epilepsy. The condition is lifelong but treatable. Its genetic relations to other IGE remain to be identified – which could clarify some of the nosological uncertainties still under discussion.

Epilepsy with myoclonic absences

Epilepsy with myoclonic absences (EMA) is characterized by a specific seizure type, *i.e.*, myoclonic absences (MA), the diagnosis of which rests on clinical observation and polygraphic and/or video recording. Rhythmic and bilateral myoclonic jerks are observed.

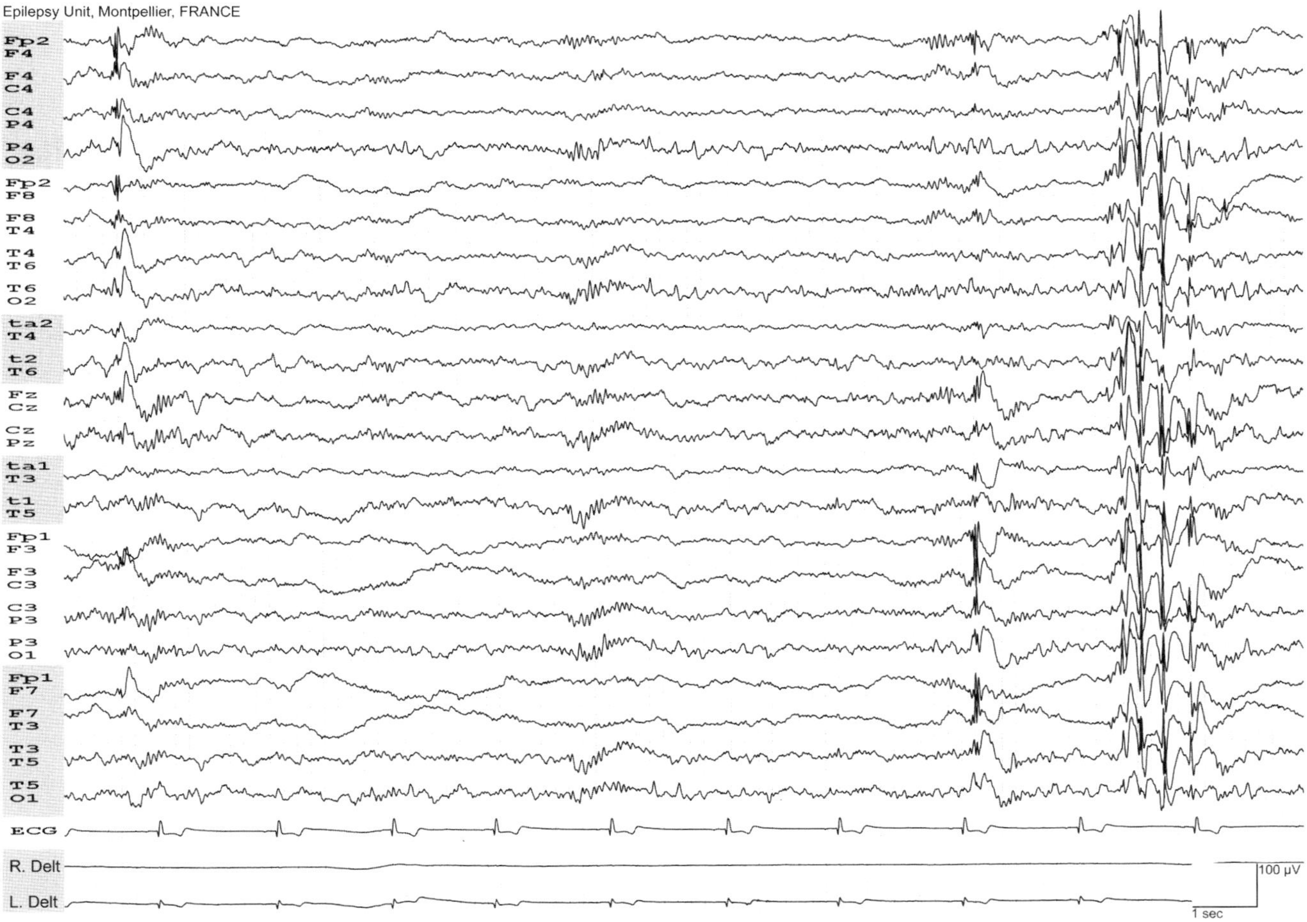

Figure 5

18-year-old man. Asymmetric changes observed independently over the right and left hemisphere. At the end of the plate, burst of generalized spike-waves.

Polygraphic recording (EEG + EMG) shows a rhythmic spike and wave (SW) discharge at 3 Hz that is bilateral, synchronous and symmetric, associated with an EMG discharge of myoclonias at 3 Hz and an increasing bilateral tonic contraction. The earliest description of MA is by Tassinari *et al.* (1969; 1971). They later (Tassinari & Bureau, 1985) stressed that MA were a particular and specific seizure type and proposed to individualize a specific syndrome in which MA were the only or the predominant seizure type. Several studies contributed to the description of EMA (Salas Puig *et al.*, 1990; Tassinari *et al.*, 1992; 1995; Tassinari & Michelucci, 1994; Manonmani & Wallace, 1994; Elia *et al.*, 1998; Capovilla *et al.*, 2001; Bureau & Tassinari, 2002; Tassinari *et al.*, 2004; Bureau & Tassinari, 2005; Genton &

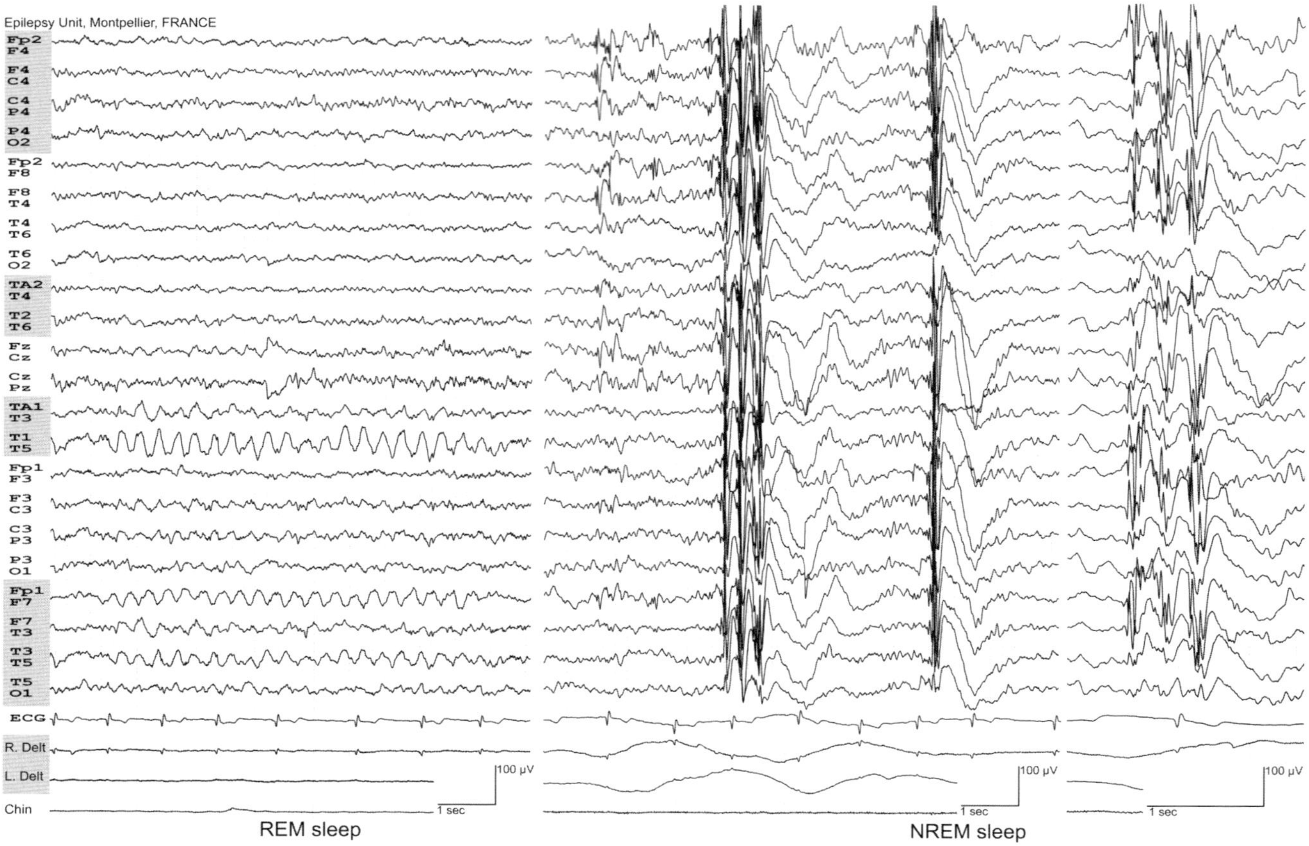

Figure 6

EEG with international 10–20-electrode system with supplementary anterior/inferior temporal electrodes (TA1, T1, TA2, T2). 29-year-old man. Onset of typical absences at adolescence. When he was evaluated, he had no treatment. On the left, the patient is in REM sleep. Rhythmic delta intermittent waves are recorded over the left temporal region. In the middle and on the right, the patient is in stage 2 NREM sleep. There are generalized polyspike-waves. Note the presence of some asymmetric changes over the right hemisphere.

Bureau, 2006). The syndrome of epilepsy with myoclonic absences described is incorporated in the ILAE Classification (1989, Scheffer *et al.*, 2017) as a rare generalized absence epilepsy with a variable prognosis.

EMA is uncommon, accounting for less than 0,5–1% of pediatric epilepsies. This condition is however recognized as a specific entity, *e.g.*, in Japan (Ikeda *et al.*, 2011), China (Yang *et al.*, 2009) or India

(Zanzmera *et al.*, 2016). There is a male preponderance (70%). A family history of epilepsy, most often of generalized type, is found in about 20%. *Aetiological factors* are present in 33% (14/42 cases of the Centre Saint-Paul): prematurity (4 cases), perinatal damage (6 cases), consanguinity (2 cases), congenital hemiparesis (1 case) and partial trisomy of the long arm of chromosome 14 (1 case). Chromosomal anomalies have been reported (Guerrini *et al.*, 1990; Elia *et al.*, 1998): Angelman syndrome, 12p trisomy, invdup (15). AGDH mutation was found in four members of a family with MA (Bahi-Buisson *et al.*, 2008) and a glucose transporter type 1 deficiency syndrome (GLUT1DS) was reported in a Turkish patient by Gökben *et al.* (2011). A balanced translocation resulting in disruption of SYNGAP1 was also found in a patient with MA and intellectual disability (Klitten *et al.*, 2011).

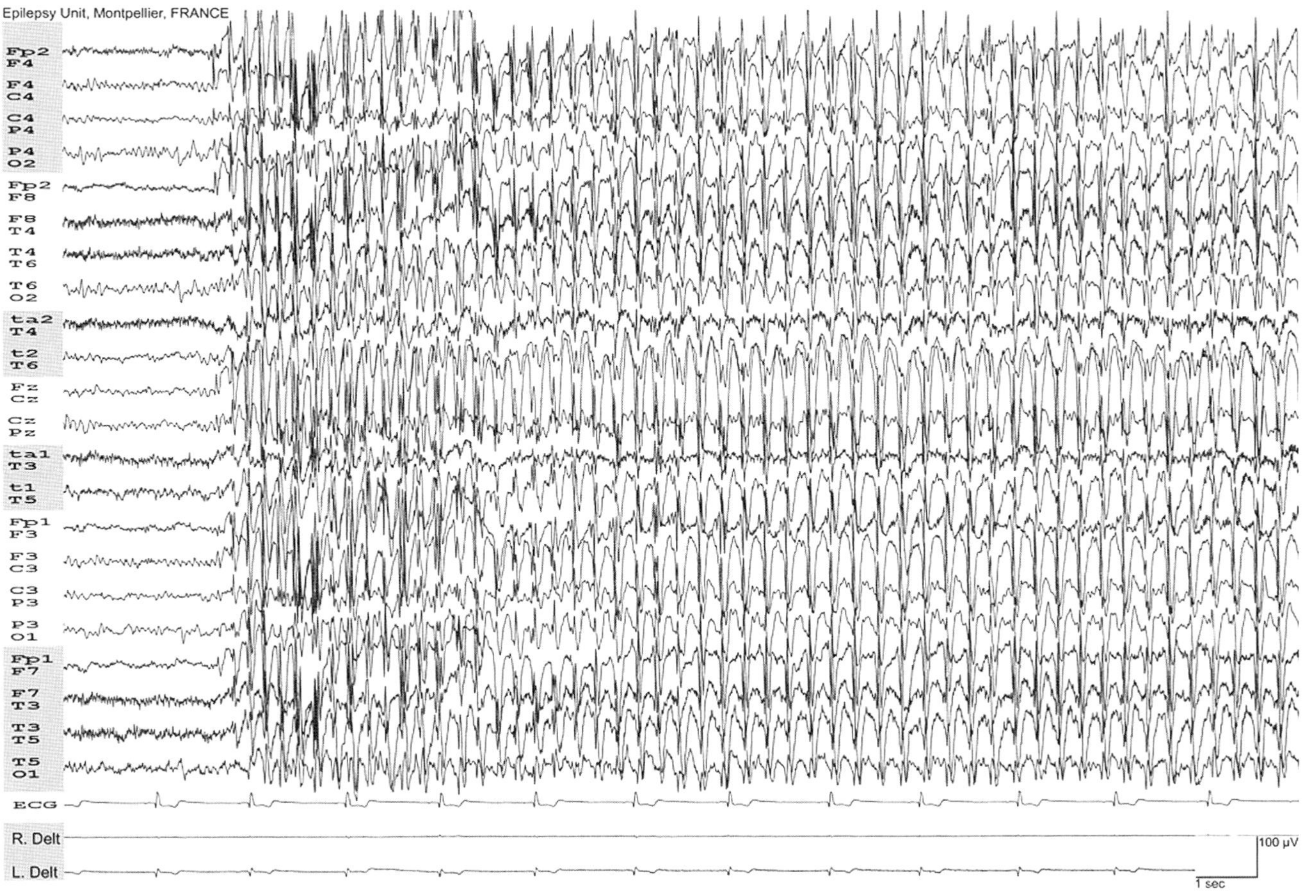

Figure 7

Same patient as in *Figure 4*. The patient is awake. Recording of a spontaneous typical absence with complete loss of contact. Sudden-onset with 3.5–4 Hz spike-waves that become slower.

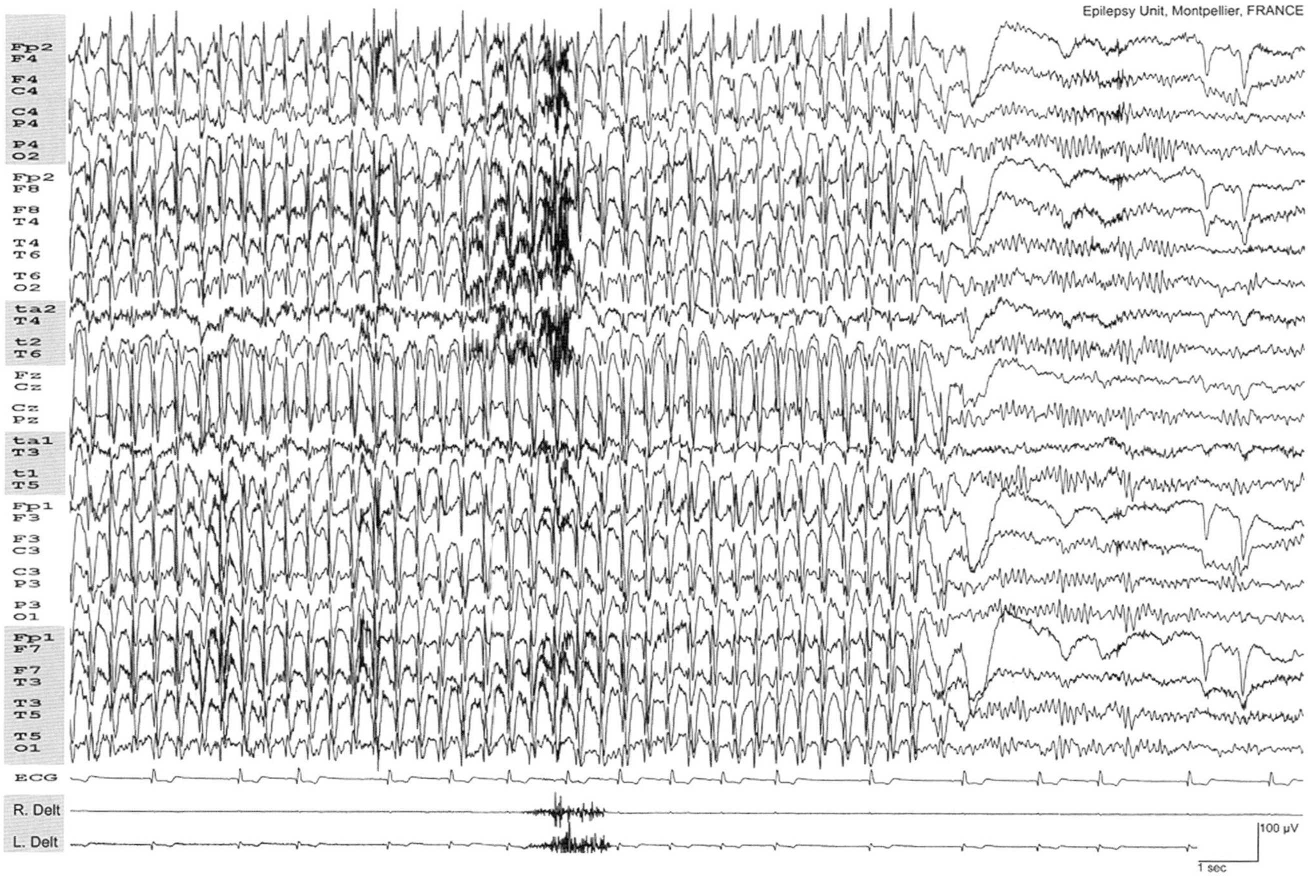

Figure 8

Same patient, end of the absence. This absence is accompanied by some simple automatims. Note the presence of chewing artefacts over the temporal regions and also note the brief slight contraction of the deltoid muscles.

Mean age at onset is 7 years (range: 1.1–12.5), but very early onset before age 1 is possible, more frequently than in CAE (Tassinari *et al.*, 1992; Aicardi, 1994; Manonmani & Wallace, 1994; Verrotti *et al.*, 1999). The neurological status is normal except in the case with congenital hemiparesis. Mental retardation is noted in 45% of the cases before onset of epilepsy. Neuroimaging is abnormal in 17% of the cases, showing mostly a slight degree of diffuse and aspecific atrophy, without focal lesions.

Myoclonic absences

Loss of contact and impairment of consciousness are of variable intensity, less pronounced than in CAE and may not cover the whole duration of the EEG discharge. The myoclonias are felt as a very disturbing experience; the subject frequently holds himself, as if to control the jerking, a "semi-automatic" behavior related to the incomplete impairment of awareness, similar to the one described as "self-oriented" automatisms in petit mal epilepsy by Penry and Dreifuss (1969). In the same way, other "object-oriented" automatisms observed in CAE are also observed in EMA (Myers & Scheffer, 2018). MA have an abrupt onset and offset. Motor manifestations are typically an association of rhythmic myoclonic jerks with axial tonic contraction, the latter occurring often progressively during the absence. The myoclonias mainly involve shoulders, arms and legs. The muscles of the face are less frequently involved: they are then more evident around the chin and the mouth, eyelid twitching is rare. Due to concomitant tonic contraction, the jerking of the arms is accompanied by a progressive elevation of the upper extremities, giving rise to a quite constant and recognizable pattern. When the patient is standing, falling is uncommon but a backward or forward oscillation is frequently seen. The myoclonic jerks may be asymmetric. Lateralized deviation of eyes, head and body during the jerks (without concomitant ocular or oculoclonic deviation) can be observed in some cases (Bureau & Tassinari, 2005; Genton & Bureau, 2006) and has also been reported by Yang *et al.* (2009). In some cases a change or an arrest of respiration that lasts as long as the tonic contraction and sometimes a loss of urine can be noted.

The duration ranges from 10 to 60 seconds (longer than in CAE). The frequency is high and MA occur at least several times per day, often tens of times per day. They are often increased by hyperventilation or awakening. In 14% of cases, they can be elicited by ILS. MA can occur during light sleep, awakening the patient. Status of MA is rare (1 case among 36 cases reported by Tassinari *et al.*, 1992).

EEG and polygraphic semiology

The interictal EEG shows a normal background activity for the age in the majority of the cases. We never observed a sinusoidal slow posterior rhythm as can be seen in CAE. Generalized spikes and waves (SW) were noted only in 1/3 of cases while focal or multifocal spikes or SW are present in about 14% of patients.

The ictal EEG consists of rhythmic SW discharges at 3 Hz that are bilateral, synchronous and symmetric as in the absences of CAE. The on- and offset of the SW are abrupt, except in rare cases in which the EEG discharge ends progressively with sometimes asymmetric delta waves over the frontal areas. Typical SW can be intermixed with polyspikes.

The polygraphic recording (as exemplified in *Figure 9)* discloses the appearance of bilateral and rhythmic myoclonias, at the same frequency as the SW, beginning about 1 second after the onset of the EEG discharge *(Figure 10)*. Later into the seizure, the myoclonias are associated with a progressive tonic contracton that is maximal on the shoulder and deltoid muscles and that is responsible for the elevation of the arms *(Figure 10)*. The tonic contraction can mask or render the myoclonias clinically less evident, the motor manifestations are thus less evident. Sometimes the myoclonias and the tonic contraction are unilateral or clearly asymmetric (with a jerky rotation of head and trunk) despite the generalized EEG pattern *(Figures 9 and 10)*. Tassinari *et al.* (1969, 1971) proved by means of high speed oscil-loscopic recording that there is a strict and constant relation between the SW discharge and the myoclonias. The detailed morphology of spikes shows a positive transient (Weir, 1965) of high amplitude in strict relationship with the appearance, latency and amplitude of the myoclonias. At times, the SW in the first second are of smaller amplitude (because the early positive component of the spike is of small amplitude) and are not accompaned by myoclonias *(Figure 9)*. Each spike on the EEG is followed on the EMG by a myoclonia with a latency of 15 to 40 ms for the more proximal muscles and of 50 to 70 ms for the more distal muscles. This myoclonia is again followed by a brief silent period (60 to 120 ms) which interrupts the tonic contraction.

Even if it may not be evident clinically, the myoclonic absence seizure may include a significant motor component of the cephalic segment, particularly of the perioral region. The EMG recordings show a clonic activation of the facial muscles corresponding to the 1–2 first SW complexes, while the successive complexes correspond to a myoclonic cascade with propagation from the cranial to the proximal limbs (Gardella *et al.*, 2002). From a physiopathological point of view, the tonic muscular contraction component that is superimposed on the myoclonic activity might be correlated to the involvement of secondary motor areas (Ikeda *et al.*, 1999).

Sleep organization is constantly normal and physiologic patterns (vertex spikes, K complexes, spindles) are present bilaterally and symmetrically. The evolution of interictal SW discharges during sleep is similar to that observed in CAE (Tassinari *et al.*, 1974). The MA may occur during drowsiness and stage I of sleep, sometimes awakening the patient *(Figure 11)*. Generalized SW discharges of variable duration (10 to 25 seconds), that are sometimes associated with bursts of myoclonias, can be observed during NREM sleep. Isolated spikes or irregular SW predominating on one or the other anterior regions are frequent during slow sleep. On the other hand no other interictal discharges are recorded and particularly no bursts of fast rhythms at 10 Hz as observed in the Lennox-Gastaut syndrome.

Seizures other than myoclonic absences

In 1/3 of cases, MA are the only seizure type observed throughout the evolution. Seizures before the onset or the diagnosis of MA were found in 38% of cases. These were above all simple absences (in some cases, in fact, these may have been MA that were not recognized), rare GTCS or other convulsive seizures, generally of a clonic type. In only one case a lasting febrile convulsion was noted. GTCS were noted in 45% of cases. They were rare in half of the cases (< 1/year) and in the other cases they were frequent (1/month) and occurred without circadian distribution. Simple absences were mentioned in 4% of cases, sometimes accompanied by eyelids myoclonias. In 33% of cases were mentioned sudden and brutal falls which have however never been recorded. Absence status without myoclonias accompanied by SW discharges on the EEG was recorded in 17% of cases. Only one patient in our series has presented a status with rhythmical myoclonias and diffuse SW discharges, which was interrupted by an intravenous injection of diazepam. About 10% of patients had more than 2 types of seizures.

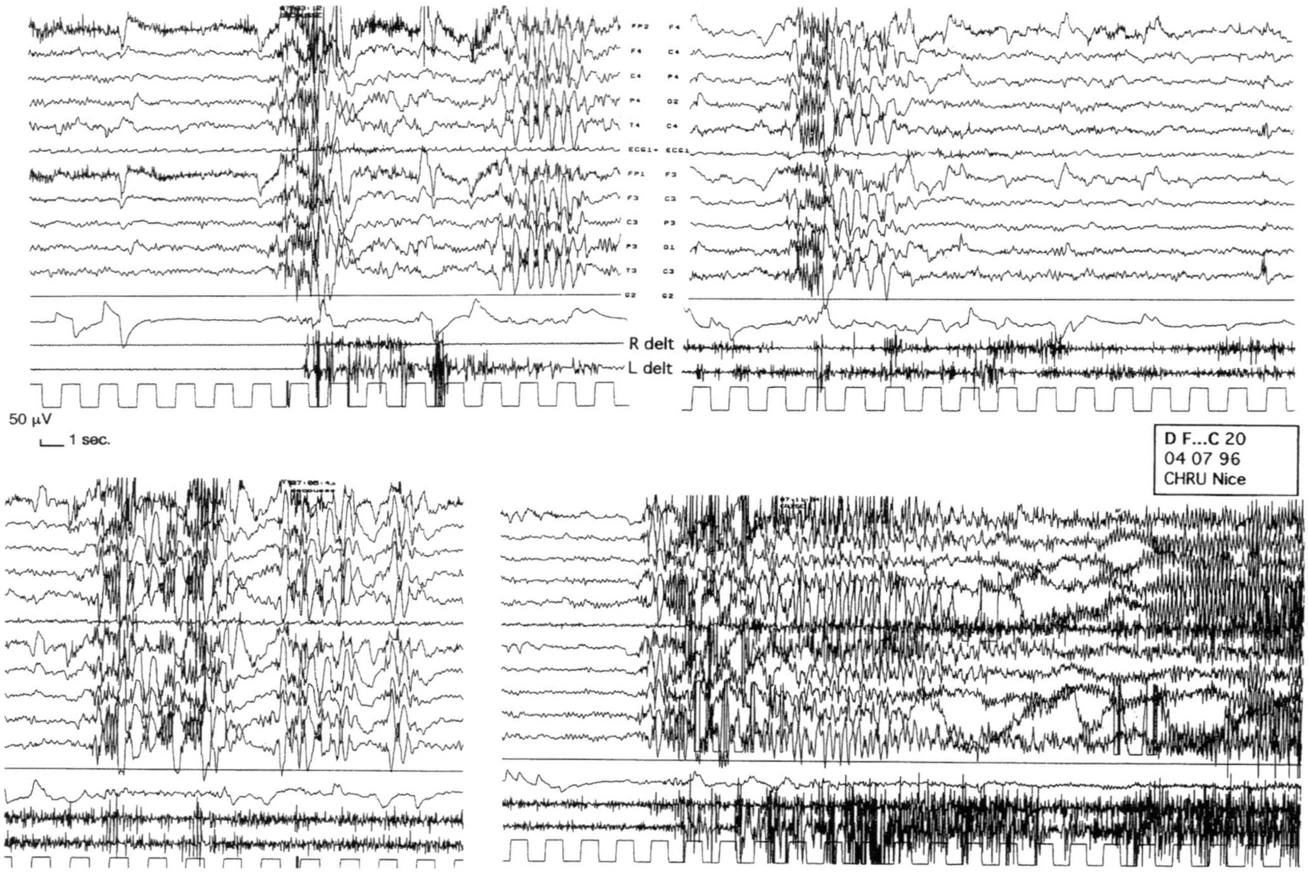

Figure 9

JME in a 20 year old woman recorded at morning awakening, after partial sleep deprivation. Several generalized PSW discharges with massive bilateral jerks are associated with the increased interictal changes, and precede by some minutes the occurrence of a GTCS. The onset of the tonic phase is preceded by a volley of massive bilateral MJ that lasts 10 seconds.

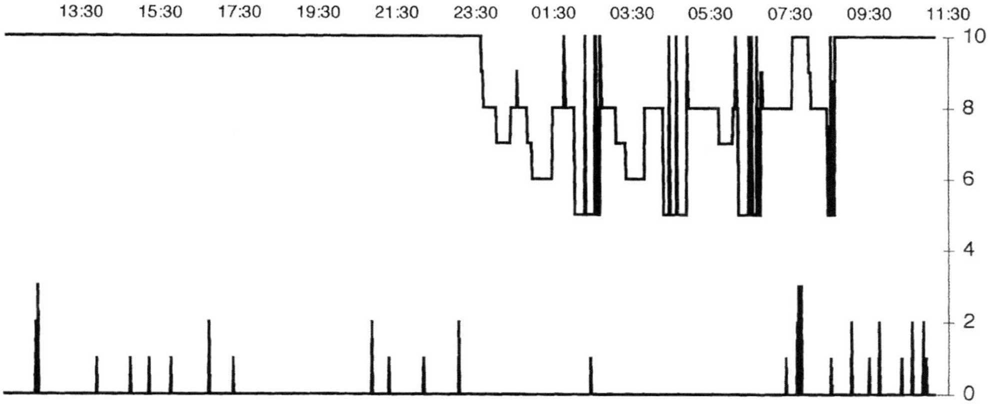

Figure 10

Activation profile of paroxysmal changes over 24 hours in a 24-year-old women with JME on VPA, 1,000 mg/d (Medilog 9000 system). Numerous PSW discharges at awakening at 7.30 AM and 8.30 AM (final awakening). Presence of isolated discharges at other times of the day, with long periods devoid of any discharge, especially in the late afternoon.

Evolution

In 1973, Lugaresi *et al.* studied the evolutive aspects. A longitudinal study of long-term prognosis performed on the 42 cases of the Centre Saint-Paul (Bureau & Tassinari, 2005) shows that MA disappear in 38% of the cases (16/42) (Group 1) and that they persist or that epilepsy changes in the other 26 cases (Group 2). The follow up of the patients after the onset of epilepsy varied from 3 years 4 months to 29 years with a median of 13 years 2 months.

In Group 1, the mean follow-up after the end of MA is of 11 years 6 months (range 4–15 years) and the follow up in Group 2 is of 12 years 5 months (7 years-23 years) after the onset of MAs. The different parameters studied show that there are more personal antecedents in Group 1 than in Group 2 (47% *vs.* 20%). A family history of epilepsy is less frequent in Group 1 than in Group 2 (13% *vs.* 33%). The age of onset of MA is approximately the same in the 2 groups (mean: 7 years). The main difference concerns the associated seizures which were present in 80% of Group 2 and only in 35% of Group 1. In Group 2, the seizures were mainly represented by GTCS, seizures with falls and absence status while in Group 1 simple absences were the main associated seizure type.

In Group 2, 5 patients have had at a certain time of the follow-up a disappearance of MA and the appearance of other seizure types such as atypical absences with slow SW and clinical or subclinical tonic seizures, particularly during wakefulness or light sleep accompanied on the EEG by fast rhythms, resulting in an electroclinical picture similar to that of the Lennox-Gastaut syndrome. This state was transitory in 2 cases; MA reappeared later and remained the only seizure type, with a comparatively benign outcome. In the 3 other cases the disappearance of the generalized SW complexes was replaced by focal frontal spikes and a frontal partial status occurred in one case controlled by phenytoin.

The appearance or worsening of psychomotor retardation was observed in both groups but it was more severe and concerned more children in Group 2.

One of the factors predictive of good or bad outcome, *i.e.*, adequate treatment as mentionned by Tassinari *et al.* (1992; 1994; 1995), is not confirmed in our long term study of 42 patients. Indeed, the association in 17 cases of sodium valproate (VPA) and ethosuximide (ESM) at appropriate doses led to a remission in only 8 cases (47%). There was no notable difference between the time when the VPA + ESM cotherapy was given and the onset of MA (4 years 2 months,

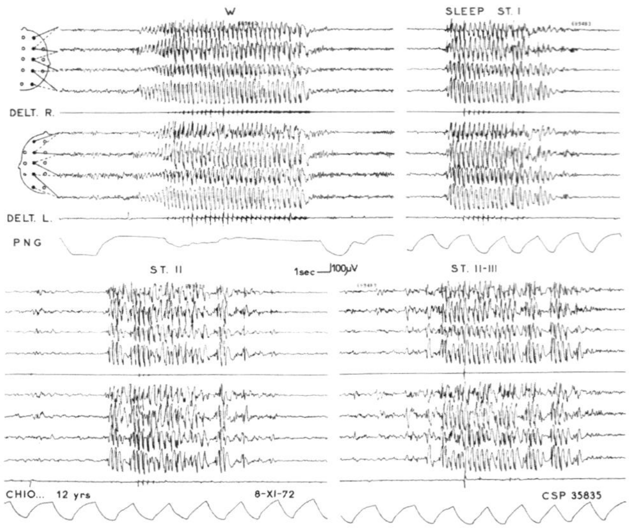

Figure 11 **Upper left: awake recording showing rhythmic myoclonic jerks with a slight tonic contraction.** Upper right: **at sleep onset (NREM stage 1), there is a decrease in the duration and intensity of the clinical manifestations.** Lower left and right: **in NREM sleep stages 2 and 3, the myoclonic jerks have practically disappeared and the EEG SW discharges are less rhythmical.**

Group 1 and 3 years 6 months, Group 2). The plasma levels in the 2 groups were quite similar (VPA: 105,5 mg/L in Group 1 *vs.* 90 mg/L in Group 2 and ESM 60 mg/L *vs.* 70 mg/L). Patients with unfavourable outcome had numerous GTCS associated with MAs. They had never received phenytoin or carbamazepine which in other 5 cases have been considered factors of worsening. Thus in our series the evolution of epilepsy seems to depend primarily on the existence of associated GTCS (as also noted by Yang *et al.*, 2009) and is not in relation with the existence of signs of encephalopathy (27% in Group 1 and 9% in Group 2).

The syndrome of EMA represents a particular form of epilepsy of childhood, because of a type of seizure that is observed exclusively in this form of epilepsy. The recognition of the specific seizure type rests on direct clinical observation and polygraphic EEG-video recording. The EEG-EMG pattern of MAs is specific and allows differential diagnosis with other generalized seizure types. The diagnosis of MAs is per se sufficient for the identification of a syndrome, namely myoclonic absence epilepsy, which stands among cryptogenic or symptomatic generalized epilepsies in the international classification of epilepsies and epileptic syndromes (Commission, 1989). In fact there are two forms: a pure form in which MAs are the only or predominant type of seizures and another form in which MAs are associated with other seizure types, particularly with frequent GTCS. The later form has a poorer prognosis. This prognosis does not depend on the treatment or on the timing of its prescription after the onset of MAs

Other absence epilepsies

Absence epilepsy of early childhood

Absence epilepsies with onset before age 3 years are considered as "early-onset" and constitute a rare and heterogeneous group, representing around 1% of all epilepsies with onset before age 3 for Chaix *et al.* (2003) and 0.7% for Caraballo *et al.* (2011). A single family with a multiplex sibship has been reported (Titomanlio *et al.*, 2007). Only a few cases may be included into well-defined epileptic syndromes, like CAE or BMEI or eyelid myoclonias with absence. In a series of 10 patients with onset before age 3 (Chaix *et al.*, 2003), 8 patients were unclassifiable. The absences in these infants and young children are often characterized by a myoclonic component: 4 out of 10 cases for Chaix *et al.* (2003), including 2 with non-rhythmic myoclonias and 2 with eyelid myoclonias; 27 out of 39 cases for Caraballo *et al.* (2011), including 6 with eyelid myoclonias and 21 with peripheral myoclonic jerks. Although some of these patients may correspond to an early form of CAE, or to a variant of early idiopathic myoclonic epilepsy, with good prognosis in both cases, there is a significant proportion of patients who develop behavioural problems or developmental delay.

A glucose-transporter 1 (GLUT-1) deficiency may be the cause (Leary *et al.*, 2003). The SYNGAP1 encephalopathy may begin with early-onset TA, but is characterized mostly by eyelid myoclonias and drop attacks (Vlaskamp *et al.*, 2019). For the latter, the ketogenic diet may be used. For the others, classical anti-absence drugs may help control the seizures, but a large proportion, much higher than in classical CAE, appears to be drug-resistant with persisting frequent absences: 5 out of 10 for Chaix *et al.* (2003), even in the absence of associated myoclonias; 15 out of 35 among those with myoclonic jerks, *vs.* 2 out of 11 among those without myoclonic components (Caraballo *et al.* (2011). In contradiction with these findings, Giordano *et al.* (2013) reported 16 cases with TA onset in the first year of life, seizure freedom in 11 with the first anti-absence drug, negative *SLC2A1* gene analysis and consider that these patients belong to the spectrum of CAE.

Eyelid myoclonias with absences

The syndrome of eyelid myoclonia with absences was first described by Jeavons in 1977 as a form of photosensitive epilepsy (Jeavons, 1977) and was confirmed by other investigators (Appleton *et al.*, 1993). It is considered more a myoclonic than an absence syndrome (Panayiotopoulos, 2005; Striano *et al.*, 2002). The following definition was proposed by Panayiotopoulos (2005): Jeavons syndrome (eyelid myoclonia with absences) is an idiopathic epileptic syndrome manifested with frequent (pyknoleptic) seizures, consisting of eyelid myoclonia often associated with absences. Onset is usually in childhood (range 2–14 years) (Panayiotopoulos, 2005) but the seizures persists into adulthood. The seizures are brief (3–6 seconds) and occur mainly after eye closure *(Figure 12)*. They consist of eyelid

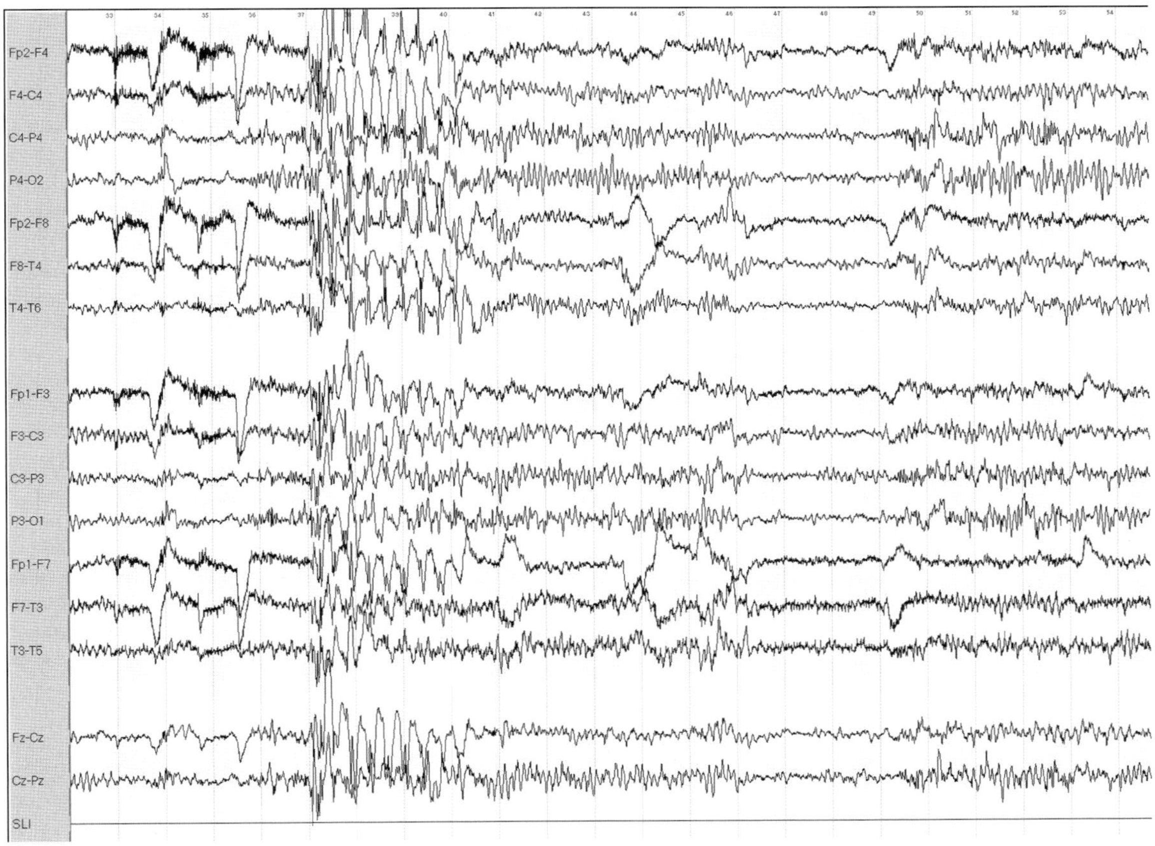

Figure 12

14-year old girl who had a history of absence seizures from age 1 year 6 months on. She had mild intellectual delay and resistant, short absences (intermittently with marked photoparoxysmal response on her EEGs). At age 14, persistance of short absences associated with eye closure and fast eyelid myoclonias. The EEG plate shows that eye closure is followed by posterior fast activities that quickly spead into a generalized discharge of 3-Hz spike and waves that lasts for 3.5 seconds.

myoclonia, which persists throughout the attack with or without absences. Absences without eyelid myoclonia do not occur. The eyelid myoclonia consists of marked, fast rhythmic jerks of the eyelids, often associated with jerky upward deviation of the eyeballs and retropulsion of the head. There is probably an associated tonic component of the involved muscles. If the seizure is prolonged, impairment of consciousness occurs. The latter is mild or moderately severe without associated automatisms. Milder seizures of eyelid myoclonia without absences are common, particularly in adults and treated patients, and may occur without EEG accompaniments.

All patients are highly photosensitive in childhood, and photoparoxysmal responses are recorded from all untreated young patients. but this declines with age. Infrequent GTCS, either induced by lights or spontaneous, are probably inevitable in the long term and are likely to occur after sleep deprivation, fatigue and alcohol indulgence. Myoclonic jerks of the limbs may occur, but are infrequent and random. Jeavons syndrome is resistant to treatment, and may be lifelong. Self-induction can occur. However, clinical absences may become less frequent with age. The EEG ictal manifestations consist mainly of generalized polyspike-waves at 3-6 Hz, which are more likely to occur after eye closure in an illuminated room. Total darkness abolishes the abnormalities related to eye closure.

Perioral myoclonia with absences

Panayiotopoulos *et al.* (1994) reported that typical absences with marked perioral myoclonia may constitute a type of seizure. However, this type of seizure is often combined with other clinical and EEG features constituting perhaps a new syndrome among IGE: perioral myoclonia with absences (PMA). The age of onset ranges from 2 to 13 years (median 10 years), but a 41-year old patient has been reported (Dearborn & Kaplan, 2014). There is a female preponderance. A family history of epilepsy is common (Panayiotopoulos, 2005). The characteristic feature consists in localized rhythmic myoclonus of the perioral facial muscles (lip myoclonus) or occasionally of the masticatory muscles (jaw myoclonus). Impairment of consciousness varies from severe to mild. Duration is usually brief, ranging from 2 to 10 seconds. PMA may be very frequent and occur many times a day. GTCS occur in all patients either early or several years after the onset of PMAs, they are infrequent and are usually heralded by clusters of PMAs.

Ictal EEG shows generalized discharges of spikes, more often irregular polyspikes and slow waves at 3–5 Hz, and may also show bilateral rhythmic contraction of the orbicularis oris and masseter associated with increased tone in the mylohyoidus (d'Orsi *et al.*, 2011). PMA are not associated with eye-closure and photosensitivity. Absence status is frequent (Agathonikou *et al.*, 1998) and can end with GTCS. The syndrome is lifelong and often resistant to medication. Accordingto Hirsh & Panayiotopoulos (2005): "lips and chin myoclonia are by themselves insufficient symptoms to justify a syndromic individualization, because of a possible moderate myoclonic component in CAE and JAE (Hirsch *et al.*, 1994; Capovilla *et al.*, 2001; Panayiotopoulos, 2005). However, a unique combination of characteristic clinico-EEG features is likely in perioral myoclonia with absences".

Absence status epilepsy

Absence status epilepsy is a distinct entity of IGE proposed by Genton *et al.* (2008) characterized by recurrent, unprovoked episodes of typical absence status *(Figure 13)* with an onset after puberty. These patients could have infrequent GTCS and rarely absences, which may remain undiagnosed or inapparent, much like the "phantom absences" described below. Similar findings have been reported as isolates cases or short series (Baykan *et al.*, 2002; Gélisse *et al.*, 2009; Iyer & Nisha, 2014). The occurrence of recurrent pure absence status has also been reported in children (Caraballo *et al.*, 2018). Diagnosis may be difficult because interictal changes are often atypical, and many patients carry a mistaken diagnosis of focal epilepsy with prolonged seizure aggravation due to inadequate drugs (Genton *et al.*, 2008).

Idiopathic generalized epilepsy with phantom absences

IGE with phantom absences was first described by Panayiotopoulos *et al.* (1997). "Phantom" means that the absences are inconspicuous and never appreciated prior the onset of GTCS usually starting in adulthood. Absence status is frequent in these patients (50% of the cases). Absences with exclusively mild or inconspicuous impairment of consciousness are exclusion criteria for JAE (Panayiotopoulos, 2010).

Differential diagnosis of absence epilepsies

The diagnosis of absence epilepsy may be difficult in some cases. Three child neurologists independently classified epilepsy syndromes in a cohort of children with newly diagnosed epilepsy and seven of 74 CAE were not diagnosed as such by one of the three (Berg *et al.*, 1999). In practical terms, a child suspected of typical absences should be asked to overbreathe for 3 minutes counting his/her breaths. Hyperventilation will provoke an absence in nearly all untreated children with CAE (Hirsch *et al.*, 1994; Wirrell *et al.*, 1996b). This procedure should preferably be video-taped for documentation of the clinical features.

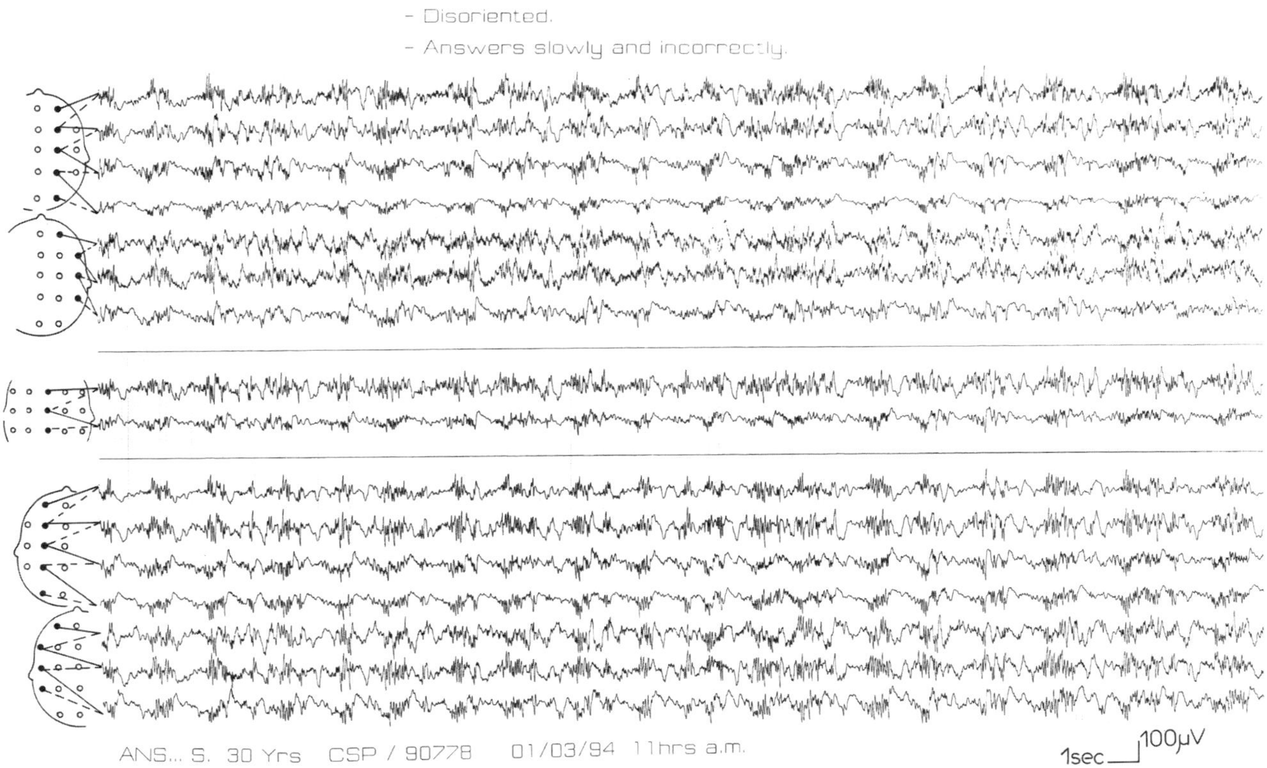

Figure 13

30-year-old woman with recurrent episodes of absence status since age 14, mostly with moderate confusion, lasting between several hours and a full day. She had had several tonic-clonic seizures when she was treated with carbamazepine. She came in the clinic by bus, accompanied by her mother, who said that she was "tired". She answered correctly, but slowly, and was slightly disoriented. The status resisted IV diazepam and stopped 2 hours after infusion of valproate.

A should be differentiated from non epileptic manifestations: attention disturbance and day-dreaming. The differential diagnosis of CAE from complex partial seizures should be easy though automatisms may be common in both.

TA seizures from frontopolar lobe origin may be concomitant to more or less regular bilateral 3-Hz spike-waves discharges (Tukel & Jasper, 1952; Fegersten & Roger, 1961; Ferrie *et al.*, 1995). Focal motor components, asymmetrical ictal discharges or stable interictal frontal foci in the EEG may help in their differentiation. MRI may demonstrate frontal abnormalities (Ferrie *et al.*, 1995) or subependymal grey matter heterotopia (Raymond & Fish, 1996). However, rare focal EEG abnormalities are possible in CAE (Beaumanoir *et al.*, 1974; Lombroso, 1997; Yoshinaga *et al.*, 2004). Some focal epilepsies especially of temporal origin may be mistaken for JAE when the absences last more than 20 seconds and are associated with automatisms *(Figures 7 and 8)*.

The major diagnostic problem is among the various syndromes of IGE with TA. There is an overlap with JAE starting earlier and CAE later than 10 years of age (Janz *et al.*, 1994). There is also a clear overlap between CAE and JME: Martinez-Juarez *et al.* (2006) studied 257 prospectively ascertained JME patients and encountered four groups: 1) classic JME (72%); 2) CAE evolving to JME (18%); 3) JME with adolescent absence (7%); and 4) JME with astatic seizures (3%). Absence seizures occur in one third of JME patients but these are usually very mild, often inconspicuous and have different EEG patterns (Panayiotopoulos *et al.*, 1989; Genton *et al.*, 2000). Absence epilepsies with a strong photosensitivity may belong to other IGE syndromes rather than JAE (Panayiotopoulos, 2010). According to this author "clinical photosensitivity, which is a consistent provocation of seizures (absences, GTCS or jerks) may be incompatible with JAE".

The "intermediate petit mal" (Lugaresi *et al.*, 1973) probably corresponds to similar situations. It was described as a borderline between CAE and more severe conditions, with slow spike-waves during absences and a comparatively poor prognosis. The presence of polyspike discharges during sleep is probably a predictor of poor prognosis with persisting seizures in adulthood (Michelucci *et al.*, 1996; Guye *et al.*, 2001). Some patients start this type of epilepsy at adolescence. They fulfill most of the criteria of IGE but they have an unusual history with GTCS, absence seizures, falls and drug resistance. The absence seizures are more or less typical. The EEGs showed generalized fast rhythms during NREM sleep similar to Lennox-Gastaut syndrome. These patients with refractory epilepsy with sleep-related fast activities are considered "intermediary" between IGE and symptomatic generalized epilepsies (Crespel *et al.*, 2006; Genton *et al.*, 2009).

In genetically predisposed individuals, brain damage may precipitate TA occurrence, most often associated with neurological signs and/or mental retardation. This category was 10% of patients with TA in a Swedish population-based study (Olsson, 1988). Ferrie *et al.* made a list of diffuse and focal cerebral pathologies in which TA have been reported (Ferrie *et al.*, 1995). In alphabetic order: arteriovenous malformations, autism, biochemical disturbances, brain tumors, cerebral abscess, congenital microcephaly, craniostenosis, Down syndrome, drugs/drug withdrawal, encephalitides, endocrine disturbances, head injury, hemiplegia, hydrocephalus, hypothalamic lesions (Mullatti *et al.*, 2003), juvenile Batten's disease, mitochondrial encephalopathies, neonatal intracranial haemorrhage, precocious puberty, progressive myoclonic epilepsy, Sturge-Weber syndrome, subacute sclerosing panencephalitis, tuberculous meningitis, and tuberous sclerosis. Most of these reports are old and, hence, poorly documented and one may wonder how many patients fitted with CAE characteristics. Subtentorial lesions are noteworthy, because they may disturb the corticothalamic oscillatory networks. Prognosis is that of the underlying patholoy. In most cases, the association is probably coincidental. However, cerebral pathology may modify the expression of a genetic seizure susceptibility (Ferrie *et al.*, 1995). In these cases, the correct diagnosis is symptomatic absence epilepsy, with a less favorable outcome.

TA with a mild clonic component (Commission,1981), in which myoclonias involve only eyelids and face, shoud not be mistaken for MA. In 2001, Cappovilla *et al.* (2001) investigated 12 patients with absence seizures associated with myoclonic manifestations and a SW dischargeat 3 Hz similar as observed in MA or in typical absences. The myoclonias in their cases were typically restricted to the facial areas (eyebrows, nostrils, perioral regions, chin) or neck muscles, contrary to the MA in which there is a constant and prominent involvement of the proximal limb muscles. They had a benign evolution: during follow-up, seven patients withdrew from treatment without relapse. This study points out the importance of plygraphic recordings to differentiate between absences with myoclonias and myoclonic absences. Giovanardi Rossi *et al.* (1988) described as *atypical* MA 4 cases in which the clinical diagnosis could be invoked because of the association, during a seizure, of loss of contact, eyelid myoclonias and myoclonias of the arms. However, there were atypical clinical phenomena, such as slow falls in 2 cases. The seizures were elicited by the opening or the closure of the eyes in 3 cases. The EEG was different, above all because of the existence of fast rhythms occurring between the SW discharges or preceding the generalized 3-Hz spike-waves discharges. Elia *et al.* (1998) studied 14 patients with MAs. Among these, 7 had chromosomal abnormalities (Angelman syndrome: 4, 12p trisomy: 2, inv dup [15]). In these cases, the MA were atypical because of their early onset, their brief duration and the mild intensity of the myoclonias and the tonic contraction.

Treatment

In the treatment of TA, the first line drugs are ethosuximide (ESM), sodium valproate (VPA) and lamotrigine (LTG), alone or in combination. A landmark double-blind, controlled study comparing VPA, ESM and LTG (Glauser *et al.*, 2010) showed that VPA and ESM were more effective than LTG and ESM was associated with fewer cognitive side-effects. Older studies had shown that VPA controls absences in 75% of patients and has the advantage also to control generalized tonic-clonic seizures (70%) and myoclonic jerks (7%). Rare cases of paradoxical aggravation in CAE with VPA are reported, this might be related to a genetic heterogeneity of CAE (Lerman-Sagie *et al.*, 2001). Similarly, LTG may control absences in possibly 50–60%, GTCS in 50–60% but may worsen myoclonic jerks; hypersensitivity immune reaction is possible (Frank *et al.*, 1999; Gericke *et al.*, 1999; Coppola *et al.*, 2004a, 2004b). ESM controls 70% of absences but is considered undesirable as monotherapy if other generalized seizures are at risk. However, Schmitt *et al.* (2007) showed that ESM and VPA carried the same risk of GTCS in patients with CAE. Minute doses of LTG added to VPA may have a dramatic beneficial effect. However, VPA may be undesirable for teenage girl and young women.

Clonazepam, clobazam, acetazolamide are second-line drugs, sharing similar risks of tolerance and adverse effects. Levetiracetam may aggravate absences, in CAE or other IGE. Syndromes (Auvin *et al.*, 2011), but may also help control resistant absences (Di Bonaventura *et al.*, 2005, Nolan *et al.*, 2019). Topiramate monotherapy was shown to be inefficient against absences in CAE (Pina-Garza *et al.*, 2011).

Despite this clear-cut evidence of anti-absence drug efficacy, many children with typical absence seizures would still be treated with inappropriate drugs (Parker *et al.*, 1998). Conversely, carbamazepine, oxcarbazepine, vigabatrin, gabapentin and tiagabine are contra-indicated because of their pro-absence effect (Parker *et al.*, 1998; Genton, 2000; Gélisse *et al.*, 2004; Thomas *et al.*, 2006). Phenytoin and phenobarbital are contra-indicated because of their usual inefficacy (Panayiotopoulos, 2001, 2005).

Thus monotherapy with sodium VPA, ESM or LTG should be the choice first-line treatment in CAE. Monotherapy should not be abandoned before making sure that maximum tolerated dose has been achieved if smaller doses have failed. There are anecdotal reports whereby children may not respond to syrup of VPA despite adequate levels but seizures stop if this is replaced by tablets or microspheres of VPA. If monotherapy fails or unacceptable adverse reactions appear, then replacement of one by the other is the alternative. The best possible combination is adding small doses of LTG to adequate doses of VPA. Gradual withdrawal of medication is recommended in patients with CAE who have been seizure-free for 1-2 years and have a normalized EEG. EEG confirmation of the seizure free state is needed during this withdrawal period.

In JAE, there is a frequent association of absences and GTCS, and the first line drug is valproate. When there is concern about teratogenicity or side effects, lamotrigine can be given (Wheless *et al.*, 2005, 2007) but lamotrigine is less effective than valproate (Marson *et al.*, 2007; Mazurkiewicz-Beidzinska *et al.*, 2010). A severe aggravation of myoclonic jerks has been reported in a patient with JAE several months after LTG titration. The drug was stopped and jerks ceased (Crespel *et al.*, 2005).

In myoclonic absences, the classical treatment associating valproate (VPA) + ethosuximide (ESM) with appropriate plasma levels is most efficient if MA are not associated with other seizures types, particularly with GTCS. MA are usually completely controlled by this cotherapy. In some cases, the association of phenobarbital, VPA and benzodiazepines leads to a good control of seizures. Manonmani *et al.* (1994) and Wallace (1998) showed that the association VPA or ESM with lamotrigine had a favorable effect in cases that resist the classical treatment. The efficacity of more recent antiepileptic drugs currently used in refractory absences or in myoclonic epilepsies, such as levetiracetam, topiramate, felbamate, zonisamide has not been properly evaluated in EMAs. Häusler *et al.* (2011) observed a favourable response to add-on rufinamide treatment on MA refractory to conventional antiepileptic drugs.

Zonisamide is an antiepileptic drug with a broad-spectrum action. Experimental studies indicate that zonisamide could be a blocker of T-type voltage-gated calcium channel (MacDonald, 2002; Matar *et al.*, 2009). Zonisamide was used in add-on therapy in 6 drug-resistant JAE patients (dose range: 175–600 mg/day; follow-up range: 28–39 months) (Da Costa Ferreira, 2009). Four patients became seizure free. Two had a significant reduction of seizures.

Levetiracetam is effective in IGE, especially JME (Noachtar *et al.*, 2008). In JAE, the responder rate for all seizure types was significantly higher for levetiracetam than placebo (53.3% *vs.* 25%; p = 0.004) (target dose of 3,000 mg/day for adults and 60 mg/kg/day for children) (Rosenfeld *et al.*, 2009). Fattore *et al.* (2011) reported that the responder rate seems to be modest in children and adolescents with newly diagnosed absence epilepsy and Auvin *et al.* (2011) reported increase of number of absences in three JAE patients with levetiracetam. In these 3 adolescents, the daily dose was quite high (more than 1,750 mg/day in all). Levetiracetam is not a drug of choice for absences but it can be proposed in association with ethosuximide or valproate or lamotrigine in order to control GTCS. The same rule can be applied to topiramate.

Other drugs have been indicated in selected cases. Sultiame brought some improvement in patients with refractory absences (Gorman & Shahwan, 2016). Two newer agents have shown broad-spectrum efficacy across epilepsy types, and are candidates for the treatment of TA. Brivaracetam, chemically related to levetiracetam but with pharmacodynamic differences, shows apparently more efficacy against myoclonias and GTCS than against absences (Strzelczyk *et al.*, 2018), although single case reports point to efficacy against refractory absences (Grande-Martin *et al.*, 2018). Perampanel, which is a non-competitive inhibitor of AMPA receptors, is indicated in GTCS, often used against myoclonias (Gil-Lopez *et al.*, 2018) and was used in a large group of IGE patients (Villanueva *et al.*, 2018): at 12 months, the seizure-free rate was 59% for all seizures (88/149), 63% for GTCS (72/115), 65% for myoclonic seizures (31/48), and 51% for absence seizures (24/47).

Conclusion

The absence epilepsies include two frequent, clinically different form of "idiopathic" generalized epilepsy, CAE and JAE, but also several other syndromes with variable clinical expression and severity. All distinct syndromes remain genetically heterogeneous (and still unresolved), and many patients with typical absences remain difficult to classify precisely in the light of our present knowledge (Guilhoto *et al.*, 2003). Most absence epilepsies are treatable, and three anticonvulsants stand out as primary anti-absence agents: valproate, ethosuximide and lamotrigine. Other drugs may exhibit an aggravating effect, increasing absences in various syndromes of IGE. The syndromic approach – clinical and EEG phenotyping – is still necessary for progress in genetic and pharmacologic studies.

REFERENCES ▶

Adie WJ (1924): Pyknolepsy: a form of epilepsy occurring in children, with a good prognosis. *Brain* 47: 96–102.

Agathonikou A, Giannakodimos S, Koutroumanidis M, *et al.* (1997): Idiopathic generalised epilepsies in adults with onset of typical absences before the age of 10 years. *Epilepsia* 38 (Suppl. 3): 213.

Agathonikou A, Panayiotopoulos CP, Giannakodimos S, Koutroumanidis M (1998): Typical absence status in adults: diagnostic and syndromic considerations. *Epilepsia* 39: 1265–1276.

Aghakhani Y, Bagshaw AP, Benar CG, *et al.* (2004): fMRI activation during spike and wave discharges in idiopathic generalized epilepsy. *Brain* 127: 1127–1144.

Agostinelli S, Accorsi P, Beccaria F, *et al* (2013): Clinical dissection of early onset absence epilepsy in children and prognostic implications. *Epilepsia* 54: 1761–1770.

Aicardi J (1994): Typical absences in the first two years of life. In: Duncan JS, Panayiotopoulos CP (eds). *Typical Absences and Related Syndromes*, pp. 284–288. London: Churchill Livingstone.

Andermann E (1980): Genetic aspects of epilepsy. In: Robb P (ed) *Epilepsy Updated: Causes and Treatment*, pp. 11–24. New York: Year Book Medical Publisher.

Appleton RE, Panayiotopoulos CP, Acomb BA, Beirne M (1993): Eyelid myoclonia with typical absences: an epilepsy syndrome. *J Neurol Neurosurg Psychiatry* 56: 1312–1316.

Audic-Gerard F, Szepetowski P, Genton P (2003): GEFS + syndrome: phenotypic variations from the newborn to the adult in a large French pedigree. *Rev Neurol* (Paris) 159: 189–195.

Auvin S, Chhun S, Berquin P, Ponchel E, Delanoë C Chiron C (2011): Aggravation of absence seizure related to levetiracetam. *Eur J Paediatr Neurol* 15: 508–511.

Bahi-Buisson N, El Sabbagh S, Soufflet C, *et al.* (2008): Myoclonic absence epilepsy with photosensitivity and a gain of function mutation in glutamate dehydrogenase. *Seizure* 17: 658–664.

Bartolomei F, Roger J, Bureau M, *et al.* (1997): Prognostic factors for childhood and juvenile absence epilepsies. *Eur Neurol* 37: 169–175.

Baykan B, Gökyğit A, Gürses C, Eraksoy M (2002): Recurrent absence status epilepticus: clinical and EEG characteristics. *Seizure* 11: 310–319.

Beaumanoir A (1976): *Les épilepsies infantiles. Problèmes de diagnostic et de traitement*. Bâle: Éditions Roche.

Beaumanoir A, Ballis T, Varfis G, Ansari K (1974): Benign epilepsy of childhood with Rolandic spikes. *Epilepsia* 15: 301–315.

Beck-Mannagetta G, Janz D, Hoffmeister U, Behl I, Scholz G (1989): Morbidity risk for seizures and epilepsy in offsprings of patients with epilepsy. In: Beck-Mannagetta G, Anderson WE, Doose H, Janz D (eds) *Genetics of the Epilepsies*, pp. 119–126. Berlin Heidelberg: Springer-Verlag.

Berg AT, Levy SR, Testa FM, Shinnar S (1999): Classification of childhood epilepsy syndromes in newly diagnosed epilepsy: interrated agreement and reasons for disagreement. *Epilepsia* 40: 439–444.

Berg AT, Shinnar S, Levy SR, Testa FM, Smith-Rapaport S, Beckerman B (2000): How well can epilepsy syndromes be identified at diagnosis? A reassessment two years after initial diagnosis. *Epilepsia* 41: 1267–1275.

Berg AT, Berkovic SF, Brodie MJ, *et al.* (2010): Revised terminology and concepts for organization of seizures and epilepsies: report of the ILAE Commission on Classification and Terminology, 2005-2009. *Epilepsia* 51: 676–685.

Bergamini L, Bram S, Broglia S, Riccio A (1965): L'insorgenza tardiva di crisi Grande Male nel Piccolo Male puro. Studio catamnestico di 78 casi. *Arch Suisses Neurol Neurochir Psychiatr* 96: 306–317.

Berkovic SF (1996): Childhood absence epilepsy and juvenile absence epilepsy. In: Wyllie E (ed) *The Treatment of Epilepsy: Principles and Practice*, pp. 461–466. Baltimore: Williams & Wilkins.

Berkovic SF, Andermann F, Andermann E, Gloor P (1987): Concepts of absence epilepsies: discrete syndromes or biological continuum? *Neurology* 37: 993–1000.

Berkovic SF, Howell RA, Hay DA, Hopper JL (1994): Epilepsy in twins. In: Wolf P (ed) *Epileptic Seizures and Syndromes*, pp. 157–164. London: John Libbey and Co.

Bergen DC, Beghi E, Medina MT. Revising the ICD-10 codes for epilepsy and seizures (2012): *Epilepsia* 53 Suppl 2: 3–5.

Bertaso F, Zhang C, Scheschonka A, de Bock F, *et al.* (2008): *PICK1* uncoupling from mGluR7a causes absence-like seizures. *Nat Neurosci* 11: 940–948.

Bianchi A and the Italian LAE Collaborative Group (1995): Study of concordance of symptoms in families with absence epilepsies. In: Duncan JS, Panayiotopoulos CP (eds) *Typical Absences and Related Epileptic Syndromes*, pp. 328–337. Edinburgh: Churchill Livingstone.

Blom S, Heijbel J, Bergfors PG (1978): Incidence of epilepsy in children: a follow-up study three years after the first seizure. *Epilepsia* 19: 343–350.

Bouma PA, Westendorp RG, van Dijk JG, Peters AC, Brouwer OF (1996): The outcome of absence epilepsy: a meta-analysis. *Neurology* 47: 802–808.

Browne TR, Dreifuss FE, PenryJK, Porter RJ, White BG (1983): Clinical and EEG estimates of absence seizure frequency. *Arch Neurol* 40: 469–472.

Bureau M, Guey J, Dravet C, Roger J (1968): Étude de la répartition des absences chez l'enfant en fonction de ses activités. *Rev Neurol* (Paris) 118: 493–494.

Bureau M, Tassinari CA (2002): The syndrome of myoclonic absences. In: Roger J, Bureau M, Dravet C, Genton P, Tassinari CA, Wolf P, (eds) *Epileptic Syndromes in Infancy, Childhood and Adolescence*, 3rd ed, pp. 305–312. Eastleigh: John Libbey & Co.

Bureau M, Tassinari CA (2005). Myoclonic absences: The seizure and the syndrome. In: Delgado-Escueta AV, Guerrini R, Medina MT, Genton P, Bureau M, Dravet C (eds). *Myoclonic Epilepsies*, pp. 185–196. Philadelphia, Lippincott Williams & Wilkins.

Callenbach PMC, Geerts AT, Arts WFM, *et al.* (1998): Familial occurrence of epilepsy in children with newly diagnosed multiple seizures: Dutch study of epilepsy in childhood. *Epilepsia* 39: 331–336.

Calmeil LF (1924): De l'épilepsie étudiée sous le rapport de son siège et de son influence sur la production de l'aliénation mentale. Paris. [*Thèse*].

Capovilla G, Rubboli G, Beccaria F, *et al.* (2001): A clinical spectrum of the myoclonic manifestations associated with typical absences in childhood absence epilepsy. A video-polygraphic study. *Epileptic Disord* 3: 57–62.

Caraballo RH, Darra R, Fontana E, Garcia R, Monese E, Dalla Bernardina B (2011): Absence seizures in the first 3 years of life: An electroclinical study of 46 cases. *Epilepsia* 52: 393–400.

Caraballo RH, Chacón S, Fasulo L, Bedoya C (2018): *De novo* absence status epilepticus in three paediatric patients: a new idiopathic epilepsy syndrome? *Epileptic Disord* 20:502–507.

Cavazzuti G.B, Ferrari F, Galli V, Benatti A (1989): Epilepsy with typical absences with onset during the first year of life. *Epilepsia* 30: 802–806.

Chaix Y, Daquin G, Monteiro F, Villeneuve N, Laguitton V, Genton P (2003): Absence epilepsy with onset before age three years: a heterogeneous and often severe condition. *Epilepsia* 44: 944–949.

Charlton MH, Yahr MD (1967): Long-term follow-up of patients with petit mal. *Arch Neurol* 16: 595–598.

Chen Y, Lu J, Pan H, Zhang Y, *et al.* (2003): Association between genetic variation of CACNA1H and childhood absence epilepsy. *Ann Neurol* 54: 239–243.

Cobb WA, Gordon N, Matthews SC, Nieman EA (1961): The occipital delta rhythm in petit mal. *Electroencephalogr Clin Neurophysiol* 13: 142–143.

Coenen AM, Van Luijtelaar EL (2003): Genetic animal models for absence epilepsy: a review of the WAG/Rij strain of rats. *Behav Genet* 33:635–655.

Commission on Classification and Terminology of the International League Against Epilepsy (1981): Proposal fora revised clinical and electroencephalographic classification of epileptic seizures. *Epilepsia* 22: 489–501.

Commission on Classification and Terminology of the International League Against Epilepsy (1989): Proposal for revised classification of epilepsies and epileptic syndromes. *Epilepsia* 30: 389–399.

Coppola G, Auricchio G, Federico F, Carotenuto M, Pascotto A (2004a): Lamotrigine *versus* valproic acid as first-line monotherapy in newly diagnosed typical absence seizures: an open-label, randomized, parallel-group study. *Epilepsia* 45: 1049–1053.

Coppola G, Licciardi F, Sciscio N, Russo F, Carotenuto M, Pascotto A (2004b): Lamotrigine as first-line drug in childhood absence epilepsy: a clinical and neurophysiological study. *Brain Dev* 26: 26–29.

Crespel A, Genton P, Berramdane M, *et al* (2005): Lamotrigine associated with exacerbation or *de novo* myoclonus in idiopathic generalized epilepsies. *Neurology* 65: 762–764.

Crespel A, Gélisse P, Bureau M, Genton P (2006): Atlas of Electroencephalography, vol. 2. *The Epilepsies. EEG and Epileptic Syndromes*. Montrouge: John Libbey Eurotext.

Crunelli V, Leresche N (2002): Childhood absence epilepsy: genes, channels, neurons and networks. *Nat Rev Neurosci* 3: 371–382.

Currier RD, Kooi KA, Saidman LJ (1963): Prognosis of pure petit mal. *Neurology* 13: 959–967.

d'Orsi G1, Demaio V, Trivisano M, *et al.* (2011): Ictal video-polygraphic features of perioral myoclonia with absences. *Epilepsy Behav* 21: 314–317.

Da Costa Ferreira J (2009): Utilisation du zonisamide dans le traitement des épilepsies généralisées idiopathiques de type absence juvénile. A propos de 6 cas. *Pharm Thesis*. University of Montpellier I.

Danober L, Deransart C, Depaulis A, Vergnes M, Marescaux C (1998): Pathophysiological mechanisms of genetic absence epilepsy in the rat. *Prog Neurobiol* 55: 27–57.

Darra F, Fontana E, Scaramuzzi V, *et al.* (1996): Typical absence seizures in the first three years of life: electroclinical study of 31 cases. *Epilepsia* 37 (Suppl. 4): 95.

Delgado-Escueta AV, Medina MT, Serratosa JM, *et al.* (1999): Mapping and positional cloning of common idiopathic generalized epilepsies: juvenile myoclonus epilepsy and childhood absence epilepsy. *Adv Neurol* 79: 351–374.

Dearborn JL, Kaplan PW (2014): Generalised electrographic seizures presenting as perioral myoclonia. *Epileptic Disord* 16: 80–83.

Depaulis A, David O, Charpier S (2016): The genetic absence epilepsy rat from Strasbourg as a model to decipher the neuronal and network mechanisms of generalized idiopathic epilepsies, *J Neurosci Methods* 260: 159–174.

Depaulis A, Charpier S (2018): Pathophysiology of absence epilepsy: Insights from genetic models. *Neurosci Lett* 22: 53–65.

Di Bonaventura C, Fattouch J, Mari F, *et al.* (2005): Clinical experience with levetiracetam in idiopathic generalized epilepsy according to different syndrome subtypes. *Epileptic Disord* 7: 231–235.

Dieterich E, Baier WK, Doose H, Tuxhorn I (1985): Long-term follow-up of childhood epilepsy with absences at onset. *Neuropediatrics* 16: 149–154.

Doose H, Völzke E, Scheffner D (1965): Verlaufsformen kindlicher Epilepsien mit Spike-Wave-Absencen. *Arch Psychiat Nervenkrankh* 207: 394–415.

Doose H, Gerken H, Horstmann T, Völzke E (1973): Genetic factors in spike wave absences. *Epilepsia* 14: 57–75.

Duncan JS (1999): Positron emission tomography receptor studies. *Adv Neurol* 79: 893–899.

Duncan JS, Panayiotopoulos CP (1995): *Typical Absences and Related Epileptic Syndromes*. Edinburgh: Churchill Livingstone.

Elia M, Guerrini R, Musumeci SA, Bonanni P, Gambardella A, Aguglia U (1998): Myoclonus absence-like seizures and chromosome abnormality syndromes. *Epilepsia* 39: 660–663.

Engel J Jr (2001): A proposed diagnostic scheme for people with epileptic seizures and with epilepsy. Report of the ILAE Task Force on Classification and Terminology. *Epilepsia* 42: 796–803.

Engel J Jr (2006): Report of the ILAE classification core group. *Epilepsia* 47: 1558–1568.

Escayg A, De Waard M, Lee DD, *et al.* (2000): Coding and noncoding variation of the human calcium-channel beta4-subunit gene CACNB4 in patients with idiopathic generalized epilepsy and episodic ataxia. *Am J Hum Genet* 66: 1531–1539.

Esquirol J (1838): De l'épilepsie. In: *Traité des maladies mentales*. Vol. I. pp. 274–355. Paris: Baillière Publishers.

Fakhoury T, Abou-Khalil B (1999): Generalized absence seizures with 10–15 Hz fast discharges. *Clin Neurophysiol* 110: 1029–1035.

Fattore C, Boniver C, Capovilla G, *et al.* (2011): A multicenter, randomized, placebo-controlled trial of levetiracetam in children and adolescents with newly diagnosed absence epilepsy. *Epilepsia* 52: 802.

Fegersten L, Roger J (1961): Frontal epileptogenic foci and their clinical correlations. *Electroencephalogr Clin Neurophysiol* 13: 905–913.

Ferrie CD, Giannakodimos S, Robinson R O, Panayiotopoulos CP (1995): Symptomatic typical absence seizures. In: Duncan JS, Panayiotopoulos CP (eds) *Typical Absences and Related Epileptic Syndromes*, pp. 241–252. Edinburgh: Churchill Livingstone.

Feucht M, Fuchs K, Pichlbauer E, *et al.* (1999): Possible association between childhood absence epilepsy and the gene encoding GABRB3. *Biol Psychiatry* 46: 997–1002.

Fisher RS, Cross JH, French JA, *et al.* (2017): Operational classification of seizure types by the International League Against Epilepsy: Position Paper of the ILAE Commission for Classification and Terminology. *Epilepsia* 58: 522–530.

Fong GC, Shah PU, Gee MN, *et al.* (1998): Childhood absence epilepsy with tonic-clonic seizures and electroencephalogram 3–4-Hz spike and multispike-slow wave complexes: linkage to chromosome 8q24. *AmJ Hum Genet* 63: 1117–1129.

Frank LM, Enlow T, Holmes GL, *et al.* (1999): Lamictal (lamotrigine) monotherapy for typical absence seizures in children. *Epilepsia* 40: 973–979.

Friedmann M (1906): Über die nichtepileptischen Absencen oder kurzen narkoleptischen Anfälle. *Dtsch Z Nervenheilk* 30: 462–492.

Gardella E, Rubboli G, Meletti S, Volpi L, Tassinari CA (2002): Polygraphic study of muscular activation pattern in myoclonic absence seizures. *Epilepsia* 43 (Suppl. 8): 98–99.

Gastaut H, Zifkin BG, Mariani E, Salas Puig J (1986): The long-term course of primary generalized epilepsy with persisting absences. *Neurology* 36: 1021–1028.

Gélisse P, Genton P, Kuate C, Pesenti A, Baldy-Moulinier M, Crespel A (2004): Worsening of seizures by oxcarbazepine in juvenile idiopathic generalized epilepsies. *Epilepsia* 45: 1282–1286.

Gélisse P, Velizarova R, Genton P, Crespel A (2009): Epilepsy with absence status: A new syndrome of idiopathic generalized epilepsy. *Rev Neurol* 165: 839–841.

Gélisse P, Serafini A, Velizarova R, Genton P, Crespel A (2011): Temporal intermittent delta activity: a marker of juvenile absence epilepsy? *Seizure* 20: 38–41.

Genton P (2000): When antiepileptic drugs aggravate epilepsy. *Brain Dev* 22: 75–80.

Genton P, Bureau M (2006): Epilepsy with myoclonic absences. *CNS Drugs* 20: 911–916.

Genton P, Gélisse P, Thomas P (2000): Juvenile myoclonic epilepsy today: current definition and limits. In: Schmitz B, Sander T (eds) *Juvenile Myoclonic Epilepsy: The Janz Syndrome*, pp. 11–32, Petersfield and Philadelphia: Wrightson Medical Publishing.

Genton P, Ferlazzo E, Thomas P (2008): Absence status epilepsy: Delineation of a distinct idiopathic generalized epilepsy syndrome. *Epilepsia* 49: 642–649.

Gericke CA, Picard F, de Saint-Martin A, Strumia S, Marescaux C, Hirsch E (1999): Efficacy of lamotrigine in idiopathic generalized epilepsy syndromes: a video-EEG-controlled, open study. *Epileptic Disord* 1: 159–165.

Giannakodimos S, Panayiotopoulos CP (1996): Eyelid myoclonia with absences in adults: a clinical and video-EEG study. *Epilepsia* 37: 36–44.

Gibberd FB (1966): The prognosis of petit mal. *Brain* 89: 531–538.

Gibbs FA, Davis H, Lennox WG (1935): The EEG in epilepsy and in conditions of impaired consciousness. *Arch Neurol Psychiatry* 34: 1134–1148.

Gibbs FA, Gibbs EL, Lennox WG (1943): Electrographic classification of epileptic patients and control subjects. *Arch Neurol Psychiatry* 50: 111–128.

Gil-López FJ, Montoya J, Falip M, *et al.* (2018): Retrospective study of perampanel efficacy and tolerability in myoclonic seizures. *Acta Neurol Scand* 138: 122–129.

Giordano L, Vignoli A, Cusmai R, *et al.* (2013): Early onset absence epilepsy with onset in the first year of life: a multicenter cohort study. *Epilepsia* 54 (Suppl. 7): 66–69.

Giovanardi Rossi P, Ricciotti A, Melideo G, Santucci M, Gobbi G (1988): Atypical myoclonic absences: clinical, electroencephalographic and neuropsychological aspects. *Clin EEG* 19: 87–94.

GlauserTA, Cnaan A, Shinnar S, *et al.* (2010): Ethosuximide, valproic acid, and lamotrigine in childhood absence epilepsy. *N Engl J Med* 362: 790–799.

Gökben S, Yilmaz S, Klepper J, Serdaroglu G, Tekgül H (2011): Video/EEG recording of myoclonic absences in GLUT1 deficiency syndrome with a hot-spot R126C mutation in the SLC2A1 gene. *Epilepsy Behav* 21: 200–202.

Gorman KM, Shahwan A (2016): Sultiame revisited: treatment of refractory absence seizures. *Epileptic Disord* 18:329–333.

Gowers WR (1881): *Epilepsies and Other Chronic Convulsive Disorders. Their Causes, Symptoms and Treatment*. London: Churchill.

Grande-Martín A, Sopelana-Garay D, Pardal-Fernández JM, *et al.* (2018): Exceptional response to brivaracetam in a patient with refractory idiopathic generalized epilepsy and absence seizures. *Epileptic Disord* 20: 60–64.

Guerrini R, Bureau M, Mattei MG, Battaglia A, Galland MC, Roger J (1990): Trisomy 12p syndrome: a chromosomal disorder associated with generalized 3-Hz spike and wave discharges. *Epilepsia* 31: 557–566.

Guye M, Bartolomei F, Gastaut JL, Chauvel P, Dravet C (2001): Absence epilepsy with fast rhythmic discharges during sleep: an intermediary form of generalized epilepsy? *Epilepsia* 42: 351–356.

Guilhoto LM, Manreza ML, Yacubian EM (2003): Syndromic classification of patients with typical absence seizures. *Arq Neuropsiquiatr* 61: 580–587.

Guiwer J, Valenti MP, De Saint-Martin A, Chassagnon S, Hirsch E (2004): Pronostic des épilepsies idiopathiques avec absences. *Epilepsies* 2: 67–74.

Guye M, Bartolomei F, Gastaut JL, Chauvel P, Dravet C (2001): Absence epilepsy with fast rhythmic discharges during sleep: an intermediary form of generalized epilepsy? *Epilepsia* 42: 351–356.

Häusler M, Kluger G, Nikanorova M (2011): Epilepsy with myoclonic absences – favourable response to add-on rufinamide treatment in 3 cases. *Neuropediatrics* 42: 28–29.

Healy L, Moran M, Singhal S, *et al.* (2018): Relapse after treatment withdrawal of antiepileptic drugs for Juvenile Absence Epilepsy and Juvenile Myoclonic Epilepsy. *Seizure* 59:116–122.

Hedström A, Olsson I (1991): Epidemiology of absence epilepsy: EEG findings and their predictive value. *Pediatr Neurol* 7: 100–104.

Hertoft P (1963): The clinical, electroencephalographic and social prognosis in petit mal epilepsy. *Epilepsia* 4: 298–314.

Hirose S, Okada M, Kanedo S, Mitsudone A (2000): Are some idiopathic epilepsies disorders of ion channels? A working hypothesis. *Epilepsy Res* 41: 191–204.

Hirsch E, Panayiotopoulos CP (2005): Childhood absence epilepsy and related syndromes. In: Roger J, Bureau M, Dravet C, Genton P, Tassinari CA, Wolf P (eds) *Epileptic Syndromes in Infancy, Childhood and Adolescence*, 4th ed, pp. 315-335. Montrouge: John Libbey Eurotext.

Hirsch E, Blanc-Platier A, Marescaux C (1994): What are the relevant criteria for a better classification of epileptic syndromes with typical absences? In: Malafosse A, Genton P, Hirsch E, Marescaux C, Broglin D, Bernasconi R (eds) *Idiopathic Generalized Epilepsies: Clinical, Experimental and Genetic Aspects*, pp. 87–93. London: John Libbey & Company Ltd.

Holmes GH, McKeever M, Adamson M (1987): Absence seizures in children: clinical and electroencephalographic features. *Ann Neurol* 21: 268–273.

Holowach J, Thurston DL, O'Leary JL (1962): Petit mal epilepsy. *Pediatrics* 30: 893–901.

Imbrici P, Cusimano A, D'Adamo MC, De Curtis A, Pessia M (2003): Functional characterization of an episodic ataxia type-1 mutation occurring in the S1 segment of hKv1.1 channels. *Pflugers Arch* 446: 373–379.

Ikeda A, Nagamine T, Kunieda T, *et al.* (1999): Clonic convulsion caused by epileptic discharges arising from the human supplementary motor area as studied by subdural recording. *Epileptic Disord* 1: 21–26.

Ikeda H, Fujiwara T, Shigematsu H, *et al.* (2011): Symptoms and clinical course of epilepsy with myoclonic absences. *No To Hattatsu* (in Japanese): 43(1): 14–18.

ILAE classification of epilepsies: its applicability and practical value of different diagnostic categories. Osservatorio Regionale per L'Epilessia (OREp), Lombardy (1996). *Epilepsia* 37: 1051–1059.

Imbrici P, Jaffe SL, Eunson LH, *et al.* (2004): Dysfunction of the brain calcium channel CaV2.1 in absence epilepsy and episodic ataxia. *Brain* 127: 2682–2692.

Iyer RS, Nisha SR (2014): Absence status epilepsy: report of a rare electroclinical syndrome. *Neurol India* 62: 224–226.

Jallon P, Latour P (2005): Epidemiology of idiopathic generalized epilepsies. *Epilepsia* 46 (Suppl. 9): 10–14.

Janz D (1969): *Die Epilepsien. Spezielle Pathologie und Therapie*. Stuttgart: Thieme.

Janz D, Christian W (1957): Impulsiv Petit-Mal. Dtsch Z Nervenheilk 176: 346–386. (English translation by Genton P. In: Malafosse A, Genton P, Hirsch E, Marescaux C, Broglin D, Bernasconi M (eds) *Idiopathic Generalized Epilepsies,* pp. 229–251. London: John Libbey.

Janz D, Beck-Mannagetta G, Spröder B, Spröder J, Waltz S (1994): Childhood absence epilepsy (pyknolepsy) and juvenile absence epilepsy: one or two syndromes? In: Wolf P (ed) *Epileptic Seizures and Syndromes*, pp. 115–126. London: John Libbey & Company.

Jasper HH, Drooglever-Fortuyn J (1947): Experimental studies on the functional anatomy of petit mal epilepsy. *Res Publ Assoc Nerv Ment Dis* 26: 272–298.

Jeavons PM (1977): Nosological problems of myoclonic epilepsies in childhood and adolescence. *Dev Med Child Neurol* 19: 3–8.

Jus A, Jus K (1962): Retrograde amnesia in Petit Mal. *Arch Gen Psychiatry* 6: 163–167.

Klitten LL, Meiler RS, Nikanorova M, Silahtarogl A, Hjalgrim H, Tommerup (2011): A balanced translocation disrupts SYNGAP1 in a patient with intellectual disability, speech impairment and epilepsy with myoclonic absences (EMA). *Epilepsia* 52: 190–193.

Kobayashi K, Ohtsuka Y, Ohmori I, *et al.* (2004): Clinical and electroencephalographic characteristics of children with febrile seizures plus. *Brain Dev* 26: 262–268.

Leary LD, Wang D, Nordli DR Jr, Engelstad K, De Vivo DC (2003): Seizure characterization and electroencephalographic features in Glut-1 deficiency syndrome. *Epilepsia* 44: 701– 707.

Lennox WG (1945): The Petit Mal epilepsies. *JAMA* 129: 1069–1073.

Lennox WG, Davis JP (1950): Clinical correlates of the fast and slow spike-wave electroencephalogram. *Pediatrics* 5: 626–644.

Lennox WG, Lennox MA (1960): *Epilepsy and Related Disorders*, pp. 546–574. Boston: Little, Brown and Co.

Lerche H, Weber YG, Baier H, *et al.* (2001): Generalized epilepsy with febrile seizures plus: further heterogeneity in a large family. *Neurology* 57: 1191–1198.

Lerman-Sagie T, Watemberg N, Kramer U, Shahar E, Lerman P (2001): Absence seizures aggravated by valproic acid. *Epilepsia* 42: 941–943.

Livingston S, Torres I, Pauli LL, Rider RV (1965): Petit Mal epilepsy. Results of a prolonged follow-up study of 117 patients. *JAMA* 194: 227–232.

Loiseau P (1992): Childhood absence epilepsy. In: Roger J, Bureau M, Dravet C, Dreifuss F, Perret A, Wolf P (eds). *Epileptic Syndromes in Infancy, Childhood and Adolescence*, 3rd ed, pp. 135–150. London: John Libbey & Company.

Loiseau P, Duché B (1995): Childhood absence epilepsy. In: Duncan JS, Panayiotopoulos CP (eds). *Typical Absences and Related Epileptic Syndromes,* pp. 152–160. Edinburgh: Churchill Livingstone.

Loiseau P, Panayiotopoulos CP (2005): Childhood absence epilepsy. In: Gilman S (ed) *Medlink Neurology*. San Diego SA: Arbor Publishing Corp.

Loiseau P, Cohadon F, Cohadon S (1966): Le petit mal qui guérit, guérit rapidement. *J Med Lyon* 1108: 1557–1565.

Loiseau P, Duché B, Pédespan JM (1995a): Absence epilepsies. *Epilepsia* 36: 1182–1186.

Loiseau P, Duché B, Pédespan JM (1995b): Splitting or lumping absence epilepsies. *Epilepsia* 36: 116.

Loiseau J, Loiseau P, Guyot M, Duché B, Dartigues JF, Aublet B (1990): Survey of seizure disorders in the French southwest. I. Incidence of epileptic syndromes. *Epilepsia* 31: 391–396.

Loiseau P, Panayiotopoulos CP (2000): Childhood absence epilepsy. In: Gilman S (ed) *Neurobase*. San Diego SA: Arbor Publishing Corp.

Loiseau P, Pestre M, Dartigues JF, Commenges D, Barberger-Gateau C, Cohadon S (1983): Long-term prognosis in two forms of childhood epilepsy: typical absence seizures and epilepsy with Rolandic (centrotemporal) EEG foci. *Ann Neurol* 13: 642–648.

Loiseau P, Panayiotopoulos CP, Hirsch E (2002): Childhood absence epilepsy and related syndromes. In: Roger J, Bureau M, Dravet C, Genton P, Tassinari CA, Wolf P (eds) *Epileptic Syndromes in Infancy, Childhood and Adolescence*; 3rd ed, pp. 285–303. Eastleigh: John Libbey & Co.

Lombroso CT (1997): Consistent EEG focalities detected in subjects with primary generalized epilepsies monitored for two decades. *Epilepsia* 38: 797–812.

Lu Y, Waltz S, Stenzel K, Muhle H, Stephani U (2008): Photosensitivity in epileptic syndromes of childhood and adolescence. *Epileptic Disord* 10: 136–143.

Lugaresi E, Pazzaglia P, Franck L, *et al.* (1973): Evolution and prognosis of primary generalized epilepsy of the petit mal type. In: Lugaresi E, Pazzaglia P, Tassinari CA (eds) *Evolution and Prognosis of Epilepsy*, pp. 2-22. Bologna: Aulo Gaggi.

Macdonald RL (2002): Zonisamide: mechanisms of action. In: Levy RH, Mattson RH, Meldrum BS, Perucca E (eds) *Antiepileptic Drugs*, 5th ed, pp. 868–872. Philadelphia: Lippincott Williams & Wilkins.

Maljevic S, Krampfl K, Cobilanschi J (2006): A mutation in the GABA(A) receptor alpha(1)-subunit is associated with absence epilepsy. *Ann Neurol* 59: 983–987.

Manonmani V, Wallace SJ (1994): Epilepsy with myoclonic absences. *Arch Dis* Child 70: 288–290.

Marini C, Harkin LA, Wallace RH, Mulley JC, Scheffer IE, Berkovic SF (2003): Childhood absence epilepsy and febrile seizures: a family with a GABA(A) receptor mutation. *Brain* 126 (Pt1): 230–240.

Marini C, Scheffer IE, Crossland KM, *et al.* (2004): Genetic architecture of idiopathic generalized epilepsy: clinical genetic analysis of 55 multiplex families. *Epilepsia* 45: 467–478.

Marson AG, Al-Kharusi AM, Alwaidh M, *et al.* (2007): The SANAD study of effectiveness of valproate, lamotrigine, or topiramate for generalized and unclassifiable epilepsy: an unblinded randomised controlled trial. *Lancet* 369: 1016–1026.

Martinez-Juarez IE, Alonso ME, Medina MT, *et al.* (2006): Juvenile myoclonic epilepsy subsyndromes: family studies and long-term follow-up. *Brain* 129 (Pt 5): 1269–1280.

Matar N, Jin W, Wrubel H, Hescheler J, Schneider T, Weiergräber M (2009): Zonisamide block of cloned human T-type voltage-gated calcium channels. *Epilepsy Res* 83: 224–234.

Mazurkiewicz-Betdzinska M, Szmuda M, Matheisel A (2010): Long-term efficacy of valproate versus lamotrigine in treatment of idiopathic generalized epilepsies in children and adolescents. *Seizure* 19: 195–197.

Medina MT, Duron RM, Alonso ME, *et al.* (2005): Childhood absence epilepsy evolving to juvenile myoclonic epilepsy: electrical and genetic features. In: Delgado-Escueta AV, Guerrini R, Medina MT, Genton P, Bureau M, Dravet C (eds) *Myoclonic epilepsies: Adv Neurol* (vol. 95), pp. 197–216. Philadelphia: Lippincott Williams & Wilkins.

Meencke HJ (1995): Pathological findings in childhood absence epilepsy. In: Duncan JS, Panayiotopoulos CP (eds) *Typical Absences and Related Epileptic Syndromes*, pp. 122–132. Edinburgh: Churchill Livingstone.

Meencke HJ, Janz D (1985): The significance of microdysgenesia in primary generalized epilepsy: an answer to the considerations of Lyon and Gastaut. *Epilepsia* 26: 368–371.

Metrakos JD, Metrakos K (1966): Childhood epilepsy of subcortical ("centrencephalic") origin. Some questions and answers for the pediatrician. *Clin Pediatr* (Phila.) 5: 536–542.

Metrakos K, Metrakos JD (1961a): Genetics of convulsive disorders. II. Genetic and electroencephalographic studies in centrencephalic epilepsy. *Neurology* 11: 474–483.

Metrakos K, Metrakos JD (1961b): Is the centrencephalic EEG inherited as a dominant? *Electroencephalogr Clin Neurophysiol* 13: 289.

Michelucci R, Rubboli G, Passarelli D, *et al.* (1996): Electroclinical features of idiopathic generalized epilepsy with persisting absences in adult life. *J Neurol Neurosurg Psychiatry* 61: 471–417.

Mirsky AF, Duncan CC, Levav ML (1995): Neuropsychological and psychophysiological aspects of absence epilepsy. In: Duncan JS, Panayiotopoulos CP (eds) *Typical Absences and Related Epileptic Syndromes*, pp. 112–121. Edinburgh: Churchill Livingstone.

Mirsky AF, Duncan CC, Myslobodsky MS (1986): Petit mal epilepsy: a review and integration of recent information. *J Clin Neurophysiol* 3:179–208.

Muccioli L, Licchetta L, Stipa C, *et al.* (2018): Juvenile absence epilepsy relapsing as recurrent absence status, mimicking transient global amnesia, in an elderly patient. *Epileptic Disord* 20:557–561.

Mullatti N, Selway R, Nashef L, *et al.* (2003): The clinical spectrum of epilepsy in children and adults with hypothalamic hamartoma. *Epilepsia* 44: 1310–1319.

Mullen SA, Berkovic SF (2018): ILAE Genetics Commission. Genetic generalized epilepsies. *Epilepsia* 59: 1148–1153.

Myers KA, Scheffer IE (2018): Myoclonic absence seizures with complex gestural automatisms. *Eur J Paediatr Neurol* 22: 532–535.

Nehlig A, Valenti MP, Thiriaux A, Hirsch E, Marescaux C, Namer IJ (2004): Ictal and interictal perfusion variations measured by SISCOM analysis in typical childhood absence seizures. *Epileptic Disord* 6: 247–253.

Ngomba RT, Santolini I, Salt TE, *et al.* (2011): Metabotropic glutamate receptors in the thalamocortical network: Strategic targets for the treatment of absence epilepsy. *Epilepsia* 52: 1211–1222.

Noachtar S, Andermann E, Meyvisch P, Andermann F, Gough WB, Schiemann-Delgado J, N166 Levetiracetam Study Group (2008): Levetiracetam for the treatment of idiopathic generalized epilepsy with myoclonic seizures. *Neurology* 70: 607–616.

Nolan D, Lester SG, Rau SM, Shellhaas RA (2019): Clinical use and efficacy of Levetiracetam for absence epilepsies. *J Child Neurol* 34: 94–98.

Obeid T (1994): Clinical and genetic aspects of juvenile absence epilepsy. *J Neurol* 241: 487–491.

Oller-Daurella L, Sanchez ME (1981): Evolucion de las ausencias tipicas. *Rev Neurol* (Barcelona) 9: 81–102.

Olsson I (1988): Epidemiology of absence epilepsy. I. Concept and incidence. *Acta Paediatr Scand* 77: 860–866.

Panayiotopoulos CP (2005): Idiopathic generalised epilepsies. In: Panayiotopoulos CP (ed) *The Epilepsies: Seizures, Syndromes and Management*, pp. 271–348. Oxford: Bladon Medical Publishing.

Panayiotopoulos CP (2005): Syndromes of idiopathic generalized epilepsies not recognized by the International League Against Epilepsy. *Epilepsia* 46 (Suppl. 9): 57–66.

Panayiotopoulos CP (2010): *A Clinical Guide to Epileptic Syndromes and their Treatment*, Revised 2nd ed. London: Springer Healthcare Ltd.

Panayiotopoulos CP, Obeid T (1989): Juvenile myoclonic epilepsy: an autosomal recessive disease. *Ann Neurol* 25: 440–443.

Panayiotopoulos CP, Obeid T, Waheed G (1989): Differentiation of typical absence seizures in epileptic syndromes. *Brain* 112: 1039–1056.

Panayiotopoulos CP (1997): Absence epilepsies. In: Engel JJ, Pedley TA (eds) *Epilepsy: a Comprehensive Textbook*, pp. 2327–2346. Philadelphia: Lippincott-Raven.

Panayiotopoulos CP (2001): The treatment of typical absence seizures and related epileptic syndromes. *Paediatric Drugs* 3: 379–403.

Panayiotopoulos CP, Ferrie CD, Giannakodimos S, *et al.* (1994): Perioral myoclonia with absences: a new syndrome. In: Wolf P (ed) *Epileptic Seizures and Syndromes*, pp. 143–153, London: John Libbey & Company Ltd.

Panayiotopoulos CP (2005): Idiopathic generalised epilepsies. In: Panayiotopoulos CP (ed) *The Epilepsies: Seizures, Syndromes and Management*, pp. 271–348. Oxford: Bladon Medical Publishing.

Panayiotopoulos CP, Obeid T, Waheed G (1989): Differenciation of typical absence seizures in epileptic syndromes. A video EEG study of 224 seizures in 20 patients. *Brain* 112: 1039–1056.

Panayiotopoulos CP, Ferrie CD, Giannakodimos S, Robinson RO (1994): Perioral myoclonia with absences: a new syndrome. In: Wolf P (ed) *Epileptic Seizures and Syndromes*, pp. 143–153. London: John Libbey and Co.

Panayiotopoulos CP, Koutroumanidis M, Giannakodimos S, Agathonikou A (1997): Idiopathic generalized epilepsy in adults manifested by phantom absences generalized tonic-clonic seizures, and frequent absence status. *J Neurol Neurosurg Psychiatry* 63: 622–627.

Panayiotopoulos CP, Ferrie CD, Koutroumanidis M, Rowlinson S, Sanders S (2001): Idiopathic generalised epilepsy with phantom absences and absence status in a child. *Epileptic Disord* 3: 63–66.

Panayiotopoulos CP, Chroni E, Daskalopoulos C, Baker A, Rowlinson S, Walsh P (1992): Typical absence seizures in adults: clinical, EEG, video-EEG findings and diagnostic/syndromic considerations. *J Neurol Neurosurg Psychiatry* 55: 1002–1008.

Parker APJ, Agathonikou A, Robinson RO, Panayiotopoulos CP (1998): Inappropriate use of carbamazepine and vigabatrin in typical absence seizures. *Dev Med Child Neurol* 40: 517–519.

Penry JK, Dreifuss RE (1969): Automatisms associated with the absence of petit mal epilepsy. *Arch Neurol* 21: 142–149.

Penry JK, Porter RJ, Dreifuss FE (1975): Simultaneous recording of absence seizures with video tape and electroencephalography. A study of 374 seizures in 48 patients. *Brain* 98: 427–440.

Peterman MG (1945): Abstract of discussion on The petit mal epilepsies: their treatment with tridione. *JAMA* 129: 1074.

Pina-Garza JE, Schwarzman L, Wiegand F, Hulihan J (2011): A pilot study of topiramate in childhood absence epilepsy. *Acta Neurol Scand* 123: 54–59.

Porter RJ (1993): The absence epilepsies. Epilepsia 34 (Suppl 3): S42–S48. Raymond AA, Fish DR (1996): EEG features of focal malformations of cortical development. *J Clin Neurophysiol* 13: 495–506.

Reynolds JR (1861): Epilepsy, its Symptoms, Treatment. London, Churchill. Robinson R, Taske N, Sander T, *et al.* (2002): Linkage analysis between childhood absence epilepsy and genes encoding GABAA and GABAB receptors, voltage-dependent calcium channels, and the ECA1 region on chromosome 8q. *Epilepsy Res* 48: 169–179.

Rocca WA, Sharbrough FW, Hauser WA, Annegers JF, Schoenberg BS (1987): Risk factors for absence seizures: a population-based case-control study in Rochester, Minnesota. *Neurology* 37: 1309–1314.

Rosenfeld WE, Benbadis S, Edrich P, Tassinari CA, Hirsch E (2009): Levetiracetam as add-on therapy for idiopathic generalized epilepsy syndromes with onset during adolescence: analysis of two randomized, double-blind, placebo-controlled studies. *Epilepsy Res* 85: 72–80.

Rudolf G, Bihoreau MT, Godfrey RF, *et al.* (2004): Polygenic control of idiopathic generalized epilepsy phenotypes in the genetic absence rats from Strasbourg (GAERS). *Epilepsia* 45: 301–308.

Ryvlin P, Mauguière F (1998): Imagerie fonctionnelle dans les épilepsies généralisées idiopathiques. Rev *Neurol* (Paris) 154: 691–696.

Salas Puig J, Acebes A, Gonzalez C, Tunon A, Guisasola LM, Lahoz CH (1990): Epilepsy with myoclonic absences. *Neurologia* (in Spanish) 5: 242–245.

Salek-Haddadi A, Lemieux L, Merschhemke M, Friston KJ, Duncan JS, Fish DR (2003): Functional magnetic resonance imaging of human absence seizures. *Ann Neurol* 53: 663–667.

Sander T, Hildmann T, Kretz R, *et al.* (1997): Allelic association of juvenile absence epilepsy with a GluR5 kainate receptor gene (GRIK1) polymorphism. *Am J Med Genet* 74: 416–421.

Sander T, Peters G, Jaliz D, *et al.* (1998): The gene encoding the 1 A-voltage-dependant calcium channel (CACN1A4) is not a candidate for causing common subtypes of idiopathic generalized epilepsy. *Epilepsy Res* 29: 115–122.

Sarkisova K, van Luijtelaar G (2011): The WAG/Rij strain: a genetic animal model of absence epilepsy with comorbidity of depression [corrected]. *Prog Neuropsychopharmacol Biol Psychiatry* 35: 854–876.

Sato S, Dreifuss FE, Penry JK (1976): Prognostic factors in absence seizures. *Neurology* 28: 788–796.

Sauer H (1916): Übergehäufte kleine Anfälle bei Kindern (Pyknolepsie). *Mschr Psychiat Neurol* 40: 276–300.

Scheffer IE, Berkovic S, Capovilla G, *et al.* (2017): ILAE classification of the epilepsies: Position paper of the ILAE Commission for Classification and Terminology. *Epilepsia* 58: 512–521.

Schmitt B, Kovacevic-Preradovic T, Critelli H, Molinari L (2007): Is ethosuximide a risk factor for generalised tonic-clonic seizures in absence epilepsy? *Neuropediatrics* 38: 83–87.

Sgro V, Paola M, Canevini M, Canger R (1996): Absence epilepsy: electroclinical study of 37 cases. *Epilepsia* 37 (Suppl 4): 106.

Siren A, Eriksson K, Jalava H, Kilpinen-Loisa P, Koivikko M (2002): Idiopathic generalized epilepsies with 3 Hz and faster spike wave discharges: a population-based study with evaluation and long-term follow-up in 71 patients. *Epileptic Disord* 4: 209–216.

Snead OCIII, Depaulis A, Vergnes M, Marescaux C (1999): Absence Epilepsy: Advances in Experimental Animal Models. In: Delgado-Escueta AV, Wilson WA, Olsen RW, Porter RJ (eds) *Jasper's Basic Mechanisms of the Epilepsies*, 3rd Edition: *Advances in Neurology*, Vol. 79, pp. 253–278. Philadelphia: Lippincott Williams & Wilkins.

Strzelczyk A, Kay L, Bauer S, *et al.* (2018): Use of brivaracetam in genetic generalized epilepsies and for acute, intravenous treatment of absence status epilepticus. *Epilepsia* 59: 1549–1556.

Striano S, Striano P, Nocerino C, *et al.* (2002): Eyelid myoclonia with absences: an overlooked epileptic syndrome? *Neurophysiol Clin* 32: 287–296.

Striano P, Weber YG, Toliat MR, *et al.* EPICURE Consortium (2012): GLUT1 mutations are a rare cause of familial idiopathic generalized epilepsy. *Neurology* 78: 557–562.

Sugimoto Y, Morita R, Amano K, *et al.* (2000): Childhood absence epilepsy in 8q24: refinement of candidate region and construction of physical map. *Genomics* 68: 264–272.

Suls A, Mullen SA, Weber YG, *et al.* (2009): Early onset absence epilepsy caused by mutations in the glucose transporter GLUT1. *Ann Neurol* 66: 415–419.

Tanaka M, Olsen RW, Medina MT, *et al.* (2008): Hyperglycosylation and reduced GABA currents of mutated GABRB3 polypeptide in remitting childhood absence epilepsy. *Am J Hum Genet* 82: 1249–1261.

Tassinari CA, Bureau M (1985): Epilepsy with myoclonic absences. In: RogerJ, Dravet C, Bureau M, Dreifuss F, Wolf P (eds) *Epileptic Syndromes in Infancy, Childhood and Adolescence*, pp. 121–129. London: John Libbey & Co.

Tassinari CA, Lyagoubi S, Santos V, *et al.* (1969): Étude des décharges de pointes ondes chez l'homme II: Les aspects cliniques et électroencéphalographiques des absences myocloniques. *Rev Neurol* 121: 379–383.

Tassinari CA, Lyagoubi S, Gambarelli F, RogerJ, Gastaut H (1971): Relationships between EEG discharge and neuromuscular phenomena. *Electroenceph Clin Neurophysiol* 31: 176.

Tassinari CA, Bureau-Paillas M, Dalla Bernardina B, *et al.* (1974): Generalized epilepsies and seizures during sleep. A polygraphic study. In: Van Praag HM, Meinardi H (eds) *Brain and Sleep*, pp. 154–166. Amsterdam: De Erven Bhon.

Tassinari CA, Bureau M, Thomas P (1992): Epilepsy with myoclonic absences. In: Roger J, Bureau M, Dravet C, Dreifuss F, Perret A, Wolf P (eds). *Epileptic Syndromes in Infancy, Childhood and Adolescence* (2nd ed), pp. 151–160. London: John Libbey & Co.

Tassinari CA, Michelucci R (1994): Epilepsy with myoclonic absences: a reappraisal. In: Wolf P (ed) *Epileptic Seizures and Syndromes*, pp. 137–141. London: John Libbey & Co.

Tassinari CA, Michelucci R, Rubboli G, *et al.* (1995): Myoclonic absence epilepsy. In: Duncan JS, Panayiotopoulos CP (eds) *Typical Absences and Related Syndromes*, pp. 187–195. London: Churchill Livingstone.

Temkin O (1971): *The Falling Sickness: A History of Epilepsy from the Greeks to the Beginning of Modern Neurology*. Baltimore: Johns Hopkins Press.

Tissot SA (1770): Traité de l'épilepsie, faisant le Tome troisième du Traité des nerfs et de leurs maladies. Lausanne: Antoine Chapuis.

Titomanlio L, Romano A, Bellini G, *et al.* (2007): Familial occurrence of early-onset childhood absence epilepsy. *Eur J Paediatr Neurol* 11: 178–180.

Thomas P (1999): Absence status epilepsy. *Rev Neurol* (Paris) 155: 1023–1038.

Thomas P, Valton L, Genton P (2006): Absence and myoclonic status epilepticus precipitated by antiepileptic drugs in idiopathic generalized epilepsy. *Brain* 129: 1281–1292.

Tissot SA (1770): *Traité de l'épilepsie*. Lausanne: Chapuis.

Trinka E, Baumgartner S, Unterberger I, *et al.* (2004): Long-term prognosis for childhood and juvenile absence epilepsy. *J Neurol* 251: 1235–1241.

Tukel K, Jasper H (1952): The EEG in parasagittal lesions. *Electroencephalogr Clin Neurophysiol* 4: 284–290.

Verrotti A, Greco R, Chiarelle F, Domizio S, Sabatino G, Morgese G (1999): Epilepsy with myoclonic absences with early onset: a follow-up study. *J Child Neurol* 14: 746–749.

Villanueva V, Montoya J, Castillo A, *et al.* (2018): Perampanel in routine clinical use in idiopathic generalized epilepsy: The 12-month GENERAL study. *Epilepsia* 59: 1740–1752.

Vlaskamp DRM, Shaw BJ, Burgess R, *et al.* (2019): SYNGAP1 encephalopathy: A distinctive generalized developmental and epileptic encephalopathy. *Neurology* 92: e96–e107.

Wallace RH, Marini C, Petrou S, *et al.* (2001): Mutant GABA(A) receptor gamma2-subunit in childhood absence epilepsy and febrile seizures. *Nat Genet* 28: 49–52.

Wallace SJ (1998): Myoclonus and epilepsy in childhood: a review of treatment with valproate, ethosuximide, lamotrigine and zonisamide. *Epilepsy Res* 29: 147–154.

Weber YG, Lerche H (2008): Genetic mechanisms in idiopathic epilepsies. *Dev Med Child Neurol* 50: 648–654.

Weir B (1965): The morphology of the spike-wave complex. *Electroencephalogr Clin Neurophysiol* 19: 284–290.

Wheless JW, Clarke DF, Carpenter D (2005): Treatment of pediatric epilepsy: expert opinion, 2005. *J Child Neurol* 20 (Suppl 1): 1–56.

Wheless JW, Clarke DF, Arzimanoglou A, Carpenter D (2007): Treatment of pediatric epilepsy: European expert opinion, 2007. *Epileptic Disord* 9: 353–412.

Winawer MR, Rabinowitz D, Pedley TA, Hauser WA, Ottman R (2003): Genetic influences on myoclonic and absence seizures. *Neurology* 61: 1576–1581.

Wirrell EC, Camfield CS, Camfield PR, Gordon KE, Dooley JM (1996a): Long-term prognosis of typical childhood epilepsy: remission or progression to juvenile myoclonic epilepsy. *Neurology* 47: 912–918.

Wirrell EC, Camfield PR, Gordon KE, Camfield CS, Dooley JM, Hanna BD (1996b): Will a critical level of hyperventilation-induced hypocapnia always induce an absence seizure? *Epilepsia* 37: 459–462.

Woermann FG, Sisodiya SM, Free SL, Duncan JS (1998): Quantitative MRI in patients with idiopathic generalized epilepsy. Evidence of widespread cerebral structural changes. *Brain* 121: 1661–1667.

Wolf P (1992): Juvenile absence epilepsy. In: Roger J, Bureau M, Dravet C, Dreifuss F, Perret A, Wolf P (eds) *Epileptic Syndromes in Infancy, Childhood and Adolescence,* 2nd ed., pp. 307-312. London: John Libbey & Co Ltd.

Wolf P (1995): Juvenile absence epilepsy. In: Duncan JS, Panayiotopoulos CP (eds) *Typical Absences and Related Epileptic Syndromes*, pp. 161–167. London: Churchill.

Wolf P, Inoue Y (1984): Therapeutic response of absence seizures in patients of an epilepsy clinic for adolescents and adults. *J Neurol* 231: 225–229.

Wolf P, Goosses R (1986): Relation of photosensitivity to epileptic syndromes. *J Neurol Neurosurg Psychiat* 49: 1386–1391.

Wolf P, Inoue Y (2005): Complex reflex epilepsies: reading epilepsy and praxis induction. In: Roger J, Bureau M, Dravet C, Genton P, Tassinari CA, Wolf P (eds) *Epileptic Syndromes in Infancy, Childhood and Adolescence*, 4th ed., pp. 347–358. Montrouge: John Libbey Eurotext.

Yalçin O, Baykan B, Agan K, *et al.* (2011): An association analysis at 2q36 reveals a new candidate susceptibility gene for juvenile absence epilepsy and/or absence seizures associated with generalized tonic-clonic seizures. *Epilepsia* 52: 975–983.

Yang Z, Liu X, Qin J, Jiang Y (2009): Neck myoclonia with absence seizures: report of 3 cases. *J Child Neurol* 24: 1026–1029.

Yang ZX, Liu XY, Qin J, Zhang YH, Wu Y, Jiang YW (2009a). Clinical and electroencephalographic characteristics of epilepsy with myoclonic absences. *Zhonghua Er Ke Za Zhi* (in Chinese) 47: 862–866.

Yoshinaga H, Ohtsuka Y, Tamai K, *et al.* (2004): EEG in childhood absence epilepsy. *Seizure* 13: 296–302.

Zanzmera P, Menon RN, Karkare K, Soni H, Jagtap S, Radhakrishnan A (2016): Epilepsy with myoclonic absences: Electroclinical characteristics in a distinctive pediatric epilepsy phenotype. *Epilepsy Behav* 64: 242–247.

WITH VIDEO SUPPLEMENTS

CHAPTER 16
ISOLATED FOCAL (FORMERLY PARTIAL) SEIZURES IN ADOLESCENCE

Roberto H. Caraballo[1] and Pierre Jallon[2]

[1] Department of Neurology, Hospital Nacional de Pediatria "Prof. Dr. Juan P. Garrahan", Buenos Aires, Argentina
[2] Thézan des Corbières, France

This chapter is dedicated to the memory of Pierre Loiseau, who was the first to describe the syndrome of isolated focal seizures.

Introduction

The concept of idiopathic, or in the new terminology genetic or probably genetic (Berg *et al.*, 2010; Scheffer *et al.*, 2016), and benign focal epilepsies in childhood is relevant not only from the theoretical point of view, but also as a practical tool because the term implies absence of a structural brain lesion. It took many years for idiopathic or probably genetic focal epileptic syndromes in childhood to become generally accepted as it was against the logical rule, *i.e.* that focal seizures arise from focal epileptogenic areas that are typically due to an underlying focal cortical lesion. Idiopathic focal epilepsies in infancy were first described in the late 1980s and started to be accepted after the report of a series of familial cases with benign evolution (Caraballo & Fejerman, 2007).

In 1972, a French study was published presenting 14 patients suffering from unprovoked isolated focal seizures with onset in adolescence who were followed up for 4–12 years (Loiseau *et al.*, 1972). A few years later, the same group published a series of 83 adolescents with the same features (Loiseau & Orgogozo, 1978). In 1992, the series was updated and 108 patients with a minimum follow-up of 5 years were reported (Loiseau & Louiset, 1992). The authors still considered the entity to be a syndrome, although they preferred the term "benign partial epileptic seizures of adolescence" because the patients usually did not present chronically recurrent seizures.

Thereafter, different series of patients were reported (Mauri *et al.*, 1996; King *et al.*, 1998, 1999; Capovilla *et al.*, 2001; Panayiotopoulos, 2005; Caraballo *et al.*, 1999, 2004, 2007). Mauri *et al.* presented 10 cases in an abstract. King *et al.* published eight cases that were part of an important first-seizure study of 300 consecutive patients over 5 years of age. Ninety-two of 300 patients between 10 and 20 years of age were enrolled and 37 of them had focal epilepsies. Of these, eight met the more strict criteria for diagnosis of benign focal seizures of adolescence, but six others (registered as "unclassified") were apparently also idiopathic and had a benign course. Capovilla *et al.* presented 37 cases, but normal EEGs were found in only 17. The authors hypothesized that other forms of idiopathic focal epilepsies might be seen in adolescents. Nevertheless, they suggested that, even though these patients presented with spikes in the interictal EEGs, they should not be medicated.

When in 1989 in the ILAE Classification (Commission, 1989) at the end of the table of "Special syndromes" a category of "Isolated seizures or isolated status epilepticus" was added, Loiseau proposed the term "isolated partial seizures of adolescence" (IPSA) for the condition (Loiseau *et al.*, 2002). The group from Buenos Aires preferred the name "benign focal seizures of adolescence" for this epileptic syndrome. In this chapter we will use the term IPSA for the entity.

Subsequently, Panayiotopoulos described 120 personal cases in a book chapter (2005). At a single center in Buenos Aires, Argentina, Caraballo *et al.* (2004) reported 15 cases with a 6-year follow-up in a first prospective study and three years later a larger series of

44 patients including the 29 previously presented patients (Caraballo *et al.*, 1999; 2004; 2007). Currently, in this latter series overall 52 cases have been seen.

Whether IPSA is an epileptic syndrome or only a single seizure event associated with a normal interictal EEG is controversial. In view of the knowledge gained since the first recognition of the entity, we believe that IPSA should be considered as a benign, age-related, self-limited epileptic syndrome starting in the second decade of life. It is a transient condition, predominantly occurring in males, with a peak of onset between 13 and 14 years of age. IPSA is characterized by simple focal motor and somatosensory seizures with secondary generalization occurring isolated or in a cluster in the first 24–48 hours after onset. The seizures occur predominantly when awake and have a benign course. The interictal EEG, neurological examination, and neuroradiological images are normal and a family history of epilepsy is rare (Loiseau & Louiset, 1992).

Epidemiology

According to Loiseau & Louiset (1992), a quarter of patients who suffer focal seizures – single or in a cluster of up to five seizures during 36 hours, never to occur again – with an onset between 12 and 18 years of age, have a benign course. IPSA may account for 7.5–22% of patients having simple focal seizures in the second decade of life (Panayiotopoulos, 1996, 2005; King *et al.*, 1999). However, to date no population-based study documents these figures. Around 220 cases have been described (Mauri *et al.*, 1996; Panayiotopoulos, 1996; King *et al.*, 1999; Capovilla *et al.*, 2001; Loiseau *et al.*, 2002; Caraballo *et al.*, 1999, 2004, 2007).

In the Buenos Aires study, at a single center 15 adolescent patients with IPSA were registered over a period of 6 years. In the same period, 17 adolescents were diagnosed with late-onset benign focal epilepsy of childhood, eight adolescents with focal epilepsy of unknown etiology and 38 adolescents with structural focal epilepsy.

IPSA may be more frequent than reported in the literature. This is because IPSA is characterized by a single seizure or cluster of seizures that are short-lived and transient and probably do not get to be controlled by an epileptologist. On the other hand, it is important that this type of patients be recognized to accurately determine the real prevalence of the entity.

Clinical features

The age at onset of the seizures ranges from 11 to 18 years, with a mean age of 13.5 and a median age of 14 years. There is a 70% male preponderance. Physical examination and mental status of the patients are normal.

Simple focal seizures are the most frequent type of seizures, characterized by eye and/or head deviation, facial tonic or clonic focal seizures, and visual symptoms followed by upper-limb clonic focal seizures. Seizures are followed by tonic-clonic seizures with secondary generalization in 50% of the cases. The motor seizures do not follow a Jacksonian march. In some cases a sensorimotor Jacksonian march was reported (Loiseau & Orgogozo, 1978) and this was an inclusion criterion selected for the eight cases presented by King *et al.* (1999). Rarely, the seizures are complex focal and characterized by motion arrest and oral automatisms, followed or not by secondarily generalized tonic-clonic seizures. In the series of Capovilla *et al.* (2001), a subgroup of patients presented with versive seizures.

The duration of the seizures is around 2 minutes, but in patients who have secondarily generalized seizures they last 5 minutes approximately (Caraballo *et al.*, 1999, 2004; King *et al.*, 1999; Capovilla *et al.*, 2001; Loiseau *et al.*, 2002). Speech difficulties, autonomic symptoms, and vertigo were reported in the cases of Loiseau *et al.* (2002). Psychological symptoms are rare (Loiseau *et al.*, 2002). Auditory, olfactory, and gustatory symptoms have never been reported. (Caraballo *et al.*, 1999, 2004; King *et al.*, 1998, 1999; Capovilla *et al.*, 2001; Loiseau *et al.*, 2002).

Although these focal motor and somatosensory seizures with or without secondary generalization may also be found in cryptogenic and symptomatic focal epilepsies, a hallmark of IPSA is that postictal signs, such as motor or psychological deficits, are extremely rare. The teenager is typically fully aware and may give a reliable account of the onset of the clinical manifestations of the simple focal seizures throughout the whole event.

The first diagnosed seizure actually may not have been the first experienced seizure of the patient (Loiseau *et al.*, 2002). Generalized convulsive seizures are easier to recognize whereas a brief focal seizure can be less impressive and more difficult to identify. In this setting, it is very important to take a detailed interview from both the parents and the teenager.

Most seizures occur when the patient is awake, but in rare cases patients also have seizures during sleep.

The event is a single seizure in 75%. In the remaining 25%, a cluster of two to four seizures occurs in less than 36–48 hours.

Romeo *et al.* (2008) described nine patients with a diagnosis of benign focal seizures of adolescence who experienced an ictal sensation of impending danger coming from behind, followed by coordinated behavior of head-turning toward the danger. This feeling was described in all patients as "a shadow behind me on one side" or "something or someone behind me". All the patients explained that they felt an early warning of a high-risk situation at the onset of the seizure. Electrophysiological data suggested a frontal origin.

Recently, the son of a colleague of the Buenos Aires group presented at 17 years of age with two focal seizures with the typical clinical manifestations characterized by somatosensory symptoms (paresthesia) in the right upper limb with secondary generalization, lasting no more than 3 minutes. There was no personal or familial history of epilepsy and neurological and neuropsychological evaluation, as well as the interictal EEG and the MRI were normal. After a two-year follow-up without medication the boy has remained event free.

In a study on the neuropsychological findings in patients with IPSA, mild dysfunctions in the attention domain, in some executive functions, such as working memory and planning, in visual memory, and in reading and writing, were described. These findings, however, may have different causes as the neuropsychological evaluation is normal in the literature. Further studies would be necessary to assess this issue.

EEG features

A normal interictal EEG or unspecified abnormalities on the same at onset and on repeated control sleep and awake EEGs are mandatory for the diagnosis of IPSA. Bilateral centro-parieto-occipital or diffuse slow waves may be found when the EEG is recorded soon after the seizure, particularly between or after a cluster of seizures (*Figure 1*). However, King *et al.* (1999) and Capovilla *et al.* (2001) found non-specific unilateral theta activities predominantly during sleep. The group from Buenos Aires found similar abnormalities with seizures occurring in clusters but when the patient was awake (Caraballo *et al.*, 2004). In the particular subgroup reported by Capovilla *et al.* (2001), the versive seizures were associated with focal spike-wave discharges over posterior regions.

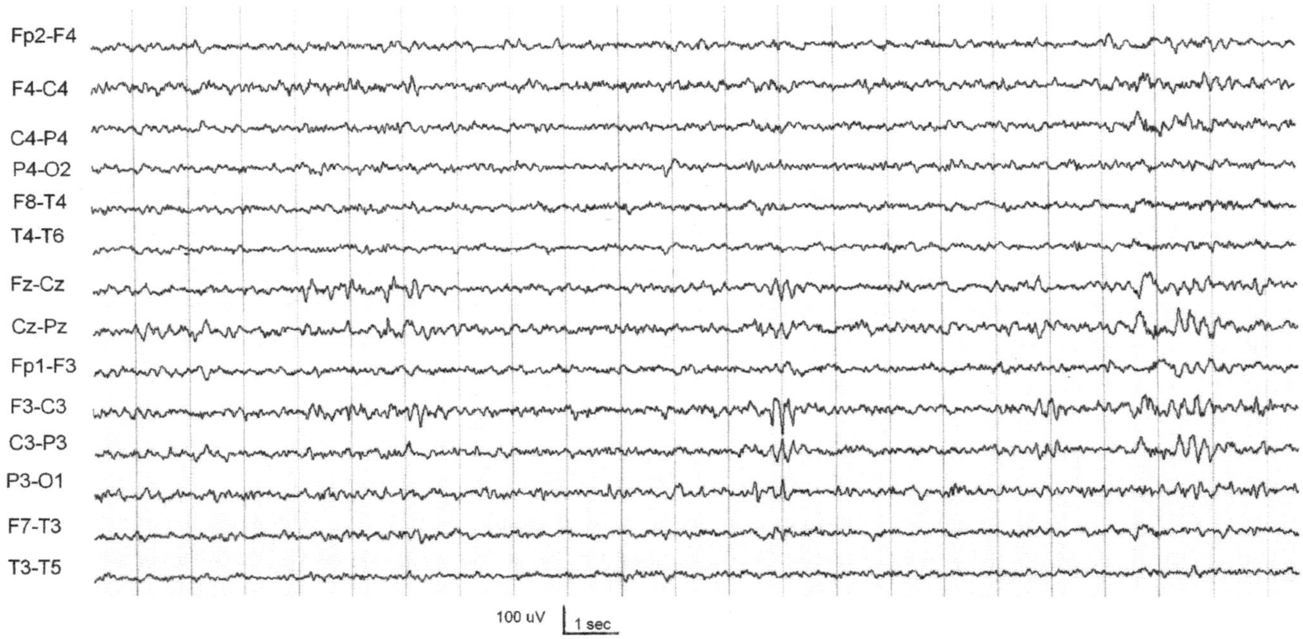

Figure 1

After a cluster of seizures, the interictal EEG shows theta activity and sharp waves in frontal regions predominantly in the left hemisphere.

EEG recordings during hyperventilation are normal or show mild slow activities. No typical spike-wave discharges were seen in any of the cases, nor were any focal or multifocal abnormalities, with the exception of the eight cases with versive seizures reported by Capovilla *et al.* (2001) and the two cases with early postictal multifocal spikes in the series of King *et al.* (1999).

In the group of nine patients published by Romeo *et al.* (2008), the seizures characterized by the sensation of impending danger were associated with uni- or bilateral sharp-wave complexes and theta activity in frontal and fronto-central regions, predominantly during sleep.

The ictal EEG recording shows unilateral frontal fast activity followed by bilateral theta-delta waves in the centrotemporal regions or fast activity in the vertex region *(Figure 2)* (Caraballo *et al.*, 2010).

In the subgroup published by Capovilla *et al.* (2001), the ictal EEG showed "arceaux-like" activity followed by rhythmic low-voltage spikes in the posterior regions. In the group of patients reported by Romeo *et al.* (2008), the ictal recordings also showed fast activity followed by rhythmic theta activity in the frontal region. In *Table I*, the different series of patients with IPSA that have been published are listed.

Etiology

A family history of epilepsy is very rare (3–5%) as is a personal history predisposing to epilepsy (Caraballo *et al.*, 1999, 2004, 2007; Loiseau *et al.*, 2002). Capovilla *et al.* (2001) found a high rate of family history of epilepsy, supporting a presumable genetic nature.

In one of the series, incidentally two patients with a personal history of another idiopathic or probably genetic focal epilepsy syndrome in infancy were found (Caraballo *et al.*, 2007), and curiously enough, in the families of these patients, two close relatives with benign childhood epilepsy with centrotemporal spikes were registered.

Acquired risk factors are found in 4% of the cases (Loiseau *et al.*, 2002). Non-specific factors provoking or precipitating seizures, such as sleep deprivation, stress, or alcohol abuse are not described by either the patients or their parents.

Pathophysiology

The pathophysiology of these particular focal seizures is still a challenge for epileptologists. The seizures are characterized by a succession of symptoms and signs implicating a stepwise involvement of primary or secondary cortical areas and very seldom of temporal structures. The absence of documented cases with ictal studies and the rare positive EEG finding in isolated cases precludes the possibility of a pathophysiological interpretation of the discharges. Other neurophysiological studies might be useful, although it is difficult to perform so many investigations in adolescents with isolated seizures.

Diagnostic work-up

In an adolescent patient who presents with a first unprovoked focal seizure, the possible presence of an underlying brain lesion should be strongly suspected. Therefore, a brain MRI should always be performed in these patients. A high probability of seizure recurrence exists, even when neuroradiologic imaging is normal and a diagnosis of cryptogenic or probably symptomatic focal epilepsy (unknown etiology) is possible in the absence of a brain lesion. Laboratory tests and brain imaging are normal. Other studies, such as karyotyping or neurometabolic investigations, are not necessary.

The EEG may show some minor, non-specific abnormalities without spikes or focal slowing. However, the early postictal waking and sleep EEG might help to find more specific focal abnormalities as shown in some cases (King *et al.*, 1999). Due to the characteristics of IPSA no thorough EEG studies have been performed in the reported series. Recording an ictal EEG in these patients is not feasible unless they are admitted after the first seizure and they happen to have a second one.

Differential diagnosis and associations with other epilepsy syndromes

The most important differential diagnosis of IPSA is cryptogenic or probably symptomatic focal epilepsy (unknown etiology), in which a normal neurological examination and normal neuroradiological imaging are often found. Electroclinical features and evolution in patients with focal epilepsy of an unknown cause are different from those found in our benign cases. Late-onset benign focal epilepsies of childhood, such as benign childhood epilepsy with centrotemporal spikes (BCECTS) or childhood epilepsy with occipital paroxysms (CEOP), may also be considered in the differential diagnosis and an interictal EEG will provide the definite answer. Adolescents with juvenile myoclonic epilepsy may sometimes present with focal myoclonic or clonic seizures. An interview regarding the presence of myoclonic movements in the hands after waking up and the EEG finding of polyspike discharges would confirm this diagnosis even before the patients start with typical generalized tonic-clonic seizures. Patients with migraine may present with a sensory march without motor seizures. However, none of the patients in the group from Buenos Aires had migraine.

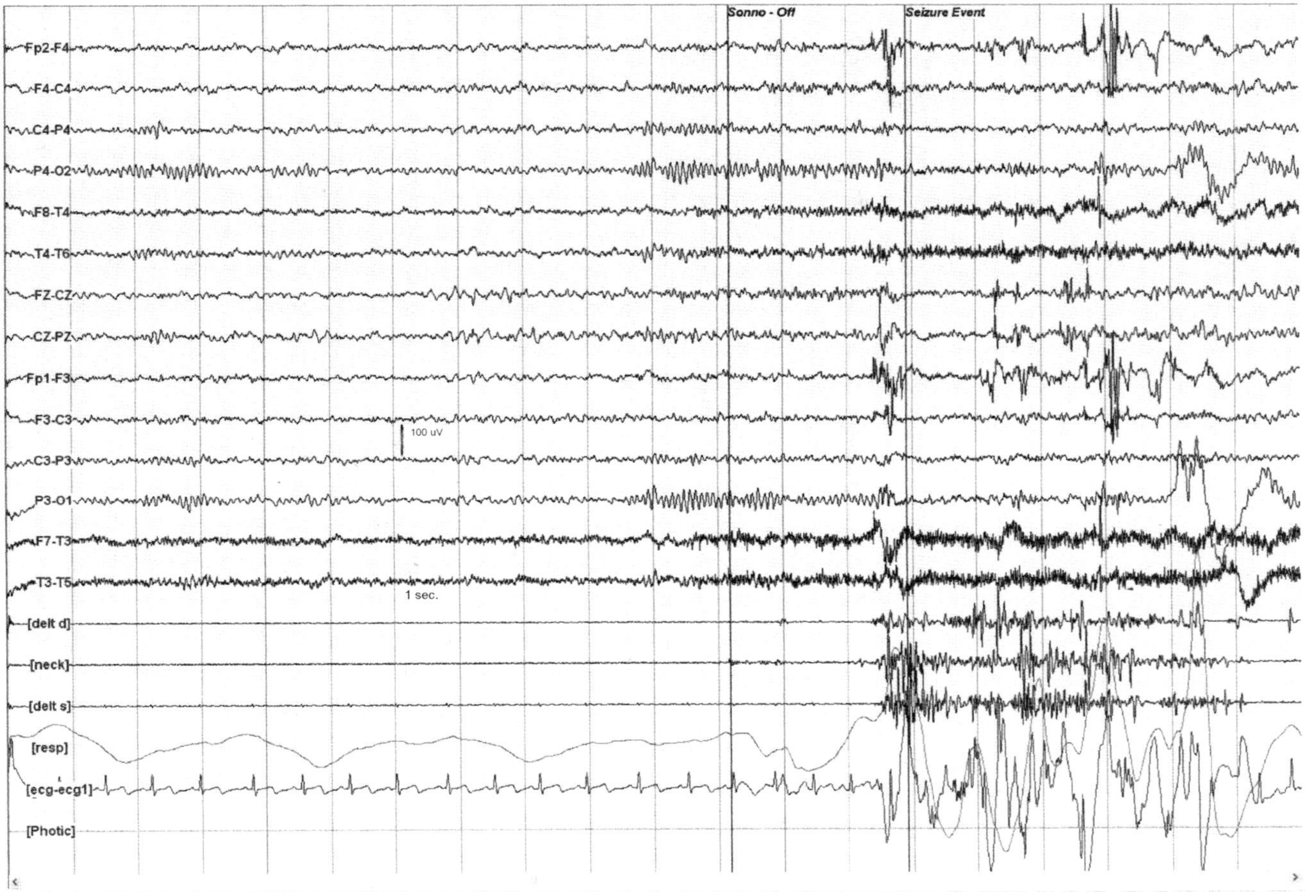

Figure 2

Ictal EEG recording of a seizure occurring during drowsiness shows beta activity in the vertex regions. This ictal discharge tends to progressively increase in amplitude and decrease in frequency. From the clinical point of view, the boy awakes, looks confused, and calls for his mother. The ictal event lasts 40 seconds and is not followed by a postictal EEG or clinical deficit.

Teenagers may present with isolated seizures symptomatic of hypoglycemia or associated with excessive alcohol intake or other drug intoxications, which must be considered as possible etiologies (Wolf, 1997). Additionally, adolescents with epilepsy are more sensitive to certain factors that facilitate the appearance of seizures, such as sleep deprivation, emotional stress, and even excessive intermittent light stimulation, than persons with epilepsy in other age periods.

Table I **Reported series of patients with IPSA**

Series of patients with IPSA	Gender (males)	Age at onset (years)	Type of seizures			Distribution		EEG
			S PS	CPS	SGTCS	Awake	Sleep	
Loiseau *et al.* (2002) (108 patients)	71.2%	Peak at 13–15	87.4%	13.6%	57.2%	87%	**13%**	Normal
Capovilla *et al.* (2001) (37 patients)	**60%**	Mean 14.5	**86%**	**27%**	**57%**	62%	**38%**	Spikes, sharp waves and theta discharges
Mauri *et al.* (1996) (10 patients)	**70%**	Range: 12 to 19	**30%**	**20%**	**50%**	?	**?**	Unspecified abnormalities
King *et al.* (1999) (8 patients)	**50%**	Mean age: 15.5	100%	-	**75%**	?	**?**	Unspecified abnormalities
Caraballo *et al.* (1999). Retrospective study (14 patients)	71.4%	Peak at 12–13	85.7%	26.7%	64.2%	93%	7%	Normal
Caraballo *et al.* (2004) Prospective study (15 patients)	66.5%	Median 14	86.6%	13.4%	**40%**	100%	13.3%	Normal or unspecified abnormalities
Caraballo *et al.* (2007) (44 patients)	54.5%	Median 14	**86%**	**24%**	47.5%	100%	11%	Normal or unspecified abnormalities
Ferreira Guilhoto *et al.* (2009)	25%	Range: 10 yrs. 9 m to 14 yrs. 3 m.	**100%**	-	100%	100%	12.5%	Normal (2) and focal spikes (6)

Table II **Differential diagnosis of IPSA**

Type of epilepsy and epileptic syndromes	Late-onset of idiopathic or probably genetic focal epilepsies of childhood (BCECTS, CEOP)
	Structural focal epilepsies
	Focal epilepsies of unknown etiology
	Juvenile myoclonic epilepsy with focal motor seizures
Other paroxysmal events and seizures in adolescence	Migraine with focal paresthesias
	Occasional seizures associated with sleep deprivation, excessive alcohol intake other intoxications
	Pseudo-seizures

SPS: Simple partial seizures; CPS: complex partial seizures; SGTCS: secondary generalized tonic-clonic seizures.

The differential diagnoses of IPSA are listed in *Table II*.

IPSA might also present with different types of seizures and interictal focal EEG discharges as do most of the idiopathic or probably genetic focal epilepsies in childhood. These functional EEG foci may be located in any part of the cerebral cortex, as long as the seizures and the EEG abnormalities show spontaneous remission or disappear after antiepileptic drug (AED) treatment. Undoubtedly, the possibility of having structural epilepsy is always a concern in benign focal epilepsy.

Regarding the association with previous or subsequent idiopathic focal epilepsy syndromes in patients with IPSA, in a series of 40 patients with benign familial infantile seizures, two developed IPSA at ages 14 and 16 years (Caraballo & Fejerman, 2007). We are not aware of any other reports on the association of IPSA with other idiopathic epilepsy syndromes.

As shown above, the diagnostic workup and differential diagnosis of IPSA may be complicated. Indeed, early diagnosis is difficult since some time of follow-up is necessary to confirm the clinical suspicion. In the face of a teenager with focal seizures, it is important to bear the possibility of this syndrome in mind. The patients and their parents should be told about the condition and that upon finding normal EEG and MRI studies, the use of antiepileptic drugs is not necessary. However, we have to be alert to the appearance of new signs or symptoms pointing to a different diagnosis.

In the diagnosis of IPSA we should no longer rely upon the old recommendations of the Commission of ILAE 1993 stating that two epileptic seizures are needed for a diagnosis of epilepsy. This concept has been reviewed by a joint committee with representatives of the ILAE and the International Bureau for Epilepsy (IBE) who concluded that an epileptic syndrome can often be identified after the first seizure (Fisher *et al.*, 2005).

Finally, in the diagnostic scheme proposed in 2001 by the Task force on Classification of ILAE, the item "Single seizures or isolated clusters of seizures" was included in the "Conditions with epileptic seizures that do not require a diagnosis of epilepsy" (Engel, 2001). Since IPSA is not mentioned in the last report of the ILAE Classification core group (Engel, 2006) there would be no room for the entity in that scheme. This is probably why this epileptic syndrome characterized by isolated seizures with a benign course is not consulted in specialized epilepsy centers. However, we believe IPSA should be considered a syndrome in order to raise awareness of the entity among pediatric neurologists.

Treatment

It is crucial to identify IPSA to avoid giving a poor prognosis at a first seizure based on the sole reason that this type of seizure occurred during adolescence. Antiepileptic treatment should be avoided in these cases as the course is benign and the seizures isolated, as has been corroborated in a prospective study (Caraballo *et al.*, 2004).

Prognosis and long-term evolution

In these patients a longer follow-up is necessary to confirm a benign course as typically occurs in IPSA. Previous studies confirm that a benign course may be seen in adolescents with focal seizures, normal neurologic examination, and normal brain imaging (King *et al.*, 1999; Capovilla *et al.*, 2001; Loiseau *et al.*, 2002; Caraballo *et al.*, 1999, 2004, 2007). Naturally, the evolution of the patient will confirm the diagnosis of this particular entity.

Longer follow-ups and future prospective electroclinical studies are necessary to confirm and define the nosologic place of this entity.

We confirm the existence of adolescents with isolated single or clusters of focal motor or somatosensory seizures, and less frequently other focal seizure types, with or without secondarily generalized seizures, with a normal EEG, normal neurologic examination, normal brain imaging, and a benign course, as previously described by Loiseau *et al.* (1972).

REFERENCES

Berg AT, Berkovic SF, Brodie MJ, *et al.* (2010): Revised terminology and concepts for organization of seizures and epilepsies: report of the ILAE Commission on Classification and Terminology, 2005–2009. *Epilepsia* 51: 676–685.

Capovilla G, Gambardella A, Romeo A, *et al.* (2001): Benign partial epilepsies of adolescence: A report of 37 new cases. *Epilepsia* 42: 1549–1552.

Caraballo R, Galicchio S, Granana N, Cersosimo R, Fejerman N (1999): Convulsiones parciales benignas de la adolescencia. *Rev Neurol* (Barc) 28: 669–671.

Caraballo R, Cersosimo R, Fejerman N (2004): Benign focal seizures of adolescents: a prospective study. *Epilepsia* 45: 1600–1603.

Caraballo R, Fejerman N (2007): Benign familial and non-familial infantile seizures. In: Fejerman N, Caraballo R (eds) *Benign Focal Epilepsies in Infancy, Childhood and Adolescence*, pp. 31–49. London: John Libbey Eurotext.

Caraballo R, Cersosimo R, Capovilla G, Fejerman N (2007): Benign focal seizures of adolescence. In: Fejerman N, Caraballo R (eds) *Benign Focal Epilepsies in Infancy, Childhood and Adolescence*, London: John Libbey, pp. 243–252.

Caraballo R, Capovilla G, Romeo A (2010): Benign focal seizures of adolescence. In: Panayiotopoulos C (ed) *Atlas of Epilepsies*, Berlin: Springer-Verlag, pp. 989–994.

Commission on Classification and Terminology of the International League Against Epilepsy (1989): Proposal for revised classification of epilepsies and epileptic syndromes. *Epilepsia* 30: 389–399.

Commission on Epidemiology and Prognosis, International League Against Epilepsy (1993): Guidelines for epidemiologic studies on epilepsy. *Epilepsia* 34: 592–596.

Engel J (2001): A proposed diagnostic scheme for people with epileptic seizures and with epilepsy: Report of the ILAE Task Force on Classification and Terminology. *Epilepsia* 42: 796–803.

Engel J Jr (2006): Report of the ILAE classification core group. *Epilepsia* 47: 1558–1568.

Ferreira Guilhoto LMF, Cruz Fernandes AD, Pasquali Pacheco S, Ballester D, Gilio AE (2009): Benign focal seizures of adolescence and neuropsychological findings in patients from community. *J Epilepsy Clin Neurophysiol* 15: 184–191.

Fisher RS, van Emde Boas W, Blume W, Elger C, Genton P, Lee P, Engel J Jr (2005): Epileptic seizures and epilepsy: definitions proposed by the International League Against Epilepsy (ILAE) and the International Bureau for Epilepsy (IBE). *Epilepsia* 46: 470–472.

King MA, Newton MR, Jackson GD, *et al.* (1998): Epileptology of the first-seizure presentation: a clinical, electroencephalographic, and magnetic resonance imaging study of 300 consecutive patients. *Lancet* 352: 1007–1011.

King MA, Newton MR, Berkovic SF (1999): Benign partial seizures of adolescence. *Epilepsia* 40: 1244–1247.

Loiseau P, Jogeix M, Lafitte M (1972): Crises épileptiques sans suite chez les adolescents. *Bordeaux Medical* 5: 2623–2629.

Loiseau P, Orgogozo JM (1978): An unrecognized syndrome of benign focal epileptic seizures in teenagers. *Lancet* 2: 1070–1071.

Loiseau P, Louiset P (1992): Benign partial seizures of adolescence. In: Roger J, Bureau M, Dravet C, *et al.* (eds) *Epileptic Syndromes in Infancy, Childhood and Adolescence*, 2nd ed, pp. 343–345. London: John Libbey.

Loiseau P, Jallon P, Wolf P (2002): Isolated partial seizures of adolescence. In: Roger J, Bureau M, Dravet C, *et al.* (eds) *Epileptic Syndromes in Infancy, Childhood and Adolescence*, 3rd ed, pp. 327–330. London: John Libbey.

Mauri JA, Iniguez C, Jerico I, *et al.* (1996): Benign partial seizures of adolescence: report of 10 cases. *Epilepsia* 37 (Suppl 4): 102.

Panayiotopoulos CP (1996): Benign partial seizures of adolescence. In: Wallace S (ed) *Epilepsy in Children*, pp. 377–378. London: Chapman & Hall.

Panayiotopoulos CP (2005): Benign (isolated) focal seizures of adolescence. In: Panayiotopoulos CP (ed) *The Epilepsies. Seizures, Syndromes and Management*, pp. 264–269. Oxfordshire: Bladon Medical Publishing.

Romeo A, Chifari R, Capovilla G, *et al.* (2008): Ictal impending danger – "sixth sense seizures" – in patients with benign focal epileptic seizures of adolescence. *Epilepsy Res* 79: 90–96.

Scheffer I E, French J, Hirsch E, *et al.* (2016), Classification of the epilepsies: New concepts for discussion and debate – Special report of the ILAE Classification Task Force of the Commission for Classification and Terminology. *Epilepsia Open* 1: 37–44.

Wolf P (1997): Isolated seizures. In: Engel J Jr, Pedley T (eds) *Epilepsy: a Comprehensive Textbook*, pp. 2475–2481. Philadelphia: Lippincott Raven.

WITH VIDEO SUPPLEMENTS

CHAPTER 17
JUVENILE MYOCLONIC EPILEPSIES

Pierre Genton[1], Pierre Thomas[2], Philippe Gélisse[3], Anna Serafini[4], Marco T. Medina[5] and Elza Márcia Yacubian[6]

[1] Centre Saint-Paul, Henri-Gastaut Hospital, Marseille, France
[2] Department of Neurology, Pasteur Hospital, Nice, France
[3] Epilepsy Unit, Montpellier, France
[4] Department of neurology and rehabilitation, University of Illinois, Chicago, USA
[5] School of Medical Sciences, University of Honduras, Tegucigalpa, Honduras
[6] Universidade Federal de São Paulo, São Paulo, Brazil

Definitions

The characteristics of juvenile myoclonic epilepsy (JME) were established by Janz & Christian in 1957. It is thus quite surprising that JME is still often misdiagnosed or diagnosed with a marked delay. In 1995, we evaluated a series of 56 consecutive JME patients, and found that the correct diagnosis had never been made prior to the referral to our specialized center (Genton *et al.*, 1995). However, the situation has changed, and half of the patients are now often referred for confirmation of the diagnosis of JME. As noted by Janz & Durner (1997), JME "is very easy for the informed physician to diagnose, and very easy to miss when not aware of its characteristics". The major symptom, which is represented by morning jerks, is rarely mentioned by patients and requires an active interview.

The 1989 International Classification of Epilepsies and Epileptic Syndromes (Commission, 1989) gave a precise definition of JME: *"Juvenile myoclonic epilepsy appears around puberty and is characterized by seizures with bilateral, single or repetitive, arrhythmic, irregular myoclonic jerks, predominantly in the arms. Jerks may cause some patients to fall suddenly. No disturbance of consciousness is noticeable. The disorder may be inherited, and sex distribution is equal. Often, there are generalized tonic-clonic seizures and, less often, infrequent absences. The seizures usually occur shortly after awakening and are often precipitated by sleep deprivation. Interictal and ictal EEGs have rapid, generalized, often irregular spike-waves and polyspike-waves; there is no close phase correlation between EEG spikes and jerks. Frequently, the patients are photosensitive. Response to appropriate drugs is good."*

The three seizure types that are characteristic of idiopathic generalized epilepsies (IGE) can be associated in JME: myoclonic jerks (MJ), generalized tonic-clonic seizures (GTCS) and typical absences (TA). MJ can remain the only seizure type in some patients, particularly in subjects who do not seek medical advice. There are no other ictal manifestations in JME, except the occasional occurrence of myoclonic status, the reflex induction of ictal phenomena by specific stimuli, or the presence of asymmetrical MJ or asymmetrical onset of GTCS. Although it is not fully specific, the combination of seizures, MJ at awakening being the most characteristic, should make the diagnosis of JME easy. JME is also characterized by copathologies, especially cognitive and behavioral, which have been particularly scrutinized in recent years, and which may be prominent in some patients – although the condition remains a fairly benign disorder in most.

The interindividual and interfamilial heterogeneity of JME has been stressed by phenotypic studies, but has not been correctly rendered in the internationally accepted definition. Progresses in the understanding of the mechanisms underlying this condition have rested in great part on genetic findings, which have confirmed the heterogeneity of this syndrome, caused by several possible mechanisms, and most probably by a combination of genetic factors.

This heterogeneity has led to the concept of a "plural" JME – hence the title of this chapter. The JMEs are a fairly homogenous syndrome, with a range of prognoses and copathologies, and remain highly treatable in a vast majority of cases.

History of juvenile myoclonic epilepsy *(Figure 1)*

The first descriptions of JME has been ascribed to Herpin, who, in 1867, described "impulsions" or "commotions": "[...] jerks that shake the whole body like an electric commotion. Most of the time, the hands open and drop whatever they are holding; some patients unwillingly throw an object [...]". According to Rabot (1899), the link between myoclonias and epilepsy was established in the early XIXth century, and Delasiauve proposed, in 1854, the term "Motor Petit Mal". Rabot (1899), who introduced the term "myoclonia", published some convincing observations, while Lundborg (1903) separated JME (which he called "intermittent myoclonic epilepsy") from the progressive myoclonus epilepsies. From a personal series of 47 patients, Janz & Christian (1957, 1994) gave the first precise description of JME, and, as a tribute to Herpin, proposed that it be named Impulsiv "Petit Mal". Nearly half a century after their publication, their thorough clinical approach has not been surpassed: *"There are epileptic equivalents that look like a sudden contraction caused by intense fright. Patients report that – mostly after getting up in the morning – during their morning wash or breakfast, they experience unprovoked jerks, causing them to drop their razor, their coffee cup or whatever they are holding"*. In Uruguay, a series of 70 JME patients was analysed in detail in 1958 by authors who were not aware of the German publication and who labelled it *"conscious and bilateral myoclonic epilepsy"* (Castells & Mendilaharsu, 1958).

Before and after these two seminal papers, other descriptions and denominations were published that did not result in a clear individualization of JME: myoclonic epilepsy (Lennox, 1945); jerk epilepsy (Lennox, 1960); myoclonic Petit Mal (Penfield & Jasper, 1954). While other authors were rediscovering JME (Gastaut & Broughton, 1972) and were giving precisions on its characteristics using large patient series (Tsuboi, 1977), it was Lund, a Danish author, who first used its present denomination in 1976, in a paper devoted to *a controlled sociological and psychological study of patients with juvenile myoclonic epilepsy* (Lund *et al.*, 1976). It took ten more years for North American to recognize JME: "benign JME" (Asconapé & Penry, 1984), "JME of Janz" (Delgado-Escueta & Enrile-Bacsal, 1984), "JME" (Dinner *et al.*, 1987). In 1989, JME was included among IGEs in the new international classification of epilepsies and epileptic syndromes (Commission, 1989; Wolf, 2000) as one of the best defined and most studied syndromes. The publication of a comprehensive monography bears witness to the major importance of JME (Schmitz & Sander, 2000). In a proposed revised diagnostic scheme for the IGE included JME in a broader group of "IGE with variable phenotypes", together with juvenile absence epilepsy and epilepsy with GTCS on awakening (Engel, 2001). The 2017 position paper of the ILAE puts JME among the genetic generalized epilepsies (Scheffer *et al.*, 2017).

There is no certain historical figure with JME, with the (probable) exception of Emperor Pedro I of Brazil (and Portugal), who had a history of infrequent GTCS with onset in adolescence, and a neuropsychological profile very evocative of JME, *e.g.* with impulsive decisions (Gomes & Chalub, 2007).

Genetics

Although most patients appear as isolated cases, a family history of epilepsy is found in approximately one third of them (Janz, 1985). In 1973, Tsuboi & Christian studied 319 index cases with JME. Among 1,618 first-degree relatives, 66 (4.1%) had epilepsy. Fifty other subjects had isolated EEG abnormalities. Janz *et al.* (1992) summarized the data collected by the Berlin group. The cumulative incidence of epilepsies in first-degree relatives of patients with JME was 5.8% (35/600), with the following distribution: parents: 3%; siblings: 7.7%; children 6.6%. The following epileptic syndromes were found in relatives: JME: 31.4%; absence epilepsies: 34.3%; epilepsies with GTCS: 28.6%; other forms of epilepsy: 5.7%. In a series of 43 index cases, 24 (10.7%) of relatives had at least one epileptic seizure (Delgado-Escueta & Enrile-Bacsal, 1984). In a study of 68 index cases (Delgado-Escueta *et al.*, 1989), an epileptic seizure was reported in first-and second-degree relatives in half of the families. For Greenberg *et al.* (1988a), around 15% of first-degree relatives had isolated EEG abnormalities. These data suggest a familial aggregation of IGE in families of JME probands, since around 5% of first-degree relatives have epilepsy, which is much higher than the prevalence in the general population. However, these rates are below those expected in case of mendelian monogenic transmission. Besides epileptic phenotypes, there may be other traits mediated by genetic mechanisms: it has been recently shown that neuropsychological changes typical of JME patients can be found in their siblings, without associated epilepsy or EEG abnormalities (Iqbal *et al.*, 2015).

Cossette *et al.* (2002, 2005) evaluated 14 family members of a large French Canadian family with an autosomal dominant JME. All the affected individuals had GTCS and MJ, four patients also had TA. The EEG showed generalized polyspike-and-waves discharges induced by photic stimulation in all affected individuals. An Ala322Asp mutation was found in *GABRA1*, encoding the $\alpha 1$ subunit of the GABA receptor subtype A (GABAA). The mutant subunit shows a lesser amplitude of GABA-activated currents *in vitro*, indicating that seizures may result from loss of function of this inhibitory ligand-gated channel (Cossette *et al.*, 2002, 2005).

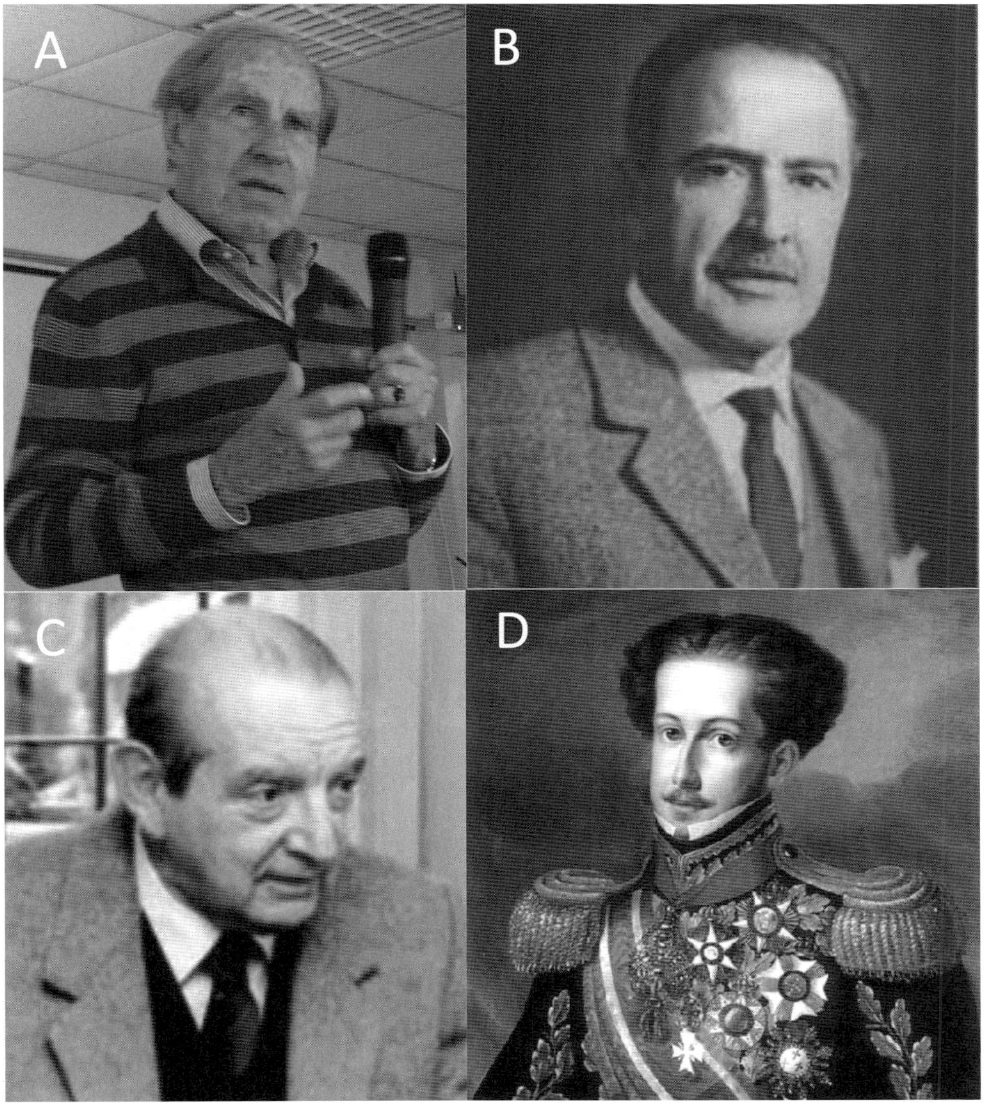

Figure 1

Historical aspects of JME.
A. **Dieter Janz in 2011 during the Avignon, meeting on JME.** B. **Constancio Castells, 1911–1964.** C. **Carlos Mendilaharsu, 1919–2001.** D. **Dom Pedro I do Brazil, Pedro de Alcantara Serafim de Bourbon e Bragança, 1798–1834.**

In 2004 Suzuki *et al.* described a new gene associated with JME, *EFHC1*, which encodes a protein with an EF-hand motif. Mutation analyses identified five missense mutations in *EFHC1* that cosegregated with epilepsy or EEG polyspike waves in affected members of six unrelated families with JME and did not occur in 382 control individuals. Overexpression of *EFHC1* in mouse hippocampal primary culture neurons induced apoptosis that was significantly lowered by the mutations. Apoptosis was specifically suppressed by SNX-482, an antagonist of R-type voltage-dependent Ca(2+) channel a(v). *EFHC1* and Ca(v)2.3 immunomaterials overlapped in mouse brain, and *EFHC1* coimmunoprecipitated with the Ca(v)2.3 C terminus. In patch-clamp analysis, *EFHC1* specifically increased R-type Ca(2+) currents that were reversed by the mutations associated with JME. Mouse models were produced, and *EFHC1* deficient mice showed myoclonus and increased seizure susceptibility (Suzuki *et al.*, 2009).

Pinto *et al.* (2006) found no mutations in the *EFHC1* gene in 112 JME Dutch patients. Stogmann *et al.* (2006) sequenced 61 Austrian patients with various IGE syndromes for mutations in the *EFHC1* gene. They detected three novel heterozygous missense mutations (I174V, C259Y, A394S) and one possibly pathogenic variant in the 3' UTR (2014t>c). The mutation I174V was also detected in 1 of 372 screened patients with temporal lobe epilepsy. Annesi *et al.* (2007) evaluated 27 Italian families with at least two affected members with JME; each exon of the *EFHC1* gene was amplified and sequenced using intronic primers. Two heterozygous mutations were identified in three unrelated families. One (R353 W) was a novel missense mutation, while the F229 L mutation was previously described. Both mutations cosegregated with the disease. In a fourth family, the variant 545GrA (resulting in the amino acid substitution R182H) cosegregated with JME.

Medina *et al.* (2008) screened 44 consecutive patients from Mexico and Honduras and 67 patients from Japan using heteroduplex analysis and direct sequencing. They found five novel mutations in transcripts A and B of *Myoclonin1/EFHC1*. Two novel heterozygous missense mutations (c.755C>A and c.1523C>G) in transcript A occurred in both a singleton from Mexico and another singleton from Japan. A deletion/frameshift (c.789del.AV264fsx280) in transcript B was present in a mother and daughter from Mexico. A nonsense mutation (c.829C>T) in transcript B segregated in four clinically and seven epileptiform-EEG affected members of a large Honduran family. The same nonsense mutation (c.829C>T) occurred as a *de novo* mutation in a sporadic case. Finally, a three-base deletion (364–362del.GAT) was found in the promoter region in a family from Japan. Nine percent of consecutive JME cases from Mexico and Honduras and 3% of patients from Japan carry mutations in *Myoclonin1/EFCH1*. However, mutations in the *EFHC1* gene remain uncommon in JME patients and families (Ma *et al.*, 2006).

De Nijs *et al.* (2006) studied the properties of *EFHC1*. They expressed EGFP-tagged protein in various cell lines. In interphase cells, the fusion protein was present in the cytoplasm and in the nucleus with specific accumulation at the centrosome. During mitosis *EGFP-EFHC1* co-localized with the mitotic spindle, especially at spindle poles and with the midbody during cytokinesis. Using a specific antibody, they demonstrated the same distribution of the endogenous protein. Deletion analyses revealed that the N-terminal region of *EFHC1* is crucial for the association with the mitotic spindle and the midbody. It was further demonstrated that *EFHC1* regulates cell division and cortical development through its action on microtubules (De Nijs *et al.*, 2009).

Heterozygous EFHC1 mutations produce subtle malformations of cortical and subcortical architecture, whereas homozygous F229L mutation induces intractable epilepsy in infancy, severe brain pathology and death (de Nijs *et al.*, 2012; Berger *et al.*, 2012). EFHC1 is a microtubule-associated protein (MAP) involved in cell division and radial migration during cerebral corticogenesis, acting in a dominant-negative manner to impair mitotic spindle organization. Mutants EFHC1 disrupt radial and tangential migration by affecting the morphology of radial glia and migrating neurons (de Nijs *et al.*, 2012). Zhao *et al.* (2016) identified domains of EFHC1 involved in ciliary localization, ciliogenesis, and the regulation of Wnt signaling.

Raju *et al.* (2017) examined the complete structure of the EFHC1 transcript from 480 JME patients and 700 controls from India by direct sequencing (Raju *et al.*, 2017); they reported on thirteen EFHC1 mutations of which 11 were previously not known in 28 JME patients. These mutations accounted for about 6% of the patients examined. Functional studies suggest that these EFHC1 mutations result in microtubule-related abnormalities during cell division. In silico analysis for a subset of mutations suggests that they may affect EFHC1 protein domains, compromising its ability to interact with other proteins.

In a reanalysis of 54 EFHC1 variants associated with JME from 17 cohorts based on National Human Genome Research Institute (NHGRI) and American College of Medical Genetics and Genomics (ACMG) guidelines for interpretation of sequence variants by Bailey *et al.* (2017), found nine variants classified as "pathogenic", 14 as "likely pathogenic", 9 as "benign", and 2 as "likely benign". Twenty variants of unknown significance had an insufficient number of ancestry-matched controls. According with the NHGRI gene-level evidence and variant-level evidence established EFHC1 is the first non-ion channel associated with JME. Thounaojam *et al.* (2017) evaluated 63 patients with JME and 80 healthy controls from India, they found three novel coding variants 661C→T, 779 G→A, and 730 C→T, which lead to R221C, R260Q, and R244STOP amino acid substitutions, respectively.

Bailey *et al.* (2018) sequenced the exomes of six members of a large JME family and confirmed cosegregation in all 37 family members. They screened an additional 310 JME patients for variants on DNA melting-curve analysis and targeted real-time DNA sequencing of the gene encoding intestinal-cell kinase (ICK). A variant, K305T (c.914A→C), cosegregated with epilepsy or polyspikes on EEG in 12 members of the family affected with JME. They identified 21 pathogenic ICK variants in 22 of 310 additional patients (7%). They performed functional tests of the effects of variants on mitosis, apoptosis, and radial neuroblast migration *in vitro* and conducted video-EEG studies in mice lacking a copy of ICK. Four strongly linked variants (K220E, K305T, A615T, and R632X) impaired mitosis, cell-cycle exit, and radial neuroblast migration while promoting apoptosis. Tonic-clonic convulsions and polyspikes on EEG resembling seizures in human JME occurred more often in knockout heterozygous mice than in wild-type mice (P = 0.02).

Several linkage and population association studies have connected the bromodomain-containing gene *BRD2* to JME. Pal *et al.* (2003) reported that *BRD2* could be a probable major susceptibility gene for common JME. They found highly significant linkage disequilibrium (LD) between JME and a core haplotype of five single-nucleotide-polymorphism (SNP) and microsatellite markersin the *BRD2 (RING3)* gene (odds ratio 6.45; 95% confidence interval 2.36–17.58). Velisek *et al.* (2011) reported that heterozygous *BRD2* mice had a lower seizure threshold compared to wild type mice and exhibited fewer GABAergic neurons cortex and basal ganglia. DNA methylation of the BRD2 promoter is associated with JME in Caucasians (Pathak *et al.*, 2018). BRD2+/- haplo insufficient mice show no cognitive impairment but have behavioral traits (recklessness, aggression) similar to those found in JME (Chachua *et al.*, 2014). However, Cavalleri *et al.* (2007) reported a multicenter study of *BRD2* as a risk factor for JME. They studied the association between the candidate causal SNP (the promoter variant rs3918149) and JME in five independent cohorts comprising in total 531 JME cases and 1,390 healthy controls, and the results did not support a strong effect for susceptibility to JME across populations of European descent.

Other loci have been proposed in IGE, specifically including JME. Helbig *et al.* (2009) reported that 15q13.3 microdeletions increase risk of IGE and other associated, *e.g.*, psychiatric phenotypes. In a report by the EPICURE consortium (2012) a meta-analysis of three genome-wide linkage datasets was carried out in 379 genetic generalized epilepsies (multiplex families of European ancestry) including 982 relatives with IGEs. They found a susceptibility locus at 2q34 for myoclonic seizures. A probable association between JME and 22q11.2 deletion syndrome (22q11DS) was found (Lemke *et al.*, 2008). Sapio *et al.* (2015) reported carboxypeptidase A6 (CPA6) mutations in patients with juvenile myoclonic and generalized epilepsy. Novel copy number variations (CNVs) were reported in a Saudi JME family with nine siblings including one male and one female affected members (Naseer *et al.*, 2017).

The genetics of JME have thus progressed; they help explain the microdysgeneses originally described by Meencke and Janz (1984). Three genes have been identified: *GABRA1*, *EFHC1* and *ICK*. Other susceptibility genes include BRD2, 15q13.3 microdeletions and carboxypeptidase A6 (CPA6) mutations. From a genetic point of view, JME appears highly heterogenous.

Clinical context

Prevalence

JME is a very common form of epilepsy, and probably the most frequent form of IGE (Genton *et al.*, 2000a). It accounts for 5–10% of all epilepsies, the rate ranging between 3.4% (Simonsen *et al.*, 1976) and 11.9% (Goosses, 1984). In institutions that select patients with severe epilepsies, the prevalence is lower 4.3% for Janz (1969); 5.4% for Tsuboi (1977); 4.1% for Genton *et al.* (2000a) than in centers with less selected referrals, where the prevalence is often twice as high (11.4% for Wolf & Goosses [1969]; 10.7% for Obeid & Panayiotopoulos [1988]; 10.2% for Panayiotopoulos *et al.* [1994]). According to Loiseau & Duché (1990), JME is more often diagnosed in the setting of a private clinic (4.8%) than in the hospital (3.5%). In Norway, JME, which had frequently remained mis- or undiagnosed, represents 9.3% of all epilepsies in subjects aged less than 30 years (Syvertsen *et al.*, 2016). Among patients with IGE, 23.3% (Numata *et al.*, 1986), 26.7% (Genton *et al.*, 2000a) or 20.6% (Goosses, 1984) has JME. The actual prevalence in the general population remains unknown, as many cases escape medical attention or are diagnosed very late after the onset.

Personal history

Simple febrile seizures are found in 5–10% (Janz & Durner, 1997; Genton *et al.*, 1994, 2000a), otherwise JME occurs in patients with no preexisting neurological history. The evolution from another type of epilepsy poses mainly nosological problems: there is indeed a subset of patients who evolve from childhood absence epilepsy (CAE) into JME (Martinez-Juarez *et al.*, 2006). It is possible to make a diagnosis of JME in patients with a brain lesion, the presence of which does not influence the clinical presentation or the prognosis of JME (Gélisse *et al.*, 2000a). The presence of minor or major neurological conditions will thus appear as purely coincidental, and should not interfere with the diagnosis of JME, as long as the main elements of the syndrome are present (Wolf, 1992a).

Sex ratio and age at onset

In our personal series and in that of Durner (1988), there is a clear female predominance (61% and 57%, ratios of 1.56 and 1.35, respectively). This female predominance is in contrast with former studies, which reported equal sex distribution (Janz, 1969; Tsuboi, 1977), or even male predominance (33 *vs.* 20, Delgado-Escueta & Enrile-Bacsal, 1984).

The onset of JME is clearly age-related. The syndrome begins between the ages of 8 and 26 years (Janz, 1969), with a strictly unimodal distribution *(Figure 2)*. Over 75% of patients have their first seizure between the ages of 12 and 18 (Obeid & Panayiotopoulos, 1988), with a mean age at onset around 14. MJ occur sooner in girls (12–14 years) than in boys (14–16), which might reflect the precocious development of hormonal maturity in females (Genton *et al.* 1994; Genton, 1999). GTCS occur somewhat later, around age 16 (Durner, 1988). Early onset before age 10, or late onset after age 20 is possible, but requires some caution in the diagnosis (Gram *et al.*, 1988). In our experience, half of the patients with onset before age 11 had photosensitivity in the EEG laboratory, *vs.* 38% of the whole sample of 170 JME cases, a fact already noted by others (Wolf & Goosses, 1986; Sundqvist, 1990). Besides this particularity, the age at onset does not constitute a factor of prognosis, nor is it associated with a particular clinical presentation.

Circumstances at first referral and precipitating factors

Patients will typically be referred following the first GTCS, which had been preceded by isolated MJ during months. This first GTCS is usually precipitated by one or several factors: for Pedersen and Petersen (1998), the most common are lack of sleep (84%) *(Figure 3)*, stress (70%), consumption of alcohol (51%). The latter factor was implicated in 40% of the patients of Janz and Christian (1957, 1994), and in 30% of the patients of Penry *et al.* (1989). Other factor may be identified less frequently: soft drugs, drug withdrawal, psychotropic drugs such as amitryptiline (Resor & Resor, 1990). There is also a report of JME being revealed by an intercurrent prescription of bupropion (Kuate *et al.*, 2004). In a study of 75 JME patients (da Silva Sousa *et al.*, 2005), triggering factors were reported by 92%

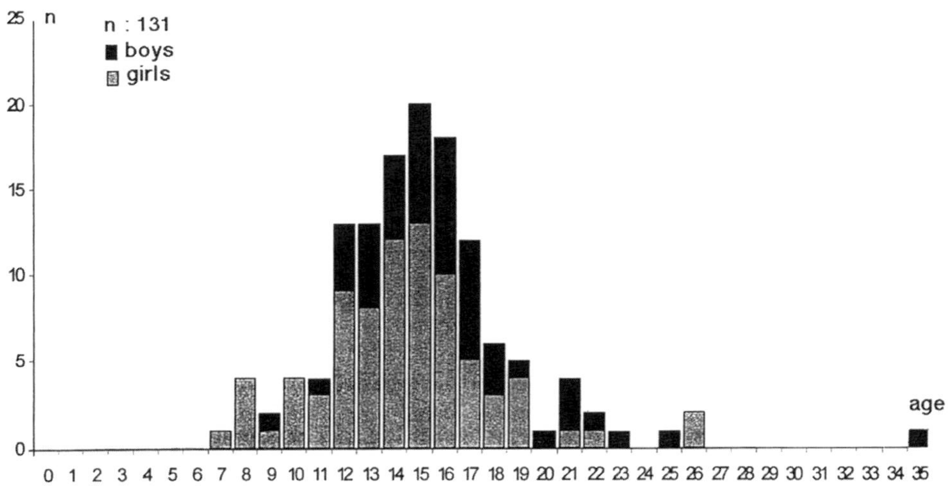

Figure 2

Age at onset of myoclonic jerks (MJ) in a population of 131 patients with JME. Mean age is 15.2 ± 3.8 years, range 7–26. Only one patient had a late apparent onset, at age 35. Onset of MJ was earlier in girls (14.5 ± 3.5 yrs) than in boys (16.4 ± 4.1 years, p < 0.01). (From Genton *et al.*, 2000a).

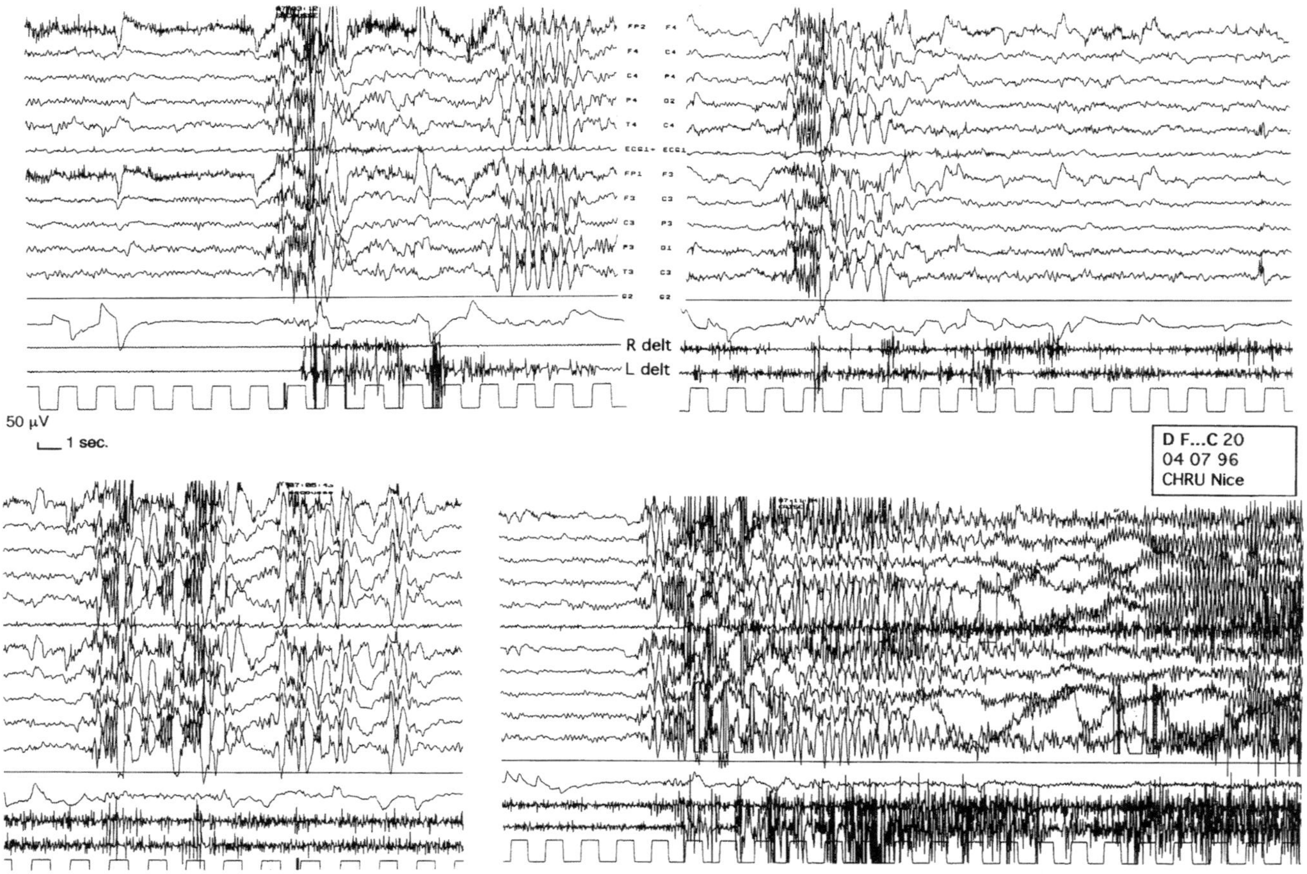

Figure 3

JME in a 20-year-old woman recorded at morning awakening, after partial sleep deprivation. Several generalized PSW discharges with massive bilateral jerks are associated with the increased interictal changes, and precede by some minutes the occurrence of a GTCS. The onset of the tonic phase is preceded by a volley of massive bilateral MJ that lasts 10 seconds.

of patients, in decreasing order: stress (83%), sleep deprivation (77%), specific thoughts/mental concentration (23%), performance of hand activities and complex finger movements (20%), flashing lights and playing games (15%), speaking out in public (11%), alcohol intake (11%), reading (7%), calculating and writing (5%), playing musical instruments (4%), drawing (3%), and specific types of music (1%); the menstrual cycle was the third most important precipitant in women (33%).

Mental tasks that imply manual activity and decision-making may thus trigger seizures (Inoue *et al.*, 1994). This evokes a relation between JME and certain reflex epilepsies in which seizures are precipitated by calculus, cards, chess, writing, decision-making, even reading. In their personal series of 132 JME cases, these authors noted that in 19 patients (14%), seizures or EEG discharges were triggered by such activities, *vs.* even 31% of the JME cases of Wolf & Mayer (2000).

Matsuoka *et al.* (2000) used brief neuropsychological tests in the routine EEG investigation of 480 patients with epilepsy. These comprised reading and speaking, mental and written calculation, writing and spatial construction. In 38 of their patients (8%), induction of epileptiform discharges by praxis or action-programming activities was found, ictal in 24 cases: the induction was most frequent in their JME cases, affecting about one half of the 45 cases. Such praxis-induced myoclonias may be unilateral or asymmetric, and may be associated with spike-waves instead of the more typical polyspike-waves (Abarrategui *et al.*, 2018). Praxis-induction is thus a frequent probably underestimated and underinvestigated reflex component in JME.

Diagnostic delays and mistakes

A precise syndromic diagnosis is rarely made at the first GTCS and JME is thus often missed (Delgado-Escueta & Enrile-Bacsal, 1984; Janz, 1985; Panayiotopoulos *et al.*, 1991; Genton *et al.*, 1994). In our series (Genton *et al.*, 2000a), the mean delay between onset of symptoms and correct diagnosis was close to eight years. When a diagnosis had been proposed by the referring physician (in 137 of 170 cases), it was JME in only 22 patients (16%). In the Southern Indian state of Kerala, only 3.3% of patients carry the diagnosis of JME at referral, and the mean delay of diagnosis was 8.6 ± 7.0 years (Vijai *et al.*, 2003). Several factors may account for the delayed diagnosis. The principal factor is lack of knowledge of this syndrome by clinicians (Panayiotopoulos *et al.*, 1991; Lancman *et al.*, 1994). Patients rarely mention MJ spontaneously, and physicians too often forget to ask about them. When the information is given, it is often considered as a minor symptom without significance. Unilateral or asymmetric MJ, adversive onset of a GTCS or asymmetric EEG changes lead to a misdiagnosis of focal epilepsy (Aliberti *et al.*, 1994; Genton *et al.*, 1995; Lombroso, 1997; So *et al.*, 1998). A normal EEG may result in the diagnosis of non-epileptic events, or of an undetermined type of epilepsy. Such mistakes may have serious consequences, as inadequate treatment may result in seizures remaining uncontrolled (Atakli *et al.*, 1998), or even aggravated (Genton & Mc Menamin, 1998) during years. Diagnostic accuracy has increased in recent years, but the situation is far from perfect, as shown by the repeat study by Atakli *et al.* (2016): in 2014–2015, 49 out of 200 JME patients were still misdiagnosed, often in spite of typical EEG findings.

Seizures

Myoclonic jerks

The cardinal symptom, necessary for the diagnosis of JME, is the occurrence of spontaneous, brief, involuntary, sudden, synchronous and grossly symmetric MJ of variable amplitude. Such MJ occur as single events, or as brief, arrhythmic clusters, and are not associated with any noticeable change of consciousness. They occur typically in the half-hour that follows morning awakening, especially when the night has been short *(Figure 2)*. MJ may also occur during an intermediary awakening or after an afternoon nap, or sporadically during the day. MJ can occur as myoclonic status (7.3% of patients in the series of Salas-Puig *et al.*, 1990). Such episodes of status are characterized by full preservation of consciousness and are sometimes triggered by the patient not stopping his activity after a series of MJ (Janz & Durner, 1997). They are clearly facilitated by acute drug withdrawal, or by the intake of inadequate anticonvulsants.

MJ predominate on the upper limbs. Video studies (Oguni *et al.*, 1994) show that proximal muscles are involved in some patients, with flexion of forearms on arms, extension of the upper spine and sometimes flexion and abduction of the thighs. In others, distal segments are more involved, with a flexion and external rotation of the forearm. Polygraphic studies show that other muscular groups are involved, *i.e.*, abdominal, paraspinal, leg muscles. These grossly symmetric jerks are visible to the onlooker and significantly interfere with activities, as they make the patient drop or more or less violently throw objects (coffee cup, toothbrush, shaver, make-up artifacts...). This apparent clumsiness is often a subject of mockery. MJ may be felt to be asymmetric or even unilateral, either because they are (Canevini *et al.*, 1992), or because their amplitude is modulated by the degree of tonic contraction of the arm that is involved. Some patients will state that only their dominant arm is more involved, which may be due either to an underutilization of the contralateral limb, or to a reflex triggering of the jerk.

The amplitude of MJ may vary. Minimal MJ are hardly seen by onlookers, and are perceived by the patient as an inner electric vibration, as an intermittent tremulation, or as an occasional clumsiness. When MJ are ample, they can involve the lower limbs, with a limited flexion of the knees. Falls occur only in selected circumstances, as when the patient is climbing up or more often down stairs (Thomas & Ostrowski, 1997). Sometimes, violent MJ may cause a sudden and traumatic fall, which is immediately preceded by a short cry, and followed by a brief sensation of fatigue that may be mistaken for loss of consciousness. The patient thus collapses "as if thunderstruck", then immediately recovers his balance (Janz & Christian, 1957, 1994).

In the course of JME, non-epileptic seizures, with factitious MJ, may occur, often in response to particular psychological events. Such events are rare and misleading (Dunac *et al.*, 1998).

Generalized tonic-clonic seizures

GTCS are present in 80–95% of patients (Janz, 1969; Tsuboi, 1977; Obeid & Panayiotopoulos, 1988, Genton *et al.*, 2000a). GTCS usually cause patients to seek medical advice. They share the same daily distribution and the same triggering factors as MJ and may help identify the latter retrospectively. The course of the GTCS is characteristic. Typically, a longer than usual cluster of MJ occurs, with increasing amplitude and frequency, until MJ melt into the initial tonic phase of the GTCS. The sequence is a *clonic*-tonic-clonic seizure (Delgado-Escueta & Enrile-Bacsal, 1984), added in the operative classification of epileptic seizures as *myoclonic*-tonic-clonic seizures (Fisher *et al.*, 2017), which is practically synonymous with JME when it occurs in this age class in an otherwise healthy subject. Less typical variants have been described, with a versive component *(Figure 4)*, or even a true rotatory seizure (Topcuoglu *et al.*, 1997; Aguglia *et al.*, 1999). GTCS are not very frequent in the natural course of JME (one or two per year at most). They may however cluster over a few weeks during certain periods of adolescence. They may be frequent and invalidating in non-compliant or mistreated patients, in cases with abnormal lifestyle, or, rarely, without any specific reason.

Typical absences

TAs found in JME are not constant, infrequent and short. They mostly appear as simple TAs with mild impairment of consciousness (Janz & Waltz, 1994). Because of this, they are often ignored by the patient and his entourage, and are diagnosed only during the EEG work-up. Their prevalence has been diversely assessed: they are found in 10% of patients by Janz (1969); 14% by Tsuboi (1977), 18% by Obeid & Panayiotopoulos (1988). A more systematic use of long-term video-EEG monitoring yields higher numbers: 38% for Panayiotopoulos *et al.* (1989); 33% in our personal experience (Genton *et al.*, 2000a). Absence status is very uncommon (Kimura & Kobayashi, 1996; Agathonikou *et al.*, 1998). However, TA may be the initial seizure type in some subsets of JME patients, who present as CAE or JAE before JME (Martinez-Juarez *et al.*, 2006).

Perioral reflex myoclonias

Single, lightning-like oro-linguo-facial myoclonias, typical for Primary Reading Epilepsy (PRE), may occur in JME. Unlike PRE, where they are precipitated by loud or silent reading but also in a minority of subjects by talking, in JME they are usually precipitated by talking and much less commonly by reading. In the investigation of Wolf & Mayer (2000), 14 out of 62 JME patients (23%) reported perioral myoclonias with talking. Perioral reflex myoclonias were not found in the study of Matsuoka *et al.* (2000) which is probably due to the brevity of the language-related tests they used. These consisted of only three short sentences in both reading and writing. When attention is paid to them, the perioral reflex myoclonias can easily be observed in prolonged talks with the patients.

Status epilepticus

Myoclonic status epilepticus (MSE) is uncommon in JME. Among 237 consecutive JME cases, Larch *et al.* (2009) found 7 cases of MSE, including 5 with associated GTCS; triggering factors were present in 6 (drug withdrawal in four, including one with sleep deprivation and alcohol intake, inappropriate treatment in two). MSE was also seen in patients with inadequate drug regimen by Thomas *et al.* (2006). MSE responds to benzodiazepines (Larch *et al.*, 2009) and to valproate (Crespel *et al.*, 2009b).

Other seizure types

In spite of the frequency of photoparoxysmal responses on the EEG, MJ and GTCS that are triggered by environmental visual stimuli (television screen, videogames, stroboscopic flashes in discos, intermittent solar light) are uncommon. No studies have specifically focused on this subject, which might concern as little as 5% of JME patients (Genton *et al.*, 1994).

The occurrence of atonic seizures in JME is controversial. In the original work of Janz and Christian (1957, 1994), as in the works of Asconapé and Penry (1984) and of Manon-Espaillat *et al.* (1987), pure atonic seizures, occurring independently from JM, were noted. Other authors (Delgado-Escueta & Enrile-Bacsal, 1984; Janz, 1985; Grunewald & Panayiotopoulos, 1993; Loiseau & Duché, 1990; Wolf, 1992a) have expressed doubts about their existence, and have stressed that no polygraphic studies have confirmed them. However, some consider JME with atonic seizures to represent a rare subtype, at 3% of all JME cases (Martinez-Juarez *et al.*, 2006). The association of JME with a focal epilepsy has been reported (Diehl *et al.*, 1998; Koutroumanidis *et al.*, 1999): two patients were successfully operated for temporal lobe epilepsy, but after surgery the characteristic clinical syndrome of JME and the generalized EEG discharges persisted.

Association of seizure types

Most patients (58.2% in our series) have frequent MJ and rare GTCS. Around one third of patients have all three seizure types (Janz & Durner, 1997). There is no particular combination according to sex, although we found a slight male predominance (36.4% in males *vs.* 26.9% in females). GTCS follow MJ after a mean delay of 1.3 (Durner, 1988) to 3.3 years (Janz, 1969). A probably sizeable

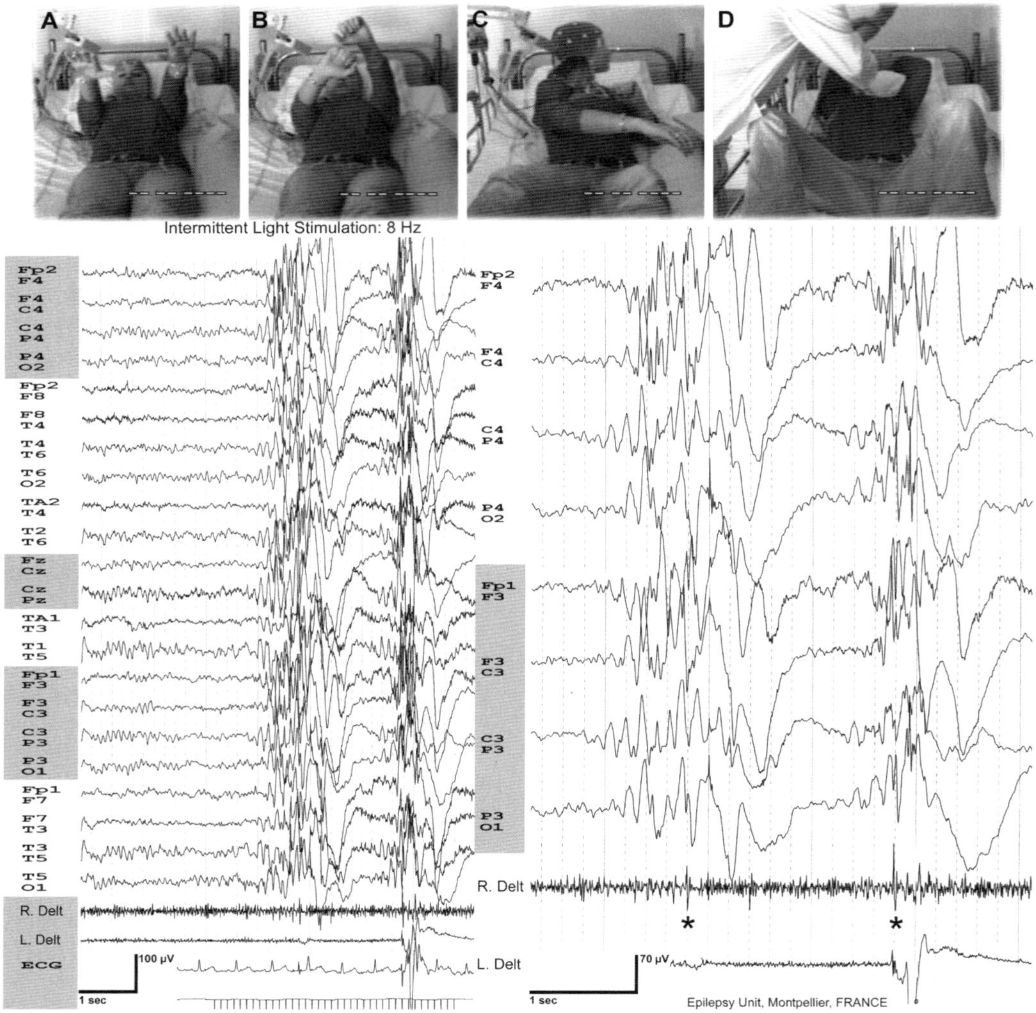

Figure 4

Young woman with JME. She had visual auras (flashes) just before GTCS, corresponding to myoclonic jerks (MJ). Top: **A: arms raised. B: intermittent light stimulation at 8 Hz triggers a myoclonic jerk. C: version of head and body to the left just before a GTCS (D).** Bottom: **EEG: on the left, recording at 15 mm/s and 10 µV/mm. On the right, same abstract at 30 mm/s and 70 µV/mm with only suprasylvian leads. Arms raised. ILS triggers two bursts of polyspike-waves associated with myoclonic jerk (*). The first MJ is clearly visible on the right deltoid. The second MJ is associated with an artifact on the EKG.**

proportion of patients have only isolated MJ, and these may escape medical attention, because they never seek medical advice (Jain *et al.*, 1997). A very small proportion of patients have the unusual association of MJ and TA (2.4% in our series).

Chronodependency

The characteristic circadian distribution of seizures is a major trait of JME. They occur mostly after morning awakening, but also after waking from a nap, and are clearly precipitated by a sudden,provoked awakening, after a short and insufficient sleep period. In the study of Touchon *et al.* (1982), seizures clearly peak after morning awakening. MJ may occur during intermediate awakenings in the night, after a nap or during a relaxation period in the afternoon or evening. The distribution of EEG changes follows the same pattern (Janz & Durner, 1997) *(Figure 5)*. The circadian distribution of seizures in JME is apparently correlated to a specific circadian pattern of personality or of general activity: compared to temporal lobe epilepsy patients, JME subjects are less likely to feel well before 10 AM (1 subject out of 20 *vs.* 16/20) and tend to be "evening" types (13 *vs.* 6) (Pung & Schmitz, 2006).

Psychological and cognitive profile

JME is a stable condition and is not associated with neurological or mental deterioration. The presence of organic neurological damage or of mental deficiency should be considered as coincidental (Gélisse *et al.*, 2000b). However, Janz and Christian (1957, 1994) noted that some patients had an "attractive but immature" personality, which resulted in some difficulties of social integration, abnormal lifestyle or less than perfect compliance, with consequences regarding the therapeutic control of their condition. Similar findings were reported by Tsuboi (1977) and by Lund *et al.* (1976). Devinsky *et al.* (1977) suggested that these might be due to a dysfunction of the prefrontal cortex.

Early observations were confirmed by studies utilizing modern psychiatric criteria. Psychological assessment of a series of JME patients using the DSM-IV criteria showed that there was a high prevalence of a variety of psychological disturbances, without any very specific profile (Gélisse *et al.*, 2001a): in 170 consecutive JME patients, 26.5%

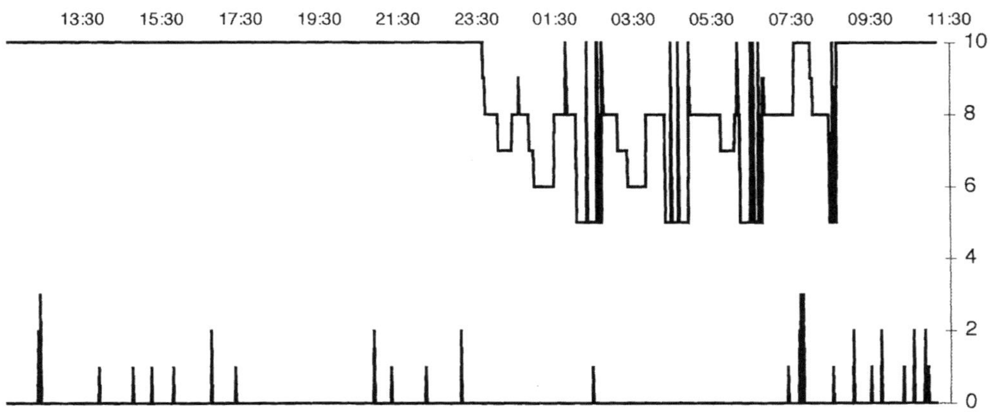

Figure 5

Activation profile of paroxysmal changes over 24 hours in a 24-year-old women with JME on VPA, 1,000 mg/d (Medilog 9000 system). Numerous PSW discharges at awakening at 7.30 AM and 8.30 AM (final awakening). Presence of isolated discharges at other times of the day, with long periods devoid of any discharge, especially in the late afternoon.

had a lifetime history of some form of psychiatric disorder. Personality disorders were the most frequent finding and were detected in 14%. A borderline personality, responsible for social maladjustment was the most frequent personality disorder (6.5%). Trinka *et al.* (2006) evaluated 43 JME patients with the Structured Clinical Interviews for DSM-IV. Thirty-five percent of the patients suffered from one or more psychiatric disorders, 19% of them reported Axis I psychiatric disorders and 23% were diagnosed with personality disorders. The lifetime prevalence of psychiatric disorders was high: 47% reported one or more. Their presence was not related to the duration of epilepsy, seizure freedom, seizure types, or compliance.

De Araújo Filho *et al.* (2007) compared 100 JME patients (age range 18–54) with 100 normal subjects. JME patients had a higher prevalence of Axis I psychiatric disorders (49% of JME patients) and psychosocial problems than controls ($p < 0.01$). Twenty patients fulfilled criteria for personality disorders (Axis II), and 85% of them were diagnosed with cluster B personalities (histrionic, borderline, passive-aggressive). The prevalence of psychiatric disorders among JME patients was higher in this study than in previous ones; the authors attributed this to the fact that nearly half of them had not been free of GTCS for at least one year. Anxiety (23%) and mood disorders (19%) were the most frequently reported. The presence of psychiatric disorders was compared with the clinical and socio-demographic characteristics and an association between the presence of psychiatric disorders and a higher seizure frequency ($p < 0.005$) was found. Treatment with AED for more than two years appeared to be a factor protecting against psychiatric disorders, especially generalized anxiety disorders. No correlations between the presence of psychiatric disorders, the type of AED and the number of AEDs were found. This might be due to the small number of patients taking more than one AED.

The difference in the prevalence of psychiatric disorders between temporal lobe epilepsy (TLE) and JME was studied by several authors. Perini *et al.* (1996) compared 18 JME patients with 20 TLE patients, 20 patients affected by type I diabetes and 20 normal subjects. The prevalence of psychiatric disorders was higher in the TLE group (80%) while JME and diabetic patients presented much lower prevalence, 22% and 10% respectively. JME was not significantly associated with any psychiatric diagnosis. However, a correlation with a higher anxiety trait was found. De Araújo Filho *et al.* (2011) compared 248 patients with refractory TLE and mesial temporal sclerosis to 124 JME patients and found a high prevalence of psychiatric disorders in both groups. Psychiatric disorders were present in 41% of TLE and in 46.7% of JME patients. Psychoses were significantly associated with TLE ($p = 0.01$), mood and anxiety disorders (25% and 21%, respectively) being the most common in JME.

The personality traits found among JME patients seemed very similar to the personality characteristics of patients with frontal lobe dysfunction. These observations led to the assessment of cognitive functions in JME patients. Sonmez *et al.* (2004) evaluated cognition in 35 JME patients and 35 healthy subjects. JME patients had a worse performance on frontal and visuospatial function. Pascalicchio *et al.* (2007) studied the factors related to the presence of cognitive dysfunction in 50 JME patients and in 50 healthy subjects. A lower performance on measures of attention, memory, naming, and verbal fluency was observed in JME. Cognitive decline and duration of epilepsy were positively related. However, when patients had more than 11 years of education this correlation was not significant. No correlations were found between the number of AEDs taken and the presence of cognitive dysfunction. Piazzini *et al.* (2008) compared frontal cognitive functions in 50 JME patients, 40 patients with TLE, 40 patients with frontal lobe epilepsy (FLE) and 40 controls. Impairment in frontal cognitive functions similar to FLE patients was found in JME, worse than in TLE and controls. The cognitive decline in JME was not related to duration of epilepsy, frequency of seizures, treatment or seizure type. Executive deficits and impulsiveness may however be masked, or compensated, by patients with higher IQ (Rzezak *et al.*, 2018). It appears that JME patients with marked reflex phenomena (*e.g.*, praxis-induction, eye-closure sensitivity and/or photosensitivity) had higher drug resistance and overall severity, including greater executive dysfunction (Carvalho *et al.*, 2016).

JME may be thus associated with some degree of cognitive dysfunction and of personality disorders. The presence of psychiatric disorders seems to be a correlate of drug resistance (Gélisse *et al.*, 2001b). These deficits may lead to social dysfunction (Giorgi *et al.*, 2016), and to long-term lack of social integration.

Other copathologies

Essential tremor seemed to be very common, noted in 35% of the JME patients studied in Saudi Arabia by Panayiotopoulos *et al.* (1994). Headache is apparently also common: among 75 patients with JME, 47 had headache, including 31 with migraine (without aura, 20; with aura, 11; with additional tension headache, 14), and 16 with tension headache, and the risk ratio for these various types of headache ranged between 3.4 and 7.3 in comparison with the general population (Schankin *et al.*, 2011); similar findings were reported by Dedey Daryan *et al.* (2018). A significant association between type 1 diabetes mellitus and IGE (including JME cases) was found by McCorry *et al.* (2006).

Several conditions may interfere with the treatment and prognosis of JME. Graves' disease may be an aggravating – or revealing-condition in patients with JME (Su *et al.*, 1993). Similarly, we have collected several observations of well-controlled JME patients who relapsed with invalidating GTCS when they developed obstructive sleep apnea syndrome, a condition causing severe sleep deprivation. In 62 patients treated with levetiracetam, sleep quality and daytime sleepiness were investigated by questionnaires and seizure control was clearly correlated with both parameters (Buratti *et al.*, 2018).

EEG

Ictal EEG

An ictal recording is best obtained by polygraphic video-EEG performed after a sudden, provoked early morning awakening during a full-night sleep recording *(Figures 5 and 6)*. In practice, however, a morning nap obtained after nocturnal sleep deprivation may be sufficient. The characteristic EEG trait is a polyspike-wave (PSW) discharge that is bilateral, synchronous and symmetric, and which immediately precedes a MJ that is recorded on polygraphic surface EMG leads (often limited to both deltoids). The EEG discharge includes 5 to 20 spikes, with a frequency between 12 and 16 Hz. The amplitude of spikes is typically increasing and is maximal over the frontal leads where it reaches 200–300 mV. Slow waves of variable frequency (3–4 Hz) and amplitude (200–350 mV) often precede or follow the polyspikes, which results in a PSW complex that lasts much longer than the MJ, around 2 to 4 seconds. The number of spikes appears to be correlated to the intensity of the MJ: there are few spikes and a more pronounced slow component when the MJ is mild. Back averaging shows that the conduction time, between the apex of the spike and the onset of the MJ, is short (20–50 msec) and characteristic of a cortical myoclonia.

In our practice, all patients suspected of having JME are recorded by video-polygraphy. In China, a long-term video-EEG has been used to confirm a firm diagnosis of JME (Wang *et al.*, 2016). Such recordings should precede the initiation of therapy. It brings resolution of diagnostic problems and validation of the phenotype for genetic studies. Given the risk of provocation of a GTCS associated with major sleep deprivation of drug withdrawal, this type of recording is ethically and practically not recommended in a well-controlled patient, *e.g.*, in order to retrospectively validate the diagnosis.

Interictal EEG

The background activity is normal during waking and sleep, except in case of drug overload or of inadequate treatment. Interictal PSW complexes are characterized by a smaller number of spikes. They may appear to be localized only over the anterior portions of the scalp. The presence of interictal changes is in favour of the diagnosis of JME but does not allow its confirmation. Conclusions on the clinical symptomatology cannot be drawn solely from this EEG pattern (Janz, 1985). These discharges are not pathognomonic of JME: they are found in about 50% of the cases, as in the interictal EEG in childhood and juvenile absence epilepsies (Janz & Waltz, 1994). PSW complexes may also be found in epilepsy with Grand Mal seizures on awakening (Janz, 1985), and in other syndromes of IGE.

As noted by Tsuboi (1977) in his large series of 381 patients with JME, other, less evocative paroxysmal changes may often be present: irregular spike-waves (SW) (11.8%), fast SW (> 3.5 Hz, 25%), "classical" SW (2.5–3.5 Hz, 11%), slow SW (< 2.5 Hz, 3.4%). In this series, 2.1% of patients had a normal waking EEG. The profitability of the interictal EEG is increased by early morning recording, sleep deprivation (Touchon *et al.*, 1982), and hyperventilation.

Focal changes are present in 15–55% of patients, and in 29% of cases on the first EEG (Aliberti *et al.*, 1994; Genton *et al.*, 1994; Lancman *et al.*, 1994). These are asymmetric ictal discharges, or focal slow waves that shift sides from one recording to the other or during the same registration. The diagnosis of focal epilepsy is eliminated because of the association of these changes with generalized SW and PSW discharges, but misdiagnosis of focal epilepsy often occurs when the more typical changes are not present during the same recording.

Sleep EEG (nap or full-night) is more often abnormal than the waking EEG, especially during intermediate awakenings (Genton *et al.*, 1994) or after provoked awakenings (Touchon *et al.*, 1982). EEG changes are also clearly activated during deep NREM sleep, while discharges tend to disappear during NREM sleep (Gigli *et al.*, 1992). The circadian activation profile of EEG changes is thus globally the same as the seizure profile.

Photosensitivity and eye-closure sensitivity

Among common epileptic syndromes, JME is the one that is most clearly associated with photosensitivity (Wolf & Goosses, 1986) *(Figure 6)*. In the EEG laboratory, a photoparoxysmal response with the PSW that are characteristic for JME is found in 30% (Janz, 1985) to 48% (Loiseau & Duché, 1990) of patients, *vs.* only 18% of patients with absence epilepsy (Wolf & Goosses, 1986). Female patients are nearly twice as often affected than males (Janz & Durner, 1997; Genton *et al.*, 1994). MJ can be easily elicited by intermittent photic stimulation in photosensitive patients. Isolated eye closure may also facilitate PSW discharges and MJ (Gigli *et al.*, 1991; Baykan-Kurt *et al.*, 1999). In JME, however, the actual prevalence of clinical photosensitivity in natural surroundings is obviously lower than that of photosensitivity in the EEG laboratory.

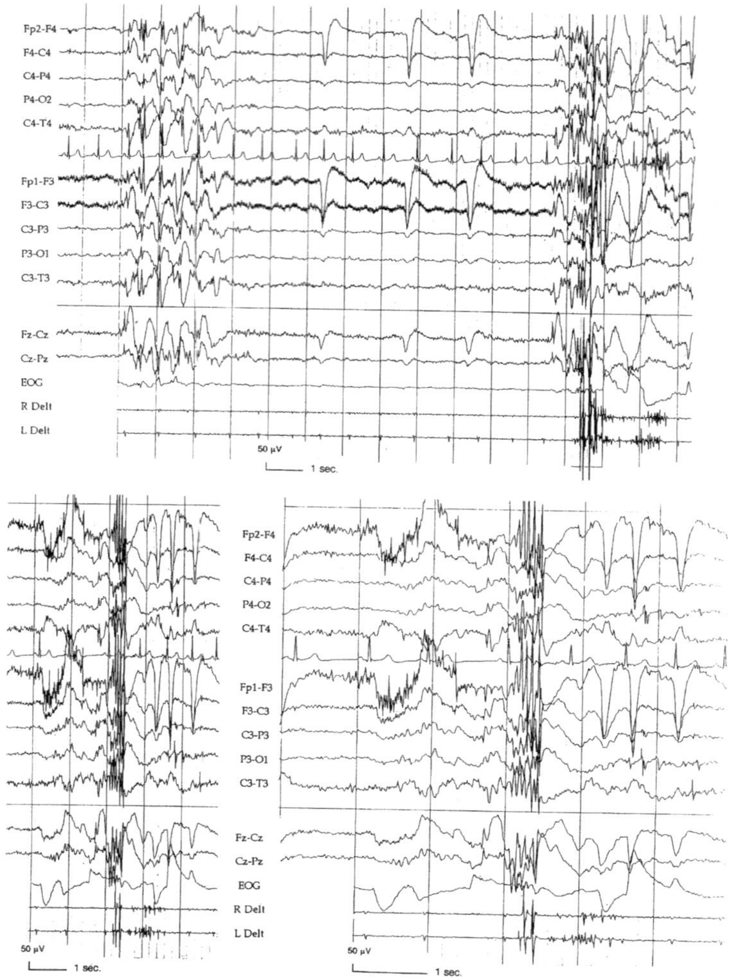

Figure 6

Typical aspects of ictal EEG in a 27-year-old patient with JME recorded in the morning after sleep deprivation.
Top: **normal background activity and a burst of generalized SW at 2 Hz, 12 seconds before a second burst of generalized PSW that is associated with MJ recorded on the deltoid muscles.**
Bottom: **volley of polyspikes with MJ. Enhancement at 30 mm/sec (on the right) shows clearly that the burst begins with an isolated spike-wave complex over the anterior vertex (Fz-Cz), which lasts 250 msec (frequency: 4 Hz) and is immediately followed by a discharge of 7 spikes lasting 400 msec (frequency: 17.5 Hz).**

Neuroimaging and pathology

Although they are frequently performed, morphological studies of the brain are not useful. JME may be fortuitously associated with minor or longstanding anatomic changes and may thus occur on a very particular background (Gélisse *et al.*, 2000a). Janz (1969) reported 1 patient out of 280 with residual hemiplegia following injury at birth. Crespel *et al.* (2009a) reported a similar case with a benign evolution *(Figure 7)*. Among 170 consecutive JME patients, neuroimaging was performed in 82 cases (Gélisse *et al.*, 2000b). Nine had non-specific lesions. In 4 subjects, specific neurological abnormalities had justified neuroimaging: severe head trauma after the onset of JME (2, both with lesions related to the trauma), multiple sclerosis with onset after JME (1, with normal MRI before the onset of multiple sclerosis and abnormal, specific findings later), severe mental retardation, with diffuse MRI changes (Gélisse *et al.*, 2000a). All patients with abnormal neuroradiological findings were fully controlled and the course of the disease was benign in all patients.

Quantified MRI may yield interesting results. Woermann *et al.* (1999) found in nearly half of their patients a thickening of the grey matter in the mesiofrontal regions, sometimes in association with abnormal cortical organization. Using voxel-based morphometry, Betting *et al.* (2006) found increased grey matter concentration in the frontobasal regions, while Pillal *et al.* (2017) found significant reduction in grey matter volume in dorsolateral prefrontal cortex in JME patients with frontal executive dysfunction. Pulsipher *et al.* (2009) found that thalamic and frontal volumes were significantly related to executive functioning. On quantitative MRI, JME patients had more frontal cerebrospinal fluid than controls and children with benign centro-temporal spikes and had significantly smaller thalamic volumes. Keller *et al.* (2011) showed combined microstructural and macrostructural putamen abnormalities, which were correlated with early age of onset and a longer duration of epilepsy. It was also shown that, compared with non-epileptic controls, JME patients had a thinner corpus callosum (Anastasopoulou *et al.*, 2017). Thus the morphologic findings are varied; Swartz *et al.* (2016) have stressed the heterogeneity of brain volume changes between individuals with JME, finding larger pulvinar nuclei or thalami, and conclude that such studies should be stringently matched to the (also heterogeneous) genetic background of JME patients.

Using flumazenil [11C] PET scans, Koepp *et al.* (1997) reported increased binding in thalamus, cerebellum and neocortex, a finding which might be correlated with the presence of microdysgenesis. Meschaks *et al.* (2005) found reductions in serotonin 1A receptor binding in the dorsolateral prefrontal cortex, raphe nuclei, and hippocampus. They suggested that the serotonin system could be affected in JME. The same team suggested that dopamine system is also altered in JME with impairment dopamine uptake in the midbrain (Odano *et al.*, 2012).

Previously, Bernasconi *et al.* (2003) had not found differences in the volume of the thalami in patients with IGE. These authors reported reduction of mean thalamic N-acetylaspartate/creatine ratio (a measure of neuronal injury) compared with normal controls, supporting the notion of abnormal thalamo-cortical circuitry. Savic *et al.* (2004) demonstrated reduced frontal lobe levels of N-acetyl aspartate in JME patients compared with GTCS patients whose values were normal. On the other hand, patients with GTCS showed significantly lower thalamic acetylaspartate than controls. This study showed partly differentiated alterations within the thalamo-cortical loop in GTCS *vs.* JME patients. Lin *et al.* (2009) investigated 60 JME patients and demonstrated a reduction of the N-acetyl aspartate/creatine ratio, in the primary motor cortex, the medial prefrontal cortex, and the thalamus.

Together with the recent genetic data, which showed predispositions to defects in neuronal migration, these morphologic and functional data seem to validate the controversial findings of Meencke (1985), who described focal microdysgenesias in the cortex of 15 patients with IGE, including 3 with JME.

Differential diagnosis and nosology

Hypnagogic MJ are frequent and normal in young subjects. Some progressive myoclonus epilepsies with onset around adolescence (Lafora's disease, Unverricht-Lundborg disease) may be mistaken for JME at their onset. Later, the severity of the myoclonic syndrome, the occurrence of intellectual decay, the slowing of the background activity on the EEG and the characteristics of the paroxysmal EEG changes will correct the diagnosis.

In clinical practice, the diagnosis of JME may be discussed against several other types of IGE and related syndromes. Age at diagnosis may play a major part: late onset of JME should lead to the discussion of other diagnoses. Some patients may exhibit the clinical features of JME in middle- or old age (Gram *et al.*, 1988). A syndrome of adult-onset myoclonic epilepsy mimicking the clinical and EEG characteristics of JME has been proposed, with possible familial aggregation (Gilliam *et al.*, 2000), and only genetic elucidation of this entity will show whether it should be separated from the classical JME. However, *adult myoclonic epilepsy* has also been used as a label to describe an often familiar condition that has been linked to a 2q locus, and should be distinguished from JME on the basis of its clinical characteristics, which include cortical tremor, and a slow clinical progression (review in Crompton *et al.*, 2012).

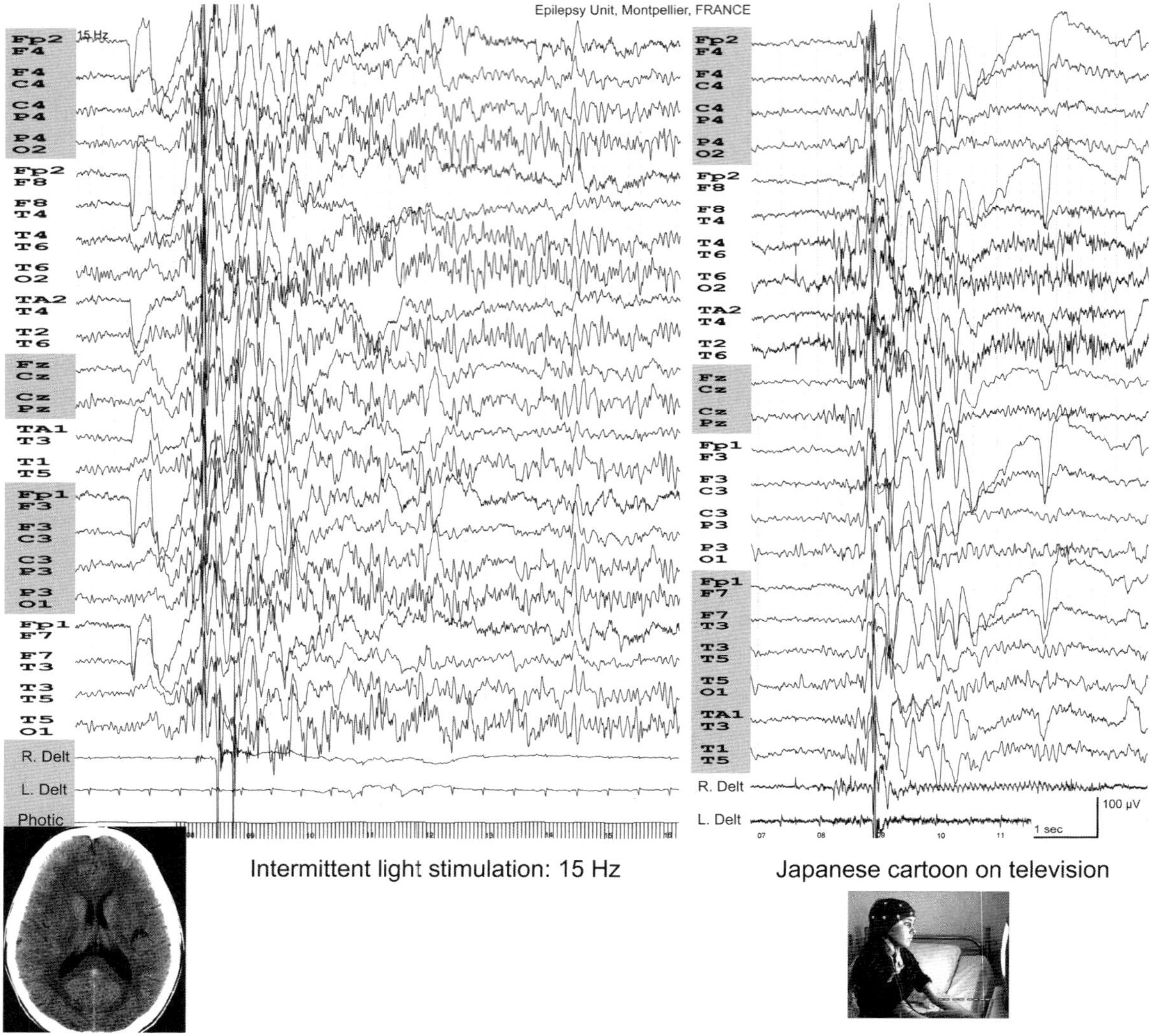

Figure 7

JME in a young woman with history of infantile hemiplegia. At adolescence, two GTCS followed by rare typical absences and myoclonic jerks. Physical examination revealed right hemiparesis. A CT scan documented a left Rolandic cerebral infarction and focal, central epilepsy was diagnosed. EEG: left: **ILS performed at awakening from an afternoon nap; generalized polyspike-wave discharge with two myoclonic jerks.** Right: **watching a Japanese cartoon on television triggers polyspikes waves associated with a myoclonic jerk.**

In primary reading epilepsy (PRE), MJ are limited to the cephalic segment, and are provoked by reading aloud. Several papers, however, have drawn attention to the occasional co-occurrence of JME and PRE (Radhakrishnan *et al.*, 1995; Mayer & Wolf, 1999), and of JME and "noogenic" epilepsies (Inoue *et al.*, 1994). In purely photosensitive idiopathic epilepsies, MJ occur only in response to visual stimuli.

The myoclonic component found in TA of absence epilepsies is much more pronounced in the syndrome of epilepsy with myoclonic absences, and in certain epilepsies with myoclonias (eyelid myoclonia with absences, perioral myoclonia with absences). In these syndromes, MJ are associated with a 3 Hz rhythmic SW discharge and with altered consciousness or contact. CAE begins earlier than JME and is characterized by the frequent, "pycnoleptic" repetition of TA. An overlap between JME and eyelid myoclonia with absence has been suggested (Destina Yalçin *et al.*, 2006).

Nosological problems are maximal among the adolescent-onset forms of IGE, which have now been clustered as "IGE with variable phenotypes", a group that includes, besides JME, juvenile absence epilepsy (JAE), with GTCS in most patients and MJ in some, and epilepsies with GTCS on awakening (AwGM), which may also include MJ and TA (Wolf, 1992c). Only the quantitative predominance of MJ, and the fact that GTCS are preceded by an increasing volley of MJ, will push the diagnosis towards JME, but a certain number of cases remain difficult to classify (Janz, 1991; Wolf, 1992b; Schmitz *et al.*, 2000).

Treatment

Lifestyle

In patients with JME, counseling on lifestyle is essential. The sleep/wake rhythm must be regulated and circumstances that interfere with normal sleep and progressive awakening in the morning must be dealt with (Janz & Durner, 1997). Alcoholic drinks will only be permitted in small quantities, on social occasions: the cumulative effects of excessive alcohol intake, sleep deprivation, photic stimulation and early awakening (*e.g.*, after a celebration like New Year's eve or a night in the disco) is very often the revealing circumstance, with a first GTCS. A permission to drive will depend on local legislation. When such legislation is liberal, patients will be advised not to drive in case of lack of sleep, and they will be informed on the risks associated with driving soon after awakening. They should also avoid visual stimuli if they are photosensitive. Such measures will certainly decrease the necessity of high-dose medical treatment, but only patients with a minor form of JME, who never experienced a GTCS and have a reasonable lifestyle, can do without medication. Even mild restrictions, *i.e.* aiming at preserving adequate sleep and avoiding excessive alcohol intake, may, however, be perceived by teenagers as tiresome limitations, as imposed "curfews", and the concept of a "Cinderella syndrome" has been proposed, as most JME youngsters will be asked to be home before midnight (Leahy *et al.*, 2018)!

Aggravation of JME due to anticonvulsants

Several authors have insisted on the possibility of aggravation of epilepsy by AEDs (Bauer, 1996; Perucca *et al.*, 1998; Genton & Mc Menamin, 1998). JME is indeed very much concerned by paradoxical effects of AEDs. The pharmacological sensitivity of JME, which it shares with other forms of IGE, is characteristic.

Phenytoin (PHT) has modest efficacy in JME. Among 18 patients exposed to PHT, 4 were better, 8 were unchanged and 6 experienced aggravation (Genton *et al.*, 2000b). In refractory patients, increasing PHT dosage clearly exacerbates MJ (Sözüer *et al.*, 1996). Carbamazepine (CBZ) is the AED with the most prominent aggravating effect in JME: among 38 patients exposed to CBZ in our series, symptoms were aggravated in 68% *(Figure 8)*; some patients even developed myoclonic status on CBZ (Genton *et al.*, 2000b; Thomas *et al.*, 2006). In spite of this, CBZ may be useful in some selected cases (Knott & Panayiotopoulos, 1994). Oxcarbazepine (OXC) also appears to have a significant potential for aggravating JME (Gélisse *et al.*, 2004). Among newer AEDs, vigabatrin was given to four of our patients in association with CBZ and triggered a myoclonic status. However, Pedersen *et al.* (1985) have reported partial efficacy in three of their patients. Tiagabine provoked a state of obtundation resembling absence status in one patient (Knake *et al.*, 1999). The efficacy of lamotrigine (LTG) in JME remains controversial, with reports of worsening of MJ or even absence status (Biraben *et al.*, 2000; Trinka *et al.*, 2002), or increased GTCS (Maiga *et al.*, 2006), while other authors recommend its use in JME (Buchanan, 1996; Wallace, 1998). It must be noted here that LTG can provoke a dose-related, early-onset aggravation of myoclonus, but that a clear aggravation can also be seen after several years at constant doses (Crespel *et al.*, 2005).

Anticonvulsants used in JME

In 1957, Janz and Christian had already noted that barbiturates controlled seizures in 86% of patients, while PHT was inefficient or aggravating in 33%. Phenobarbital (PB) and primidone (PRM) were thus the treatment of choice, until valproate (VPA) was shown to have a very specific potency in JME.

The first North American reports on JME already stated that VPA was the choice treatment: only 4/43 patients were not controlled on VPA (Delgado Escueta & Enrile-Bacsal, 1984); 47/50 patients received VPA

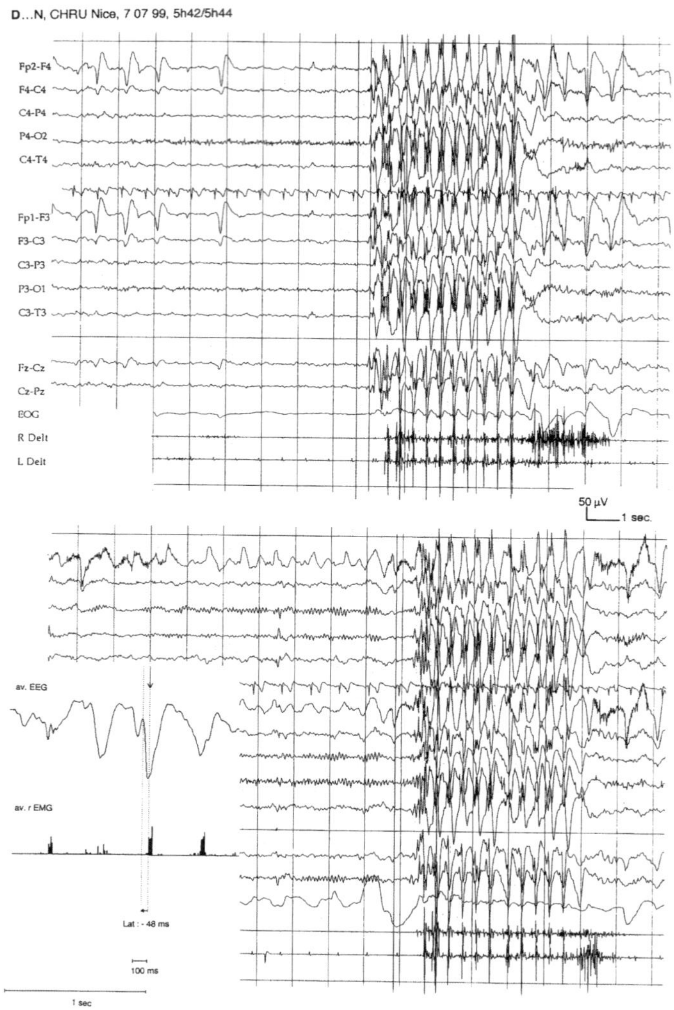

Figure 8

Aggravation in a 17-year-old man with JME, inadequately treated with carbamazepine (CBZ). Normal background activity, volleys of rhythmic MJ lasting 5 sec, without alteration of consciousness, preceded by regular generalized PSW discharges at 3 Hz. Backaveraging on the EMG, which was made easy by the unusual regularity of the PSW discharges, shows a latency of 48 msec between the peak of the last spike and the onset of the MJ. All symptoms remitted when CBZ was replaced by VPA at 1,000 mg/d. av.
EEG: averaged EEG; av r EMG: averaged rectified EMG; lat.: latency.

(Penry *et al.*, 1989): total control of seizures on VPA monotherapy was obtained in 86% of their patients (Penry *et al.*, 1989) and in 84.5% of our patients (Genton *et al.*, 2000a). Daily dosage ranges in adults between 1,000 and 2,000 mg. Persistence of interictal EEG changes does not appear to have a bad prognostic significance (Sundqvist *et al.*, 1999). The whole daily dose may be given in the evening, after dinner. In case of resistance to VPA, increasing dosage until side-effects show does not appear very efficient (Sundqvist *et al.*, 1998). Thus VPA is widely considered the first-line treatment in JME, even very recently (Chowdhury & Brodie, 2016), with restrictions in younger women, and the actual question may be: what if VPA fails (Nicolson & Marson, 2010)?

Other older drugs that have some efficacy in JME are clonazepam, which may be associated with VPA (Obeid & Panayiotopoulos, 1989), acetazolamide (Resor & Resor, 1990) and methsuximide (Hurst, 1996). An obese adult female patient without GTCS for many years received piracetam 3,200 mg/d with sustained antimyoclonic efficacy (Khani *et al.*, 2005).

Several among the newer AEDs have been used in JME

Lamotrigine (LTG) has been often used, in open studies, often in association with VPA (Buchanan, 1996; Wallace, 1998), and has been recommended in younger women because of the potential teratogenicity of VPA. LTG has been evaluated in patients who failed VPA: 13.6% of these achieved seizure remission, but only if VPA had failed because of side-effects and not because of lack of efficacy; moreover, LTG achieved a 2-year remission rate of 7.7%, *vs.* 41.2% for VPA (Nicolson *et al.*, 2004), while the combination therapy of LTG with VPA did not seem very efficient, with a 3-year remission rate of 8.3% in the same study. Bodenstein-Sachar *et al.* (2011) found that LTG was helpful in patients who had failed VPA because of side-effects, and who had JME without GTCS. Clearly, LTG is useful in JME, but perhaps not as a first-line option, because of potential aggravation, which may occur after a long delay.

Levetiracetam (LEV) is increasingly used in JME. There had been early reports of its efficacy against myoclonus (Genton & Gélisse, 2000c) and photoparoxysmal responses (Kasteleijn-Nolst-Trénité *et al.*, 1996). Specific efficacy in JME was shown in open studies: among 8 patients on LEV monotherapy, 5 achieved remission, 1 was improved, 1 unchanged and 1 aggravated (Labate *et al.*, 2006); 5/10 patients on monotherapy and 11/38 on polytherapy with LEV became seizure-free (Specchio *et al.*, 2006). In an open study of LEV as the first monotherapy in 32 patients with new onset JME (mean age 13.2 years), 29 were seizure-free and 3 responders at 12 months (Verrotti *et al.*, 2008). Similarly, the retrospective study of Sharpe *et al.* (2008) found that 80% (24/32) patients became seizure-free on LEV monotherapy. Controlled studies confirmed the effect of LEV in JME: of 54 patients with JME among 164 uncontrolled IGE patients, 24 received LEV, which was significantly better than placebo on seizure outcomes, but specific responses in the JME group were not provided (Berkovic *et al.*, 2007); among 122 patients with IGE and myoclonias (JME, juvenile absence epilepsy or awakening Grand Mal), who had resisted a first AED, 62 were treated with LEV and 60 with placebo, with a very significant effect of LEV on myoclonic seizures (Noachtar *et al.*, 2008). A further analysis of the two latter studies showed that 61% of JME patients responded and 20.8% became seizure-free on LEV (*vs.* 24.7% and 3.4%, respectively, on placebo) (Rosenfeld *et al.*, 2009). LEV has thus become a clear alternative to VPA in patients with JME, especially women of childbearing age: a head-to-head comparison showed, however, that VPA was more efficient, with better control of GTCS (Sala-Padro *et al.*, 2016).

Topiramate (TPM) appeared promising (Kellett *et al.*, 1999; Prasad *et al.*, 2003). In their retrospective analysis of a subgroup of 22 JME patients collected among 160 with "primary" GTCS in two prospective, double-blind add-on studies of TPM *vs.* placebo, Biton & Bourgeois (2006) showed that TPM reduced GTCS. In their randomized, open-label study comparing adolescent and adult patients, 19 on TPM *vs.* 9 on VPA, both drugs titrated to the optimal doses. Levisohn & Holland (2007) found that TPM (at a median dose of 250 mg/d) was slightly more efficient than VPA (at a median dose of 750 mg/d). An open study of TPM in uncontrolled JME (15 patients with uncontrolled seizures, 4 controlled but with side-effects and 3 newly diagnosed), showed that TPM was efficient, especially against GTCS and MJ, and reasonably well tolerated (Sousa *et al.*, 2005). Thus TPM appears to constitute a good alternative to VPA, perhaps especially in patients who have had unacceptable weight gain on VPA. However, TPM is associated with neuropsychiatric side-effects, and compares unfavourably with VPA in JME, especially in terms of attention, short-term memory, processing speed and verbal fluency (de Araújo Filho *et al.*, 2006).

Interesting results have also been reported using zonisamide (ZNS) in monotherapy in 13 patients (Kothare *et al.*, 2004), but the number of totally controlled cases was not reported. ZNS markedly reduces the EEG changes in JME (Szaflarski, 2004). Kothare *et al.* (2004) reported on 15 patients, of whom 13 received ZNS as first drug on monotherapy, and 2 as add-on to VPA: 69%, 62% and 38% were free of GTCS, myoclonic, and absence seizures, respectively. A retrospective evaluation of 7 patients with refractory JME showed that ZNS had decreased by 83.3%, 100% and 100% GTCS, MJ, and TA respectively, with two patients becoming seizure-free (O'Rourke *et al.*, 2007). Marinas *et al.* (2009) reported on ZNS in IGE: 6 had JME, 3 were seizure-free (including one on monotherapy), 2 were unchanged and one stopped ZNS due to side effects. Thus ZNS has been used in JME with success, but controlled studies are clearly missing.

Lacosamide (LCM) was marketed as add-on treatment in resistant focal epilepsy. Three JME patients were reported, two receiving LCM as monotherapy and one as add-on, with a good effect (Afra & Adamolekun, 2012), but LCM may provoke exacerbation of myoclonus (Birnbaum & Koueissi, 2016). Perampanel (PER), a novel inhibitor of AMPA receptor, has shown promising efficacy against various types of myoclonus and myoclonic epilepsies, *e.g.* in Lafora's disease (Goldsmith & Minassian, 2016) and might be a new, powerful tool for the treatment of resistant forms of JME.

Vagal nerve stimulation (VNS) has been used in various types of refractory, including generalized, epilepsies: Ng and Devinsky (2005) reported that, among 14 patients with IGE, VNS achieved a mean seizure reduction of 72.9%, 5 patients experiencing a more than 50% reduction in seizure frequency while one was aggravated; these authors did not state how many patients had JME. Kostov *et al.* (2007) reported on 12 patients with resistant IGE, including 7 with JME: 5 of the latter responded with > 50% seizure reduction, with one remaining on VNS alone with > 75% reduction in GTCS, and > 50% in TA and MJ. These data are not sufficient for VNS to qualify as a recommended treatment for JME.

In summary, the first line treatment of JME remains VPA; LEV is the alternative, TPM and ZNS can be considered second-line drugs, PER is promising, and LTG, PB and PRM, piracetam, acetazolamide and methsuximide can be used in special situations. Benzodiazepines may have an adjunctive role for short periods. Most other drugs are likely to produced aggravation; however, in individual patients, they may still be beneficial and can be tried with proper warning, or can be maintained if the patient has benefited from them.

Drug treatment of JME may pose a problem in girls and young women; one should keep in mind, however, that none of the alternative drugs is devoid of teratogenic effects, with the possible exception of LEV. Although no strict consensus is available, we share the opinion expressed by Montouris & Abou-Khalil (2009): taking into consideration copathologies, one can recommend LEV as a first-line agent if MJ are the dominant seizure type; LTG may be tried if TA are prominent; TPM may be chosen in case of associated migraine, TPM or ZNS in overweight patients; low-dose VPA definitely remains an option in female patients if JME is difficult to control with other agents.

Evolution and prognosis

JME had been described as "benign" JME (Asconapé & Penry, 1984; Wolf, 1985), a qualification withdrawn later, when it became apparent that relapses were very common after withdrawal of treatment: JME is thus considered a longlasting, potentially "lifetime" condition. Even after years of full seizure control, withdrawal of AEDs nearly always results into recurrence of seizures (Delgado-Escueta & Enrile-Bacsal, 1984; Baruzzi *et al.*, 1988). Nevertheless, clinical experience has shown that JME is seldom very active in middle-aged to elderly patients, which might be in part explained by changes in lifestyle. However, the true long-term prognosis, in terms of seizures and of social outcome, was not adequately documented until recently.

JME remains indeed a condition with a good seizure prognosis in most patients, as 80–90% are fully controlled by treatment. Symptoms tend to remit during pregnancies (Asconapé & Penry, 1984), but certain patients relapse in the post-partum, possibly due to the sleep deprivation that is associated with this period.

Pharmacoresistance may be a problem in patients with JME. A group of patients with intractable seizures was identified by Camfield & Camfield (2009) in their long-term study: among 24 patients, 3 were therapy-resistant in the long term, among 12 who were kept on medication. It is important, however, to distinguish pseudo-resistant cases (in whom persistence of seizures is associated with inadequate lifestyle, poor compliance or suboptimal drug regimen) from truly resistant cases. Pseudo-resistant cases represent between 9.7% (Gélisse *et al.*, 2001b) and 16.7% (Baykan *et al.*, 2008) of all resistant cases. Truly pharmacoresistant cases represent 15.1% (Desai *et al.*, 2016), 15.5% (Gélisse *et al.*, 2001a) or 16.7% (Baykan *et al.*, 2008). For Dasheiff & Ritaccio (1993), these patients are characterized by a longer duration of epilepsy, diagnostic delay, and inefficient initial treatment. Among 33 JME patients who were not controlled on VPA, Fernando-Dongas *et al.* (2000) identified several factors of drug resistance: low IQ, atypical EEG aspects, and atypical clinical features, *e.g.*, auras or postictal confusion. For Gélisse *et al.* (2001a), clinical factors of resistance are, independently, either the association of all 3 seizure types (62.5% are resistant) or the presence of psychiatric problems (58% are resistant); the coexistence of overt psychiatric symptoms was also noted by Baykan *et al.* (2008) in association with pharmacoresistance, which was also more common in patients with copathologies. Among factors of refractoriness and poorer prognosis: sleep disorders (Buratti *et al.*, 2018); longer, > 3 sec runs of paroxysmal EEG activity (Arntsen *et al.*, 2007); praxis-induction (Matsuoka, 1992; Inoue *et al.*, 1994; Inoue & Kubota, 2000; Guaranha *et al.*, 2009; Guaranha *et al.*, 2011; Uchida *et al.*, 2015; Abarrategui *et al.*, 2018); photosensitivity (Inoue & Kubota, 2000); language-sensitive patients (Guaranha *et al.*, 2011).

The long-term seizure outcome has been assessed in three studies. For Camfield & Camfield (2009), although 35% of their patients experienced status epilepticus, 39% were able to discontinue medication: 26% were totally seizure-free and 13% had persisting mild myoclonus (while 8% had discontinued treatment but still had rare GTCS). For Martinez-Juarez *et al.* (2006), the prognosis depends on the JME subtype: in classic JME, 5% of patient can stop medication without recurrence of seizures, while 40% have persistent seizures under treatment; in JME evolving from childhood absence epilepsy, apparently a more severe condition, only 8% achieve total seizure control on medication, and none has remission without medication; in the smaller groups with adolescence-onset absences or with atonic seizures, 44% and 37%, respectively, have persistent seizures. Baykan *et al.* (2008) showed that myoclonic jerks abate with age, especially after age 30 years, becoming less frequent and less intense; more than 10% of their patients were able to stop medication without relapse.

The social outcome of JME patients has not been extensively evaluated. One can suspect that, due to persisting seizures in some, to associated psychologic and cognitive problems, it might not be optimal. This has been confirmed by Camfield & Camfield (2009): after a follow-up of 25 to 43 years, 31% were unemployed, 61% had taken a psychotropic drug, and overall 74% had at least one measure of negative social outcome.

Patients with JME are exposed to the risk of sudden unexplained death (SUDEP, Nashef *et al.*, 1995). Among three cases with premature death, two died suddenly and unexpectedly, probably in association with a major seizure (Genton & Gélisse, 2001). Baykan *et al.* (2008) also reported a morbidly obese, well-controlled patient with probable SUDEP.

In summary, JME cannot be considered a truly benign condition, although it may remit, at least partially, with age. Some patients are pharmacoresistant, and the social outcome is clearly below expectancy in many. A logical therapeutic attitude is to maintain treatment in most patients beyond early adulthood, but with low-dose VPA, with a single evening intake (de Toffol & Autret, 1996).

Conclusion

JME was discovered in France, described in Germany (and Uruguay), named in Denmark, rediscovered in the US, and is now universal. JME, or Janz syndrome, is an epileptic condition that is frequent and particularly easy to identify and treat. The electro-clinical, syndromic approach should protect clinicians from mistakes in diagnosis and treatment of JME. As some other epileptic syndromes, and contrary to many others, JME looks a lot like a disease, but is not, as the underlying genetic mechanisms are multiple, and still far from fully elucidated. JME is a treatable, "manageable" form of epilepsy that should, under optimal conditions, have few consequences on a patient's potentials. However, JME may be associated with refractoriness to treatment, with significant social and behavioural handicap, and thus covers a range of situations: this justifies, in our opinion, the widening of the concept to one of "JMEs", or juvenile myoclonic "*epilepsies*", which is coherent with the concept of JME as a "spectrum disorder" (Baykan & Wolf, 2017), and with the conclusion of studies pointing to the existence of distinct phenotypes, including subsets of more severely affected patients, in terms of drug resistance, psychological and cognitive profile, and social outcome (Valente *et al.*, 2016).

REFERENCES ▶

Abarrategui B, De Marchi LR, Guaranha MSB, Yacubian EMT (2018): Praxis-induced myoclonia: From the neurophysiologist to the patient perspective. *Seizure* 60: 184–189.

Afra P, Adamolekun B (2012): Lacosamide treatment of juvenile myoclonic epilepsy. *Seizure* 21: 202–204.

Agathonikou A, Panayiotopoulos CP, Giannakodimos S, Koutroumanidis M (1998): Typical absence status in adults: diagnostic and syndromic considerations. *Epilepsia* 39: 1265–1276.

Aguglia U, Gambardella A, Le Piane E, *et al.* (1999): Idiopathic generalized epilepsies with versive or circling seizures. *Acta Neurol Scand* 99: 219–224.

Aliberti V, Grünewald RA, Panayiotopoulos CP (1994): Focal EEG abnormalities in juvenile myoclonic epilepsy. *Epilepsia* 35: 297–301.

Arntsen V, Sand T, Syvertsen MR, Brodtkorb E (2017): Prolonged epileptiform EEG runs are associated with persistent seizures in juvenile myoclonic epilepsy. *Epilepsy Res* 134: 26–32.

Anastasopoulou S, Kurth F, Luders E, Savic I (2017): Generalized epilepsy syndromes and callosal thickness: Differential effects between patients with juvenile myoclonic epilepsy and those with generalized tonic-clonic seizures alone. *Epilepsy Res* 129: 74–78.

Annesi F, Gambardella A, Michelucci R, *et al.* (2007): Mutational analysis of *EFHC1* gene in Italian families with juvenile myoclonic epilepsy. *Epilepsia* 48: 1686–1690.

Asconapé J, Penry JK (1984): Some clinical and EEG aspects of benign juvenile myoclonic epilepsy. *Epilepsia* 25: 108–114.

Atakli D, Sozuer D, Atay T, Baybas S, Arpaci B (1998): Misdiagnosis and treatment in juvenile myoclonic epilepsy. *Seizure 7:* 63–66.

Atakli D, Senadim S, Baslo SA, *et al.* (2016): Misdiagnosis in JME: Still a problem after 17 years? *Seizure* 36: 27–30.

Bailey JN, Patterson C, de Nijs L, *et al.* (2017): EFHC1 variants in juvenile myoclonic epilepsy: reanalysis according to NHGRI and ACMG guidelines for assigning disease causality. *Genet Med* 19: 144–156.

Bailey JN, de Nijs L, Bai D, *et al.* (2018): Variant Intestinal-Cell Kinase in Juvenile Myoclonic Epilepsy. *N Engl J Med* 378: 1018–1028.

Baykan-Kurt B, Gokyigit A, Parman Y, Kinay D, Gurses C (1999): Eye closure related spike and wave discharges: clinical and syndromic associations. *Clin Electroencephalogr* 30: 106–110.

Baykan B, Wolf P (2017): Juvenile myoclonic epilepsy as a spectrum disorder: A focused review. *Seizure* 49: 36–41.

Bauer J (1996): Seizure-inducing effect of antiepileptic drugs: a review. *Acta Neurol Scand* 94: 367–377.

Baruzzi A, Procaccianti G, Tinuper P, Lugaresi E (1988): Antiepileptic drug withdrawal in childhood epilepsies: preliminary results of a prospective study. In: Faienza C, Prati GL (eds) *Diagnostic and Therapeutic Problems in Pediatric Epileptology*, pp. 117–123. Amsterdam: Elsevier.

Baykan B, Altindag EA, Bebek N, *et al.* (2008): Myoclonic seizures subside in the fourth decade in juvenile myoclonic epilepsy. *Neurology* 70: 2123–2129.

Berger I, Dor T, Halvardson J, *et al.* (2012): Intractable epilepsy of infancy due to homozygous mutation in the EFHC1 gene. *Epilepsia* 53: 1436–1440.

Berkovic SF, Knowlton RC, Leroy RF, Schiemann J, Falter U; Levetiracetam N01057 Study Group (2007): Placebo-controlled study of levetiracetam in idiopathic generalized epilepsy. *Neurology* 69: 1751–1760.

Bernasconi A, Bernasconi N, Natsume J, Antel SB, Andermann F, Arnold DL (2003): Magnetic resonance spectroscopy and imaging of the thalamus in idiopathic generalized epilepsy. *Brain* 126: 2447–2454.

Betting LE, Mory SB, Li LM, *et al.* (2006): Voxel-based morphometry in patients with idiopathic generalized epilepsies. *NeuroImage* 32: 498–502.

Biraben A, Allain H, Scarabin JM, Schuck S, Edan G (2000): Exacerbation of juvenile myoclonic epilepsy with lamotrigine. *Neurology* 55: 1758.

Birnbaum D, Koubeissi M. (2016): Unmasking of myoclonus by lacosamide in generalized epilepsy. *Epilepsy Behav* 7: 28–30.

Biton V, Bourgeois BFD (2006): Topiramate in patients with juvenile myoclonic epilepsy. *Arch Neurol* 62: 1705–1708.

Bodenstein-Sachar H, Gandelman-Marton R, Ben-Zeev B, Chapman J, Blatt I (2011): Outcome of lamotrigine treatment in juvenile myoclonic epilepsy. *Acta Neurol Scand* 124: 22–27.

Buchanan N (1996): The use of lamotrigine in juvenile myoclonic epilepsy. *Seizure* 5: 149–151.

Buratti L, Natanti A, Viticchi G, *et al.* (2018): Impact of sleep disorders on the risk of seizure recurrence in juvenile myoclonic epilepsy. *Epilepsy Behav* 80: 21–24.

Camfield CS, Camfield PR (2009): Juvenile myoclonic epilepsy 25 years after seizure onset: a population-based study. *Neurology* 73: 1041–1045.

Canevini MP, Mai R, Di Marco C, *et al.* (1992): Juvenile myoclonic epilepsy of Janz: Clinical observations in 60 patients. *Seizure* 1: 291–298.

Carvalho KC, Uchida CG, Guaranha MS, *et al.* (2016): Cognitive performance in juvenile myoclonic epilepsy patients with specific endophenotypes. *Seizure* 40: 33–41.

Castells C, Mendilaharsu C (1958): La epilepsia mioclonica bilateral y consciente. *Acta Neurol Latinoamer* 4: 23–48.

Cavalleri GL, Walley NM, Soranzo N, *et al.* (2007): A multicenter study of BRD2 as a risk factor for juvenile myoclonic epilepsy. *Epilepsia* 48: 706–712.

Chachua T, Goletiani C, Maglakelidze G *et al.* (2014): Sex-specific behavioral traits in the Brd2 mouse model of juvenile myoclonic epilepsy. *Genes Brain Behav* 13: 702–712.

Chowdhury A, Brodie MJ (2016): Pharmacological outcomes in juvenile myoclonic epilepsy: Support for sodium valproate. *Epilepsy Res* 119: 62–66.

Commission on Classification and Terminology of the International League Against Epilepsy (1989): Proposal for revised classification of epilepsies and epileptic syndromes. *Epilepsia* 30: 389–399.

Cossette P, Liu L, Brisebois K, *et al.* (2002): Mutation of GABRA1 in an autosomal dominant form of a juvenile myoclonic epilepsy. *Nat Genet* 31: 184–189.

Cossette P, Lortie A, Vanasse M, Saint-Hilaire JM, Rouleau GA (2005): Autosomal dominant juvenile myoclonic epilepsy and GABRA1. *Adv Neurol* 95: 255–263.

Crespel A, Genton P, Berramdane M, *et al.* (2005): Lamotrigine associated with exacerbation or *de novo* myoclonus in idiopathic generalized epilepsies. *Neurology* 65: 762–764.

Crespel A, Genton P, Coubes P, Gélisse P (2009a): Juvenile myoclonic epilepsy in a patient with history of infantile hemiplegia. *Rev Neurol (Paris)* 165: 189–193.

Crespel A, Velizarova R, Genton P, Gélisse P (2009b): Juvenile myoclonic epilepsy with recurrent myoclonic status: efficacy of valproate. *Therapie* 64: 321–323.

Crompton DE, Sadleir LG, Bromhead CJ, *et al.* (2012): Familial adult myoclonic epilepsy: recognition of mild phenotypes and refinement of the 2q locus. *Arch Neurol* 69: 474–481.

da Silva Sousa P, Lin K, Garzon E, Sakamoto AC, Yacubian EM (2005): Self-perception of factors that precipitate or inhibit seizures in juvenile myoclonic epilepsy. *Seizure* 14: 340–346.

Dasheiff RM, Ritaccio AL (1993): Characterization of intractable juvenile myoclonic epilepsy: new perspectives on primarily generalized seizures. *Seizure* 2: 11–19.

de Araujo Filho GM, Pascalicchio TF, Lin K, Sousa PS, Yacubian EM (2006): Neuropsychiatric profiles of patients with juvenile myoclonic epilepsy treated with valproate or topiramate. *Epilepsy Behav* 8: 606–609.

de Araujo Filho GM, Pascalicchio TF, Sousa Pda S, Lin K, Ferreira Guilhoto LM, Yacubian EM (2007): Psychiatric disorders in juvenile myoclonic epilepsy: a controlled study of 100 patients. *Epilepsy Behav* 10: 437–441.

de Nijs L, Lakaye B, Coumans B, *et al.* (2006): EFHC1, a protein mutated in juvenile myo-clonic epilepsy, associates with the mitotic spindle through its N-ter-minus. *Exp Cell Res* 312: 2872–2879.

de Nijs L, Léon C, Nguyen L, *et al.* (2009): EFHC1 interacts with microtubules to regulate cell division and cortical development. *Nat Neurosci* 12: 1266–1274.

de Nijs L, Wolkoff N, Coumans B, *et al.* (2012): Mutations of EFHC1, linked to juvenile myoclonic epilepsy, disrupt radial and tangential migrations during brain development. *Hum Mol Genet.*21: 5106–5117.

de Toffol B, Autret A (1996): Treatment of juvenile myoclonic epilepsy with low-dose sodium valproate. *Rev Neurol* 152: 708–710.

Dedei Daryan M, Güveli BT, Baslo SA, *et al.* (208): Prevalence and clinical characteristics of headache in juvenile myoclonic epilepsy: experience from a tertiary epilepsy center. *Neurol Sci* 39(3): 519–525.

Delasiauve LJF (1854): *Traité de l'épilepsie*. Paris: Masson. Delgado-Escueta AV, Enrile-Bacsal F (1984): Juvenile myoclonic epilepsy of Janz. *Neurology* 34: 285–294.

Delgado-Escueta AV, Greenberg DA, Treiman L, *et al.* (1989): Mapping the gene for juvenile myoclonic epilepsy. *Epilepsia* 30 (Suppl 4): 8–18.

Desai D, Desai S, Jani T (2016): Juvenile Myoclonic Epilepsy in Rural Western India: Not Yet a Benign Syndrome. *Epilepsy Res Treat* 2016: 1435150.

Destina Yalçin A, Forta H, Kiliç E (2006): Overlap cases of eyelid myoclonia with absences and juvenile myoclonic epilepsy. *Seizure* 15: 359–365.

Devinsky O, Gershengorn J, Brown E, Perrine K, Vazquez B, Luciano D (1997): Frontal functions in juvenile myoclonic epilepsy. *Neurol Neuropsychol Behav Neurol* 10: 243–246.

Diehl B, Wyllie E, Rothner AD, Bingaman W (1998): Worsening seizures after surgery for focal epilepsy due to emergence of primary generalized epilepsy. *Neurology* 51: 1178–1180.

Dinner DS, Lüders H, Morris HH, Lesser RP (1987): Juvenile myoclonic epilepsy. In: Lüders H, Lesser RP (eds). *Epilepsy: Electroclinical Syndromes*, pp. 131–149. Berlin: Springer Verlag.

Dunac A, Thomas P, Hirsch E, Marescaux C, Chatel M (1998): Psychogenic seizures in juvenile myoclonic epilepsy: a video-EEG study. *J Neurol* 245 (Suppl 1): 389.

Durner M (1988): *HLA und Epilepsie mit Impulsiv-Petit mal*. [Dissertation].Berlin: Freie Universitat Berlin.

Engel J (2001): A proposed diagnostic scheme for people with epileptic seizures and with epilepsy: report of the ILAE Task Force on Classification and Terminology. *Epilepsia* 42: 796–803.

EPICURE Consortium, Leu C, de Kovel CG, Zara F, *et al.* (2012): Genome-wide linkage meta-analysis identifies susceptibility loci at 2q34 and 13q31.3 for genetic generalized epilepsies. *Epilepsia* 53: 308–318.

Fernando-Dongas MC, Radtke RA, Van Landingham KE, Husain AM (2000): Characteristics of valproic acid resistant juvenile myoclonic epilepsy. *Seizure* 9: 385–388.

Filho GM, Mazetto L, da Silva JM, Caboclo LO, Yacubian EM (2011): Psychiatric comorbidity in patients with two prototypes of focal *versus* generalized epilepsy syndromes. *Seizure* 20: 383–386.

Fisher RS, Cross JH, French JA, *et al.* Operational classification of seizure types by the International League Against Epilepsy: Position Paper of the ILAE Commission for Classification and Terminology. *Epilepsia* 2017; 58: 522–530.

Gastaut H, Broughton R (1972): *Epileptic Seizures, Clinical and Electrographic Features, Diagnosis and Treatment*. Springfield: CC Thomas.

Gélisse P, Genton P, Raybaud C, Thomas P, Bartolomei F, Dravet C (2000a): Is it juvenile myoclonic epilepsy? *Epileptic Disord* 2: 27–32.

Gélisse P, Genton P, Raybaud C, Thomas P, Dravet C (2000b): Structural brain lesions do not influence the prognosis of juvenile myoclonic epilepsy. *Acta Neurol Scand* 102: 188–191.

Gélisse P, Genton P, Samuelian JC, Thomas P, Bureau M (2001a): Troubles psychiatriques dans l'épilepsie myoclonique juvénile. *Rev Neurol* 157: 297–302.

Gélisse P, Genton P, Thomas P, Rey M, Samuelian JC, Dravet C (2001b): Clinical factors of drug resistance in juvenile myoclonic epilepsy. *J Neurol Neurosurg Psychiatry* 70: 240–243.

Gélisse P, Genton P, Kuate C, *et al.* (2004): Worsening of seizures by oxcarbazepine in juvenile idiopathic generalized epilepsies. *Epilepsia* 45: 1282–1286.

Genton P, Salas Puig J, Tunon A, Lahoz C, Gonzalez Sanchez M (1994): Juvenile myoclonic epilepsy and related syndromes: clinical and neurophysiological aspects. In: Malafosse A, Genton P, Hirsch E, Marescaux C, Broglin D, Bernasconi R (eds). *Idiopathic Generalized Epilepsies: Clinical, Experimental and Genetic Aspects*, pp. 253–265. London: John Libbey.

Genton P, Gonzales Sanchez MDS, Saltarelli A, Bureau M, Dravet C, Roger J (1995): Aspects trompeurs de l'EEG standard dans l'épilepsie myoclonique juvénile: étude rétrospective de 56 cas consécutifs. *Neurophysiol Clin* 25: 285–290.

Genton P, Gélisse P (2001): Premature death in juvenile myoclonic epilepsy. *Acta Neurol Scand* 104: 125–129.

Genton P, McMenamin J (1998): Aggravation of seizures by antiepileptic drugs: what to do in clinical practice. *Epilepsia* 38 (Suppl 3): 26–29.

Genton P (1999): Limites du concept d'épilepsie généralisée idiopathique. *Rev Neurol* 155: 121–128.

Genton P, Gélisse P,Thomas P (2000a): Juvenile myoclonic epilepsy today: current definitions and limits. In: Schmitz B, Sander T (eds) *Juvenile Myoclonic Epilepsy: the Janz Syndrome*, pp. 11–32. Petersfield: Wrightson Biomedical Publishing.

Genton P, Gélisse P, Thomas P, Dravet C (2000b): Do carbamazepine and phenytoin aggravate juvenile myoclonic epilepsy? *Neurology* 55: 1106–1109.

Genton P, Gélisse P (2000c): Antimyoclonic effect of levetiracetam. *Epileptic Disord* 2: 209–212.

Gigli GL, Calia E, Luciani L, Diomedi M, De La Pierre L, Marciani MG, Sasanelli F (1991): Eye closure sensitivity without photosensitivity in juvenile myoclonic epilepsy: polysomnographic study of electroencephalographic epileptiform discharge rates. *Epilepsia* 32, 677–683.

Gigli GL, Calia E, Marciani MG, Mazza S, Mennuni G, Diomedi M, Terzano MG, Janz D (1992): Sleep microstructure and EEG epileptiform activity in patients with juvenile myoclonic epilepsy. *Epilepsia* 33: 799–804.

Gilliam F, Steinhoff BJ, Bittermann HJ, Kuzniecky R, Faught E, Abou-Khalil B (2000): Adult myoclonic epilepsy: a distinct syndrome of idiopathic generalized epilepsy. *Neurology* 55: 1030–1033.

Giorgi FS, Guida M, Caciagli L, *et al.* (2016): Social cognition in Juvenile Myoclonic Epilepsy. *Epilepsy Res* 28: 61–67.

Goldsmith D, Minassian BA (2016): Efficacy and Tolerability of Perampanel in Ten Patients with Lafora Disease. *Epilepsy Behav* 62: 132–135.

Gomes Mda M, Chalub M (2007): Dom Pedro I of Brazil and IV of Portugal: epilepsy and peculiar behavior. *Arq Neuropsiquiatr* 65: 710–715.

Goosses R (1984): *Die Beziehung der Fotosensibilität zu den verschiedenen epileptischen Syndromen*. [Med Diss Thesis] Berlin: Freie Universitat Universität Berlin.

Gram L, Alving J, Sagild JC, Dam M (1988): Juvenile myoclonic epilepsy in unexpected age groups. *Epilepsy Res* 2: 137–140.

Greenberg DA, Delgado-Escueta AV, Maldonado HM, Widelitz H (1988a): Segregation analysis of juvenile myoclonic epilepsy. *Genetic Epidemiol* 5: 81–94.

Grünewald RA, Panayiotopoulos CP (1993): Juvenile myoclonic epilepsy: a review. *Arch Neurol* 50: 594–598.

Guaranha MS, Da Siva Sousa P, De Araújo-Filho GM, *et al.* (2009): Provocative and inhibitory effects of a video-EEG neuropsychologic protocol in juvenile myoclonic epilepsy. *Epilepsia* 50: 2446–2455.

Guaranha MS, Filho GM, Lin K, Guilhoto LM, Caboclo LO, Yacubian EM (2011): Prognosis of juvenile myoclonic epilepsy is related to endophenotypes. *Seizure* 20: 42–48.

Helbig I, Mefford HC, Sharp AJ, *et al.* (2009): 15q13.3 microdeletions increase risk of idiopathic generalized epilepsy. *Nat Genet* 41: 160–162.

Herpin T (1867): *Des accès incomplets d'épilepsie.* Paris, Baillère.

Hurst DL (1996): Methsuximide therapy of juvenile myoclonic epilepsy. *Seizure* 5: 47–50.

Inoue Y, Kubota H (2000): Juvenile myoclonic epilepsy with praxis-induced seizures. In: Schmitz B, Sander T (eds). *Juvenile Myoclonic Epilepsy: the Janz Syndrome*. Petersfield: Wrightson Biomedical, pp. 73–81.

Inoue Y, Seino M, Kubota H, Yamakaku K, Tanaka M, Yagi K (1994): Epilepsy with praxis-induced seizures. In: Wolf P (ed) *Epileptic Seizures and Syndromes*, pp. 81–91. London: John Libbey.

Iqbal N, Caswell H, Muir R, *et al.* Neuropsychological profiles of patients with juvenile myoclonic epilepsy and their siblings: An extended study. *Epilepsia* 56: 1301–1308.

Jain S, Padma MV, Maheshwari MC (1997): Occurrence of only myoclonic jerks in juvenile myoclonic epilepsy. *Acta Neurol Scand* 95: 263–267.

Janz D (1969): *Die Epilepsien*. Stuttgart: Thieme.

Janz D (1985): Epilepsy with impulsive petit mal (juvenile myoclonic epilepsy). *Acta Neurol Scand* 72: 449–459.

Janz D (1991): Juvenile myoclonic epilepsy. In: Dam M, L Gram L (eds) *Comprehensive Epileptology*, pp. 171–185. New York: Raven Press.

Janz D, Beck-Mannageta G, SanderT (1992): Do idiopathic generalized epilepsies share a common susceptibility gene? *Neurology* 42 (Suppl 5): 48–55.

Janz D, Christian,W (1957): Impulsiv Petit Mal. *Dtsch Z. Nervenheilk* 176: 346–386.

Janz, D, Christian, W (1994): Impulsive Petit Mal (traduction anglaise par P. Genton). In: Malafosse A, Genton P, Hirsch E, Marescaux C, Broglin D, Bernasconi R (eds) *Idiopathic Generalized Epilepsies: Clinical, Experimental and Genetic Aspects*, pp. 229–251. London: John Libbey.

Janz D, Durner M (1997): Juvenile myoclonic epilepsy. In: Engel T, Pedley TA (eds) *Epilepsy: a Comprehensive Textbook*, pp. 2389–2400. Philadelphia: Lippincott-Raven.

Janz D, Waltz S (1994): Juvenile myoclonic epilepsy with absences. In: Duncan JS, Panayiotopoulos CP (eds) *Typical Absences and Related Epileptic Syndromes*, pp. 174–183. London, Churchill-Livingstone.

Kasteleijn-Nolst Trénité DGA, Marescaux C, Stodieck S, Edelbroek PM, Oosting J (1996): Photosensitive epilepsy: a model to study the effects of antiepileptic drugs. Evaluation of the piracetam analogue, levetiracetam. *Epilepsy Res* 25: 225–230.

Keller SS, Ahrens T, Mohammadi S, Möddel G, Kugel H, Ringelstein EB, Deppe M (2011): Microstructural and volumetric abnormalities of the putamen in juvenile myoclonic epilepsy. *Epilepsia* 52: 1715–1724.

Kellett MW, Smith DF, Stockton PA, Chadwick DW (1999): Topiramate in clinical practice: first year's post-licensing experience in a specialist epilepsy clinic. *J Neurol Neurosurg Psychiatry* 66: 759–763. Khani YA, Andermann F, Andermann E (2005): Antimyoclonic efficacy of piracetam in idiopathic generalized epilepsy. *Epilepsia* 46: 1145–1146.

Kimura S, Kobayashi T (1996): Two patients with juvenile myoclonic epilepsy and nonconvulsive status epilepticus. *Epilepsia* 37: 275–279.

Knake S, Hamer HM, Schomburg U, Oertel WH, Rosenow F (1999): Tiagabine-induced absence status in idiopathic generalized epilepsy. *Seizure* 8: 314–317.

Knott C, Panayiotopoulos CP (1994): Carbamazepine in the treatment of generalized tonic-clonic seizures in juvenile myoclonic epilepsy. *J Neurol Neurosurg Psychiatr* 57: 503.

Koepp MJ, Richardson MP, Brooks DJ, Cunningham VJ, Duncan JS (1997): Central benzodiazepine/gamma-aminobutyric acid A receptors in idiopathic generalized epilepsy: an [11C] flumazenil positron emission tomography study. *Epilepsia* 38: 1089–1197.

Kostov H, Larsson PG, Reste GK (2007): Is vagus nerve stimulation a treatment option for patients with drug-resistant idiopathic generalized epilepsy? *Acta Neurol Scand* (Suppl) 187: 55–58.

Kothare SV, Valencia I, Khurana DS, Hardison H, Melvin JJ, Legido A (2004): Efficacy and tolerability of zonisamide in juvenile myoclonic epilepsy. *Epileptic Disord* 6: 267–270.

Koutroumanidis M, Hennessy MJ, Elwes RD, Binnie CD, Polkey CE (1999): Coexistence of temporal lobe and idiopathic generalized epilepsies. *Neurology* 53: 490–495.

Kuate C, Gélisse P, Baldy-Moulinier M, Crespel A (2004): Crises épileptiques induites par le bupropion. *Rev Neurol* 160: 701–703.

Labate A, Colosimo E, Gambardella A, Leggio U, Ambrosio R, Quattrone A (2006): Levetiracetam in patients with generalised epilepsy and myoclonic seizures: an open label study. *Seizure* 15: 214–218.

Lancman ME, Asconape JJ, Penry JK (1994): Clinical and EEG asymmetries in juvenile myoclonic epilepsy. *Epilepsia* 35: 302–306.

Larch J, Unterberger I, Bauer G, Reichsoellner J, Kuchukhidze G, Trinka E (2009): Myoclonic status epilepticus in juvenile myoclonic epilepsy. *Epileptic Disord* 11: 309–314.

Leahy T, Hennessy MJ, Counihan TJ (2018): The "Cinderella Syndrome": A narrative study of social curfews and lifestyle restrictions in juvenile myoclonic epilepsy. *Epilepsy Behav* 78: 104–108.

Lemke JR, Beck-Wödl S, Zankl A, *et al.* (2009): Juvenile myoclonic epilepsy with photosensitivity in a female with Velocardiofacial syndrome (del(22)(q11.2)) – causal relationship or coincidence? *Seizure* 18: 660–663.

Lennox WG (1945): The petit mal epilepsies. *JAMA* 129: 1069–1973.

Lennox WG (1960): *Epilepsy and Related Disorders*. Boston: Little, Brown &Co.

Levisohn PM, Holland KD (2007): Topiramate orvalproate in patients with juvenile myoclonic epilepsy: a randomized open-label comparison. *Epilepsy Behav* 10: 547–552.

Lin K, Carrete H Jr, Lin J, *et al.* (2009): Magnetic resonancespectroscopy reveals an epileptic network in juvenile myoclonic epilepsy. *Epilepsia* 50: 1191–1200.

Loiseau P, Duché B (1990): Épilepsie myoclonique juvenile. *Rev Neurol* 146: 719–725.

Lombroso CT (1997): Consistent EEG focalities detected in subjects with primary generalized epilepsies monitored for two decades. *Epilepsia* 38: 797–812.

Lund M, Reintoft M, Simonsen N (1976): Eine kontrollierte soziologische und psychologische Untersuchung von Patienten mit juveniler myoklonischer Epilepsie. *Nervenarzt* 47: 708–712.

Lundborg M (1903): *Die progressive Myoklonus-Epilepsie (Unverrichts Myoklonie)*. Upsala: Almquist und Wiksell.

Ma S, Blair MA, Abou-Khalil B, Lagrange AH, Gurnett CA, Hedera P (2006): Mutations in the GABRA1 and EFHC1 genes are rare in familial juvenile myoclonic epilepsy. *Epilepsy Res* 71: 129–134.

Maiga Y, Nogues B, Guillon B (2006): Exacerbation of tonico-clonic seizures in a juvenile myoclonic epileptic taking lamotrigine. *Rev Neurol* 162: 1125–1127.

Manon-Espaillat R, Osorio I, Badour R, Remler B (1987): Epileptic drop attacks in juvenile myoclonic epilepsy. *Epilepsia* 28: S614.

Marinas A, Villanueva V, Giraldez BG, Molins A, Salas-Puig J, Serratosa JM (2009): Efficacy and tolerability of zonisamide in idiopathic generalized epilepsy. *Epileptic Disord* 11: 61–66.

Martinez-Juarez IE, Alonso ME, Medina MT, *et al.* (2006): Juvenile myoclonic epilepsy subsyndromes: family studies and long-term follow-up. *Brain* 129: 1269–1280.

Matsuoka H (1992): The seizure prognosis of juvenile myoclonic epilepsy. *Jpn J Psychiatry Neurol*46: 293–296.

Matsuoka H, Takahashi T, Sasaki M, *et al.* (2000): Neuropsychological EEG activation in patients with epilepsy. *Brain* 123: 318–330.

Mayer T, Wolf P (1999): Reading epilepsy: clinical and genetic background. In: Berkovic S, Genton P, Hirsch E, Picard F (eds) *Genetics of Focal Epilepsies*, pp. 159–168. London: John Libbey.

McCorry D, Nicolson A, Smith D, Marson A, Feltbower RG, Chadwick DW (2006): An association between type 1 diabetes and idiopathic generalized epilepsy. *Ann Neurol* 59: 204–206.

Medina MT, Suzuki T, Alonso ME, *et al.* (2008): Novel mutations in Myoclonin1/EFHC1 in sporadic and familial juvenile myoclonic epilepsy. *Neurology* 70: 2137–2144.

Meencke HJ (1985): Neurodensity in the molecular layer of the frontal cortex in primary generalized epilepsy. *Epilepsia* 26: 450–454.

Meschaks A, Lindstrom P, Halldin C, Farde L, Savic I (2005): Regional reductions in serotonin 1A receptor binding in juvenile myoclonic epilepsy. *Arch Neurol* 62: 946–950.

Montouris G, Abou-Khalil B (2009): The first line of therapy in a girl with juvenile myoclonic epilepsy: should it be valproate or a new agent? *Epilepsia* 50 (Suppl 8): 16–20.

Nashef L, Fish DR, Sander JWAS, Shorvon SD (1995): Incidence of sudden unexpected death in an adult outpatient cohort with epilepsy at a tertiary referral centre. *J Neurol Neurosurg Psychiatry* 58: 462–464.

Naseer MI, Rasool M, Chaudhary AG, *et al.* (2017): Chromosomal microaberration in a Saudi Family with Juvenile Myoclonic Epilepsy. *CNS Neurol Disord Drug Targets* 16: 1010–1017.

Ng M, Devinsky O (2004): Vagus nerve stimulation for refractory idiopathic generalised epilepsy. *Seizure* 13: 176–178.

Nicolson A, Marson AG (2010): When the first antiepileptic drug fails in a patient with juvenile myoclonic epilepsy. *Pract Neurol* 10: 208–218.

Nicolson A, Appleton RE, Chadwick DW, Smith DF (2004): The relationship between treatment with valproate, lamotrigine, and topiramate and the prognosis of the idiopathic generalised epilepsies. *J Neurol Neurosurg Psychiatry* 75: 75–79.

Noachtar S, Andermann E, Meyvisch P, Andermann F, Gough WB, Schiemann-Delgado J; N166 Levetiracetam Study Group (2008): Levetiracetam for the treatment of idiopathic generalized epilepsy with myoclonic seizures. *Neurology* 70: 607–616.

Numata Y, Inoue Y, Hamanaka K, Yagi K, Seino M (1986): Clinical characteristics of 25 patients with juvenile myoclonic *epilepsy. Jpn J Psychiatr Neurol* 40: 421–422.

O'Rourke D, Flynn C, White M, Doherty C, Delanty N (2007): Potential efficacy of zonisamide in refractoryjuvenile myoclonic epilepsy: retrospective evidence from an Irish compassionate-use case series. *Ir Med J* 100: 431–433.

Obeid T, Panayiotopoulos CP (1988): Juvenile myoclonic epilepsy: a study in Saudi Arabia. *Epilepsia* 29: 280–282.

Obeid T, Panayiotopoulos CP (1989): Clonazepam in juvenile myoclonic epilepsy. *Epilepsia* 30: 603–606.

Odano I, Varrone A, Savic I, *et al.* (2012): Quantitative PET analyses of regional [11C]PE2I binding to the dopamine transporter – application to juvenile myoclonic epilepsy. *NeuroImage* 59: 3582–3593.

Oguni H, Mukahira K, Oguni M, *et al.* (1994): Video-polygraphic analysis of myoclonic seizures in juvenile myoclonic epilepsy. *Epilepsia* 35: 307–316.

Pal DK, Evgrafov OV, Tabares P, Zhang F, Durner M, Greenberg DA (2003): BRD2 (RING3) is a probable major susceptibility gene for common juvenile myoclonic epilepsy. *Am J Hum* Genet 73: 261–270.

Panayiotopoulos CP, Obeid T, Waheed G (1989): Absences in juvenile myoclonic epilepsy: a clinical video-EEG study. *Ann Neurol* 25: 391–397.

Panayiotopoulos CP, Tahan AR, Obeid T (1991): Juvenile myoclonic epilepsy: factors of error involved in the diagnosis and treatment. *Epilepsia* 32: 672–676.

Panayiotopoulos CP, Obeid T, Tahan AR (1994): Juvenile myoclonic epilepsy: a 5-year prospective study. *Epilepsia* 35: 285–296.

Pascalicchio TF, de Araujo Filho GM, da Silva Noffs MH, *et al.* (2007): Neuropsychological profile of patients with juvenile myoclonic epilepsy: a controlled study of 50 patients. *Epilepsy Behav* 10: 263–267.

Pedersen SA, Klosterskov P, Gram L, Dam M. (1985): Long-term study of gamma-vinyl GABA in the treatment of epilepsy. *Acta Neurol Scand* 72: 295–298.

Pathak S, Miller J, Morris EC, Stewart WCL, Greenberg DA (2018): DNA methylation of the BRD2 promoter is associated with juvenile myoclonic epilepsy in Caucasians. *Epilepsia* 59: 1011–1019.

Pedersen SB, Petersen KA (1998): Juvenile myoclonic epilepsy: clinical and EEG features. *Acta Neurol Scand* 97: 160–163.

Penfield W, Jasper H (1954): *Epilepsy and the Functional Anatomy of the Human Brain*. Boston: Little, Brown & Co.

PenryJK, Dean JC, Riela AR (1989): Juvenile myoclonic epilepsy: long-term response to therapy. *Epilepsia* 30 (Suppl4): 19–23.

Perini GI, Tosin C, Carraro C, *et al.* (1996): Interictal mood and personality disorders in temporal lobe epilepsy and juvenile myoclonic epilepsy. *J Neurol Neurosurg Psychiatry* 61: 601–605.

Perucca E, Gram L, Avanzini G, Dulac O (1998): Antiepileptic drugs as a cause of worsening seizures. *Epilepsia* 39: 5–17.

Piazzini A, Turner K, Vignoli A, Canger R, Canevini MP (2008): Frontal cognitive dysfunction in juvenile myoclonic epilepsy. *Epilepsia* 49: 657–662.

Pillai SH, Raghavan S, Mathew M, *et al.* (2017): Juvenile Myoclonic Epilepsy with Frontal Executive Dysfunction is Associated with Reduced Gray Matter Volume by Voxel-based Morphometry. *Ann Indian Acad Neurol* 20: 270–273.

Pinto D, Louwaars S, Westland B, *et al.* (2006): Heterogeneity at the JME 6p11–12 locus: absence of mutations in the *EFHC1* gene in linked Dutch families. *Epilepsia* 47: 1743–1746.

Prasad A, Kuzniecky RI, Knowlton RC, *et al.* (2003): Evolving antiepileptic drug treatment in juvenile myoclonic epilepsy. *Arch Neurol* 60: 1100–1105.

Pulsipher DT, Seidenberg M, Guidotti L, *et al.* (2009): Thalamofrontal circuitry and executive dysfunction in recent-onset juvenile myoclonic epilepsy. *Epilepsia* 50: 1210–1219.

Pung T, Schmitz B (2006): Circadian rhythm and personality profile in juvenile myoclonic epilepsy. *Epilepsia* 47 (Suppl 2): 111–114.

Rabot (1899): De la myoclonie épileptique. [Thèse]. Paris.

Radhakrishnan K, Silbert PL, Klass DW (1995): Reading epilepsy: an appraisal of 20 patients diagnosed at the Mayo Clinic, Rochester, Minnesota, between 1949 and 1989, and delineation of the epileptic syndrome. *Brain* 118: 75–89.

Raju PK, Satishchandra P, Nayak S, *et al.* (2017): Microtubule-associated defects caused by EFHC1 mutations in juvenile myoclonic epilepsy. *Hum Muta* 38: 816–826.

Resor SR, Resor LD (1990): The neuropharmacology of juvenile myoclonic epilepsy. *Clin Neuropharmacol* 13: 465–491.

Rosenfeld WE, Benbadis S, Edrich P, Tassinari CA, Hirsch E (2009): Levetiracetam as add-on therapy for idiopathic generalized epilepsy syndromes with onset during adolescence: analysis of two randomized, double-blind, placebo-controlled studies. *Epilepsy Res* 85: 72–80.

Rzezak P, Moschetta SP, Mendonça M, *et al.* (2018): Higher IQ in juvenile myoclonic epilepsy: Dodging cognitive obstacles and "masking" impairments. *Epilepsy Behav* 17: S1525–5050.

Sala-Padró J, Toledo M, Santamarina E, *et al.* (2016): Levetiracetam and Valproate Retention Rate in Juvenile Myoclonic Epilepsy. *Clin Neuropharmacol* 39: 299–301.

Salas-Puig X, Camara da Silva AM, Dravet C, Roger J (1990): L'épilepsie myoclonique juvénile dans la population du Centre Saint-Paul. *Epilepsies* 2: 108–113.

Sapio MR, Vessaz M, Thomas P, *et al.* (2015): Novel carboxypeptidase A6 (CPA6) mutations identified in patients with juvenile myoclonic and generalized epilepsy. *PLoS One* 10(4): e0123180.

Savic I, Osterman Y, Helms G (2004): MRS shows syndrome differentiated metabolite changes in human-generalized epilepsies. *NeuroImage* 21: 163–172.

Schankin CJ, Rémi J, Klaus I, *et al.* (2011): Headache in juvenile myoclonic epilepsy. *J Headache Pain* 12: 227–233.

Schmitz B, Sailer U, Sander T, Bauer G, Janz D (2000): Clinical genetics in subtypes of idiopathic generalized epilepsies. In: Schmitz B, Sander T (eds) *Juvenile Myoclonic Epilepsy: the Janz Syndrome*, pp. 129–144, Petersfield: Wrightson Biomedical Publishing.

Scheffer IE, Berkovic S, Capovilla G, *et al.* (2017): ILAE classification of the epilepsies: Position paper of the ILAE Commission for Classification and Terminology. *Epilepsia* 58: 512–521.

Schmitz B, Sander T (2000): *Juvenile Myoclonic Epilepsy: the Janz Syndrome*. Petersfield: Wrightson Biomedical Publishing.

Sharpe DV, Patel AD, Abou-Khalil B, Fenichel GM (2008): Levetiracetam monotherapy in juvenile myoclonic epilepsy. *Seizure* 17: 64–68.

Simonsen M, Mollgaard V, Lund M (1976): A controlled clinical and electro-encephalographic study of myoclonic epilepsy (Impulsiv-Petit mal). In: Janz D (ed) *Epileptology*. Stuttgart: Thieme.

So GM, Thiele EA, Sanger T, Schmid R, Riviello JJ (1998): Electroencephalogram and clinical focalities in juvenile myoclonic epilepsy. *J ChildNeurol* 13: 541–545.

Sonmez F, Atakli D, Sari H, Atay T, Arpaci B (2004): Cognitive function in juvenile myoclonic epilepsy. *Epilepsy Behav* 5: 329–336.

Sousa Pda S, Araiijo Filho GM, Garzon E, Sakamoto AC, Yacubian EM (2005): Topiramate for the treatment of juvenile myoclonic epilepsy. *Arq Neuropsiquiatr* 63: 733–737.

Sözüer DT, Atakli D, Atay T, Baybas S, Arpaci B (1996): Evaluation of various antiepileptic drugs in juvenile myoclonic epilepsy. *Epilepsia* 37 (Suppl 4): S77.

Specchio LM, Gambardella A, Giallonardo AT, *et al.* (2006): Open label, long-term, pragmatic study on levetiracetam in the treatment of juvenile myoclonic epilepsy. *Epilepsy Res* 71: 32–39.

Stogmann E, Lichtner P, Baumgartner C, *et al.* (2006): Idiopathic generalized epilepsy phenotypes associated with different EFHC1 mutations. *Neurology* 67: 2029–2031.

Su YH, Izumi T, Kitsu M, Fukuyama Y (1993): Seizure threshold in juvenile myoclonic epilepsy with Graves' disease. *Epilepsia* 34: 488–492.

Sundqvist A (1990): Juvenile myoclonic epilepsy: Events before diagnosis. *J Epilepsy* 3–4: 189–192.

Sundqvist A, Tomson T, Lundkvist B (1998): Valproate as monotherapy for juvenile myoclonic epilepsy: dose-effect study. *Ther Drug Monit* 20: 149–157.

Sundqvist A, Nilsson BY, Tomson T (1999): Valproate monotherapy in juvenile myoclonic epilepsy: dose-related effects on electroencephalographic and other neurophysiologic tests. *Ther Drug Monit* 21: 91–96.

Suzuki T, Delgado-Escueta AV, Aguan K, *et al.* (2004): Mutations in EFHC1 cause juvenile myoclonic epilepsy. *Nat* Genet 36: 842–849.

Suzuki T, Miyamoto H, Nakahari T, *et al.* (2009): Efhc1 deficiency causes spontaneous myoclonus and increased seizure susceptibility. *Hum Mol Genet* 18: 1099–1109.

Swartz BE, Spitz J, Vu AL *et al.* (2016): Heterogeneity of anatomic regions by MR volumetry in juvenile myoclonic epilepsy. *Acta Neurol Scand* 134: 300–308.

Syvertsen M, Hellum MK, Hansen G, *et al.* (2016): Prevalence of juvenile myoclonic epilepsy in people < 30 years of age-A population-based study in Norway. *Epilepsia* 58: 105–112.

Szaflarski JP (2004): Effects of zonisamide on the electroencephalogram of a patient with juvenile myoclonic epilepsy. *Epilepsy Behav* 5: 1024–1026.

Thomas P, Valton L, Genton P (2006): Absence and myoclonic status epilepticus precipitated by antiepileptic drugs in idiopathic generalized epilepsy. *Brain* 129: 1281–1292.

Thomas P, Ostrowsky K (1997): Falls in epileptic syndromes of adolescence. In: Beaumanoir A, Andermann F, Avanzini G, Mira L (eds) *Falls in Epileptic and non Epileptic Seizures of Adolescence*, pp. 13–123. London: John Libbey.

Thounaojam R, Langbang L, Itisham K, *et al.* (2017): EFHC1 mutation in Indian juvenile myoclonic epilepsy patients. *Epilepsia* 58: 84–89.

Topcuoglu MA, Saygi S, Ciger A (1997): Rotatory seizures in juvenile myoclonic epilepsy. *Clin Neurol Neurosurg* 99: 248–251.

Touchon J, Besset A, Billiard M, Baldy-Moulinier M (1982): Effects of spontaneous and provoked awakening on the frequency of polyspike and wave discharges. In: Akimoto H, Kazamatsuri M, Seino M, Ward M (eds) *Bilateral Massive Epileptic Myoclonus*, Advances in Epileptology, Vol. 13, pp. 269–272. New York: Raven Press.

Trinka E, Dilitz E, Unterberger I, *et al.* (2002): Non convulsive status epilepticus after replacement of valproate with lamotrigine. *J Neurol* 249: 1417–1422.

Trinka E, Kienpointner G, Unterberger I, *et al.* (2006): Psychiatric comorbidity in juvenile myoclonic epilepsy. *Epilepsia* 47: 2086–2091.

Tsuboi T (1977): *Primary Generalized Epilepsy with Sporadic Myoclonias of Myoclonic Petit Mal Type*. Stuttgart: Thieme.

Tsuboi T, Christian W (1973): On the genetics of primary generalized epilepsy with sporadic myoclonias, or impulsive Petit Mal: a clinical and electroencephalographic study of 399 probands. *Humangenetik* 19: 155–182.

Uchida CG, de Carvalho KC, Guaranha MS, *et al.* (2015): Phenotyping juvenile myoclonic epilepsy. Praxis induction as a biomarker of unfavorable prognosis. *Seizure* 32: 62–68.

Valente KD, Rzezak P, Moschetta SP, *et al.* (2016): Delineating behavioral and cognitive phenotypes in juvenile myoclonic epilepsy: Are we missing the forest for the trees? *Epilepsy Behav* 54: 95–99.

Velisek L, Shang E, Veliskovâ J, *et al.* (2011): GABAergic neuron deficit as an idiopathic generalized epilepsy mechanism: the role of BRD2 haploinsufficiency in juvenile myoclonic epilepsy. *PLoS One* 6 (8): e23656.

Verrotti A, Cerminara C, Coppola G, *et al.* (2008): Levetiracetam in juvenile myoclonic epilepsy: long-term efficacy in newly diagnosed adolescents. *Dev Med Child Neurol* 50: 29–32.

Vijai J, Cherian PJ, Stlaja PN, Anand A, Radhakrishnan K (2003): Clinical characteristics of a South Indian cohort of juvenile myoclonic epilepsy probands. *Seizure* 12: 490–496.

Wallace SJ (1998): Myoclonus and epilepsy in childhood: a review of treatment with valproate, ethosuximide, lamotrigine and zonisamide. *Epilepsy Res* 29: 147–154.

Wang L, Jiang Z, Chen BB, *et al.* (2016): Electroclinical aspects and therapy of Han patients with juvenile myoclonic epilepsy in northern China. *Epilepsy Behav* 62: 204–208.

Woermann FG, Free SL, Koepp MJ, Sisodiya SM, Duncan JS (1999): Abnormal cerebral structure in juvenile myoclonic epilepsy demonstrated with voxel-based analysis of MRI. *Brain* 122: 2101–2108.

Wolf P (1985): Benign juvenile myoclonic epilepsy. In: Roger J, Bureau M, Dravet C, Dreifuss FE, Wolf P (eds) *Epileptic Syndromes in Infancy, Childhood and Adolescence*, pp. 242–246. London: John Libbey.

Wolf P (1992a): Juvenile myoclonic epilepsy. In: Roger J, Bureau M, Dravet C, Dreifuss FE, Perret A, Wolf P (eds) *Epileptic Syndromes in Infancy, Childhood and Adolescence*, 2nd ed, pp. 313–327. London: John Libbey.

Wolf P (1992b): Juvenile absence epilepsy. In: Roger J, Bureau M, Dravet C, Dreifuss FE, Perret A, Wolf P (eds) *Epileptic Syndromes in Infancy, Childhood and Adolescence*, 2nd ed, pp. 307–312. London: John Libbey.

Wolf P (1992c): Epilepsy with Grand Mal on awakening. In: Roger J, Bureau M, Dravet C, Dreifuss FE, Perret A, Wolf P (eds) *Epileptic Syndromes in Infancy, Childhood and Adolescence*, 2nd ed, pp. 329–341. London: John Libbey.

Wolf P (2000): Dieter Janz and the Janz syndrome: gestalt perception and analysis. In: Schmitz B, Sander T (eds) *Juvenile Myoclonic Epilepsy: the Janz Syndrome*, pp. 1–3. Petersfield: Wrightson Biomedical Publishing.

Wolf P, Goosses R (1986): Relation of photosensitivity to epileptic syndromes. *J Neurol Neurosurg Psychiatry* 49: 1368–1391.

Wolf P, Mayer T (2000): Juvenile myoclonic epilepsy: a syndrome challenging syndromic concepts? In: Schmitz B, Sander T *(eds) Juvenile Myoclonic Epilepsy: the Janz Syndrome*, pp. 33–39. Petersfield: Wrightson Biomedical Publishing.

Zhao Y, Shi J, Winey M, Klymkowsky MW (2016): Identifying domains of EFHC1 involved in ciliary localization, ciliogenesis, and the regulation of Wnt signaling. *Dev Biol* 411: 257–265.

Epileptic Syndromes in Infancy, Childhood and Adolescence (6th ed), M. Bureau, P. Genton, C. Dravet, A. V. Delgado-Escueta, R. Guerrini, C.A. Tassinari, P. Thomas & P. Wolf

WITH VIDEO SUPPLEMENTS

CHAPTER 18

RASMUSSEN ENCEPHALITIS

Tiziana Granata[1], Flavio Villani[2] and Frederick Andermann[3]

[1] Department of Pediatric Neuroscience, Neurological Institute Foundation "Besta", Milan, Italy
[2] Epilespy Monitoring Unit "Paolo Zorzi", Divison of Clinical and Experimental Epileptology, Neurological Institute Foundation "Besta", Milan, Italy
[3] Montreal Neurological Hospital and Institute, McGill University, Montreal, Quebec, Canada

Introduction

Rasmussen encephalitis (RE) is a rare, chronic inflammatory unilateral brain disease which typically occurs in children. Clinically, RE is characterized by intractable focal seizures, worsening unilateral motor deficits and cognitive decline. Histopathology is consistent with a T-cell dominated encephalitis with activated microglial cells and reactive astrogliosis which progressively evolves into extensive neuronal cell death. The disease was first described by Theodore Rasmussen, Jerzy Olszewski & Donald Lloyd-Smith in three children referred to the Montreal Neurological Institute for the management of intractable focal epilepsy (Rasmussen *et al.*, 1958). In this description, the peculiar clinical imaging and pathological characteristics of the disease as well as etiologic and therapeutic issues were masterly pointed out *(Figure 1)*. Since then, increasing reports of RE patients confirmed the original description and widened the clinical spectrum of the disease manifestations and course. RE may have atypical features such as late or very early onset, may coexist with a second pathology and may show a persistently focal or protracted course. In more recent years, moreover, new insights have been added to our understanding of the aetiology, pathophysiology and management of this condition (Granata & Anderman, 2013).

Etiopathogenesis

The etiology of RE is still unknown, though it has been identified as a chronic inflammatory process since its original description. Suggested mechanisms include chronic viral infection, acute viral infection leading to an abnormal immune response, or an immune-mediated mechanism not linked to infection. A possible viral etiology has been originally suggested by Rasmussen, based on the constituents of the immune reaction in the brain such as lymphocytic infiltration and microglial nodules (Rasmussen *et al.*, 1958). However, virological studies aimed at detecting viral particles or genetic evidence of viral material in brain tissue taken from RE patients gave inconsistent results (Walter & Renella, 1989; Power *et al.*, 1990; Farrell *et al.*, 1991; McLachlan *et al.*, 1993; Vinters *et al.*, 1993; Jay *et al.*, 1995; Atkins *et al.*, 1995). Findings of a crucial role of T-cell immunity focus the attention on the potential role of a virus antigen as the initiating event in the complex pathogenetic mechanism leading to the brain damage of RE. A cytotoxic T-cell response is in fact compatible with a viral infection and a viral infection could explain the peculiar hemispheric distribution with centrifugal expansion observed in RE (see Bauer in Granata *et al.*, 2011). However, the hypothesis that cytotoxic T-cells found in RE are directed against a specific viral protein present in both the neurons and astrocytes, still requires confirmation.

In the nineties the possibility of antibody-mediated pathogenesis for RE was raised by Rogers *et al.* who observed that rabbits immunized with a recombinant fragment of the glutamate receptor (GluR3) developed seizures and brain pathology with inflammatory changes similar to those of RE. The authors also detected anti-GluR3 antibodies in two out of four children with RE and observed clinical improvement after plasma exchange in one of them (Rogers *et al.*, 1994; Andrews *et al.*, 1996). Later, however, the pathogenetic role of anti-GluR3 antibodies was challenged by the observation that these antibodies may be found in other severe forms of epilepsy (Wiendl *et al.*, 2001; Mantegazza *et al.*, 2002), and that other antibodies directed against antigens of brain resident cells (presynaptic protein Munc18-1, NMDA-GluRε2, and anti-α7nAChR) could be found in RE patients (Yang *et al.*, 2000; Takahashi *et al.*, 2005; Watson *et al.*,

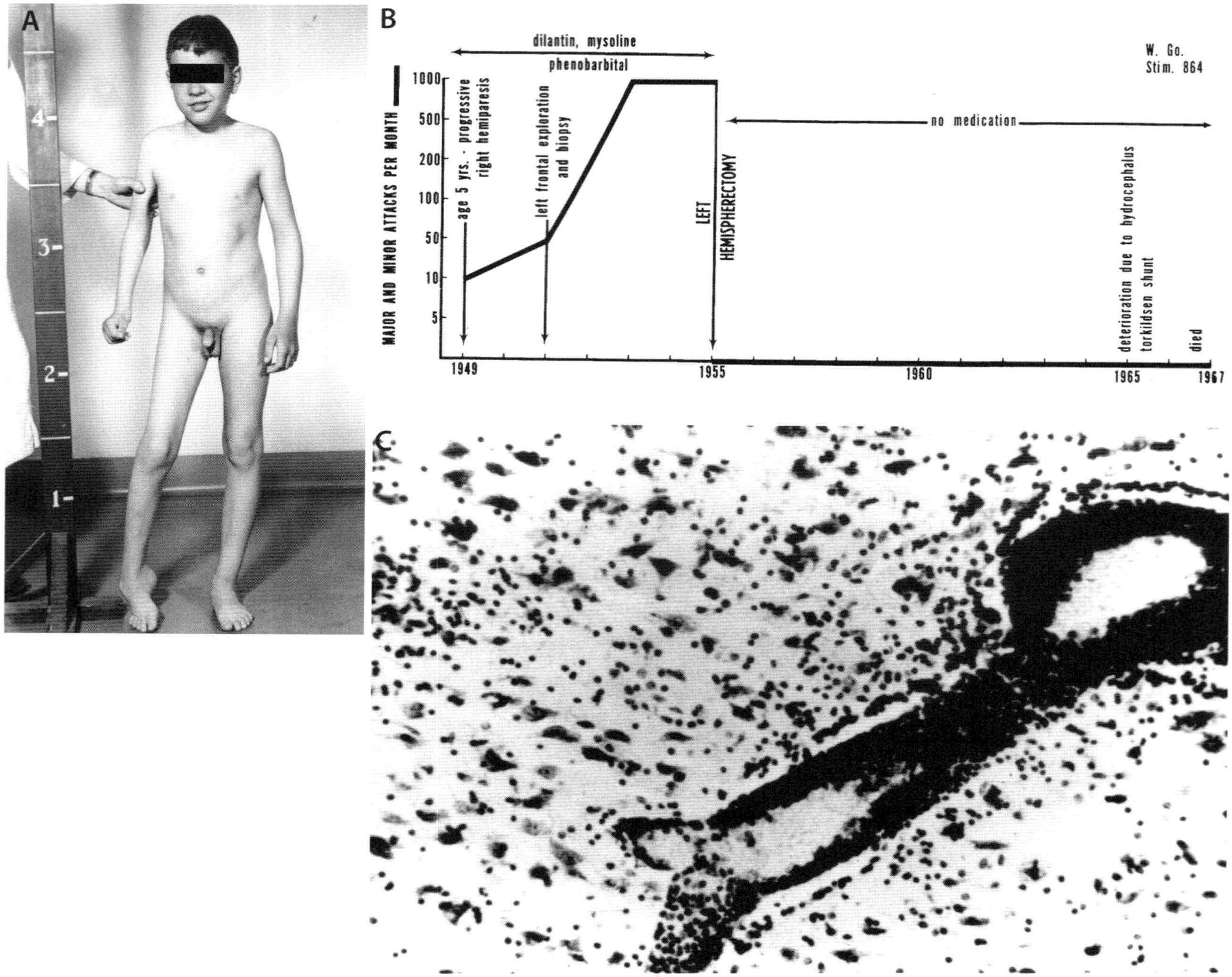

Figure 1

A. The original patient of Penfield and Rasmussen suffering from intractable epilepsy and progressive hemiparesis. B. The clinical course, response to surgery, and outcome in this patient. C. Pathological changes in resected tissue: perivascular infiltrates and microglial nodules.

2005). Moreover, it became evident that the presence of circulating antibodies could be secondary to cerebral damage and that humoral immunity, albeit involved in RE, is not the primary factor.

Actually, evidences accumulated in the last decades definitely clarified the pivotal role of cell-mediated immunity, and related the pathogenesis of RE to the cytotoxic T-cells causing apoptotic cell death. The main pathological features of RE are brain inflammation dominated by T-cells, microglial activation and microglial nodules, followed by neuronal loss and astrogliosis restricted to the affected hemisphere. Infiltrating T-cells have been characterized as $CD8^+$ cells containing granules positive for granzyme B^+ and part of these cells were in close contact with MHC class I positive neurons. Granzyme B is a protease released by activated cytotoxic T cells into target cells that undergo apoptosis (Bien *et al.*, 2002a; Bauer *et al.*, 2002). The importance of astrocytes has been underscored by the observation of astrocytic apoptosis and loss within cortex and white matter. Indeed, granzyme B^+ lymphocytes were found in close contact with astrocytes, with granules polarized toward the astrocytic membranes suggesting that astrocytes might be a target for T-cells leading to astrocytic degeneration. The apoptotic astrocytes and astrocyte deficient lesions were not present in other forms of epilepsy such as those due to Ammon's horn sclerosis or focal cortical dysplasia. This suggests that T-cell mediated death of astrocytes is a specific feature of RE (Bauer *et al.*, 2007). Spectratyping analysis of clonal composition and T- cell receptor repertoire (TCR) of $CD4^+$ and $CD8^+$ T cells demonstrated that $CD8^+$ T-cell clones found in the RE brain are also expanded in the periphery (Schwab *et al.*, 2009). This provides further evidence for an antigen-driven MHC Class I restricted T- cell attack against neurons and astrocytes. Analysis of biospecimens (brain, CSF, and blood), taken from RE patients and from children with epilepsy of different etiologies confirmed that RE patients present a peripheral $CD8^+$ T cells expansion correlating with disease severity. This prominent T-cell expansion in CNS was present only in RE patients (Schneider-Hohendorf *et al.*, 2016) who also shared common clones and MHC-I alleles (Schneider-Hohendorf *et al.*, 2016; Dadenkar *et al.*, 2016). Recent studies demonstrated that the brain infiltrating T- cells include, beside $CD8^+$, also clonally expanded CD4 T-cells and $\gamma\delta$ T-cells that secrete Interferon γ (IFN-γ) and tumor necrosis factor (TNF). This suggests a more complex T-cell immunity in RE (Al Nimer *et al.*, 2017).

Finally, Owens *et al.* (2016) demonstrated the presence of resident memory T-cells (TRM) in the parenchyma of RE brain tissue. TRM cells are a population of memory cells that develop *in situ* from T-cells that enter an inflamed tissue during the effector stage of an immune response and persist in non-lymphoid tissues long after the resolution of an immune response. In RE, TRM were detected irrespective of the duration of the disease at the time of surgery, suggesting that cellular immune response occurs early and may precede the clinical presentation. The authors hypothesize that local reactivation of TRM cells recruits antigen-experienced or newly primed T-cells into the brain, thus perpetuating the inflammation and the ensuing progressive destruction of brain tissue (Owens *et al.*, 2016).

From a therapeutic perspective, the evidence of a peripheral $CD8^+$ T cells expansion together with the known role of adhesion molecules (*e.g.*, chemokine) in governing migration of lymphocytes into different organs (Mirones *et al.*, 2013; Guillaume Martin-Blondel *et al.*, 2016), suggest that modulating the trafficking of immune cells to restrict their entry to the CNS might be a valuable therapeutic strategy. On the other hand, treatments designed to block T-cell entry into the brain might not be completely effective given the involvement of reactivated TRM cells in the progression of the disease. Moreover, increasing evidence for a concurrent role of cytokine network in the pathogenesis of RE, also suggests that these molecules could be a further target for treatment.

Pathology

The pathological hallmarks of RE, namely chronic inflammatory changes of cortex and white matter, neuronal loss, and gliosis confined to one hemisphere were masterly documented in Rasmussen's original papers (Rasmussen *et al.*, 1958; Aguilar & Rasmussen, 1960) *(Figure 1c)*. In the following years Robitaille (1991) defined the changes in greater detail and recognized that the pathology of RE could be quite variable from patient to patient, according to the activity of the disease. In patients with the most active disease, the predominant features were those of an ongoing inflammatory process, with numerous microglial nodules, perivascular round cells, and glial scarring. In patients with "active and remote disease", there were several microglial nodules, perivascular round cell cuffing, and at least one gyral segment of complete necrosis and cavitation including full-thickness cortex. Samples from patients with less active or "remote" disease showed neuronal loss, gliosis, a few microglial nodules, but moderately abundant perivascular round cells. Finally, samples from patients with less active disease showed nonspecific changes, with mild perivascular inflammation, few or no microglial nodules, and varying degrees of neuronal loss and gliosis. In the following years the heterogeneity in the stages of cortical damage was confirmed by the study of Pardo *et al.* (2004) who demonstrated that the pathological changes varied from early inflammation defined by infiltration of T lymphocytes and neuroglial reactions, to severe extensive neuronal cell death and cavitation of the cerebral cortex. The authors demonstrated that different stages of the destructive process coexist in each patient with a multifocal distribution suggesting an ongoing disease process affecting different parts of the brain at different times. In the same study, the authors found that the burden of pathology was similar in all brain regions except the occipital lobe, where it was significantly lower, and that greater burden of pathology was significantly associated with an earlier age at onset and longer duration of disease (Pardo *et al.*, 2004). Interestingly, regional differences, and correlation between early age at onset and the burden of pathology, were also observed in volumetric MRI studies (Wagner *et al.*, 2012).

Clinical features of typical RE

The disease is sporadic, affecting both males and females. RE typically starts in childhood or early adolescence, with a mean age at presentation of 5 years. The previous personal history is uneventful, but in about half of the patients, a seemingly trivial febrile illness in the months preceding the onset of seizures or a remote head trauma has been reported. Onset in almost all cases is characterized by seizures. Exceptionally, seizure onset is preceded by slowly progressive hemiparesis, or more rarely, by hemidystonia or hemiathetosis (Frucht *et al.*, 2002; Korn Lubetzki *et al.*, 2004; Bien *et al.*, 2007; Samanta *et al.*, 2016). Hemiparesis, cortical sensory loss and aphasia (when the dominant hemisphere is affected) together with cognitive impairment invariably develop during the course of the disease. The natural history of RE was summarized by Oguni *et al.* who reviewed a series of 48 patients observed at the Montreal Neurological Institute (Oguni *et al.*, 1992) and in a report by Bien *et al.*, who correlated the clinical course with the development of brain damage as documented by serial MRIs (Bien *et al.*, 2002b). Both groups recognize three stages that are virtually comparable. In the "prodromal stage", lasting from 0 month to 8 years, seizures manifest at low frequency and, rarely, mild hemiparesis may be present. The "acute stage" that in a significant number of cases appears to be the initial clinical manifestation, lasts 4 to 8 months and is characterized by frequent seizures, epilepsia partialis continua (EPC) in more than half the cases, and rapid neurological deterioration. In this stage, MR shows changes consistent with inflammation, which will be followed by progressive unilateral atrophy. Finally, the patient enters the "residual stage" with stable neurological deficits, and persisting, albeit less frequent, seizures. In a number of patients this "residual stage" may be followed, years later, by relapse of severe epilepsy and further worsening of neurological deficits.

Epilepsy

Seizures are the initial neurological manifestation of RE in the majority of patients. In up to 20% epilepsy onset is marked by status epilepticus. As the disease progresses, most patients demonstrate more than one seizure type: beside simple motor seizures, virtually all types of focal seizures may be present. This polymorphism *(Figure 2)* can be due to multifocal – though hemispheric – origin of seizures, or to progressive enlargement of the original epileptic zone (Oguni *et al.*, 1992; Granata *et al.*, 2003a). Seizures are refractory to antiepileptic (AE) treatment, their frequency usually increases rapidly, and SE may recur.

Epilepsia partialis continua

Although *epilepsia partialis continua* (EPC) *(Figure 3)* has been considered to be a hallmark of RE, it occurred in 56 to 92% of the patients according to different series (Oguni *et al.*, 1992; Bien *et al.*, 2002b; Granata *et al.*, 2003a). EPC is defined as spontaneous regular or irregular clonic muscle twitching of cortical origin, sometimes aggravated by action or sensory stimuli, confined to one part of the body, and continuing for a period of hours, days or week (Obeso *et al.*, 1985). EPC is refractory to AE drugs, mostly involves distal muscles or the face, and, differently from other movement disorders persists during sleep. Surface EEG may fail to detect ictal epileptic activity because the cortical area involved may be very small or because the dipole of the discharge is oriented in an unfavorable angle with respect to the recording scalp electrodes (Mameniskiene & Wolf 2017).

Neurologic symptoms other than epilepsy

Hemiparesis invariably develops during the course of the disease. As already mentioned, the motor deficit may be the initial symptom, and exceptionally remains the one and only manifestation of RE (Bien *et al.*, 2007). In the first stages of the disease, hemiparesis may be limited to the postictal phase, but rapidly becomes persistent, albeit fluctuating in severity as it worsens with increasing seizure activity. Fixed neurological deficits occur later with the neurological deterioration beginning within the first year after seizure onset in 40%, and in the second or third years in another 40% (Rasmussen & Andermann, 1991). In an Italian series of 12 patients, focal motor deficits appeared from 15 days to 24 months after the first seizure and invariably worsened to severe hemiparesis leading three patients to be wheelchair bound within three years of onset (Granata *et al.*, 2003 a). Hemiparesis is often associated with a dystonic component;

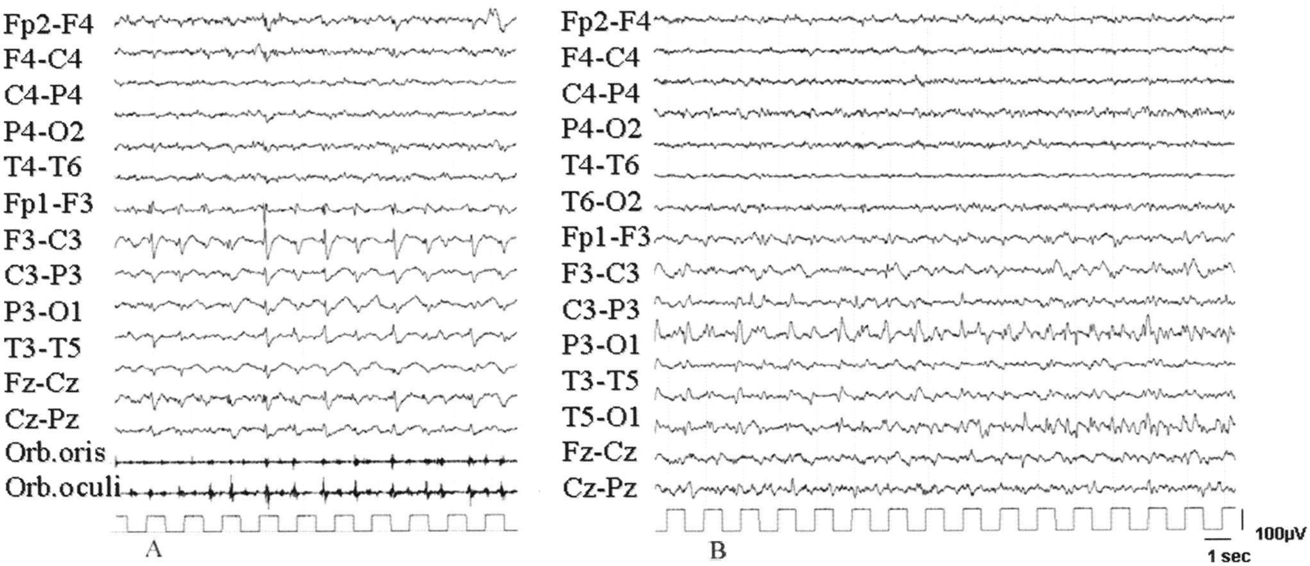

Figure 2

Left hemisphere RE. EEG recorded from the patient in two consecutive days, showing the polymorphic seizure activity: clonic jerks involving the right side of the face are associated with focal epileptic activity over the left central leads (A). A brief versive seizure is associated with an ictal discharge over the left posterior region (B). (EMG1: left orbicularis oris; EMG2: left orbicularis oculi).

more rarely hyperkinetic ipsilateral movement disorders may also be observed. Additional neurological symptoms include progressive speech deficits, cortical sensory loss and hemianopia. Eventually, often after several years, the neurological deficit seems to plateau, but usually only after significant deterioration has occurred.

Cognitive impairment is another constant feature of RE and, as for motor deficits, its appearance may be subtle. Behavioral changes, with irritability, emotional lability or hyperactivity often herald the first signs of mental decline, that consist mainly of memory and attention disorders, and learning difficulties. In the Italian series, these symptoms were detected within 4 to 36 months after the first seizure, and progressively worsened until surgery. At the time of surgery, performed between 7 months and 14 years after disease onset, the mean IQ was 61.3 ± 15.1 (range 44–87) (Granata *et al.*, 2003a). The progression of mental impairment in most cases parallels with the severity of epilepsy and seems to correlate with the bilateral spreading of epileptic EEG abnormalities (Longaretti *et al.*, 2012).

Less common and atypical forms of Rasmussen encephalitis

Late-onset RE

Although the outbreak of RE characteristically occurs in childhood, a late-onset form, affecting adolescent and adult patients, has been increasingly recognized and accounts for about 10% of all cases (Oguni *et al.*, 1992; Hart *et al.*, 1997; Bien 2002b; Villani *et al.*, 2006; Dupont *et al.*, 2017). A recent literature review (Dupont *et al.*, 2017) identified 102 late-onset RE patients with a sex ratio of 8 women for 2 men. Although only a 67% of late-onset RE patients fulfill the consensus diagnostic criteria for RE (Bien *et al.*, 2005), these patients share similar histopathological, clinical, electrophysiological and neuroimaging findings with childhood RE. The main difference consists in the more frequent occurrence of focal unaware seizures, less frequent EPC throughout evolution, and a milder, more protracted,

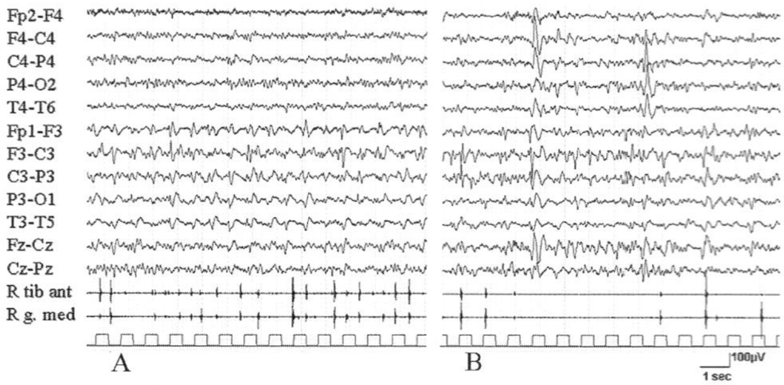

Figure 3 **Wake (A) and sleep (B) EEG recorded from a 5-year-old patient, four months from the first seizure. EPC involving the right lower limb is shown. The rhythmic myoclonic jerks are continuous while awake, and persist, albeit at lower frequency, during sleep. Note the asymmetry of EEG tracing: rhythmic background activity during wakefulness and sleep spindles are evident over the right hemisphere. On the left hemisphere the EEG is dominated by slow activity and continuous epileptic discharges over the central region.**

clinical course: motor and mental deterioration are less severe than in typical childhood RE, hemispheric damage is less pronounced, and patients tend to respond better to immunological treatment (Leach *et al.*, 1999; Villani *et al.*, 2001; Dupont *et al.*, 2017). However, in a number of cases late-onset RE takes a malignant course, comparable to that of childhood-onset disease. Hart *et al.* (1997) described thirteen patients developing seizures in adolescence or adulthood with a pathological appearance of chronic encephalitis: the patients who developed seizures in adulthood bore considerable resemblance to the childhood form, whereas in patients who developed seizures in adolescence, the disease appeared to pursue a more benign course. Villani *et al.* (2006), identified two distinct patterns of disease presentation, one characterized by focal motor seizures (the "epileptic" phenotype), and the other by focal cortical myoclonus (the "myoclonic" phenotype). Unilateral neurological deficits and brain atrophy were progressive in both phenotypes, but they were more prominent and detected earlier in the "epileptic" phenotype. Whatever the subtype of adult-onset RE, its slow and torpid course and the complex, heterogeneous symptomatology make the treatment timing (*i.e.*, the timing for starting an immunosuppressive or surgical treatment) of these cases particularly challenging. Deleo *et al.* (2015) have proposed an instrument that allows a prospective evaluation of these patients, a bedside tool to evaluate late-onset RE progression called "adult-onset RE severity scale" (aRESS). Based on medical history and neurological examination, this scale measures different parameters and is organized in three axes: the first axis relates to focal deficits, like motor deficits and aphasia; the second entails epilepsy-related symptoms, such as drug-refractory seizures, status epilepticus and EPC; the third axis pertains to cognitive and behavioral changes. The number represented by the sum of the scores obtained from the evaluation of each parameter reflects the overall clinical status of the patient and constitutes a useful practical resource for the follow-up of late-onset RE patients.

Persistent focal non-progressive RE

The suggestion that a mild, non-progressive form of RE exists dates back to the pioneering clinical-pathologic study of Aguilar & Rasmussen (1960) and has been confirmed by a number of case reports. In such patients, the disease starts during adolescence or adulthood and may remain circumscribed, without development of severe motor deficits, nor episodes of EPC or convulsive status epilepticus. The relatively benign clinical course is in line with the slow progression of brain damage that may remain circumscribed or involve a restricted area (Gambardella *et al.*, 2008).

RE with no seizures or delayed seizure onset

Drug-refractory epilepsy, with EPC and frequent episodes of status epilepticus, is the clinical hallmark of RE in established cases. Samanta *et al.* (2016) reported a child with histopathologically proven RE who presented with progressive cerebral hemiatrophy, unilateral cortical deficits, but no history of seizures. This case and similar others in which progressive cerebral hemiatrophy has already been noted at epilepsy onset (Korn-Lubetzki *et al.*, 2004; Bien *et al.*, 2007; Villani, personal observation) or in patient without seizure (Ravindra *et al.*, 2017) suggest that inflammation may be latent and precede epilepsy by few months to several years. This, excludes, at least in these patients, that progressive brain atrophy was induced by seizures.

RE with prominent basal ganglia involvement and predominant movement disorders

Deep gray matter is almost invariably involved in RE, therefore a certain degree of dystonia or choreo-athetosis is usually associated with the hemiparesis. In some instances, extensive and early damage to the basal ganglia (including putamen and globus pallidus) may occur and result in disease presenting with hemidystonia or hemiathetosis, associated or followed by EPC and other symptoms of RE (Frucht *et al.*, 2002). Awareness of the possibility of movement disorder as a presenting symptom of RE is important because it may lead to misdiagnosis, particularly in the less common adolescent or adult patients. The diagnosis of RE must be considered when choreic and hemidyskinetic movements are strictly unilateral, and associated with MRI and EEG changes in the contra-lateral hemisphere.

RE with brainstem involvement

Quesada *et al.* (2007) described a 37-year-old woman who developed, four years after RE onset and two years after epilepsy onset, difficulties in swallowing and speech. Brain MRI showed progressive supratentorial left-sided hemiatrophy associated with a signal increase, extending subcortically to the left mesencephalon and pons, without contrast enhancement. Cerebral biopsy was consistent with the diagnosis of RE. Immunomodulatory therapy resulted in the regression of the swallowing and speech problems, while follow-up MRI did not show any substantial changes after one year of treatment. Even if ipsilateral or contralateral involvement of the infratentorial cerebellar structures with no clinical sign had previously been observed in childhood-onset cases (Chiapparini *et al.*, 2003), a demonstrated affection of the brainstem has never been described before in RE. The upper left brainstem lesion was in continuity with the supratentorial disease, and clearly delineated from the right side, in line with the puzzling RE feature of respecting the midline of cerebral structures. Nevertheless, it could not be ruled out that Wallerian degeneration secondary to the supratentorial pathology contributed to this MRI presentation.

Bilateral RE

The hallmark of RE is the unilaterality of brain damage, and this distinctive and unique characteristic is mandatory for diagnosis. True bilateral, pathologically proven, RE is extremely rare and includes a familial (Silver *et al.*, 1998) and a few sporadic cases with early onset of malignant epilepsy and neuropathology consistent with chronic encephalitis (Tobias *et al.*, 2003), as well as rare adult-onset cases (McLachlan, 1993). It should be noted that in bilateral RE, symptoms, and when available, MRI findings pointed to bilateral brain damage within the first months of the disease (Chinchilla *et al.*, 1994). Secondary involvement of the unaffected hemisphere, compatible with the diagnosis of RE, is frequently observed in long standing disease. It consists of the appearance of contralateral interictal epileptic abnormalities (presumably by a mechanism of secondary epileptogenesis) and by the mild brain atrophy, that most probably results from wallerian degeneration of commissure fibers (Larionov, 2005).

RE associated with other diseases (double pathology)

The term double-pathology is employed to define about 10% of all RE cases, in which the clinical and imaging characteristics are fully consistent with the diagnosis, but in which histopathology confirms the coexistence of preexisting brain lesions. This dual pathology has been documented in low-grade tumors, focal cortical dysplasia (FCD), tuberous sclerosis, vascular malformations, or old ischemic lesions (Yacubian *et al.*, 1996; Hart *et al.*, 1998; Palmer *et al.*, 1999; Firlik *et al.*, 1999). Possible explanations for the coexistence of the two pathologies include the suggestion that the structural lesion may cause a breakdown in the blood-brain barrier, increasing the risk of viral infection, or the entry of other compounds with immunogenic or inflammatory potential.

Several studies have focused on the association of RE and FCD. It has been suggested that the expression of antigens within the dysplastic cortex (for example, through major histocompatibility complex molecules) could activate $CD8^+$ T-cells, which are responsible for the immunological attack against neurons and astrocytes in Rasmussen encephalitis (Schwab *et al.*, 2009). Further studies on surgical specimens demonstrated that identical $\gamma\delta$ T-cell clones may traffic to the brain in both FCD and RE but only enter the brain parenchyma in appreciable numbers in RE. Moreover, at the time of surgery, there was evidence of T-cells trafficking into brain parenchyma, whereas T-cells were confined to the perivascular spaces and did not cross the glia limitans in FCD (Owens *et al.*, 2015). A further difference between RE and FCD pathology refers to the presence of tissue resident memory T-cells (TRM) in a significantly high proportion in RE compared to FCD (see paragraph on etiology) (Owens *et al.*, 2016). Further studies on specimens taken from patients with FCD associated with RE might clarify whether this association is the result of a persisting and self-maintaining inflammation around the cortical dysplasia, possibly depending on the host immunological asset.

Clinical and imaging features suggestive of Rasmussen syndrome have been described in patients with gliomatosis, granulomatosis and porphyria, but pathological proof of their association is lacking (Goyal *et al.*, 2007; Ghostine *et al.*, 2007; Tziperman *et al.*, 2007).

Few authors reported disorders resembling RE in patients with autoimmune diseases, such as vasculitis, linear scleroderma, and Parry Romberg syndrome (Shah *et al.*, 2003; Carreno *et al.*, 2007; Damasceno *et al.*, 2009; Seifert *et al.*, 2011). Furthermore, recent isolated reports identified the presence of different autoantibodies directed to surface neuronal antigens (like N-methyl-D-aspartate receptor and voltage-gated potassium channels VGKC), and with the onconeural Anti-Hu antibodies in patients with Rasmussen-like encephalitis (Gurcharran &

Karkare, 2017; Spitz *et al.*, 2014; Aravamuthan, 2015). The co-occurrence of RE with other autoimmune diseases, as well as the recent finding that some RE patients carry HLA alleles that are known to confer susceptibility to different autoimmune diseases (Dandekar *et al.*, 2016) are of interest as they provide new indirect evidence that RE onset may be conditioned by an immunogenetic predisposition. This could interact with a yet undefined environmental factors but it should be stressed that the relationship between RE and these other autoimmune diseases is still unclear. The disease course in these patients may be different (often less severe compared to that of typical RE), and the inflammation potentially involve both hemispheres. It is conceivable that these are different diseases that mimic RE, and this must be considered in planning medical or surgical treatment.

Diagnosis

The diagnosis of RE is based on clinical and laboratory findings that, taken together, support the hypothesis of a lateralized progressive brain disease. In 2005, a European consensus panel proposed formal diagnostic criteria *(Table I)* (Bien *et al.*, 2005) based on clinical (presence of focal seizures, with or without EPC and unilateral cortical deficits) and paraclinical (EEG, MRI and histopathology) findings.

The proposed clinical criteria include a two-step diagnostic approach: i) if all the highly characteristic clinical, EEG and imaging criteria are fully met, the diagnosis can be established without the need for brain biopsy (part A in *Table I*); ii). If the criteria are not fulfilled, the progression of clinical deficits must be associated with progressive hemispheric atrophy, as documented by sequential MRIs or, alternatively, by histopathologically proven T-cell mediated encephalitis, with activated microglial cells and astrogliosis (part B in *Table I*). Making the diagnosis also requires: i) at least two sequential examinations to assess the progression of a neurological deficit and the worsening of unilateral brain damage; ii) MRI with gadolinium and CT scan to rule out a unihemispheric vasculitis; and iii) an accurate work-up to rule out all the conditions characterized by unilateral neurological syndromes or EPC, as well as inflammatory diseases mimicking RE. A study to evaluate the sensitivity, specificity, and positive (PPV) and negative (NPV) predictive values, using pathology as the gold standard, was carried out on a series of 87 patients with biopsy reports (35 evaluated for RE and 52 controls) observed at the Boston Children's Hospital between 1993 and 2011. The authors found that the European diagnostic criteria had a high sensitivity (81%), specificity, PPV and NPV. Nevertheless, strict application of the criteria resulted in four false negatives (criteria-negative, biopsy-positive) and five false positives (criteria-positive, biopsy-negative, with demonstrated alternative diagnosis in 3 patients). The investigators therefore suggest that the 2005 diagnostic criteria could be refined to avoid false negatives; they specifically suggest that the diagnosis can be made when the biopsy is positive, and two of the three criteria of part A are satisfied (Olson *et al.*, 2013).

Table I Diagnosis of RE

RE can be diagnosed if either all 3 criteria of Part A or 2 out of 3 criteria of Part B are present. Check first for the features of Part A. Then, if these are not fulfilled, of Part B. In addition: if no biopsy is performed, MRI with administration of gadolinium and cranial CT needs to be performed to document the absence of gadolinium enhancement and calcifications to exclude the differential diagnosis of a unihemispheric vasculitis (Derry *et al.*, 2002). (From Bien *et al.*, 2005, with permission.)

Part A	
1. Clinical	Focal seizures (with or without EPC) and unilateral cortical deficits
2. EEG	Unihemispheric slowing with or without epileptiform activity and unilateral seizure onset
3. MRI	Unihemispheric focal cortical atrophy and at least one of the following: Grey or white matter T2/FLAIR hyperintense signal Hyperintense signal or atrophy of the ipsilateral caudate head
Part B	
1. Clinical	EPC or progressive* unilateral cortical deficit(s)
2. MRI	Progressive* unihemispheric focal cortical atrophy
3. Histopathology	T cell dominated encephalitis with activated microglial cells (typically, but not necessarily forming nodules) and reactive astrogliosis Numerous parenchymal macrophages, B cells or plasma cells or viral inclusion bodies exclude the diagnosis of RE

RE: Rasmussen encephalitis; EPC: epilepsia partialis continua.

* Progressive means that at least 2 sequential clinical examinations or MRI studies are required to meet the respective criteria. To indicate clinical progression, each of these examinations must document a neurological deficit, and this must increase over time. To indicate progressive hemiatrophy, each of these MRIs must show hemiatrophy, and this must increase over time.

Overall, the 2005 diagnostic criteria are still useful in most patients with typical RE, particularly during the first stage of disease and before the start of immunosuppressive treatment which might slow the disease course and the progression of MRI changes. Nevertheless, reports of further series of patients, together with advances in imaging techniques and better characterization of pathologic findings (namely, the involvement of specific T-cell subsets and of microglia) will hopefully lead to the refinement of criteria to prompt an early diagnosis and to avoid missing patients who could benefit of targeted treatment.

Diagnostic tests

Blood and CSF studies

No laboratory test is available to positively support the diagnosis of RE. Blood tests are unrevealing. Cerebrospinal fluid (CSF) may be normal or show non-specific abnormalities, such as a mild increase in the white cell count (predominantly lymphocytes) and proteins. Oligoclonal bands are found in about half the patients (Grenier *et al.*, 1991; Hart *et al.*, 1994; Granata *et al.*, 2003a). Overall, either a normal or abnormal CSF examination does not exclude or confirm the diagnosis of RE, but must be carried out to exclude CNS infections or other disorders. The presence of anti-glutamate receptor 3 (GluR3) antibodies, should not be considered as a clue to diagnosis since it is now well established that GluR3 antibodies do not discriminate between RE and other epilepsies (Wiendl *et al.*, 2001; Mantegazza *et al.*, 2002). Similarly, the inconsistent finding of other antibodies (Yang *et al.*, 2000; Takahashi *et al.*, 2005; Watson *et al.*, 2005) is not a marker of RE. The potential role of immune molecules (namely IgG, CD4+ T- cells, TNFa, and Granzyme B levels in CSF) as biomarkers for early diagnosis and evolution of RE has been only preliminarily evaluated (Takahashi *et al.*, 2009).

EEG

EEG changes at onset are confined to the affected hemisphere and consist of slowing of background activity and sleep disorganization, focal slow and epileptic abnormalities, early evidence of ictal and interictal hemispheric multifocal abnormalities, and the appearance of subclinical ictal discharges. With time, the EEG shows further deterioration, the epileptic activity increases and tends to spread, and involves the unaffected hemisphere as well. The seizure onset, however, though multifocal, remains clearly unilateral; recordings of early seizures from the unaffected hemisphere should lead to questioning the diagnosis of RE (So & Gloor 1991; Granata *et al.*, 2003a).

The most extensive study of the electroencephalographic changes seen in RE has been that of So & Gloor (1991) at The Montreal Neurological Hospital who studied 339 electroencephalograms (EEGs) and 58 electrocorticograms from 49 patients with a disease duration at the time of recording ranging from a few weeks to 16 years. The abnormalities seen varied widely, and were partly dependent on the stage of the disease at the time of the EEG, with early traces tending to show unilateral abnormalities and later EEGs, bilateral changes with more widespread epileptiform abnormalities. Background activity was normal in only a single patient: in the others, the abnormality was unilateral in 10 patients, bilateral in 4, and bilateral with lateralized predominance in 32. The range of abnormalities described by So & Gloor included slowing or irregularity of the background activity, irregularities in the morphology and frequency of waveforms, and asymmetrical voltage depression of background activity, which occurred in 45%.

Abnormal slow wave activity occurred in all patients, usually consisting of polymorphic delta activity but sometimes comprising polymorphic and intermittent bilateral rhythmic delta activity *(Figure 4)*. Slow wave disturbances were unilateral in 19% and bilateral but with unilateral predominance in 68%: in the remainder, they were symmetrical. Unilateral disturbances of background activity and unilateral slow wave abnormalities were more likely to occur in patients with mild clinical disease prior to the development of hemiparesis than in those with very early disease and those studied at a later stage, after the development of a hemiparesis: in both these groups, the abnormalities were more likely to be bilateral. Forty-four of the Montreal patients showed interictal epileptiform discharges in their EEG. There was a well-localized focus in only 6%: in a further 6% bilaterally synchronous discharges occurred. Thirty per cent had multiple independent foci lateralized to one hemisphere, and a further 13% had a similar picture but with bilaterally synchronous discharges *(Figure 5)*. In 13% there were bilateral multiple independent foci, with bilaterally synchronous discharges being seen in a further 21%. In 2 (4%) patients only bilaterally synchronous discharges were seen. In the 32 patients in whom seizures were recorded, a strictly localized onset was recorded in only 5 (16%). The onset could be lateralized in 22 (69%), the picture usually being one of multifocal onset. Among patients in the Montreal series followed up with serial EEGs, six showed progressively more widespread interictal or ictal epileptiform abnormalities, while three showed the development of independent epileptiform abnormalities over the contralateral hemisphere. By the time that hemiparesis and radiographic abnormalities had occurred, bilateral disturbance of background activity was present in 76%, bilateral slow wave abnormalities in 81%, and bilateral multiple independent interictal epileptiform discharges in 34%, while 6% had seizures arising independently from the two hemispheres.

EPC *(Figure 3)*, like in other conditions, is often not clearly related to EEG changes recorded by scalp electrodes that may just record uncharacteristic, often polyphasic slow waves. In the Montreal series EEG examination was carried out during a period of epilepsia partialis

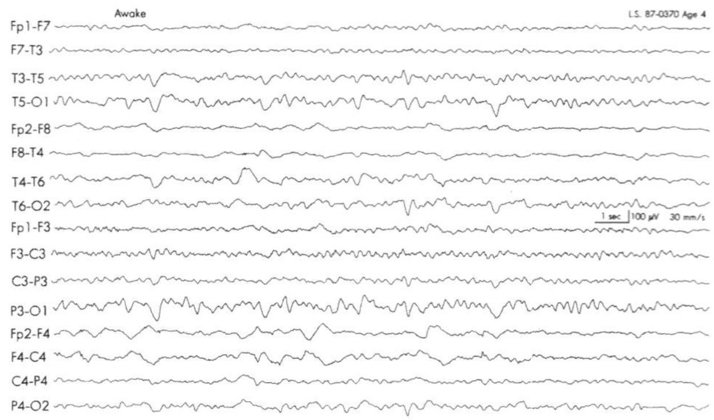

Figure 4 **Asymmetrical disturbance of background activity showing more severe polymorphic delta activity and relative depression of background rhythms over the right hemisphere. From So & Gloor, 1991 with permission.**

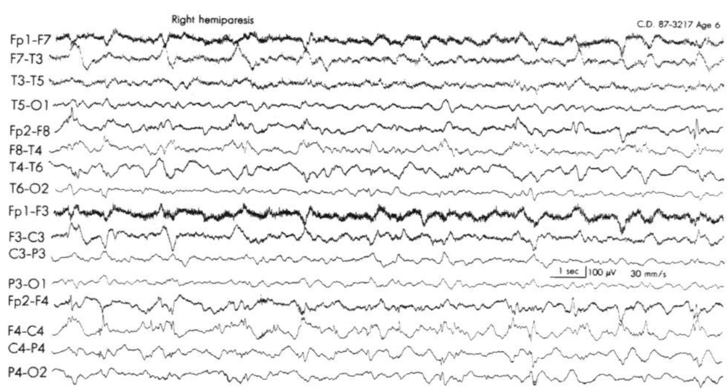

Figure 5 **Multiple independent epileptiform discharges over the right hemisphere, maximally involving the right fronto-centro-parietal regions. Some irregular repetitive slow sharp wave complexes appear to be approximately synchronous over both frontal regions. From So and Gloor, 1991 with permission.**

continua in 17 patients: no electroclinical correlation was seen in nine; in three, there was correlation between the muscle jerks and EEG discharges on some occasions, while in five, the relationship was uncertain (So & Gloor, 1991).

Auxiliary neurophysiologic techniques may contribute to define the cortical origin of the jerks. Jerked-locked back-averaging study, eliminating the ongoing background EEG noise, may identify the small hidden spikes preceding the motor phenomena.

Magnetoencephalography (MEG) may be particularly useful in localizing focal epileptic activity, since it can detect epileptiform abnormalities that are not revealed by EEG (Barkley & Baumgartner, 2003). Recently, Rossi Sebastiano *et al.* (2017) used MEG to evaluate five children with RE in two distinct assessments, each one separated from the other by a six-month period. They showed that epileptic foci were located in different areas of the affected hemisphere in all RE patients, supporting the idea that the multifocal pattern of epileptic generators is probably unrelated to the duration or the disease stage. The different distribution of epileptic abnormalities in each subject and their changes in location over a period of about six months led to the hypothesis of a "migratory" behavior of spike generators in RE, which probably reflects the patchy progression of the inflammatory/degenerative process. Furthermore, the limited correlation between spike generation and local progression of the atrophic changes revealed by MRI, suggests that functional changes causing epileptogenesis do not precisely match the morphological changes (Rossi Sebastiano *et al.*, 2017). Hence, serial MEG assessments may reveal periods of fast or slow disease progression, helping clinicians in the modulation of the therapy and in the decision-making of neurosurgery. Guan *et al.* (2017) also recognized that MEG may have a role in managing RE patients who are candidates for hemispheric disconnection, because it can clarify the cortical sources of interictal epileptic spikes and assist postoperative care.

Neuroimaging

The original patients described by Rasmussen were studied by pneumoencephalography (PEG) which detected unilateral atrophy with ventricular dilatation. The advent of computerized tomography and, later, of MRI confirmed that the progressive cerebral hemiatrophy was the main characteristic of the disease (Tampieri *et al.*, 1991; Bien *et al.*, 2002b; Chiapparini *et al.*, 2003). Starting from the nineties, the widespread use of MRI better characterized the pathologic changes that occur in RE, contributed to the diagnosis even in the early stages of the disease, and allowed longitudinal evaluation of the brain damage *(Figure 6)* (Bien *et al.*, 2002c; Chiapparini *et al.*, 2003). In most cases, within the first few months, RE patients disclose a combination of changes, that, albeit not diagnostic, are sufficiently characteristic to raise the suspicion of RE. In the early stages of the disease, the mild focal cortical atrophy mainly involves the temporo-insular region associated with enlargement of the ipsilateral temporal horn and Sylvian fissure and with an abnormal cortical and/or subcortical hyperintense signal in T2 and FLAIR images. A further change,

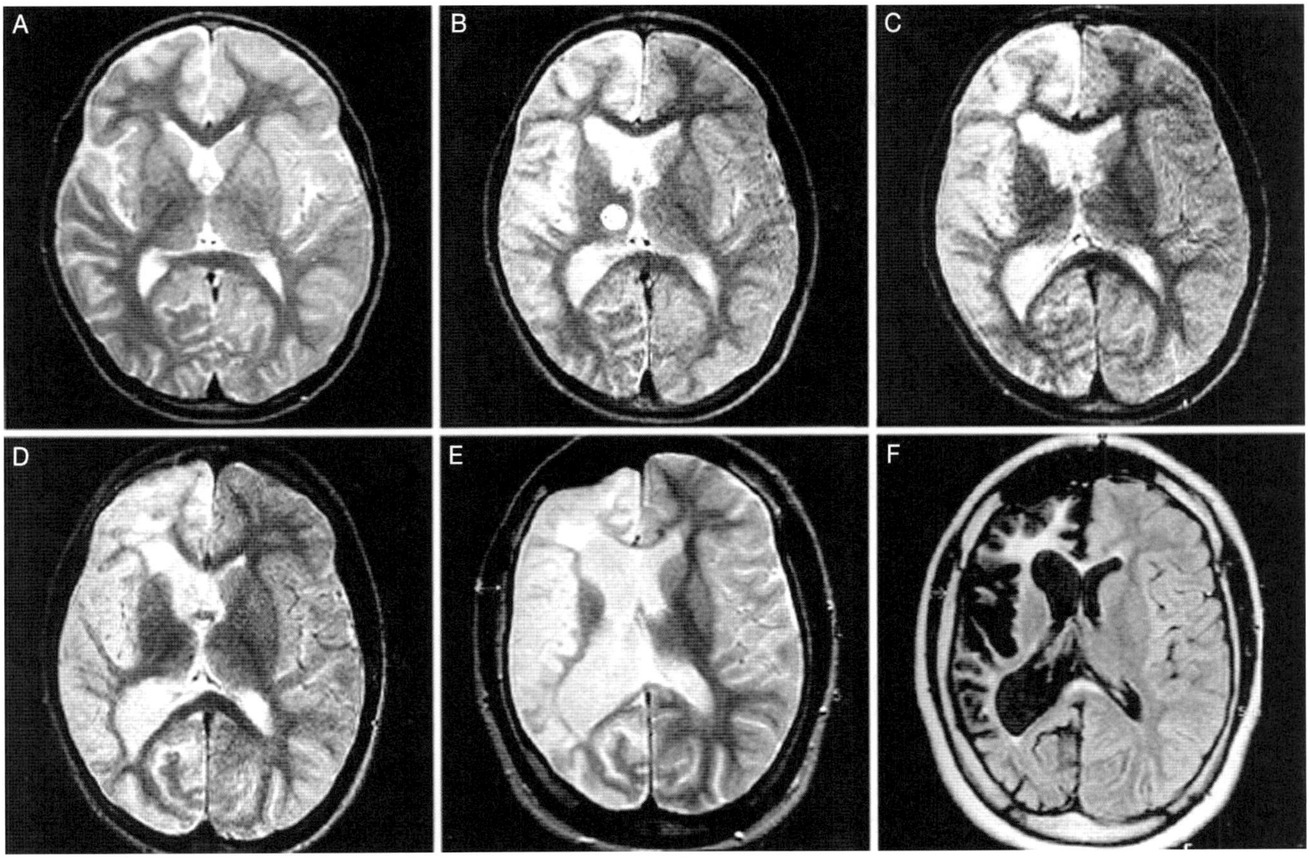

Figure 6 **MRI showing the progression of the disease in a patient with right sided RE. Axial T-2w images taken at 10 days (A), 9 months (B), 12 months (C), 18 months (D) after the onset show the progression of cortical atrophy and ventricular enlargement, spreading of abnormal signal and progression of atrophy of the basal ganglia. The disease mainly progressed during the first 18 months, although further damage occurred in the following years as shown in axial T-2w (E) and FLAIR (F) images taken 8 years after the disease onset. (Reproduced from Chiapparini *et al.*, 2003, with permission.)**

frequently observed in the early phases of the disease is T2 hyperintensity or atrophy of the head of the caudate nucleus, as well as of putamen (Bhatjiwale *et al.*, 1998; Chiapparini *et al.*, 2013; Rajesh *et al.*, 2006). Transient focal cortical swelling may occasionally precede the above-described findings. Gadolinium enhancement is not observed. During the course of the disease, the caudate atrophy worsens and the unilateral cortical atrophy spreads to involve the rest of the hemisphere. In a study comparing MRI and histopathology findings, Bien *et al.* demonstrated that increased MRI signal correlates with an active inflammatory process, as witnessed by the high density of inflammatory cells and reactive astrocytes, *i.e.* with the presence of T-cells, microglial nodules, and GFAP-positive astrocytes.

Conversely, MRI atrophic areas without signal abnormalities correlate with tissue loss that mostly occurs during the first year after the "acute disease stage" (Bien *et al.*, 2002c). The supratentorial tissue loss is accompanied by atrophy of the contralateral, but seldom global, cerebellar hemisphere, the brain stem, and thinning of the corpus callosum. The more recent MRI volumetry studies confirm that the highest rate of volume loss is in the first months of disease, and that among the subcortical structures the temporo-mesial region and the putamen are the mainly involved areas (Wagner *et al.*, 2012). A further study (Wang *et al.*, 2016) compared the volumetric MRIs of 19 RE patients with those of 42 patients with epilepsy and 42 health controls to determine the predictive value of lobar volumetric measures. The authors demonstrated that volumetric measures, particularly interhemispheric and frontal lobe ratios had a high degree of accuracy to separate RE patients from non-RE epilepsy patients with the same disease duration. The authors suggest that this technique, in an appropriate clinical setting, may aid the diagnosis in the early phases of the disease, and serve as marker of disease progression and treatment effectiveness (Wang *et al.*, 2016).

Studies involving magnetic resonance spectroscopy (MRS), which provide an index of neuronal loss or damage by measuring the relative resonance intensity of N-acetyl-D-aspartate (NAA) to choline (NAA/Cho) have shown decreased relative NAA signal intensity over the entire affected hemisphere involving both cortex and white matter (Cendes *et al.*, 1995; Chiapparini *et al.*, 2003). The MRS changes tended to worsen progressively with time, but did not affect the contralateral hemisphere. MRS may detect increased lactate peaks, resulting from seizure activity.

Functional imaging demonstrates, even in the early stages, areas of glucose hypometabolism on fluorodeoxyglucose-positron emission tomography (FDG-PET), interictal hemispheric hypoperfusion and ictal multifocal hyperperfusion on single photon emission computed tomography (SPECT) (Burke *et al.*, 1992; Banati *et al.*, 1999; Fiorella, 2001; Fogarasi, 2003).

The role of functional imaging has been recently studied in a series of 23 patients, 12 of whom also had a histological diagnosis (Kuki *et al.*, 2018). Cerebral blood flow single photon emission computed tomography (CBF-SPECT) detected hypoperfusion areas in 16 of 22 patients by interictal SPECT, and in 10 of 12 patients by ictal SPECT, which correlated with ictal onset area by ictal EEG. Lowered glucose metabolism was observed in affected areas in all five patients examined by FDG-PET, also when the MR images were unrevealing. In summary, functional studies provide valuable information, including early detection of affected areas, and target for biopsy site. Nonetheless, in clinical practice data obtained by these techniques must be cautiously interpreted and integrated with clinical and MRI findings.

Brain biopsy

Histopathology study is usually not necessary in RE cases because clinical and imaging findings allow the correct diagnosis in most cases, even in the early stages. However, in uncertain or atypical cases brain biopsy can help to reach a diagnosis. In this case an open biopsy is recommended to avoid false negative results given that normal and abnormal tissue elements (with different degrees of pathologic changes) may be located in very close apposition. The tissue samples must be taken in a non-eloquent area where there is an increased T2/FLAIR signal on MRI and must be large enough to include meninges, gray and white matter to demonstrate the multifocal changes of the T-cell-dominated encephalitis with activated microglia and reactive gliosis (Robitaille, 1991; Pardo *et al.*, 2004). The characterization of specific T-cells subset might help in differentiating RE by other chronic inflammatory disease.

Differential diagnosis

Early in the disease, RE may be confused with a number of other conditions characterized by focal or unilateral brain damage, or by EPC. Differential diagnosis includes: i) epileptic conditions with possible unihemispheric presentation such as focal or hemispheric dysplasia, neoplasia, and neurocutaneous syndromes (tuberous sclerosis, and Sturge-Weber), stroke, and Hemiconvulsion Hemiplegia-Epilepsy (HHE); ii) progressive diseases such as MELAS, POLG1 and other mitochondriopathies, lipofuscinosis and Alpers disease; iii) cerebral vasculitis in systemic diseases, such as lupus erythematosus, or Derry's vasculitis; iv) rare infective disorders such as cat scratch disease, but also HIV infection.

The most common differential diagnosis is with epilepsy due to cortical dysplasia, particularly when the epilepsy onset is with high-frequency seizures in an otherwise normal child. In these cases, the first MR examination may be misleading. In fact, the white matter signal abnormalities that may be associated with cortical dysplasia could be confused with the initial inflammatory changes seen in RE. However, characteristically in cortical dysplasia there is no progressive loss of tissue, and the MR follow-up will confirm a stable image. Furthermore, Longaretti *et al.* (2012) indicate EEG features, such as early lateralized slow activity and the consecutive emergence of contralateral epileptiform abnormalities, as highly suggestive of RE and important features in the differential diagnosis between RE and focal cortical dysplasia.

In children a frequent cause of EPC and status epilepticus are the mitochondriopathies. In such diseases, EPC may involve either one or both sides and is often associated with focal seizures of predominantly occipital onset. Moreover, MRI shows progressive brain atrophy or multifocal abnormalities which are different from what is usually seen in RE. A comprehensive review of causes of EPC has been recently published by Mameniskiene and Wolf (2017).

RE must be differentiated from the autoimmune encephalitides increasingly reported to occur also in children and adolescents, more frequently as non-paraneoplastic syndromes (Dalmau & Graus 2018). The explosive onset of seizures, with neuropsychiatric decline, together with focal signal abnormalities on MRI may mimic the clinical and imaging features of RE and lead to misdiagnosis (Greiner *et al.*, 2011; Gurcharran *et al.*, 2017). Similarly, clinical and laboratory features observed in RE, especially in those patients with a late onset or limited chronic focal variant, may mimic those observed in autoimmune limbic encephalitis in which the typical presentation is with subacute onset of confusion, behavioural changes and psychosis, short-term memory loss and seizures.

Treatment

RE is an inflammatory disease with a progressive course in which the key symptoms are seizures and motor and mental deficits. The management of RE should therefore include the treatment of symptoms and of the underlying inflammation. The efficacy of treatment must consider both seizure reduction and motor and cognitive improvement, weighted against the side effects. Moreover, treatment planning requires a differentiated approach at different ages: the disease presentation and course, and the load of the cardinal symptoms may be different; awareness of the disease increases with age; and the role of the patient in the decision making, usually negligible in children, becomes crucial in adolescents and adults. The latter implies a different way of communicating and may require the management of different points of view within the family (see the dedicated paragraph in Nabbout *et al.*, 2017)

Further issues that must be kept in mind during decision making are the following: i) the use of immunomodulatory treatment also in children can result in delaying surgery also in patients who could benefit from an early intervention; ii) in successfully operated children, inevitable post-op motor deficits, may lead to behavioural and mood disturbances, once the child grows up and becomes aware of her/his disability; iii) in patients who have not been operated or with non- optimal post-op outcome, issues related to the motor deficits, neuropsychological disabilities, and behavioral disorders may become disruptive at the time of adolescence. The reduced ability to comprehend his/her disability together with the behavior problems (which may include aggressiveness, lack of inhibition, and iterative behaviors), may result in social maladjustment and exclusion (see the dedicated paragraph in Thiele *et al.* 2014).

In summary, given that the severity of symptoms is different in different patients and phases, the therapeutic strategy must be tailored to the need of each patient, and must consider, besides the management of seizures and neurological deficits, short and long term psychological and social concerns.

Antiepileptic drugs

Seizures, particularly EPC and focal motor attacks, are almost invariably resistant to conventional AEDs and no drug regimen has been shown to be superior to any other. A realistic goal of AED treatment is therefore the suppression of the more disabling attacks avoiding heavy polytherapy to limit side effects and drug interactions. In patients given immunotherapy it is preferable to use non enzyme-inducing or inhibiting AED.

Surgical treatment

RE was first described in surgically treated patients, and 60 years later, despite advances in understanding the pathogenesis of the disease, surgery remains inevitable in most patients. It is now widely accepted that the hemispheric disconnection (hemispherectomy or hemispherotomy, consisting in deafferentation of the hemisphere with very limited removal of tissue) is effective in halting seizures, as well as motor and mental deterioration, in over 80% of patients (Vining *et al.*, 1993; Kossoff *et al.*, 2003; Thomas *et al.*, 2003; Pulsifer *et al.*, 2004; Tubbs *et al.*, 2005; Villemure *et al.*, 2006; Marras *et al.*, 2010). Recent outcome data from a series of sixteen RE patients submitted to hemispherotomy and followed for a median of 9.5 years (range 3–20 years) showed a complete seizure control in 81% of cases at last follow-up, with antiepileptic drugs withdrawn in 76% of seizure-free patients (Granata *et al.*, 2014). A notable postoperative improvement of motor and cognitive functions was observed in most of the patients, despite the inevitable sequelae (hemianopia, loss of fine motor skills, hemiparesis, aphasia). Cognitive outcomes were strongly influenced by the time from disease onset to surgery, cognitive improvement being more pronounced in patients operated soon after RE onset as compared to patients operated on later, in line with previous experiences (Jonas *et al.*, 2004; Thomas *et al.*, 2012). These long-term results provide an important support to early hemispherotomy as the first choice surgical treatment for RE, especially in younger children.

The awareness of the inevitable progression of the disease and the known positive outcome after hemispherectomy/hemispherotomy should theoretically lead to surgery in virtually all patients once the diagnosis is established. However, when dealing with each individual patient, concerns always arise not only in the family but also in the referring physician.

If the patient is a young child, the procedure is rather easy to propose and to be accepted given the high potential of brain plasticity that will limit surgery sequelae even in patients with involvement of the dominant hemisphere. The potential ability of the right hemisphere to functionally reorganize language is well known in very young children, and recently demonstrated over a long period of time in children operated on at the age of 4–8 years, even when aphasia had worsened post-operatively (Bulteau *et al.*, 2015). By contrast, reluctance is almost the rule in school-aged children, adolescents and adults, particularly in the early stages and when the dominant hemisphere is affected. In these cases, the expected surgically induced hemianopia, hemiparesis (albeit with preserved walking), loss of fine motor skills and aphasia, make the decision regarding indication and timing of surgery quite difficult. In selected late-onset patients conservative surgical options may represent a choice in the treatment of RE. Villani *et al.* (2014) reported two adult-onset RE patients with super-refractory EPC and SE who underwent limited cortectomy. Surgery resulted in complete control of epilepsy and improvement of quality of life. The authors suggest, in line with few other reports (Ramesha *et al.*, 2009; Abd-El-Barr *et al.*, 2011) that limited cortical resection can be feasible in highly selected clinical settings. and propose prognostic parameters, necessary to decide among surgical techniques. These parameters, represented by motor seizure with an easily recognizable and possibly spatial limited epileptogenic zone, a late onset, and a slower disease progression, would be predictive of a good seizure outcome for limited cortical resections, at least on the temporal span of the available follow-up (three to five years).

When surgery is not feasible or ineffective or not accepted by patients and family, other treatment strategies may be attempted in RE patients. Anecdotally, two RE cases treated, at least temporarily, with vagus nerve stimulation (VNS) have been described in the literature. VNS is a neuromodulation treatment classically performed in patients with drug-resistant epilepsy. Grujic *et al.* (2011) described a 41-year-old RE patient with sub-continuous, drug resistant, motor seizures and slowly progressive cognitive impairment, who rejected surgery to avoid permanent deficits and underwent VNS implantation. After 6 months, a significant reduction in seizure frequency, associated with neurocognitive improvement, was reported. De Benedictis *et al.* (2013) described a 3-year-old patient, who experienced motor seizures at age 24 months and later developed a severe, disabling EPC, resistant to intravenous medical treatment (steroids, IVIg and midazolam). Due to the atypical early severe motor impairment and the presence of slow EEG activity over the unaffected hemisphere, a diagnosis of RE was only contemplated. In the meantime, at age of 3 years, VNS was implanted with a progressive benefit on EPC. Two years later a cortectomy confirmed the RE diagnosis and hemispherotomy was then performed.

Medical treatment

Immunomodulatory treatments

An increasing number of reports on the use of immunomodulatory treatments have accumulated in the last decade, indicating their potential role in selected patients and circumstances. The mechanisms by which these treatments may act in RE are probably complex, and include, besides the anti-inflammatory and immunomodulating effects, the regulation of blood brain barrier permeability and a direct antiepileptic effect. Corticosteroids and intravenous immunoglobulin (IVIg) are the older and more widely used treatments. More recently, following new insights on the role of humoral and cellular immunity in the pathogenesis of RE, different immunomodulatory treatments have been proposed, including plasma exchange, monoclonal antibodies, and immunosuppressants.

Several issues limit the correct evaluation of the effect of immunomodulation. Existing studies are mainly based on case reports or small patient series; the patients have been treated at different stages of the disease, according to different schedules, and often with multiple drugs. Moreover, the effect of treatment is usually defined as "a whole", separate data on seizure outcome and motor/cognitive outcome are rarely available, and adequate measures of outcome are rarely defined.

Corticosteroids

Corticosteroids probably remain the most effective medical treatment (Hart *et al.*, 1994; Granata *et al.*, 2003b; Bahi-Buisson *et al.*, 2007) at least in the short term. Hart *et al.* (1994) reported 19 children treated with high-dose steroids, intravenous immunoglobulin, or both. Although just over half the patients showed some improvement in seizure control with high-dose steroids, in most the improvement was transient. The patients reverted to their previous state within a few days or weeks of the cessation of treatment, and they usually had prominent steroid side effects. However, in many patients the treatments were not started until late in the disease: fourteen already had mild hemiparesis and four showed cognitive impairment. The effect of intravenous methylprednisolone (MPN) was reported to produce a dramatic improvement in one patient given this treatment at the age of 29, 14 years after onset of RE (Krauss *et al.*, 1996). The short-term effect of IV MPN in a proportion of patients was confirmed in two retrospective series (Granata *et al.*, 2003b; Bahi-Buisson *et al.*, 2007). Bahi-Buisson *et al.* (2007), reported 11 children treated 1–36 months after the diagnosis with MPN 400 mg/mq (3 boli on alternate days every 2 months) followed by 2 mg/kg/day of oral prednisone. The effect of the steroid treatment, that had a mean duration of 24 ± 15 months, was assessed on a clinical basis. One patient exhibited total cessation of seizures after steroid treatment for 3 years, but seizures progressively recurred although the frequency was moderate. Four children had significant reduction of seizure frequency with disappearance of EPC, and improved motor function, but the efficacy was not confirmed during long term follow-up: two patients died of unexpected sudden death 5 and 7 years after seizure control, two others with initial response experienced progressive recurrence of seizures, 1 to 4 years after the end of steroid therapy and required hemispherotomy.

Intravenous immunoglobulin

Intravenous immunoglobulin (IVIg), usually employed at monthly doses of 2.0 g/kg, has been reported to be effective in a proportion of patients with RE (Granata *et al.*, 2003c). In the series of Hart *et al.* (1994) seven of nine patients treated with IVIg showed improvement in seizure control, at least initially, though this was only transient in three. Any improvement in neurological function which accompanied the improvement in seizure frequency was similarly transient. Caraballo *et al.* (1998) likewise reported a transient cessation of progression of the neurological deterioration and control of seizures in seven of their 12 patients with Rasmussen syndrome treated with IVIg, and Leach *et al.* (1999), noted striking improvement in seizure control, hemiparesis and cognition in two patients with adult-onset RE treated with intravenous immunoglobulin. Granata *et al.* (2003b) reported that seizures decreased by 50% and neurological conditions improved in 4 out of 12 patients treated with monthly infusion of IVIg 2 g/kg. However, the effect was transient and all patients eventually underwent surgery.

Taken together the literature data suggest that sequential IV courses of high doses MPN (alone or combined with chronic oral prednisone) can help stop epileptic status and decrease the intensity of EPC. Chronic steroid treatment, repeated IVIg administration, or the combination of the two may have some effect on seizure reduction and neurological improvement, but the effect on disease progression is limited, as most reported patients required delayed hemispheric disconnection.

Monoclonal antibodies

Several monoclonal antibodies have been tested in RE in the attempt to modulate the immune response against neurons and astrocytes.

Rituximab is a chimeric mouse-human monoclonal antibody that binds to surface glycoprotein CD20 and coats B cells, causing their depletion. The drug has been reported to be highly effective on epileptic activity in a 20 years old patient who had been previously treated with steroids, IVIg, tacrolimus and immunoadsorption (Thilo *et al.*, 2009). The rationale underlying the use of a B-cell-depleting therapy was, according to the authors, to suppress the role of B cells in activating T-cell through their antigen-presenting and cytokine-producing activities. Additional therapeutic effects might be related to the control of humoral immunity that probably has a role, although not pivotal, in RE. A pilot study based on a multi-centre, open label, uncontrolled trial investigated the safety, tolerability and efficacy of rituximab, given as IV infusion (375 mg/mq) weekly for four doses (Laxer *et al.*, 2008). Of the nine patients treated eight showed some improvement in seizure severity and frequency, with three becoming seizure free (including two with EPC). One patient had no change in seizure frequency. Some patients had marked improvements in motor deficits. There is little information about long-term efficacy and tolerability of rituximab in RE patients. El Tawil *et al.* (2016) reported the case of an adult-onset RE patient, with peculiar reflex language-induced seizures who significantly benefited from rituximab infusions. However, other Authors reported that rituximab is not, or only very partially, effective, and that relapse may occur after initial improvement using the drug (Villani, personal communication; Bittner *et al.*, 2013; Liba *et al.*, 2017).

Natalizumab is a humanized monoclonal antibody against the α4-integrin (α4-integrin antagonist), a glycoprotein expressed on the surface of lymphocytes and monocytes, which facilitates the adhesion of these cells to the endothelial vessel wall. Its mechanism consists in selectively blocking T-cell entry into the CNS. The assumption that peripheral lymphocytes invading the CNS may contribute to disease activity and seizure generation (Fabene *et al.*, 2008) led to try this drug in a RE patient, already given several other immunomodulants (dexamethasone, IVIg, plasma exchange), and immunosuppressant the Infusion of 300 mg IV monthly, resulted, after 18-month treatment period, in a significant reduction of seizure frequency and optimal EPC control (Bittner *et al.*, 2013).

Adalimumab is a fully humanized monoclonal antibody with elevated affinity for the tumor necrosis factor alpha (TNF-α), a cytokine known to contribute in perpetuating hyperexcitability and increasing sensitivity to seizures (Balosso *et al.*, 2009; Balosso *et al.*, 2013; Weinberg *et al.*, 2013). Following the serendipitous observation of a significant improvement in seizure control and neurologic function in a patient with RE who was given Adalimumab for the treatment of the associated juvenile idiopathic arthritis, a multicenter, uncontrolled, open-label study was carried out (Lagarde *et al.*, 2016). The study included 11 RE patients, aged 1.5–37 years, who did not benefit from previous immunotherapy (corticosteroids, immunoglobulins, azathioprine) and who were not eligible for surgery. Adalimumab (24 mg/mq administered *via* subcutaneous injection every 14 days for a median period of 12 months) was started after a median delay of 31 months after the first seizure, and the patients have been followed for a median of 18 months. The authors report a significant decrease of seizure frequency following treatment in all patients: 5 patients experienced a sustained decrease in seizure frequency (by at least 50% compared to the baseline), with stabilization of functional decline in 3 of them. The five responder patients were aged 4–37 years at the time of seizure onset, 4 of them had a slow disease course, and 2 of them had comorbid autoimmune disease (uveitis, juvenile arthritis). These preliminary data are certainly of interest, but as for other studies on extremely rare diseases, the lack of a control group, the low number of enrolled patients, and the wide heterogeneity in age and clinical course, require further confirmation

Alemtuzumab: there is a single case report, with unsatisfactory results, on the use of this monoclonal humanized antibody directed against CD52 glycoprotein expressed on the surface of both T and B-lymphocytes and other immune cells (Liba *et al.*, 2017).

Plasmapheresis

Plasmapheresis (PEX) or Protein A Immunoadsorption (PAI) have been used with the rationale of removing potentially pathogenic circulating antibodies. The first experience with PEX followed the discovery of an association between antibodies to GluR3 in some patients with Rasmussen's syndrome by Andrews *et al.* (1996) who treated four patients (two of them previously described by Rogers *et al.* (1994). Three responded dramatically, with repeated though transient clinical improvement in seizure control and neurological function, while the fourth showed only a slight response. They suggested a protocol for the use of plasma exchange, with 5 or 6 single volumes of plasma exchange initially (using albumin and saline replacement) over 10 to 12 days, an infusion of 1 g/kg of IVIg being given to the patient the day after. The aim is to prolong the improvement after each plasma exchange and to limit expense. In the following years, a dramatic effect of PEX or PAI (that consists in the selective removal of circulating Igs from the patient's plasma) in blocking status epilepticus and neurological deterioration has been reported (Antozzi *et al.*, 1998; Granata *et al.*, 2003b; Thilo *et al.*, 2009). However, in no cases has the plasma treatment been effective as a long-term therapy (Granata *et al.*, 2003b; Bien, personal communication; Villani, personal communication on a series of 5 adult patients). Plasma treatment should therefore be reserved to phases of acute deterioration, or to assess residual motor and mental function before surgery.

Immunosuppressive drugs

Tacrolimus, a T-cell inhibiting drug has been used, based on the growing evidence of the role of granzyme β mediated T-cell cytotoxicity. An open trial was conducted on seven patients followed for a median of 22.4 months. The outcome of the patients with regard to seizure frequency, motor and cognitive functions, and the ratio of hemispheric brain tissue loss, was compared with that of 12 "historical" patients. The study demonstrated that tacrolimus treated patients had a superior outcome compared to historical controls with respect to neurological function and progression of cerebral atrophy to the point that none was treated surgically; by contrast, tacrolimus had no effect on seizures (Bien *et al.*, 2004).

Years later, a randomized controlled trial compared two immunotherapy regimens in patients with RE. Sixteen patients were enrolled over a 6-year period, randomized to tacrolimus (9 cases) or IVIg (7 cases) and followed for at least one year. Seven untreated patients were used as historical controls for the effectiveness of immunotherapy. Motricity Index (MI); and serial MRIs were used to score the motor abilities and the hemispheric ratio (HR). Both immunotherapies slowed down tissue and functional loss with no differences between the two groups, but had limited effect on seizures: no immune-treated but several control patients developed intractable epilepsy, neither therapy was effective in controlling seizures in patients with established drug resistant seizures (Bien *et al.*, 2013).

Conflicting and limited results, precluding any definite conclusion, have been reported for cyclophosphamide, azathioprine, mycophenolate mofetil and other immunosuppressants.

Cyclophosphamide was reported to be ineffective in a small series of four patients (Granata *et al.*, 2003b). Another anecdotal experience with cyclophosphamide confirmed the previous observation (Liba *et al.*, 2015).

Mycophenolate mofetil was used as long-term secondary-choice immunosuppressant in a few RE cases with still uncertain long-term efficacy (Thilo *et al.*, 2009; Liba *et al.*, 2015, 2017). Recently, other immunosuppressive agents have been employed. Intrathecal methotrexate, combined with alemtuzumab or alone, was used in a RE case by Liba *et al.* (2017) with a transitory positive effect on seizures, motor and cognitive performances; mitoxantrone demonstrated to be effective in two late-onset RE patients, leading to a significant reduction in seizure frequency and SE-related hospitalization (Stabile *et al.*, 2018).

In the search for new immunological treatments for RE, different drugs directed to other cells involved in the pathophysiology of this disease, such as microglia, have been proposed, at least theoretically. Mynocicline and perindopril have been cited as molecules capable of inhibiting microglial cells, but experiences with these drugs in RE are still absent in the literature (Varadkar *et al.*, 2014).

To summarize, the available evidence suggests that steroids, plasma treatment, and IVIg appear to be effective in acute phases of RE when seizures are frequent and status epileptics recurs, whereas immunomodulants andimmunosuppressive treatments may be effective in slowing motor and to some extent cognitive decline as well as tissue loss, but have minimal or no effect on seizure activity. However, the effectiveness of current treatments is limited: this may be due the frequent delay between the onset of RE and the start of treatment, and, most probably to the still limited understanding of the complex pathogenesis of the disease. Finally, the use of immunomodulatory treatment, beside new hopes, has opened new issues. To date it is not known to what extent the endpoint of the disease has been modified; by contrast, the effectiveness of some drugs in preventing motor deterioration and brain atrophy has made a decision for surgical treatment much more difficult in patients with persisting, often disabling, seizures. Given the transient and partial effect of immunomodulatory treatment on seizure activity and progression of symptoms, it should be limited to patients who are not, or not yet, suitable candidates for surgery. These include: late-onset (adolescent or adult patients) RE with slow and mild course; patients with dominant hemisphere involvement and slow progression when the risks of motor and language decline by surgery are not accepted by patient and family; suspected RE in which neurologic deterioration and hemispheric atrophy have not yet occurred; proven or suspected bilateral RE.

Antiviral treatment

Antiviral and interferon treatment has been reported in a few papers in the 1990s, but the paucity of data do not allow any conclusions about their effect. The use of antiviral medication is currently not included in the therapeutic algorithm of RE patients. However, for the sake of completeness, we summarize the limited experience with antiviral treatments reported in the literature.

Because of the observation that cytomegalovirus had been isolated from some patients with Rasmussen syndrome, McLachlan *et al.* (1996), treated four patients with ganciclovir. Cytomegalovirus genome had been sought in three of these, and found in two. There was no benefit in one patient; two, treated 34 and 72 months after the start of the disease, showed some benefit, and the other child, who had very frequent seizures developing over 3 months, became seizure free 5 days after treatment was started, with improvement in cognitive function and EEG changes, and resolution of focal neurological signs. Maria *et al.* (1993) and Dabbagh *et al.* (1997) have each published case reports of the use of intraventricular interferon in patients with Rasmussen's syndrome, the rationale for this treatment being both the fact that interferons have immunomodulating effects and also inhibit virus replication in infected cells. Both patients showed improvement in seizure control with treatment, at least in the short term. The patient described by Dabbagh *et al.*, required repeated courses of treatment to maintain the improvement.

Acknowledgements

The Authors wish to thank Andrea Stabile, MD, for his help in revising the manuscript.

Research activity on Rasmussen Encephalitis at the Neurological Institute "Besta" are partly supported by the "Paolo Zorzi" Association for Neuroscience and by the "Pierfranco and Luisa Mariani Foundation".

REFERENCES ▶

Abd-El-Barr MM, Wub B, Rahman M, Yachnis AT, Roper SN, Eisenschenk S (2011): Atypical Rasmussen's encephalitis treated with temporal lobectomy. *J Clin Neurosci* 18: 287–290.

Aguilar MJ, Rasmussen T (1960): Role of encephalitis in pathogenesis of epilepsy. *Arch Neurol* 2: 633–676.

Al Nimer F, Jelcic I, Kempf C, *et al.* (2018): Phenotypic and functional complexity of brain-infiltrating T cells in Rasmussen encephalitis. *Neurol Neuroimmunol Neuroinflamm* 5: e419.10.1212

Andermann F (1991): *Chronic Encephalitis and Epilepsy: Rasmussen Syndrome.* Boston, MA: Butterworth Heinemann.

Andrews PI, Dichter MA, Berkovic SF, Newton MR, McNamara JO (1996): Plasmapheresis in Rasmussen's encephalitis. *Neurology* 46: 242–246.

Antozzi C, Granata T, Aurisano N, *et al.* (1998): Long-term selective IgG immuno-adsorption improves Rasmussen's encephalitis. *Neurology* 51: 302–305.

Aravamuthan BR, Sánchez Fernández I, Zurawski J, Olson H, Gorman M, Takeoka M. (2015): Pediatric anti-Hu-associated encephalitis with clinical features of Rasmussen encephalitis. *Neurol Neuroimmunol Neuroinflamm* 2(5): e150.

Atkins MR, Terrell W, Hulette CM (1995): Rasmussen's syndrome: a study of potential viral etiology. *Clin Neuropathol* 14: 7–12.

Bahi-Buisson N, Villanueva V, Bulteau C, *et al.* (2007): Long term response to steroid therapy in Rasmussen encephalitis. *Seizure* 16: 485–492.

Balosso S, Ravizza T, Pierucci M, *et al.* (2009): Molecular and functional interactions between tumor necrosis factor-alpha receptors and the glutamatergic system in the mouse hippocampus: implications for seizure susceptibility. *Neuroscience* 161: 293–300.

Balosso S, Ravizza T, Aronica E, Vezzani A (2013): The dual role of TNF-alpha and its receptors in seizures. *Exp Neurol* 247: 267–271.

Banati RB, Goerres GW, Myers R, *et al.* (1999): [11C](R)-PK11195 positron emission tomography imaging of activated microglia *in vivo* in Rasmussen's encephalitis. *Neurology* 53: 2199–2203.

Barkley GL, Baumgartner C (2003): MEG and EEG in epilepsy. *J Clin Neurophysiol* 20: 163–178.

Bauer J, Bien CG, Lassmann H (2002): Rasmussen's encephalitis: a role for autoimmune cytotoxic T lymphocytes. *Curr Opin Neurol* 15: 197–200.

Bauer J, Elger CE, Hans VH, *et al.* (2007): Astrocytes are a specific immunological target in Rasmussen's encephalitis. *Ann Neurol* 62: 67–80.

Bhatjiwale MG, Polkey C, Cox TC, Dean A, Deasy N.(1998): Rasmussen's encephalitis: neuroimaging findings in 21 patients with a closer look at the basal ganglia. *Pediatr Neurosurg* 29(3): 142–148.

Bien CG, Bauer J, Deckwerth TL, *et al.* (2002a): Destruction of neurons by cytotoxic T cells: a new pathogenic mechanism in Rasmussen's encephalitis. *Ann Neurol* 51: 311–318.

Bien CG, Widman G, Urbach H, *et al.* (2002b): The natural history of Rasmussen's encephalitis. *Brain* 125: 1751–1759.

Bien CG, Urbach H, Deckert M, *et al.* (2002c): Diagnosis and staging of Rasmussen's encephalitis by serial MRI and histopathology. *Neurology* 58: 250–256.

Bien CG, Gleissner U, Sassen R, Widman G, Urbach H, Elger CE (2004): An open study of tacrolimus therapy in Rasmussen encephalitis. *Neurology* 62: 2106–2109.

Bien CG, Granata T, Antozzi C, *et al.* (2005): Pathogenesis, diagnosis and treatment of Rasmussen encephalitis: a European consensus statement. *Brain* 128: 454–471.

Bien CG, Elger CE, Leitner Y, *et al.* (2007): Slowly progressive hemiparesis in childhood as a consequence of Rasmussen encephalitis without or with delayed-onset seizure. *Eur J Neurol* 14: 387–390.

Bien CG, Tiemeier H, Sassen R, *et al.* (2013): Rasmussen encephalitis: Incidence and course under randomized therapy with tacrolimus or intravenous immunoglobulins. *Epilepsia* 54: 543–550.

Bittner S, Simon OJ, Göbel K, Bien CG, Meuth SG. (2013): Rasmussen encephalitis treated with natalizumab. *Neurology* 81: 395–398.

Bulteau C, Grosmaitre C, Save-Pédebos J, *et al.* (2015): Language recovery after left hemispherotomy for Rasmussen encephalitis. *Epilepsy Behav* 53: 51–57.

Burke GJ, Fifer SA, Yoder J (1992): Early detection of Rasmussen's syndrome by brain SPECT imaging. *Clin Nucl Med* 17: 730–731.

Caraballo R, Tenembaum S, Cersosimo R, *et al.* (1998): Rasmussen syndrome. *Rev Neurol (Madrid)* 26: 978–983.

Carreno M, Donaire A, Barcelo MI, *et al.* (2007): Parry Romberg syndrome and linear scleroderma in coup de sabre mimicking Rasmussen encephalitis. *Neurology* 68: 1308–1310.

Cendes F, Andermann F, Silver K, Arnold DL (1995): Imaging of axonal damage *in vivo* in Rasmussen's syndrome. *Brain* 118: 753–758.

Chiapparini L, Granata T, Farina L, *et al.* (2003): Diagnostic imaging in 13 cases of Rasmussen's encephalitis: can early MRI suggest the diagnosis? *Neuroradiology* 45: 171–183.

Chinchilla D, DulacO, Robain O, *et al.* (1994): Reappraisal of Rasmussen's syndrome with special emphasis on treatment with high doses of steroids. *J Neurol Neurosurg Psychiatry* 57: 1325–1333.

Dabbagh O, Gascon G, Crowell J, Bamoggodam F (1997): Intraventricular interferon-stops seizures in Rasmussen's encephalitis: a case report. *Epilepsia* 38: 1045–1049.

Dalmau J, Graus F. (2018): Antibody-Mediated Encephalitis. *N Engl J Med.* 378: 840–851.

Dandekar S, Wijesuriya H, Geiger T, Hamm D, Mathern GW, Owens GC. (2016): Shared HLA Class I and II Alleles and Clonally Restricted Public and Private Brain-Infiltrating $\alpha\beta$ T Cells in a Cohort of Rasmussen Encephalitis Surgery Patients. *Front Immunol* 7: 608.

Damasceno A, França M Jr, Queiroz LS, Cendes F, Nucci A, Damasceno BP (2009): Adult onset chronic unihemispheric vasculitis resembling Rasmussen encephalitis. *Neurologist* 15: 285–288.

De Benedictis A, Freri E, Rizzi M, *et al.* (2013): Vagus nerve stimulation for drug-resistant Epilepsia Partialis Continua: Report of four cases. *Epilepsy Res* 107: 163–171.

Deleo F, Matricardi S, Didato G, Pappalardo I, Villani F (2015): The dilemma of adult-onset Rasmussen encephalitis clinical assessment: Proposal for a new bedside tool to evaluate disease progression. *Epilepsy Behav* 46: 249–251.

Dupont S, Gales A, Sammey S, Vidailhet M, Lambrecq V (2017): Late-onset Rasmussen Encephalitis: A literature appraisal. *Autoimmun Rev* 16: 803–810.

El Tawil S, Morris R, Mullatti N, Nashef L, Rajakulendran S (2016): Adult onset Rasmussen's encephalitis associated with reflex language induced seizures responsive to Rituximab therapy. *Seizure* 42: 60–62.

Fabene PF, Navarro Mora G, Martinello M, *et al.* (2008): A role for leukocyte-endothelial adhesion mechanisms in epilepsy. *Nat Med* 14: 1377–1383.

Farrell M, Cheng L, Cornford ME, Grody WW, Vinters HV (1991): Cytomegalovirus and Rasmussen's encephalitis. *Lancet* 337: 1551–1552.

Fiorella DJ, Provenzale JM, Edward CR, Crain BJ, Al Sugair A (2001): 18Ffluorodeoxyglucose positron emission tomography and MR imaging findings in Rasmussen encephalitis. *Am J Neuroradiol* 22: 1291–1299.

Firlik KS, Adelson PD, Hamilton R (1999): Coexistence of a gangioglioma and Rasmussen's encephalitis. *Pediat Neurosurg* 30: 278–282.

Fogarasi A, Hegyi M, Neuwirth M, *et al.* (2003): Comparative evaluation of concomitant structural and functional neuroimages in Rasmussen's encephalitis. *J Neuroimaging* 13: 339–345.

Frucht S (2002): Dystonia, athetosis, and epilepsia partialis continua in a patient with late-onset Rasmussen's encephalitis. *Mov Disord* 17: 609–612.

Fukuda T, Oguni H, Yanagaki S, *et al.* (1994): Chronic localized encephalitis (Rasmussen's syndrome) preceded by ipsilateral uveitis: a case report. *Epilepsia* 35: 1328–1321.

Gambardella A, Andermann F, Shorvon S, Le Piane E, Aguglia U (2008): Limited chronic focal encephalitis: another variant of Rasmussen syndrome? *Neurology* 70: 374–377.

Goyal M, Cohen ML, Bangert BA, Robinson S, Singer NG (2007): Rasmussen syndrome and CNS granulomatous disease with NOD2/CARD15 mutations. *Neurology* 69: 640–643.

Ghostine S, Raghavan R, Michelson D, *et al.* (2007): Gliomatosis cerebri mimicking Rasmussen encephalitis. Case report. *J Neurosurg* 107: 143–146.

Granata T, Gobbi G, Spreafico R, *et al.* (2003a): Rasmussen's encephalitis: early characteristics allow diagnosis. *Neurology* 60: 422–425.

Granata T, Fusco L, Gobbi G, *et al.* (2003b): Experience with immunomodulatory treatments in Rasmussen's encephalitis. *Neurology* 61: 1807–1810.

Granata T (2003c): Rasmussen's syndrome. *Neurol Sci* 24 (S4): 239–243.

Granata T, Cross H, Theodore W, Avanzini G (2011): Immune-mediated epilepsies. *Epilepsia* (Suppl 3): 5–11.

Granata T, Andermann F. (2013): Rasmussen encephalitis. *Handb Clin Neurol* 111: 511–519.

Granata T, Matricardi S, Ragona F, *et al.* (2014): Hemispherotomy in Rasmussen encephalitis: Long-term outcome in an Italian series of 16 patients. *Epilepsy Res* 108: 1106–1119.

Grenier Y, AntelJP, Osterland CK (1991): Immunologic studies in chronic encephalitis of Rasmussen. In: Andermann F (ed) *Chronic Encephalitis and Epilepsy: Rasmussen's Syndrome*, pp. 125–134. Boston: Butterworth-Heinemann.

Greiner H, Leach JL, Lee KH, Krueger DA (2011): Anti-NMDA receptor encephalitis presenting with imaging findings and clinical features mimicking Rasmussen syndrome. *Seizure* 20: 266–270.

Grujic J, Bien CG, Pollo C, Rossetti AO (2011): Vagus nerve stimulator treatment in adult-onset Rasmussen's encephalitis. *Epilepsy Behav* 20: 123–125.

Guan Y, Chen S, Liu C, *et al.* (2017): Timing and type of hemispherectomy for Rasmussen's encephalitis: analysis of 45 patients. *Epilepsy Res* 132: 109–115.

Gurcharran K, Karkare S (2017): Anti-N-Methyl-D-Aspartate Receptor Encephalitis and Rasmussen-like Syndrome: An Association? *Pediatr Neurol* 66: 104–107.

Hart YM, Cortez M, Andermann F, *et al.* (1994): Medical treatment of Rasmussen's syndrome (chronic encephalitis and epilepsy); effect of high-dose steroids or immunoglobulins in 19 patients. *Neurology* 44: 1030–1036.

Hart YM, Andermann F, Fish DR, *et al.* (1997): Chronic encephalitis and epilepsy in adults and adolescents: a variant of Rasmussen's syndrome? *Neurology* 48: 418–424.

Hart YM, Andermann F, Robitaille Y, Laxer KD, Rasmussen T, Davis R (1998): Double pathology in Rasmussen's syndrome: A window on the etiology? *Neurology* 50: 731–735.

Harvey AS, Andermann F, Hopkins IJ, Kirkham TH, Berkovic SF (1992): Chronic encephalitis (Rasmussen's syndrome) and ipsilateral uveitis. *Ann Neurol* 32: 826–829.

Jay V, Becker LE, Otsubo H, *et al.* (1995): Chronic encephalitis and epilepsy (Rasmussen's encephalitis): detection of cytomegalovirus and herpes simplex virus 1 by the polymerase chain reaction and in situ hybridization. *Neurology* 45: 108–117.

Jonas R, Nguyen S, Hu B, *et al.* (2004): Cerebral hemispherectomy: hospital course, seizure, developmental, language, and motor outcomes. *Neurology* 62: 1712–1721.

Korn-Lubetzki I, Bien CG, Bauer J, *et al.* (2004): Rasmussen encephalitis with active inflammation and delayed seizures onset. *Neurology* 62: 984–986.

Kossoff EH, ViningEP, Pillas DJ, *et al.* (2003): Hemispherectomy for intractable unihemispheric epilepsy etiology *vs.* outcome. *Neurology* 61: 887–890.

Kozhevnikov AY (translated by Asher DM) (1991): A particular type of cortical epilepsy (epilepsia corticalis sive partialis continua): In: Andermann F (ed) *Chronic Encephalitis and Epilepsy: Rasmussen's Syndrome*, pp. 245–261. Boston: Butterworth-Heinemann.

Krauss GL, Campbell ML, Roche KW, Huganir RL, Niedermeyer E (1996): Chronic steroid-responsive encephalitis without autoantibodies to glutamate receptor GluR3. *Neurology* 46: 247–249.

Kuki I, Matsuda K, Kubota Y, *et al.* (2018): Functional neuroimaging in Rasmussen syndrome. *Epilepsy Res.* 140: 120–127.

Lagarde S, Villeneuve N, Trébuchon A, *et al.* (2016): Anti-tumor necrosis factor alpha therapy (adalimumab) in Rasmussen's encephalitis: An open pilot study. *Epilepsia* 57: 956–966.

Larionov S, König R, Urbach H, Sassen R, Elger CE, Bien CG (2005): MRI brain volumetry in Rasmussen encephalitis: the fate of affected and "unaffected' hemispheres. *Neurology* 64: 885–887.

Laxer KD, Wilfong A, Morris GL, Andermann F (2008): Pilot study of rituximab to treat chronic focal encephalitis. *Epilepsia* 49 (Suppl 7): 121.

Leach JP, Chadwick DW, Miles JB, Hart IK (1999): Improvement in adult-onset Rasmussen's encephalitis with long-term immunomodulatory therapy. *Neurology* 52: 738–742.

Liba Z, Muthaffar O, Tang J, *et al.* (2015): Rasmussen encephalitis: Response to early immunotherapy in a case of immune-mediated encephalitis. *Neurol Neuroimmunol NeuroInflamm* 2: e69.

Liba Z, Sedlacek P, Sebronova V, *et al.* (2017): Alemtuzumab and intrathecal methotrexate failed in the therapy of Rasmussen encephalitis. *Neurol Neuroimmunol NeuroInflamm* 4: e354.

Longaretti F, Dunkley C, Varadkar S, Vargha-Khadem F, Boyd SG, Cross H (2012): Evolution of the EEG in children with Rasmussen's syndrome. *Epilepsia* 53: 1539–1545.

Mameniškienė R, Wolf P (2017): Epilepsia partialis continua: A review. *Seizure* 44: 74–80.

Mantegazza R, Bernasconi P, Baggi F, *et al.* (2002): The Italian Rasmussen's Encephalitis Study Group. Antibodies against GluR3 peptides are not specific for Rasmussen's encephalitis but are also present in epilepsy patients with severe, early onset disease and intractable seizures. *J Neuroimmunol* 131: 179–185.

Maria BL, Ringdahl DM, Mickle JP, *et al.* (1993): Intraventricular alpha interferon therapy for Rasmussen's syndrome. *Can J Neurological Sci* 20: 333–336.

Marras CE, Granata T, Franzini A, *et al.* (2010): Hemispherotomy and functional hemispherectomy: indications and outcome. *Epilepsy Res* 89: 104–112.

Martin-Blondel G, Brassat D, Bauer J, Lassmann H, Liblau RS (2016): CCR5 blockade for neuroinflammatory diseases – beyond control of HIV. *Nature Rev Neurol* 12: 95–105.

McLachlan RS, Levin S, Blume WT (1996): Treatment of Rasmussen's syndrome with ganciclovir. *Neurology* 47: 925–928.

Mirones I, de Prada I, Gómez AM, *et al.* (2013); A role for the CXCR3/CXCL10 axis in Rasmussen encephalitis. *Pediatr Neurol.* 49: 451–457.

Nabbout R, Andrade DM, Bahi-Buisson N, *et al.* (2017): Outcome of childhood-onset epilepsy from adolescence to adulthood: Transition issues. *Epilepsy Behav.* 69: 161–169.

Obeso JA, Rothwell JC, Marsden CD (1985): The spectrum of cortical myoclonus. From focal reflex jerks to spontaneous motor epilepsy. *Brain* 108: 193–224.

Oguni H, Andermann F, Rasmussen TB (1992): The syndrome of chronic encephalitis and epilepsy. A study based on the MNI series of 48 cases. *Adv Neurol* 57: 419–433.

Olson HE, Lechpammer M, Prabhu SP *et al.* (2013): Clinical application and evaluation of the Bien diagnostic criteria for Rasmussen encephalitis. *Epilepsia* 54: 1753–1760.

Owens GC, Erickson KL, Malone CC, *et al.* (2015): Evidence for the involvement of gamma delta T cells in the immune response in Rasmussen encephalitis. *J Neuroinflammation* 12: 134.

Owens GC, Chang JW, Huynh MN, Chirwa T, Vinters HV, Mathern GW. (2016): Evidence for Resident Memory T Cells in Rasmussen Encephalitis. *Front Immunol* 7: 64.

Palmer CA, Geyer JD, Keating JM, *et al.* (1999): Rasmussen's encephalitis with concomitant cortical dysplasia: the role of GluR3. *Epilepsia* 40: 242–247.

Pardo CA, Vining EP, Guo L, Skolasky RL, Carson BS, Freeman JM (2004): The pathology of Rasmussen syndrome: stages of cortical involvement and neuropathological studies in 45 hemispherectomies. *Epilepsia* 45: 516–526.

Power C, Poland SD, Blume WT, Girvin JP, Rice GPA (1990): Cytomegalovirus and Rasmussen's encephalitis. *Lancet* 336: 1282–1284.

Pulsifer MB, Brandt J, Salorio CF, Vining EP, Carson BS, Freeman JM (2004): The cognitive outcome of hemispherectomy in 71 children. *Epilepsia* 45: 243–254.

Quesada CM, Urbach H, Elger CE, Bien CG. (2007): Rasmussen encephalitis with ipsilateral brain stem involvement in an adult patient. *J Neurol Neurosurg Psychiatry*. 78: 200–201.

Rajesh B, Kesavadas C, Ashalatha R, Thomas B (2006): Putaminal involvement in Rasmussen encephalitis. *Pediatr Radiol* 36: 816–822.

Ramesha KN, Rajesh B, Ashalatha R, *et al.* (2009): Rasmussen's encephalitis: experience from a developing country based on a group of medically and surgically treated patients. *Seizure* 18: 567–572.

Rasmussen T, Olszewski J, Lloyd-Smith D (1958): Focal seizures due to chronic localised encephalitis. *Neurology* 8: 435–445.

Rasmussen T, McCann W (1968): Clinical studies of patients with focal epilepsy due to "chronic encephalitis". *Trans Am Neurol Assoc* 93: 89–94.

Rasmussen T, Andermann F (1991): Rasmussen's syndrome. Symptomatology of the syndrome of chronic encephalitis and seizures: 35-year experience with 51 cases. In: Luders H (ed) *Epilepsy Surgery*. New York: Raven Press Ltd, pp. 173–182.

Ravindra VM, Mazur MD, Mohila CA, Sweney MT, Hersh A, Bollo RJ. (2015) Rasmussen encephalitis with dual pathology in a patient without seizures: case report and literature review. *Childs Nerv Syst* 31: 2165–2171.

Robitaille Y (1991): Neuropathologic aspects of chronic encephalitis. In: Andermann F (ed) *Chronic Encephalitis and Epilepsy: Rasmussen's Syndrome*. Boston: Butterworth-Heinemann, pp. 79–110.

Rogers SW, Andrews PI, Gahring LC, *et al.* (1994): Autoantibodies to glutamate receptor GluR3 in Rasmussen's encephalitis. *Science* 265: 648–651.

Rossi Sebastiano D, Visani E, Duran D, *et al.* (2017): Epileptic spikes in Rasmussen's encephalitis: Migratory pattern and short-term evolution. A MEG study. *Clin Neurophysiol* 128: 1898–1905.

Samanta D, Gokden M, Albert GW (2016): Absence of seizures in Rasmussen encephalitis with active inflammation. *J Clin Neurosci*. 28: 175–178.

Schneider-Hohendorf T, Mohan H, Bien CG, *et al.* (2016): CD8(+) T-cell pathogenicity in Rasmussen encephalitis elucidated by large-scale T-cell receptor sequencing. *Nat Commun*. 7: 11153.

Schwab N, Bien CG, Waschbisch A, *et al.* (2009): CD8+ T-cell clones dominate brain infiltrates in Rasmussen encephalitis and persist in the periphery. *Brain* 132: 1236–1246.

Seifert F, Bien CG, Schellinger PD, *et al.* (2011): Parry-Romberg syndrome with chronic focal encephalitis: two cases. *Clin Neurol Neurosurg* 113: 170–172.

Shah JR, Juhâsz C, Kupsky WJ, *et al.* (2003): Rasmussen encephalitis associated with Parry-Romberg syndrome. *Neurology* 61: 395–397.

Silver K, Andermann F, Meagher-Villemure K (1998): Familial alternating epilepsia partialis continua with chronic encephalitis: another variant of Rasmussen syndrome? *Arch Neurol* 55: 733–736.

So NK, Gloor P (1991): Electorencephalographic and electorcorticographc findings in chronic encephalitis of the Rasmussen type. In: Andermann F (ed) *Chronic Encephalitis and Epilepsy: Rasmussen's Syndrom*. Boston: Butterworth-Heinemann, pp. 37–45.

Spitz MA, Dubois-Teklali F, Vercueil L, *et al.* (2014): Voltage-gated potassium channels autoantibodies in a child with Rasmussen encephalitis. *Neuropediatrics* 45: 336–340.

Stabile A, Deleo F, Didato G, *et al.* (2018): Adult-onset Rasmussen encephalitis treated with mitoxantrone. *Eur J Neurol* 25: e126.

Takahashi Y, Mori H, Mishina M, *et al.* (2005): Autoantibodies and cell-mediated autoimmunity to NMDA-type GluRepsilon2 in patients with Rasmussen's encephalitis and chronic progressive epilepsia partialis continua. *Epilepsia* 46 (S5): 152–158.

Takahashi Y, Mine J, Kubota Y, Yamazaki E, Fujiwara T (2009): A substantial number of Rasmussen syndrome patients have increased IgG, CD4+ T cells, TNFalpha, and Granzyme B in CSF. *Epilepsia* 50: 1419–1431.

Tampieri D, Melanson D, Ethier R (1991): Imaging of chronic encephalitis. In: Andermann F (ed) *Chronic Encephalitis and Epilepsy: Rasmussen's Syndrome*. Boston: Butterworth-Heinemann, pp. 47–60.

Thiele EA, Granata T, Matricardi S, Chugani HT (2014): Transition into adulthood: tuberous sclerosis complex, Sturge-Weber syndrome, and Rasmussen encephalitis. *Epilepsia*. 55 S 3: 29–33.

Thilo B, Stingele R, Knudsen K, *et al.* (2009): A case of Rasmussen encephalitis treated with rituximab. *Nat Rev Neurol* 5: 458–462.

Thomas P, Zifkin B, Ghetâu G, Delalande O (2003): Persistence of ictal activity after functional hemispherectomy in Rasmussen syndrome. *Neurology* 60: 140–142.

Thomas SG, Chacko AG, Thomas MM, Babu KS, Russell PS, Daniel RT (2012): Outcomes of disconnective surgery in intractable pediatric hemispheric and subhemispheric epilepsy. *Int J Pediatr* 2012: 527891.

Tobias SM, Robitaille Y, Hickey WF, Rhodes CH, Nordgren R, Andermann F (2003): Bilateral Rasmussen encephalitis: postmortem documentation in a five-year-old. *Epilepsia* 44: 127–130.

Tubbs RS, Nimjee SM, Oakes WJ (2005): Long-term follow-up in children with functional hemispherectomy for Rasmussen's encephalitis. *Childs NervSyst* 21: 461–465.

Tziperman B, Garty BZ, Schoenfeld N, *et al.* (2007): Acute intermittent porphyria, Rasmussen encephalitis, or both? *J Child Neurol* 22: 99–105.

Varadkar S, Bien CG, Kruse CA, *et al.* (2014): Rasmussen's encephalitis: Clinical features, pathobiology, and treatment advances. *Lancet Neurol* 13: 195–205.

Villani F, Spreafico R, Farina L, *et al.* (2001): Positive response to immunomodulatory therapy in an adult patient with Rasmussen's encephalitis. *Neurology* 56: 248–250.

Villani F, Pincherle A, Antozzi C, *et al.* (2006): Adult-onset Rasmussen's encephalitis: anatomical-electrographic-clinical features of 7 Italian cases. *Epilepsia* 47 (S5): 41–46.

Villani F, Didato G, Deleo F, *et al.* (2014): Long-term outcome after limited cortical resections in two cases of adult-onset Rasmussen encephalitis. *Epilepsia* 55: e38-e43.

Villemure JG, Andermann F, Rasmussen TB (1991): Hemispherectomy for the treatment of epilepsy due to chronic encephalitis. In: Andermann F (ed) *Chronic Encephalitis and Epilepsy: Rasmussen's Syndrome*. Boston: Butterworth-Heinemann, pp. 235–241.

Villemure JG, Daniel RT (2006): Peri-insular hemispherotomy in paediatric epilepsy. *Childs Nerv Syst* 22: 967–981.

Vining EP, Freeman JM, Brndt J, Carson BS, Uematsu S (1993): Progressive unilateral encephalopathy of childhood (Rasmussen's syndrome): a reappraisal. *Epilepsia* 34: 639–650.

Vinters HV, Wang R, Wiley CA (1993): Herpes viruses in chronic encephalitis associated with intractable childhood epilepsy. *Hum Pathol* 24: 871–879.

Wagner J, Schoene-Bake JC, Bien CG, Urbach H, Elger CE, Weber B. (2012) Automated 3D MRI volumetry reveals regional atrophy differences in Rasmussen encephalitis. *Epilepsia* 53: 613–621.

Walter GF, Renella RR (1989): Epstein-Barr virus in brain and Rasmussen's encephalitis. *Lancet* I: 279–280.

Wang ZI, Krishnan B, Shattuck DW, *et al.* (2016): Automated MRI Volumetric Analysis in Patients with Rasmussen Syndrome. *AJNR Am J Neuroradiol* 37: 2348–2355.

Watson R, Jepson JE, Bermudez I, *et al.* (2005): Alpha7-acetylcholine receptor antibodies in two patients with Rasmussen encephalitis *Neurology* 65: 1802–1804.

Weinberg MS, Blake BL, McCown TJ (2013): Opposing actions of hippocampus TNF alpha receptors on limbic seizure susceptibility. *Exp Neurol* 247: 429–437.

Wiendl H, Bien CG, Bernasconi P, *et al.* (2001): GluR3 antibodies: Prevalence in focal epilepsy but no specificity for Rasmussen's encephalitis. *Neurology* 57: 1511–1514.

Yacubian EM, Rosemberg S, Marie SK, Valerio RM, Jorge CL, Cukiert A (1996): Double pathology in Rasmussen's encephalitis: etiologic considerations. *Epilepsia* 37: 495–500.

Yang R, Puranam RS, Butler LS, *et al.* (2000): Autoimmunity to munc-18 in Rasmussen's encephalitis. *Neuron* 28: 375–383.

WITH VIDEO SUPPLEMENTS

CHAPTER 19

EPILEPSY WITH GENERALIZED TONIC-CLONIC SEIZURES ALONE

Philippe Gélisse[1], Arielle Crespel[1], Greta Macorig[1], Maria Del Socorro Gonzalez Sanchez[2], Pierre Thomas[3] and Pierre Genton[2]

[1] Epilepsy Unit, Montpellier Hospital, Montpellier, France
[2] Centre Saint-Paul, Henri-Gastaut Hospital, Marseille, France
[3] Department of Neurology, Pasteur Hospital, Nice, France

Introduction

The concept of awakening epilepsy was developed by Janz (1953). It is commonly accepted that awakening epilepsies are similar to idiopathic generalized epilepsy (IGE). Epilepsy with "Grand Mal" on awakening (EGMA) was included in the 1989 classification (Commission, 1989). However, it appears that some patients cannot be classified into any known category of IGE because they have generalized tonic-clonic seizures (GTCS) only under certain circumstances like sleep deprivation, excessive intake of alcohol, or illicit substance abuse. Other patients have only rare GTCS occurring either only during sleep or in wakefulness or both during sleep and wakefulness, without specific triggering mechanisms, and with no special relationship with the awakening period.

In a proposed diagnostic scheme for people with epilepsy published in 2001 after intense debate within the ad hoc committee of the International League Against Epilepsy (Engel, 2001), a larger group of IGEs with variable phenotypes was proposed, that includes juvenile myoclonic epilepsy (JME), juvenile absence epilepsy, and epilepsies with GTCS only (which supposedly include EGMA besides other, less well-defined entities). But the ILAE classification core group in 2006 mentioned that *"Epilepsy with Generalized Tonic-Clonic Seizures only is not a syndrome"* (Engel *et al.*, 2006). The ILAE Commission on Classification and Terminology, 2005-2009 revised this position and added this epilepsy under the name "Epilepsy with GTCS alone" among the syndromes that start at adolescence-adulthood (Berg *et al.*, 2010) and this term was confirmed by the last revision of the Classification (Scheffer *et al.*, 2017) which also maintained the term of IGE as an alternative for "generalized genetic epilepsy".

Thus epilepsy with GTCS alone is not a clear entity and does not represent a definite syndrome, but rather, for most cases, a constellation of different subtypes of IGE. One of the questions is whether we can accept in the description of these patients mild myoclonic jerks or infrequent, mild absence seizures. A precise diagnosis of the epilepsy type is probably of little interest for clinicians but represents a challenge for epidemiologic and genetic studies. The aim of this chapter is to review, in a very practical perspective, the diagnostic characteristics and practical management of patients with EGMA. Other denominations are commonly used: awakening Grand Mal, epilepsy with generalized tonic-clonic seizures (GTCS) on awakening. The main issue, to us, is whether one applies a strict definition to EGMA, limiting the diagnosis to patients with proven or highly probable IGE and a characteristic association between seizures and awakening from a sleep period, or whether one accepts many cases with GTCS, whatever the possible etiology and whatever the exact chronodependency of seizures; such epilepsies may be referred to as IGE with random GTCS.

Epilepsy with Grand Mal on awakening

Historical background

The study of large epileptic patient cohorts during the XIXth and XXth centuries led some authors to propose a classification of epilepsies in function of seizure occurrence in the wake/sleep cycle. These authors defined epilepsies with seizures occurring in sleep as sleep epilepsies, epilepsies with seizures occurring in wakefulness as diurnal epilepsies and the epilepsies with seizures occurring either in sleep or in wakefulness as diffuse epilepsies. In 1885, Gowers studied seizure distribution of 840 patients living in an institution and found 24% of sleep epilepsies, 43% of diurnal epilepsies and 33% of diffuse epilepsies. Langdon-Down & Brain (1928) described the same distribution in 66 patients. In sleep, seizure peaks were observed at the beginning of the night towards 10-11 p.m. and at the end of the night around 4-5 a.m. The diurnal seizure peaks were observed during awakening at around 7-8 a.m. and a second peak at around 2-3 p.m.

Although the preferential occurrence of GTCS soon after awakening had been noted by early authors from various countries, the "awakening epilepsies" *(Aufwachepilepsien)* were especially well presented by Janz in 1953 as a special, fairly common group of epilepsies with clinically evident triggering factors, mostly a benign course and no apparent etiology. Out of this group, he singled out the very typical and recognizable *"Impulsiv Petit Mal"* (Janz & Christian, 1957), better known nowadays as juvenile myoclonic epilepsy (JME). Janz (1953, 1962, 1974) had an etiologic approach and showed that sleep epilepsies corresponded to focal epilepsies, awakening epilepsies corresponded to IGE and diffuse epilepsies corresponded to symptomatic epilepsies. In awakening epilepsies, he defined the Grand Mal epilepsies of awakening and established their clinical characteristics. These patients present by definition their GTCS in the two hours which follow awakening but they also have seizures in the evening hours of relaxation.

In his review, Loiseau (1964) proposed that an awakening syndrome could exist. The patients had GTCS with generalized EEG discharges and sometimes myoclonic seizures or absences. Billiard *et al.* (1982) studied the nycthemeral distribution of seizures under continuous 24-hour EEG monitoring in 320 patients: 141 patients had IGE. Among them, 77 had only GTCS which occurred in wakefulness (36%), in sleep (28.5%) and on awakening (16.8%). The concept of awakening epilepsies remained very popular, although it covered heterogenous entities, and epilepsy with "Grand Mal" on awakening was included in the 1989 Classification proposal as an officially sanctioned syndrome (Commission, 1989).

Definition

In the 1989 International Classification of Epilepsies and Epileptic Syndromes, EGMA was classified as an IGE with age-related onset: *"Epilepsy with GTCS on awakening is a syndrome with onset occurring mostly in the second decade of life. The GTCS occur exclusively or predominantly (> 90 per cent of the time) shortly after awakening regardless of the time of day or in a second seizure peak in the evening period of relaxation. If other seizures occur, they are mostly absence or myoclonic, as in JME. Seizures may be precipitated by sleep deprivation and other external factors. Genetic predisposition is relatively frequent. The EEG shows one of the patterns of IGE. There is a significant correlation with photosensitivity"* (Commission, 1989).

According to Janz & Wolf (1997), the diagnosis of EGMA depends on the occurrence of at least six GTCS exclusively or predominantly after awakening or while at leisure. Subjects with less than six seizures may be classified as epilepsy with rare GTCS (Janz & Wolf, 1997).

Physiopathology and genetic factors

A genetic basis is acknowledged for the IGEs. A family history of epilepsy is found in about 10% of the patients with EGMA (Janz, 1969; Tsuboi & Christian, 1976) *vs.* 36% in first and second-degree relatives in a cohort study of 168 consecutive JME patients (Gélisse *et al.*, 2001a).

A mutation of the chloride channel CLCN2 was implicated in a large family with different subtypes of IGEs including EGMA (Haug *et al.*, 2003) but this study was not confirmed and the authors published a retraction (Haug *et al.*, 2009). Hempelmann *et al.* (2006) performed a genome-wide nonparametric linkage scan in IGE-multiplex families and confirmed linkage to the chromosomal region 6p12 in JME/EGMA families. They found evidence for two loci on chromosome 5q34 and 19q13 that confer susceptibility to myoclonic jerks and GTCS on awakening. Recurrent microdeletions on chromosome 15 (15q13.3, 15q11.2) and chromosome 16 (16p13.11) were shown in subtypes of IGEs including patients with GTCS alone and constitute a genetic risk factor for common IGE syndromes rather than causative alleles (Mullen & Berkovic, 2018). These copy number variants are also risk factors for other neurodevelopmental disorders (Mullen & Berkovic, 2018).

Variants in the gene *VRK2* located at 2p16.1 have been found in IGE patients. *VRK2* is a serine-threonine protein kinase involved in signal transduction and apoptosis. Variation in this gene has been previously suggested as a risk factor for schizophrenia. However, one of the single nucleotide polymorphisms forming the association signal in this gene has one allele that predisposes to IGE while being simultaneously protective against schizophrenia (Mullen & Berkovic, 2018).

Patients are very sensitive to sleep deprivation which facilitates seizure occurrence after awakening. Polygraphic sleep studies showed that the sleep of these patients is particularly unstable (Janz & Wolf, 1997).

Epidemiology

The prevalence of EGMA was estimated at around 33% among all patients with GTCS in the classical work of Janz (1969) but using strict criteria (patients with more than six GTCS occurring only or predominantly after awakening), the same author reported EGMA in 17% of patients having GTCS with additional seizures (mild absences and myoclonic jerks) and in 10% of patients having GTCS only (Janz, 1998). The incidence of EGMA has been estimated at 1.8 per 100,000 in a population-based study (Loiseau *et al.*, 1990). ECMA is less frequent than JME and childhood absence epilepsy, accounting for approximately 0.75 to 1% of all epilepsies. Of 2,841 consecutive newly referred patients first seen between 1986 and 1997 at the Centre Saint-Paul in Marseille (center specialized in epilepsy for children and adults), the group of IGE represented 15.3% of all cases. JME was the most frequent form of IGE (26.7% of IGE; 4.1% of all epilepsies), preceding childhood absence epilepsy (23.3% of IGE; 3.6% of all epilepsies); juvenile absence epilepsy (11% of IGE; 1.7% of all epilepsies); photogenic epilepsy (9.1% of IGE; 1.4% of all epilepsies) and EGMA (6.2% of IGE; 0.96% of all epilepsies) (Genton *et al.*, 2000a). Among 2,783 consecutive patients seen at Montpellier in a center specialized in epilepsy evaluating adolescents and adults, we identified 961 patients with IGE (34.5%), 21 EGMA (2.75% of IGE; 0.75% of all epilepsies). However, "benign" epilepsies are underrepresented in specialized clinics, and both EGMA and other IGEs with only rare GCTS are probably less often referred than JME cases, which are also highly treatable but are likely to pose more problems.

The sex ratio is close to 1, with a slight male preponderance in some series especially in EGMA without absences or myoclonic jerks (Janz & Wolf, 1997) whereas in JME the sex-ratio was 1.33 for females in a metaanalysis of 1,660 patients (Gélisse *et al.*, 2001a). In our series of 21 patients with EGMA seen at Montpellier, we found 13 males (62%) and 8 females (38%).

Clinical presentation

The age at the first GTCS, which can be considered as the age at onset of EGMA, spans a longer range than other forms of IGE: 5 to 25 years in our experience. All large series point to a wide range, with 78-90% of patients experiencing their first seizure between the ages of 6 and 26 (review in Wolf, 1992).

The clinical characteristics of 41 patients with EGMA seen at the Centre Saint-Paul (Marseille) between 1986 and 2002 are summarized in *Table I*. Few seizures have been recorded. In our point of view,

Table I Clinical characteristics of 41 patients with epilepsy with Grand Mal on awakening diagnosed at the Centre Saint-Paul between 1986 and 2002. Neuroimaging was performed in 14 cases and consistently normal

Clinical features	
Age at onset (years)	Mean: 15, range 5–25
Sex ratio (M/F)	19/22
Seizure types: GTCS Typical absences Myoclonic jerks	 41 (100%) 4 (9.8%) 9 (22%)
Photosensitivity in the EEG laboratory	10 (24.4%; 7 F, 3 M)
Frequency of GTCS before adequate therapy	< 1 per year: 21 (51.2%) > one per month: 8 (19.5%)
Total number of GTCS	One single GTCS: 2 2–5: 23 (56.1%) 6–10: 10 (24.4%) 11–30: 5 (12.2%) more than 30: 1
EEG (poly) SW on routine EEG normal routine EEG, (poly)SW on sleep EEG only no evidence of SW (routine only) no evidence of SW (with sleep)	41 (100%) 18 (44%) 13 (31.7%) 4 (9.8%) 6 (14.6%)

M: Male; F: Female; GTCS: generalized tonic-clonic seizure; SW: spike-waves.

the GTCS may have a slightly more complex presentation than expected (see *Figure 1*). A rare example of a GTCS recorded in a patient with EGMA is provided in the video supplement to this volume. Other seizure types typical of IGE may be found in EGMA: in our experience, 4/41 patients reported typical absences that were rare (spanioleptic), and 9/41 reported myoclonic jerks. The latter have the same triggering factors as GTCS, and may immediately precede GTCS.

Classically, there is no aura in IGE but Boylan *et al.* (2006) reported than among 5 patients with IGE and GTCS alone, 3 (60%) had auras. Gélisse *et al.* (2009) reported very brief visual auras in one patient with GTCS alone and photosensitivity and in two JME patients with photosensitivity just before the GTCS. Visual auras were confirmed latter in different subtypes of IGEs, especially in patients with photosensitivity (Gungor-Tuncer *et al.*, 2012).

Sleep deprivation represents a major triggering factor of GTCS in EGMA, often in association with sudden arousal, and excessive alcohol intake or, in women, the premenstrual period may also be associated with a higher seizure risk.

EEG

It typically shows spike-wave (SW) and polyspike-wave (pSW) discharges that have frequencies between 2 and 4 Hz, and are also typically irregular (Loiseau, 1964). However, such changes are not found in all patients on routine EEGs: only 44% had SW or pSW on their first routine EEG, while 26% of our patients failed to exhibit any EEG abnormality, even during or after a sleep recording. However, among the 23/41 patients with normal routine EEG, 19 had a sleep recording and this produced significant EEG abnormalities in 13. The sleep recording we used in most patients was a sleep-deprived afternoon nap, and this procedure should be recommended in case of diagnostic doubts. Full-night polygraphic recordings may also be productive, especially when early morning awakening is imposed to the patient *(Figure 2)*: in patients with EGMA, SW discharges are most likely to be recorded soon after awakening from a sleep period. Ictal EEG recordings are rare. *Figure 1* shows the onset of a GTCS of the patient whose seizure is included in the video supplement of this volume. *Figure 3* shows the onset of a GTCS in another patient. Both ictal recordings demonstrate the generalized onset of the seizure.

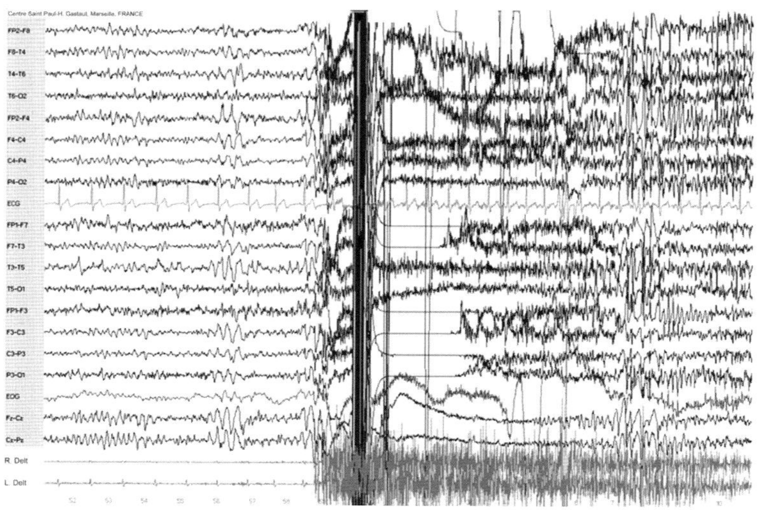

Figure 1

Onset of generalized tonic-clonic seizure (seizure shown in video supplement). A short burst of slow waves precedes by seconds the onset of a diffuse tonic contraction that masks most of the EEG, which shows diffuse fast activities. The onset can be considered as truly generalized. I 15 mm/s – 1 cm/100 µv.

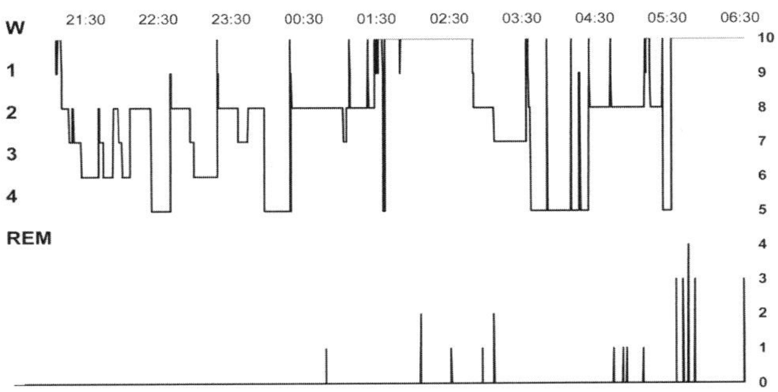

Figure 2 **Full-night EEG with quantification of SW discharges in a 20-year-old male untreated patient with EGMA.** Top: **hypnogram.** Bottom: **spike-wave (SW) discharges. Note the clustering of SW discharges during intermediate awakenings, and especially after the early morning awakening at 5.30 am (scale on the lower right: seconds with SW per 30-second epoch).**

Among the IGEs, EGMA is also an important provider of photosensitive patients, with around 13% (mostly females) exhibiting photoparoxysmal responses (PPR) in the laboratory (Janz & Wolf, 1997), 10/41 (24%) in our experience (7 females and 3 males) and 23/31 (74%) (13 females and 10 males) according to Lu *et al.* (2008). However, few patients report clinical photosensitivity, and PPRs can be considered a biological, but not a clinical marker.

Diagnosis

The diagnosis of EGMA is mainly clinical. EGMA should be suspected when there have been GTCS upon awakening, without hints of frequent myoclonic jerks, and often in relation to triggering factors such as sleep deprivation. A familial context of IGE, or of rare GTCS, is also an element of diagnosis. It is common but far from constant: it is reported by 12.5% of patients in the classical study of Janz (1969), thus being much more frequent than in patients with random GTCS. Unterberger *et al.* (2001) stressed the difference between EGMA and IGE with only random GTCS, in that probands with random GTCS never had relatives with EGMA, and that the reverse was also nearly true.

The EEG plays an important role in the diagnosis of EGMA. Standard EEG recordings are not likely to show many spontaneous changes. Long-term EEG recordings with sleep periods are more likely to show generalized SW discharges, both during sleep and after awakening *(Figure 4)*. Indeed, interictal EEG changes may be much more prominent in patients who exhibit clear seizure aggravation following the use of an inadequate antiepileptic drug *(Figure 5)*.

Neurological examination and brain MRI are normal.

Prognosis

A major issue in EGMA is the frequency of seizures that is low in most patients. Most patients experience rare GTCS before seizure control is reached: a majority of our patients had only 2-5 GTCS. The overall frequency of seizures appears to be intermediate between that found in patients with JME and that found in patients with IGE and random GTCS.

The prognosis of EGMA is favorable, as seizures remain spontaneously rare, and response to treatment is good. A recent study on 57 patients with EGMA and a long follow-up period (median 37 years) showed that the prognosis was good: 63% of patients achieved 5-year terminal seizure remission (Vorderwülbecke *et al.*, 2017). In our series of 21 consecutive patients seen at Montpellier and followed for at least 1 year (median 20 years), 15 (71.4%) were seizure free on antiepileptic drugs. Drug resistance should raise doubts about diagnosis, lifestyle, compliance, and insufficient or inadequate treatment. In our experience *(Table I)*, patients with numerous seizures (6/41 had more than 10 GTCS) have raised problems of compliance or refuse treatment for many years.

Early seizures onset (age < 13), long-time epilepsy, history of status epilepticus, EEG with generalized epileptiform activity, mainly polyspikes, and side effects with AED are negative prognostic factors for patients with EGMA (Gomez-Ibañez *et al.*, 2017). In JME, the presence of psychiatric problems and independently, the presence of all three seizures (GTCS, myoclonic jerks and absences) were a risk factor for true drug resistance (15.5% of the cases) in a large series of 155 consecutive patients seems between 1981 and 1998 (Gélisse *et al.*, 2001b). It is not clear whether associated seizure types (absences and myoclonic jerks) worsen the prognosis in EGMA. Some patients may evolve into EGMA from other forms of IGE with earlier onset, especially from childhood absence epilepsy. The main, clinically relevant fact is that, not unlike in JME, many patients with EGMA experience relapse when efficient medication is withdrawn: such relapse occurred in 16 out of 57 patients (59%) in the study of Vorderwülbecke *et al.* (2017) and in 83% of cases in the large serie of Janz *et al.* (1983). Thus patients with EGMA may need long-term treatment. The evolution in middle age and beyond has not been documented.

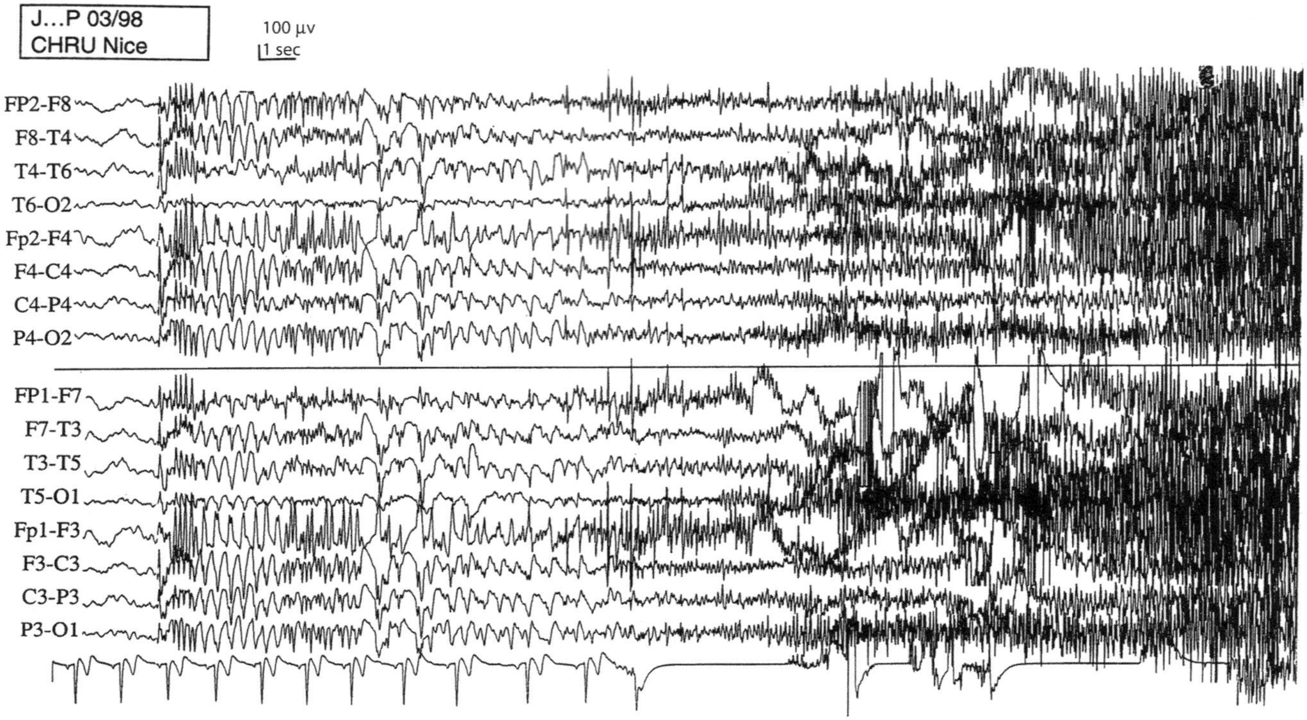

Figure 3

Onset of generalized tonic-clonic seizure. The tonic contraction is preceded by a burst of polyspikes and irregular slow waves. In spite of this peculiar onset, there is no hint of any focal change.

Management of patients

When clear triggering factors, such as sleep deprivation and excessive alcohol intake have been identified, specific measures should be adopted. The counseling should be the same as in JME. The pharmacological sensitivity is probably the same as in JME, with better response to phenobarbital and bromides than to phenytoin in older studies (review in Genton *et al.*, 2000a). Recent studies and guidelines stress the first-line place of valproate in IGE in males and menopausal women, while its use is not recommended in women of childbearing age. Lamotrigine, levetiracetam, topiramate and zonisamide can be reasonably considered valid alternatives. Recently available drugs like perampanel or lacosamide can be used as adjunctive treatment. Few data are available for the use of brivaracetam (Coppola *et al.*, 2017). In case of resistance, combination of these different drugs can be proposed.

In epilepsy with GTCS alone, as with other IGEs, there is, a significant risk of seizure aggravation associated with the use of improper anticonvulsants, such as carbamazepine in JME (Genton *et al.*, 2000b) and most probably oxcarbazepine (Gélisse *et al.*, 2004). In some patients, inappropriate drugs may change the clinical presentation, increasing in particular myoclonic jerks, and these patients may thereafter be diagnosed with JME. This has been seen in three patients with IGE with isolated GTCS who experienced *de novo* myoclonic

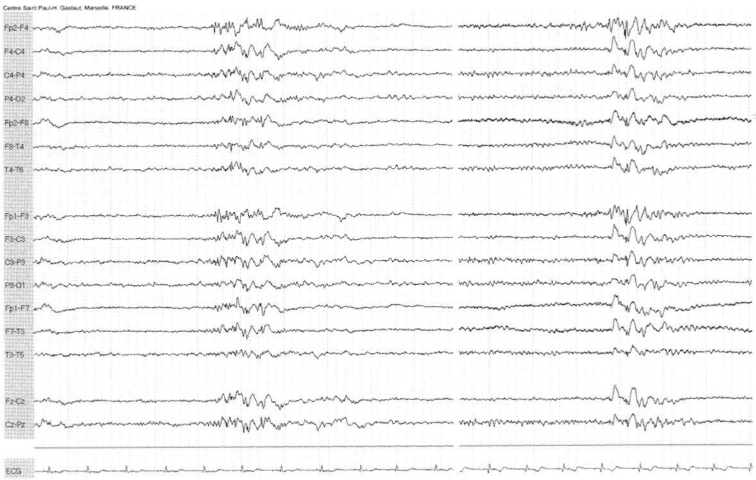

Figure 4 EEG recorded during an afternoon nap after sleep deprivation in a 24-year-old woman after a first GTCS that occurred on awakening after a shortened sleep period: a short, subclinical burst of blunted polyspike-waves was recorded during sleep, and again minutes after awakening.
I 15 mm/s – 1 cm/100 µv.

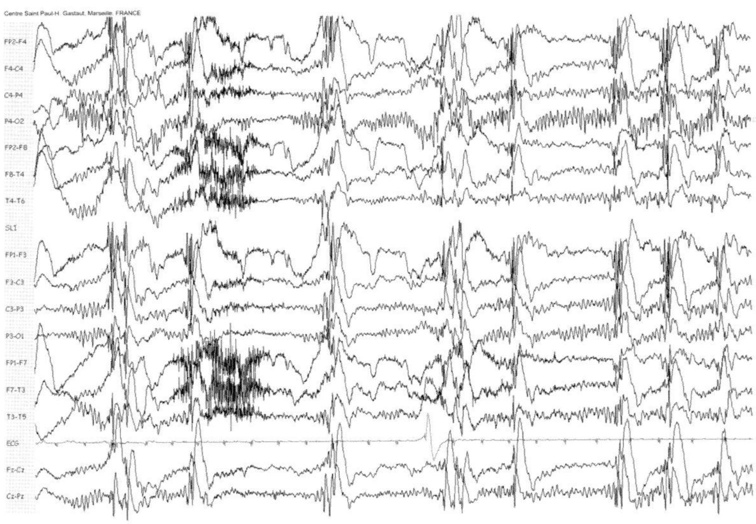

Figure 5 18-year-old woman who had had rare GTCS (less than 1/year), mostly after awakening, with normal standard EEGs and no treatment; when she received lamotrigine, progressively increased to 200 mg/d, there was a marked increase in seizure frequency (at least one per month). In this context, the EEG showed numerous polyspike-wave discharges at awakening from an afternoon nap. The situation resolved after tapering of lamotrigine and the patient chose to remain without treatment.
I 15 mm/s – 1 cm/100 µv.

jerks under lamotrigine (Crespel *et al.*, 2005). In two patients, myoclonic jerks appeared during titration and ceased when lamotrigine was decreased. In one patient, myoclonic jerks appeared one year after the introduction and evolved into myoclonic status requiring cessation of the drug. Thomas *et al.* (2006) reported two patients with EGMA who developed atypical absence status when valproate was decrease and carbamazepine was increased in a patient also treated with vigabatrin, and when carbamazepine was increased and gabapentin was added in the other one.

Nosology and conclusion

The controversies about the individualization or regrouping of IGE with onset around adolescence focus on the category of patients with GTCS seizures alone (or predominantly). Unterberger *et al.* (2001) brought evidence for the existence of separate entities among "pure Grand Mal" epilepsies belonging to the IGE: compared with patients experiencing "random" GTCS, patients with EGMA had longer duration of active epilepsy and were more sensitive to provocative factors; the familiarity was also fairly homogenous, with EGMA in families of EGMA probands and random GTCS in families of the other probands.

Indeed, if limited to patients with positive diagnosis of IGE (with proof of generalized discharges on the EEG), or at least without any evidence against IGE (no element in favor of focal seizures, for instance), EGMA stands as a recognizable syndrome. It is on the benign side of JME, with fewer seizures, less sensitivity to the same seizure precipitants, but the same pharmacological sensitivity and pharmacodependency. Typical EGMA can thus in practice be considered a minor form of JME, with a good to excellent overall prognosis. JME remains the prototype of awakening epilepsies (Janz, 2000), and whether EGMA must be kept as an entity separate from JME remains an open question.

Contrary to such typical cases, patients with only GTCS that are not clearly linked to the awakening period may or may not belong to the IGEs. Most of them will exhibit (often only after repeated EEGs and recordings of nocturnal sleep + awakening) generalized EEG changes, in others either focal epilepsy can be suspected on the basis of focal EEG changes, or no EEG changes at all can be found. The management of such cases, that are usually associated with mild epilepsy and rare seizures, is unproblematic in most.

However, not all patients with GTCS that occur at awakening have IGE. Clinical evaluation should help sort out those who are suspected of having focal epilepsy, in order to evaluate them carefully, looking for brain pathology or other etiological factors. Keeping such patients in a same category with those who have clear-cut IGE, based only on the preferred occurrence of GTCS at awakening, is certainly confusing and should be avoided.

REFERENCES ▶

Berg AT, Berkovic SF, Brodie MJ, *et al.* (2010): Revised terminology and concepts for organization of seizures and epilepsies: report of the ILAE Commission on Classification and Terminology, 2005-2009. *Epilepsia* 51: 676–685.

Billiard M. (1982): Epilepsies and the sleep-wake cycle. In: Sterman MB, Shouse MN, Passouant P (eds) *Sleep and Epilepsy*. Academic Press, New York, pp. 269–286.

Boylan LS, Labovitz DL, Jackson SC, Starner K, Devinsky O (2006): Auras are frequent in idiopathic generalized epilepsy. *Neurology* 67: 34–345.

Commission on Classification and Terminology of the International League Against Epilepsy (1989): Proposal for revised classification of epilepsies and epileptic syndromes. *Epilepsia* 30: 389–399.

Coppola G, Piccorossi A, Operto FF, Verrotti A (2017): Anticonvulsant drugs for generalized tonic-clonic epilepsy. *Expert Opin Pharmacother* 18: 925–936.

Crespel A, Genton P, Berramdane M, *et al.* (2005): Lamotrigine associated with exacerbation or *de novo* myoclonus in idiopathic generalized epilepsies. *Neurology* 65: 762–764.

Engel J (2001): A proposed diagnostic scheme for people with epileptic seizures and with epilepsy: report of the ILAE Task Force on Classification and Terminology. *Epilepsia* 42: 796–803.

Engel J Jr (2006): Report of the ILAE classification core group. *Epilepsia* 47: 1558–1568.

Gélisse P, Malafosse A, Genton P, Thomas P, Moulard B, Baldy-Moulinier M (2001a): Aspects génétiques de l'épilepsie myoclonique juvénile. *Epilepsies* 13: 97–102.

Gélisse P, Genton P, Thomas P, Rey M, Samuelian JC, Dravet C (2001b): Clinical factors of drug resistance in juvenile myoclonic epilepsy. *J Neurol Neurosurg Psychiatry* 70: 240–243.

Gélisse P, Genton P, Kuate C, Pesenti A, Baldy-Moulinier M, Crespel A (2004): Worsening of seizures by oxcarbazepine in juvenile idiopathic generalized epilepsies. *Epilepsia* 45: 1282–1286.

Gélisse P, Coubes P, Crespel A (2008): Visual auras in idiopathic generalized epilepsy. *Rev Neurol* (Paris) 164: 258–263.

Genton P, Gélisse P, Thomas P (2000a): Juvenile myoclonic epilepsy today: current definition and limits. In Schmitz B, Sander T (eds) *Juvenile myoclonic epilepsy: The Janz Syndrome*, pp. 11-32. Petersfield and Philadelphia: Wrightson Medical Publishing.

Genton P, Gélisse P, Thomas P, Dravet C (2000b): Do carbamazepine and phenytoin aggravate juvenile myoclonic epilepsy? *Neurology* 55: 1106–1109.

Gomez-Ibañez A, McLachlan RS, Mirsattari SM, Diosy DC, Burneo JG (2017): Prognostic factors in patients with refractory idiopathic generalized epilepsy. *Epilepsy Res* 130: 69–73.

Gowers WR (1885): *Epilepsy and Other Chronic Convulsive Diseases*. London: William Wood and Co.

Gungor-Tuncer O, Baykan B, Altindag E, Bebek N, Gurses C, Gokyigit A (2012): Prevalence and characteristics of visual aura in idiopathic generalized epilepsy. *Epilepsy Behav* 25: 573–576.

Haug K, Warnstedt M, Alekov AK, *et al.* (2003): Mutations in CLCN2 encoding a voltage-gated chloride channel are associated with idiopathic generalized epilepsies. *Nat Genet* 33: 527–532.

Haug K, Warnstedt M, Alekov AK, *et al.* (2009): Retraction. *Nat Genet* 41: 1043.

Hempelmann A, Taylor KP, Heils A, *et al.* (2006): Exploration of the genetic architecture of idiopathic generalized epilepsies. *Epilepsia* 47: 1682–1690.

Janz D (1953): "Aufwach"-Epilepsien. (Als Ausdruck einer den "Nacht" -oder "Schlaf" - Epilepsien gegenüberzustellenden Verlausform epileptischer Erkrankungen). *Arch Psychiat Nervenkrh* 191: 73–98.

Janz D, Christian W (1957): Impulsiv Petit-Mal. *Dtsch Z Nervenheilk* 176: 346–386. (English translation by Genton P. In: Malafosse A, Genton P, Hirsch E, Marescaux C, Broglin D, Bernasconi M (eds) *Idiopathic generalized epilepsies*. John Libbey, London, pp. 229–251.

Janz D (1962): The grand mal epilepsies and the sleeping-waking cycle. *Epilepsia* 3: 69–109.

Janz D (1969): *Die Epilepsien. Spezielle Pathologie und Therapie*. Stuttgart: Thieme.

Janz D (1974): Epilepsy and the sleep waking cycle. In: Vinken PJ, Bruyn GW (eds) *Handbook of Clinical Neurology*, vol. 15, pp. 457-490. Amsterdam: North Holland Publishing Co.

Janz D, Kern A, Mössinger HJ, Puhlmann HU (1983): Rückfallprognose während und nach Reduktion der Medikamente bei Epilepsiebehandlung. In: Remschmidt H, Rentz R, Jungmann J (eds), *Epilepsie 1981, Verlauf und Prognose, neuropsychologische und psychologische Aspekte*. Thieme, Stuttgart, pp. 17–24.

Janz D, Wolf P (1997): Epilepsy with Grand Mal on awakening. In: Engel J, Pedley TA (eds). *Epilepsy. A comprehensive textbook*. Lippincott-Raven, Philadelphia, pp. 2347–2354.

Janz D (1998): *Die Epilepsien. Spezielle Pathologie und Therapie. 2nd ed.* Stuttgart: Thieme.

Janz D (2000): Epilepsy with grand mal on awakening and sleep-waking cycle. *Clin Neurophysiol* 111 (Suppl 2): 103–110.

Langdon-Down M, Brain W (1928): The relationship of time of day sleep, and other factors to the incidence of epileptic seizures. *Lancet* 1: 1029–1032.

Loiseau P (1964): Crises épileptiques survenant au réveil et épilepsie du réveil. *Sud Médical et Chirurgical* 99: 11492–11502.

Loiseau J, Loiseau P, Guyot M, Duche B, Dartigues JF, Aublet B (1990): Survey of seizure disorders in the French southwest. I. Incidence of epileptic syndromes. *Epilepsia* 31: 391–396.

Lu Y, Waltz S, Stenzel K, Muhle H, Stephani U (2008): Photosensitivity in epileptic syndromes of childhood and adolescence. *Epileptic Disord* 10: 136–143.

Mullen SA, Berkovic SF (2018): ILAE Genetics Commission. Genetic generalized epilepsies. *Epilepsia* 59: 1148–1153.

Scheffer IE, Berkovic S, Capovilla G, *et al.* (2017): ILAE classification of the epilepsies: Position paper of the ILAE Commission for Classification and Terminology. *Epilepsia* 58: 512-521.

Thomas P, Valton L, Genton P (2006): Absence and myoclonic status epilepticus precipitatedby antiepileptic drugs in idiopathic generalized epilepsy. *Brain* 129: 1281–1292.

Tsuboi T, Christian W (1976): *Epilepsy: a Clinical, Electroencephalographic and Statistical Study of 466 Patients.* New York: Springer.

Unterberger I, Trinka E, Luef G, Bauer G (2001): Idiopathic generalized epilepsies with pure grand mal: clinical data and genetics. *Epilepsy Res* 44: 19–25.

Vorderwülbecke BJ, Kowski AB, Kirschbaum A, *et al.* (2017): Long-term outcome in adolescent-onset generalized genetic epilepsies. *Epilepsia* 58: 1244–1250.

Wolf P (1992): Epilepsy with grand mal on awakening. In: Roger J, Bureau M, Dravet C, Dreifuss F, Perret A, Wolf P (eds) *Epileptic Syndromes in Infancy, Childhood and Adolescence*, 2nd ed, pp. 329–341. London: Libbey & Co Ltd.

WITH VIDEO SUPPLEMENTS

CHAPTER 20

THE SYNDROMES OF MESIO-TEMPORAL LOBE EPILEPSY WITH HIPPOCAMPAL SCLEROSES AND TEMPORAL PLUS EPILEPSIES

Jerome Aupy[1], Elinor Ben-Menachem[2], Patrick Chauvel[3], Antonio V. Delgado-Escueta[4]

[1] Bordeaux University Hospital, Department of Clinical Neurosciences, Bordeaux, France
[2] Institute for Clinical Neurosciences, Sahlgrenska Academy, Goteborg, Sweden
[3] Cleveland Clinic and Aix-Marseille Université, Marseille (AMU), France
[4] Department of Neurology, David Geffen School of Medicine, University of California, Los Angeles, USA; Epilepsy Genetics and Genomics Labs, Neurology and Research Services, Veterans Affairs Greater Los Angeles Healthcare System, West Los Angeles, USA

History: The concept of the electro-clinical-neuropathologic syndrome of mesio-temporal lobe epilepsy with hippocampal scleroses

The concept of a mesio-Temporal Lobe Epilepsy (mTLE) was introduced by Bancaud *et al.* in 1965, when their team in INSERM UNITE 97, Hôpital Sainte-Anne, described in French the anatomical-stereoelectroencephalographic-clinical features of mTLE under the term "primary rhinencephalic epilepsy" in their classic book La Stéréo-Electroencephalographie dans l'Epilepsie. It took 18 years before confirmation of this syndrome appeared in English when Delgado-Escueta & Walsh presented videotaped seizures of "amygdalar-hippocampal epilepsy" during the 1983 Proceedings of the Association for Research in Nervous and Mental Disorders. In the decade of the 1980s, Delgado-Escueta in Los Angeles (1983, 1984, 1985, 1988), Wieser in Zurich (1983, 1987), Williamson & Spencer in New Haven (1983, 1987) Wada in Vancouver (1984, 1987) and Chauvel in Paris and then in Rennes (1986, 1987, 1992) all contributed to clinically separate mTLE (described under different terms of "primary rhinencephalic," "medio-basal limbic," or "amygdalar-hippocampal epilepsy") from neocortical-posterior temporal lobe epilepsy, from temporal-opercular epilepsy and from frontal lobe epilepsy.

The syndrome of mTLE with hippocampal scleroses (mTLE with HS) acquired further clarity, in 1990, when Houser, Miyashiro, Swartz *et al.* described for the first time, altered patterns of dynorphin immunoreactivity and mossy fiber reorganization in human temporal lobe epilepsy. The wide band of immunoreactive material in the inner molecular layer and in terminals in the granule cells and adjacent supragranular regions plus dispersion of granule cells meant that sprouting of mossy fibers or their axon collaterals had occurred in human hippocampal epilepsy as suggested by Sutula in experimental epilepsy in 1988 and 1989. In each of the TLE specimens examined, some neurons in the CA3 field appeared to receive a mossy fiber input, as indicated by the presence of dynorphin-like immunoreactivity and Timm's staining near their cell bodies and proximal dendrites. Furthermore, the presence of Dyn-IR structures within the CA2 field of some cases further suggested that additional aberrant connections might exist. Houser, Miyashiro, Swartz *et al.* (1990) also connected the human hippocampal epilepsy syndrome to febrile seizures in infancy, implying complex febrile seizures had something to do with epileptogenesis of temporal lobe epilepsy as championed earlier by Falconer (1974).

Since then, the syndrome of mTLE with hippocampal scleroses has been accepted to start as complex febrile seizures (febrile convulsive status or convulsive status with focal onset or hemiconvulsive status or prolonged obtundations status) in infancy and early childhood. A silent interval- a long latent period of years without seizures usually follows before recurrent clinically detectable psychomotor seizures (ILAE classification by Merlis group, 1970) or complex partial seizures (ILAE classification by Gastaut group, 1970) or focal seizures with loss of awareness seizures or FSLA (ILAE classification by Fisher group, 2018) appear in late childhood or early adolescence. Because granule dispersion is present in hippocampal scleroses and because asymptomatic siblings of probands with mesial temporal lobe epilepsy can have MRI evidence of hippocampal scleroses (Kobayashi *et al.*, 2004), genetic factors and possible neurogenesis are also considered important in establishing epileptogenesis in mesial temporal lobe epilepsy with hippocampal scleroses (Baulac *et al.*, 2004).

The present conceptual synthesis that explains the long silent latent period preceding established epileptogenesis and clinically detectable seizures in mTLE consists of an initial hippocampal injury produced by the complex febrile seizures of infancy and early childhood. Extensive dentate hilar neuron loss specifically of mossy cells, reduce translammelar dentate granule cell inhibition, causing granule cell hyperexcitability when afferent input from entorhinal cortex arrives (Sloviter, 1994). When entorhinal cortex is damaged and entorhinal hyperexcitability input arrives at the dentate granule cells, more in series excitation of disinhibited granule cells result. This in turn led to spontaneous granule cell-onset seizures. The long latency is explained by the time it takes for entorhinal cortex discharges to overcome granule cell inhibition and for the time it takes for granule cell hyperexcitability to overcome cortical and subcortical barriers to spread of electrographic dentate gyrus seizures and appearance of clinically detectable psychomotor seizures (Sloviter, 2012).

Networks and systems: semiology, pre-ictus, interictus and ictus

Mesio-temporal lobe epilepsy (mTLE) associated with hippocampal sclerosis (HS) in its clear-cut classical presentation (see below) is a distinctive syndrome (No *et al.*, 2017). Nevertheless, special attention must be given to any clinical, electrophysiological or radiological ***atypical*** features as they can attest to a larger epileptogenic network than expected.

Pre-ictus

The initial assault is usually characterized by a generalized or prolonged focal seizure often linked to complex febrile seizure during the infancy or early childhood (Cendes *et al.*, 1993a, b). This first seizure is usually followed by a silent interval/latent period of several years before clinically detectable focal seizures reoccur during late childhood or adolescence. Then, seizures are often pharmaco-resistant and epilepsy tends to become intractable (Semah *et al.*, 1998).

Interictus: interictal physical and neuropsychological examination

Neurological examination is classically normal. However, neuropsychological findings commonly demonstrate memory dysfunctions, which are material-specific according to the hemisphere involved, and have been related to the degree of hippocampal sclerosis (Jones-Gotman, 1991; 1993; Trenerry *et al.*, 1996). Longer duration of seizure is related to greater memory and behavioural disturbances suggesting that ***mesial temporal lobe epilepsy may be a progressive epileptic disorder***. Children's neuropsychological deficits can be less specific. Impairment of both verbal and non-verbal learning as well as long-term recall, independent of the side of HS is not uncommon.

Ictal classical picture

Frequency of seizures is highly variable, from several times a week to every month. Secondary generalizations or status epilepticus are uncommon. Precipitating factors can include stress, sleep deprivation, and, in women, hormonal changes associated with the menstrual cycle. Seizures usually start with auras that can be isolated. Typically, they consist of a rising epigastric sensation, potentially associated with emotional feelings such as anxiety or fear, familiarity (déjà-vu, déjà-vécu) unfamiliarity (jamais-vu) and autonomic symptoms (flushing, palor, mydriasis, tachycardia...). Olfactory hallucinations are also possible but raise the question of an extratemporal involvement such as orbitofrontal cortex (Bancaud & Talairach, 1992). When interrogating patients, it appears that auras can precede for years, the first appearance of focal seizure with loss of awareness.

When the psychomotor symptomatology develop, patients usually exhibit an arrest of their ongoing activity with a motionless stare and oroalimentary automatisms (*e.g.*, lip smacking, chewing) (Aupy *et al.*, 2018; Maillard *et al.*, 2004). Manual automatisms are also frequent and preferentially ipsilateral to seizure. They are usually associated with distal dystonic posturing contralateral to seizure (Kotagal *et al.*, 1989). Alteration of consciousness is common, but patients may remain responsive, even during automatisms (Aupy *et al.*, 2018; Ebner *et al.*, 1995; Park *et al.*, 2001). A clearly intelligible speech during seizure or immediate postictally is highly suggestive of a non-dominant hemisphere involvement (Gabr *et al.*, 1989). Seizures usually last less than 2 minutes but can be prolonged and followed by transient postictal confusion with some degree of postictal aphasia depending on the lateralization of seizures. Postictal nose wiping performed with the ipsilateral hand has been recognized as a frequent symptom

(Catenoix *et al.*, 2004; Leutmezer *et al.*, 1998). Patients are usually amnestic of the seizure even though they may have semi-appropriate responses to the environment during it. The aura, however, is usually remembered.

Electrophysiological findings

Interictal scalp EEG findings usually consist in ipsilateral anterior or mid temporal spikes (Cascino *et al.*, 1996; Gambardella *et al.*, 1995; Gilliam *et al.*, 1997) *(Figure 1)*. Contralateral independent spikes can also be observed without necessarily questioning the seizure lateralization. On the contrary, frequent extratemporal, temporal posterior or synchronous bilateral interictal paroxysms may indicate wider epileptogenic network. In infants and children, however, the topography of the interictal EEG abnormalities is much less defined and may have a multilobar - often temporo-frontal – or bilateral distribution (Franzon *et al.*, 2016; Mohamed *et al.*, 2001).

Ictal scalp EEG recordings are usually characteristic. Ictal pattern consists of regular well-lateralized sharply contoured rhythmic theta (> 5 Hz) activity within the temporal region (especially on the anterior-mid and infero-mesial temporal electrodes) either at onset or emerging later within 30s (Assaf & Ebersole, 1999; Ebersole & Pacia, 1996; Risinger *et al.*, 1989; Wieser & Siegel, 1991) *(Figure 2)*. If sustained, it is found to correlate with the lobe of seizure onset. This may be followed by a fast propagation of ictal discharges to the ipsilateral temporal neocortex. It may also diffusely propagate to both hemispheres (Spanedda *et al.*, 1997). However, this pattern is found in only 50 to 60% of seizures in patients with verified mTLE. In addition it is not strictly pathognomonic and can be seen as the result of spread from another lobe. This should be considered before any final surgical decision.

Imaging the epileptogenic zone

Brain MRI visual analysis efficiently allows the recognition of HS (Jackson *et al.*, 1990). HS is usually characterized by unilateral hippocampus atrophy associated with decrease T1 signal intensity and T2 increased signal intensity (Berkovic *et al.*, 1991; Cheon *et al.*, 1998; Heinz *et al.*, 2013; Van Paesschen *et al.*, 1995) *(Figure 3)*. Volumetric MRI seems to improve the detection rate of mild unilateral HS (Ho *et al.*, 1998; Jack *et al.*, 1992; Watson *et al.*, 1997). On the other side, bilateral hippocampal atrophy suggests bilateral hippocampal sclerosis and is associated with poorer surgical outcome (Berkovic *et al.*, 1995; Jack *et al.*, 1992; 1995). In the same way, single proton magnetic resonance spectroscopy and magnetic resonance spectroscopic imaging (MRSI) have demonstrated a reduction in temporal lobe N-acetylaspartate to choline-creatine ratios in up to 75% of mTLE patients, correctly lateralizing in 55%. Bilateral abnormalities, however, have also been reported using MRSI techniques in 45% of mTLE patients (Kuzniecky *et al.*, 1999; Li *et al.*, 2000). Thus, to date, these time-consuming brain MRI quantitative analysis cannot be use to identify the extent of the seizure onset zone.

Interictal brain metabolic imaging using ^{18}F-fluorodeoxyglucose (FDG) positron emission tomography (PET) is usually associated with mesio-temporal hypometabolism (Hajek *et al.*, 1993) that could extent to the temporal pole or the lateral temporal neocortex (Semah *et al.*, 1995). Interestingly, PET has demonstrated that extensive hypometabolism outside the resected regions is associated with poorer surgical outcome. Thus, extratemporal hypometabolism (Arnold *et al.*, 1996; Chassoux, 2004; Henry *et al.*, 2016) should raise the question of an extend of the epileptogenic zone outside the mesio-temporal regions. The same is demonstrated with Ictal-interictal single photon emission computed tomography (SPECT) studies (Ho *et al.*, 1997; Kazemi *et al.*, 2010). SPECT changes usually consist of hyperperfusion in a temporal lobe but also within the extratemporal region or even subcortical structures (Aupy *et al.*, 2018; Duncan *et al.*, 1997; Shin *et al.*, 2002) depending on the networks involved and the time of injection. Nevertheless it could be useful for defining the epileptogenic zone and improving stereoEEG intracranial implantation (Kaiboriboon *et al.*, 2005; Newey *et al.*, 2013; Van Paesschen *et al.*, 2003).

Thus, to date, no morphologic or metabolic imaging is considered sufficiently accurate to define the epileptogenic zone well enough to determine the extent and borders of the surgical resection. In addition, the size and extent of epileptic networks, as defined by electrophysiological recording, may increase with time and with more seizures (Bartolomei *et al.*, 2008). Imaging studies may confirm these findings by showing that temporal lobe epilepsy are observed with grey matter atrophy that in turn associate with frequent seizures (Coan *et al.*, 2014). However, gray matter atrophy is also seen in seizure free patients (Alvim *et al.*, 2016), which would make epilepsy a progressive disease regardless of seizure activity.

Networks, systems and SEEG contribution

The above characteristics of this electro-clinical syndrome, when complete, is highly suggestive of mesio-temporal lobe seizures (Hoffmann *et al.*, 2010). Nevertheless, any atypical feature (including clinical, electrophysiological or imaging findings), should make the clinician rethink and consider the possibility of a wider epileptogenic zone that could encompasses not only the mesial temporal structures but, also the temporal pole and lateral temporal cortex, or different parts of ventro-medial frontal lobe, perisylvian areas or parietal-occipital regions, according to the individual cases. Indeed, none of these features is specific of HS but can be seen in non-lesional case or

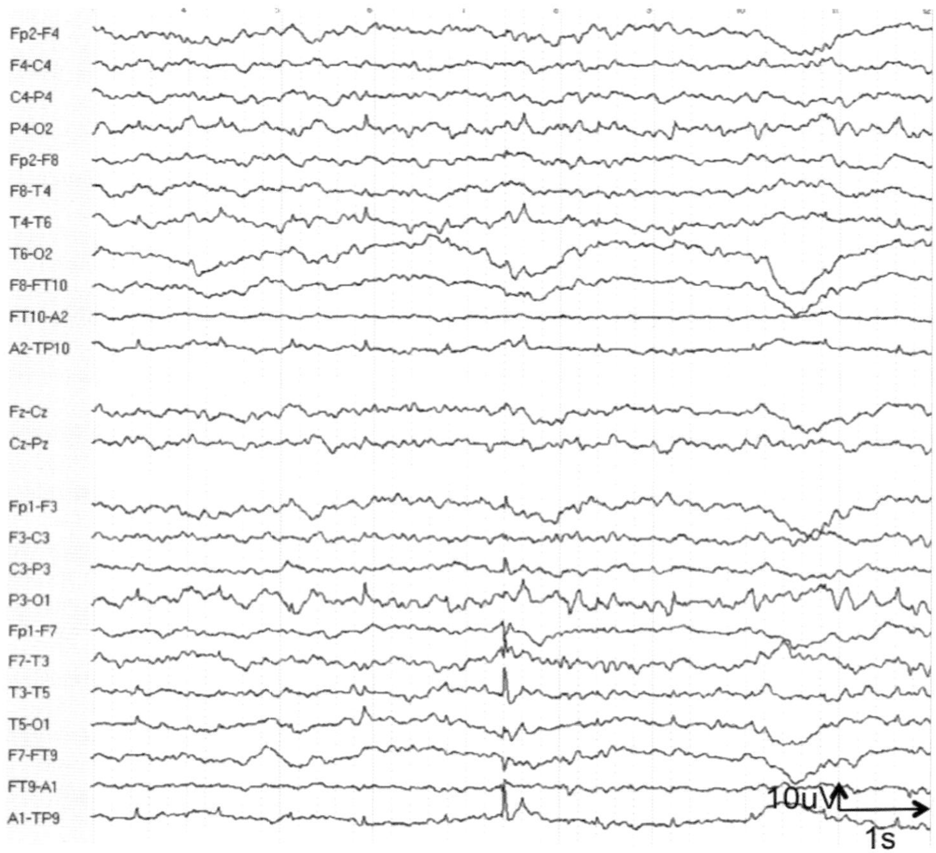

Figure 1

Interictal scalp EEG recordings of a patient with left mesio-temporal epilepsy associated with hippocampal sclerosis (10/20 longitudinal bipolar montage, 70 Hz, 0.3s, sampling 512 Hz) showing interictal spike over the left anterior temporal and basal temporal region maximum on F7-T3 et FT9-A1.

with other mesio-temporal lesions. Furthermore, classical mesio-temporal ictal symptomatology may be due to spreading ictal discharges from other temporal or extratemporal regions (Ludwig & Marsan, 1975; Schneider *et al.*, 1965) (Degado-Escueta, 1991; Hirsch *et al.*, 1991; Isnard *et al.*, 2000; Palmini *et al.*, 1999). Conversely, mesio-temporal seizures can also manifest with somehow atypical clinical features such as hypermotor behaviours (Nobili *et al.*, 2002; Vaugier *et al.*, 2009).

Defining the epileptogenic zone for surgical resection in mesio-temporal seizures with hippocampal sclerosis may not always require invasive explorations (Cascino *et al.*, 1996; Cendes *et al.*, 2000). However, any atypical electro-clinical features mandate additional long-term SEEG intracranial recordings. Even if subdural strips or grids and foramen ovale electrodes are used, stereoelectroencephalographic recordings remain the gold standard. Indeed, stereoEEG

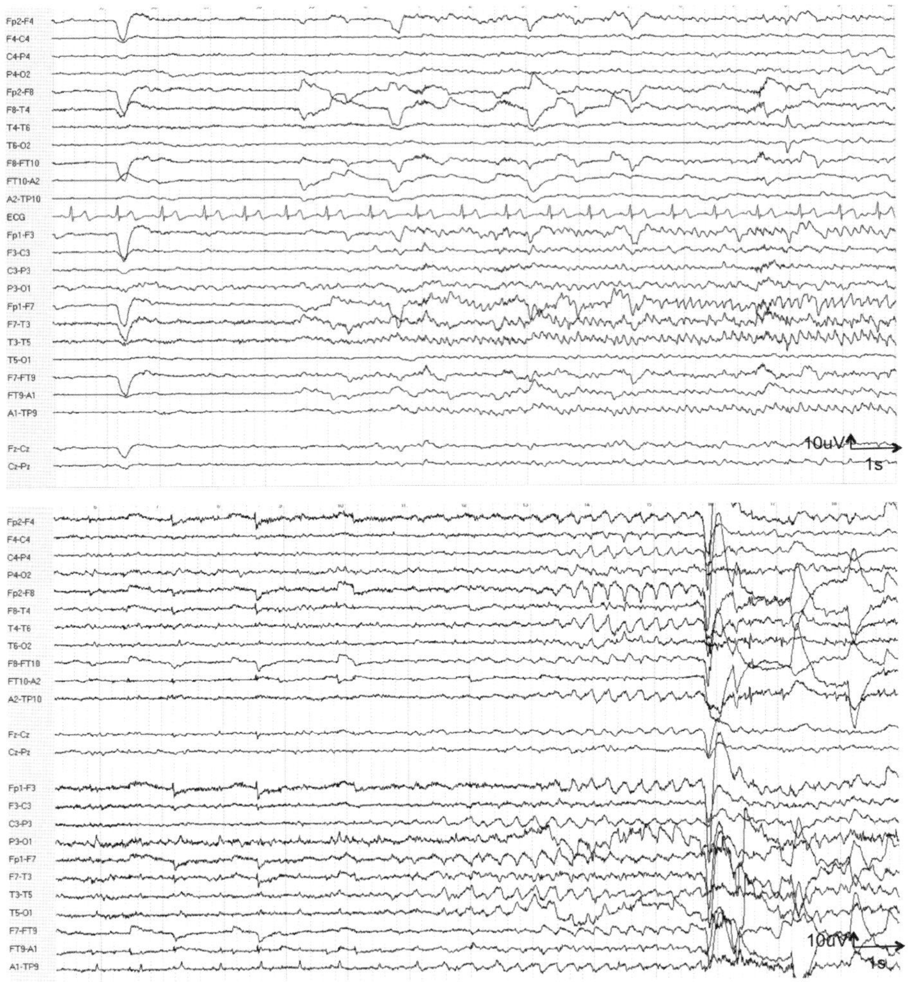

Figure 2

Ictal scalp EEG recordings of temporal lobes epilepsies (10/20 longitudinal bipolar montage, 70 Hz, 0.3 s, sampling 512 Hz). Top epoch: ictal EEG of a patient with left mesio-temporal epilepsy showing a build-up of theta rhythmic activity over the left anterior temporal regions (F7-T3) that rapidly spread to the basal temporal regions and secondarily to the anterior frontal regions. Bottom epoch: ictal EEG of a patient with bilateral mesio-temporal epilepsy showing a progressive build-up of delta/theta activity maximum over the left anterior temporal region that almost immediately spread to the posterior and basal temporal regions then to the anterior frontal and controlaterally.

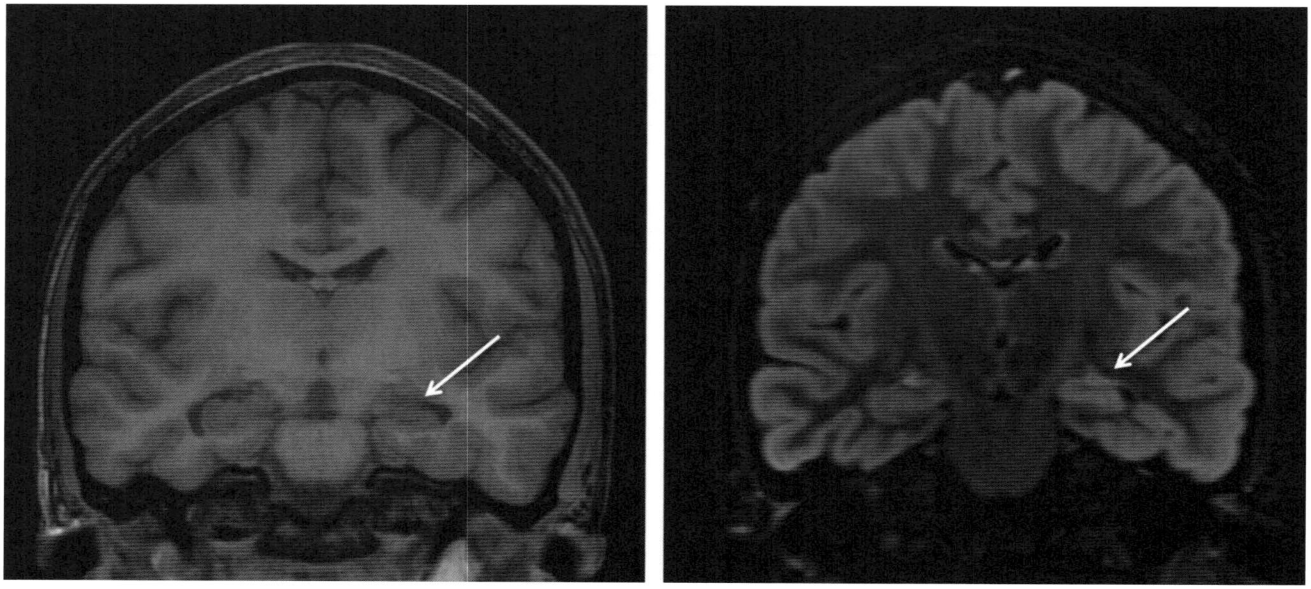

Figure 3

Brain imaging of a patient with left mesio-temporal seizure associated with hippocampal sclerosis. On the left, high resolution T1-weighted MRI (coronal slice) showing left hippocampal atrophy with flattening and loss of internal structure (arrow). T1-weighted MRI allows correct hippocampal morphologic evaluation (volume, shape and orientation). Hippocampal atrophy (arrow) is the most specific and the most reliable single indicator of MTS in patients with TLE. Coronal slices are useful to qualitatively compare both sides. A sclerotic hippocampus is usually flattened with a loss of internal structure, consequence of neuronal loss and gliosis with a collapse of pyramidal cell layers. On the right, T2 fluid attenuated inversion recovery (FLAIR) of the same patient (coronal slice) showing a hyperintense flattened and inclined downward left hippocampus (arrow). T2-weighted MRI allows the recognition of abnormal signal intensity. A hyperintense T2-weighted signal is usually easy to identify, caused by an increased concentration of free water in the abnormal tissue and potentially related to glial cell density.

gives more accurate anatomical localization and direct access to deeper structures such as hippocampus or amygdala and allows studying large-scale network configuration of seizures with an accurate time and space resolution (Bartolomei *et al.*, 2017; Bulacio *et al.*, 2016; Talairach *et al.*, 1962). Thus, SEEG studies demonstrate that the epileptogenic zone is not always confined to the sole sclerotic hippocampus, but frequently involve a complex and potentially vast epileptogenic network including close and distant regions such as the amygadala, the parahippocampal gyrus or the entorhinal cortex (Bartolomei *et al.*, 2001; Spanedda *et al.*, 1997; Spencer and Spencer, 1994; Wennberg *et al.*, 2002), the temporo-polar region (Chabardès *et al.*, 2005), or even the perisylvian cortex and the insula (Isnard *et al.*, 2000) (Aupy *et al.*, 2018; Ostrowsky *et al.*, 2000) *(Figure 4)*. Epileptogenic networks including both mesiotemporal structures and extratemporal regions (orbito-frontal cortex, insula, frontal and parietal operculum) have been defined as "TEMPORAL PLUS

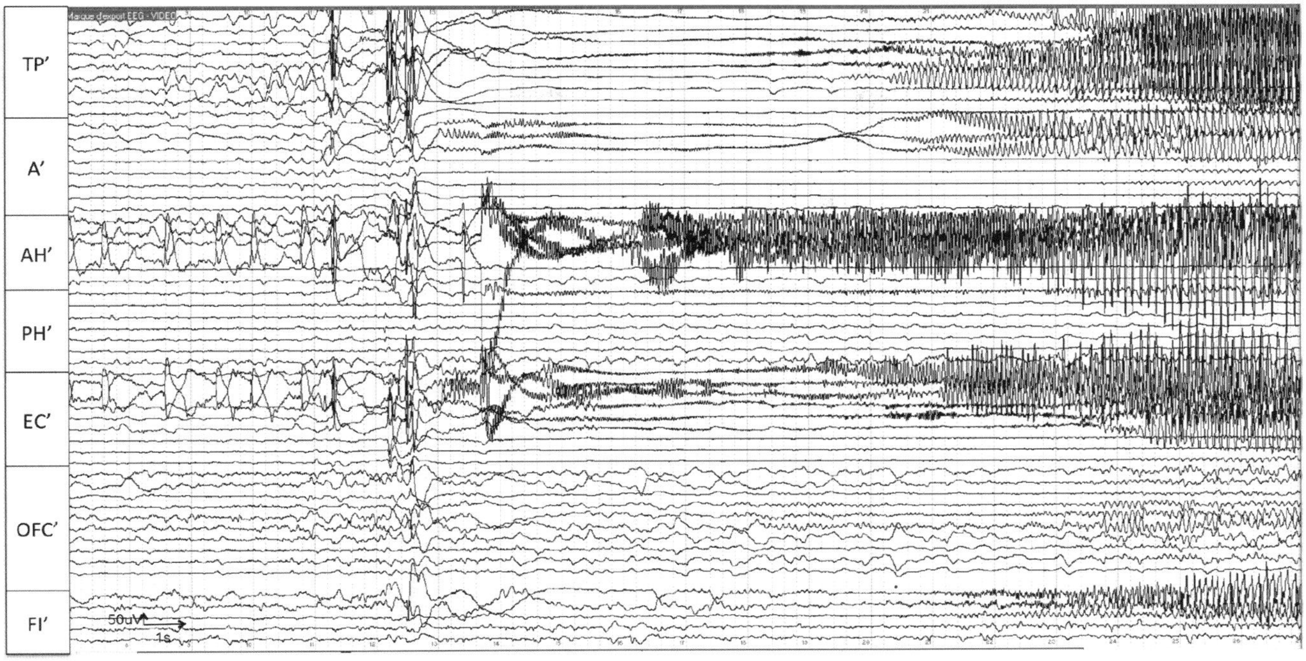

Figure 4

Ictal SEEG recordings of a patient with left mesio-temporal epilepsy associated with hippocampal sclerosis (bipolar montage, 120 Hz, 0.3 s, sampling 512 Hz) showing pre-ictal spiking over the anterior hippocampus (HA') and enthorinal cortex (EC') contacts followed by a low-voltage fast activity. A similar low-voltage fast activity was found on the amygdalar (A') and temporal pole (TP') contacts while the fronto-insular (FI') and orbitofrontal cortex (OFC') were later involved. Epileptogenic zone was not confined to the sole sclerotic hippocampus, but involved a more complex and vast epileptogenic network including the amygdala, the entorhinal cortex and the temporal pole. Patient remains seizure free after left anterior temporal lobe resection with amygdalo-hipocampectomy.

EPILEPSIES" (Barba *et al.*, 2007; Bartolomei *et al.*, 2010) and remain a major determinant of temporal lobe surgery failures (Barba *et al.*, 2016).

Pharmacological approach

The syndromes of i) MesioTemporal Epilepsy with Hippocampal Scleroses and ii) Temporal Plus Epilepsies belong to the more refractory focal epilepsy types. However, there is no special pharmacological treatment for these syndromes that differs from the treatment for other focal epilepsies (Glauser *et al.*, 2013). Clinical trials for the determination of efficacy for refractory focal onset seizures have historically included patients who have had unknown, single or multifocal locations in the brain. In these trials some patients with seizures due to mesial temporal scleroses (MTS) will become seizure-free with AED monotherapy and go into remission (Brodie & Mohanraj, 2003 ; Androsova *et al.*, 2017). However, others, despite treatment with a range of AEDs used singly and in combination, will develop refractory epilepsy (Schilller & Najjar, 2008). Another significant group of people will be controlled initially and subsequently relapse (Berg *et al.*, 2003; Schiller, 2009).

With this variety of possible outcomes, an aggressive pharmacological plan should be formulated for each patient when initiating treatment in an effort to try to prevent the development of refractory epilepsy, rather than waiting until the seizure disorder becomes chronic with all the negative problems associated with it such as cognitive deterioration and psychosocial dysfunction (Kwan & Brodie, 2002). Therefore the initial endpoint for each patient should be seizure-freedom with no or minimal drug side-effects.

The choice of the first AED will determine the subsequent strategy and should be made according to the ILAE analysis of initial monotherapy (Glauser *et al.*, 2013) or subsequent analyses in guideline form (Kanner *et al.*, 2018). Based on the results of these meta-analyses and monotherapy comparison trials in new onset epilepsy (Lattanzi *et al.*, 2019), most would now choose as a first drug either one that blocks voltage-dependent Na+ channels or a SV2A receptor modulator like levetiracetam. Recently a decision by the FDA to approve most new AEDs for use as initial monotherapy when shown to be effective against placebo in add-on trials for refractory focal onset seizures has greatly widen the choice of AEDs to use.

The first choice of an AED will be influenced by cost, results of efficacy studies, side effect profiles, age (elderly are more sensitive), gender (potential hormonal and teratogenic effects), metabolism and potential drug interactions of each drug, weight issues, general health, concomitant medication, likely compliance, availability of an intravenous formulation and cost. The dose of any AED should be titrated slowly, starting at a low dose and increasing to what is the most effective dose for the particular patient without causing undue side effects. Each patient is different, and while some tolerate high doses of a given AED, others will not.

If seizures continue unabated despite tolerability, another AED, usually with a different mechanism(s) of action should be substituted or added (Brodie & Kwan, 2002). There is no consensus as to which method is better, *i.e.* to add on to a single AED or to switch. Here again it depends on the individual patient (Beghi *et al.*, 2003).

It is estimated that seizures will not be fully controlled with INITIAL pharmacotherapy in about 20–30% of patients with focal onset seizures including MTS (Glauser *et al.*, 2013) The likelihood of success using combination therapy with the established drugs are rated as small (Schmidt & Gram, 1995; Beghi *et al.*, 2003). However, the mechanistic diversity of the newer AEDs provides a wider number of pharmacological options (Androsova *et al.*, 2017).

Some patients respond to drugs with different or overlapping mechanisms of action (Brodie & French, 2000). Whether these positive interactions are synergistic or additive remains to be determined (Deckers *et al.*, 2000).

Still to this date, the best data support rational polytherapy is the efficacy of sodium valproate in combination with lamotrigine (Brodie *et al.*, 1997; Pisani *et al.*, 1999), but note that these studies were underpowered. The other problem is that today we try to avoid the use of valproate, especially in women of childbearing potential because of the serious teratogenic effects of valproate. (Tomson *et al.*, 2019). Nevertheless, the general consensus when combing AEDs is to try to combine a drug with one mechanism to another with another mechanism of action (Santulli *et al.*, 2016). For example sodium channel antagonists can be combined with AEDs like levetiracetam, (SV2A modulator), perampanel (AMPA receptor inhibitor), zonisamide (T-type calcium channel blocker), clobazam (GABA receptor), lacosamide (slow sodium channel receptor modulator) and so forth. Today there are 25 AEDs to choose from and the number is increasing constantly. Therefore there are unlimited combinations. The main principle, however, is that if two adequate AEDs do not produce seizure freedom, then surgical evaluation with the goal of surgical resection is to be favored. Besides combining different AEDs in an attempt to reach seizure freedom, neurostimulators such as vagus nerve stimulation, deep brain stimulation and responsive neurostimulation (RNS) offer palliative help and sometimes, but infrequently, seizure freedom (Kwon, 2018; Markert, 2018).

Surgical approach

The landscape for surgical treatment of epilepsy has changed over the last two decades impacting presurgical evaluation and methods of surgical resection of epileptogenic zones and networks (Schmeiser *et al.*, 2018; Aull-Watschinger *et al.*, 2008) *(Figure 5)*.

For mTLE with unilateral hippocampal scleroses, the choices are (a) open craniotomy followed by Falconer's "en bloc" standard anterior temporal lobectomy (sATL) which includes removal of 1.5 cm of anterior hippocampus, *versus* (b) selective amygdala-hippocampectomy (sAH), *versus* (c) combination of sATL and complete AH *versus* (d) MRI-guided stereotactic selective laser interstitial thermal AH which does not require a craniotomy. For mTLE with bilateral hippocampal scleroses and time independent bilateral ictal onset zones, the choice is between brain RNS and deep brain stimulation (DBS).

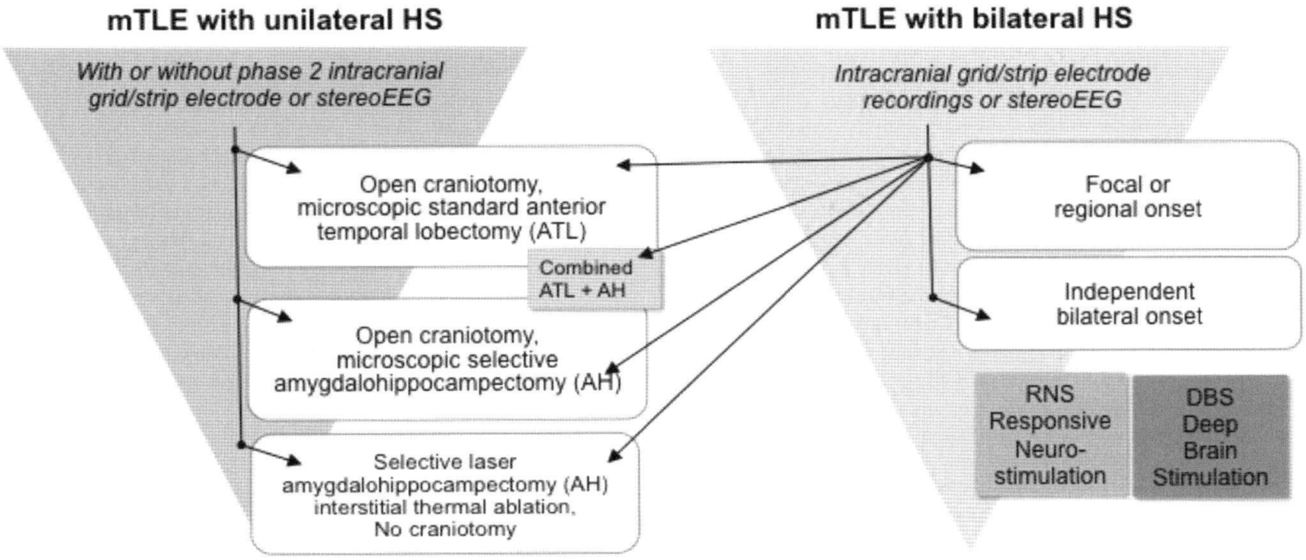

Figure 5

2019 algorithm for epilepsy surgery: medial temporal lobe epilepsy (mTLE) with hippocampal sclerosis (HS).

Mesio-temporal lobe epilepsy with unilateral hippocampal scleroses

Standard Anterior Temporal Lobectomy (sATL) versus selective Amygdalo-Hippocampectomy (sAH)

In 2001, Wiebe and colleagues provided a landmark randomized, controlled (RC) trial of surgery in temporal lobe epilepsy, assigning 40 patients to surgery and 40 patients to medical treatment. Phase 2 intracranial recordings were skipped if "the origin of a unilateral or mostly unilateral temporal-lobe seizure was determined by interictal and ictal indexes on the EEG". When the origin of seizures were unclear, phase 2 intracranial EEG was performed using bitemporal subdural strips of electrodes and extratemporal electrodes. One of three neurosurgeons experienced in surgery for epilepsy modified Falconer's sATL and combined resection of "a maximum of 6.0 to 6.5 cm of the anterior lateral nondominant temporal lobe or 4.0 to 4.5 cm of the dominant temporal lobe with partial mesial resection (AH) which included the amygdala and, at a minimum, the anterior 1.0 to 3.0 cm of the hippocampus (most commonly, 4.0 cm)".

At one year, the cumulative proportion of patients who were free of seizures that impair awareness was 58% in the surgical group while only 8 percent were free of seizures in the medical group. The surgical group has a significantly better quality of life ($P < 0.001$) than the medical group. One patient in the medical group died presumably from SUDEP while none did in the surgical group.

Almost two decades after the randomized controlled trial of Wiebe *et al.* (2001), comparable results from surgical centers worldwide have reported seizure free outcomes ranging from 52% to 85% 2 years after surgery compared to 5% to 8% with antiepileptic drug therapy. In these past two decades, longer follow up of 5 to 18 years (Hemp *et al.*, 2013) of these surgically operated epilepsy patients have also yielded freedom from seizures and better quality of life in 50% to 80% arguing for a sustained benefit in the majority of patients.

Selective amydalo-hippocampactomy (sAH)

Because of the results reported by Wyler *et al.* in 1995, arguing for complete resection of the hippocampus, a debate continued into the first decade of this millennium on whether standard anterior temporal lobectomy (sATL) could compare to sAH and whether sATL was resecting enough hippocampal tissue sufficient in stopping seizures of mesio-temporal lobe epilepsy with unilateral HS. Fortunately, in this second decade of this millennium, several groups have provided long term follow-ups from 5 to 18 years post-surgery that addressed this issue. Wendling *et al.* (2013) compared selective amygdalahippocampactomy (sAH) in 46 patients with standard anterior temporal lobectomy (sATL) in 49 patients. Seventy eight percent (27 patients) that underwent sAH were seizure free while 85.7% (33 patients) were seizure free after sATL seven years after surgery. Quality of life had improved in 95.6% of the sAH patients and 89.8% of the sATL patients. These differences were not statistically significant. Left-sided TLE patients had a significantly worse verbal memory outcome irrespective of the surgical method. However, sAH patients had a significantly better outcome concerning visual encoding, verbal and visual short-term memory and visual working memory.

These results on sAH by Wendling *et al.* (2013) are similar to the recent reports by Dorfer *et al.* (2018) who studied 158 patients (mean age 37 years) that underwent trans-sylvian sAH. Ten years after surgery, Engel class I was 78.4% and Engel class II was an additional 10.5%. Eighty-four percent were free of seizures (including re-operations) ten years after surgery. These results are also similar to the seminal series of 369 patient (151 with HS) by Wieser *et al.* (2003) on trans-sylvian sAH. Sixty-six (66.9%) percent of patients were free of seizures but had auras (Engel class I) while 57% were free of seizures and free of auras (ILAE class I) five to 24 years after surgery. These results on trans-sylvian sAH are further confirmed by the experience of Schmeiser *et al.* (2018).

Standard anterior temporal lobectomy (sATL) and sATL combined with sAH

Comparable success in standard ATL was reported by Jeong *et al.* (2005) in 227 patients. The seizure free rate was 81% ay one year and had decreased to 75% at 5 years after surgery. Generalized estimation equation model for longitudinal multiple logistic regression of the 5-year follow-up period revealed that younger age at surgery, absence of secondarily generalized tonic-clonic seizure and hippocampal sclerosis on MRI were significant predictors of a good surgical outcome. Jeong *et al.* (2005) also concluded that HS was a progressive disorder.

Other reports on sATL had lower and unsustained success rates 5 to 10 years after surgery. Jeha *et al.* (2006) reviewed 371 patients who underwent sATL. Fifty three percent of patients were free of seizures at 10 years. McIntosh *et al.* (2004) reported on 325 patients who underwent sATL who had a mean follow up period of 9.5 years (+/-4 years). Fifty-five percent were free of seizures at two years, 47.7% at five years and 41% at ten years.

Spencer *et al.* (2005) reported on a seven center observational study of 396 patients; 269 underwent mesial resection (Spencer method of combined anterior lateral temporal resection and complete AH). Sixty-eight percent (183 patients) were free of seizures but not of auras, two years after surgery. Fourteen of these 183 patients relapsed and seizures returned after two years. A longer follow up is provided in later publications with 68% free of seizures 5 years after surgery. Savitr Sastri *et al.* (2014) had similar results on 87 patients who underwent combined ATL and AH. Eighty nine percent were free of seizures one year after surgery and 76% were seizure free 5 years after surgery. Hembet *et al.* (2013) studied 108 patients with mesio-temporal lobe epilepsy and unilateral HS and used combined ATL and AH to resect epileptogenic zones. Sixty-five percent were seizure free 12 years after surgery and 62% were free of seizures 18 years after surgery.

Elliot *et al.* (2018) argue against using sAH in pediatric patients. A total of 79 patients were treated initially with sAH (n = 18) or sATL (n = 61) with a mean follow-up of 5.3 ± 4 years (range 1–16 years). The patients' average age at initial surgery was 10.6 ± 5 years. Seizure freedom (Engel I) following the initial operation was significantly more likely following ATL (47/61, 77%) than sAH (8/18, 44%; p = 0.017, Fisher's exact test). There was no statistically significant difference in the proportion of patients with postoperative neuropsychological deficits following SelAH (8/18, 44%) or ATL (21/61, 34%). However, reoperation was significantly more likely following SelAH (8/18, 44%) than after ATL (7/61, 11%; p = 0.004) and was more likely to result in Engel I outcome for ATL after failed SelAH (7/8, 88%) than for posterior extension after failed ATL (1/7, 14%; p = 0.01). Reoperation was well tolerated without significant neuropsychological deterioration. Ultimately, including 15 reoperations, 58 of 79 (73%) patients were free from disabling seizures at the most recent follow-up.

Laser interstitial thermal therapy (LITT) for selective amygdala-hippocampectomy or stereotactic laser amygdala-hippocampactomy (SLAH)

MRI-guided laser ablation of mesial temporal structures or stereotactic laser amygdala-hippocampactomy (SLAH) or Laser guided Interstitial Thermal Therapy (LITT) was first used to treat mesio-temporal lobe epilepsy in 2010. The development of magnetic resonance thermography and its application to LITT have allowed for real-time thermal imaging and feedback control during laser energy delivery, allowing for precise and accurate provision of tissue hyperthermia. Improvements in laser probe design, surgical stereotactic targeting hardware, and computer monitoring software have accelerated acceptance and clinical utilization of LITT as a neurosurgical treatment alternative.

Considered minimally invasive since a craniotomy is not required, the LITT procedure immediately destroys that target tissues like amygdala and hippocampus unlike radiosurgical gamma knife AH where late complications of cerebral edema at 6 to 12 months can be troubling and a seizure free state can arrive 6 to 18 months and as long as two years post resection (Bezchlibnyk *et al.*, 2018). Since 2010, there have been approximately 187 patients with mTLE reported in six separate series of SLAH. These patients have been followed for a minimum of 6 months to as long as 4 years and Engel class 1 seizure free states are reported to range at 53% to 65% at the 2 years follow up (Hoppe & Helmstaedter, 2018).

Drane *et al.* (2015) compared 19 patients who underwent SLAH with 39 patients who had standard anterior temporal lobectomy (sATL) and addressed naming and recognition of common nouns and famous persons. Patients with dominant TLE who underwent open craniotomy resection and sATL declined performance for naming famous faces and common nouns. Patients with nondominant TLE undergoing open craniotomy resection and sATL declined scores for recognizing famous faces. When examined on an individual subject basis, no SLAH patients experienced any performance declines on these measures. In contrast, 32 of the 39 patients undergoing standard ATL declined on one or more measures for both object types ($p < 0.001$, Fisher's exact test). Twenty-one of 22 left (dominant) TLE patients declined on one or both naming tasks after open resection, while 11 of 17 right (nondominant) TLE patients declined on face recognition. Crane *et al.* (2015) suggested that i) naming and recognition functions can be spared in TLE patients undergoing SLAH, and ii) the hippocampus does not appear to be an essential component of neural networks underlying name retrieval or recognition of common objects or famous faces.

Kang *et al.* (2016) prospectively tracked seizure outcome in 20 patients at Thomas Jefferson University Hospital with drug-resistant mTLE who underwent MRI-guided LiTT from December 2011 to December 2014. Patients who were free of seizures impairing consciousness (including those with auras only) are as follows: 8 of 15 patients (53%) after 6 months, 4 of 11 patients (36.4%) after 1 year, 3 of 5 patients (60%) at 2-year follow-up. Median follow-up was 13.4 months after LiTT (range 1.3 months to 3.2 years). Four patients had anterior temporal lobectomy (ATL) after LiTT; three are seizure-free. Kang *et al.* (2016) concluded that MRI-guided stereotactic LiTT is a safe alternative to ATL in patients with medically difficult mTLE.

Waseem *et al.* (2017) evaluated seizure freedom, neuropsychological performance, and complications, in 38 patients with mTLE who underwent MRI guided stereotactic LITT for AH. Eighteen (53%) had an Engel class I outcome. 10 patients had repeat procedures/operations, and 12 post-procedural complications occurred. Follow-up time ranged from 6 to 38.5months. There was decreased length of procedure time, hospitalization time, and analgesic requirement when compared to open surgery. In cases of well-localized mTLE this procedure may offer similar (albeit slightly lower) rates of seizure freedom versus traditional sATL.

Le *et al.* (2017) described seizure outcomes and complications after LITT in a cohort of 30 patients with intractable mesial temporal lobe epilepsy (MTLE) that were studied from October 2014 to October 2017. Mesial temporal sclerosis was present in 23/30 (77%) patients. Median follow-up was 18 ± 12 months (range: 6–44 months). Engel Class I outcome was achieved in 18/29 (62%) patients; with complete seizure freedom in 9/29 (31%) patients (Engel Class IA). Three (10%) patients have had only focal aware seizures (Engel Class 1B). Seizures only occurred with medication withdrawal in 6/29 (21%) patients (Engel Class ID). Class II was achieved by 6/29 (21%) and Class III by 5/29 (17%) patients. Complications included perioperative seizures in 10/29 (34%) and nonseizure complaints in 6/29 (21%) patients. Three (10%) patients had neurological deficits including one permanent superior quadrantanopsia, one transient trochlear, and one transient oculomotor nerve palsy.

Youngerman *et al.* (2018) also reported on seizure outcomes and complications in 30 patients with drug resistant mTLE who underwent LITT-AH between January 2013 and December 2016. Patients who required SEEG to confirm mesial temporal onset were compared with those treated based on imaging evidence of MTS and without use of SEEG. Twelve patients with SEEG-confirmed, non-medial temporal scleroses and 18 patients with MRI-confirmed medial temporal scleroses underwent MRI guided LITT-AH. Patients with mesial temporal scleroses were older (median age 50 *vs.* 30 years) and had longer standing epilepsy (median 40.5 *vs.* 5.5 years) than non-mesial temporal scleroses. Engel class I seizure freedom was achieved in 7 of 12 patients with no medial temporal lobe scleroses (58%) and 10 of 18 patients with medial temporal lobe scleroses (56%) with no significant difference between groups (odds ratio [OR] 1.12, 95% CI 0.26-4.91, $P = 0.88$). Length of stay was 1 day for most patients (range 0–3 days). Procedural complications were rare and without long-term sequelae. Youngermann *et al.* (2018) concluded that rates of seizure freedom in patients with SEEG confirmed mesial temporal scleroses and non SEEG-confirmed, non-mTLE were similar. Consistent with early literature, these rates are slightly lower than typically observed with sATL (60%–80%). However, LITT-AH is less invasive than open craniotomy surgery, with shorter hospital stays and recovery, and severe procedural complications are rare. Youngerman *et al.* (2018) further concluded that LITT-AH may be a reasonable first-line surgical option for patients with SEEG confirmed mTLE and mesial temporal lobe scleroses and patients with SEEG confirmed mTLE who do not have mTLE.

Donos *et al.* (2018) evaluated seizure outcomes in 43 consecutive patients undergoing LITT-AH for mTLE for MTL epilepsy and the relationships between ablation volumes and surgical or cognitive outcomes. A median of 73.7% of amygdala, 70.9% of hippocampus, and 28.3% of entorhinal cortex was ablated. Engel class I surgical outcome was obtained in 79.5% and 67.4% of the 43 patients at 6 and 20.3 months of follow-up, respectively. No significant differences in surgical outcomes were found across patient subgroups (hemispheric dominance, hippocampal sclerosis, or need for intracranial evaluation). Furthermore, no significant differences in volumes ablated were found between patients with Engel class IA *vs.* Engel class II-IV outcomes. In patients undergoing LITT in the dominant hemisphere, a decline in verbal and narrative memory, but not in naming function was noted. Donos *et al.* (2018) concluded that seizure-free outcomes following LITT-AH may be comparable in carefully selected patients with and without MTS, and these outcomes are comparable with outcomes following open craniotomy microsurgical resection. Failures may result from non-mesial components of the epileptogenic network that are not affected by LITT-AH. Cognitive declines following LITT-AH are modest, and principally affect memory processes.

Grewal *et al.* (2018a, b) also addressed ablation volume and relations to seizure outcome as well as safety and complications in 23 patients that underwent LITT across Mayo Clinic's three surgical centers. Pre-ablation and post-ablation follow-up volumes of the hippocampus were measured using FreeSurfer, and the volume of ablated tissue was also measured on intraoperative MRI using a supervised spline-based edge detection algorithm. Fifteen patients (65%) had left-sided procedures. The median follow-up was 34 months (range 12–70 months). At last follow-up, 11 (48%) of these patients were seizure free. The mean ablation volume was 6,888 mm^3. Median hippocampal ablation was 65%, with a median amygdala ablation of 43%. There was no correlation between ablation volume and seizure freedom ($p = 0.69$). There was also no correlation between percent ablation of the amygdala ($p = 0.28$) or hippocampus ($p = 0.82$) and seizure outcomes. Twelve patients underwent formal testing with computational visual fields. Visual field changes were seen in 67% of patients who underwent testing. Comparing the 5 patients with clinically noticeable visual field deficits to the rest of the cohort showed no significant difference in ablation volume between those patients with visual field deficits and those without ($p = 0.94$). There were 11 patients with follow-up neuropsychological testing. Within this group, verbal learning retention was 76% in the patients with left-sided procedures and 89% in those with right-sided procedures. Grewal *et al.* concluded that there was no significant correlation between ablation volume after LiTT and seizure outcomes. Visual field deficits were common in formally tested patients, much as in patients treated with open temporal lobectomy. Jermakowicz *et al.* (2018) also considered ablation dynamics during laser interstitial thermal therapy for mesiotemporal epilepsy.

Recently, Carminucci *et al.* (2019) presented 2 cases of delayed onset cyst formation occurring more than 1 year following LITT ablation. In the first case, a 59-year-old female who previously underwent LITT for a radiation induced cavernoma developed a 2 cm cystic lesion 18 months following ablation, resulting in recurrent seizure. In the second case, 53-year-old female with a recurrent left frontal cerebral metastasis developed a large cystic lesion 30 months post ablation. Both patients required craniotomies and resection of their cystic lesions. In both cases pathology demonstrated reactive gliosis and blood vessel sclerosis. Carminucci *et al.* hypothesized that chronic gliosis following LITT therapy results in blood vessel sclerosis leading to blood-brain-barrier breakdown and resulting delayed cyst formation.

Tatum *et al.* (2019), meanwhile, may have recently provided us a biomarker for failures of LITT-AH in drug resistant mTLE. Tatum *et al.* retrospectively identified 40 consecutive cases of LITT and examined EEGs for the prevalence of postoperative Transient Intermittent Rythmic Delta Activity (TIRDA). Median duration of follow-up was 15 months. Ten patients had post-LITT ipsilateral TIRDA, another two demonstrated post-operative TIRDA but they occurred contralateral to the side of ablation. None of the patients with TIRDA on their post-LITT EEG became seizure-free. Six out of 29 patients (21%) eventually required anterior temporal lobectomy (ATL), and of those 6 patients. Four (66%) had evidence of TIRDA on their post-LITT follow up EEG. The sensitivity and specificity of post-LITT TIRDA in predicting surgical failure was 57.14% and 100% respectively.

In contrast to Tatum *et al.* Caligas *et al.* with Ibrahim *et al.* (2019) examined for presurgical hyperconnectivity of the potential ablation volume in LITT hoping to find a biomarker for successful treatment in LITT. Presurgical fMRI and intraoperatively volumetric structural imaging were obtained, from which the ablation volume was segmented. The network properties of the ablation volume within the brain's large-scale brain networks were characterized using graph theory and compared between children who were and were not rendered seizure-free. Of the seventeen included children, five achieved seizure freedom following MRgLITT. Greater functional connectivity of the ablation volume to canonical resting-state networks was associated with seizure-freedom ($p < 0.05$, FDR-corrected). The ablated volume in children who subsequently became seizure-free following LITT had significantly greater strength, and "eigenvector centrality" within the large-scale brain network.

The above reports and data on LITT-AH are still limited and continued collection of data with long-term 5 to 10 years seizure outcomes have yet to be reached. Insights through the use of graph theory examining interactions between epileptogenic ablation volume cortex and large-scale brain networks should be obtained for presurgical planning and patient stratification. Post-resection EEGs searching for TIRDA and delayed complications require a long surveillance program. More investigations, therefore, are required to understand the full potential of this minimally invasive technique for mTLE with hippocampal scleroses.

Mesio-temporal lobe epilepsy with bilateral hippocampal scleroses

Evidence of gross bilateral hippocampal scleroses on Magnetic Resonance Imaging (MRI) correlate with lower success rate after sATL or sAH, 58% seizure free 2 years post-surgery compared to 78% seizure freedom when hippocampal scleroses is unilateral on MRI (Jehi, 2008). Bitemporal or extratemporal hypometabolism on 2-FDG PET drops the percentage of seizure freedom to 50% compared to 86% seizure freedom when 2FDG PET shows unilateral temporal lobe hypometabolism (Casse *et al.*, 2002; Choi *et al.*, 2003).

When time independent interictal or ictal anterior temporal and midtemporal spikes on surface EEG are bilateral, further exploration with stereoEEG should still be done. Sixty four percent can still achieve seizure freedom if SEEG recorded ictus is exclusively focal or regional and brain imaging, neuropsychological tests and WADA test support the focalization/regionalization of SEEG results (Holmes *et al.*, 2003). Surface scalp EEG can be helpful when posterior temporal (T5 or T6) interictal spikes or ictal onset, as well as extra-temporal (frontal or parietal) interictal spikes, are observed in MRI proven bilateral hippocampal scleroses. These T5 or T6 interictal spikes or ictal onsets suggest pathology and epileptogenicity may extend beyond the mesial temporal structures (Hennessy *et al.*, 2001).

Brain responsive neurostimulation

In a significant number of mesiotemporal lobe epilepsy with bilateral hippocampal scleroses, who are drug-resistant and for whom open craniotomy resective procedures are not possible, neuromodulation is an option, including closed-loop stimulation, such as brain RNS. This system was approved by the FDA in 2013 for patients 18 years and older. Developed and manufactured in Silicon Valley by NEUROPACE, the clinical trials have been led by Martha Morrell from Stanford, RNS is a programmable and responsive device that consists of intracranial leads that are placed in two seizure onset epileptogenic zones, a pulse generator, and an external programmer. An algorithm detects specific patterns of intracranial ictal activity and triggers focal self-stimulation to interrupt a seizure. One clinical trial, led by Martha Morrell, in adults with medically intractable mesio-temporal lobe epilepsy treated with RNS reduced the frequency of disabling seizures by 70 to 79% after 9 years of treatment (Skarpaas *et al.*, 2019; Geller *et al.*, 2017).

The first of several clinical trials supported by NEUROPACE and led by Martha Morrell was a pivotal trial by Heck *et al.* in 2014. One hundred ninety one patients with medically intractable partial onset seizures were implanted with the RNA system. One month post-implant, patients were randomized to active or sham stimulation. Five months post-implant, responsive neurostimulation was started to continue for two years as an open label study. The percent change in seizures at the end of the blinded period was -37.9% in the active and -17.3% in the sham stimulation group ($p = 0.012$, Generalized Estimating Equations). The median percent reduction in seizures in the open label period was 44% at 1 year and 53% at 2 years, which represents a progressive and significant improvement with time ($p < 0.0001$).

In 2015, Bergey *et al.* transitioned from the pivotal study of Heck *et al.* (2014), 230 patients into an ongoing 7 years study. The median age of patients were 34 (± 11.4) years old and epilepsy had been present for 19.6 (± 11.4) years. The median pre-implant frequency of disabling partial or generalized tonic-clonic seizures was 10.2 seizures a month. Seizure frequency dropped in this randomized blinded controlled trial by 44% at 1 year and 53% at 2 years ($p < 0.0001$, generalized estimating equation) and ranged from 48% to 66% over post-implant years 3 through 6 in the long-term study.

Three years after the pivotal study of Heck *et al.* (2014), Geller *et al.* (2017) focused on 111 patients with medically intractable mesio-temporal lobe epilepsy, 72% of which had bilateral ictal onsets. Seizure frequency was measured over 2 to 6 years post-implant. The mean follow-up was 6.1 ± (standard deviation 2.2 years). Seizure frequency dropped by 70% (median percent at last observation carried forward). Twenty-nine percent of subjects experienced at least one seizure-free period of 6 months or longer, and 15% experienced at least one seizure-free period of 1 year or longer. There was no difference in seizure reduction in subjects with and without mesial temporal sclerosis (MTS), bilateral MTL onsets, prior resection, prior intracranial monitoring, and prior vagus nerve stimulation.

In the same year of 2017, Jobst *et al.* turned attention to 126 patients with drug resistant neocortical epilepsy including eloquent areas. Patients with frontal or parietal lobe epilepsy dropped seizure frequency by 70% (median frequency) temporal neocortical epilepsy by 58% and multilobar epilepsy by 51%. Twenty-six percent of patients experienced at least one seizure-free period of 6 months or longer and 14% experienced at least one seizure-free period of 1 year or longer. Patients with lesions on magnetic resonance imaging (77% reduction) and those with normal MRI findings (45% reduction) benefitted, although treatment response was more robust in patients with an MRI lesion (p = 0.02, generalized estimating equation [GEE]). There were no differences in the seizure reduction in patients with and without prior epilepsy surgery or vagus nerve stimulation.

Some centers are also using the RNS system for long-term electrocorticography recording in the patient's normal ambulatory home environment to determine the primary ictal zones in bilateral hippocampal scleroses (Di Lorenzo *et al.*, 2014). In 5 study patients, the notion of resective surgery was revisited in light of information from the chronic intracranial recordings obtained from RNS. Four patients who had previously been considered not to be candidates for surgery did undergo resective surgery, and all have achieved seizure freedom. A fifth patient, who had a double-band heterotopia, underwent surgery but did not achieve significant seizure reduction.

The most frequent serious device-related adverse events were soft tissue implant-site infection (overall rate, including events categorized as device-related, uncertain, or not device-related: 0.017 to 0.03 per patient implant year) and perioperative hemorrhage (0.8%) were not greater than with other neurostimulation devices.

Treatment with responsive cortical stimulation is also associated with improvement in quality of life and cognitive function related to the functional area being treated.

Deep brain stimulation

Deep brain stimulation (DBS) to control seizures was first applied to the cerebellum by Cooper *et al.* (1973). Since the study of Cooper *et al.* (1973), 52 clinical studies of brain stimulation to decrease seizures in 817 patients are documented in literature with the stimulating electrodes implanted in the caudate, locus coeruleus, subthalamic nucleus, mammillary bodies, centromedian thalamus, anterior nucleus of thalamus, hippocampus and amygdala, hippocampal commissure, corpus callosum, and neocortex. A wide variety of stimulation parameters have been employed in multiple different combinations of frequencies, amplitudes, and durations.

Two large, randomized, and controlled studies of DBS have been conducted, one in the anterior nucleus of thalamus and another at the cortical or hippocampal seizure focus. Both of these studies showed efficacy and tolerability of stimulation. Many questions remain about DBS. We do not know the mechanisms, the best stimulation parameters, the best patient population, or how to predict benefit in advance. We do not know why benefit of neurostimulation for epilepsy seems to increase over time or whether there are long-term deleterious effects. All of these questions may be answerable with a combination of laboratory research and clinical experience.

The first such large randomized, controlled trial was organized in 2010 by Robert Fisher (1992; 2010) of Stanford (SANTE trial). This trial involved 17 surgical epilepsy centers that followed 110 patients who had had electrical wires placed in anterior thalamus. These 110 patients suffered from medication-resistant focal-onset seizures that occurred, on average, about 20 times per month. Half of these 110 patients were randomized to active stimulation and half to placebo stimulation. Patients could not feel the stimulation so could not tell which group they were in. Active stimulation reduced seizures by 40%, whereas placebo reduced seizures by 15% – a significant difference. There were fewer seizure injuries in the active group. This was the first proof in a large, controlled trial that electrical brain stimulation could reduce seizures.

In 2015, Salanova *et al.* representing the same SANTE trial led by Robert Fisher, reported on the long-term efficacy and safety of deep brain stimulation of anterior nucleus of the thalamus (ANT) for treatment of focal epilepsy. Long-term follow-up began 13 months after device implantation and seizure frequency was determined using daily seizure diaries. Seizure frequency dropped 41% (median percent seizure reduction from baseline) at 1 year and 69% at 5 years. The responder rate (≥ 50% reduction in seizure frequency) at 1 year was 43%, and 68% at 5 years. In the 5 years of follow-up, 16% of subjects were seizure-free for at least 6 months. There were no reported unanticipated adverse device effects or symptomatic intracranial hemorrhages. The Liverpool Seizure Severity Scale and 31-item Quality of Life in Epilepsy measure showed statistically significant improvement over baseline by 1 year and at 5 years ($p < 0.001$). Salanova *et al.* (2015) concluded that ANT deep brain stimulation has sustained efficacy and safety in a treatment-resistant population. The SANTE trial has provided Class IV evidence that anterior thalamic stimulation is associated with a 69% reduction in seizure frequency and a 34% serious device-related adverse event rate at 5 years in patients with drug-resistant partial epilepsy,

In April 2018, the FDA approved the DBS device's use for epilepsy. DBS entails sending electrical signals to electrodes implanted in the anterior thalamus. Power is supplied to these implanted electrodes through fine wires threaded to a pulse-generating device placed under the skin of the patient's chest.

Concluding remarks: The concept of temporal plus epilepsies

Ideally, optimal reconstruction of the epileptic network/system in unilateral mesial temporal lobe epilepsy with hippocampal scleroses during SEEG and complete resection of the crucial seizure generating epileptogenic network should result in freedom from seizures (including freedom from auras) that is sustained through the patient's life.

But many questions still remain challenging in surgery of mTLE with unilateral HS. Examples of questions are the following: i) what explains the wide disparity of seizure free outcomes reported by surgical centers – from 52% to 85% two years after surgery and from 50% to 80% ten years after surgery? ii) Why do seizure free states decline and seizures recur after 5 years and after 10 years of follow up? iii) Are these differences explained by a more systematic SEEG mapping of systems and networks followed by tailored surgery versus the use of "skip of phase 2 protocols" followed by standard anterior temporal lobectomy? iv) If the presence of febrile seizures in infancy (better prognosis), the presence of secondarily generalized tonic-clonic convulsions (worse prognosis), early age of onset and younger age at time of surgery (better prognosis) and long duration of epilepsy (worse prognosis) are controlled for, does extent of mesial temporal hippocampal resection make a difference?

Different factors may explain the wide disparity of seizure free outcomes reported by surgical centers and the decline of seizure free states after 5 years and after 10 years of follow up? The neuropathologist would argue that the etiologic pathology of the surgical specimen is most important. Nonspecific Chaslin's gliosis is associated with 44% seizure free states at 8 years follow up compared to 64% when hippocampal scleroses was present (Jeha *et al.*, 2006) and at even at higher rates of 84% when hippocampal scleroses was most severe (LoPinto-Khoury *et al.*, 2012; Wieser *et al.*, 2003).

The neurosurgeon, on the other hand, would point out that complete resection of the crucial seizure generating epileptogenic network, and eliminating all components of the epileptogenic network and any parts that can re-ignite excitation in the reorganized mossy fiber network and its connectomes should support sustainability of a seizure free state during a lifetime post-surgery. This is exemplified by posterior hippocampal epilepsy and how the extent of posterior hippocampus resection can impact postsurgical freedom from seizures. Thirty percent of hippocampal epilepsy have their crucial epileptogenic networks in its posterior third and tail. Wyler *et al.* (1995) showed that 69% of patients were seizure free if the resection of the hippocampus were taken as far back as the level of the superior colliculus. Contrast this to only 38% of patients who attained seizure freedom because their hippocampectomies were limited posteriorly by the lateral mesencephalic sulcus.

Even if standard anterior temporal lobectomy is combined with sAH, the epileptologist would add that the disparity of seizure free states reported by different epilepsy centers and the late recurrence of seizures after 5 to 10 years of follow up, are also linked to inaccuracies in mesial temporal epilepsies topographical diagnosis and linked to misdiagnosis and missing the concept of temporal plus epilepsies. In fact, the concept of "temporal plus epilepsies", rather than "temporal lobe epilepsies" are multiple and many of their networks and pathology are not limited to the boundaries of the anatomical temporal lobe. As Jean Bancaud use to argue and now Patrick Chauvel – "pathology does not respect anatomical borders of the temporal lobe". This has been well illustrated by the term "temporal plus epilepsies". This term is too imprecise, but it means that the epileptogenic network (*i.e.* the epileptogenic zone – EZ) encompasses not only the mesial temporal structures but also temporal pole and lateral temporal cortex, and different parts of ventro-medial frontal lobe, perisylvian areas or parietal-occipital regions, according to specific cases. The best example is given by the temporal-perisylvian epilepsies where opercular and insular cortices are part of the epileptogenic zone or are the sites of epileptogenic zones themselves. While the diagnosis of hippocampal sclerosis from MRI or temporal hypometabolism from PET are generally easy to make, the exact and full extent of the EZ is much more difficult (Bartolomei *et al.*, 2018; Maillard *et al.*, 2004) without the help of intracerebral SEEG recordings. The difficulty is increased by the fact, as demonstrated by classical and recent studies (Penfield & Faulk, 1955; Van Buren, 1963; Aupy *et al.*, 2017), that most of the elements of the semiological pattern of the so-called "mesial temporal seizures" are generated outside the temporal lobe, especially in the perisylvian areas. The recurrence of seizures after anterior temporal lobe surgery may simply be the re-emergence of perisylvian semiology hidden by AEDs maintained long after operation. The latter observation explains late seizure recurrence as drugs are being tapered off after years of a seizure free state.

In the same way, the presence of secondary generalized seizures, the early age at surgery, the long duration of epilepsy (Bartolomei *et al.*, 2008; Coan *et al.*, 2014) as they represent major factors of prognosis, bear the same meaning. Extension of the network space with time is actually a basic feature of the "temporal plus epilepsies" which are progressive diseases. (Coan *et al.*, 2009, 2014; Alvim *et al.*, 2016; Conz *et al.*, 2011).

REFERENCES ▶

Alvim MKM, Coan AC, Campos BM, *et al.* (2016): Progression of gray matter atrophy in seizure-free patients with temporal lobe epilepsy. *Epilepsia* 57: 621–629.

Androsova G, Krause R, Borghei M, *et al.* (2017): Comparative effectiveness of antiepileptic drugs in patients with mesial temporal lobe epilepsy with hippocampal sclerosis. *Epilepsia* 58: 1734–1741.

Arnold S, Schlaug G, Niemann H, *et al.* (1996): Topography of interictal glucose hypometabolism in unilateral mesio-temporal epilepsy. *Neurology* 46: 1422–1422.

Assaf BA, Ebersole JS. (1999): Visual and Quantitative Ictal EEG Predictors of Outcome After Temporal Lobectomy. *Epilepsia* 40: 52–61.

Aull-Watschinger S, Pataraia E, Czech T, Baumgartner C (2008): Outcome predictors for surgical treatment of temporal lobe epilepsy with hippocampal sclerosis. *Epilepsia* 49: 1308–1136.

Aupy J, Noviawaty I, Krishnan B, *et al.* (2018): Insulo-opercular cortex generates oroalimentary automatisms in temporal seizures. *Epilepsia* 72: 603–612.

Aupy J, Wongwiangjunt S, Wang ZI, Wu G, Alexopoulos A (2018): Subcortical SISCOM hyperperfusion: Should we pay more attention to it? *Seizure* 62: 43–48.

Bancaud J, Talairach J (1992): Clinical semiology of frontal lobe seizures. *Adv Neurol* 57: 3–58.

Bancaud J, Talairach J, Bonis A, *et al.* (1965): *La Stéréoélectroencéphalographie dans l'épilepsie.* Paris, Masson.

Barba C, Barbati G, Minotti L, Hoffmann D, Kahane P (2007). Ictal clinical and scalp-EEG findings differentiating temporal lobe epilepsies from temporal plus' epilepsies. *Brain* 130: 1957–1967.

Barba C, Rheims S, Minotti L, *et al.* (2016): Temporal plus epilepsy is a major determinant of temporal lobe surgery failures. *Brain* 139: 444–451.

Bartolomei F, Chauvel P, Wendling F (2008): Epileptogenicity of brain structures in human temporal lobe epilepsy: a quantified study from intracerebral EEG. *Brain* 131: 1818–1830.

Bartolomei F, Cosandier-Rimele D, McGonigal A, *et al.* (2010): From mesial temporal lobe to temporoperisylvian seizures: A quantified study of temporal lobe seizure networks. *Epilepsia* 51: 2147–2158.

Bartolomei F, Lagarde S, Wendling F, *et al.* (2017): Defining epileptogenic networks: Contribution of SEEG and signal analysis. *Epilepsia* 58: 1131–1147.

Bartolomei F, Nica A, Valenti-Hirsch MP, Adam C, Denuelle M (2018): Interpretation of SEEG recordings. *Neurophysiol Clin* 48: 53–57.

Bartolomei F, Wendling F, Bellanger JJ, Regis J, Chauvel P (2001): Neural networks involving the medial temporal structures in temporal lobe epilepsy. *Clin Neurophysiol* 112: 1746–1760.

Baulac S, Gourfinkel-An I, Nabbout R, *et al.* (2004): Fever, genes, and epilepsy. *Lancet Neurology* 3: 421–430.

Beghi E, Gatti G, Tonini C, *et al.* (2003): Adjunctive therapy *vs.* alternative monotherapy in patients with partial epilepsy failing on a single drug: a multicenter, randomisedpragmatic trial. *Epilepsy Res* 57: 1–13.

Berg AT, Langfitt J, Shinnar S, *et al.* (2003): How long does it take for partial epilepsy to become intractable? *Neurology* 60: 186–190.

Bergey GK, Morrell MJ, Mizrahi EM, *et al.* (2015): Long-term treatment with responsive brain stimulation in adults with refractory partial seizures. *Neurology* 84: 810–817.

Bergey GK, Morrell MJ, Mizrahi EM, *et al.* (2015): Long-term treatment with responsive brain stimulation in adults with refractory partial seizures. *Neurology* 24; 84: 810–817.

Berkovic SF, Andermann F, Olivier A, *et al.* (1991): Hippocampal sclerosis in temporal lobe epilepsy demonstrated by magnetic resonance imaging. *Ann Neurol* 29: 175–182.

Berkovic SF, McIntosh AM, Kalnins RM, *et al.* (1995): Preoperative MRI predicts outcome of temporal lobectomy: An actuarial analysis. *Neurology* 45: 1358–1363.

Bezchlibnyk YB, Willie JT, Gross RE (2018): A neurosurgeon's view: Laser interstitial thermal therapy of mesial temporal lobe structures. *Epilepsy Res* 142: 135–139.

Brodie MJ, French JA (2000): Management of epilepsy in adolescents and adults. *Lancet* 356: 323–329.

Brodie MJ, Kwan P (2002): Staged approach to epilepsy management. *Neurology* 58(suppl 5): S2–S8.

Brodie MJ, Mohanraj R (2003): Response to treatmentin newly diagnosed epilepsy. *Epilepsia* 44 (Suppl 9): 14.

Brodie MJ, Yuen AWC; and the 105: study group (1997): Lamotrigine substitution study: evidence for synergism with sodium valproate? *Epilepsy Res* 26: 423–432.

Bulacio JC, Chauvel P, McGonigal A (2016): Stereoelectroencephalography. *J Clin Neurophysiol* 33: 503–510.

Cajigas I, Kanner AM, Ribot R, *et al* (2019): Magnetic Resonance-Guided Laser Interstitial Thermal Therapy for Mesial Temporal Epilepsy: A Case Series Analysis of Outcomes and Complications at 2-Year Follow-Up. *World Neurosurg* [Epub ahead of print].

Carminucci A, Parr M, Bitar M, Danish SF (2019): Delayed Onset Cyst Formation After Laser Interstitial Thermal Therapy: An Unreported Long-term Complication. *World Neurosurg* [Epub ahead of print].

Cascino GD, Trenerry MR, So EL, *et al.* (1996): Routine EEG and temporal lobe epilepsy: relation to long-term EEG monitoring, quantitative MRI, and operative outcome. *Epilepsia* 37: 651–656.

Catenoix H, Guénot M, Isnard J, Fischer C, Mauguiere F, Ryvlin P (2004): Intracranial EEG study of seizure-associated nose wiping. *Neurology* 63: 1127–1129.

Cendes F, Andermann F, Dubeau F, *et al* (1993a): Early childhood prolonged febrile convulsions, atrophy and sclerosis of mesial structures, and temporal lobe epilepsy: An MRI volumetric study. *Neurology* 43: 1083–1083.

Cendes F, Andermann F, Gloor P, *et al.* (1993b): Atrophy of mesial structures in patients with temporal lobe epilepsy: Cause or consequence of repeated seizures? *Ann Neurol* 34: 795–801.

Cendes F, Li LM, Watson C, Andermann F, Dubeau F, Arnold DL (2000): Is Ictal Recording Mandatory in Temporal Lobe Epilepsy: Not When the Interictal Electroencephalogram and Hippocampal Atrophy Coincide. *Arch Neurol* 57: 497–500.

Chabardès S, Kahane P, Minotti L, *et al.* (2005): The temporopolar cortex plays a pivotal role in temporal lobe seizures. *Brain* 128: 1818–1831.

Chassoux F (2004): Metabolic changes and electro-clinical patterns in mesio-temporal lobe epilepsy: a correlative study. *Brain* 127: 164–174.

Chauvel P, Trottier S, Bancaud J (1988): Seizures from the precentral and the premotor areas II: Neurophysiological Analysis. *Epilepsia* 29: 207.

Cheon JE, Chang KH, Kim HD, *et al.* (1998): MR of hippocampal sclerosis: comparison of qualitative and quantitative assessments. *AJNR Am J Neuroradiol* 19: 465–468.

Coan AC, Appenzeller S, Bonilha L, Li LM, Cendes F (2009): Seizure frequency and lateralization affect progression of atrophy in temporal lobe epilepsy. *Neurology* 15;73: 834–842.

Coan AC, Campos BM, Yasuda CL, *et al.* (2014): Frequent Seizures Are Associated with a Network of Gray Matter Atrophy in Temporal Lobe Epilepsy with or without Hippocampal Sclerosis. *PLoS ONE* 9: e85843–9.

Cooper IS, Amin I, Gilman S (1973): The effect of chronic cerebellar stimulation upon epilepsy in man. *Trans Am Neurol Assoc* 98: 192–196.

Deckers CLP, Czuczwar SJ, Hekster YA, *et al.* (2000): Selection of antiepileptic drugs polytherapy based on mechanisms of action: the evidence reviewed. *Epilepsia* 41: 1364–1374.

Delgado-Escueta AV (1991): Frontal lobe seizures and epilepsies in neurobehavioral disorders. *Adv Neurol* 55: 317–340.

Delgado-Escueta AV, Walsh GO (1983): The Selection Process for surgery of intractable complex partial seizures: surface EEG and depth electrocorticography. In: Ward AA Jr, Penry JK, Purpura DP (eds): *Epilepsy Proceedings of the Association for Research in Nervous and Mental Disorders*. vol 61, pp 295–326, Raven Press, New York.

Delgado-Escueta AV, Walsh GO (1985): Type I Complex Partial Seizures of Hippocampal origin: excellent results of anterior temporal lobectomy. *Neurology* 35: 143–154.

DiLorenzo DJ, Mangubat EZ, Rossi MA, Byrne RW (2014): Chronic unlimited recording electrocorticography-guided resective epilepsy surgery: technology-enabled enhanced fidelity in seizure focus localization with improved surgical efficacy. J *Neurosurg* 120: 1402–1414.

Donos C, Breier J, Friedman E, *et al.* (2018): Laser ablation for mesial temporal lobe epilepsy: Surgical and cognitive outcomes with and without mesial temporal sclerosis. *Epilepsia* 59: 1421–1432.

Dorfer C, Czech T, Aull-Watschinger S, *et al.* (2018): Mesial temporal lobe epilepsy: long-term seizure outcome of patients primarily treated with transsylvian selective amygdalohippocampectomy. *J Neurosurg* 129: 174–181.

Drane DL, Loring DW, Voets NL, *et al.* (2015): Better object recognition and naming outcome with MRI-guided stereotactic laser amygdalohippocampotomy for temporal lobe epilepsy. *Epilepsia* 56: 101–113.

Duncan R, Patterson J, Hadley D, Roberts R (1997): Ictal regional cerebral blood flow in frontal lobe seizures. *Seizure* 6: 393–401.

Ebersole JS, Pacia SV (1996): Localization of Temporal Lobe Foci by Ictal EEG Patterns. *Epilepsia* 37: 386–399.

Ebner A, Dinner DS, Noachtar S, Luders H (1995): Automatisms with preserved responsiveness: A lateralizing sign in psychomotor seizures. *Neurology* 45: 61–64.

Elliott CA, Broad A, Narvacan K, *et al.* (2018): Seizure outcome in pediatric medically refractory temporal lobe epilepsy surgery: selective amygdalohippocampectomy *vs.* anterior temporal lobectomy. *J Neurosurg Pediatr* 22: 276–282.

Falconer MA (1974): Mesial temporal (Ammon's horn) sclerosis as a common cause of epilepsy. Aetiology, treatment, and prevention. *Lancet* 2(7883): 767–70.

Fisher R, Salanova V, Witt T, *et al.* (2010): Electrical stimulation of the anterior nucleus of thalamus for treatment of refractory epilepsy. *Epilepsia* 51: 899–908.

Fisher RS, Uematsu S, Krauss GL, *et al.* (1992): Placebo-controlled pilot study of centromedian thalamic stimulation in treatment of intractable seizures. *Epilepsia* 33: 841–851.

Franzon RC, Montenegro MA, Guimarães CA, Guerreiro CAM, Cendes F, Guerreiro MM (2016): Clinical, Electroencephalographic, and Behavioral Features of Temporal Lobe Epilepsy in Childhood. *J Child Neurol* 19: 418–423.

Gabr M, Lüders H, Dinner D, Morris H, Wyllie E (1989): Speech manifestations in lateralization of temporal lobe seizures. *Ann Neurol* 25: 82–87.

Gambardella A, Gotman J, Cendes F, Andermann F (1995): The relation of spike foci and of clinical seizure characteristics to different patterns of mesial temporal atrophy. *Arch Neurol* 52: 287–293.

Gilliam F, Bowling S, Bilir E, *et al.* (1997): Association of combined MRI, interictal EEG, and ictal EEG results with outcome and pathology after temporal lobectomy. *Epilepsia* 38: 1315–1320.

Glauser T, Ben-Menachem E, Bourgeois B, *et al.* (2013): ILAE Subcommission on AED Guidelines: Updated ILAE evidence review of antiepileptic drug efficacy and effectiveness as initial monotherapy for epileptic seizures and syndromes. *Epilepsia*. 54: 551–563.

Grewal SS, Gorny KR, Favazza CP, Watson RE, Kaufman TJ, Van Gompel JJ (2018a). Safety of laser interstitial thermal therapy in patients with pacemakers. *Open Neurosurg* (Hagerstown) 15(5): E69–E72.

Grewal SS, Zimmerman RS, Worrell G, *et al.* (2018b): Laser ablation for mesial temporal epilepsy: a multi-site, single institutional series. *J Neurosurg* 1: 1–8.

Hajek M, Antonini A, Leenders KL, Wieser HG (1993): Mesiobasal *vs.* lateral temporal lobe epilepsy: Metabolic differences in the temporal lobe shown by interictal 18F-FDG positron emission tomography. *Neurology* 43: 79–86.

Heck CN, King-Stephens D, Massey AD, *et al.* (2014): Two-year seizure reduction in adults with medically intractable partial onset epilepsy treated with responsive neurostimulation: final results of the RNS System Pivotal trial. *Epilepsia* 55: 432–441.

Heinz ER, Crain BJ, Radtke RA, *et al.* (2013): MR imaging in patients with temporal lobe seizures: correlation of results with pathologic findings. *AJR Am j roentgenology* 155: 581–586.

Hemb M, Palmini A, Paglioli E, *et al.* (2013): An 18-year follow-up of seizure outcome after surgery for temporal lobe epilepsy and hippocampal sclerosis, *J Neurol Neurosurg Psychiatry* 84: 800–805.

Henry TR, Mazziotta JC, Jerome Engel J, *et al.* (2016): Quantifying Interictal Metabolic Activity in Human Temporal Lobe Epilepsy. *J Cereb Blood Flow Metab* 10: 748–757.

Hirsch LJ, Spencer SS, Williamson PD, Spencer DD, Mattson RH (1991): Comparison of bitemporal and unitemporal epilepsy defined by depth electroencephalography. *Ann Neurol* 30: 340–346.

Ho SS, Kuzniecky RI, Gilliam F, Faught E, Morawetz R (1998): Temporal lobe developmental malformations and epilepsy: Dual pathology and bilateral hippocampal abnormalities. *Neurology* 50: 748–754.

Ho SS, Newton MR, McIntosh AM, *et al.* (1997): Perfusion patterns during temporal lobe seizures: relationship to surgical outcome. *Brain* 120: 1921–1928.

Hoffmann JM, Elger CE, Kleefuss-Lie AA (2010): Analysis of the initial ictal phenomenon in patients with temporal lobe epilepsy. *Seizure* 19: 217–221.

Hoppe C, Helmstaedter C (2018): Laser interstitial thermotherapy (LiTT) in pediatric epilepsy surgery. *Seizure* pii: S1059-1311(18)30575-2.

Houser CR, Miyashiro JE, Swartz BE, Walsh GO, Rich JR, Delgado-Escueta AV (1990): Altered patterns of dynorphin immunoreactivity suggest mossy fiber reorganization in human hippocampal epilepsy. *J Neurosci* 10: 267–282.

Isnard J, Guénot M, Ostrowsky K, Sindou M, Mauguière F (2000): The role of the insular cortex in temporal lobe epilepsy. *Ann Neurol* 48: 614–623.

Jack CR, Sharbrough FW, Cascino GD, Hirschorn KA, O'Brien PC, Marsh WR (1992): Magnetic resonance image–based hippocampal volumentry: Correlation with outcome after temporal lobectomy. *Ann Neurol* 31: 138–146.

Jack CR, Trenerry MR, Cascino GD, Sharbrough FW, So EL, O'Brien PC (1995): Bilaterally symmetric hippocampi and surgical outcome. *Neurology* 45: 1353–1358.

Jackson GD, Berkovic SF, Tress BM, Kalnins RM, Fabinyi GCA, Bladin PF (1990): Hippocampal sclerosis can be reliably detected by magnetic resonance imaging. *Neurology* 40: 1869–1869.

Jeha LE, Najm IM, Bingaman WE, *et al.* (2006): Predictors of outcome after temporal lobectomy for the treatment of intractable epilepsy. *Neurology* 27;66: 1938–1940.

Jeong SW, Lee SK, Hong KS, Kim KK, Chung CK, Kim H (2005): Prognostic factors for the surgery for mesial temporal lobe epilepsy: longitudinal analysis. *Epilepsia* 46: 1273–1279.

Jermakowicz WJ, Cijigas I, Dan L, *et al.* (2018): Ablation dynamics during laser interstitial thermal therapy for mesio-temporal epilepsy. *PLoS One* 13: e0199190.

Jobst BC, Kapur R, Barkley GL, *et al.* (2017): Brain responsive neurostimulation in patients with medically intractable seizures arising from eloquent and other neocortical areas. *Epilepsia* 58: 1005–1014.

Jones-Gotman M (1991). Presurgical neuropsychological evaluation for localization and lateralization of seizure focus. In Luders H (ed). *Epilepsy Surgery* pp. 469–475. New York: Raven Press.

Jones-Gotman M (1993): Word and design list learning deficits related to side of hippocampal atrophy as assessed by volumetric MRI measurement. *Epilepsia* 34: 71.

Kaiboriboon K, Bertrand ME, Osman MM, Hogan RE (2005): Quantitative analysis of cerebral blood flow patterns in mesial temporal lobe epilepsy using composite SISCOM. *J Nucl Med* 46: 38–43.

Kang JY, Wu C, Tracy J, Lorenzo M, Evans J (2015): Laser interstitial thermal therapy for medically intractable mesial temporal lobe epilepsy. *Epilepsia* 24.

Kanner AM, Ashman E, Gloss D, *et al.* (2018): Practice guideline update summary: Efficacy and tolerability of the new antiepileptic drugs II: Treatment-resistant epilepsy: Report of the American Epilepsy Society and the Guideline Development, Dissemination, and Implementation Subcommittee of the American Academy of Neurology. *Epilepsy Curr* 18: 269–278.

Kazemi NJ, Worrell GA, Stead SM, *et al.* (2010): Ictal SPECT statistical parametric mapping in temporal lobe epilepsy surgery. *Neurology* 74: 70–76.

Kobayashi E, Li LM, Lopes-Cendes I, Cendes F (2002): Magnetic resonance imaging evidence of hippocampal sclerosis in asymptomatic, first-degree relatives of patients with familial mesial temporal lobe epilepsy. *Arch Neurol* 59: 1891–1894.

Kotagal P, Lüders H, Morris HH, *et al.* (1989): Dystonic posturing in complex partial seizures of temporal lobe onset: A new lateralizing sign. *Neurology* 39: 196–201.

Kuzniecky R, Hugg J, Hetherington H, *et al.* (1999): Predictive value of 1H MRSI for outcome in temporal lobectomy. *Neurology* 53: 694–694.

Kwan P, Brodie MJ (2002): Refractory epilepsy; a progressive, intractable but preventable condition? *Seizure* 11: 77–84.

Kwon CS, Ripa V, Al-Awar O, Panov F, Ghatan S, Jetté N (2018): Epilepsy and Neuromodulation-Randomized Controlled Trials. *Brain* 8: 8.

Lattanzi S, Zaccara G, Giovannelli F, *et al.* (2019): Antiepileptic monotherapy in newly diagnosed focal epilepsy. A network meta-analysis. *Acta Neurol Scand* 139: 33–41.

Le S, Ho AL, Fisher RS, *et al.* (2018): Laser interstitial thermal therapy (LITT): Seizure outcomes for refractory mesial temporal lobe epilepsy. *Epi Behav* 89: 37–41.

Leutmezer F, Serles W, Lehrner J, Pataraia E, Zeiler K, Baumgartner C (1998): Postictal nose wiping: A lateralizing sign in temporal lobe complex partial seizures. *Neurology* 51: 1175–1177.

Li LM, Cendes F, Antel SB, *et al.* (2000): Prognostic value of proton magnetic resonance spectroscopic imaging for surgical outcome in patients with intractable temporal lobe epilepsy and bilateral hippocampal atrophy. *Ann Neurol* 47: 195–200.

Ludwig BI, Marsan CA (1975): Clinical ictal patterns in epileptic patients with occipital electroencephalographic foci. *Neurology* 25: 463–463.

Maillard L, Vignal J-P, Gavaret M, *et al.* (2004): Semiologic and electrophysiologic correlations in temporal lobe seizure subtypes. *Epilepsia* 45: 1590–1599.

Maldonado HM, Delgado-Escueta AV, Walsh GO, Swartz BE, Rand RW (1988): Complex Partial Seizures of hippocampal and amygdalar origin. *Epilepsia* 29: 420–433.

Markert MS, Fisher RS (2018): Neuromodulation - Science and Practice in Epilepsy: Vagus Nerve Stimulation, Thalamic Deep Brain Stimulation, and ResponsiveNeuroStimulation. *Expert Rev Neurother* 11: 1–13.

McIntosh AM, Kalnins RM, Mitchell LA, Fabinyi GC, Briellmann RS, Berkovic SF (2004): Temporal lobectomy: long-term seizure outcome, late recurrence and risks for seizure recurrence. *Brain* 127(Pt 9): 2018-2030. Epub 2004 Jun 23.

Mohamed A, Wyllie E, Ruggieri P, *et al.* (2001): Temporal lobe epilepsy due to hippocampal sclerosis in pediatric candidates for epilepsy surgery. *Neurology* 56: 1643–1649.

Newey CR, Wong C, Irene Wang Z, Chen X, Wu G, Alexopoulos AV (2013): Optimizing SPECT SISCOM analysis to localize seizure-onset zone by using varying z scores. *Epilepsia* 54: 793–800.

No YJ, Zavanone C, Bielle F, *et al.* (2017): Medial temporal lobe epilepsy associated with hippocampal sclerosis is a distinctive syndrome. *J Neurol* 264: 875–881.

Nobili L, Francione S, Cardinale F, Lo Russo G (2002): Epileptic nocturnal wanderings with a temporal lobe origin: a stereo-electroencephalographic study. *Sleep* 25: 669–671.

Ostrowsky K, Isnard J, Ryvlin P, Guénot M, Fischer C, Mauguiere F (2000): Functional mapping of the insular cortex: clinical implication in temporal lobe epilepsy. *Epilepsia* 41: 681–686.

Palmini A, Andermann F, Dubeau F, *et al.* (1999): Occipitotemporal relations: evidence for secondary epileptogenesis. *Adv Neurol* 81: 115–129.

Park SA, Heo K, Koh R, Chang JW, Lee BI (2001): Ictal automatisms with preserved responsiveness in a patient with left mesial temporal lobe epilepsy. *Epilepsia* 42: 1078–1081.

Penfield W, Faulk ME (1955): The insula; further observations on its function. *Brain* 78: 445–470.

Pisani F, Otero G, Russo MF, Di Perri R, Perucca E, Richens A (1999): The efficacy of valproate-lamotrigine comedication in refractory complex partial epilepsy: evidence for a pharmacodynamics interaction. *Epilepsia* 40: 1141–1146.

Risinger MW, Engel J, Van Ness PC, Henry TR, Crandall PH (1989): Ictal localization of temporal lobe seizures with scalp/sphenoidal recordings. *Neurology* 39: 1288–1293.

Salanova V, Witt T, Worth R, *et al.* (2015): Long-term efficacy and safety of thalamic stimulation for drug-resistant partial epilepsy. *Neurology* 84: 1017–1025.

Santulli L, Coppola A, Balestrini S, Striano S (2016): The challenges of treating epilepsy with 25 antiepileptic drugs. *Pharmacol Res* 107: 211–219.

Savitr Sastri BV, Arivazhagan A, Sinha S, *et al.* (2014): Clinico-pathological factors influencing surgical outcome in drug resistant epilepsy secondary to mesial temporal sclerosis. *J Neurol Sci* 340: 183–190.

Schiller Y (2009): Seizure relapse and development of drug resistance following long-term seizure remission. *Arch Neurol* 66: 1233–1239.

Schiller Y, Najjar Y (2008): Quantifying the response to antiepileptic drugs: effect of past treatment history. *Neurology* 70: 54–65.

Schmeiser B, Wagner K, Schulze-Bonhage A, *et al.* (2017): Transsylvian Selective Amygdalohippocampectomy for Mesio-temporal Epilepsy: Experience with 162 Procedures. *Neurosurg* 80: 454–464.

Schmeiser B, Wagner K, Schulze-Bonhage A, *et al.* (2018): Surgical Treatment of Mesio-temporal Lobe Epilepsy: Which Approach is Favorable? *Neurosurgery* 81: 992–1004.

Schmidt D, Gram L (1995): Monotherapy *vs.* polytherapy in epilepsy. A reappraisal. *CNS Drugs* 3: 194–208.

Schneider RC, Crosby EC, Farhat SM (1965): Extratemporal Lesions Triggering the Temporal-Lobe Syndrome: The Role of Association Bundles. *J Neurosurg* 22: 246–263.

Semah F, Baulac M, Hasboun D, *et al.* (1995): Is Interictal Temporal Hypometabolism Related to Mesial Temporal Sclerosis? A Positron Emission Tomography/Magnetic Resonance Imaging Confrontation. *Epilepsia* 36: 447–456.

Semah F, Picot MC, Adam C, *et al.* (1998): Is the underlying cause of epilepsy a major prognostic factor for recurrence? *Neurology* 51: 1256–1262.

Shin WC, Hong SB, Tae WS, Kim SE (2002): Ictal hyperperfusion patterns according to the progression of temporal lobe seizures. *Neurology* 58: 373–380.

Skarpaas TL, Jarosiewicz B, Morrell MJ (2019): Brain-responsive neurostimulation for epilepsy (RNS System). *Epilepsy Res* [Epub ahead of print].

Spanedda F, Cendes F, Gotman J (1997): Relations Between EEG Seizure Morphology, Interhemispheric Spread, and Mesial Temporal Atrophy in Bitemporal Epilepsy. *Epilepsia* 38: 1300–1314.

Spencer S, Huh L (2008): Outcomes of epilepsy surgery in adults and children. *Lancet Neurol* 7: 525–537.

Spencer S, Spencer D, Williamson P, Mattson R (1983): Sexual Automatisms in complex partial seizures. *Neurology* 33: 527–533.

Spencer SS, Spencer DD (1994): Entorhinal-Hippocampal Interactions in Medial Temporal Lobe Epilepsy. *Epilepsia* 35: 721–727.

Sutula G, Xiao-Xian H, Cavazos J, Scott G (1988): Synaptic reorganization in the hippocampus induced by abnormal functional activity. *Science* 239: 1147–1150.

Sutula, T, Cascino G, Cavazos J, Parada I, and Ramirez L (1989): Mossy fiber synaptic reorganization in the epileptic human temporal lobe. *Ann Neurol* 26: 321–330.

Talairach J, Bancaud J, Bonis A, Szikla G, Tournoux P (1962): Functional stereotaxic exploration of epilepsy. *SFN* 22: 328–331.

Tatum WO, Thottempudi N, Gupta V, Feyissa AM, Grewal SS, Wharen RE, Pizzi MA (2019): *De novo* temporal intermittent rhythmic delta activity after laser interstitial thermal therapy for mesial temporal lobe epilepsy predicts poor seizure outcome. *Clin Neurophysiol* 130: 122–127.

Tomson T, Battino D, Perucca E (2019): Teratogenicity of antiepileptic drugs. *Curr Opin Neurol* 32: 246–252.

Trenerry MR, Jack CR, Cascino GD, Sharbrough FW, So EL (1996): Bilateral Magnetic Resonance Imaging-Determined Hippocampal Atrophy and Verbal Memory Before and After Temporal Lobectomy. *Epilepsia* 37: 526–533.

Van Paesschen W, Dupont P, Van Driel G, Van Billoen H, Maes A (2003): SPECT perfusion changes during complex partial seizures in patients with hippocampal sclerosis. *Brain* 126: 1103–1111.

Van Paesschen W, Sisodiya S, Connelly A, *et al.* (1995): Quantitative hippocampal MRI and intractable temporal lobe epilepsy. *Neurology* 45: 2233–2240.

Vaugier L, Aubert S, McGonigal A, *et al.* (2009): Neural networks underlying hyperkinetic seizures of temporal lobe' origin. *Epilepsy Res* 86: 200–208.

Wada JA, Purves SJ (1984): Oral and bimanual-bipedal activity as ictal manifestations of frontal lobe epilepsy. *Epilepsia* 25: 668.

Walsh GO, Delgado-Escueta AV (1984): Type II complex partial seizures: poor results of anterior temporal lobectomy. *Neurology* (Cleveland) 34: 1–13.

Waseem H, Vivas AC, Vale FL (2017): MRI-guided laser interstitial thermal therapy for treatment of medically refractory non-lesional mesial temporal lobe epilepsy: Outcomes, complications, and current limitations: A review. *J Clin Neurosci* 38: 1–7.

Waterman L, Purves SJ, Kosaka B, Strauss E, Wada J (1987): An epileptic Syndrome caused by mesial frontal lobe foci. *Neurology* 7: 577–582.

Watson C, Jack CR, Cendes F (1997): Volumetric Magnetic Resonance Imaging: Clinical Applications and Contributions to the Understanding of Temporal Lobe Epilepsy. *Arch Neurol* 54: 1521–1531.

Wendling AS, Hirsch E, Wisniewski I, *et al.* (2013): Selective amygdalohippocampectomy *vs.* standard temporal lobectomy in patients with mesial temporal lobe epilepsy and unilateral hippocampal sclerosis. *Epilepsy Res* 104: 94–104.

Wennberg R, Arruda F, Quesney LF, Olivier A (2002): Preeminence of Extrahippocampal Structures in the Generation of Mesial Temporal Seizures: Evidence from Human Depth Electrode Recordings. *Epilepsia* 43: 716–726.

Wiebe S, Blume WT, Girvin JP, Eliasziv M (2001): Effectiveness and Efficiency of Surgery for Temporal Lobe Epilepsy Study Group. A randomized, controlled trial of surgery for temporal-lobe epilepsy. *N Engl J Med* 345: 311–318.

Wieser HG (1983): *Electroclinical Features of the Psychomotor Seizure*. Gustav Fisher, Butterworths, Stuttgart, London.

Wieser HG and Kausel W (1987): Limbic Seizures In: Wieser HG, Elger CE (eds): *Presurgical Evaluation of Epileptics*. pp 227–248. Berlin, Springer.

Wieser HG, Ortega M, Friedman A, Yonekawa Y (2003): Long-term seizure outcomes following amygdalohippocampectomy. *J Neurosurg* 98: 751–763.

Wieser HG, Siegel AM (1991): Analysis of Foramen Ovale Electrode-Recorded Seizures and Correlation with Outcome Following Amygdalohippocampectomy. *Epilepsia* 32: 838–850.

Wlliamson PD, Spencer SS (1986): Clinical and EEG features of complex partial seizures of extratemporal origin. *Epilepsia* 27 (Suppl. 2): S46–S63.

Wyler AR, Hermann BP, Somes G (1995): Extent of medial temporal resection on outcome from anterior temporal lobectomy: a randomized prospective study. *Neurosurgery* 37: 982–990; discussion 990–991.

Youngerman BE, Oh JY, Anbarasan D, Billakota S, *et al* (2018): Laser ablation is effective for temporal lobe epilepsy with and without mesial temporal sclerosis if hippocampal seizure onsets are localized by stereoelectroencephalography. *Epilepsia* 59: 595–606.

WITH VIDEO SUPPLEMENTS

CHAPTER 21

FRONTAL LOBE EPILEPSY SYNDROMES

Stefano Francione[1], Lino Nobili[2], Barbara Swartz[3], Laura Tassi[1], Roberto Mai[1], Massimo Cossu[1], Carlo Alberto Tassinari[4] and Antonio V. Delgado Escueta[5,6]

[1] Department of Neurosciences, Center for Epilepsy Surgery "C. Munari", Hospital Niguarda, Milan, Italy
[2] Child Neuropsychiatry Unit, IRCCS G. Gaslini Institute, DINOGMI-Department of Neurosciences, Rehabilitation, Ophthalmology, Genetics, Maternal and Child Health, University of Genoa, Genova, Italy
[3] Hoag Memorial Hospital Presbyterian, Newport Beach, California, and Children's Hospital of Orange County, Orange, USA
[4] University of Bologna, Bologna, Italy
[5] Epilepsy Genetics/Genomics Lab, Neurology and Research Services, VA Greater Los Angeles Healthcare System (VA GLAHS), University of California, Los Angeles, United States
[6] Department of Neurology, David Geffen School of Medicine, University of California, Los Angeles, USA

Introduction

Among patients with refractory or drug resistant focal epilepsies, frontal lobe epilepsy (FLE) accounts for about 20 to 30%. Such a percentage is mainly derived from surgical series, since reliable localization of FLE should be based on data obtained from a complex and complete diagnostic work-up, in general, utilized only for surgical aims (Jeha *et al.*, 2007). Moreover, an absolute certainty of localization is best reached when the patient is cured of epilepsy after surgical resection of its localized epileptogenic zones (EZ) (Kellinghaus & Lüders, 2004). Unfortunately, only few published series report data concerning frontal lobe epilepsy surgery in children (Kral *et al.*, 2001). Actually, data about frontal lobe epilepsy surgery in children can be derived from surgical series concerning frontal lobe epilepsy regardless of the age of the patients (Talairach *et al.*, 1992; Olivier, 1995; Laskowitz *et al.*, 1995; Jobst *et al.*, 2000; Jeha *et al.*, 2007; Nobili *et al.*, 2007; Kim *et al.*, 2010), or from surgical paediatric series regardless of the localization of the epilepsy (Fish *et al.*, 1993; Wyllie *et al.*, 1998; Paolicchi *et al.*, 2000; Francione *et al.*, 2003a; Sinclair *et al.*, 2004a; Cossu *et al.*, 2008; Krsek *et al.*, 2008, 2009a).

Bancaud & Talairach (1992), Fogarasi *et al.* (2001), Kellinghaus & Lüders (2004) collected very important information about general clinical features, seizure semiology, neuroimaging and histological findings in patients affected by FLE. From these series, it can be argued that FLE is frequent in children – probably even more than temporal lobe epilepsy (Lawson *et al.*, 2002) –, and that surgical results in children with FLE are, in general, more favourable than surgical results in adults with FLE (see Spencer & Huh, 2008 for a review).

Another interesting finding coming from these frontal lobe surgical series, is that the mean age at onset of epilepsy is most frequently in childhood, even if patients are operated on in adulthood (Kim *et al.*, 2010). Starting from this consideration – which depicts FLE as a prevalent paediatric disorder – and with the aim of providing a more comprehensive picture of this syndrome, we selected for this study a population of FLE patients who arrived at surgery at different ages, but had an epilepsy onset before the age of 16 years. Indeed, this selection criterion would also provide evidence of different surgical outcomes in relation to different durations of the illness.

Patients and methods

We reviewed retrospectively 643 patients who underwent resective surgery in the "Claudio Munari" Epilepsy Surgery Centre from May 1996 to December 2006 for drug-resistant focal epilepsy. We identified 125 cases (19.4%) in which surgery was performed in the frontal lobe, excluding the motor strip. Within these 125 cases, we selected 106 patients (84.8%) in which epilepsy onset was before the age of 16 years. This group of 106 patients was analyzed as a whole and then analyzed as two separate groups, namely, (a) patients who underwent surgery when they were below 16 years of age and (b) patients who underwent surgery after 16 years of age *(Table I)*.

Table I General clinical characteristics of the patients included in the study as a whole (Total pop) and subdivided in patients operated on before 16 years of age (group A) and after (group B)

	Total pop (106 pts)	Group A (51 pts)	Group B (55 pts)
Sex: m/f	57/49	26/25	31/24
Age at surgery	19.8 ± 11.9 yrs	9.8 ± 4.0 yrs	29.2 ± 8.8 yrs
Age at onset	4.6 ± 4.4 yrs	2.7 ± 3.0 yrs	6.4 ± 4.7 yrs
Duration	15.2 ± 10.8 yrs	7.1 ± 3.8 yrs	22.8 ± 9.5
▼ Seizure frequency			
Low	16 (15.1%)	6 (11.7%)	10 (18.2%)
Mid	21 (19.8%)	7 (13.7%)	14 (25.4%)
High	69 (65.1%)	38 (74.6%)	31 (56.4%)
Family history	29 (27.3%)	16 (31.4%)	13 (23.6%)
Prenatal ATCD	13 (12.2%)	12 (23.5%)	1 (1.8%)
Perinatal ATCD	16 (15.1%)	2 (3.9%)	14 (25.4%)
Febrile convulsions	2 (1.9%)	0	2 (3.6%)
Other ATCD	2 (1.9%)	2 (3.9%)	0
Neurological Ex.	6 (5.7%)	3 (5.9%)	3 (5.4%)
Cognitive problems	33 (31.1%)	22 (43.1%)	11 (20%)

Pts: patients; m: male, f: female; Seizure frequency: Low: till 8 seizures per month, Mid: 9 to 30 seizures per month, High: more than 30 seizures per month. ATCD: antecedents (see text for explanation). Percentages in brackets refer to the number of patients in each column.

All subjects were submitted to an individualized presurgical diagnostic protocol including:

(1) Accurate analysis of historical data, with particular attention to subjective and objective manifestations of ictal and possible postictal deficits.

(2) Interictal EEG and, when needed, long-term monitoring with video-taped clinical seizures and simultaneous ictal EEG recorded using scalp electrodes.

(3) High-resolution MRI, customized according to main electroclinical information employing a 1.5-tesla ACS-NT unit (Philips Medical Systems, Best, The Netherlands). Since in this population of patients, the electroclinical data pointed to a frontal lobe origin of seizures, the images were acquired parallel with and perpendicular to the antero-posterior commissure line, according to a previously reported protocol (Colombo *et al.*, 2003).

(4) Full neuropsychological testing, utilizing age-related protocols.

(5) For patients with inconclusive anatomo-electroclinical data as to the localization of the epileptogenic zone (EZ), stereo-electro-encephalography (SEEG) with stereotactically placed intracerebral electrodes was performed (Munari *et al.*, 1994; Cossu *et al.*, 2005), for a better definition of the EZ. An individualized arrangement of electrodes (exploration) was employed, according to a predefined localization hypothesis based on non-invasive findings. Following recording of spontaneous seizures, intracerebral electrical stimulations were used, when needed, to provide a functional mapping of motor and speech eloquent structures and to induce seizure or parts of seizure, with the aim of better defining the EZ.

At the end of presurgical evaluation, resective microsurgery was conducted according to the results of the anatomo-electroclinical investigations. Surgery was aimed at removal of the EZ, taking potential functional constraints into account to avoid new neurological deficits. All surgical specimens were routinely processed to obtain a histological diagnosis. Seizure outcome was assessed according to Engel's classification (Engel *et al.*, 1993). On the occasion of a first follow-up visit, EEG, neuropsychological testing and postoperative MRI examination were performed 6 months after surgery and then repeated at least every year for the first 5 years following surgery. Tapering of preoperative antiepileptic drug regimen was almost never considered before 12 months following surgery.

The following variables were analyzed in relation to the postoperative outcome on seizure frequency.

(1) Seizure frequency: three groups were identified: low frequency (less than 8 seizures/month), mid frequency (8–25 seizures/month), high frequency (more than 26 seizures/month).

(2) Preoperative MRI: normal (non-informative); doubtful (without a clearly defined lesion); multi-focal (with multiple lesions); positive unifocal (with a well-defined unique lesion independent of its size).

(3) Seizure type: considering the dominant signs of the most frequently presented episodes in each patient and classified, according to the International League Against Epilepsy (ILAE) glossary (Blume *et al.*, 2001) and other study concerning ictal semiology of frontal lobe seizures (Lüders *et al.*, 1999; Jobst & Williamson, 2005), in: (a) hypertonic (regardless mono or bilateral component), (b) hypokinetic (otherwise defined as "pseudoabsences" or "dialeptic" seizures), (c) hyperkinetic (otherwise defined as "hypermotor" or "bizarre hyperactive seizure"), (d) spasms, (e) clonic.

(4) Localization of surgery: (a) mesial (involving only the mesial aspect of the frontal lobe ± including the superior frontal gyrus and regardless the antero-posterior extension of the resection), (b) dorsolateral (involving the lateral aspect of the frontal lobe regardless the antero-posterior extension of the resection), (c) mesial + dorso-lateral (involving both mesial and lateral aspect of the frontal lobe for a limited extension), (d) orbito-polar (involving orbital cortex and/or the frontal pole), (e) lobar (involving the great majority of the frontal lobe both on the mesial and the lateral aspect).

(5) Histological result: (a) type I focal cortical dysplasia, or isolated lesions which present either as radial or tangential dyslamination of neocortex identified in one or multiple lobes; (b) type II focal cortical dysplasia, or isolated lesion characterized by cortical dyslamination and dysmorphic neurons with or without balloon cells (Palmini *et al.*, 2004; Blumcke *et al.*, 2011); (c) neoplastic lesions; (d) cortical tubers; (e) various pathologies.

Results

General characteristics of the studied population are presented in *Table I*. The total population of 106 patients was divided into two subgroups, namely those operated on in paediatric age (group A: 51 patients) and those operated on in adulthood (group B: 55 patients). Age at onset, by definition, shows that frontal lobe epilepsy starts in childhood, in general at 4.6 years of age. It is lower in group A (2.7 years) than in group B (6.4 years). Both groups showed a high seizure frequency, though higher in the pediatric age (74.6% group A; 56.4% in group B; NS: Fisher exact test). A family history was present in about one fourth of the whole group. Frequency of prenatal antecedents (mainly threatened miscarriage) was higher in the pediatric group (23.5 group A *vs.* 1.8% group B); an opposite distribution was evident for the presence of perinatal antecedents which is statically associated with patients operated on after 16 years of age (3.9% group A *vs.* 25.4% group B, $p = 2 \times 10^{-5}$; Fisher exact test). Frequency of febrile seizures was extremely low. Frequency of cognitive disturbances was statistically higher ($p = 0.01$; Fisher exact test) in the pediatric group (43.1% group A *vs.* 20% group B).

Considering seizure type (data are reported as a part of *Table II*), 40 patients presented with hypertonic seizures without differences between group A and B. Hypokinetic seizures occurred in 24 patients with a similar distribution in the two groups while hyperkinetic seizures showed a prevalence in the adult population (17 *vs.* 5 cases, $p = 0.02$; Fisher exact test). Spasms were observed only in group A and clonic seizures occurred in 7 patients, 2 in group A and 5 in group B.

Diagnostic and surgical features are reported in *Table III*. MRI showed a clear focal lesion in the majority of patients of both groups. Negative MRI prevailed in adults, while multiple lesions and doubtful abnormalities were slightly more frequent in group A (NS). A minority of patients, all lesional, underwent surgery without ictal recordings due to a clear coherence between the site of the lesion and the anamnestic data; it is possible to note a slight difference between group A and B concerning stereo-EEG exploration, more often performed in group B. There is a global prevalence, without intergroup difference, of surgery performed in the right hemisphere. Globally the most frequent localization of the resection was in the mesial structures, and this is the case also in group B, while in group A, dorsolateral resections prevailed ($p = 0.08$; Fisher exact test). Only transient postoperative morbidity was observed and it consisted in the vast majority of cases in motor deficits contralateral to the side of surgery, ascribable to resection of the supplementary motor area (Krainik *et al.*, 2001).

Type II FCD was the commonest histological diagnosis overall and in each group. Tumoral pathology, slightly more frequent in group B, in detail consisted in: dysembryoplastic neuroepithelial tumor in 10 cases, pilocytic astrocytoma in 6 cases, ganglioglioma and grade II oligodendroglioma in one case each. Other pathologies included: gliosis in 6 cases, cortical scar in 2 patients and cavernous angioma in one. The great majority of cortical tubers was found in group A.

After a mean follow-up period of 93.4 months, surgical outcome following Engel's classification is listed in *Table IV*: overall 72.4% were seizure-free with a slightly better outcome in group A (74.5 *vs.* 70.4%; NS); class II outcome seems to prevail slightly more in group B and no statistically significant difference appears. Forty nine percent of children in group A had already stopped medical treatment *vs.* 37% of adults, in group B, where the majority of the cured patients is still tapering their antiepileptic drugs.

Table II **Analysis of seizure outcome in relation to different pre- and post-surgical variables of the patients included in the study as a whole (Total pop) and subdivided in patients operated on before 16 years of age (group A) and after (group B)**

		Total pop	Group A			Group B		
		Tot. (% class I)	Tot A	Class I	Non class I	Tot B	Class I	Non class I
Seizure frequency	Low	16 (87.5)	6	6 (100)	–	10	8 (80)	2 (20)
	Mid	20 (70)	7	6 (85.7)	1 (14.3)	13	8 (61.5)	5 (38.5)
	High	69 (69.5)	38	26 (68.4)	12 (31.6)	31	22 (70.9)	9 (29.1)
MRI	Norm	16 (50)	5	3 (60)	2 (40)	11	5 (45)	6 (65)
	Doubt	10 (50)	7	4 (57)	3 (43)	3	1 (33.4)	2 (66.6)
	Multi	7 (29)	4	0	4 (100)	3	2 (66.6)	1 (33.4)
	Pos	72 (85)	35	31 (89)	4 (11)	37	30 (81)	7 (19)
Seizure semiology	HyperT	40 (57.5)	21	14 (66.7)	7 (33.3)	19	9 (47.4)	10 (52.6)
	HypoK	24 (91.3)	10	10 (100)	0	14	11 (78.6)	3 (21.4)
	HyperK	22 (81.8)	5	3 (60)	2 (40)	17	15 (88.2)	2 (11.8)
	Spasm	13 (76.9)	13	10 (76.9)	3 (23.1)	–	–	–
	Clonic	7 (57.1)	2	1 (50)	1 (50)	5	3 (60)	2 (40)
Surgery localisation	Mes	33 (66.7)	11	8 (72.7)	3 (27.3)	22	14 (63.6)	8 (36.4)
	DL	26 (73.1)	16	11 (68.7)	5 (31.3)	10	8 (80)	2 (20)
	Mes+DL	19 (68.4)	7	6 (85.7)	1 (14.3)	12	7 (58.3)	5 (41.7)
	Orb	10 (90)	7	6 (85.7)	1 (14.3)	3	3 (100)	–
	Lob	17 (76.5)	10	7 (70)	3 (30)	7	6 (85.7)	1 (14.3)
Histology	T I FCD	18 (44.4)	10	6 (60)	4 (40)	8	2 (25)	6 (75)
	T II FCD	47 (89.4)	22	18 (81.8)	4 (18.2)	25	24 (96)	1 (4)
	Tumoral	18 (77.7)	7	6 (85.7)	1 (14.3)	11	8 (72.7)	3 (27.3)
	Tubers	13 (61.5)	11	7 (63.6)	4 (36.4)	2	1 (50)	1 (50)
	Other	9 (44.4)	1	1	–	8	3 (37.5)	5 (62.5)

Seizure frequency: see legend *Table I*; MRI: see text for explanation; Seizure Semiology: HyperT: hypertonic, HypoK: hypokinetic, HyperkK: hyperkinetic; Surgery Localisation: see text for explanation. For the column Total pop, percentages in brackets refer to the number of patients in each single cell; for the columns group A and group B, numbers in brackets are percentages referring to the number of patients in the corresponding raw.

Table III Diagnostic and surgical variables of the patients included in the study as a whole (total pop) and subdivided in patients operated on before 16 years of age (group A) and after (group B)

	Total pop	Group A	Group B
▼ MRI			
Negative	17 (16.1%)	5 (9.8%)	12 (21.8%)
Doubtful	10 (9.4%)	7 (13.7%)	3 (5.5%)
Multiple	7 (6.6%)	4 (7.8%)	3 (5.5%)
Focal lesion	72 (67.9%)	35 (68.6%)	37 (67.2%)
▼ Presurg. investigation			
No ictal recordings	7 (6.6%)	3 (5.9%)	4 (7.2%)
Video-EEG	34 (32.1%)	19 (37.2%)	15 (27.3%)
Stereo-EEG	65 (61.3%)	29 (56.9%)	36 (65.5%)
Side of surgery: R/L	61/45	30/21	31/24
▼ Localisation of surgery			
Mesial	33 (31.1%)	11 (21.6%)	22 (40%)
Dorsal	26 (24.5%)	16 (31.4%)	10 (18.2%)
Mesial + dorsal	19 (17.9%)	7 (13.7%)	12 (21.8%)
Orbito-polar	11 (10.4%)	7 (13.7%)	4 (7.3%)
Lobar	17 (16.1%)	10 (19.6%)	7 (12.7%)
▼ Histology:			
Type I FCD	18 (17.0%)	10 (19.6%)	8 (14.5%)
Type II FCD	48 (45.3%)	22 (43.2%)	26 (47.3%)
Tumoral	18 (17.0%)	7 (13.7%)	11 (20.0%)
Tubers	13 (12.2%)	11 (21.6%)	2 (3.7%)
Other	9 (8.5%)	1 (1.9%)	8 (14.5%)

R: right; L: left. Percentages in brackets refer to the number of patients in each column.

In *Table II* some clinical, morphological, surgical and histological variables are reported in relation to the surgical outcome.

In the overall population, seizure frequency seems to be inversely correlated with surgical results, and this is particularly evident in group A patient but no difference between group A and group B with respect to outcome was statistically significant.

The presence of a focal MRI abnormality is correlated with a better outcome in both groups, while a negative MRI or the presence of multiple lesions seems to negatively influence the post-surgical outcome.

Concerning seizure semiology, hypertonic seizures show a lower percentage of cured patients than other seizure types ($p = 0.02$; Fisher exact test), with consistently better results in group A. Conversely, hypokinetic seizures were related to a very good surgical outcome, compared to other seizure types ($p = 0.04$; Fisher exact test), especially in group A. Hyperkinetic seizures show a high percentage of surgical success in group B. Seizures appearing as spasms also had surgical success and was observed only in group A. No differences were noted between group A and group B as far as clonic seizures were concerned and an unsatisfactory outcome was present in both groups.

Considering resection topography, good results were obtained in orbito-polar localization in the whole population; mesial + dorsolateral surgery showed a good outcome only in group A while lobectomies seemed to be related with a better outcome in group B.

Histological findings illustrate a statistically significant observation, namely, that surgical resection of Type II FCD is more successful in relieving seizures compared to surgery of Type I FCD ($p = 0.0003$; Fisher exact test). In general, a relatively bad outcome is present for surgery in Type I FCD in the total population, although apparently better in group A (NS). Type II FCD are linked to the best surgical results in both groups, again apparently better in group B (NS). As far as tumour pathology, a better outcome seems to be present in group A but the number of patients is too small (NS).

Table IV **Follow-up, seizure outcome following Engel's Classification and post-operative drug treatment of the patients included in the study as a whole (total pop) and subdivided in patients operated on before 16 years of age (group A) and after (group B)**

	Total population	Group A	Group B
Follow-up	93.4 ± 32.8 months	92.0 ± 33.4 months	94.7 ± 32.1 months
▼ Engel's Class			
I	76 (72.4%)	38 (74.5%)	38 (70.4%)
Ia	68 (64.7%)	34 (66.7%)	34 (62.9%)
II	7 (6.6%)	1 (1.9%)	6 (11.1%)
III	13 (12.4%)	7 (13.7%)	6 (11.1%)
IV	9 (8.6%)	5 (9.8%)	4 (7.4%)
▼ Drugs			
Unchanged	26 (24.8%)	13 (25.5%)	13 (24.1%)
On tapering	34 (32.4%)	13 (25.5%)	21 (38.9%)
Stopped	45 (42.8%)	25 (49.0%)	20 (37.0%)

Discussion

FLE is relatively frequent in surgical series, and this is confirmed by our population which accounts for *circa* 20% of the total "operated on" patients in the Claudio Munari Epilepsy Surgery Centre in the same period. The difference between our series and other reported surgical populations (in which such a percentage can reach 30%) could be due to the exclusion from the studied population of the patients where part of the motor strip has also been removed.

From the present study, conducted in a large population of drug-resistant FLE patients, clearly emerges the concept that FLE is mainly a paediatric syndrome. Eighty-four percent of the whole population started having seizure under the age of 16 years. Moreover, the mean age at which seizures started in the 106 patients was 4.4 years. This indicates prepubertal onset in the majority of cases.

The overall surgical results on seizure frequency (72.4% of Class I patients), can be considered more than satisfactory if not close to excellent. A slightly better outcome obtained in group A patients (74.5 *vs.* 70.4%; NS) is not statistically significant but the trend seems to suggest that an earlier indication to surgery could increase the percentage of success in this localization. The approach we choose for this study can probably give some suggestion for explaining this difference. Also considering that the global features of our population seem to be superimposable to those reported in literature, even if comparative studies have never been attempted before.

As expected and largely reported in literature (Lawson *et al.*, 2002; Sinclair *et al.*, 2004b), seizure frequency is considerably high, with 65.1% of cases presenting with at least one seizure per day. It looks even higher in the patients who had surgery in childhood.

Even if a clear interpretation is lacking, it seems important to underline the great difference in pre and perinatal antecedents' distribution in the two groups. In fact, the only study dealing with pre and perinatal antecedents we found in literature (Krsek *et al.*, 2010) was limited to children having a cortical dysplasia, without comparison with adults, and without taking early pregnancy problems into account. These authors find that a perinatal adverse event is correlated with the presence of a "low grade focal cortical dysplasia", but the data emerging from our study underline a correlation between early pregnancy problems (mainly threatened miscarriage) and surgery performed in childhood, thus suggesting a more severe picture of the epilepsy in these cases. Therefore, we suggest that pregnancy course and perinatal variables should be better specified and analyzed in further studies on FLE.

Our data stress how febrile convulsions have a very low incidence in FLE, especially when compared to temporal lobe epilepsy (Fish *et al.*, 1993; Lawson *et al.*, 2002).

The high percentage of cognitive disturbances in group A patients could be linked to the severity of the illness and could, in part, explain their earlier surgical indication. In fact, the few available literature data report a high frequency of attention deficits, executive functions and motor coordination disturbances in both the pre-operative evaluation of children suffering from FLE (Lendt *et al.*, 2002; Chieffo *et al.*, 2011), and also in a population of children with FLEs not specifically studied in a surgical perspective (Braakman *et al.*, 2011). The lower incidence of these deficits in group B cases probably has multiple reasons: part of these deficits (mainly the motor) could be compensated during the development even with the persistence of seizures; the presence of a higher epilepsy severity with a greater impact on cognition in group A patients; finally, we can hypothesize that the indication for surgical treatment is not retained in adult patients with a strong cognitive impairment.

Our findings on seizure semiology confirm literature data about hyperkinetic seizures which are not common in the paediatric age, whereas spasms are an almost exclusive ictal pattern of even younger patients (Fogarasi *et al.*, 2001).

Largely more than half of our patients underwent an invasive neurophysiologic study by means of intracerebral electrodes, thus confirming the difficulties for a precise localization diagnosis in FLE cases (Bancaud & Talairach, 1992; Swartz *et al.*, 1998; Jobst *et al.*, 2000; Jeha *et al.*, 2007). Nonetheless it must be noted, as already suggested in previous studies (Mariottini *et al.*, 2001; Kim *et al.*, 2010), that even in this particularly difficult population, very selected patients can undergo surgery just after a careful anamnestic and neuroimaging evaluation, more or less corroborated by ictal Video-EEG monitoring (see *Figures 1 and 2* for examples).

Histological findings in our series correspond well to previously reported surgical populations (Frater *et al.*, 2000), in particular FCD (classified following Palmini *et al.*, 2004) is the most frequent pathological entity (with a strong prevalence of Type II FCD) followed by neoplastic lesions and, only in group A patients, by cortical tubers.

On the basis of two previous studies that looked at the recurrence of seizures after frontal lobe surgery (Jeha *et al.*, 2007; Kim *et al.*, 2010), we defined a minimum post-surgical follow-up of 4 years. In fact, both Jeha *et al.* and Kim *et al.* show that recurrence of postoperative seizures is maximal in the first 3 years after surgery, and do not significantly vary after this time span. Consequently our surgical results could be considered as, almost, definitive.

As a whole, seizure outcome in our population is quite good with 72.4% of patients in Engel's class I. Taking the long follow-up period into account, our results are consistently better than those reported in most of the previous FLE surgical series. In particular, considering the two previously quoted papers with a long follow-up, the percentage of Engel class I patients after at least 3 years of follow up in these two series is about 50%. Our data further suggest a better result from surgery when performed in childhood, since the percentage of "cured" patients is higher in group A cases. Moreover, a greater number of children reached "drug-freedom" after surgery compared to patients who were operated on when adults: 49% *vs.* 37%. The drug withdrawal issue is not specifically addressed in the literature in terms of surgery localisation and age at surgery (see Schmidt *et al.*, 2004 for a review); in this view our data suggest that also in FLE patients, a complete drug discontinuation can be achieved after surgery, especially when facing a relatively short illness duration.

Data reported in *Table IV* seem to suggest that some anatomo-electroclinical variables have a prognostic significance on the surgical outcome. A high seizure frequency is, in general, considered to be related to a poorer surgical outcome. Nonetheless, when analyzed in frontal lobe surgical series, this data never reach a statistically significant level. Indeed, in the present population, the high seizure frequency category (both in group A and B) show less seizure freedom, although even in this highly seizing patients, the percentage of Class I outcome is about 70%.

One of the most frequently considered prognostic variable in literature is MRI, and there is an almost global consensus about its importance in defining the surgical prognosis. When neuroimaging data are not informative (*i.e.*, negative, or doubtful or multiple lesion/foci) surgical results are consistently less favourable (Mosewich *et al.*, 2000; Chapman *et al.*, 2005; Lee *et al.*, 2005; Bien *et al.*, 2009). This is also the case in our population where just about 50% of patients with a non-focal MRI abnormality reached seizure freedom. This data must be carefully interpreted, since it could lead to an oversimplified conclusion that the epileptogenic zone is always within and about the lesion (Awad *et al.*, 1991; Bourgeois *et al.*, 1999; Aubert *et al.*, 2009). This is probably the fact in cases of very focal lesions with a high epileptogenic potential such as single cortical tubers (Teutonico *et al.*, 2008) or Type II focal cortical dysplasia (Tassi *et al.*, 2002; 2012), where concordance and coherence of electro-clinical data with the lesional site is verified. In most of the cases, the MRI abnormality is useful in guiding the diagnostic steps, including, as it is often the case in our series, the realisation of a more targeted intracerebral exploration, aimed at defining the real extension and borders of the epileptogenic zone (Francione *et al.*, 2003b; McGonigal *et al.*, 2007). A good example of the prognostic role of the MRI is given in *Figure 1*. It compares two patients with cortical tubers, the first with an isolated tuber, and the second with multiple tubers. In the first case, complete seizure-free outcome has been obtained after lesionectomy, while in the second case, seizures persist, despite the complete resection of the tuber whose etiologic role for seizures generation was established on the basis of apparently coherent/concordant clinical and electrical video-EEG data.

Seizure semiology is strictly linked with the localisation of the epileptogenic zone (Bancaud & Talairach, 1992; Lüders *et al.*, 1993; Bartolomei & Chauvel, 2000). In this sense, the unsatisfactory results in patients with hypertonic seizures could be explained by the early involvement of the motor region, by definition spared by surgical resection. It seems particularly interesting to underline, however, that group A patients with hypertonic seizures show a significantly better outcome. An explanation of this finding could be the longer duration the motor region is exposed, in group B patients, to the epileptogenic effect of ictal and interictal discharges – possibly originating from the premotor cortex of the mesial frontal lobe (Baumgartner *et al.*, 1996; Morris *et al.*, 1998; Nobili *et al.*, 2003). This prolonged exposure could induce a secondary, stable and autonomous, epileptogenicity of this area. These assumptions may also be true in clonic seizures, where, in fact, a poor surgical outcome has been obtained in both groups of patients.

Spasms, a type of seizure that has undergone a long debate on its etiopathogenetic mechanisms (see Holmes & Vigevano, 1997 and Wong & Trevathan, 2001 for a review), are now more and more frequently considered for surgical treatment (Kramer *et al.*, 1997; Asano *et al.*, 2001). We can underline how young patients suffering from these seizures, can reach very good results. The surgical failures in patients with spasms are probably not determined by their semiology, but by their underlying pathology, in particular multiple cortical tubers (Teutonico *et al.*, 2008) or Type I focal cortical dysplasia (Krsek *et al.*, 2008, 2009a).

Very good results have also been obtained in patients, especially in adults, with hyperkinetic/hypermotor seizures. In the context of "frontal" syndromes, these seizures represent a peculiar condition and were referred to as hypermotor (Luders *et al.*, 1999) or hyperkinetic (Blume *et al.*, 2001) with a complex semiology (Wash & Delgado-Escueta, 1984; Wada & Purves, 1984; Williamson *et al.*, 1985; Wada, 1989; Fusco *et al.*, 1990; Montagna, 1992; Swartz, 1994; Hirsch *et al.*; 1994, Oldani *et al.*, 1998; Provini *et al.*, 1999).
a) In 1972, Tharp reported: "Three children had strikingly similar seizures" with abrupt appearance, frightened facial expression, with stamping of the feet or running; frequent nocturnal episodes during which a 11 years old boy abruptly sit up in the bed, rock back and forth scream loudly... call for a family member and return promptly to sleep". One child had a resection of the right frontal lobe with gliotic tissue in the lateral orbitofrontal region and remained seizure free and resumed regular schooling.
b) Wada and Purves (1984) described these seizures in adults as follows: "Clinical episodes, often nocturnal, recur repetitively with short intervals, displaying screaming, yelling, coughing, whining, labored breathing, and bimanual-bipedal activity, in addition to occasional versive movements, laughter, oral automatisms, and genital manipulation, while retaining intact awareness, intermittent responsiveness, or becoming totally nonresponsive. Interictal epileptiform abnormality may be completely absent."

Such events when occurring during wakefulness can be misdiagnosed as psychogenic seizures and during sleep can be confounded with parasomnias posing difficult diagnostic problems (Scheffer *et al.*, 1994; Biraben *et al.*, 2001; Proserpio *et al.*, 2001; Bartolomei *et al.*, 2004; Mai *et al.*, 2005; Gardella *et al.*, 2006; Tinuper *et al.*, 2007; Derry *et al.*, 2009; Gibbs *et al.*, 2019 a, b). Common shared semiological features of some epileptic seizures (see infra) and parasomnias might be explained by the activation of the same neuronal network, the "Central Pattern Generators (CPG). CPG are functional neuronal aggregates present in all vertebrates, located from brain stem to pons, down to lumbar spinal cord subserving automatic rhythmic motor sequences (respiration, swallowing locomotion, reproduction, emotion (Tassinari *et al.*, 2003), *i.e.* specific behaviors, responsible for the survival (Grillner & Wallen, 1985). The CPG system is under control – so to say – "bracked" by the cortical neomammalian brain. When such cortical control is transitorily disrupted by an epileptic seizure, or a sleep related arousal disorder, as in parasomnias (Parrino *et al.*, 2006), or by an anoxic event (Iani *et al.*, 1996; Ambrosetto *et al.*, 2009), then released CPG produce motor automatic sequences.

Such interpretation (Tassinari *et al.*, 2005,2006,2009) is supported by the following data:
1. PET studies (Guedj *et al.*, 2012) "aimed at the identification of selective brain regions involved in hyperkinetic seizures have documented a specific subcortical hypometabolism in bilateral midbrain and caudate systems involved in generation of primitive motor program", such as CPG;
2. Ictal SPECT evidence of hyperperfusion during hypermotor seizures leading to the conclusion that "certain areas in the brain stem are involved in the pathogenesis of hypermotor seizures which could be referred to CPG" (Masuda *et al.*, 2012).
3. The report of a video-SEEG, revealing in hyperkinetic seizures a "bifocal organization of the epilepsy with two distinct cortical origins of seizures: right temporal pole and left temporal lateral and perisylvian cortex. Irrespective of the cortical pattern of seizure onset the hyperkinetic semiology is extremely similar. This supports a major role for "final common pathway" subcortical circuits in the genesis of hyperkinetic semiology" (Vaugiers *et al.*, 2009, 2017).

Along the same line, should be considered that hyperkinetic seizures were already observed, the epileptogenic zone being the temporal lobe (Swartz, 1994; Nobili *et al.*, 2002, 2004), or the insula (Ryvlin *et al.*, 2006) or the parietal lobe (Swartz, 1995). Accordingly, an expert consensus suggested to drop the terminology "Frontal" to refer to hyperkinetic seizures, suggesting alternatively the terminology "Sleep related Hypermotor Epilepsy" or SHE (Tinuper *et al.*, 2016). Different epileptogenic zones give the same symptomatologic expression: this leads to the "carillon theory": independently from either the topography of the epileptogenic zone or the etiology,when the lid of the carillon is open the same motor symphony will flow.

The long term (16 years) outcome of sleep related hypermotor epilepsy (SHE) in a retrospective study of a large cohort (139 patients) is poor (Lichetta *et al.*, 2017) rendering surgical therapy more relevant.

Finally, the efficacy of surgical treatment in cases of hypokinetic seizures, also known as frontal lobe pseudoabsences or dialeptic seizures, especially in children is really impressive. In accordance with literature (Munari & Bancaud, 1992; Munari *et al.*, 1995), the most probable origin of this kind of seizures is in the anterior part of the frontal lobe and this is also our experience. This is well confirmed, indeed, by the fact that in orbito-polar resections, the results are almost as satisfying. A clear example of this kind of patients is reported in *Figure 2* where the pre and postoperative MRI of 2 different patients, both suffering from hypokinetic seizures and both with a tumour lesion (dysembryoplastic neuroepithelial tumor) of the fronto-polar cortex, are shown; the first one, a 14 years old girl, has been cured, after a relatively short epilepsy history, by a complete lesionectomy, whereas the adult patient, operated on more than 40 years after the beginning of the illness, is still presenting seizures (even if reduced in number and intensity) despite a complete removal of the tumour and the adjacent dysplastic cortex. Also in this case, as for the hypertonic type of seizures, we could hypothesize a role of the duration of the epilepsy in the induction of epileptogenetic phenomena inside the extralesional tissues.

Concerning the localization of the resection, the optimal results obtained in the orbito-polar region should probably be ascribed to the absence of eloquent cortex in this area, which allows a more confident surgical approach. On the other hand, both in the posterior part of the mesial aspect (close to the paracentral lobule) and in the dorso-lateral part of the dominant frontal lobe, functional reasons could induce a less extensive resection, thus explaining worse results (Lee *et al.*, 2005; Kim *et al.*, 2010). The functional limitation plays a less important role in children, especially when youngest, since it is well known that brain plasticity could help in avoiding, or rapidly recovering, the functional deficits eventually caused by surgery (Freitag & Tuxhorn, 2005; Loddenkemper *et al.*, 2007).

In accordance with literature and the consensus classification proposed by an ILAE task force (Blumcke *et al.*, 2011), our results confirm that histological substrate of focal epilepsy exerts a big influence on surgical outcome. Paradigmatic in this sense, is the difference between surgical outcome of Type I and Type II FCD, where the latter shows an optimal outcome with twice as many cured patients. This issue has been largely discussed in literature (Tassi *et al.*, 2002; Krsek *et al.*, 2008, 2009a) and there is an almost complete agreement on the widespread nature of Type I FCD, whereas Type II FCD could be considered as the "template" of the "focal" epileptogenic lesion.

Why could Type I FCD be less successfully removed by surgical resection? In Type I FCD, part of the pathological tissue could have been left behind. The incomplete removal of the "lesion", however, seems to play a less important role in group A patients who had surgery before 16 years of age. Class I surgical outcome, though less satisfactory than in other pathological entity, is around 60% in group A patients against 25% in group B cases. Obviously, the pathological process of Type I FCD, being widespread in both groups A and B, and given the same the diagnostic and surgical approaches, it is difficult to hypothesize that a more complete lesion removal only occurred in children. Instead, we could infer that not all lesional tissues have the same epileptogenic potential. Early surgery, removing the "core" of the dysplasia, could have greatly reduced the probability of the remaining pathological cortex to be autonomous in seizures generation (see the case report in *Figures 4 to 7* for an example).

A different scenario is present in Type II FCD where, starting from a very good outcome for both groups, better surgical results were obtained when surgery was performed after 16 years of age (group B cases). Multiple reasons must be taken into account when trying to explain why some patients did not achieve surgical success when surgery was performed earlier before 16 years of age. Indeed, incomplete cortical maturation could reduce the ability of the pre-operative MRI in precisely defining the actual limits of the dysplasia, which can become evident only once the maturation phenomena are achieved. This limitation could probably prevent the total removal of the lesion in a higher percentage of group A patients. Total removal is always mandatory for reaching seizure freedom in this type of lesions (Krsek *et al.*, 2009b). It is also possible that when FCD is located in the vicinity of eloquent cortex, the level of collaboration of adult patients probably plays a major role. In fact, fMRI especially for language function, is not feasible in the majority of children, while in adults, this relatively simple and non invasive methodology gives reliable and determinant information for a successful surgical approach. An example of this eventuality is given in *Figure 3*, where the effective localization of the frontal language area was realized by fMRI in the adult patient, allowing the complete resection of the dysplasia with a class I surgical outcome without any residual deficit. Whereas, for the other patient in the same figure, a 6 years old boy at the moment of the first surgery, the impossibility of individualizing the frontal language areas by fMRI and electrical stimulations during the stereo-EEG exploration led to a conservative surgical strategy, unavoidably inducing a bad surgical outcome, for which the patient had to be further reconsidered for surgery.

Finally, the better results obtained in group A patients with tumour pathology could confirm the important role of illness duration in the enlargement of the brain area responsible of seizure generation (Bourgeois *et al.*, 1999).

In conclusion, literature data, well corroborated by the results of the present series, confirm that FLE is a disorder of children and a common pathological entity in childhood. Even if these data are extracted from surgical series, they represent an objective picture of the clinical and anatomo-electrical features of the patients suffering from epilepsies with this peculiar localization. Considering the high frequency of drug-resistance in these cases, our results suggest that surgery should be considered an effective, if not close to excellent treatment option. Moreover, as clearly appears from our "comparative" analysis of surgery before and after 16 years of age, a more precocious and early surgical work-up has to be done in order to give these patients the actual possibility of antiepileptic drug withdrawal and a cure, thus reducing the negative impact of frontal lobe epilepsy on global development and quality of life.

Cases Figure 1

The first case (a, b) is a right-handed girl operated on at almost 7 years of age, without relevant familial and personal antecedents. Her seizures started when she was 11 months old, with brief and very frequent episodes of psychomotor arrest followed by a left deviation of the eyes. A first EEG showed left fronto-temporal spikes, and a treatment by Valproate was started inducing seizures freedom till the age of 2 years. After the reappearance, despite multiple changes in drug treatment, seizures will never be controlled for prolonged periods. Numerous ictal events have been recorded in different Video-EEG recordings during the evolution; they were not completely identical under a clinical point of view (the only common element being a long-lasting staring with left orientation of the head at the beginning), but always showed a clear ictal discharge localized in the left anterior frontal region. Interictal EEG showed a progressive worsening with abundant abnormalities mainly expressed over the left frontal region, as both slow waves and spikes, but also with very frequent long-lasting bursts of spike-and-waves complexes with a diffuse localization, especially during sleep. The first MRI, performed in 2000, showed a lesion in the anterior part of the left superior frontal gyrus. At the time of surgery (May, 2003), seizures had a daily frequency, with predominance at the awakening. Despite the age, the child was not yet going to the primary school and the cognitive evaluation showed a global delay in cognitive development with an IQ at the lower limit of the normal range and, mainly, a clear deficit in language functions with no writing and reading capabilities. MRI (a) confirmed the presence of a T2 and FLAIR hyper-intense and T1 and IR hypo-intense nodular lesion in the anterior part of the left superior frontal gyrus, whose MRI features could recall a cortical tuber. No other sign of tuberous sclerosis were found at the clinical examination, at the echography of the heart, liver and kidneys and at the ophthalmologic examination. Surgery consisted in a complete lesionectomy of the MRI visible lesion; histological examination revealed, in fact, a cortical tuber. The patient is seizure free from surgery, drugs started to be tapered at 1 year follow-up and stopped at 4 years

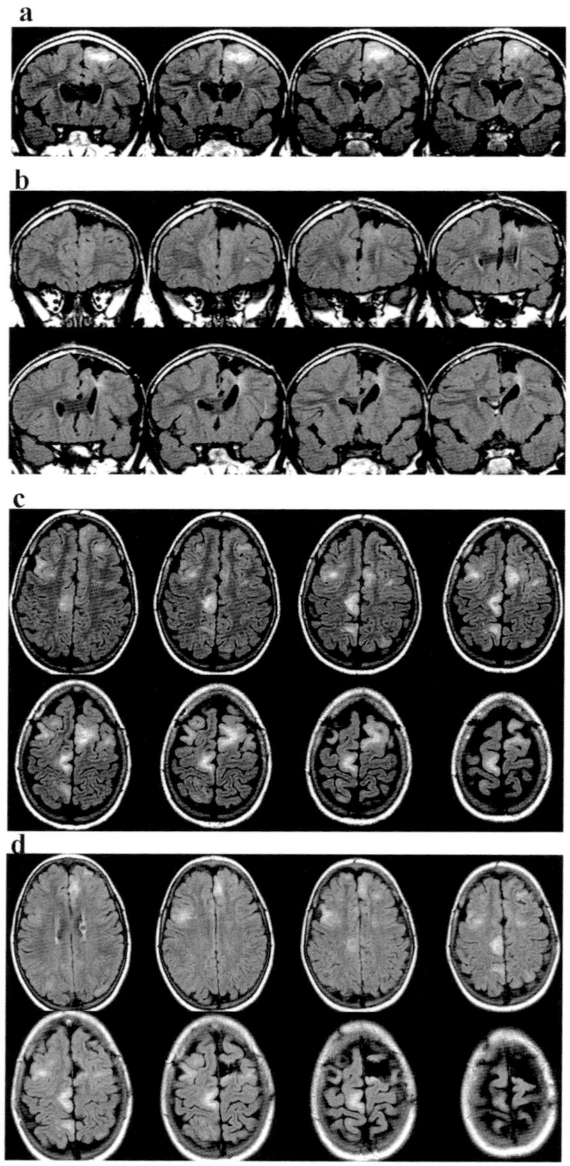

Figure 1 **Pre-operative** (a, c) **and postoperative** (b, d) **MRI of 2 operated on patients (FLAIR sequences).**

follow-up. The child is now going at the secondary school, with a good recovery in cognitive functions. Post-operative MRI at 6 months follow-up (b) showed the complete removal of the lesion.

The second case (c, d) is a right-handed girl operated on at the age of 13 years. In the family, one cousin was reported to have tuberous sclerosis, while the patient did not show any personal antecedent for epilepsy. The first seizure occurred at 10 months: long-lasting episode mainly characterized by jerks of the right limbs associated with right deviation of the head and the eyes. Drug treatment was started at that moment, but no clear effect on seizures was evident, they were reported to continue with a daily frequency, mainly nocturnal; this situation went on till the moment of surgery despite numerous modifications of the medical treatment. Seizure semiology was almost constant during all this period: the patient reports a sensation of diffuse tingling without predominance in any part of the body, in general she is able to warn calling the parents with no more than a single word. After the sensation a brief psychomotor arrest is present, followed by a global stiffening, clearly more marked on the right part of the body. Seizures are in general shorter than 30", without a complete loss of contact and a clear postictal language deficit, but followed by an hypostenia of the right part of the body; presentation in clusters is at least montly. Diagnosis of tuberous sclerosis was made after the first CT scan (showing multiple calcified lesions in both hemispheres) corroborated by the presence of multiple hypochromic skin lesions and of a Pringle's adenoma around the nose. Echography showed lesions also in both kidneys and in the hart. Cognitive evaluation showed a global IQ of 70 with a better performance in visual than in verbal tests. Video-EEG recordings, performed in different moments of the evolution, last at 4 months before surgery, showed the semeiological features described above, confirming in particular the absence of loss of contact during the episode, and of a long lasting language deficit after it. Interictal EEG showed a good background activity, better represented on the right posterior region; abnormalities mainly consisted in spikes and sharp-waves, constantly present on the left pre-central region (F3-C3 and F3-Fz). Ictal discharges were preceded by the increase in frequency of the left pre-central spikes, and consisted in a flattening followed by a rhythmic spike activity always localized over the same region but involving also the contra lateral leads. MRI (c) confirmed the presence of multiple bilateral lesion with the features of cortical tubers, one of which in the left superior frontal gyrus also involving the superior part of the mesial aspect of the frontal lobe. Anatomo-electro-clinical correlations pointed to this lesion, and surgery was realized in December 2000, with the aim of removing the pre-central superomesial left frontal tuber. Postoperative MRI (d) demonstrated the complete removal of that tuber (with histological confirmation of the diagnosis), but the patient continued to present seizures with daily frequency, mainly at the awakening. Post-operative seizures are shorter, and the patient and the family, who report less drowsiness and better cognitive functioning, positively judge the global situation of the patient; although his impression is not confirmed by neuropsychological testing who were not substantially modified at the 5 years follow-up. Patient is consequently categorized as Engel's class IVa.

Cases Figure 2

The first case (a, b) is a right-handed girl operated on at 14 years of age. Her seizures started at the age of 9 years with a not better specified abrupt fall without warning. No diagnosis was made after this first episode, but the patient did not present any other fit for circa 1 year. After a second seizure (long lasting staring), epilepsy was diagnosed, and a drug treatment by carbamazepine was started. Despite this, and 3 other drug essays, no seizure-free period has been reported afterwards. At surgery, she was having seizures at a weekly frequency (2–4 fits per week) with the following semiology: no subjective manifestations, and no warning, immediate loss of consciousness with staring and minimal gestural automatisms, lasting 20–30 seconds, without postictal deficits. EEG, only interictal, showed slow waves and spike-and-waves over the right anterior frontal region, with a normal background activity on the posterior regions. A lesion was discovered in the anterior and mesial part of the right frontal lobe since the first CT-scan has been realized. MRI showed a T2 and FLAIR hyper-intense abnormality, whose probable diagnosis was that of a glioneuronal tumour, without contrast enhancement and without size modifications in the subsequent follow-ups. The pre-operative sagittal FLAIR sequence (a) shows the lesion in the mesial and orbital part of the right anterior frontal lobe. No cognitive deficit was discovered in the pre-operative neuropsychological evaluation. Surgery was realised in December 2004; histological examination demonstrated a dysembrioplastic neuroepithelial tumour (DNt) with free margins and without associated cortical dysplasia. The patient is seizure-free from surgery; anti-epileptic drugs have been tapered since the first post-operative follow-up at 6 months and stopped after the 2 years follow-up. Cognitive profile remained normal after surgery (6 months) and showed an improvement especially in verbal scores in the subsequent follow-ups at 2 and 5 years. The patient completed the secondary school, got her driving license, and is now attending the University. Post-operative MRI follow-ups at 6 months, 2 and 5 years (c), did not show any tumour relapse.

The second case (c, d) is a right-handed man, operated on at the age of 57 years. His seizures started when he was 15 years old, mainly nocturnal and described as secondarily generalized, after a left head version. A long seizure-free interval was obtained after the introduction of Phenobarbital, and even when seizures started again (around

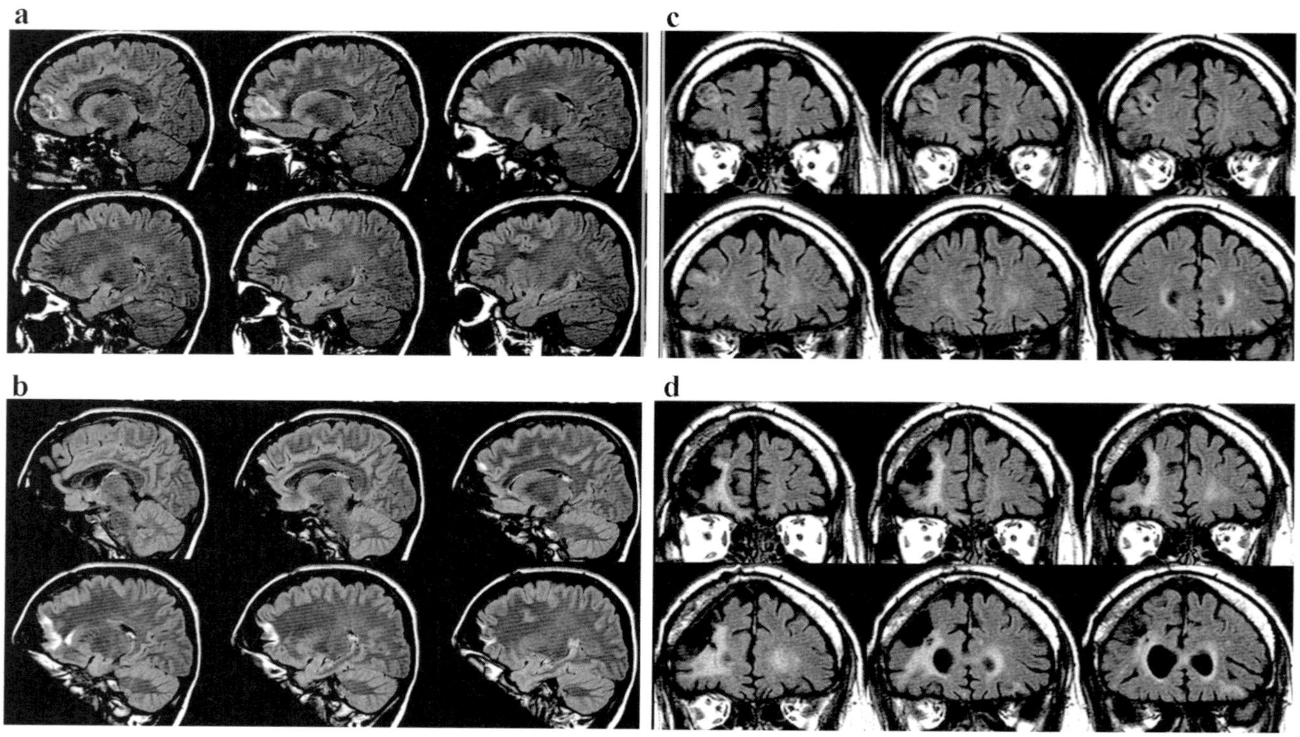

Figure 2

Pre-operative (a, c) **and post-operative** (b, d) **MRI of 2 operated on patients (FLAIR sequences).**

the age of 20 years) their frequency has been relatively low till he was 55 years old. Only at that moment, when seizures frequency showed a significant increase, an MRI was realized, demonstrating a lesion, probably a glioneuronal tumour, in the dorsal pre-frontal cortex of the right hemisphere. Seizures at the moment of surgery presented with at least daily frequency with the following characteristics: abrupt psychomotor arrest, without warning, and initial complete staring, without automatisms, possibly limited to this or followed by head and trunk deviation to the right and by a generalized clonic phase. No postictal deficits were reported when seizures stopped before generalization. Interictal EEG showed long lasting burst of rhythmic delta waves, mimicking spike-and-wave sequences, over the right frontal region and several infraclinical paroxysmal activities characterized by a flattening followed by rhythmic theta-delta activity over the same region but involving also the fronto-central and the anterior temporal derivations. Pre-operative MRI (b) shows, in coronal FLAIR sequences, the lesion in the anterior dorso-lateral part (F2-F3 sulcus and the two surrounding convolutions) of the right frontal lobe. Pre-surgical cognitive evaluation (the patient was a lawyer, still practising the profession) showed a clear deficit in long and short term visuo-spatial memory, and in visuo-constructive praxis functions, together with a reduction in executive functions concerning verbal production, working memory and visuo-motor planning. After the first evaluation in our Centre, possible diagnostic and therapeutics procedures were discussed with the patient, including a stereo-EEG exploration of the right frontal, central and anterior fh temporal region. The patient preferred to undergo a direct surgical resection of the tumour lesion and of the surrounding cerebral parenchyma, without invasive procedures, and was operated on in November 2005. Histological diagnosis showed a DNt, with free margins and with an associated Type I cortical dysplasia of the F2 convolution immediately behind the tumour lesion. At the 6 month follow-up the patient reported only 2 seizures, in concomitance with an autonomous reduction of the AED; MRI confirmed the complete resection of the tumour and cognitive evaluation showed an improvement of the executive functions with persistence of visuo-spatial and praxis deficits. Nonetheless, in the following months seizures re-appeared with a low frequency and lesser duration and intensity. At the five years follow-up MRI (coronal FLAIR sequences in d) did not show any tumour relapse, cognitive evaluation was stable and seizure outcome was definitively classified as Engel's Class IIb.

Cases Figure 3

The first patient is a left-handed boy aged 8 years at the moment of the first surgery. In the personal history there is a threatened miscarriage in the first trimester of pregnancy.

The first seizure occurred at 4 years of age, with a sensation of "shivers" in all the body followed by bilateral blinking and language problem (dysarthria? expressive aphasia?). In the following days other episodes are reported, also with clonic jerks of the right face. Medical treatment was started by carbamazepine few days after the first episode, but did never show a complete efficacy in suppressing the seizures, who presented at pluri-weekly frequency till the moment of the first evaluation at our Centre, at the age of 6 years. The MRI, realized at that moment, showed a probable dysplastic lesion (a) in the left inferior frontal gyrus (pars opercularis). Despite the left-handedness, neuropsychological testing showed a clear reduction in phonemic fluency and in verbal comprehension, thus suggesting left hemisphere language dominance. A stereo-EEG exploration was planned and realised when the boy was 7 years and a half, with the twofold aim of demonstrating the epileptogenicity of the discovered lesion and defining its anatomical relationships with the frontal language areas. Stereo-EEG ictal and interictal recordings, in fact, showed a typical EEG activity in the leads exploring the lesion thus letting hypothesize a good prognosis for a lesionectomy. Unfortunately, electrical stimulation induced a language disturbance in the vicinity of the lesion, and the realised lesionectomy (December 2001) was forcedly incomplete: see the first postoperatory FLAIR sagittal sequences (b). Histological examination demonstrated a Type II FCD, still present on the infero-anterior margins of the resection. Seizures re-appeared short time after surgery, but with reduced frequency and intensity, with free-intervals following modification of drug treatment. For this reason a re-evaluation of the patient in a surgical perspective was delayed till 2008, when a bilateral Wada test was realized, confirming the left hemispheric dominance for language, and, finally an fMRI for language function could be performed by the patient in a reliable way. This last showed no clear activation in the proximity of the residual dsyplastic lesion. For this reason, after having recorded the seizures in Video-EEG, it has been decided to complete the lesionectomy planned years before. The second surgery, completing the lesionectomy (c), was realized in June 2009, and the patient is seizure free since that moment. In fact, as we included for the outcome analysis only the patients with more than 4 years follow-up, this boy is considered as an Engel's class IVa, but the realization of the complete lesionectomy has been able to render seizure free also this patient.

The second patient illustrated in this figure is a right-handed woman operated on at the age of 23 years. The first seizure, in this patient without familial and personal antecedents for epilepsy, appeared at the age of 3 years. It was characterised by a sudden rotation of the body to the right followed by hypertonic elevation of the right arm. Since the beginning seizures showed a very high frequency, but the introduction of Carbamazepine induced an immediate arrest of them, lasting till the age of 7 years. After the reappearance, nonetheless, no other drug has been able to give an enduring positive effect on seizures, which persisted at a very high daily frequency. She came at our observation at the age of 21, when a Video-EEG recording was realized and an MRI showed a clear lesion in the triangular part of the left inferior frontal gyrus. On the basis of the Video-EEG recordings (sub-continuous spiking over the electrode F7, where also the ictal discharges were shown to start, accompanied by a fear expression without any warning, and followed by a kind of hypermotor seizure with a long lasting postictal aphasia), the possible dysplastic lesion was considered to be the cause of the epilepsy and a lesionectomy could be indicated. Nonetheless, both postictal aphasia and cognitive testing (deficit in verbal functions) suggested a left hemispheric dominance for the language, and the Wada test confirmed it. For this reason an fMRI for language was realized. The results of the verbal fluency paradigm are shown in *Figure 3e*, and clearly demonstrate no activation inside the possible dysplasia even if 2 clear areas of increased BOLD signal are present both in front and behind the lesion. This was one of our first fMRI for the language, and we needed a confirmation for a so interesting finding. For this reason a Stereo-EEG exploration was realized with completely satisfying results: clear dysplastic ictal and interictal EEG patterns inside the lesion, where electrical stimulation were not able to induce any language disturbances, while inducing a clear speech arrest immediately behind the lesion itself. A total resection of the lesion (see postoperatory MRI in *Figure 3f*) was realized in December 2003 and the patient is completely seizure free since that moment. Histological examination discovered a cortical tuber (without any other sign of tuberous sclesosis) and the patient did not show any language disturbance, not even in the immediate post-operatory period, with a cognitive testing at 5 years which clearly support a recovery in verbal functions.

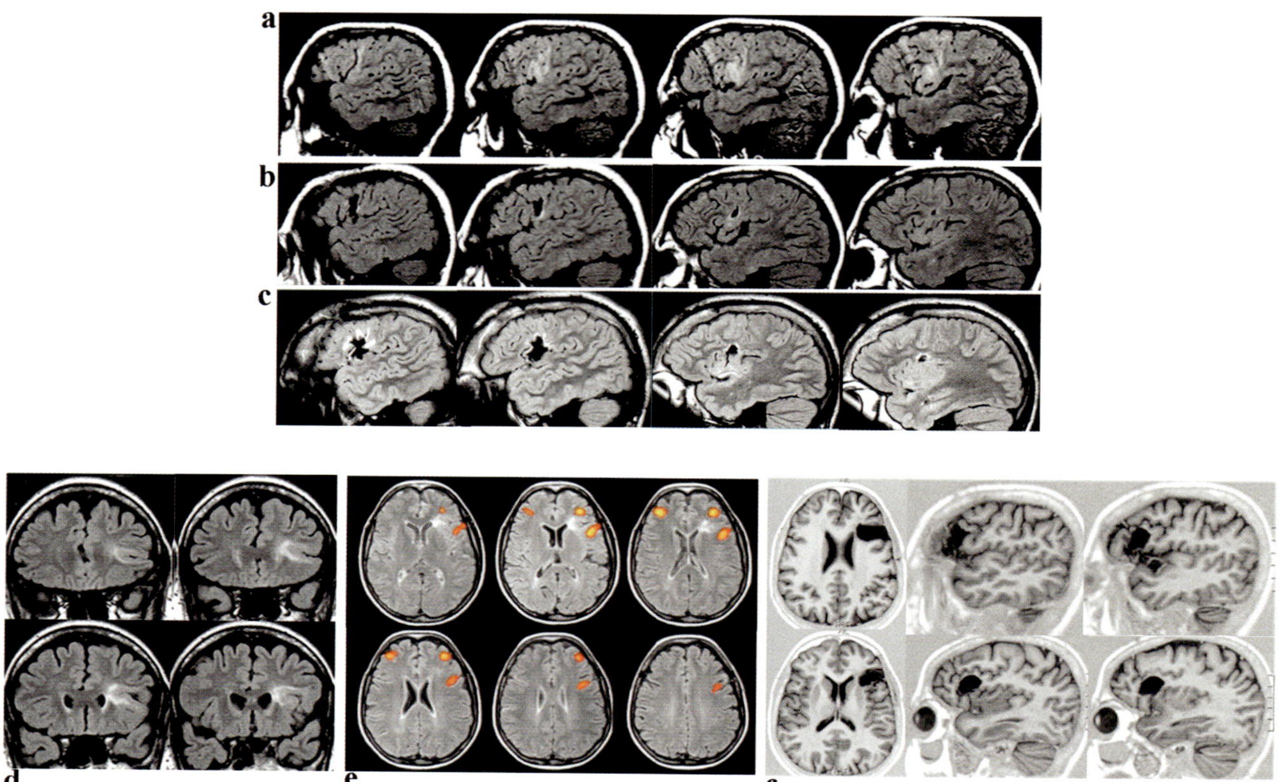

Figure 3

a, b, c. **Pre-operative** (a) **and post-operative** (b, c) **MRI of a patient operated on two times, in childhood;** d, e, f. **Pre-operative MRI** (d) **and fMRI for verbal fluency** (e), **and postoperative MRI of a patient operated on in adulthood.**

Case Figures 4 to 7

This patient is a young girl operated on at the age of 3 years and a half, with no familial and personal antecedents for epilepsy. The history of this patient is quite simple and typical: onset of seizures at 4 months of age with clusters of spasms associated with an hypsarrhytmic EEG pattern, immediately diagnosed as West syndrome, and treated by ACTH with disappearance of spasms. At 18 months of age, reappearance of seizures with short lasting moment of "absence" but also with new clusters of spasms at the awakening, EEG begins showing spike-and-wave abnormalities over the right frontal region. Valproate is started without effects and also another cycle of ACTH showed a limited efficacy during one month. At the end of this short free-interval not only spasms and "absences" restarted, but also abrupt falls induced by a left leg hypotonic fit. The patient was evaluated for the first time in our Centre when she was exactly 3 years old, and presented with several clusters of spasms at each awakening, characterized by minimal signs, such as a brief

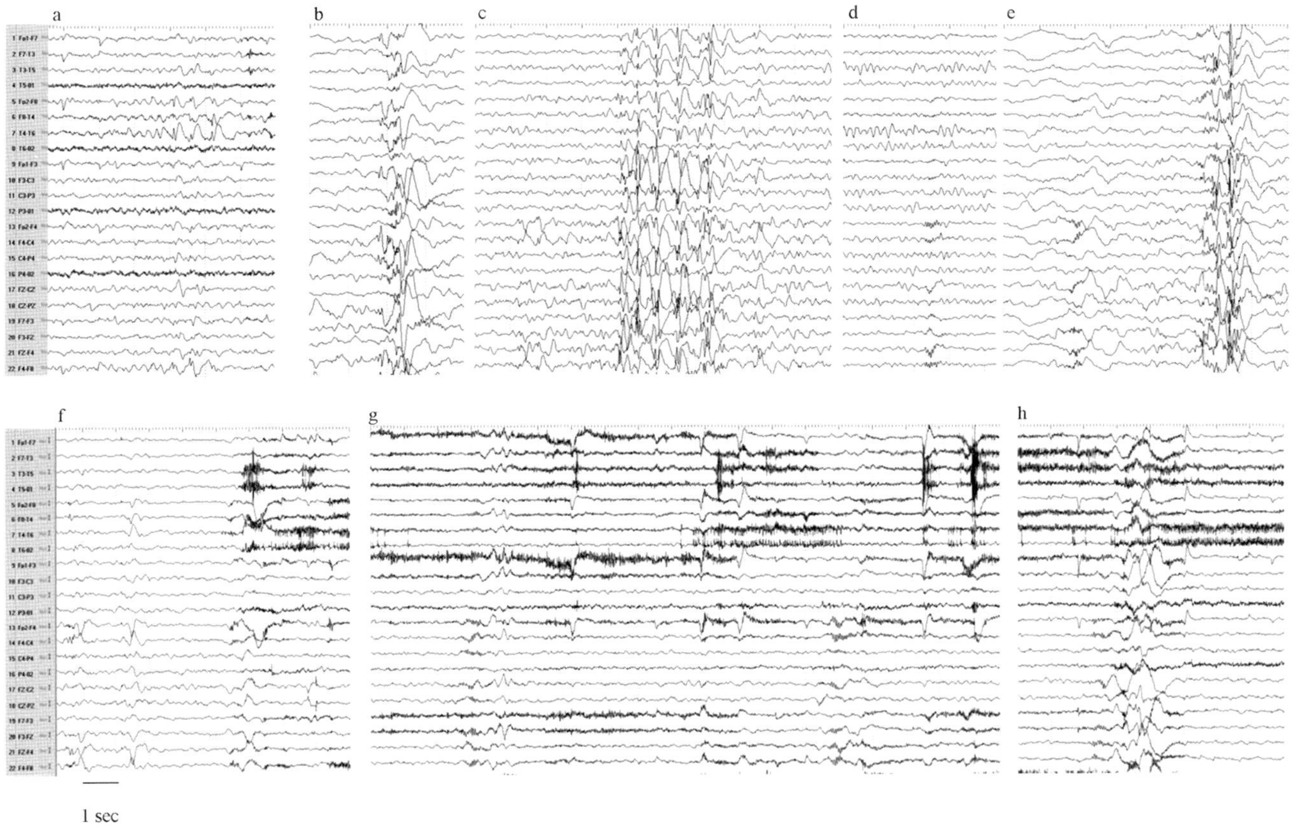

Figure 4

Interictal (a, b, c, d, e) **and ictal** (f, g, h) **scalp EEG features of a patient with Type I FCD and spasms, operated on in childhood.**

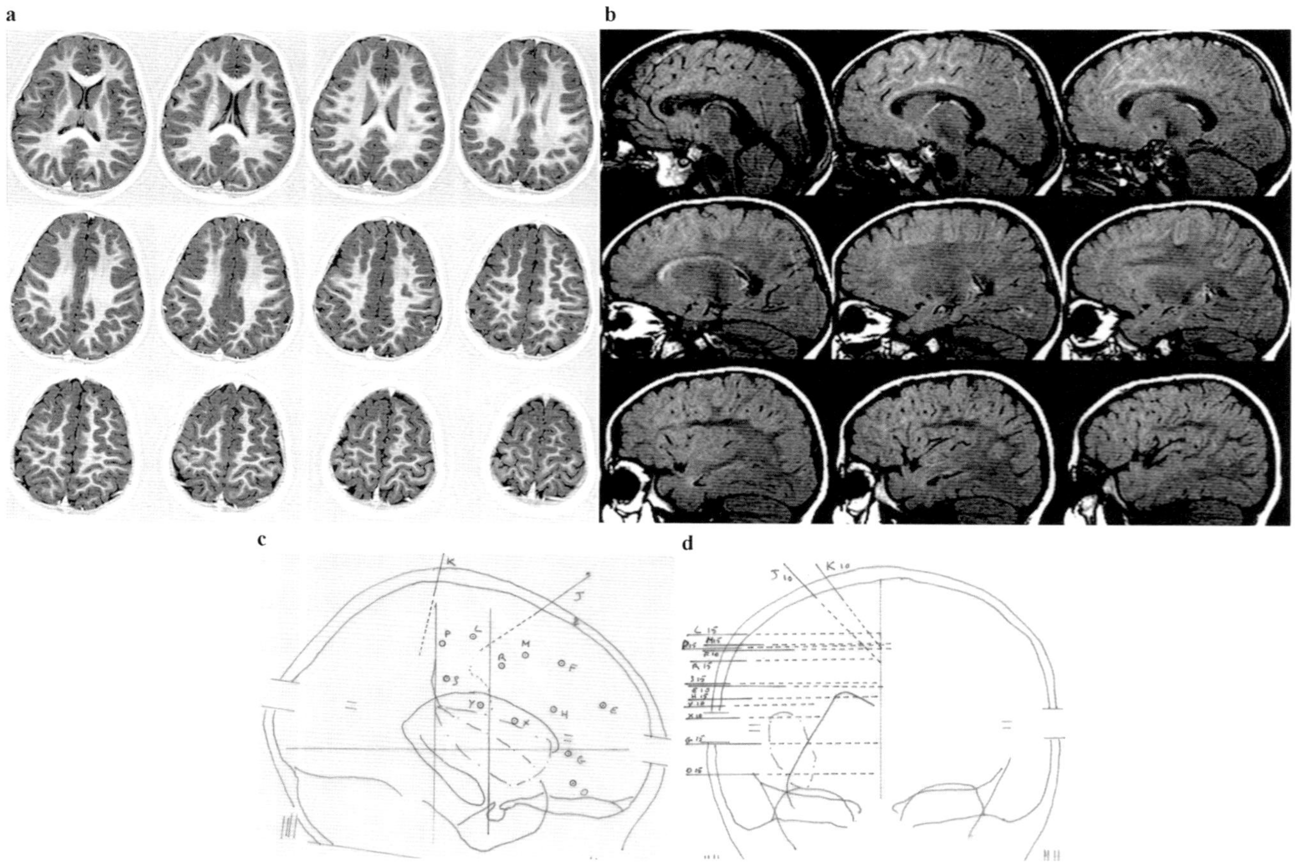

Figure 5

Pre-operative MRI in axial IR (a) and sagittal FLAIR (b) planes, and stereotactic scheme (sagittal, c; and coronal, d) of the implantation of the stereo-EEG electrodes in the patient illustrated in *Figure 4*.

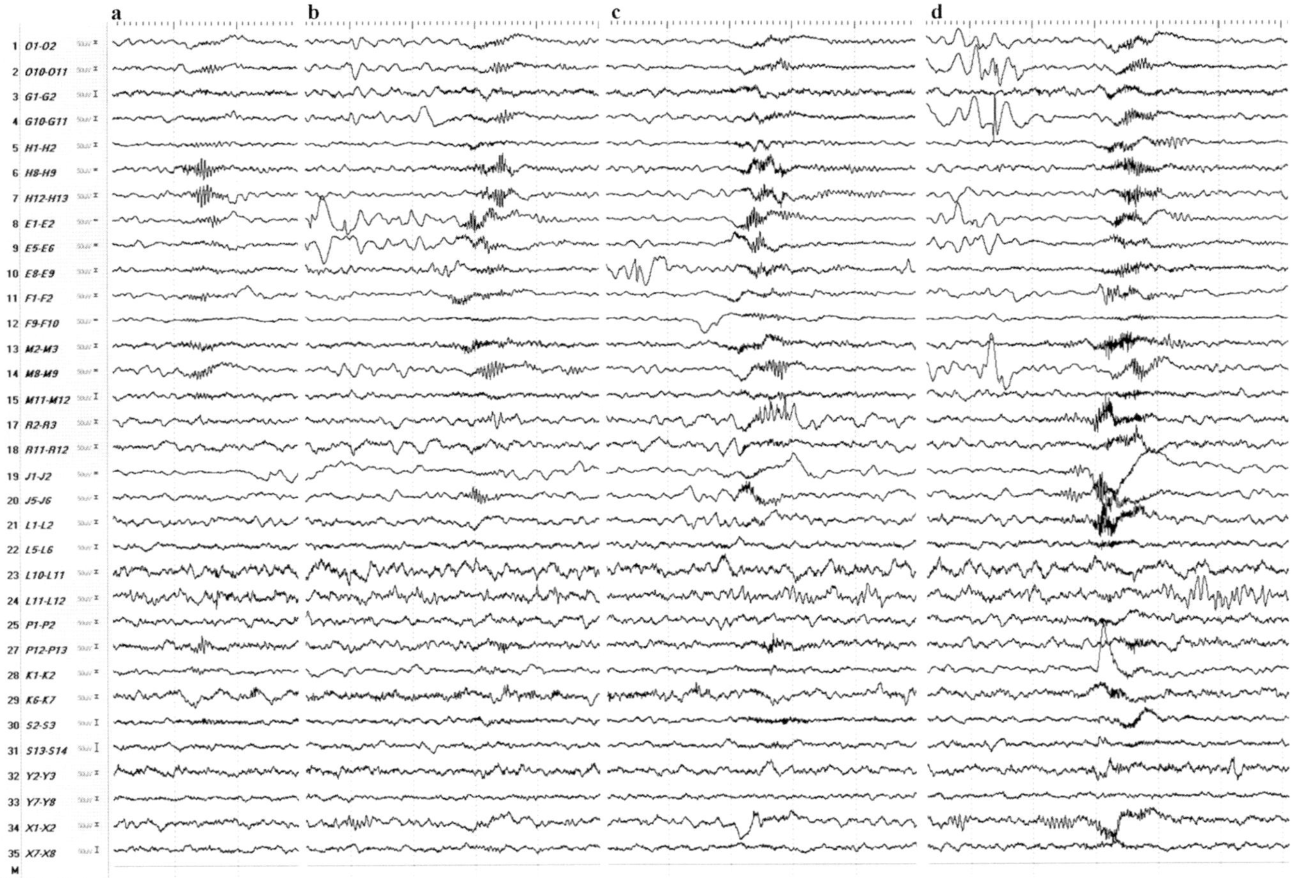

Figure 6

Stereo-EEG recordings (different frames) of a cluster of spasms in the same patient as *Figures 4 and 5*.

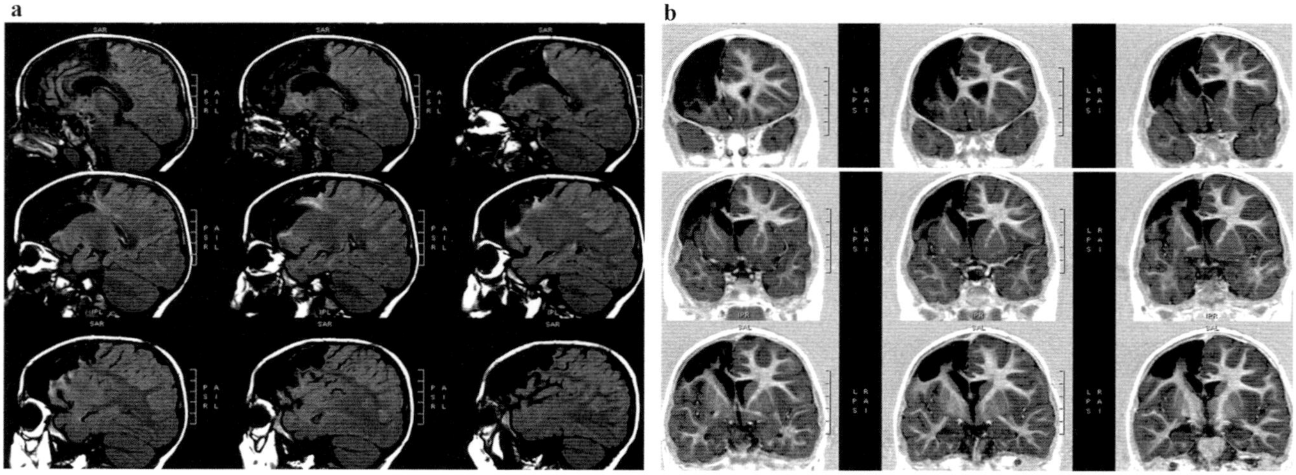

Figure 7

Postoperative MRI of the same patient as *Figures 4, 5 and 6*, in sagittal FLAIR (a) and coronal IR (b) sequences.

orientation of the eyes to the left, progressively worsening in the course of the cluster to become a typical spasm in flexion. Under a cognitive point of view there was a slight but clear delay in development, without language capabilities. A video-EEG monitoring was realized together with a new MRI. Video-EEG showed a slow background activity, better represented on the left posterior derivations, together with delta and slow spike-and-wave complexes on the right posterior temporal region (a). During sleep, the great majority of the abnormalities seemed to be very well localised on the right fronto-central region, in terms of spikes (b), slow waves (c) and low voltage rhythmic activities (d, e), but very frequently they tended to involve all the right hemisphere and also the left hemisphere was often the site of burst of rhythmic spike-and wave, apparently synchronous, however, with the right ones (b, c, e). Several clusters of spasms have been recorded, both during the night and in occasion of morning and afternoon awakenings. They were all super imposable under a clinical point of view with a "crescendo" of ictal signs from a simple deviation of the eyes to the left to a complete anterior flexion of the trunk associated with the elevation of both arms, more marked on the left side. During the entire cluster the behaviour of the patient changed: she became slower, whining and less responsive. Also the EEG pattern was almost constant: the beginning of each cluster was characterized by the appearance of short burst of low amplitude rhythmic activity well localized over F4-C4 and the anterior vertex (f), and progressively increasing in amplitude, rapidity and extension (g); the strongest clinical signs were associated to the classical EEG marker of spasms: an high amplitude burst of slow waves preceded by runs of fast activity, this last also visible superimposed to the succeeding slow waves (h). MRI realized during that hospitalization is shown in *Figure 5*.

MRI showed a clear asymmetry in the cortical mantle of the frontal lobe in axial IR sequences (a) with a hyper intense signal in FLAIR sequences on the right side, which in sagittal planes (b) seemed to involve also the region of the paracentral lobule. On the basis of the Video-EEG findings (see *Figure 4*) and of the MRI presented in this Figure we discussed with the parents two different diagnostic and therapeutic options: immediate surgery with a complete right frontal lobectomy, with reasonable chances to be cured but with a serious doubt about the paracentral lobule of the patient, which seemed dysplasic on the MRI, consequently submitting the girl to the risk of a second surgery if the seizure would not disappear after the first surgical intervention; a Stereo-EEG exploration of the whole right frontal lobe with the twofold aim of ascertaining the real position of the right motor strip, especially for the left leg, and confirming, or excluding, the real dysplastic nature of the right para-central lobule, on the basis of the depth EEG features of that region. The parents choose the second option and the Stereo-EEG exploration was realized 3 months later. It comprised 14 electrodes in the frontal and central region of the right hemisphere, exploring: the orbital cortex (mesial and lateral, electrode O), the pre-frontal region both mesial and lateral (electrodes G, E, H and F from infero-anterior to postero-superior part), the opercular region and the insula (electrodes X and Y), the pre-motor frontal cortex both mesial and lateral (electrodes M, R, J and L from anterior to posterior) and the probable central and post-central region (electrodes S, P and K). Results of the Stereo-EEG recordings are detailed in *Figure 6*.

Global results of the Stereo-EEG recordings can be summarized as follow: The great majority of interictal abnormalities, especially, in fact, slow waves and slow spike-and-waves complexes, have been recorded in the orbital and pre-frontal cortex (electrodes F, E, H, G and O) with a clear antero-posterior gradient. Hundreds of infra-clinical paroxystic fast activities were found, in wake but mainly in sleep, over the same region but simultaneously involving the pre-motor cortex explored by the electrodes M, R, J and the mesial contacts of L. As in scalp recordings the clusters of spasm showed a gradually increasing complexity, with short burst of rhythmic low voltage activity starting from the orbital leads, the pre-frontal cortex and the mesial part of the pre-motor cortex (a), progressively involving also the superior part of the pre-motor cortex and the opercular region (b, c) and finally interesting almost all the leads (d), with the only exception of the external contacts of the electrode L. Electrical stimulations allowed us to define that the motor region for the hand was in correspondence of the external leads of the electrode L, no motor response for the leg was found during the stimulations. However, following the anatomic borders of the so identified pre-central gyrus we arrived to define that none of our electrodes was placed in the possible motor area of the leg, being the mesial contacts of M, J and also L in the supplementary sensori-motor area, and being the probable motor area of the leg situated posteriorly to those contacts. These findings gave us the possibility to propose to the parents of the patient a sub-total frontal lobectomy, sparing the opercular region and mainly the motor cortex.

Surgery was done in September 2006, and as shown in this figures respected the plan made after the Stereo-EEG recordings. The patient had a slight motor deficit, linked to the resection of the SSMA, who regressed in few weeks after surgery. Seizures immediately disappeared and at the last postoperatory follow up (4 years after surgery) anti-epileptic drugs were almost completely reduced (100 mg/day of carbamazepine) and neuropsychological testing showed a good recovery in both verbal and non verbal functions, tough still under the level of her age, especially in visual praxis.

REFERENCES ▶

Ambrosetto G, Montagna P, Vetrugno R, Cortelli P (2009): Paroxysmal bipedal activity during syncope related to carotid body tumor. *Epilepsy Behav* 15: 338–390.

Asano E, Chugani DC, Juhász C, Muzik O, Chugani HT (2001): Surgical treatment of West syndrome. *Brain Dev* 23: 668–676.

Aubert S, Wendling F, Regis J, *et al.* (2009): Local and remote epileptogenicity in focal cortical dysplasias and neurodevelopmental tumours. *Brain* 132: 3072–3086.

Awad IA, Rosenfeld J, Ahl J, Hahn JF, Lüders H (1991): Intractable epilepsy and structural lesions of the brain: mapping, resection strategies, and seizure outcome. *Epilepsia* 32: 179–186.

Bancaud J, Talairach J (1992): Clinical semiology of frontal lobe seizures. *Adv Neurol* 57: 3–58.

Bartolomei F, Chauvel P (2000): Seizure symptoms and cerebral localization: frontal and Rolandic seizures. In: Oxbury JM, Polkey CE, Duchowny M (eds) *Intractable Focal Epilepsy*, pp. 55–62. London: Saunders.

Bartolomei F, Guye M, Wendling F, Gavaret M, Regis J, Chauvel P (2002): Fear, anger and compulsive behavior during seizure: involvement of large scale frontotemporal neural networks. *Epileptic Disord* 4: 235–241.

Baumgartner C, Flint R, Tuxhorn I, *et al.* (1996): Supplementary motor area seizures: propagation pathways as studied with invasive recordings. *Neurology* 46: 508–514.

Bien CG, Szinay M, Wagner J, Clusmann H, Becker AJ, Urbach H (2009): Characteristics and surgical outcomes of patients with refractory magnetic resonance imaging–negative epilepsies. *Arch Neurol* 66: 1491–1499.

Biraben A, Taussig D, Thomas P, *et al.* (2001): Fear as the main feature of epileptic seizures. *J Neurol Neurosurg Psychiatry* 70: 186–191.

Blumcke I, Thom M, Aronica E, *et al.* (2011): The clinico-pathologic spectrum of focal cortical dysplasias: A consensus classification proposed by an ad hoc Task Force of the ILAE Diagnostic Methods Commission. *Epilepsia* 52: 158–174.

Blume WT, Lüders HO, Mizrahi E, Tassinari CA, van Emde Boas W, Engel J (2001): Glossary of descriptive terminology for ictal semiology: report of the ILAE task force on classification and terminology. *Epilepsia* 42: 1212–1218.

Bourgeois M, Sainte-Rose C, Lellouch-Tubiana A, *et al.* (1999): Surgery of epilepsy associated with focal lesions in childhood. *J Neurosurg* 90: 833–842.

Braakman HM, Vaessen MJ, Hofman PA, *et al.* (2011): Cognitive and behavioral complications of frontal lobe epilepsy in children: A review of the literature. *Epilepsia* 52: 849–856.

Chapman K, Wyllie E, Najm I, *et al.* (2005): Seizure outcome after epilepsy surgery in patients with normal preoperative MRI. *J Neurol Neurosurg Psychiatry* 76: 710–713.

Chieffo D, Lettori D, Contaldo I, *et al.* (2011): Surgery of children with frontal lobe lesional epilepsy: neuropsychological study. *Brain Dev* 33: 310–315.

Colombo N, Tassi L, Galli C, *et al.* (2003): Focal cortical dysplasias: MR imaging, histopathologic, and clinical correlations in surgically treated patients with epilepsy. *AJNR Am J Neuroradiol* 24: 724–733.

Cossu M, Cardinale F, Castana L, *et al.* (2005): Stereoelectroencephalography in the presurgical evaluation of focal epilepsy: a retrospective analysis of 215 procedures. *Neurosurgery* 57: 706–718.

Cossu M, Lo Russo G, Francione S, *et al.* (2008): Epilepsy surgery in children: results and predictors of outcome on seizures. *Epilepsia* 49: 65–72.

Derry CP, Harvy AS, Wallace MG, Duncan JS, Berkovic SF (2009): NREM arousal parasomnias and their distinction from nocturnal frontal lobe epilepsy. A video EEG analysis. *Sleep* 32: 1637–1644.

Engel J, Van Ness P, Rasmussen T, Ojemann L (1993): Outcome with respect to epileptic seizures. In: Engel J Jr (ed) *Surgical Treatment of the Epilepsies*, 2nd ed, pp. 609–621. New York: Raven Press.

Fish DR, Smith SJ, Quesney LF, Andermann F, Rasmussen T (1993): Surgical treatment of children with medically intractable frontal or temporal lobe epilepsy: results, highlights of 40 years' experience. *Epilepsia* 34: 244–247.

Fogarasi A, Janszky J, Faveret E, Pieper T, Tuxhorn I (2001): A detailed analysis of frontal lobe seizure semiology in children younger than 7 years. *Epilepsia* 42: 80–85.

Francione S, Vigliano P, Tassi L, *et al.* (2003a): Surgery for drug resistant partial epilepsy in children with focal cortical dysplasia: anatomical-clinical correlations and neurophysiological data in 10 patients. *J Neurol Neurosurg Psychiatry* 74: 1493–1501.

Francione S, Nobili L, Cardinale F, Citterio A, Galli C, Tassi L (2003b): Intra-lesional stereo-EEG activity in Taylor's focal cortical dysplasia. *Epileptic Disord* 5: S105–S114.

Frater JL, Prayson RA, Morris HH III, Bingaman WE (2000): Surgical pathologic findings of extratemporal-based intractable epilepsy: a study of 133 consecutive resections. *Arch Pathol Lab Med* 124: 545–549.

Freitag H, Tuxhorn I (2005): Cognitive function in preschool children after epilepsy surgery: rationale for early intervention. *Epilepsia* 46: 561–567.

Fusco L, Iani C, Fredda MT, *et al.* (1990): Mesial frontal epilepsy: a clinical entity not sufficiently described. *J. Epilepsy* 3: 123–135.

Gardella E, Rubboli G, Francione S, *et al.* (2008): Seizure-related automatic locomotion triggered by intracerebral electrical stimulation. *Epileptic Disord* 10: 247–252.

Gardella E, Tassinari CA, Rubboli G (2006): Video analysis of ictal repetitive grasping in "frontal hyperkinetic seizures". *Epileptic Disord* 8: 1–8.

Gibbs SA, Proserpio P, Francione S, *et al.* (2018): Seizure duration and latency of hypermotor manifestations distinguish frontal from extra-frontal onset in sleep-related hypermotor epilepsy. *Epilepsia* 59: 130–134.

Gibbs S.A., Proserpio P, Francione S, *et al.* (2019): Clinical features of sleep-related hypermotor epilepsy in relation to the seizure -onset zone. A review of 135 surgically treated cases. *Epilepsia* 60: 1–11.

Grillner S, Wallen P (1985): Central Pattern Generators for locomotion with special reference to vertebrate. *Ann Rev Neurosci* 8: 233–261.

Guedj E, Mc Gonigal A, Vaugier L, Mundler O, Bartolomei F (2012): Metabolic brain PET underlying hyperkinetic seizures. *Epilepsy Res* 181: 237–245.

Hirsch E, Sellal F, Maton B, Rumbach L, Marescaux C (1994): Nocturnal paroxysmal dystonia: a clinical form of focal epilepsy. *Neurophysiol Clin* 24: 207–217.

Holmes GL, Vigevano F (1997): Infantile spasms. In: Engel Jr J, Pedley TA (eds) *Epilepsy: a Comprehensive Textbook*, pp. 627–642. Philadelphia, PA: Lippincott-Raven.

Iani C, Attanasio A, Manfredi M (1996): Paroxysmal staring and masticatory automatisms during postural hypotension in a patient with multiple system atrophy. *Epilepsia* 37: 690–693.

Jeha LE, Najm I, Bingaman W, Dinner D, Widdess-Walsh P, Lüders H (2007): Surgical outcome and prognostic factors of frontal lobe epilepsy surgery. *Brain* 130: 574–584.

Jobst BC, Siegel AM, Thadani VM, Roberts DW, Rhodes HC, Williamson PD (2000): Intractable seizures of frontal lobe origin: clinical characteristics, localizing signs, and results of surgery. *Epilepsia* 41: 1139–1152.

Jobst BC, Williamson PD (2005): Frontal lobe seizures. *Psychiatr Clin North Am* 28: 635–651.

Kellinghaus C, Lüders HO (2004): Frontal lobe epilepsy. *Epileptic Disord* 6: 223–239.

Kim CH, Chung CK, Lee SK (2010): Longitudinal change in outcome of frontal lobe epilepsy surgery. *Neurosurgery* 67: 1222–1229.

Krainik A, Lehericy S, Duffau H, *et al.* (2001): Role of the supplementary motor area in motor deficit following medial frontal lobe surgery. *Neurology* 57: 871–878.

Kral T, Kuczaty S, Blümcke I, *et al.* (2001): Postsurgical outcome of children and adolescents with medically refractory frontal lobe epilepsies. *Childs Nerv Syst* 17: 595–601.

Kramer U, Sue WC, Mikati MA (1997): Focal features in West syndrome indicating candidacy for surgery. *Pediatr Neurol* 16: 213–217.

Krsek P, Maton B, Korman B, *et al.* (2008): Different features of histopathological subtypes of pediatric focal cortical dysplasia. *Ann Neurol* 63: 758–769.

Krsek P, Pieper T, Karlmeier A, *et al.* (2009a): Different presurgical characteristics and seizure outcomes in children with focal cortical dysplasia type I or II. *Epilepsia* 50: 125–137.

Krsek P, Maton B, Jayakar P, *et al.* (2009b): Incomplete resection of focal cortical dysplasia is the main predictor of poor postsurgical outcome. *Neurology* 72: 217–223.

Krsek P, Jahodova A, Maton B, *et al.* (2010): Low-grade focal cortical dysplasia is associated with prenatal and perinatal brain injury. *Epilepsia* 51: 2440–2448.

Laskowitz DT, Sperling MR, French JA, O'Connor MJ (1995): The syndrome of frontal lobe epilepsy: characteristics and surgical management. *Neurology* 45: 780–787.

Lawson JA, Cook MJ, Vogrin S, *et al.* (2002): Clinical, EEG, and quantitative MRI differences in pediatric frontal and temporal lobe epilepsy. *Neurology* 58: 723–729.

Lee SK, Lee SY, Kim KK, Hong KS, Lee DS, Chung CK (2005): Surgical outcome and prognostic factors of cryptogenic neocortical epilepsy. *Ann Neurol* 58: 525–532.

Lendt M, Gleissner U, Helmstaedter C, Sassen R, Clusmann H, Elger CE (2002): Neuropsychological outcome in children after frontal lobe epilepsy surgery. *Epilepsy Behav* 3: 51–59.

Lichetta L, Bisulli F, Vignatelli L, Zenesini C, Di Vito L (2017): Sleep related hypermotor epilepsy . Long Term outcome in a large cohort. *Neurology* 88: 1–8.

Loddenkemper T, Holland KD, Stanford LD, Kotagal P, Bingaman W, Wyllie E (2007): Developmental outcome after epilepsy surgery in infancy. *Pediatrics* 119: 930–935.

Lüders HO, Engel J Jr, Munari C (1993): General principles. In: Engel J Jr (ed) *Surgical Treatment of the Epilepsies*, 2nd ed, pp. 137–153. New York: Raven Press.

Lüders H, Acharya J, Baumgartner C, Benbadis S, Bleasel A, *et al.* (1999): A new epileptic seizure classification based exclusively on ictal semiology. *Acta Neurol Scand* 99: 137–141.

Mai R, Sartori I, Francione S, *et al.* (2005): Sleep related hyperkinetic seizures: always a frontal onset? *Neurol Sci* 26: s220–224.

Mariottini A, Lombroso CT, De Girolami U, *et al.* (2001): Operative results without invasive monitoring in patients with frontal lobe epileptogenic lesions. *Epilepsia* 42: 1308–1315.

Masuda H, Sharif E, Tohyam J, Murakami H, Kameyama S (2012): Clinical patterns and pathophysiology of hypermotor seizures: an ictal SPECT study. *Epileptic Disord* 14: 32–40.

McGonigal A, Bartolomei F, Régis J, *et al.* (2007): Stereoelectroencephalography in presurgical assessment of MRI-negative epilepsy. *Brain* 130: 3169–3183.

Montagna P (1992): Nocturnal paroxysmal dystonia and nocturnal wandering. *Neurology* 42: S61–S67.

Morris HH, Dinner DS, Lüders HO, Wyllie E, Kramer R (1988): Supplementary motor seizures: clinical and electroencephalographic findings. *Neurology* 38: 1075–1082.

Mosewich RK, So EL, O'Brien TJ, *et al.* (2000): Factors predictive of the outcome of frontal lobe epilepsy surgery. *Epilepsia* 41: 843–849.

Munari C, Bancaud J (1992): Electroclinical symptomatology of partial seizures of orbital frontal origin. *Adv Neurol* 57: 257–265.

Munari C, Hoffmann D, Francione S, *et al.* (1994): Stereo-electroencephalography methodology: advantages and limits. *Acta Neurol Scand* Suppl 152: 56–67.

Munari C, Tassi L, Di Leo M, *et al.* (1995): Video-stereo-electroencephalographic investigation of orbitofrontal cortex: ictal electroclinical patterns. *Adv Neurol* 66: 273–295.

Nobili L, Francione S, Cardinale F, Lo Russo G (2002): Epileptic nocturnal wanderings with a temporal lobe origin: a stereo-electroencephalographic study. *Sleep* 25: 669–671.

Nobili L, Francione S, Mai R, *et al.* (2003): Nocturnal frontal lobe epilepsy: intracerebral recordings of paroxysmal motor attacks with increasing complexity. *Sleep* 26: 883–886.

Nobili L, Cossu M, Mai R, *et al.* (2004): Sleep-related hyperkinetic seizures of temporal lobe origin. *Neurology* 62: 482–485.

Nobili L, Francione S, Mai R, *et al.* (2007): Surgical treatment of drug-resistant nocturnal frontal lobe epilepsy. *Brain* 130: 561–573.

Oldani A, Zucconi M, Asselta R, *et al.* (1998): Autosomal dominant nocturnal frontal lobe epilepsy. A videopolysomnographic and genetic appraisal of 40 patients and delineation of the epileptic syndrome. *Brain* 121: 205–223.

Olivier A (1995): Surgery of frontal lobe epilepsy. *Adv Neurol* 66: 321–348.

Palmini A, Najm I, Avanzini G, *et al.* (2004): Terminology and classification of the cortical dysplasias. *Neurology* 62 (6 Suppl 3): S2–S8.

Paolicchi JM, Jayakar P, Dean P, *et al.* (2000): Predictors of outcome in pediatric epilepsy surgery. *Neurology* 54: 642–647.

Parrino L, Halasz P, Tassinari CA, Terzano MG (2006): CAP, epilepsy and motor events during sleep: the unifying role of arousal. *Sleep Med Rev* 10: 267–285.

Proserpio P, Cossu M, Francione S, *et al.* (2011): Insular-Opercular seizures manifesting with sleep-related paroxysmal motor behaviors: a stereo EEG study. *Epilepsia* 52: 1781–1791.

Provini F, Plazzi G, Tinuper P, Vandi S, Lugaresi E, Montagna P (1999): Nocturnal frontal lobe epilepsy. A clinical and polygraphic overview of 100 consecutive cases. *Brain* 122: 1017–1031.

Ryvlin P, Minotti L, Demarquay G, *et al.* (2006): Nocturnal hypermotor seizures, suggesting frontal lobe epilepsy, can originate in the insula. *Epilepsia* 47: 755–765.

Scheffer IE, Bhatia KP, Lopes-Cendes I, *et al.* (1994): Autosomal dominant frontal epilepsy misdiagnosed as sleep disorder. *Lancet* 343: 515–517.

Schmidt D, Baumgartner C, Löscher W. (2004): Seizure recurrence after planned discontinuation of antiepileptic drugs in seizure-free patients after epilepsy surgery: a review of current clinical experience. *Epilepsia* 45: 179–186.

Schramm J, Kral T, Kurthen M, Blumcke I (2002): Surgery to treat focal frontal lobe epilepsy in adults. *Neurosurgery* 51: 644–655.

Sinclair DB, Aronyk K, Snyder T, McKean JD, Wheatley M, *et al.* (2004a): Extratemporal resection for childhood epilepsy. *Pediatr Neurol* 30: 177–185.

Sinclair DB, Wheatley M, Snyder T (2004b): Frontal lobe epilepsy in childhood. *Pediatr Neurol* 30: 169–176.

So NK (1998): Mesial frontal epilepsy. *Epilepsia* 39: S49–S61.

Spencer S, Huh L (2008): Outcomes of epilepsy surgery in adults and children. *Lancet Neurol* 7: 525–537.

Swartz BE (1994): Electrophysiology of bimanual bipedal automatisms. *Epilepsia* 35: 264–274.

Swartz BE (1995): Unusual seizure types. *Semin Neurol* 15: 151–157.

Swartz BE, Delgado-Escueta AV, Walsh GO, *et al.* (1998): Surgical outcomes in pure frontal lobe epilepsy and foci that mimic them. *Epilepsy Res* 29: 97–108.

Talairach J, Bancaud J, Bonis A, *et al.* (1992): Surgical therapy for frontal epilepsies. *Adv Neurol* 57: 707–732.

Tassi L, Colombo N, Garbelli R, *et al.* (2002): Focal cortical dysplasia: neuropathological subtypes, EEG, neuroimaging and surgical outcome. *Brain* 125: 1719–1732.

Tassi L, Garbelli R, Colombo N, *et al.* (2012): Electroclinical, MRI and surgical outcomes in 100 epileptic âtients with type II FCD. *Epileptic Disord* 14: 257–266.

Tassinari CA, Gardella E, Rubboli G, *et al.* (2003): Facial Expression of Emotion in Human Frontal and Temporal Lobe Epileptic seizures. In: Ekman P, Campos JJ, Davidson RJ, de Waal F (eds). "Emotions inside out: 130 years after Darwin's". The expression of emotions in man and animals. *Ann NY AcadSci* 1000: 393–394.

Tassinari CA, Rubboli G, Gardella E, *et al.* (2005): Central pattern generators for a common semiology in fronto-limbic seizures and in parasomnias. A neuroethologic approach. *Neurol Sci* 26: S225–S232.

Tassinari CA, Meletti S, Gardella E, *et al.* (2006): Emergence des comportements moteurs communs aux crises frontales nocturnes et aux parasomnies. Approche etologique. In: Amman JP, Chiron C, Dulac O, Fagot-Largeault A (eds). *Epilepsie, Connaissance du cerveau et Societé* . Collège de France. pp. 81–91. Quebec: Presse Laval.

Tassinari CA, Cantalupo G, Högl B, *et al.* (2009): Neuroethological approach to frontolimbic epileptic seizures and parasomnias: the same central pattern generators for the same behaviours. *Rev Neurol* 165: 762–768.

Teutonico F, Mai R, Devinsky O, *et al.* (2008): Epilepsy surgery in tuberous sclerosis complex: early predictive elements and outcome. *Childs Nerv Syst* 24: 1437–1445.

Tharp BR (1972): Orbitofrontal seizures. A unique electroencephalographic and clinical syndrome. *Epilepsia* 13: 627–642.

Tinuper P, Bisulli F, Cross JH, *et al.* (2016): Definition and diagnostic criteria of sleep-related hypermotor epilepsy. *Neurology* 86: 1–9.

Tinuper P, Provini F, Bisulli F, *et al.* (2007): Movement disorders in sleep: Guidelines for differentiating epileptic from non epileptic motor phenomena arising from sleep. *Sleep Medicine Review* 11: 255–267.

Vaugier L, Aubert S, Mc Gonigal A, *et al.* (2009): Neural networks underlying hyperkinetic seizures of "temporal lobe" origin. *Epilepsy Res* 86: 2000–2008.

Vaugier L, Mc Gonigal A, Lagarde S, *et al.* (2017): On the origin of hyperkinetic motor behavior: same semiology produced by two different cortical seizure zones. *Epileptic Disord* 19: 362–366.

Wada JA, Purves SI (1984): Oral and Bimanual Bipedal activity as Ictal Manifestations of Frontal lobe Epilepsy. *Epilepsia* 25: 668.

Wada JA (1989): Predominantly nocturnal recurrence of intensely affective vocal and facial expression associated with powerful bimanual, bipedal and axial activity as ictal manifestations of mesial frontal lobe epilepsy. *Adv Epileptol* 17: 261–277.

Walsh GO, Delgado-Escueta (1984): Type II complex partial seizures: poor results of anterior temporal lobectomy. *Neurology* 34: 1–13.

Williamson PD, Jobst BC (2000): Frontal lobe epilepsy. *Adv Neurol* 84: 215–242.

Williamson PD, Spencer DD, Spencer SS, Novelly RA, Mattson RH (1985): Complex partial seizures of frontal lobe origin. *Ann Neurol* 18: 497–504.

Wong M, Trevathan E (2001): Infantile spasms. *Pediatr Neurol* 24: 89–98.

Wyllie E, Comair YG, Kotagal P, Bulacio J, Bingaman W, Ruggieri P (1998): Seizure outcome after epilepsy surgery in children and adolescents. *Ann Neurol* 44: 740–748.

Epileptic Syndromes in Infancy, Childhood and Adolescence (6th ed), M. Bureau, P. Genton, C. Dravet, A. V. Delgado-Escueta, R. Guerrini, C.A. Tassinari, P. Thomas & P. Wolf

WITH VIDEO SUPPLEMENTS

CHAPTER 22
PHOTOSENSITIVITY AND SYNDROMES

Dorothée Kasteleijn-Nolst Trenité[1], Stefano Meletti[2], Stephan Waltz[3] and Guido Rubboli[4]

[1] Department of Functional Neurosurgery and Epilepsy, University Medical Center Utrecht, the Netherlands and Faculty of Medicine and Psychology Sapienza, Rome, Italy
[2] Department of Biomedical, Metabolic, and Neural Science, University of Modena and Reggio Emilia, Italy; Neurology Unit, Azienda Ospedaliera-Universitaria Modena, Italy
[3] Child Neurology, Children's Hospital of Cologne, Cologne, Germany
[4] Danish Epilepsy Center, Epilepsihospitalet, Dianalund, Filadelfia, Denmark; University of Copenhagen, Copenhagen, Denmark

Introduction

At the end of the xixth century, Gowers wrote a clear clinical description of a patient sensitive to bright sunshine, since then many more patients have been described. Although seizures are mainly provoked by flickering sunlight and artificial light, television and striped patterns, in the last few decades, computer monitors, programs and video games are also known to be provocative. The importance of color in provoking seizures was noticed in 1997 after transmission of the Pocket-Monster (Pokemon) cartoon in Japan. More recently, a trailer for the summer Olympic Games in London 2012 contained similar type of flashing colors and was no longer shown after complaints of patients with photosensitive epilepsy. In today's world it has become more difficult for an individual patient to recognize provocative visual stimuli: modern city environment is full of different screens, patterns (clothing, architecture, etc.), disco lights and programs. EEG diagnostics with standardized photic stimulation (European guidelines 2012, see website ILAE) is thus more and more important to detect and monitor photosensitivity.

After the invention of the EEG, it was demonstrated that intermittent photic stimulation (IPS) evoked specific occipital rhythms (photic driving) in most patients and generalized epileptiform discharges in some. Because of the divergence in EEG diagnostics and availability of concurrent clinical information, there is some confusion about the significance of a generalized epileptiform reaction to IPS (the "classical" photoparoxysmal response or PPR) regarding the diagnosis of epilepsy, in general, and having visually induced seizures in daily life, in particular. A growing interest in visually induced epilepsy has led to recognition of occipital photosensitive epilepsy with PPRs confined to the occipital area and often occurring after prolonged visual stimulation. Both occipital seizures and myoclonic jerks can occur in the same patient. Especially in children, migraine features can be the only symptom of visually induced occipital epileptiform discharges. The pathophysiology of photosensitivity becomes more and more clear: pathological synchronization plays a crucial role.

An increasing number of different types of photic stimulators are used even within the same laboratory, with also different methodology and interpretation of results: thus it is difficult to compare the outcomes even within an individual patient. Moreover, a lack of consistency in the use of terminology makes it difficult to have a good comparison between the various patient groups. European Guidelines try not only to improve detection and confirmation of photosensitivity, but also to standardize it (Kasteleijn- Nolst Trenité *et al.*, 2001; 2012- see ILAE website). Genetic research seems to confirm the diversity in phenomenology of clinical history and EEGs of visual sensitive patients and their relatives.

Terminology

Here we have tried, as much as possible, to distinguish between the epileptiform EEG-responses to IPS, the so-called photoparoxysmal responses (PPRs), and the clinical signs and symptoms either evoked by IPS or by visual stimuli in daily life (visually induced seizures). Thus, if a PPR is found, the patient is considered IPS-positive or photosensitive. Visual sensitivity is defined as having seizures evoked by the physical characteristics of a visual stimulus in daily life (flickering sunlight, monitors, striped patterns, etc.) or by IPS. The PPRs can be restricted to the occipital area (occipital spikes, sharp waves and spike waves) or be generalized (regular and irregular poly-spikes and waves). These different types can occur in the same patient depending on the flash frequency used, age at investigation, and use of medication, although some patients tend to have more focal PPRs and others a more generalized response (fast secondary generalization). Family members and those with clinical photosensitive occipital epilepsy without clear, observable seizures can have exclusively focal PPRs. Much more is therefore known about the patients who produce generalized PPRs at certain or all flash frequencies and in the following discussion we consider a PPR to be generalized, unless otherwise stated.

Epidemiology

Most data on the epidemiology of visual sensitivity and PPRs are retrospective prevalence studies and are related to specific patient groups. In general routine EEG populations, prevalence rates of generalized PPRs were found in 6% of Australian children between 5 and 18 years of age and in 1% in all ages in the Boston area (Nagarajan *et al.*, 2003; Jayakar & Chiappa, 1990).

The only population-based incidence study was done in the UK after reports of seizures being provoked by the Nintendo video game, Mario World, in 1992 (Quirk *et al.*, 1995). This was a prospective nationwide study to determine the incidence of visually induced seizures and PPRs in newly diagnosed epilepsy patients over a three-month period. They identified 191 cases, 143 of which had a generalized PPR. Since not all children had an EEG recorded and different IPS methods were used, some estimations had to be made. The annual incidence of cases of epilepsy with this abnormality was conservatively estimated to be 1.1 per 100,000, representing approximately 2% of all new cases of epilepsy. If the age range was restricted to 7–19 years, the annual incidence rose to 5.7 per 100,000 (10% of all new cases).

After the Pokemon incident in December 1997 in Japan, epidemiological studies were performed based on all the visits to outpatient clinics within a two-month period after the broadcast: about 1% had seizures (in about 75% it was the first seizure) and 10% had symptoms of headache, nausea, blurred vision, vertigo, etc. (Takada *et al.*, 1999; Furusho *et al.*, 2002). PPRs were found in about 40% of cases.

Although different definitions, populations and methods have been used in many studies, some overall estimates can be made on the prevalence of abnormal, epileptiform EEG responses to IPS and its relation to visually induced seizures in daily life as is described below.

Sex

Both in studies based on the prevalence of PPRs, and of a clinical history of visually induced seizures, there is a clear female preponderance of about 60% in children, adolescents and adults (Herrlin, 1954; Jeavons & Harding, 1975; Wolf & Goosses, 1986; Kasteleijn-Nolst Trenité, 1989; Clement & Wallace, 1990; Obeid *et al.*, 1991; Familusi, 1998; Nagarajan *et al.*, 2003). Video game epilepsy is more often found in males than females, possibly because boys play with video games more often than girls. However, there are also studies that indicate that, at certain ages, more boys than girls are photosensitive (Kasteleijn-Nolst Trenité, 1989; Anyanwu *et al.*, 2003).

Most epilepsy syndromes do not show a sex difference: in those that do, there is commonly a male preponderance of 60% (West syndrome, Dravet syndrome, epilepsy with myoclonic absences, idiopathic focal epilepsy with centro-temporal spikes). A female preponderance is exclusively found in childhood absence epilepsy (CAE) and in juvenile myoclonic epilepsy (JME) patients, who are photosensitive. However, the sex difference in CAE cannot be explained by the photosensitivity trait, since the 20% of IPS-sensitive CAE patients are equal in this respect to those without it (Wolf & Goosses, 1986). Surprisingly, JME patients without a PPR do not show any sex difference, whereas another syndrome characterized by myoclonias – epilepsy with myoclonic absences – shows a male preponderance. In patients with "grand mal on awakening", about 10% are photosensitive, and most of these are female.

Until today no clear explanation for this difference has been found; it seems that hormonal changes, genetic differences and epigenetics play a role (Taylor *et al.*, 2007).

In summary: There is a female preponderance (3:2) in patients with a history of visually induced seizures or a PPR. However, not only the prevalence of photosensitivity is higher in females, but also the median photosensitivity range is greater *(Figure 1)*.

Age

Photosensitivity can appear at different ages depending on the epilepsy syndrome. In Dravet patients (Dravet *et al.*, 2005) the very early appearance of PPRs at 2 or even 1 year of age and in about 40% of patients is remarkable. In the Genetic generalized epilepsies (CAE, JAE and JME) photosensitivity starts in early puberty and show their maximum photosensitivity generally at puberty (Clement &Wallace, 1990; Kasteleijn-Nolst Trenité, 1989; Shiraishi *et al.*, 2001). An example of PPRs and concomitant complaints are given in a 14 years old girl *(Figure 2)*. Koutroumanidis *et al.* (2015) described a cohort of patients in whom photosensitivity first appeared in adulthood, manifesting itself either as idiopathic photosensitive occipital epilepsy or idiopathic generalized epilepsy.

Harding *et al.* (1997) did not find a decline with age, whereas others found a clear decrease after the age of 25 (Shiraishi *et al.*, 2001; Kasteleijn-Nolst Trenité *et al.*, 1994; Jeavons *et al.*, 1986) or even

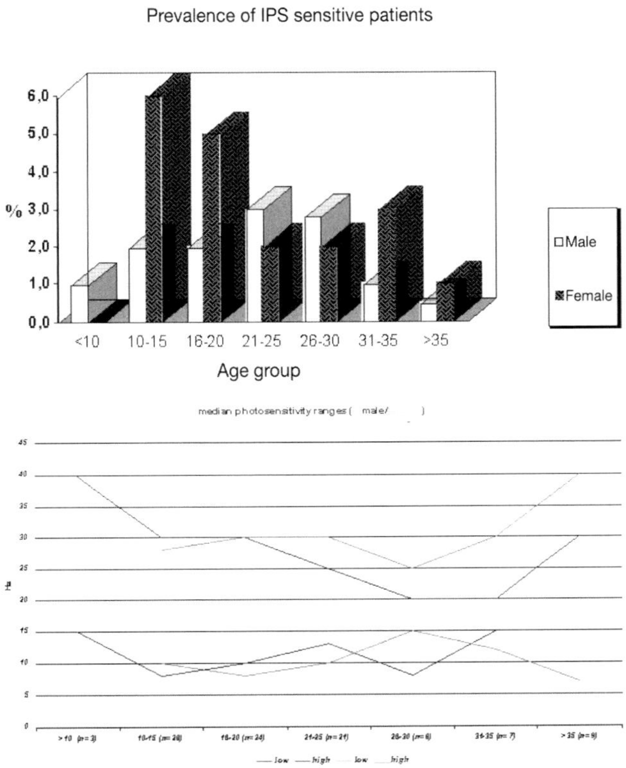

Figure 1 Prevalence of photoparoxysmal responses (PPR) in an EEG population referred to an epilepsy centre, per age and sex. Median photosensitivity ranges (upper and lower thresholds of an epileptiform reaction to IPS) per age group and per sex in the same population as (a). There are differences depending on age at investigation. In the age range 16–25 years, females become more sensitive than males. The sex differences are not explained by use of medication. Note however that the age groups < 10 and > 25 years are relatively small.
These data were originally published in 1989 in the *Acta Neurologica Scandinavica* 1989, vol. 80, Suppl 125.

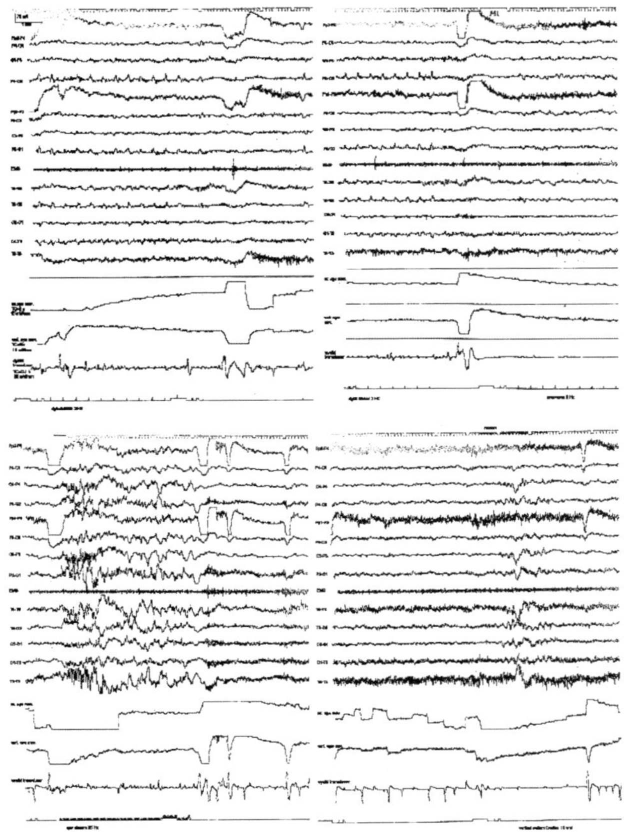

Figure 2 A 14-year-old girl, known to have had one tonic-clonic seizure at the age of 13 in a discothèque, after which she was put on valproate 600 mg. Normal (a) and epileptiform (b, c) EEG reactions to IPS and black-and-white striped patterns. No clinical signs were seen nor noted by the patient. She did not respond to television (50 Hz, 100 Hz, with various programmes). (a) Photic following or driving response; this was most prominent in the eyes closed condition. (b) Generalized irregular spikes and slow waves at IPS 25 Hz on eye closure; she felt dizzy and felt as if she was falling asleep; no clinical signs (jerks) were visible. (c) Epileptiform abnormalities over the posterior region on stimulation with a black-and-white pattern, radius 13 cm and vertical orientation.

after the age of 15 years (Melsen, 1959; Verrotti *et al.*, 2004). Some female adolescent patients with GGE stay photosensitive till at least about 70 years of age (personal data). Interestingly, a 74-year-old lady with an 8-week history of episodic myoclonic jerking with unresponsiveness showed a generalized PPR between 16 and 22 Hz with eyes open. She appeared to have had a GTCS at the age of 10 and had remained asymptomatic for 64 years (Jacob *et al.*, 2006). In a population of visually sensitive patients with a family history of visual sensitivity, no disappearance of PPRs was seen (Anyanwu *et al.*, 2003).

The expression of the disease (trait) might thus depend on different genes and thus syndromes (see below).

PPRs in normal subjects

In 1976, Papatheophilou & Turland studied the EEGs of normal school boys aged between 12 and 16 years; they restricted the study to boys to exclude the possible effect of hormonal variations. They investigated 223 boys from different social classes in the Birmingham area, UK. A photo stimulator was used with a grid with 0.12 joule intensity per flash. Three boys of 12, 14 and 15 years of age showed generalized poly-spike waves during photic stimulation; two of them suffered from recurrent headaches and pain while watching television, the other only reported suffering from migraine and possible fainting at school when 8 years old (1.3% prevalence). A similar prevalence rate was found in a study performed in Teof ilo Otoni (Brazil), where seven out of 510 school children of both sexes (1.4%) showed a PPR without relation to age (Kasteleijn-Nolst Trenité *et al.*, 2003).

Scandinavian studies in 20 normal girls and 50 normal boys revealed a prevalence of 1.4% IPS-positive reactions in one study, and in 8.9% of 389 girls and 184 boys of the same age range (0–15 years) (Herrlin, 1954; Eeg-Olofsson *et al.*, 1971). Apart from a sex difference, this large difference in results can only be explained by differences in patient selection (age, history of diseases, birth problems, etc.), methodology of stimulation (photic stimulator, flash frequencies, sleep recording, etc.) and interpretation of results (type and localization of waves included).

Other studies in "normal" populations involved studies in male candidates for aircrew training in the Netherlands, USA, UK and India, which gave PPR rates of 0.5, 2, 0.5 and 0.7% respectively (Hendriksen & Elderson, 2001; Robin *et al.*, 1978; Gregory *et al.*, 1993; Roy *et al.*, 2003). Roy *et al.* (2003) also tested established cases of epilepsy (723 men and 277 women, age range 8–20 years) using the same methodology for comparison purposes. In the epilepsy group they found 30 cases (3%) with a PPR.

PPRs in non-epileptic patients

PPRs have been found in 3% of psychiatric patients, with a 5 times higher incidence in females. No particular psychiatric diagnosis or use of drugs was associated (Small, 1971).

Although exact numbers are lacking, a PPR can often be found in migraine patientsIn EEG studies in children and adolescents with headache, a PPR was found in about 30% in the migraine with aura subgroup; in 7 out of 17 patients with both migraine and PPR, photogenic stimuli were the most frequent triggering factors of the migraine attack, compared with 10 out of 100 controls ($p < 0.01$) (Piccinelli *et al.*, 2006).

Complaints of headache are found significantly more often in photosensitive patients (twice as often) and is also a regular finding during a PPR (Kasteleijn-Nolst Trenité *et al.*, 1987; Kasteleijn-Nolst Trenité, 1989; Papetti *et al.*, 2013). Headache can thus also be the sole manifestation of an epileptic event and be the remaining complaint after AED treatment (Parisi *et al.*, 2007) especially in families with both migraine and epilepsy (Piccioli *et al.*, 2009).

PPRs have also been described in individual cases of Parkinson's disease, hypothyroidism and encephalitis, brain tumor, cerebral vascular disorder, Kleine-Levin syndrome, anti-depressants, alcoholism and trauma (Gerken & Doose, 1969; Hegedüs & Csibia, 1982; Papacostas, 2003; Solomon, 1960; Scarpino *et al.*, 1990; De Keyser *et al.*, 1984). In these cases the abnormal reaction to photic stimulation disappeared after spontaneous recovery or treatment of the underlying disease.

An illustration of the above was found in the reasons for recording an EEG in 33 patients with PPRs who had not had an epileptic seizure before or after the diagnosis (So *et al.*, 1993). In half the cases, the main reason was headache, dizziness or fainting 20%, learning disability 10%, memory disturbance 10%, brain tumor 5%, weakness 5%, psychiatric disorders 5%, head injury 5%, febrile seizures 5% and unknown in 10%.

PPRs in epileptic patients of different ethnic (genetic) backgrounds

Over the years, many prevalence studies have been performed in various countries worldwide. If we select those studies that used the same Grass photic stimulator and more or less the same methodology, we see different prevalence rates of generalized PPRs found in randomly admitted patients with suspected epilepsy. A PPR is found in 5–8% of patients in the Netherlands, Germany, the UK, South Africa and Australia (Kasteleijn-Nolst Trenité, 1989; Danesi, 1985; Doose & Gerken, 1973; De Graaf, 1995; Nagarajan *et al.*, 2003) but in only 1–2% of patients in India, Japan, Nigeria and Zimbabwe (Saleem *et al.*, 1994; Shiraishi *et al.*, 2000; Danesi, 1985; Familusi *et al.*, 1998).

Both De Graaf *et al.* (1995) and Familusi *et al.* (1998) compared different ethnic groups living in the same area. In Namibia, of 1,493 patients with suspected epilepsy referred to the EEG laboratory (80% blacks, 10% coloreds and 8% whites), PPRs were found in 0.4% of blacks, 4% of coloreds and 5.2% of whites. In Zimbabwe, in 9,082 persons aged 0–25 years with a roughly equal number of white and black people (about 48%), there were again significantly higher prevalences of PPRs among the whites (2.1%) and Asians (2.1%) than in the black people (0.2%), while the colored had an intermediate prevalence (0.6%). Interestingly, Asians living in Zimbabwe had a higher prevalence than the Asians in India. This can be explained by the genetic intermingling in Zimbabwe. Neither sunshine duration, sunlight intensity, nor the amount of pigmentation of the eyelids and retina (albino black people) can account for this difference (Familusi *et al.*, 1998; Bental, 1979; Scott *et al.*, 1985; Danesi, 1985), thus PPRs seem to depend primarily on genetic factors. Because the prevalence of epilepsy in the various countries is roughly similar, PPRs are thought to be a separate trait, adding to or modifying the other epilepsy genes (see also Genetics section).

In summary: a PPR is in general an age and sex-related phenomenon, clearly related to epilepsy and its various syndromes. It can, however, be found in normal children and adolescents with no or only minor symptoms such as headache or related diseases (see also below). Caucasians have the highest prevalence of PPRs (5–8%).

Genetics

The prevalence of the PPR trait in the general population of pediatric age was found to be 7.6% and 8.3% (Eeg-Olofsson *et al.*, 1971; Doose & Gerken, 1973). Females are significantly more often affected than males. The photoparoxysmal response is age-dependent, with a maximum penetrance and expression between 5 und 15 years of age (Waltz, 1994).

Family studies

Case reports of monozygotic twins show almost 100% concordance (Daly & Bickford, 1951; Davidson & Watson, 1956; Herrlin, 1960), but systematic twin studies comparing monozygotic and dizygotic twins have not been performed.

Large family studies in photosensitive index cases provide evidence for genetic transmission of the photoparoxysmal response. They showed a sibling's risk of 26.2% (Doose *et al.*, 1969), 22.0% (Rabending & Klepel, 1970) and 22.9% (Doose & Gerken, 1973). At the age of maximum penetrance up to 50% of siblings were affected (Doose *et al.*, 1969; Doose & Gerken, 1973; Waltz *et al.*, 1992). Parents were found to be affected in 10.2% (Rabending & Klepel, 1970). Index cases in these studies all had a photoparoxysmal response in the EEG, the epilepsy phenotype of the index cases however, was not well defined. Waltz & Stephani (2000) investigated two different groups of siblings. In families with a photosensitive parent 50% of siblings were affected. In the other group only 15% of siblings showed the trait (Waltz & Stephani, 2000). These data point towards an autosomal dominant mode of inheritance with age and sex-dependant penetrance in selected cases (Davidson & Watson, 1956; Waltz & Stephani, 2000).

A clinical study investigated families in which at least two members suffered from idiopathic epilepsy and either EEG or clinical photosensitivity. Three main photosensitive phenotypes were found: i) genetic (idiopathic) generalized epilepsies (GGE); ii) idiopathic photosensitive occipital epilepsy (IPOE); iii) mixed (GGE/IPOE). Overall the conclusion of this study was that GGE, IPOE and photosensitivity are on a continuous genetic spectrum and that the complex pattern of inheritance of these disorders likely includes shared genetic determinants (Taylor *et al.*, 2013).

Linkage studies

Based on descriptions of transient abolition of photosensitivity with apomorphine, and bromocriptine and parenteral L-dopa (Quesney *et al.*, 1980; 1981), a candidate linkage study on the five dopamine receptors gene regions of DRD1 to DRD5 was performed in a sample of 37 PPR-nuclear pedigrees. In the same study, analysis of previously reported loci concerning progressive myoclonus epilepsy EPM1 (21q22.3), EPM2 (6q24) and IGE (1p, 2q36, 3p14, 3q26, 4p, 6p11, 6p21.3, 8p11, 15q14) were analyzed. None of the loci were found to be linked to the PPR (Neubauer *et al.*, 2005).

A genome-wide linkage scan was conducted in 16 predominantly Dutch PPR multiplex families with an important background of myoclonic seizures using a broad model (inclusion of all patients with PPR types I-IV) and a narrow model (exclusion of PPR types I and II and the occipital epilepsy cases) of affectedness for PPR (Pinto *et al.*, 2005). Evidence for linkage on chromosomes 7q32 and 16p13 was found (Pinto *et al.*, 2005).

Another genome-wide linkage scan was performed by Tauer *et al.* (2005), using two family subgroups of mostly German origin. These were 19 families with predominantly pure PPR and photosensitive seizures (PPR families) and 25 families, in which PPR was strongly associated with IGE (PPR/IGE families). They found significant evidence for linkage to the region 6p21.2 in the PPR families and suggestive evidence for linkage to the region 13.q31.3 in the PPR/IGE families.

In a mega-analysis, both studies (Pinto *et al.*, 2005; Tauer *et al.*, 2005) were combined and augmented by additional families (de Kovel *et al.*, 2010). The combination of the different family subsets did not strengthen the linkage to the previously found loci. Evidence for linkage was reduced or disappeared completely. Three regions suggestive of linkage were identified, 16 p13.3, 5q35.3 and 8q 21.13 and only 16p13.3 had been found before (Pinto *et al.*, 2005). The authors found that different subsets were responsible for different peaks, indicating genetic heterogeneity. These findings might be partially explained admitting candidate loci harbouring multiple genes potentially playing a role in epileptogenesis (Tauer *et al.*, 2005).

Monogenic epileptic syndromes with photosensitivity

The description of different monogenic epileptic syndromes with a high rate of photosensitivity provides evidence for pathophysiological und genetic heterogeneity of photosensitivity.

Photosensitivity is a characteristic finding in Dravet syndrome (Verbeeketal, 2017), which is caused by mutations in the *SCN1A* gene, that encodes brain voltage-gated sodium channel type-1. Photosensitivity is also found in most cases of myoclonus epilepsy with ataxia due to a potassium channel mutation (Oliver *et al.*, 2017).

An interesting combination of two forms of reflex epilepsies, speaking induced jaw-jerks and flickering sunlight induced limb jerks, in a large family has been recently described. All photosensitive family members shared a heterozygous R129C mutation in the *SCNM1* gene that regulates splicing of voltage gated ion channels. Mutation screening of 134 unrelated patients with epilepsy and PPR and in 95 healthy controls, did not replicate these findings (Kasteleijn-Nolst Trenité *et al.*, 2015).

Mutations in the chromodomain helicase DNA-binding protein 2 (CHD2) have been found in an epileptic encephalopathy sharing some features with Dravet syndrome (Carvill *et al.*, 2013; Thomas *et al.*, 2015). 7 out of 10 patients showed extreme clinical photosensitivity with 6 patients showing self-induced seizures. A study of CHD2 mutations in a GGE cohort found an over-representation of unique CHD2 variants in eyelids myoclonia with absences and photosensitivity (Jeavons syndrome) whereas this was not present in subjects with PPR without seizures (Galizia *et al.*, 2015). In the CHD2 mutant zebrafish model, a significant increase in spontaneous abnormal burst discharge during a light "ON" state compared to light "OFF" state was observed (Galizia *et al.*, 2015). Interestingly, CHD2 does not encode for an ion channel and this finding might open new perspectives in the investigation and comprehension of cortical hyperxcitability.

In a novel animal model, Wielaender *et al.* (2017) described photosensitive seizures in Rhodesian ridgebacks with a generalized myoclonic epilepsy with photosensitivity due to a fully penetrant recessive 4-bp deletion in the DIRAS family GTPase 1 (DIRAS1) gene leading an altered expression pattern of DIRAS1 protein in the affected brain. This gene has a proposed role in cholinergic transmission.

A study on a cohort of patients with mutations within the alpha1 subunit of $GABA_A$ receptors (GABRA1) has reported a PPR response in 50% of them. The PPR was associated with clinically heterogenous epileptic disorders suggesting that the pathophysiology of PPR may be shared with other disorders of GABA inhibition (Johannesen *et al.*, 2016). The present data thus show, that no single gene is responsible for the PPR trait (de Kovel *et al.*, 2010). Furthermore, some data may contribute to further comprehend the pathophysiology of photosensitivity (Galizia *et al.*, 2015; Johannesen *et al.*, 2016) Further molecular analysis will need clinically and electroencephalographically well-defined homogenous groups to identify the various genes responsible for PPR and clinical photosensitivity.

Precipitating factors

Clinical factors

Sunlight has been recognized as an important provocative factor since classical antiquity (Radovicci *et al.*, 1932) and television as another, since the introduction of television sets in the 1950s (Pantelakis *et al.*, 1962). By 1964, fifty cases of television-related seizures had been reported in Europe (50 Hz mains frequency), with far fewer in the USA (60 Hz mains frequency) (Charlton & Hoefer, 1964). Furthermore, different types of *flickering sunlight* were reported as being provocative, *e.g.* sunlight shining through trees or rotating helicopter blades, sunlight reflections on snow, water (Van Gijn, 2001), car bumpers, etc. *Artificial lights* that have been recognized as epileptogenic include discotheque lights (Berney *et al.*, 1981), arc lights that suddenly begin to flicker (Cobb, 1947), and lights with interrupted flickers in a physics laboratory. Although normal fluorescent lighting (100 Hz tubes do not provoke epileptiform discharges in the laboratory) (Binnie *et al.*, 1979), old, dysfunctioning fluorescent lighting with irregular flashing in shops and classrooms have been reported consistently and repeatedly by some photosensitive patients as causing seizures (Specchio *et al.*, 2010). *Flickering* of fluorescent and, gas discharge lamps, in general, can be avoided by applying electronic, high frequency, lamp drivers and by proper maintenance, especially in industry and school classrooms. Movies in general do not evoke seizures or complaints, which could be due to the 24 Hz frequency of the movie images, in combination with the relatively great distance to the screen (Gastaut & Bert, 1954).

Many children had their first *television seizures* during a faulty channel broadcast or while changing channels in combination with getting close to the screen, or during specific flashing commercials, programs or video games (Ricci *et al.*, 1998; Demarco & Ghersini, 1985). Nowadays, it is common to have a variety of new and old (TV) monitors in house and also in children's bedrooms; old screens produce less stable images and the children watch cartoons and music programs with bright, flashing lights and high-contrast patterns at a close distance seizures can easily be provoked. Television screens can also be used for self-induction; the children may be found in a trance in front of the television set (Aso *et al.*, 1994). This behavior is often not recognized easily, because of children's general tendency to want to sit close to the television screen and becoming absorbed in the program. A 100 Hz television is much less provocative than a common 50 Hz, although playing special video games like *Super Mario World* can still be provocative in IPS-sensitive children (Badinand-Hubert *et al.*, 1998; Kas-teleijn-Nolst Trenité *et al.*, 2002). Computer screens (cathode ray tube) have also been shown to be provocative if the refresh rate of the screen is below 70 Hz (Kasteleijn-Nolst Trenité *et al.*, 1994b). Modern displays like LCD (Liquid Crystal Display), TFT, (Thin Film Transistor), OLED (Organic Light Emitting Diode), PolyLED (Polymer Light Emitting Diode), and PDP (Plasma Driven Panel) all generate their light output in a different way, and are therefore expected to have a specific effect on visually sensitive people- some will be more provocative (size, contrast and colors) and others less (60 and 70 Hz flicker of the mains electricity). Changing a 50 Hz television to a plasma screen reduced self-induction behavior drastically in a 9-year-old girl (Sharma & Cameron, 2007).

Display flicker may occur for numerous reasons. Overall, the chance of provoking an epileptic seizure can be minimized by using small displays, adjusting the luminance and contrast, and respecting the prescribed viewing distances: 0.7 m for computer monitors and 6 times the height of the screen for television sets (see Kasteleijn-Nolst Trenité *et al.*, 2004 for more details).

The *ambient lighting* in a room does not seem to have much additional influence on a person's sensitivity to the television, although there are differences in opinion about this (Jeavons & Harding, 1975; Binnie *et al.*, 1980).

Colored light seems to have a strong effect on some individuals; some patients benefit from blue glasses, others from red, green or smoke-tinted glasses, as confirmed by investigations with IPS and selected colored glasses (Rao & Prichard, 1955; Andermann, 1971; Takahashi Tsukahara, 1992; Wilkins *et al.*, 1999; Capovilla *et al.*, 1999; Kepecs *et al.*, 2004). In practice, children usually do not like to wear glasses for longer periods of time, but they can be very useful in specific circumstances.

In our current world, children and adolescents are increasingly being confronted with a variety of potentially epileptogenic visual stimuli and we expect many more children to have seizures at an early age. This will also necessitate anticonvulsant prophylactic treatment in a larger number of patients, since it is very hard to avoid potentially provocative visual stimuli.

In summary: Flickering sunlight (shining through trees, reflecting on snow, water, etc., rotating helicopter blades), artificial lights (discotheque, arcades, dysfunctioning fluorescent lighting), television screens (old screens, viewing close to set, special programs with colored and white flashing lights, certain video games and programmes), striped black and white patterns (Venetian blinds, rolling walkways and escalators, clothes, buildings, etc.) are the most provocative visual stimuli in daily life. Computer screens are also provocative. Modern displays like liquid crystal, organic and polymer light emitting diodes, and plasma-driven panels, all generate their light output in a different way, and it will probably depend on the size of the screen, the contrast, colors and luminance as to whether these provoke seizures in photosensitive patients.

Pathophysiology

Although visual-sensitive epilepsies are the commonest and longest known forms of reflex epilepsies, their pathophysiological mechanisms are still incompletely understood. Indeed, several approaches have been used to study human photosensitivity, either by investigating the mechanisms triggering epileptiform EEG abnormalities and visual-sensitive seizures, in particular in pattern-sensitive subjects, or by using techniques that explored the cortical mechanisms underlying the abnormal response to light, without eliciting paroxysmal EEG activities (Rubboli *et al.*, 2004).

Pathophysiological mechanisms of human photosensitivity admit that:

– *the seizure trigger is in the occipital cortex*; in pattern-sensitive patients, exposure to bright, large, continuously illuminated patterns of high contrast stripes evokes a PPR; several properties of pattern stimuli, crucial to elicit a PPR, such as length of line contour of striped patterns, pattern orientation, spatial frequency, pattern motion and the effect of binocularity, are consistent with the involvement of cortical neurons. In particular, the observation that neurons originating from the abnormal response display a spatial tuning independent of visual field position support the participation of complex cells of the visual cortex (Wilkins *et al.*, 2004). In addition, the different topographic distributions of scalp EEG responses following pattern stimuli positioned in the upper or lower hemi- field, or in lateral hemi-fields are in agreement with a trigger located in the visual cortex (Wilkins *et al.*, 2004). Regional hyperexcitability of the primary visual cortex in photosensitive epileptic patients is supported also by transcranial magnetic stimulations studies showing a rapid recovery of excitability in the visual cortex and persistent transcallosal contralateral disinhibition (Bocci *et al.*, 2016), and a lower threshold to magnetic stimuli-induced phosphenes (Brigo *et al.*, 2013);

– *abnormal functionality of occipital neurons may result in impaired contrast gain-control mechanisms:* in idiopathic photosensitive occipital epilepsy, investigation of cortical mechanisms responsible of epileptic activity have been studied by pattern visual evoked potentials with specific parameters: the results demonstrated that patterns with relatively low temporal frequency and high contrast are effective in unveiling cortical hyperexcitability possibly because of an impairment of contrast gain-control mechanisms (Porciatti *et al.*, 2000). Recent data obtained with different kinds of visual stimuli furtherly suggested enhanced cortical excitability possibly due to changes in excitatory neurotransmission (Shepherd & Siniatchkin, 2009; Moeller *et al.*, 2009);

– *seizure onset occurs on one cerebral hemisphere or both hemispheres independently:* asymmetries of responses to stimulations of lateral hemifields and also to diffuse intermittent photic stimulation have been consistently observed, supporting the hypothesis that one hemisphere might be more susceptible to produce abnormal responses. In these subjects, the PPR originates and may remain confined in one hemisphere. On the other hand, in patients without these asymmetries it can be observed that the seizure discharge can originate alternatively in one hemisphere or in the other, suggesting an equipotentiality of both hemispheres to trigger independently epileptic activity (Wilkins *et al.*, 2004). The observation of a time lag between photic myoclonus-related cortical potentials in the two hemispheres further lends support to this conclusion (Rubboli *et al.*, 1999);

– *the activation of a critical mass of cortical tissue is required to elicit an epileptiform response:* any area of the visual cortex can trigger a PPR, provided that a sufficient amount of cortical tissue is stimulated. Although the probability of obtaining an abnormal response to pattern stimuli exposure may vary in each patient, each patient's threshold can be expressed in terms of the area of cortex necessary to elicit a discharge;

– *physiologic activity of large neuronal aggregates must be synchronized to trigger seizure activity:* the synchronization of the neuronal firing such as that provoked by patterns vibrating back and forth orthogonally to the stripes is critical to initiate the seizure discharge (Wilkins *et al.*, 2004). In addition, enhancement of synchronized activity in the gamma band preceding the onset of the PPR has been demonstrated by magnetoencephalograhic investigations: this finding may indicate a loss of control over high-frequency oscillatory processes that normally intervene in a transient fashion to connect neural assemblies possibly implicated in perceptual functions (Parra *et al.*, 2003). In normal subjects, exposure to pattern stimuli able to induce visual discomfort may enhance gamma oscillations at approximately the same spatial frequencies that may trigger a PPR (Adjamian *et al.*, 2004);

– *magnocellular and parvocellular systems may contribute either synergistically or independently to elicit a PPR:* changes in pure luminance or quantity of light (black and white) are processed by the magnocellular pathway whereas the differences in wavelength of the visual stimuli are processed by the parvocellular division. Magnocellular involvement for stimuli characterized by pure luminance variations (such as pattern stimuli) is supported by extensive data demonstrating that magnocellular neurons do not generally process color, are directionally coded, are tuned for binocular disparity, and have lower spatial and higher temporal resolution than parvocellular cells (Wilkins *et al.*, 1979). Participation of the parvocellular pathway is suggested by experimental findings documenting that low-luminance, highly saturated red lights with a wavelength around 700 nm can be more provocative than black and white flickers (Takahashi *et al.*, 1999a). A similar stimulation, produced by red and blue flashes at 12 Hz, occurred in the Pokemon incident that precipitated seizures in an unexpected large number subjects, most of them non-epileptics.

EEG studies have confirmed the strong provocative effect of these colored Pokemon sequences *(Table I)*. This phenomenon might have been caused by a pronounced stimulation of red cones, the most numerous in the retina, not compensated by stimulation of complementary cones, associated with an induced color-contrast effect that produced color combinations particularly effective in inducing a PPR (Harding, 1998; Shirakawa *et al.*, 2001). It has been reported that color sensitivity depends on two mechanisms: one related to color modulation, that intervenes at frequency lower than 30 Hz, the other dependent on single-color light intensity modulation and related to white light sensitivity, that is activated at higher frequencies (Parra *et al.*, 2007). Selective activation of parvocellular or magnocellular divisions has been proposed to trigger different types of PPR: excitation of the parvocellular system by colored stimuli would be more epileptogenic eliciting a generalized PPR, whereas stimulation of the magnocellular system would result in a milder PPR, represented by occipital spikes (Harding & Fylan, 1999):

– *abnormal visuomotor integration can facilitate the anterior spread of the visually-induced epileptic activity:* overactive visuomotor connections and increased functional responsivity of the motor cortex in photosensitive epileptic patients (Strigaro *et al.*, 2015; Suppa *et al.*, 2015) and in animal models (Szabo *et al.*, 2016) might underlie the generation of photic-induced motor manifestations (such as myoclonus) (Rubboli *et al.*, 1999; Mukundan *et al.*, 2014);

– *cognitive processes and action programming may play a role:* absence of photosensitivity in some subjects who suffered from TV-or videogame-induced seizures (Kasteleijn-Nolst Trenité *et al.*, 2002) has suggested a major role in triggering seizures of intense cognitive processes and possibly of cortical activity involved in action programming (Zifkin & Inoue, 2004).

Table I Visual stimulation in the EEG laboratory in 12 patients, ranked 1 (highly sensitive) to 6 (not sensitive)
Ranking order in sensitivity (1 to 5; 6 = not sensitive) in terms of generalization and duration of discharges per patient to various visual stimuli in the laboratory: IPS, black & white striped pattern, 50 Hz TV and 100 Hz TV (Pokemon cartoon in colour and in black and white). IPS was the most provocative stimulus in all 12 patients; patterns and the black and white Pokemon cartoon on the 100 Hz TV were the least provocative. Note, however, the individual differences regardless of the antiepileptic medication. Five other patients with a history of possibly visually induced seizures were investigated with all above stimuli, but were not sensitive to any of them

Sex	IPS	Pattern	TV 50 Hz White screen Stable image Video clip Red/blue	TV 100 Hz Pokemon in black & white	TV 100 Hz Pokemon in color	Antiepileptic drugs
M	1	5	3	4	2	LTG
M	1	6	6	6	2	LTG
M	1	5	2	4	2	LTG
F	1	6	6	6	2	-
F	1	2	2	6	6	-
F	1	6	6	6	2	VPA+ESM
F	1	6	6	6	2	-
F	1	6	6	6	6	VPA
F	1	6	2	4	2	LTG
F	1	2	2	6	2	LTG+ES M
F	1	6	1	4	1	-
F	1	6	2	2	2	LTG + VPA
Total 9F/3M	**12**	**62**	**44**	**60**	**31**	
Average score	**1**	**5.17**	**3.67**	**5.0**	**2.58**	

Contribution of neuroimaging studies in elucidating the pathophysiological mechanisms underlying photosensitivity

Although hyperexcitability of the visual cortex explains some ictal and EEG findings, it does not entirely elucidate the range of photosensitivity-associated EEG and clinical correlates. Indeed, photoparoxysmal responses are often generalized, and photic stimulation ultimately can elicit seizures with motor components, which are a particularly frequent reflex trait in patients with IGE. Indeed, a dysfunction extending beyond the visual system has been supported by previous studies using transcranial magnetic stimulation that documented increased visuomotor hyperexcitability during photic stimulation in IGE patients (Strigaro *et al.*, 2012, 2015; Groppa *et al.*, 2008) and even in healthy individuals with PPR (Siniatchkin *et al.*, 2007). In this line, previous EEG-correlated functional MRI (EEG-fMRI) studies have detected photoparoxysmal-related activation in parietal and premotor cortices (Moeller *et al.*, 2009 a,b; Bartolini *et al.*, 2014).

Most studies in photosensitive epilepsy to date have focused on measuring cortical responses to visual stimuli. However, studies of resting brain rhythms in the absence of external stimuli could also shed light on neural mechanisms of photosensitive epilepsy. Vaudano and colleagues recently reported findings from simultaneous EEG and functional MRI studies in photosensitive epilepsy at rest (Vaudano *et al.*, 2017). First, they studied the hemodynamic correlates of the spontaneous EEG alpha rhythm. Fluctuations in posterior alpha power during the EEG-functional MRI scan session were extracted. Then the alpha frequency and its respective power fluctuation over time were calculated, convolved with a hemodynamic response function and used as a regressor of the functional MRI signal analysis. The main EEG findings were of a greater mean alpha power in the IGE photosensitive epilepsy group compared to controls and other epilepsy groups *(Figure 3)*. The functional MRI analysis revealed alpha-related blood oxygen level-dependent (BOLD) changes with a similar distribution to previous reports in healthy participants (Laufs *et al.*, 2003; Liu *et al.*, 2012) and in patients without photosensitivity, with decreases of BOLD signal in broad areas of cerebral cortex, including the superior and inferior parietal lobule, occipital cortex, precuneus, and premotor and motor areas. Conversely, in photosensitive patients *(Figure 3)* the anticorrelation between alpha power fluctuation and the BOLD signal was weaker or absent in the occipital lobe and an increased positive correlation was evident in the basal ganglia and anterior cingulate gyrus. Then, Vaudano *et al.* selected anatomical "seed regions" based on their EEG-functional MRI analysis and previous reports, in the medial dorsal thalamic nucleus and the pulvinar. They found that there was a significant difference in the IGE photosensitive epilepsy group compared to controls and other epilepsy groups. Specifically, the IGE photosensitive epilepsy group showed an increased correlation between resting state BOLD activity in the medial dorsal thalamic nucleus and the bilateral orbitofrontal cortex, and between resting state activity in the pulvinar nucleus and the basal ganglia (putamen and caudate), anterior cingulate cortex, dorsolateral prefrontal and parietal cortices. Despite these inherent difficulties in interpreting the BOLD response, these findings show that resting brain measures can indicate the presence of photosensitive epilepsy and link the neuronal processes involved in alpha generation and those involved in photosensitive epilepsy. Moreover, these findings add to the growing literature indicating hyperexcitability not only of occipital areas in photosensitive epilepsy but of a wider network involving subcortical (thalamic structures) and frontal motor areas. This mirrors clinical manifestations of photosensitive epilepsy, with different routes of seizure spread in the various syndromes. Notably, the occipital – premotor areas were involved in the abnormal response to eye-closure in patients with eyelid myoclonia with absences (EMA) (Vaudano *et al.*, 2014), even in the absence of paroxysmal activity on EEG *(Figure 4)*. Among the reflex epileptic traits, eye-closure sensitivity (ECS) represents the archetypal of photosensitive epilepsy. The fact that ECS and PS coexist in EMA as cardinal features of the syndrome documents the existence of a strict

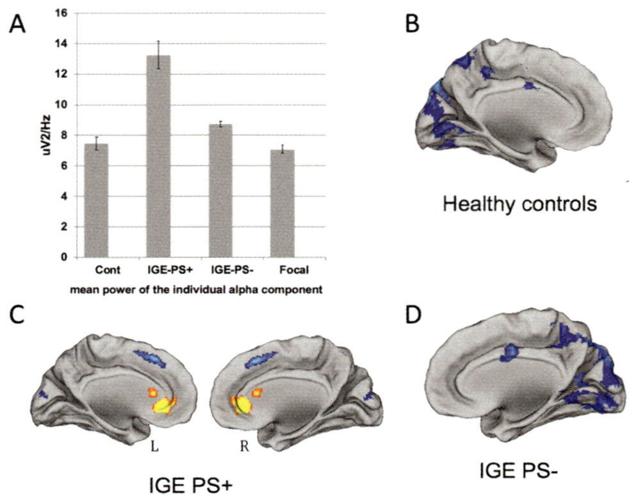

Figure 3 **Alpha rhythm and related hemodynamic changes in photosensitive epilepsy.**
A. Histograms display the mean alpha power in different subgroups of patients and in controls. The IGE PS+ shown significantly higher alpha power compared to other groups ($P < 0.01$). The bars represent the Standard Error. B, C, D. Alpha-BOLD correlation maps related to each group ($P < 0.05$, FDR corrected). The functional maps have been warped to the PALS-B12 atlas in caret (mesial and dorsal view) for right (R) and left (L) hemisphere. The yellow-red color identifies the positive correlations to alpha power, the light-blue color the negative correlations. The alpha power correlated negatively with activity in broad areas of cerebral cortex, including the superior and inferior parietal lobule, the occipital cortex (middle occipital gyrus and lingual gyrus), the precuneus, the premotor and motor regions in healthy controls (B), and in IGE without photosensitivity (D). Conversely, in photosensitive patients (C) the anticorrelation between alpha power fluctuation and the BOLD signal was weaker or absent in the occipital lobe and an increased positive correlation was evident in the basal ganglia and anterior cingulate gyrus. Adapted from Vaudano *et al.*, 2017.
Cont: controls; IGE PS+: idiopathic generalized epilepsy with photosensitivity; IGE PS-: idiopathic generalized epilepsy without photosensitivity.

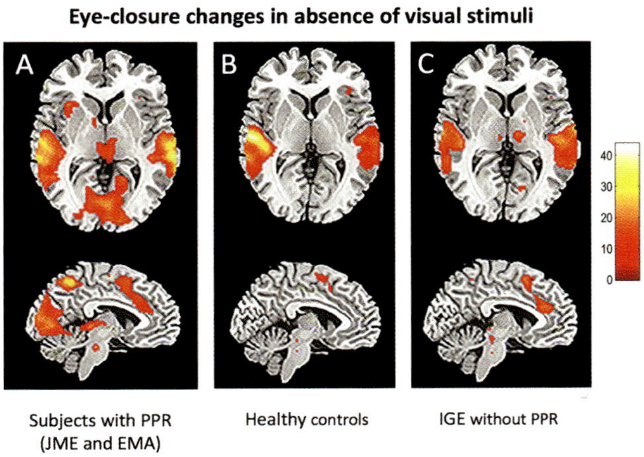

Figure 4 **Eye closure sensitivity in eyelid myoclonia with absences in the absence of photic stimulation.** Eye-closure second-level fMRI results. Group analysis results ($P < 0.05$ corrected for FWE) showing the transient BOLD signal changes immediately after the closure of the eyes in EMA and JME (A), healthy controls (B) and IGE without photoparoxysmal response (C). The BOLD changes are overlaid onto the canonical T1-Image, axial and sagittal slices, as implemented in SPM8. No decreases in BOLD signal were detected in the three populations. The random-effect model at eye-closure showed common BOLD signal increments in the bilateral temporal cortex (due to the processing of the acoustic command). Subcortical regions including the thalamus and brainstem; and the anterior cingulate/supplementary motor area bilaterally showed an increased BOLD signal change in EMA/JME. Moreover, only EMA/JME demonstrated BOLD increases at the parietal cortex adjacent to the intraparietal sulcus, and a positive BOLD involvement of the occipital cortex. Notably, this finding was observed independently of the appearance, after eye-closure, of paroxysmal EEG activities. Adapted from Vaudano *et al.* 2014.

link between these reflex epileptic traits. In accordance with this view the BOLD response to eye-closure in EMA and the BOLD response to intermittent photic stimulation in patients with PPR is characterized by the involvement of substantially the same brain circuits (Moeller *et al.*, 2009 a,b; Vaudano *et al.*, 2014). The network involves the posterior visual areas, the parietal cortex (the intraparietal sulcus), and the prefrontal cortex (namely SMA, cingulate gyrus, frontal eye filed). Interestingly, both the study of Vaudano *et al.* (2014) and the studies of Moeller *et al.* (2009 a,b) document the presence of an abnormal increase of BOLD signal before the appearance of spikes and waves discharges. Given that the increases in BOLD signal are correlated with increase in the gamma frequency range, these fMRI data are complementary to MEG/EEG observation that demonstrated gamma band synchronization preceding the photoparoxysmal response (Parra *et al.*, 2003; Perry *et al.*, 2014). One important difference between ECS phenomenon in EMA and PPR is that the BOLD signal alteration observed in ECS was present even in the absence of any subsequent epileptic discharge thus underscoring that it might be linked to an intrinsic dysfunction of this network independently of the appearance of any subsequent EEG paroxysmal activity.

Overall, the current findings obtained by multimodal imaging and neurophysiological techniques confirm the hypothesis of an intrinsic "visuo-motor hyperexcitability" in photosensitive epilepsy. The fact that this up-regulation is present under resting (unstimulated) conditions and even during the alpha rhythm, which is considered a hallmark of the brain resting state, indicates a probable genetic predisposition to generate synchronous paroxysmal activity.

As a general conclusion, the "enduring propensity" to generate seizures and/or epileptic activity in patients with photosensitivity is related to the intrinsic susceptibility of the visual system, not only limited to the occipital cortex, but expressed as an extended and functional system.

Clinical correlates of the photoparoxysmal response evoked by IPS

In 1953 Bickford, Daly & Keith described in detail the overall spectrum of clinical signs and symptoms that can be evoked by IPS in 27 children (2–13 years of age, six mentally retarded): absence seizures (Petit Mal); myoclonic jerks in the arms, head, eyelids, or upper limbs; speech arrest; turning of the eyes to the left or right-side or a generalized clonic-tonic seizure (GTCS) after head-turning to the left (subsequent build-up of occipital epileptiform activity (EA) on the right-side with generalization afterwards). Two children only had complaints of dizziness. Twenty children had spontaneous generalized or focal EA, often confined to the occipital area, and 18 had a history of seizures or self-induced seizures (two) in daily life. This study, performed more than 50 years ago, demonstrates the variability in clinical and EEG phenomena in photosensitive patients.

In a similar type of laboratory study in 36 photosensitive patients (Kasteleijn-Nolst Trenité *et al.*, 1987), clinical symptoms were seen in 75%, the most common being myoclonic jerks, but also spontaneous opening of the eyes, and loss of consciousness. No relationship was found between duration of evoked discharges and *type* of clinical symptoms. A roughly equal number of patients reported pain or awkward feelings in the eyes, head or stomach. Remarkably, only two of the 16 patients who showed clear myoclonus of the eyelids, noticed this symptom. Overall, 20 patients (56%) showed clinical signs without being aware of them *(Figure 3)*. A video-EEG study in IPS and video-game-sensitive patients has even revealed clinical signs in 100% of patients (Piccioli *et al.*, 2003). Although the most reported evoked seizures were tonic-clonic seizures, in many patients only absence seizures or myoclonic seizures in the arms were seen. Headache may be the patient's only complaint (Tozzi *et al.*, 1998). Eyestrain and pain in the eyes is a complaint that has often been found during IPS-evoked epileptiform activity. In clinical practice it can, however, be difficult to discriminate between migraine, common headache or visually induced epileptogenic headache (Kasteleijn *et al.*, 2010).

Thus, photosensitive patients may well have clinical seizures in daily life, but not notice them or, if noticed, they may under-report them, as seen in family studies: jerks and complaints about visual stimuli ran in the family and were considered normal. Patients commonly seek help only when they have had a tonic-clonic seizure, whereas case histories often reveal a preceding period of myoclonic jerks or staring. In addition, it is feasible that some patients who experience a tonic-clonic seizure do not know whether the seizure was visually induced, either because of amnesia or because there was a longer period between provocative factor and seizure. Especially children with occipital photosensitive epilepsy show this pattern. The latter situation seems to occur more often nowadays, and is most likely due to longer stimulation of a variety of provocative visual stimuli both at work and leisure. It is no surprise that the number of patients with a history of visually induced seizures has increased over the years, as evidenced in epidemic outbreaks of seizures caused by video games, commercials or cartoons (Graf *et al.*, 1994; Ricci *et al.*, 1998; Takahashi, 1999b). Bickford, Daly & Keith (1953) were the first to distinguish three separate classes in the 27 photosensitive patients they investigated, to indicate to the clinician the severity of the patient's sensitivity to light: i) "a clinically sensitive group in which light of the intensity encountered in daily life is capable of inducing clinical attacks"; ii) "a less sensitive group in which clinical seizures can be induced only under conditions of high intensity of illumination and rapid flicker"; and iii) "a group in which the only evidence of sensitivity is the occurrence of EA on IPS, unaccompanied by any detectable clinical evidence of a seizure". This distinction has also been used by others (Wadlington & Riley, 1965; Jeavons & Harding, 1975; Kasteleijn-Nolst Trenité *et al.*, 1987), but with differences in results due to referral bias, differences in methodology and whether the patient was looking into the lamp (Jeavons *et al.*, 1971). See *Table II*.

After the Pokemon incident, an epidemiological study was performed in the southern area of Tokyo (Furusho *et al.*, 2002): 14 pediatric clinics held a survey among all the parents who had visited the outpatient clinic over a two-month period. Only 30% of the parents filled in the questionnaire (1,373 children), but 80% of the children had watched the program and 67 (6.1%) of them had neurological problems: 10 (0.9%) had seizure symptoms during the program; 28 (2.6%) had complaints like headache, nausea, blurred vision, or vertigo around the cartoon broadcasting time, and in 29 (2.7%) children the symptoms and signs started within 30 minutes of the cartoon.

Table II IPS-sensitive patients with and without visually induced seizures in daily life
Distribution of IPS-sensitive patients (PPRs) among those with symptoms in daily life (group A), those with seizures during photic stimulation in the laboratory only (group B), and without any clinical signs (group C)

Number of patients	Published study	Group A		Group B		Group C	
		Visually induced seizures in daily life		*Seizures* during IPS only		PPR only No clinical signs	
27	Bickford *et al.* (1953)	**5**	**18%**	15	56%	7	26%
250	Wadlington and Riley (1965)	**8**	**3%**	17	7%	225	90%
460	Jeavons & Harding (1975)	232	**51%**	222	48%	6	1%
205	Fujiwaraet *al.* (1983)	**16**	**8%**	31	15%	158	77%
36	Kasteleijn *et al.* (1987)	**22**	**61%**	5	14%	9	25%

Distribution of IPS-sensitive patients (PPRs) among those with symptoms in daily life (group A), those with seizures during photic stimulation in the laboratory only (group B), and without any clinical signs (group C).

The children with seizures were older (over 8 years old) and more often had an individual- or family history of seizures. A clear PPR was found in only 3 of the 10 children who had seizures. In research carried out by the Japanese Ministry of Health, in a survey including older children and adolescents, up to 10.4% of viewers had symptoms and 1.4% seizures.

In another multicenter Pokemon study in 61 hospitals in Japan, questionnaires filled in by the doctors revealed that in the vast majority of the patients admitted (78 of 103; 76%) the provoked seizure was the patient's first. PPRs were found in 43% of these patients and was seen not only in those with a history of epilepsy (54%) but also in those with no history of epilepsy (38%) (Takada *et al.*, 1999; Ishiguro *et al.*, 2004). Short-term outcome after 3 years indicated that recurrence of seizures was reported in about 30% of these children. Further, there was no clear relationship found with finding a PPR. However, this study had many flaws and its results were influenced by differences in reporting, prescription of medication, and EEG methodology.

Out of 28,215 EEGs in Rochester, USA, all the patients with a PPR (188) were selected and 75% have had a seizure at some time (So *et al.*, 1993). Follow-up was possible in 33 of the 188 patients (18%) with a PPR without a seizure history (age range 3–44 years), but with complaints of headache, dizziness, brain tumor, etc., for 6–12 years (average 9 years) and none of these developed seizures. Similar results were found in another American study of 3,557 patients and 48 normal subjects (Jayakar & Chiappa, 1990). PPRs were seen in 35 (1%) patients, 27 (77%) of these had a definite history of epilepsy, 3 (9%) had a questionable history, and 5 (14%) had had no seizures.

In a prospective study in a Dutch epilepsy center, 94 of 100 patients with a generalized PPR outlasting the stimulus had a seizure history, compared to 84 of those without a PPR. In these 94 IPS-positive patients, 55 (59%) had a clear history of visually induced seizures in daily life (Kasteleijn-Nolst Trenité, 1989).

Another study in 21 Australian PPR positive children showed that 86% of them had epilepsy compared to 18% of the same hospital EEG sample, but without a PPR. Fifty percent of the photosensitive ones had a generalized PPR (Nagarajan *et al.*, 2003).

Although Reilly & Peters (1973) emphasized the predictive value of an epileptiform response that continues after the train of flashes, others did not find a difference in outcome between those with and without self-sustaining PPRs (Jakayar & Chiappa, 1990; Puglia *et al.*, 1992; Nagarajan *et al.*, 2003). In idiopathic occipital photosensitive epilepsy (focal seizures), PPRs are often confined to the occipital area. Thus clinical correlates can be found in patients with localized and generalized PPRs.

Spontaneous epileptiform abnormalities occur in up to 60% of patients with a PPR. Apart from being significantly associated with a history of seizures ($p < 0.0001$), seizure classification has been shown to be strongly associated with type of spontaneous discharge (focal *vs.* generalized $p < 0.0001$; Gilliam & Chiappa, 1995). Patients with focal discharges tended to have focal seizures, while patients with generalized discharges tended to have only generalized tonic-clonic or absence seizures.

In summary: 75% or more of patients with a PPR in their EEG will show clinical signs in the laboratory, 60–90% will have a history of epilepsy, and about 50% will have a history of seizures evoked by visual stimuli in daily life. Not all patients with a PPR will notice their clinical symptoms (or the photosensitivity range is so minimal that it is very unlikely to have provocation by stimuli within that particular range in daily life). The majority of reported evoked seizures are tonic-clonic seizures, but absence seizures and myoclonic seizures in the arms are seen in many patients and are related to the spontaneous epileptiform discharges. Headache, dizziness and nausea may be the only complaint and are indications that the patient has an occipital seizure.

Syndromes

General considerations

Because photic stimulation in the laboratory evokes mainly absence seizures and myoclonic jerks, "photogenic" and later "photosensitive" epilepsy was considered to be a genetic (idiopathic) generalized epilepsy (Penfield & Jasper, 1954; Gastaut, 1969). These patients often have exclusively visually provoked GTCS and myoclonic jerks in daily life. In patients with other epilepsy syndromes/types, the abnormal reaction to IPS regularly seems to be found by coincidence and is only one of the factors precipitating epileptic seizures. To our knowledge, no epidemiological studies have been done to determine the incidence and prevalence of photosensitivity and visually induced seizures in an *un*selected and *un*biased population with regard to syndromic classification. However, there have been some studies in cohorts of photosensitive patients: Wolf & Goosses (1986) compared 103 patients of all ages showing a PPR in the EEG with those without the trait and subsequently classified them. Of the generalized epilepsies, 15% was photosensitive, compared to only 3% of the localization-related epilepsies. Among the different syndromes, the highest prevalence of a PPR was found in juvenile myoclonic epilepsy (JME 30%) followed by childhood absence epilepsy (CAE 18%), and cryptogenic generalized syndromes (17%). In juvenile absence epilepsy 8% showed a PPR.

Shiraishi *et al.* (2001) studied a similar type of cohort and applied the 1989 syndromic classification: among a total of 2,187 unselected patients from a Japanese epilepsy centre (age range 1–81; mean 24.2 yrs;

56% male) 37 patients (1.7%) were found to have a self-sustaining generalized PPR at 18 Hz and/or other frequencies. Most PPR-positive patients were found among idiopathic generalize epilepsy (IGE) patients (5.6%) compared to localization-related epilepsy (0.7%). Within the IGE group, both JME (17.4%) and Grand Mal on awakening (7.6%) were significantly over-represented, while in the localization-related epilepsy group this was the case for occipital lobe epilepsy (6.1%). Of the patients with symptomatic generalized epilepsy, 2.0% had a PPR. Although the overall prevalence rate in Japan is lower, the distribution among the various syndromes thus appeared to be more or less the same.

In another Japanese study (Aso *et al.*, 1994), 17 children with visually induced seizures were classified: both JME and severe myoclonic epilepsy in infancy (SMEI) and localization-related epilepsies were found. However, this study did not include a control group and selection bias is highly likely to be present. The results stress, however, that visually induced seizures and a PPR can also be found in focal and other epilepsy types, as also demonstrated by many other authors (Tassinari *et al.*, 1988; Brinciotti *et al.*, 1994).

In summary, the majority of patients with visually induced seizures or PPRs can be found in the genetic (idiopathic) generalized and focal epilepsies (occipital) as well as in the severe epilepsies of childhood like Dravet syndrome (Verbeek *et al.*, 2017). In the last mentioned category the seizure frequency and severity is such that the existence of a provocative visual factor is often overlooked.

Classification systems

In the International Classification of Epilepsies and Epileptic Syndromes (1989), reflex epilepsies including visual sensitivity, were classified as a special syndrome like other situation-related seizures such as febrile convulsions and seizures, precipitated by alcohol or drugs. The diagnostic scheme proposed by the ILAE taskforce (Engel, 2001) changed this concept and proposed restricting a reflex epilepsy syndrome to those patients with seizures exclusively precipitated by sensory stimuli. Furthermore, the reflex epilepsies have been subdivided into idiopathic photosensitive occipital lobe epilepsy, other visually sensitive epilepsies, primary reading epilepsy, and startle epilepsy. The ILAE report concerning classification and terminology in 2010 (Berg *et al.*, 2010), however reduced the reflex seizures and epilepsies to just "Reflex epilepsies" under the heading: "Electroclinical syndromes and other epilepsies with a less specific age relationship". Similarly, the recent proposals of the ILAE Commission for Classification and Terminology on Classification of seizure types (Fisher *et al.*, 2017) and epilepsies (Scheffer *et al.*, 2017) failed to recognize this large group of epilepsies. Both Shorvon (2011) and Panayiotopoulos (2012), commenting the 2010 ILAE proposal (Berg *et al.*, 2010), noticed this omission: "The report fails to consider reflex epileptic seizures, which are not cited even by name, although they should be classified and precisely defined (Panayiotopoulos, 2012)".

The International Classification of Diseases of the World Health Organization (1991) did not include reflex epilepsy or visually induced epilepsy.

Since the expression of the photosensitivity genetic trait can be initiated in different ways, influenced by age, sex, concomitant cerebral states, and provocative visual stimuli in the surroundings, we would advise using the PSE trait as an extra sub-classification. Because the most frequent association of IPS sensitivity, visually induced seizures and epilepsy occurs in IGE, we propose that a separate category called Visually Sensitive IGE (to include pure photosensitive absences and absences with eyelid myoclonia) should be included under IGE.

In summary: There is no unequivocal place reserved yet for visually sensitive epilepsy or the EEG trait: PPR. Therefore, the proposed classification and terminology for Visual Sensitivity and Epilepsy, with its clear division into clinical and EEG phenomenology, will help to discriminate photosensitive from non-photosensitive patients, make collaborative research possible. This will help us learn more about the underlying mechanisms, the various subtypes of photosensitive patients, and their respective prognoses in relation to therapy, leading to a more specific and diverse position in the overall epilepsy classification system of the future (Kasteleijn-Nolst Trenité *et al.*, 2001). Given the current confusion in official classification and terminology, we consider it wise to build up a multi-level classification as is used for the purpose of genetic studies: seizure types, visually induced seizures, PPR types, specific syndromes like CAE, JME and epilepsy types like GGE.

Genetic (idiopathic) generalized epilepsies

PPRs are especially related with the IGEs and are found in up to 50% of GGE syndromes; ~10–40% of subjects with myoclonic epilepsies of infancy, in 30–40% of subjects with juvenile myoclonic epilepsy (JME) and in 13–18% of subjects with absence epilepsies of childhood (CAE) or juvenile-onset (JAE). This high degree of co-morbidity compared to a 0.5–7.6% prevalence in the general population, together with the lower comorbidity with focal syndromes such as temporal lobe epilepsy (4%), support its involvement in the predisposition to GGE (see also the genetics section).

Photosensitivity and visually induced seizures are found predominantly in the following subsyndromes of GGE.

Benign myoclonic epilepsy in infancy

This is the earliest presenting form of idiopathic generalized epilepsy associated with this rare condition (less than 0.5% of myoclonic epilepsy occurs in infancy). Benign myoclonic epilepsy in infancy (BMEI) was described for the first time in 1981 (Dravet & Bureau, 1981). These children start having massive myoclonic jerks between the age of four months and three years. The myoclonic jerks are always associated with generalized spike- and wave discharges and can be elicited in about 10% of cases by photic stimulation (Aird, 1984). Sodium valproate is effective and prevents the child from developing psychomotor retardation (Dravet *et al.*, 1992); often high AED plasma levels are necessary (Capovilla *et al.*, 1997). Although the syndrome is considered "benign", especially the cases that are photosensitive need ongoing treatment and this should be continued past the age of 6 years (Guerrini & Aicardi, 2003).

Childhood absence epilepsy

CAE is clearly associated with photosensitivity in 2–15% of patients (Wolf & Goosses, 1986; Shiraishi *et al.*, 2001). Studies have shown that up to 80% of the photosensitive CAE children are of female sex and 64% with a history of visually induced seizures (Baykan *et al.*, 2005). It is still being debated whether children with a PPR have a worse prognosis than those without (Loiseau & Duché, 1995), although the Turkish study indicates that remission is difficult to obtain (Baykan *et al.*, 2005). It is also known that absences in childhood can be the first symptom of later JME (6%) (Janz & Durner, 1991).

Juvenile onset absence epilepsy

Unlike childhood absence epilepsy, the overall sex distribution in JAE is equal and this could explain that a PPR is found in only 8% of patients at most (Wolf & Goosses, 1986). On the other hand, one would expect to have a higher number of photosensitive patients since the highest prevalence is around 13 years of age. Sixteen percent of patients with JAE go on to develop JME (Janz & Waltz, 1995) but whether relatively more of these patients will have PPRs is unknown.

Juvenile myoclonic epilepsy

This form of idiopathic generalized epilepsy has the closest association with PPR and albeit less, visually induced seizures. From 12% (in Japan and India; Shiraishi *et al.*, 2001; Mehndiratta & Aggarwal, 2002) up to 50% of JME patients (Caucasians: 40–75% of females; Wolf & Goosses, 1986; Panayiotopoulos *et al.*, 1994; Sofia *et al.*, 1999) or even 67% in Brazilian patients (De Araujo, 2009), show a PPR. When IPS is performed continuously for up to 5 minutes, a PPR was provoked in even 90% of JME patients (Appleton *et al.*, 2000). In a study of 57 cases of JME (Panayiotopoulos *et al.*, 1994), visual sensitivity was reported by 21 patients and confirmed with a PPR in 8 (14%). Ten other patients with no clinical history of visual sensitivity exhibited a PPR to IPS. Thus 31 patients (54.4%) had clinical or laboratory evidence of photosensitivity. Treatment with VPA is much more effective in patients with a PPR (Jain *et al.*, 2003), which explains some of the variability found in prevalence of PPR. Another factor might be the timing of the day of the EEG as has been observed in some Italian JME patients: 5 out of 8 PPR positive JME patients did not show a PPR anymore in the afternoon (Labate *et al.*, 2007). Although knowing that JME patients are having jerks mainly in the morning (Kasteleijn Nolst-Trenité' *et al.*, 2013), this is nevertheless remarkable. Firstly, because JME patients with a PPR usually do not complain about a greater sensitivity to lights in the early morning and secondly because in studies over the past 20 years, with hourly photic stimulation during the day in patients with a PPR, a similar overall effect has not been seen. Last mentioned studies have been done under placebo control in a laboratory environment with determination of the photosensitivity ranges and use of a photic stimulator delivering flashes between 2 and 60 Hz (Grass PS 22) in three eye conditions. About 10–20% of those have a diagnosis of JME (Binnie *et al.*, 1986; Trenité *et al.*, 2007; Kasteleijn-Nolst Trenité *et al.*, 2007). Thus, only in some JME patients, greater sensitivity in the early morning might be the case.

JME patients with a PPR (n = 72) tend to have more myoclonic jerks only and more first- degree family members with IGE compared to those without (Sofia *et al.*, 1999). No clear differences in provocative factors such as sleep deprivation, have been found (Sofia *et al.*, 1999), nor differences in personality disorders (De Araujo *et al.*, 2009).

Recently, diffusion tensor imaging studies have demonstrated widespread white matter microstructural abnormalities in particular in PPR positive JME cases. PPR positive patients showed increased fractional anisotropy in the ascending reticular activating system and ventromedial thalamus compared to PPR negative patients and healthy controls, suggesting a role of thalamo-premotor connections in the pathogenesis of photosensitivity (von Podewils *et al.*, 2015). EEG studies in JME patients with and without PPR suggested an increased posterior cortical hyperexcitability in JME with PPR subjects that could be related to structural and physiological abnormalities not present in JME without PPR (Bauer *et al.*, 2017). Subcortical microstructural changes in precentral, parietal and occipital regions and in the thalamus and precuneus have been reported also in IGE with PPR (Groppa *et al.*, 2012).

In general, different inclusion criteria are being used in JME studies: the more important EEG criteria are considered, the more PPRs will be found (see for example the study by De Araujo *et al.*, 2009).

There is a clear overlap between JME and visually sensitive patients; however, when a photosensitive patient with or without a history of visually induced seizures shows nearly exclusively myoclonic jerks in eyelids and arms evoked by IPS or other visual stimuli, they are visually sensitive patients.

Generalized tonic-clonic seizures (GTCS) on awakening

Just as in childhood absence epilepsy, about 7–13% of patients show a PPR. The incidence of PPRs is higher than in GTCS in general (Janz & Wolf, 1997; Shiraishi *et al.*, 2001).

Primary reading epilepsy

Reading epilepsy is not a variant of photosensitivity, although interestingly in a minority some kind of visual or ocular manifestation has been described in addition to typically motor seizures in the muscles involved in reading and talking. The visual symptoms can be both simple and complex, and 9% of patients show a PPR. It is possible that in the cases in which this is the only focal seizure type, the patients belong to a pattern-sensitive group and not to a specific reading epilepsy group (Wolf, 1994; Wilkins, 1995).

Visually sensitive IGE, eyelid myoclonia with absences and self-induction behavior

In this subgroup of GGE, patients have predominantly visually induced seizures or IPS-evoked clinical signs, including the "pure" photosensitive group. The first recognized seizure is usually tonic-clonic in origin and may occur in front of the television or in the discothèque, although myoclonic jerks have often occurred before. Other very common seizure types are absence seizures with or without myoclonic jerking or absences with eyelid myoclonia. Jeavons (1977) described this phenomenon for the first time as follows: "Eyelid myoclonia and absences (EMAs) show a marked jerking of the eyelids immediately after eye closure and there is an associated brief bilateral spike and wave activity in the EEG. The discharges do not occur in the dark. These patients are clearly photosensitive". Indeed, the cardinal features of this condition are: i) frequent occurrence of eyelid myoclonia, with or without absences, related to EEG generalized epileptiform activity and triggered by eye closure; ii) generalized photoparoxysmal EEG response, often in combination with a history of visually induced seizures; iii) onset in childhood, with a peak at 6–8 years. Generalized tonic-clonic seizures, although rare, can occur in most of the patients, often in relation to precipitating factors such as sleep deprivation, alcohol abuse, poor drug compliance, television or video-game exposure. Generalized tonic-clonic seizures and seizure types other than absences have been recently reported to predict poor response to antiepileptic treatment (Smith *et al.*, 2018). Myoclonic jerks other than eyelid myoclonia have been rarely described (Covanis, 2005). Photosensitivity usually decreases with age and it can be suppressed by antiepileptic drugs, whereas eyelid myoclonia persist (Striano *et al.*, 2002; Panayiotopoulos, 2005). Mental status is usually normal, although some cases with mental retardation have been described (Scuderi *et al.*, 2000). A genetic component, although not clearly defined yet, is likely, as suggested by evidences of identical twins affected (Parker *et al.*, 1996; Striano *et al.*, 2002; Adachi *et al.*, 2005). Recent studies have emphasized the occurrence of posterior focal interictal and ictal abnormalities preceding the generalized epileptic discharge, further suggesting that the ictogenic process in EMA originates in the occipital cortex (Viravan *et al.*, 2012; Dragoumi *et al.*, 2018).

The discussion about EMA is ongoing (Striano *et al.*, 2009; Nar Senol *et al.*, 2015). At least part of these patients are self-inducing (Duncan & Panayiotopoulos, 1996; Binnie, 1996).

The phenomenon of self-induction in photosensitive patients has been recognized since 1932 (Radovicci *et al.*, 1932) and because of the intriguing phenomenon, many cases have been described. Many patients admit their behavior when they report getting a nice feeling by doing it or using it as a way of relaxation or escape (Kasteleijn-Nolst Trenité, 1989; Tassinari *et al.*, 1989). One of the most typical findings in self-induction patients is that they do not complain about their photosensitivity, although they are some of the most sensitive among the photosensitive patients (Kasteleijn-Nolst Trenité *et al.*, 1989; 1998). They are furthermore very reluctant to discuss their behavior and resistant to treatment, mainly due to non-compliance. Some children and adults, with whom a good relationship has been built up, confide their pleasurable feelings. On the other hand, it can be very difficult to discriminate between self-inducing behavior and spontaneous eyelid myoclonia, especially in extremely sensitive children who show epileptiform discharges as soon as they close their eyes. It is widely accepted that patients who wave their hand in front of their eyes to produce a flickering light are self-inducers. Many skip this unpractical and obvious behavior to provoke eyelid myoclonia with absences. Up to 30% of photosensitive patients can be regarded as self-inducing, although the ultimate proof lies in personal information on doing it deliberately. Detection depends largely on the duration of the EEG registration, intensity of surrounding light (preferably sunlight), registration while seated (the eyes can be turned upwards toward the lights – "sunflower syndrome") and boredom.

Fixation-off sensitivity

Although fixation-off sensitivity (FOS) is the opposite to visual sensitivity, with occurrence of epileptiform discharges only when the eyes are closed or central vision and fixation is eliminated, a combination of both types has been described (Agathonikou *et al.*, 1998). Self-induction of seizures by fixation-off sensitivity has been recently reported in CHD2-related epilepsy (Caputo *et al.*, 2018).

Other epilepsies with or without encephalopathies

In the majority of cases, children with myoclonic-astatic epilepsy (MAE) have shown a PPR between the age of 5 and 15 years (Doose, 1992). In patients with severe myoclonic epilepsy in infancy or Dravet syndrome (DS), 40% of 31 children between the age of 3 months and 6 years were found to have a PPR. It persisted in only 8 of these patients. In addition, a provocative effect of eye closure (or self-induction) was seen (Dravet *et al.*, 2005). A recent study in DS confirmed the occurrence of PPR in more than 40% of patients and it seems to predict a more severe course of the disease (Verbeek *et al.*, 2017).

Mutations in the voltage-gated sodium channel subunit *SCN1A* gene have been reported in Dravet syndrome (Fujiwara *et al.*, 2003; Sugawara *et al.*, 2003; Ohmori *et al.*, 2003; Mulley *et al.*, 2005) and to a lesser extent in MAE (Ebach *et al.*, 2005). Nonpenetrant mutation carriers and variable expression presented by the affected carriers suggest, however, that other factors may act as modifiers. For example, there have been familial cases reported where parents carrying a mutation are asymptomatic or have a less severe phenotype. A putative modifier is the presence of PPR. However, thus far, the number of PPR-positive *vs.* PPR-negative patients with and without *SCN1A* mutations is too low to draw any definitive conclusions. A large screen of Dravet patients for the presence of PPR and *SCN1A* mutations would help to elucidate a possible correlation between Dravet syndrome PPR and *SCN1A* mutations.

Progressive myoclonus epilepsies

Visually induced seizures and PPR are a common feature in the progressive myoclonus epilepsies (PME). One of the diagnostic features in the neuronal ceroid lipofuscinosis (late infantile and adult forms) is the occurrence of huge evoked responses to low flash frequencies and even single flashes of light. In the other PMEs, such as Unverricht-Lundborg disease (ULD), the myoclonus epilepsy with ragged-red fibers and Lafora disease, a clear provocative effect of IPS can be found up to a certain stage of the disease. Treatment of photosensitivity and visual sensitivity is generally as difficult as treatment of spontaneous myoclonic jerks, thus distinguishing this type of epilepsy from the idiopathic generalized epilepsies. In some cases of ULD, the disease starts with a picture of familial idiopathic generalized visual sensitive type of epilepsy (Roger *et al.*, 1983), the clinical picture can then be very mild but the PPR persists (personal communication de Haan). PPRs and clinical photosensitivity have also been described in other rare, degenerative disorders (Harbord *et al.*, 1990; Rubboli *et al.*, 2011; Boisse Lomax *et al.*, 2013; Albert *et al.*, 2016; Specchio *et al.*, 2017) and in type III Gaucher disease (Nishimura *et al.*, 1980). A rare form of myoclonic epilepsy with autosomal dominant transmission, labelled as "myoclonic occipital photosensitive epilepsy with dystonia (MOPED)", whose clinical features include various phenotypes such as JME, IPOE, PME with paroxysmal dystonia has been recently described. In the more severe cases, status dystonicus, status epilepticus, ataxia, and progressive ophthalmoplegia could be observed, and premature death could occur (Sadleir *et al.*, 2015).

Focal seizures and syndromes

In about 20% of patients with a PPR, the diagnosis of localization-related epilepsy can be made; they have a history of focal seizures and the EEG shows interictal, predominantly temporal (50%) and frontal epileptiform discharges (25%). In *Table III* some well documented cases are presented of patients with a history of focal epileptic seizures, showing clear focal fronto-temporal or temporal EEG abnormalities and even clinical signs and symptoms of temporal lobe involvement during a generalized PPR.

The IPS evoked seizures do however not *necessarily* differ from those evoked in patients with a generalized type of epilepsy (tonic-clonic seizures, loss of consciousness or asymmetrical jerks) (Kasteleijn-Nolst Trenité, 1989).

As seen in the EEG recording, most visually evoked seizures have their onset in the temporo-parietal-occipital area, and spread to other areas. The spreading determines the type of clinical signs and symptoms. It is even likely that all visually induced seizures are, in principle, focal but that very rapid secondary generalization prohibits recognition in the EEG or the patient being able to remember the initial visual symptom. Brain SPECTS of photosensitive children with exclusively visually induced seizures have shown that the frontal lobe is often involved (secondarily): hypoperfusion of the frontal lobes was seen in six of seven patients in the interictal state and hyperperfusion during IPS (Kapucu *et al.*, 1996).

Idiopathic photosensitive occipital lobe epilepsy

In some patients the evoked epileptiform discharges can remain limited to the occipital lobe for many minutes, independent of the stimulus duration (self-sustaining). During this period, symptoms such as blurring of vision or blindness, elementary visual hallucinations with bright, flashing, white or colored lights are noticed by

Table III Documented single cases of ictal focal symptomatology during generalized PPR in patients with focal temporal lobe epilepsy
(Reprinted from Kasteleijn-Nolst Trenité D, Genton P, Brandt C, Reed RC. *Epilepsy Res* 2017 with permission from Elsevier)

Author	Country	Patient	History	Basic EEG	During PPR
Seddigh *et al.*, 1999	Germany	F, 44 yr	For 33 yrs CPS sometimes evolving into GTCS MRI normal CBZ failed	Spikes RF	Onset antero-temporal region with secondarily generalization and oro-alimentary automatisms identical to history
Seddigh *et al.*, 1999	Germany	F, 19 yr	For 2 yrs CPS (fear and automatisms) followed by GTCS Once clearly elicited by flashing lights in the disco. MRI normal PET: focus in R T and P- T region VPA failed	Focal slowing RT	1. generalized spikewaves with max F and eyelid myoclonia 2. R T onset with fear and word repetition, then evolving to GTCS
Inoue *et al.*, 2000	Japan	F, 16 yr	For 1 yr epigastric aura and headache followed by manual and oro-buccal automatisms MRI normal SPECT: RT focus VPA failed	Spikes RT	Spike and waves predominantly RT-O with some spreading.
Benbadis *et al.*, 1996	USA	F, 28 yr	For 7 yrs after minor head trauma, aura (funny feeling) followed by loss of awareness and manual and oro-buccal automatisms, sometimes evolving into GTCS MRI normal PET: focus in R T region CBZ, PHT, FBM, VPA, CLZ and PB failed	Spikes RT	Depth EEG recording: Focal fast epileptic activity in R mesio-basal anterior temporal lobe with some spreading
Lee *et al.*, 2014	Korea	F, 12 yr	For 1 yr 3x GTCS	Normal	1. Generalized SW at IPS 15 Hz 2. LT start with head turning to R then evolving to GTCS

CPS: complex partial seizures (new classification focal seizures with with loss of awareness; CBZ: carbamazepine; VPA: valproate; PHT: phenytoin; FBM: felbamate; CLZ: clonazepam; PB: phenobarbital; RF: right frontal; RT: right temporal; RP-: = right parietotemporal; RT-O: right temporo-occipital; F: frontal.

the patient (Ricci *et al.*, 1998; Tassinari *et al.*, 1988; Guerrini *et al.* 1998). Only after generalization of the discharges does the patient lose consciousness followed eventually by a tonic-clonic seizure. Concurrent epigastric discomfort and vomiting, before loss of consciousness, has also been described as a typical sign and symptom for occipital seizures (Guerrini *et al.*, 1995; 1998). Together with the visual signs, often of long duration, and the lack of myoclonic jerks in the eyelids and arms, this can help in differentiating this type of epilepsy from more common visually induced seizures. Some patients develop this type of epilepsy after having had typical benign Rolandic epilepsy (Guerrini *et al.*, 1997). The occipital seizures can be difficult to distinguish from migraine, since both have visual aura and headache as symptoms (Andermann & Zifkin, 1998). In migraine, the visual aura is usually in black and white, whereas the occipital seizure consists of colored, simple or complex, visual phenomena (Panayiotopoulos, 1999). Postictal headache is different from ictal headache (Lortie *et al.*, 1993).

Although these typical occipital, focal seizures have been observed and described in individual patients since the 1950s, the separate identity and clinical relevance has been recognized only since the 1990s (Guerrini *et al.*, 1998). The term idiopathic photosensitive occipital lobe epilepsy (IPOE) was introduced for the subset of patients with an idiopathic epilepsy (Guerrini *et al.*, 1995) and not only so-called visual or occipital seizures evoked by IPS, but also by television and video games (Tassinari *et al.*, 1988; Yalcin *et al.*, 2000; Aso *et al.*,

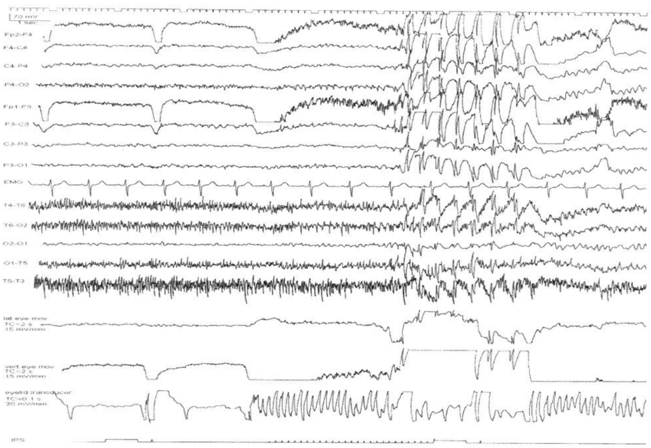

10 Hz eye closure

Girl 14 yr, GTCS, myoclonus TV, no AED
myoclonus in eyelids and trunk; glassy, no complaints

Figure 5 **A 14-year-old girl who had a tonic-clonic seizure and myoclonic jerks while close to the TV. She was not taking any medication. She is IPS-sensitive between 10 and 30 Hz in the eye-conditions: eye closure and eyes closed, but not with eyes open. The following clinical signs were seen during the above evoked epileptiform discharges: eyelid myoclonia and upwards movement of eyeballs, with mild myoclonic movement in the upper trunk and arms. She looked "glassy". She did not notice anything herself. The same EEG responses and clinical manifestations were found when she sat at a distance of 1 meter from a 50 Hz TV set, regardless of the program.**

1987; Demarco *et al.*, 1985). Overlap or better coexistence between IPOE and other forms of occipital epilepsy and even JME, or evolution to IGE has been described recently (Yalcin *et al.*, 2000; Taylor *et al.*, 2004; Bonini *et al.*, 2014).

Non-idiopathic photosensitive occipital epilepsy

IPS-evoked visual seizures were described in patients with symptomatic epilepsy, with occipital calcifications in celiac disease (Ambrosetto *et al.*, 1992) and in probably symptomatic and progressive myoclonic epilepsy of Lafora type (Tinuper *et al.*, 1983; Guerrini *et al.*, 1998).

These photically induced visual, occipital seizures have only recently been recognized and systematic epidemiological studies are lacking; an estimation of the prevalence in epileptic children is 0.6%, compared to 3% with generalized IPS-evoked seizures in the same population of 2,104 children (Guerrini *et al.*, 1998). Age at onset of the occipital seizures is between 5 and 17 years with a peak around puberty, as in the generalized photosensitive group. Prognosis depends on EEG background abnormalities and interictal discharges (Michelucci & Tassinari, 1993).

Because of the time lag between seizure symptomatology and the trigger, these focal visual seizures are often not recognized as being visually sensitive seizures. A precise differentiation between spontaneous and visually evoked occipital seizures is still lacking.

Self-induction behavior has not been described or noticed in patients with occipital photosensitive epilepsy. As far as we know, a possible explanation could be the self-sustaining nature of the occipital seizure in combination with the frightening experience of hallucinations and loss of vision. Self-inducing visually sensitive children and adults provoke short-lasting (3–6 sec) generalized discharges, with a minimal impact on their daily activities and maximal effect of feelings of pleasure and escape (Kasteleijn-Nolst Trenité, 1989).

Treatment

Often avoidance (discotheque, Venetian blinds) or altering the triggering stimulus (use of specific television- or video screens, colored glasses, etc.) is not sufficient and additional antiepileptic prophylaxis is necessary. This is especially the case when a child or adolescent is too sensitive (wide range of frequencies), has spontaneous discharges as well or does not notice the minor clinical symptoms during PPRs.

If a child shows a PPR without clear concomitant clinical symptomatology, still in 50% of them the PPR will cause delay in a simple motor task (Fallah & Nair, 2009), equal to spontaneous generalized epileptiform discharges (Kasteleijn-Nolst Trenité *et al.*, 1990). Having a PPR is thus not only an indication of having increased risk of provoked and spontaneous seizures, but also of transitory cognitive impairment.

Non-pharmacological treatment

The literature on non-pharmacological preventative measures is mostly limited to descriptions of practical experience and results from EEG studies in the same patients using different devices. Since most advice seems to work in clinical practice and is based on the pathophysiology (see above), we give some recommendations below:

– monocular occlusion of the dominant eye: If an aura is experienced, or when the patient is close to the television set or inadvertently exposed to flicker (in a discotheque, etc.);

– dark, preferably polarized, glasses: In some patients cross-polarized lenses seem to be more effective (Jain *et al.*, 2001);

– Colored glasses: Specially tinted blue glasses (Zeiss Clarlt F133Z1) have been proven successful (Capovilla *et al.*, 2006; Kepecs *et al.*, 2004). Interestingly, different colors can be beneficial for different individuals and testing with IPS is necessary to be sure that the chosen lens color is the best for a patient (Wilkins *et al.*, 1999);

– television and other displays: use small TV screens, preferably of 100 Hz or LCD/TFT or plasma type; watch the TV from at least 2 meters and use a remote control. A video-hazard blocker (VHB) on individual displays can prevent seizures evoked by programmes. In Japan these new devices have been shown to prevent flicker- and pattern-induced seizures effectively (Takahashi *et al.*, 2001).

Pharmacological treatment

Antiepileptic prophylaxis (AED) can easily be evaluated with control EEGs, ideally with measurement of lower and upper thresholds (the so called photosensitivity range). Diminishment of range equals an antiepileptic protective effect. It is not necessary to have a complete abolishment of photosensitivity to yet establish a clinically important effect.

In practice, visually induced seizures respond best to drugs effective against generalized seizures, notably valproate (VPA) and levetiracetam (LEV), with ethosuximide (ESM), lamotrigine (LTG) and the benzodiazepines as agents of second choice (Jeavons & Harding, 1975; Covanis *et al.*, 2004). Phenobarbitone (PB) showed only a minor effect (Harding & Jeavons, 1994). LTG has been shown to be effective in monotherapy in eight patients with visual epilepsy with complete seizure control in five (Covanis *et al.*, 2004). In another study, a prospective, video-EEG-controlled study with LTG in 47 patients with various types of IGE, 11 became seizure-free and 3 of the 11 had purely visually sensitive epilepsy (Gericke *et al.*, 1999). The effect of newer antiepileptic drugs for other types of generalized epilepsies such as topiramate (TPM), zonisamide (ZNS), lacosamide (LSM), rufinamide (RFM), brivaracetam (BRV) and perampanel (PER) is limited. TPM has proven to be effective in JME patients (Wheless, 2000). ZNS is effective in various types of seizures in monotherapy in children and adults (Wilfong, 2005) and has proven efficacy in patients with PME (Kinrions *et al.*, 2003). A patient with Unverricht-Lundborg Disease showed complete PPR suppression with ZNS (Kagitani-Shimono *et al.*, 2002). Broad-spectrum antiepileptic drugs such as VPA, LTG and TPM are extremely effective at controlling a variety of seizures without causing excessive seizure aggravation (Bourgeois, 2003). Slow titration is important however, especially in children and adolescents, and it seems that visually sensitive patients benefit even from relatively low dosages (Albsoul-Younes *et al.*, 2004; Kasteleijn & Hirsch, 2003). All the above drugs are potentially good medication for visually sensitive patients. The choice must primarily depend on the underlying epilepsy syndrome.

Treatment of self-induction

Although, in some cases, it is possible to treat self-inducing children successfully in an early stage with high dosages of VPA (2,000–3,000 mg/day), the compulsive behavior of hand waving and deliberate eye blinking is usually difficult to stop (Singhi & Bansal, 2004). Fewer than 10% of visually sensitive patients are therapy-resistant, but most of these engage in self-induction, and may be non-compliant as well (Duncan & Panayiotopoulos, 1996). Other neuro-active agents have been shown to be effective in self-inducing photosensitive children and adults, such as pimozide, a dopamine-receptor antagonist (Kasteleijn-Nolst Trenité *et al.*, 1989) and fenfluramine, a serotonergic agonist (Boel & Casaer, 1996), even if the drug itself is aggravating the sensitivity to IPS. Thus, it seems useful to combine these type of drugs with valproate (Boel & Casaer, 1996). It might be worthwhile using dark colored or tinted contact lenses, especially in self-inducing patients. In a 2-year-old patient with Dravet syndrome, who induced absences and myoclonic jerks by waving hand movements and forced eye closures, blue-tinted contact lenses gradually reduced photosensitivity and inhibited the hand movements (Takahashi *et al.*, 1995).

Monitoring of the drug effect, both acute and in steady state

One of the big advantages of reflex epilepsies is that standardized repeated measurements are possible and thus the drug effect can be evaluated. Photosensitivity (EEG trait) is suppressed by acute administration of all major antiepileptic drugs. Drugs more effective in treatment of focal epilepsies (carbamazepine, phenytoine, gabapentine) are of little value in long-term treatment of visual sensitivity, yet they might temporarily suppress this condition for some hours after short-term administration (Hirsch *et al.*, 2000). Levetiracetam and its analogue, brivaracetam, have shown efficacy both in abolishing the PPR as well as in concomitant and spontaneous myoclonic jerks (Kasteleijn-Nolst Trenité *et al.*, 1996; 2007).

In clinical practice the effects of the drug (in steady state) can be evaluated in combination with the patient's clinical-historical information. Photosensitivity can be monitored by determining the photosensitivity range before and after drug treatment. The drug dosage can even be titrated in the individual patient using the photosensitivity ranges (Jeavons & Harding, 1975). Many patients, especially children, can be adequately treated with a relatively low dosage of an antiepileptic drug. During adolescence, the prescribed dosage usually needs to be raised, partly because of the greater body weight and partly due to an increase in the photosensitivity trait. Therapy usually needs to be maintained until the age of about 25 years. In some patients the photosensitivity can continue until the age of 70 even. IPS in the laboratory can then help predict the relapse rate after partial or total withdrawal of the drug. Early withdrawal of VPA gives a high risk of seizure recurrence (Matricardi *et al.*, 1989).

Future

The inevitability of patients being confronted with television and computer screens and fluorescent lighting at school, work, home and leisure means the subject of visual sensitivity will become more and more important. Many questions still need to be answered, both in terms of genetics, pathophysiology, classification of the types of sensitivity, and prognosis. In order to gain more information about this subject, from a relatively limited number of affected patients, it is very important that research is conducted in a uniform manner with respect to both methodology and terminology.

Acknowledgements

D.G.A. Kasteleijn-Nolst Trenité was supported by the EU FP6 program: Marie Curie Excellence Grant MEXC-CT2005- 24224: Visual Sensitivity.

REFERENCES ▶

Agathonikou A, Koutroumanidis M, Panayiotopoulos CP (1998): Fixation-off (Scoto) sensitivity combined with photosensitivity. *Epilepsia* 39: 552–555.

Aird RB (1983): The importance of seizure-inducing factors in the control of refractory forms of epilepsy. *Epilepsia* 24: 567–583.

Albert DV, Yin H, De Los Reyes EC, Vidaurre J (2016): Unique characteristics of the photoparoxysmal response in patients with neuronal ceroid lipofuscinosis type 2: Can EEG Be a Biomarker? *J Child Neurol* 31: 1475–1482.

Albsoul-Younes AM, Salem HA, Ajlouni SF, Al-Safi SA (2004): Topiramate slow dose titration: improved efficacy and tolerability. *Pediatr Neurol* 31: 349–352.

Ambrosetto G, Antonini L, Tassinari CA (1992): Occipital lobe seizures related to clinically asymptomatic celiac disease in adulthood. *Epilepsia* 33: 476–481.

Andermann F (1971): Self-induced television epilepsy. *Epilepsia* 12: 269–275.

Andermann F, Zifkin B (1998): The benign occipital epilepsies of childhood: an overview of the idiopathic syndromes and of the relationship to migraine. *Epilepsia* 39 S4: 9–23.

Anyanwu EC, Ehiri JE, Jones J (2003): Photosensitive epilepsy beyond adolescence: is freedom from photosensitivity age-dependent? *Int J Adolesc Med Health* 5: 125–132.

Appleton R, Beirne M, Acomb B (2000): Photosensitivity in juvenile myoclonic epilepsy. *Seizure* 9: 108–111.

Aso K, Watanabe K, Negoro T, *et al.* (1994): Photosensitivity epilepsy in children, *Seizure* 3: 67–71.

Badinand-Hubert N, Bureau M, Hirsch E, *et al.* (1998): Epilepsies and video games: results of a multicentric study. *Electroenceph Clin Neurophysiol* 107: 422–427.

Bartolini E, Pesaresi I, Fabbri S, *et al.* (2014): Abnormal response to photic stimulation in juvenile myoclonic epilepsy: an EEG-fMRI study. *Epilepsia* 55: 1038–1047.

Bauer PR, Gorgels K, Spetgens W, *et al.* (2017): The topographical distribution of epileptic spikes in juvenile myoclonic epilepsy with and without photosensitivity. *Clin Neurophysiol* 128: 176–182.

Baykan B, Matur Z, Gürses C, Aykutlu E, Gökyiğit A (2005): Typical absence seizures triggered by photosensitivity. *Epilepsia* 46: 159–163.

Benbadis SR, Gerson WA, Harvey JH, Lüders HO (1996): Photosensitive temporal lobe epilepsy. *Neurology* 46: 1540–1542. Review.

Bental EL (1979): Observations on the electroencephalogram and photosensitivity of South African Black Albinos. *Epilepsia* 22: 593–597.

Berney TP, Osselton W, Kolvin I, Day MJ (1981): Effect of discothèque environment on epileptic children. *Brit Med J* 282: 180–182.

Berg AT, Berkovic SF, Brodie MJ, *et al.* (2010): Revised terminology and concepts for organization of seizures and epilepsies: report of the ILAE Commission on Classification and Terminology, 2005–2009. *Epilepsia* 51: 676–685.

Bickford RG, Daly D, Keith HM (1953): Convulsive effects of light stimulation in children. *Am J Dis Child* 86: 170.

Binnie CD, De Korte RA, Wisman T (1979): Fluorescent lighting and epilepsy. *Epilepsia* 20: 725–727.

Binnie CD, Darby, E, De Korte RA, Veldhuizen R, Wilkins AJ (1980): EEG sensitivity to television effects of ambient lighting, *Electroenceph Clin Neurophysiol* 50: 329–331.

Binnie CD, Kasteleijn-Nolst Trenité DG, De Korte R (1986): Photosensitivity as a model for acute antiepileptic drug studies. *Electroenceph Clin Neurophysiol* 63: 235–241.

Binnie CD (1996): Differential diagnosis of eyelid myoclonia with absences and self-induction by eye closure. In: Duncan JS, Panayiotopoulos CP (eds) *Eyelid Myoclonia with Absences*, London: John Libbey & Co, pp. 89–92.

Bocci T, Caleo M, Restani L, Barloscio D, Rossi S, Sartucci F (2016): Altered recovery from inhibitory repetitive transcranial magnetic stimulation (rTMS) in subjects with photosensitive epilepsy. *Clin Neurophysiol* 127: 3353–3361.

Boel M, Casaer P (1996): Add-on therapy of fenfluramine in intractable self-induced epilepsy. *Neuropediatrics* 27: 171–173.

Boissé Lomax L, Bayly MA, Hjalgrim H, *et al.* (2013): "North Sea" progressive myoclonus epilepsy: phenotype of subjects with GOSR2 mutation. *Brain* 136: 1146–1154.

Bonini F, Egeo G, Fattouch J, *et al.* (2014): Natural evolution from idiopathic photosensitive occipital lobe epilepsy to idiopathic generalized epilepsy in an untreated young patient. *Brain Dev* 36: 346–350.

Bourgeois BF (2003): Chronic management of seizures in the syndromes of idiopathic generalized epilepsy. *Epilepsia* 44S 2: 27–32.

Brigo F, Bongiovanni LG, Nardone R, *et al.* (2013): Visual cortex hyperexcitability in idiopathic generalized epilepsies with photosensitivity: a TMS pilot study. *Epilepsy Behav* 27: 301–306.

Brinciotti M, Matricardi M, Pelliccia A, Trasatti G (1994): Pattern sensitivity and photosensitivity in epileptic children with visually induced seizures. *Epilepsia* 35: 842–849.

Capovilla G, Beccaria F, Gambardella A, Montagnini A, Avantaggiato P, Seri S (1997): Photosensitive benign myoclonic epilepsy in infancy, *Brain Dev* 19: 473–479.

Capovilla G, Beccaria F, Romeo A, Veggiotti P, Canger R, Paladin F (1999): Effectiveness of a particular blue lens on photoparoxysmal response in photosensitive epileptic patients. *Ital J Neurol Sci* 20: 161–166.

Capovilla G, Gambardella A, Rubboli G, *et al.* (2006): Suppressive efficacy by a commercially available blue lens on PPR in 610 photosensitive epilepsy patients. *Epilepsia* 47: 529–533.

Caputo D, Trivisano M, Vigevano F, Fusco L (2018): CHD2-epilepsy: Polygraphic documentation of self-induced seizures due to fixation-off sensitivity. *Seizure* 57: 8–10.

Carvill GL, Heavin SB, Yendle SC, *et al.* (2013): Targeted resequencing in epileptic encephalopathies identifies *de novo* mutations in CHD2 and SYNGAP1. *Nat Genet* 45: 825–830.

Charlton MH, Hoefer PFA (1964): Television and epilepsy. *Arch Neurol* 11: 239–247.

Clement MJ, Wallace SJ (1990): A survey of adolescents with epilepsy. *Dev Med Child Neurol* 32: 849–857.

Cobb S (1947): Photic driving as a cause of clinical seizures in epileptic patients. *Arch Neurol Psychiat* 58: 239–247.

Commission on Classification and Terminology of the International League Against Epilepsy (1989): Proposal for revised classification of epilepsies and epileptic syndromes. *Epilepsia* 30: 389–399.

Covanis A, Stodieck SR, Wilkins AJ (2004): Treatment of photosensitivity. *Epilepsia* 45 S1: 40–45.

Daly D, Bickford RG (1951): Electroencephalographic studies of identical twins with photo-epilepsy. *Electroenceph Clin Neurophysiol* 3: 245–249.

Danesi MA (1985): Geographical and seasonal variations in the incidence of epileptic photosensitivity. *Electroenceph Clin Neurophysiol* 61: S216.

Davidson S, Watson CW (1956): Hereditary light sensitive epilepsy. *Neurology* 6: 235–261.

De Araujo Filho GM, Lin K, Lin G, Peruchi MM, Caboclo LOSF, Guaranha MSB, Guilhoto LMFF (2009): Are personality traits of juvenile myoclonic epilepsy related to frontal lobe dysfunctions? A proton MRS study. *Epilepsia* 50: 1201–1209.

De Graaf AS, Lombard CJ, Claassen DA (1995): Influence of ethnic and geographic factors on the classic photoparoxysmal response in the electroencephalogram of epilepsy patients. *Epilepsia* 36: 219–223.

De Keyser J, Michotte A, Ebinger G (1984): Television induced seizures in alcoholics. *Br Med J Clin Res* 289: 1191–1192.

De Kovel CGF, Pinto D, Tauer U, *et al.* (2010): Whole-genome linkage scan for epilepsy-related photosensitvity: a mega-analysis. *Epilepsy Res* 89: 286–294.

De Marco P, Ghersini L (1985): Video games and epilepsy, *Dev Med Child Neurol* 27: 519–521.

Donnet A, Bartolomei F (1997): Migraine with visual aura and photosensitive epileptic seizures. *Epilepsia* 38: 1032–1034.

Doose H (1992): Myoclonic astatic epilepsy of early childhood, In: Roger J, Bureau M, Dravet C, Dreifuss FE, Perret A, Wolf P (eds) *Epileptic Syndromes in Infancy, Childhood and Adolescence.* (2nd ed) London: John Libbey, pp. 103–114.

Doose H, Gerken H, Hien-Volpel K F, Volzke E (1969): Genetics of photosensitive epilepsy. *Neuropadiatrie* 1: 56–73.

Doose H, Gerken H (1973): On the genetics of EEG anomalies in childhood, IV: photoconvulsive reaction. *Neuropädiatria* 4: 162–171.

Dragoumi P, Emery J, Chivers F, Brady M, Desurkar A, Cross JH, Das KB (2018): Crossing the lines between epilepsy syndromes: a myoclonic epilepsy variant with prominent eyelid myoclonia and atonic components. *Epileptic Disord* 20: 35–41.

Dravet C, Bureau M (1981): L'épilepsie myoclonique bénigne du nourrisson. *Rev EEG Neurophysiol* 11: 438- 444.

Dravet C, Bureau M, Roger J (1992): Benign myoclonic epilepsy in infants, In: Roger J, Bureau M, Dravet Ch, Dreifuss FE, Perret A, Wolf P (eds) *Epileptic Syndromes in Infancy, Childhood and Adolescence.* (2nd ed) London: John Libbey, pp. 67–74.

Dravet C, Bureau M, Oguni H, Fukuyama Y, Cokar O (2005): Severe myoclonic epilepsy in infancy (Dravet Syndrome). In: Roger J, Bureau M, Dravet C, Genton P, Tassinari CA, Wolf P (eds) *Epileptic Syndromes in Infancy, Childhood and Adolescence* (4th ed) London: John Libbey, pp. 89–113.

Duncan JS, Panayiotopoulos CP (1996): The differentiation of "eye closure" from "eyes-closed" EEG abnormalities and their relation to photo- and fixation-off sensitivity, In: Duncan JS, Panayiotopoulos CP (eds) *Eyelid Myoclonia with Absences.* London: John Libbey & Co pp. 77–87.

Ebach K, Joos H, Doose H, *et al.* (2005): *SCN1A* mutation analysis in myoclonic astatic epilepsy and severe idiopathic generalized epilepsy of infancy with generalized tonic-clonic seizures. *Neuropediatrics* 36: 210–213.

Eeg-Olofsson O, Petersén I, Selldén U (1971): The development of the electroencephalogram in normal children from the age of 1 through 15 years: paroxysmal activity. *Neuropaediatrie* 2: 375–404.

Engel J (2001): A proposed diagnostic scheme for people with epileptic seizures and with epilepsy: report of the ILAE Task Force on Classification and Terminology. *Epilepsia* 42: 796–803.

Fallah A, Ramachandran Nair R (2009): Does photoparoxysmal response in children represent provoked seizure? Evidence from simultaneous motor task during EEG. *Clin Neurol Neurosurg* 111: 147–150.

Familusi JB, Adamolekun B, Olayinka BA, Muzengi D, Levy LF (1998): Electroencephalographic photosensitivity among Zimbabwean youths. *Ann Trop Paediatr* 18: 267–274.

Fisher RS, Cross JH, French JA, *et al.* (2017): Operational classification of seizure types by the International League Against Epilepsy: Position Paper of the ILAE Commission for Classification and Terminology. *Epilepsia* 58: 522–530.

Fujiwara T, Sugawara T, Mazaki-Miyazaki E, *et al.* (2003): Mutations of sodium channel alpha subunit type 1 (SCN1A) in intractable childhood epilepsies with frequent generalized tonic-clonic seizures. *Brain* 126: 531–546.

Furusho J, Suzuki M, Tazaki I, *et al.* (2002): A comparison survey of seizures and other symptoms of Pokémon phenomenon. *Pediatr Neurol* 27: 350–355.

Galizia EC, Myers CT, Leu C, *et al.* (2015): CHD2 variants are a risk factor for photosensitivity in epilepsy. *Brain* 138: 1198–207.

Gastaut H (1969): Classification of the epilepsies: proposal for an international classification, *Epilepsia* 10: S14–21.

Gastaut H, Bert J (1954): EEG changes during cinematographic presentation (Moving picture activation of the EEG). *Electroenceph Clin Neurophysiol* 6: 433–444.

Gastaut H, Tassinari CA (1966): Triggering mechanisms in epilepsy: the electroclinical point of view. *Epilepsia* 7: 85–138.

Gericke CA, Picard F, de Saint-Martin A, Strumia S, Marescaux C, Hirsch E (1999): Efficacy of lamotrigine in idiopathic generalized epilepsy syndromes: a video-EEG-controlled open study. *Epileptic Disord* 1: 159–165.

Gerken H, Doose H (1969): Encephalitis and photosensitivity. *Neuropädiatrie* 2: 235–238.

Gilliam FG, Chiappa KH (1995): Significance of spontaneous epileptiform abnormalities associated with a photoparoxysmal response. *Neurology* 45: 453–456.

Graf WD, Chatrian GE, Glass ST, Knauss TA (1994): Video game-related seizures: a report on 10 patients and a review of the literature. *Pediatrics* 93: 551–556.

Gregory RP, Oates T, Merry RT (1993): Electroencephalogram epileptiform abnormalities in candidates for aircrew training. *Electroenceph Clin Neurophysiol* 86: 75–77.

Groppa S, Moeller F, Siebner H, *et al.* (2012): White matter microstructural changes of thalamocortical networks in photosensitivity and idiopathic generalized epilepsy. *Epilepsia* 53: 668–676.

Guerrini R, Aicardi J (2003): Epileptic encephalopathies with myoclonic seizures in infants and children (severe myoclonic epilepsy and myoclonic-astatic epilepsy). *J Clin Neurophysiol* 20: 449–461.

Guerrini R, Dravet C, Genton P, *et al.* (1995): Idiopathic photosensitive occipital lobe epilepsy. *Epilepsia* 36: 883–891.

Guerrini R, Belmonte A, Veggiotti P, Mattia D, Bonanni P (1997): Delayed appearance of interictal EEG abnormalities in early onset childhood epilepsy with occipital paroxysms. *Brain Dev* 19: 343–346.

Guerrini R, Bonanni P, Parmeggiani L, *et al.* (1998): Induction of partial seizures by visual stimulation, Clinical and electroencephalographic features and evoked potential studies, In: Zifkin BJ, Andermann F, Beaumanoir A, Rowan AJ (eds) *Reflex Epilepsies and Reflex Seizures, Advances in Neurology*, 75, Philadelphia: Lippincott-Raven Publishers, pp. 159–176.

Harbord MG, Harden A, Harding B, Brett EM, Baraitser M (1990): Megalencephaly with dysmyelination spasticity ataxia seizures and distinctive neurophysiological finding in two siblings. *Neuropediatrics* 21: 164–168.

Harding GFA, Jeavons M (1994): *Photosensitive epilepsy*. London: Mac-Keith Press.

Harding GFA, Edson A, Jeavons PM (1997): Persistence of photosensitivity. *Epilepsia* 38: 663–669.

Harding GFA, Fylan F (1999): Two visual mechanisms for photosensitivity. *Epilepsia* 40: 1446–1451.

Hegedüs, Csibia L (1982): Photosensitive epilepsy and responses, *Electroenceph Clin Neurophysiol* 53: 14.

Hendriksen IJ, Elderson A (2001): The use of EEG in aircrew selection. *Aviat Space Environ Med* 72: 1025–1033.

Hennessy MJ, Binnie CD (2000): Photogenic partial seizures. *Epilepsia* 41: 59–64.

Herrlin KM (1954): EEG with photic stimulation: a study of children with manifest or suspected epilepsy. *Electroenceph Clin Neurophysiol* 6: 573–589.

Herrlin KM (1960): Epilepsy, light-sensitivity and left-handedness in a family with monozygotic triplets. *Pediatrics* 25: 385–399.

Hirsch E, de Saint-Martin A, Arzimanoglou A (2000): New insights into the clinical management of partial epilepsies. *Epilepsia* 41 S5: S13–17.

Inoue K, Mimori Y, Harada T, Oshita T, Kumagai R, Nakamura S (2000): The relationship between photosensitive temporal lobe epilepsy and eye closure activity. *Seizure* 9: 347–351.

Ishiguro Y, Takada H, Watanabe K, Okumura A, Aso K, Ishikawa T (2004): A follow-up survey on seizures induced by animated cartoon TV program "Pocket Monster". *Epilepsia* 45: 377–383.

Jacob S, Martin D, Rajabally YA (2006): Juvenile myoclonic epilepsy in an elderly patient. *Age Ageing* 35: 194–196.

Jain S, Woodruff G, Bissessar EA (2001): Cross polarized spectacles in photosensitive epilepsy. *J Pediatr Ophthalmol Strabismus* 38: 331–334.

Jain S, Tripathi M, Srivastava AK, Narula A (2003): Phenotypic analysis of juvenile myoclonic epilepsy in Indian families. *Acta Neurol Scand* 107: 356–562.

Janz D, Wolf P (1997): Epilepsy with grand mal on awakening. In: Engel J Jr, Pedley TA (eds) *Epilepsy, A Comprehensive Textbook*. Philadelphia, Lippincott-Raven: pp. 2347–2354.

Janz D, Durner M (1991): Verlauf und Genetik der Juvenilen Myoklonischen Epilepsie. In: Jacobi G, Meier-Ewert K (eds) *Epilepsien im Kindesalter, Therapie und Prognose*, Stuttgart: Fischer, pp. 67–82.

Janz D, Waltz S (1995): Juvenile myoclonic epilepsy with absences. In: Duncan JS, Panayiotopoulos DP. *Typical Absences and Related Epileptic Syndromes*. London: Churchill Livingstone, pp. 174–183.

Jayakar P, Chiappa KH. (1990) Clinical correlations of photoparoxysmal responses. *Electroenceph Clin Neurophysiol* 75: 251–254.

Jeavons PM (1977): Nosological problems of myoclonic epilepsies in childhood and adolescence. *Dev Med Child Neurol* 19: 3–8.

Jeavons PM, Harding GFA (1975): *Photosensitive Epilepsy*. London: Heinemann.

Jeavons PM, Harding GFA, Panayiotopoulos CP (1971): Photosensitive epilepsy and driving. *Lancet* 1: 1125.

Jeavons PM, Bishop A, Harding GFA (1986): The prognosis of photosensitivity. *Epilepsia* 27: 569–575.

Johannesen K, Marini C, Pfeffer S, *et al.* (2016): Phenotypic spectrum of GABRA1: From generalized epilepsies to severe epileptic encephalopathies. *Neurology* 87: 1140–1151.

Kagitani-Shimono K, Imai K, Okamoto N, Ono J, Okada S (2002): Unverricht-Lundborg disease with cystatin B gene abnormalities. *Pediatr Neurol* 26: 55–60.

Kapucu LO, Gucuyener K, Vural G, *et al.* (1996): Brain SPECT evaluation of patients with pure photosensitive epilepsy. *J Nucl Med* 37: 1755–1759.

Kasteleijn-Nolst Trenité DGA (1989): Photosensitivity in epilepsy: electrophysiological and clinical correlates, *Acta Neurol Scand* 80 S25: 1–150.

Kasteleijn-Nolst Trenité DGA (1994): Video-game epilepsy. *Lancet* 344: 1102–1103.

Kasteleijn-Nolst Trenité DGA (1998): Reflex seizures induced by intermittent light stimulation. In: Zifkin BJ, Andermann F, Beaumanoir A, Rowan AJ (eds) *Reflex Epilepsies and Reflex Seizures*, *Advances in Neurology* Vol. 75. Philadelphia: Lippincott-Raven Publishers, pp. 99–121.

Kasteleijn-Nolst Trenité DGA, Binnie CD, Meinardi H (1987): Photosensitive patients: symptoms and signs during intermittent photic stimulation and their relation to seizures in daily life. *J Neurol Neurosurg Psychiat* 50: 1546–1549.

Kasteleijn-Nolst Trenité DGA, Binnie CD, Overweg J, Oosting J, Van Emde Boas W (1989): Treatment of self-induction in epileptic patients –Who wants it? In: Beaumanoir A, Gastaut H, Naquet R (eds) *Reflex Sseizures and Reflex Epilepsy*. Geneva: Médecine et Hygiène, pp. 439–445.

Kasteleijn-Nolst Trenité, DGA, Smit AM, Velis DN, Willemse J, Van Emde Boas W(1990): On-line detection of transient neuropsychological disturbances during EEG-discharges in children with epilepsy. *Dev Med Child Neurol* 32: 46–50.

Kasteleijn-Nolst Trenité DGA, Van Emde Boas W, Binnie CD (1994): Photosensitive epilepsy as an age-related genetic disorder. In: Wolf P (ed) *Epileptic Seizures and Syndromes*. London: John Libbey & Co, Ltd, pp. 41-48.

Kasteleijn-Nolst Trenité DG, Marescaux C, Stodieck S, Edelbroek PM, Oosting J (1996): Photosensitive epilepsy: a model to study the effects of antiepileptic drugs, Evaluation of the piracetam analogue, levetiracetam. *Epilepsy Res* 25: 225–230.

Kasteleijn-Nolst Trenité DGA, Binnie CD, Harding GFA, Wilkins A (1999a): Photic stimulation: standardization of screening methods. *Epilepsia* 40 (S4): 75–79.

Kasteleijn-Nolst Trenité DGA, Binnie CD, Harding GFA, *et al.* (1999b): Medical technology assessment, Photic stimulation – Standardization of screening methods. *Neurophysiol Clin* 29: 318–324.

Kasteleijn-Nolst Trenité DGA, Guerrini R, Binnie CD, Genton P (2001): Visual sensitivity and epilepsy: A proposed terminology and classification for clinical and EEG phenomenology. *Epilepsia* 42: 692–701.

Kasteleijn-Nolst Trenité DGA, Martins da Silva A, Ricci S, Rubboli G, Tassinari CA, Segers JP (2002): Video games are exciting. *Epileptic Disord* 4: 121–128.

Kasteleijn-Nolst Trenité DG, Silva LCB, Manreza MLG (2003): Prevalence of photoparoxysmal EEG responses in normal children and adolescents in Teofile Otoni, Brazil: 2001–2002. *Epilepsia* 44 (S8): 48.

Kasteleijn-Nolst Trenité DGA, Hirsch E (2003): Levetiracetam: preliminary efficacy in generalized seizures, *Epileptic Disord* 5 (S1): 39–44.

Kasteleijn-Nolst Trenité DG, Van Der Beld G, Heynderickx I, Groen P (2004): Visual stimuli in daily life. *Epilepsia* 45 (Sl): 2–6.

Kasteleijn-Nolst Trenité D, Genton P, Parain D, *et al.* (2007): Evaluation of brivaracetam, a novel SV2A ligand, in the photosensitivity model. *Neurology* 69: 1027–1034.

Kasteleijn-Nolst Trenité DG, Verrotti A, Di Fonzo A, *et al.* (2010): Headache, epilepsy and photosensitivity: how are they connected? *J Headache Pain* 11: 469–476.

Kasteleijn-Nolst Trenité DG, Schmitz B, Janz D, *et al.* (2013): Consensus on diagnosis and management of JME: From founder's observations to current trends. *Epilepsy Behav* 28: S87–S90.

Kasteleijn-Nolst Trenité DG, Volkers L, Strengman E, *et al.* (2015): Clinical and genetic analysis of a family with two rare reflex epilepsies. *Seizure* 29: 90–96.

Kasteleijn-Nolst Trenite D, Genton P, Brandt C, Reed RC (2017): The "Photosensitivity Model" is (also) a model for focal (partial) seizures. *Epilepsy Res* 133: 113–120.

Kepecs MR, Boro A, Haut S, Kepecs G, Moshe SL (2004): A novel nonpharmacologic treatment for photosensitive epilepsy: a report of three patients tested with blue cross-polarized glasses. *Epilepsia* 45: 1158–1162.

Kinrions P, Ibrahim N, Murphy K, Lehesjoki AE, Jarvela I, Delanty N (2003): Efficacy of levetiracetam in a patient with Unverricht-Lundborg progressive myoclonic epilepsy. *Neurology* 60: 1394–1395.

Koutroumanidis M, Tsirka V, Panayiotopoulos C (2015): Adult-onset photosensitivity: clinical significance and epilepsy syndromes including idiopathic (possibly genetic) photosensitive occipital epilepsy. *Epileptic Disord* 17: 275–286.

Labate A, Ambrosio R, Gambardella A, Sturniolo M, Pucci F, Quattrone A (2007): Usefulness of a morning routine EEG recording in patients with juvenile myoclonic epilepsy. *Epilepsy Res* 77: 17–21.

Laufs H, Kleinschmidt A, Beyerle A, *et al.* (2003): EEG-correlated fMRI of human alpha activity. *Neuroimage* 19: 1463–1476.

Lee CY, Jeon JY, Cho YW, Moon HJ (2014): A case of temporal onset partial seizure induced by photic stimuli. *J Epilepsy Res* 30: 18–20.

Liu Z, de Zwart JA, Yao B, van Gelderen P, Kuo LW, Duyn JH (2012): Finding thalamic BOLD correlates to posterior alpha EEG. *Neuroimage* 63: 1060–1069.

Loiseau P, Duché B (1995): Childhood absence epilepsy. In: Duncan JS, Panayiotopoulos CP (eds) *Typical Absences and Related Epileptic Syndromes*. London: Churchill Livingstone, pp. 152–160.

Lortie A, Plouin P, Pinard JM, Dulac O (1993): Occipital epilepsy in neonates and infants, In: Andermann F, Beaumanoir A, Mira L, Roger J, Tassinari CA (eds). *Occipital Seizures and Epilepsies in Children*. London: John Libbey & Co, Ltd, pp. 121–132.

Matricardi M, Brinciotti M, Benedetti P (1989): Outcome after discontinuation of antiepileptic drug therapy in children with epilepsy. *Epilepsia* 30: 582–589.

Mehndiratta MM, Aggarwal P (2002): Clinical expression and EEG features of patients with juvenile myoclonic epilepsy (JME) from North India. *Seizure* 11: 431–436.

Melsen S (1959): The value of photic stimulation in the diagnosis of epilepsy. *J Nerv Ment Dis* 128: 508–519.

Michelucci R, Tassinari CA (1993): Television-induced occipital seizures, In: Andermann F, Beaumanoir A, Mira L, Roger J, Tassinari CA (eds)

Occipital Seizures and Epilepsies in Children. London: John Libbey & Co, Ltd pp. 165–171.

Moeller F, Siebner HR, Ahlgrimm N, *et al.* (2009): fMRI activation during spike and wave discharges evoked by photic stimulation. *Neuroimage* 48: 682–695.

Moeller F, Muthuraman M, Stephani U, Deuschl G, Raethjen J, Siniatchkin M (2013): Representation and propagation of epileptic activity in absences and generalized photoparoxysmal responses. *Hum Brain Mapp* 34: 1896–1909.

Mukundan L, Lie OV, Leary LD, Papanastassiou AM, Morgan LC, Szabó CÁ (2014): Subdural electrode recording of generalized photoepileptic responses. *Epilepsy Behav Case Rep* 3: 4–7.

Mulley JC, Scheffer IE, Petrou S, Dibbens LM, Berkovic SF, Harkin LA (2005): SCN1A mutations and epilepsy. *Hum Mutat* 25: 535–542.

Nagarajan L, Kulkarni A, Palumbo-Clark L, *et al.* (2003): Photoparoxysmal responses in children: their characteristics and clinical correlates. *Pediatr Neurol* 29: 222–226.

Nar Senol P, Tezer FI, Saygi S (2015): Eyelid myoclonia seizures in adults: An alternate look at the syndrome paradox. *Epilepsy Behav* 45: 265–270.

Neubauer BA, Waltz S, Grothe M, *et al.* (2005): Photosensitivity: genetics and clinical significance, *Adv Neurol* 95: 217–226.

Nishimura R, Omos-Lau N, Ajmone-Marsan,C, Barranger JA (1980): Electroencephalographic findings in Gaucher disease. *Neurology* 30: 152–159.

Obeid T, Daif AK, Waheed G, *et al.* (1991): Photosensitive epilepsies and photoconvulsive responses in Arabs. *Epilepsia* 32: 77–81.

Ohmori I, Ohtsuka Y, Ouchida M, *et al.* (2003): Is phenotype difference in severe myoclonic epilepsy in infancy related to *SCN1A* mutations? *Brain Dev* 25: 488–493.

Oliver KL, Franceschetti S, Milligan CJ, *et al.* (2017): Myoclonus epilepsy and ataxia due to *KCNC1* mutation: Analysis of 20 cases and K+ channel properties. *Ann Neurol* 81: 677–689.

Panayiotopoulos CP, Obeid T, Tahan AR (1994): Juvenile myoclonic epilepsy: a 5-year prospective study. *Epilepsia* 35: 285–296.

Panayiotopoulos CP (1999): Elementary visual hallucinations, blindness and headache in idiopathic occipital epilepsy: differentiation from migraine. *J Neurol Neurosurg Psych* 66: 536–540.

Pantelakis S, Bower BD, Jones HD (1962): Convulsions and television viewing. *Brit Med J* ii: 633–637.

Papacostas SS (2003): Photosensitivity during the hypersomnic phase in a patient with Kleine-Levin syndrome. *J Child Neurol* 18: 432–433.

Papatheophilou R, Turland DN (1976): The electroencephalogram of normal adolescent males: visual assessment and relationship with other variables. *Dev Med Child Neurol* 18: 603–619.

Papetti L, Nicita F, Parisi P, Spalice A, Villa MP, Kasteleijn-Nolst Trenité DG (2013): "Headache and epilepsy"–how are they connected? *Epilepsy Behav* 26: 386–393.

Parisi P, Kasteleijn-Nolst Trenité DGA, Piccioli M, *et al.* (2007): A case with atypical childhood occipital epilepsy "Gastaut type": an ictal migraine manifestation with a good response to intravenous diazepam. *Epilepsia* 48: 2181–2186.

Parra J, Kalitzin SN, Iriarte J, Blanes W, Velis DN, Lopes da Silva FH (2003): Gamma-band phase clustering and photosensitivity: is there an underlying mechanism common to photosensitive epilepsy and visual perception? *Brain*126: 1164–1172.

Parra J, Lopes da Silva FH, Stroink H, Kalitzin S (2007): Is colour modulation an independent factor in human visual photosensitivity? *Brain* 130: 1679–1689.

Perry G, Brindley LM, Muthukumaraswamy SD, Singh KD, Hamandi K (2014): Evidence for increased visual gamma responses in photosensitive epilepsy. *Epilepsy Res* 108: 1076–1086.

Piccinelli P, Borgatti R, Nicoli F, *et al.* (2006): Relationship between migraine and epilepsy in pediatric age. *Headache* 46: 413–421.

Piccioli M, Ricci S, Vigevano F, Buttinelli C, Kasteleijn-Nolst Trenité DGA (2003): Visual sensitive children: symptoms and signs during intermittent photic stimulation and video game playing. *Epilepsia* 44 S9: 307.

Piccioli M, Parisi P, Tisei P, Villa MP, Buttinelli C, Kasteleijn-Nolste Trenité DGA (2009): Ictal Headache and Visual Sensitivity. *Cephalalgia* 29: 194–203.

Pinto D, Westland B, de Haan GJ, *et al.* (2005): Genome-wide linkage scan of epilepsy-related photoparoxysmal electroencephalographic response: evidence for linkage on chromosomes 7q32 and 16p13. *Hum Mol Genet* 14: 171–178.

Pinto D, Kasteleijn-Nost Trenité DG, Coerdell HJ, *et al.* (2007): Explorative two-locus linkage analysis suggests a multiplicative interaction between the 7q32 and 16p13 myoclonic seizures-relates photosensitivity loci. *Genet epidemiol* 31: 42–50.

Porciatti V, Bonanni P, Fiorentini A, Guerrini R (2000): Lack of cortical contrast gain control in human photosensitive epilepsy. *Nat Neurosci* 3: 259–263.

Puglia JF, Brenner RP, Soso MJ (1992): Relationship between prolonged and self-limited photoparoxysmal responses and seizure incidence: study and review. *J Clin Neurophysiol* 9: 137–144.

Quesney LF, Andermann F, Gloor P (1981): Dopaminergic mechanism in generalized photosensitive epilepsy. *Neurology* 31: 1542–1544.

Quesney LF, Andermann F, Lal S, Prelevic S (1980): Transient abolition of generalized photosensitive epileptic discharge in humans by apomorphine, a dopamine-receptor agonist. *Neurology* 30: 1169–1174.

Quirk JA, Fish DR, Smith SJ, Sander JW, Shorvon SD, Allen PJ (1995): Incidence of photosensitive epilepsy: a prospective national study. *Electroencephalogr Clin Neurophysiol* 95: 260–267.

Rabending G, Klepel H (1970): Photoconvulsive and photomyoclonic reactions: age-dependent, genetically determined variants of enhanced photosensitivity. *Neuropadiatrie* 2: 164–172.

Radovicci A, Misirliou V, Gluckman M (1932): Epilepsie réflexe provoquée par excitations optiques des rayons solaires. *Rev Neurol (Paris)* 1: 1305–1308.

Rao KS, Prichard JS (1955): Photogenic epilepsy. *J Pediatr* 47: 619–623.

Reilly EL, Peters JF (1973): Relationship of some varieties of electroencephalographic photosensitivity to clinical convulsive disorders. *Neurology* 23: 1050–1057.

Ricci S, Vigevano F, Manfredi M, Kasteleijn-Nolst Trenité DGA (1998): Epilepsy provoked by television and video games: Safety of 100 Hz screens. *Neurology* 50: 790–793.

Robin JJ, Tolan GD, Arnold JW (1978): Ten-year experience with abnormal EEGs in asymptomatic adult males. *Aviat Space Environ Med* 49: 732–736.

Roger J, Pellissier JF, Bureau M, Dravet C, Revol M, Tinuper P (1983): Le diagnostic précoce de la maladie de Lafora, importance des manifestations paroxystiques visuelles et intérêt de la biopsie cutanée. *Rev Neurol* 139: 115–124.

Roy AK, Pinheiro L, Rajesh SV (2003): Prevalence of photosensitivity- an Indian experience. *Neurol India* 51: 241–243.

Rubboli G, Meletti S, Gardella E, *et al.* (1999): Photic reflex myoclonus: a neurophysiological study in progressive myoclonus epilepsies. *Epilepsia* 40 S4: 50–58.

Rubboli C, Parra J, Seri S, Takahashi T, Thomas P (2004): EEG diagnostic procedures and special investigations in the assessment of photosensitivity. *Epilepsia* 45 (S1): 35–39.

Rubboli C, Franceschetti S, Berkovic SF, *et al.* (2011): Clinical and neurophysiologic features of progressive myoclonus epilepsy without renal failure caused by SCARB2 mutations. *Epilepsia* 52: 2356–2363.

Sadleir LG, Paterson S, Smith KR, *et al.* (2015): Myoclonic occipital photosensitive epilepsy with dystonia (MOPED): A familial epilepsy syndrome. *Epilepsy Res* 114: 98–105.

Saleem SM, Thomas M, Jain S, Maheshwari MC (1994): Incidence of photosensitive epilepsy in unselected Indian epileptic population. *Acta Neurol Scand* 89: 5–8.

Scarpino O, Pelliccioni G, Guidi M, Mauro AM, Mercante O (1990): Parkinson disease and photosensitive epilepsy. *Rev Neurol* 146: 36–40.

Scheffer IE, Berkovic S, Capovilla G, *et al.* (2017): ILAE classification of the epilepsies: Position paper of the ILAE Commission for Classification and Terminology. *Epilepsia* 58: 512–521.

Scott DF, Furlong PF, Moffett AM, Harding GFA (1985): Is sunshine protective in photosensitive epilepsy? *Electroenceph Clin Neurophysiol* 61: S216.

Seddigh S, Thömke F, Vogt TH (1999): Complex partial seizures provoked by photic stimulation. *J Neurol Neurosurg Psych* 66: 801–802.

Sharma A, Cameron D (2007): Reasons to consider a plasma screen TV-photosensitive epilepsy. *Epilepsia* 48: 2003.

Shepherd AJ, Siniatchkin M (2009): Visual pattern adaptation in subjects with photoparoxysmal EEG response: evidence for increased visual cortical excitability. *Invest Ophthalmol Vis Sci* 50: 1470–1476.

Shiraishi H, Fujiwara T, Inoue Y, Yagi K (2001): Photosensitivity in relation to epileptic syndromes: a survey from an epilepsy center in Japan. *Epilepsia* 42: 393–397.

Shirakawa S, Funatsuka M, Osawa M, Fujita M, Oguni H (2001): A study of the effect of color photostimulation from a cathode-ray tube (CRT) display on photosensitive patients: the effect of alternating red-cyan flicker stimulation. *Epilepsia* 42: 922–929.

Singhi PD, Bansal D (2004): Self-induced photosensitive epilepsy. *Indian J Pediatr* 71 (7): 649–651.

Small JG (1971): Photoconvulsive and photomyoclonic responses in psychiatric patients. *Clin Electroencephal* 2: 78–88.

Smith KM, Youssef PE, Wirrell EC, *et al.* (2018): Jeavons Syndrome: Clinical Features and Response to Treatment. *Pediatr Neurol* 86: 46–51.

So EL, Ruggles KH, Ahmann PA, Olson KA (1993): Prognosis of photoparoxysmal response in non-epileptic patients. *Neurology* 43: 1719–1722.

Sofia V, Proietto M, Poidomani A, *et al.* (1999): Ruolo della fotosensibilita nell'epilessia mioclonica giovanile. *Boll lega It Epil* 106/7: 175–176.

Specchio N, Trenité DG, Piccioli M, *et al.* (2010): Diagnosing photosensitive epilepsy: Fancy new *versus* old fashioned techniques in patients with different epileptic syndromes. *Brain Dev* 33: 294–300.

Specchio N, Bellusci M, Pietrafusa N, Trivisano M, de Palma L, Vigevano F (2017): Photosensitivity is an early marker of neuronal ceroid lipofuscinosis type 2 disease. *Epilepsia* 58: 1380–1388.

Striano S, Capovilla G, Sofia V, *et al.* (2009): Eyelid myoclonia with absences (Jeavons syndrome), a well-defined idiopathic generalized epilepsy syndrome or a spectrum of photosensitive conditions? *Epilepsia* 50 (S5): 15–19.

Strigaro G, Prandi P, Varrasi C, Monaco F, Cantello R (2012): Defective visual inhibition in photosensitive idiopathic generalized epilepsy. *Epilepsia* 53: 695–704.

Strigaro G, Falletta L, Varrasi C, Rothwell JC, Cantello R (2015): Overactive visuomotor connections underlie the photoparoxysmal response. A TMS study. *Epilepsia* 56: 1828–1835.

Sugawara T, Mazaki-Miyazaki E, Fukushima K, *et al.* (2002): Frequent mutations of SCN1A in severe myoclonic epilepsy in infancy. *Neurology* 58: 1122–1124.

Suppa A, Rocchi L, Li Voti P, *et al.* (2015): The photoparoxysmal response reflects abnormal early visuomotor integration in the human motor cortex. *Brain Stimuli* 8: 1151–1161.

Szabó CA, Salinas FS, Li K, *et al.* (2016): Modeling the effective connectivity of the visual network in healthy and photosensitive, epileptic baboons. *Brain Struct Funct* 221: 2023–2033.

Takada H, Aso K, Watanabe K, Okumura A, Negoro T, Ishikawa T (1999): Epileptic seizures induced by animated cartoon, "Pocket Monster". *Epilepsia* 40: 997–1002.

Takahashi T, Tsukahara Y (1992): Usefulness of blue sunglasses in photosensitive epilepsy. *Epilepsia* 33: 517–521.

Takahashi T, Nakasato N, Yokoyama H, Tsukahara Y (1999a): Low luminance visual stimuli compared to stroboscopic IPS in eliciting PPR in photosensitive patients. *Epilepsia* 40 (S4): 44–9.

Takahashi T, Tsukahara Y, Nomura M, Matsuoka H (1999b): Pokemon seizures. *Neurol J Southeast Asia* 4: 1–11.

Takahashi Y, Shigematsu H, Fujiwara T, Yagi K, Seino M (1995): Self-induced photogenic seizures in a child with severe myoclonic epilepsy in infancy: optical investigations and treatments. *Epilepsia* 36: 728–732.

Takahashi Y, Sato T, Goto K, *et al.* (2001): Optical filters inhibiting television-induced photosensitive seizures, *Neurology* 57: 1767–1773.

Tassinari CA, Rubboli G, Plasmati R, *et al.* (1988): Television-induced epilepsy with occipital seizures, A variety of idiopathic partial seizures. In: Beaumanoir A, Gastaut H, Naquet R (eds) *Reflex Seizures and Reflex Epilepsies.* Geneva: Médecine et Hygiène, pp. 241–243.

Tassinari CA, Michelucci R, Rubboli G, *et al.* (1989): Self-induced seizures, In: Beaumanoir A, Gastaut H, Naquet R. (eds) *Reflex Seizures and Reflex Epilepsies*, Geneva: Médecine et Hygiène, pp. 363–368.

Taylor I, Marini C, Johnson MR, Turner S, Berkovic SF, Scheffer IE (2004): Juvenile myoclonic epilepsy and idiopathic photosensitive occipital lobe epilepsy: is there overlap? *Brain* 127: 1878–1886.

Taylor I, Berkovic SF, Scheffer IE (2013): Genetics of epilepsy syndromes in families with photosensitivity. *Neurology* 80: 1322–1329.

Tauer U, Lorenz S, Lenzen KP, *et al.* (2005): Genetic dissection of photosensitivity and its relation to idiopathic generalized epilepsy. *Ann Neurol* 57: 866–873.

Thomas RH, Zhang LM, Carvill GL, *et al.* (2015): CHD2 myoclonic encephalopathy is frequently associated with self-induced seizures. *Neurology* 84: 951–958.

Tinuper P, Aguglia U, Pellissier JF, Gastaut H (1983): Visual ictal phenomena in a case of Lafora diseas proved by skin biopsy. *Epilepsia* 24: 214–218.

Tozzi E, Florio I, Mesturino A, Marrelli A, Criscione S (1998): Hemicrania and photosensitive epilepsy in pediatric age. *Clin Ter* 149: 357–360.

Trenité DG, French JA, Hirsch E, *et al.* (2007): Evaluation of carisbamate, a novel antiepileptic drug, in photosensitive patients: An exploratory, placebo-controlled study. *Epilepsy Res* 74: 193–200.

Van Gijn J (2001): The uses of error: Sharing with colleagues. *Lancet* 357: 2128.

Vaudano AE, Ruggieri A, Tondelli M, *et al.* (2014): The visual system in eyelid myoclonia with absences. *Ann Neurol* 76: 412–427.

Vaudano AE, Ruggieri A, Avanzini P, *et al.* (2017): Photosensitive epilepsy is associated with reduced inhibition of alpha rhythm generating networks. *Brain* 140: 981–897.

Verbeek NE, Kasteleijn-Nolst Trenité D, Wassenaar M, *et al.* (2017): Photosensitivity in patients with SCN1A-related Dravet Syndrome is underrecognized and related to prognosis. *Clin Neurophysiol* 128: 323–330.

Verrotti A, Trotta D, Salladini C, *et al.* (2004): Photosensitivity and epilepsy: a follow-up study. *Dev Med Child Neurol* 46: 347–351.

Viravan S, Go C, Ochi A, Akiyama T, Carter Snead O 3rd, Otsubo H (2011): Jeavons syndrome existing as occipital cortex initiating generalized epilepsy. *Epilepsia* 52: 1273–1279.

Von Podewils F, Runge U, Krüger S, *et al.* (2015): Diffusion tensor imaging abnormalities in photosensitive juvenile myoclonic epilepsy. *Eur J Neurol* 22: 1192–1200.

Wadlington WB, Riley HD (1965): Light-induced seizures. *J Pediat* 66: 300–312.

Waltz S (1994): Photosensitivity and epilepsy: a genetic approach. In: Malafosse A, Genton P, Hirsch E, Marescaux C, Broglin D, Bernasconi R (eds) *Idiopathic Generalized Epilepsies: Clinical, Experimental and Genetic Aspects*. London: John Libbey and Co Ltd, pp. 317–328.

Waltz S, Christen HJ, Doose H (1992): The different patterns of the photoparoxysmal response – a genetic study, *Electroenceph Clin Neurophysiol* 83: 138–145.

Waltz S, Stephani U (2000): Inheritance of photosensitivity. *Neuropediatrics* 31: 82–85.

Wheless JW (2000): Use of topiramate in childhood generalized seizure disorders. *J Child Neurol* 15 (S1): 7–13.

Wielaender F, Sarviaho R, James F, *et al.* (2017): Generalized myoclonic epilepsy with photosensitivity in juvenile dogs caused by a defective DIRAS family GTPase 1. *Proc Natl Acad Sci USA* 114: 2669–2674.

Wilfong AA (2005): Zonisamide monotherapy for epilepsy in children and young adults. *Pediatric Neurol* 32: 77–80.

Wilkins A. (1995): *Visual Stress*. Oxford Psychology Series, no 24.

Wilkins AJ, Baker A, Amin D, *et al.* (1999): Treatment of photosensitive epilepsy using coloured filters. *Seizure* 8: 444–449.

Wilkins AJ, Bonanni P, Porciatti P, Guerrini R (2004): Physiology of human photosensitivity. *Epilepsia* 45 (S1): 7–13.

Wolf P (1994): Reading epilepsy, In: Wolf P (ed) *Epileptic seizures and syndromes*, London: John Libbey & Co, Ltd, pp. 67–73.

Wolf P, Goosses R (1986): Relation of photosensitivity to epileptic syndromes. *J Neurol Neurosurg Psychiatry* 49: 1386–1391.

World Health Organisation (1991): International classification of diseases. Geneva: WHO.

Yalcin AD, Kaymaz A, Forta H (2000): Reflex occipital lobe epilepsy. *Seizure* 9: 436–441.

Zifkin B, Inoue Y (2004): Visual reflex seizures induced by complex stimuli. *Epilepsia* 45 (S1): 27–29.

Epileptic Syndromes in Infancy, Childhood and Adolescence (6th ed), M. Bureau, P. Genton, C. Dravet, A. V. Delgado-Escueta, R. Guerrini, C.A. Tassinari, P. Thomas & P. Wolf

WITH VIDEO SUPPLEMENTS

CHAPTER 23

EPILEPTIC SYNDROMES IN THE ELDERLY

Javier Salas-Puig

Epilepsy Unit, Neurology Department, Hospital Universitari Vall d'Hebron, Autonoma University, Barcelona, Spain

Introduction

Epilepsy was long thought to be a disease of infancy, childhood, adolescence and young adulthood. Nevertheless, epidemiological studies have demonstrated that epilepsy is even most common among persons aged 65 and older (Hauser, 1993). In old age, epilepsy is the third most common brain disease after stroke and dementing diseases.

As compared to the younger population epilepsy in elderly has different etiological causes and presents with different diagnostic and therapeutic challenges and with higher susceptibility to adverse effects of the pharmacological treatment. Furthermore the outcome includes a higher incidence of status epilepticus and mortality. In addition a higher possibility of physical injury due to falls and seizures provokes a deeper social and familial dependency and a poorer quality of life. Among the frequent epilepsy situations found in elderly patients, some may indeed qualify as syndromes. We shall try to highlight these in this chapter.

Differential diagnosis and seizure types

The different types of seizures depend mainly on their etiology. Generalized tonic-clonic seizures (GTCS) dominate for metabolic or toxic etiologies although generalized seizures related to generalized idiopathic epilepsies can occur. Epileptic seizures in the elderly are almost always focal (Mc Bride, 2002) and belong to a focal symptomatic epilepsy *(Table I)*. Epileptic seizures are frequently not recognized and are misdiagnosed as mental changes of uncertain origin, confusion, syncope, memory disorders, vertigo, somnolence or parasomnia. Premonitory symptoms (auras) are rare in older patients. The lack of an aura makes epileptic seizures difficult to recognize and to classify (Silveira *et al.*, 2011). GTCS are rare in the elderly. So, the less frequent evolution of focal seizure evolving to generalized convulsive seizure, the common lack of motor phenomena such as automatisms and the rare auras, are all reasons to explain the difficult diagnosis in some patients. Furthermore, postictal confusion can last during several hours and even days leading to a wrong diagnosis (Abubark & Wambacq, 2005). When an elderly patient presents with acute confusion, neuroimaging does not reveal any structural lesion and there are no other explanations such as metabolic disorder or infection, an epileptic seizure or nonconvulsive status epilepticus must be considered and an EEG should be performed as soon as possible (Sheth *et al.*, 2006).

Some detailed studies about semiology of seizures in the elderly have shown that focal simple motor seizures as well as bilateral simple motor seizures were seen less frequently in the elderly in comparison with younger adults (Kellinghaus *et al.*, 2004; Silveira *et al.*, 2011).

Table I **Etiology of acute symptomatic seizures and epilepsy in the elderly (Seang Lim & Tin Tan, 2010)**

Epilepsy		Acute symptomatic seizures	
Cryptogenic	33–50%	Acute stroke	40–54%
Stroke	33–40%	Toxic – metabolic	15–30%
Dementia	11–16%	Neoplasm	8–10%
Neoplasm	4–6%	Trauma	4–10%
Trauma	1–3%	Alcohol	3–5%
		CNS infection	2–3%

One of the most difficult diagnosis is transient epileptic amnesia. Transient amnesia is an arresting clinical phenomenon. The patient is temporarily unable to form new memories (anterograde amnesia), to retrieve established memories (retrograde amnesia) or both. Recognized causes of transient amnesia include transient global amnesia (TGA), transient ischemic attack, migraine, drug effects. Several authors have proposed that transient amnesia can be a unique manifestation of epileptic seizure (Butler *et al.*, 2007). Transient epileptic amnesia is characterized by brief (less than 30 minutes), recurrent attacks of amnesia in the majority of cases in elderly patients, often occurring on waking. In addition, patients with transient epileptic amnesia frequently report two varieties of persistent interictal memory disturbances: i) the accelerated forgetting, over days or weeks, of newly acquired information and ii) a patchy loss of memories for salient autobiographical events in the more remote past. In 2007, it was reported a series of 50 patients with transient epileptic amnesia perfectly defining the main characteristics of this clinical situation (Butler *et al.*, 2007): The male/female ratio was 2:1. The amnestic attacks were a mixed anterograde and retrograde amnesia, sometimes with repetitive questioning. Attacks commonly occur on waking, a helpful diagnostic clue. Some episodes may be accompanied by olfactory hallucinations, automatisms or a brief loss of contact. The duration was usually less than one hour but could be longer. Transient epileptic amnesia was responsive to antiepileptic drug treatment. Nevertheless, many patients reported persistent memory deficits after the cessation of the attack.

In contrast, TGA is characterized by an episode of dense anterograde amnesia often triggered by emotional or physical stress, which usually lasts 4–10 hours and rarely recurs. It is not associated with persistent memory impairment. Epileptiform discharges on the EEG, other features of epileptic seizures such as automatisms, olfactory hallucinations, déjà-vu, or loss of contact and a response to antiepileptic treatment support the diagnosis of transient epileptic amnesia. The mesial temporal lobes are particularly susceptible to hypoxic damage and it is possible that the cause of this particular kind of partial seizures is ischemic cerebrovascular disease. Nevertheless in the above mentioned study, cardiovascular disease was not prominent comparing this particular patients with a control group (Butler *et al.*, 2007). In a recent series of 30 patients an autoimmune context was found in 30% (Mosbah *et al.*, 2016).

One of the main characteristics of patients with transient epileptic amnesia is the autobiographical amnesia, the topographic amnesia and the accelerated forgetting which means abnormallly rapid forgetting of material learned to a demanding criterion and it suggests an impairment of long-term processes of memory consolidation (Butler *et al.*, 2009). A dysfunction of a hippocampal-neocortical network sustaining episodic memory has been hypotesized (Mosbah *et al.*, 2016). Despite the clinical findings that distinguish transient epileptic amnesia from other etiologies of amnesia in the elderly, differential diagnosis may be very difficult in the individual patient (Bilo *et al.*, 2009).

Etiology

Epilepsy in old age is an expression of an underlying disease of the brain. The etiology is an important prognostic factor. We need to distinguish between acute symptomatic seizures, very frequent in the elderly, and epilepsy (Loiseau, 1997).

Acute symptomatic seizures

Acute stroke is the commonest etiological cause. Between 2.3% and 10.5% of patients experiende a seizure following stroke (Stefan, 2011). Mortality is higher for stroke in patients with acute symptomatic seizures compared with those without seizures. Metabolic disturbances (hypoglycemia, hyperglycemia, hyponatremia, hypocalcemia, uremia, hepatic failure, hypothiroidism) are also common causes of acute symptomatic seizures. Alcohol abuse and withdrawl are seldom toxic causes of seizures in the elderly.

One of the most identifiable clinical syndromes in the elderly is focal reflex seizures induced by movement related to non ketotic hyperglycemia. This frequently occurs in an elderly patient as the first clinical manifestation of this metabolic disorder; treatment consists in improving the metabolic disorder with insulin and no antiepileptic drugs are usually needed. Movement-induced seizures are so characteristic that reflex epilepsy and non-ketotic hyperglycemia in the elderly have been proposed as a specific neuroendocrine syndrome (Brick *et al.*, 1989). Realization that the seizures are movement-induced is a critical diagnostic clue (Suarez-Moro *et al.*, 1999). Most authors attribute the focal seizures to a preexisting structural lesion, activated by hyperglycemia, mild hyperosmolarity, hyponatremia and lack of cetoacidosis. Focal venous thrombosis could also be a consequence of metabolic derangement. A small cerebral infarct provoked by such thrombosis could be triggered by hyperglycemia and provoke seizures.

Acute symptomatic seizures related to infectious disease are less common but may be occur in encephalitis or meningoencephalitis *(Figure 1)*.

A wide range of drugs can precipìtate seizures *(Table II)*.

Epilepsy

Stroke is the most important factor for the development of epilepsy in elderly *(Table III)*. The risk of epilepsy increases up to 20-fold in the first year after a stroke and aproximately 8% of patients

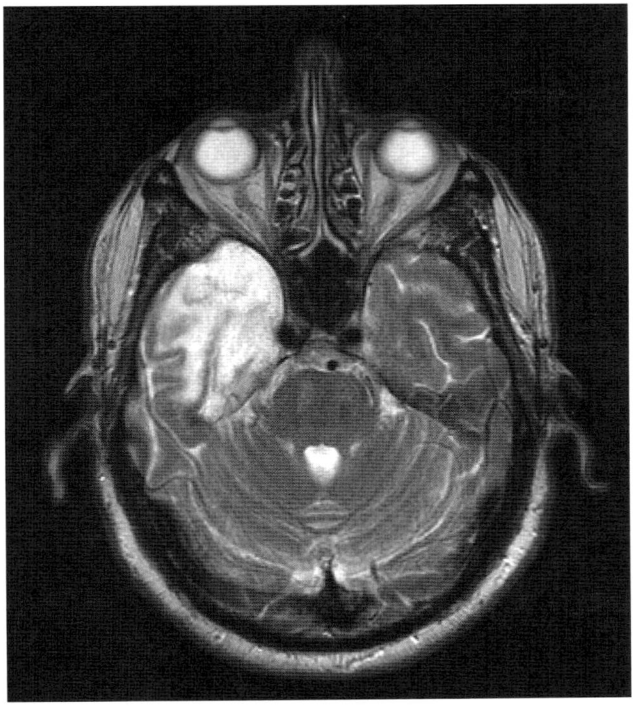

Figure 1 **Acute symptomatic seizures of infectious etiology. 71-year-old woman. Nonconvulsive status and fever. Herpes encephalitis.**

Table II **Drugs reported to potentially cause seizures**

▼ Psychotropic drugs: Tricyclic, tetracyclic antidepressants Serotonin reuptake inhibitors Neuroleptics (phenotiazines, haloperidol, clozapine) Lithium Bupropion
Methylxanthines (theophylline)
Narcotic analgesics (meperidine, propoxyphene)
▼ Antimicrobials: Penicillins, cephalosporins Imipenen Isoniazid Antimalarials Cyclosporine Nalidixic acid
Chemotherapeutic agents (methotrexate, chlorambucil)
General anesthetics (ketamine, enflurane)
Local anesthetics (lidocaine
Stimulants (amphetamines, cocaine)
Antiarrhythmics (verapamil, mexiletine, procainamide, propranolol overdose)
Antihistamines (diphenydramine)
Baclofen
Antiemetics (chlorpromazine)

with stroke will develop epilepsy (So *et al.*, 1996). Stroke is the cause of 50% of cases in whom an etiology can be identified. The majority of poststroke recurrent seizures occurs within one year after the onset of stroke *(Figure 2)*. There is higher incidence of epilepsy following cortical, large and multiple stroke, or following acute symptomatic seizures (Pitkänen *et al.*, 2016). A higher incidence after haemorraghic stroke has been reported (Brodie *et al.*, 2009).

Epileptic seizures in old age can also be the first signs of cerebrovascular disease. In a study of 4,709 patients with epilepsy over age 60 without any history of known prior cerebrovascular events, trauma, dementia or alcoholism, it was shown that they had a five-year risk of stroke that was 2.89 times higher than 4,709 people in a control group (Cleary *et al.*, 2004). For that reason any elderly person with new-onset seizures should undergo assessment for the presence of cerebrovascular risk factors and be treated accordingly for stroke prevention. In some rare ocasions, a seizure may herald ischemic or hemorraghic stroke. To make a diagnosis of heralding seizures a temporal and a topographic relationship between both events is necessary (García-García *et al.*, 2004).

Neurodegenerative disorders with cognitive impairment are a frequent etiology of epilepsy in elderly patients. Patients with Alzheimer's disease are up to ten times more likely to develop epileptic seizures than those without it. The cumulative incidence of epilepsy at 7 years of follow-up in a prospective study, was nearly 8%. The incidence per person-year was markedly higher in young patients with Alzheimer's disease (age 50 to 59: 4.3%) than in patients who developped the disease in old age (over age 80: 0.55%). Further risk factors for epilepsy were the severity of dementia and the presence of epileptiform discharges on the EEG (Amatniek *et al.*, 2006). Dementia accounts for 10–20% of epilepsies in older patients. Seizures can

Table III Etiology of epilepsy in 279 consecutive patients older than 65 years seen during the year 2010 in the Epilepsy Unit of University Hospital Vall d'Hebron, Barcelona, Spain

Focal symptomatic	193 (69.1%)	
	Vascular	108
	Tumor	25
	Trauma	20
	Infection CNS	11
	Mesial temporal sclerosis	7
	Cortical Development Dis.	4
	Other	18
Focal cryptogenic	50 (17.9%)	
Generalized idiopathic	14 (5%)	
Undetermined (pure sleep)*	9 (3.2%)	
Unclassifiable	12 (4.3%)	
Symptomatic generalized	1	

* **Undetermined:** patients with convulsive seizures exclusively during sleep with normal EEG and MRI studies.

occur at any stage of the disease but are more frequent in more advanced disease (Scaldaferri *et al.*, 2010). Recognition of seizures and adverse effects of treatment might be more challenging after several years of evolution.

Patients with Down syndrome frequently suffer epileptic seizures when they are older. A characteristic epilepsy syndrome called senile myoclonic epilepsy has been reported as typical of ageing and dementing Down syndrome patients (De Simone *et al.*, 2010). In these patients, the onset of myoclonic seizures is related to cognitive decline corresponding with Alzheimer's type dementia. Massive, bilateral myoclonic jerks, sometimes leading to falls, are the major feature of epileptic seizures. The EEG shows slow background activity, generalized spike, polyspike-waves with a photoparoxysmal response in some patients. At the beginning, the myoclonic seizures occur predominantly on awakening and later on during awake periods. GTCS may occur later during the progression of dementia.

Recent findings show that older patients with new-onset epilepsy are more likely to suffer from cognitive decline and epilepsy is considered a risk factor for dementia. There is increasing knowledge of some shared mechanisms of cerebrovascular disease, Alzheimer disease and epilepsy (Sen *et al.*, 2018).

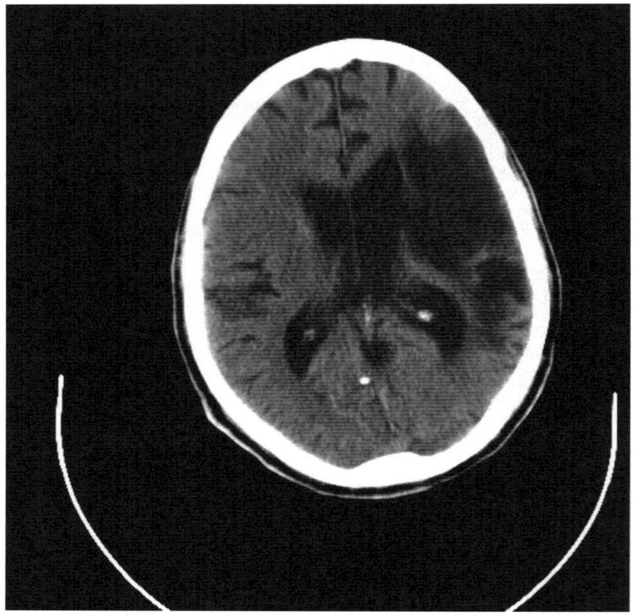

Figure 2 Focal symptomatic epilepsy of vascular etiology. 78-year-old male. Middle cerebral artery ischemic infarction. Focal motor right hand seizures after 7 months. Good response to levetiracetam 1,000 mg/day.

Between 10 and 30% of seizures are associated with tumours, especially gliomas, meningiomas and brain metastases.

Inmune encephalitis are an increasing cause of seizures and epilepsy of late-onset including elderly. There have been recently reports of antiNMDA encephalitis in patients over 65 years of age. LGI1 encephalitis also can occur in elderly. Hashimoto encephalopathy is another etiology which responds to steroids and inmune therapy.

Head injury predominantly brain contusion with subdural haematoma, skull fracture with loss of conciousness is a common cause of epilepsy in elderly patients *(Figure 3)*.

In older patients sleep-related seizures are relatively common *(Figure 4)*. Among so called *pure sleep seizures* there is a group whose seizures begin after 65 years of age (Benavente & Salas-Puig, 2007). They can belong to focal symptomatic epilepsy, focal cryptogenic epilepsy or undetermined epilepsy which means patients with

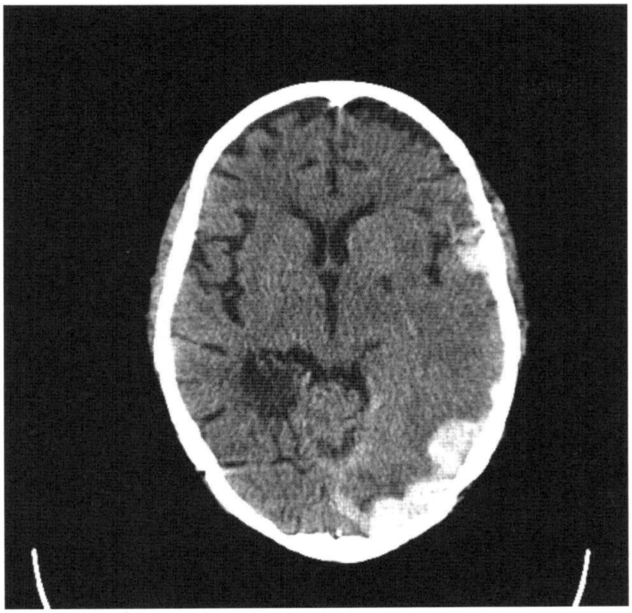

Figure 3 **Acute symptomatic seizures of traumatic etiology.** 81-year-old male. Antecedents of embolic ictus. Warfarin treatment. Cranial trauma. Loss of concioussness and convulsive seizures. CT scan: Subdural haematoma.

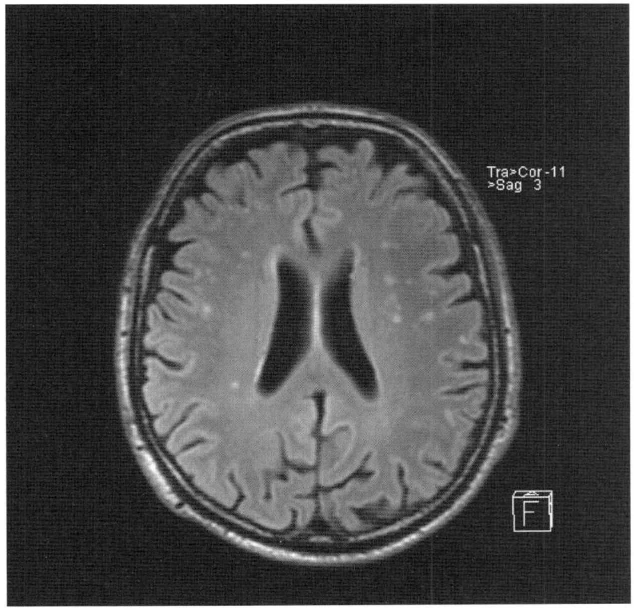

Figure 4 **Pure sleep epilepsy.** 75-year-old male. At the age of 69, apparently generalized convulsive seizures during sleep which occurred 2–3 times per year. Normal neurological examination. MRI: small vessel ischemic lesions. Good response to oxcarbazepine 900 mg/day.

apparently generalized convulsive seizures with no abnormalities on the EEG and no pathological findings in neuroimaging. This latter group have a good prognosis with more than 75% of seizure-free patients on monotherapy. However, relapse and the possibility to suffer seizures during waking after withdrawl of antiepileptic treatment is high (D'Alessandro *et al.*, 2004; Benavente & Salas-Puig, 2007).

Idiopathic generalized epilepsies appear mainly in childhood or adolescence. Nevertheless they can be found also or even appear in the elderly. Among more than 1,000 geriatric patients referred for EEG over 30 month period, there were 10 patients with idiopathic generalized epilepses. Eight begun their seizures in childhood or adolescence and two other patients had a late-onset (Michel *et al.*, 2011).

It is important to take into account the possibility of psychogenic seizures also in the elderly (Kawai *et al.*, 2007).

Status epilepticus in the elderly

Status pilepticus (SE) in not infrequent in elderly patients. The incidence of SE in the elderly population is 90 per 100,000 and it is almost twice that of the general population. It is the mode of presentation of epilepsy in aproximately 30% of elderly individuals. Mortality is high with 38% in those over 60 and 50% in those over 80 years. Stroke, either acute or remote, is the most common etiology of SE. Convulsive status has been described in 1% of stroke patients and SE occurs within the first week following stroke in 0.1–0.2% (Santamarina *et al.*, 2018).

Nonconvulsive status epilepticus (NCSE) is a particularly common and challenging diagnosis in elderly patients (Veran *et al.*, 2010). NCSE in the elderly may represent 10% of all SE across the ages.

NCSE may present as a focal cognitive disturbance with aphasia or a neglect syndrome or can manifest as a confusional state, behavior disorder, lethargy or also coma. This nonspecific presentation can be associated with a delay in the diagnosis. EEG correlates of NCSE include focal rythmic discharges, often of frontal or temporal origin, or generalized spike or sharp and slow wave activity. In a prospective study during one year, 16% of patients aged 60 or older with a confusional state had a NCSE (Veran *et al.*, 2010). More than a half of NCSE occur in the setting of acute medical conditions such as organ failure, drug toxicity, alcohol or benzodiazepine withdrawl and other metabolic disturbances. Two situations are relatively frequent in the elderly: *de novo* absence status epilepticus which occurs as a confusional state with generalized spike-wave discharges in the EEG (Thomas *et al.*, 1992) and a confusional state with periodic lateralized epileptiform discharges in the EEG (PLEDs). Many of the cases of *de novo* absence status occurred after withdrawl from benzodiazepines or psychotropic drugs.

As with absence status in patients with idiopathic generalized epilepsies, behavior during the episodes may range from subtle behavioral changes to profound stupor. The EEG typically shows diffuse, bilaterally symmetric spike and wave discharges at 1–4 Hz frequency. Intravenous benzodiazepines is almost always effective at normalizing both the patient's behavior and the EEG. Status does not recur unless there are other episodes of drug withdrawl (Thomas *et al.*, 1992).

Confusional status epilepticus with PLEDs is a disorder characterized by usually prolonges episodes of confusion associated with periodic, sometimes lateralized epileptiform discharges on the EEG. Normalization of behavior and the EEG coincide. The great majority appears in the elderly (Terzano *et al.*, 1986). Neuroimaging studies indicate that PLEDs may arise from a variety of structural chnages including cortical and subcortical lesions. Nevertheless, they can occur in patients without any demonstrable brain lesion (Kalamangalam *et al.*, 2007). Hyperperfusion found in the SPECT adds further to the evidence that PLEDs may be related to a form of focal status epilepticus (Assal *et al.*, 2001).

NCSE is also quite frequent in the setting of severe medical illness in intensive care units. Electroclinical differences have been reported to distinguish patients with NCSE proper (ambulatory form) and coma. The authors found that a previous history of epilepsy was more frequent in cases with NCSE proper. The NCSE in comatose patients as more frequent in the elderly and had a poorer prognosis (Fernandez-Torre *et al.*, 2012).

Treatment

There are several changes with aging that may have effects on the pharmacokinetics of antiepileptic drugs: reductions in the absorption, perfusion and motility at the gastrointestinal level; reduction in the liver volume with a decrease in protein production and variations in metabolic activity. In the kidneys, the normal aging process is accompanied by physiologic changes at glomerular and tubular levels producing a decrease of renal elimination of some antiepileptic drugs (Krämer, 2001). In addition, elderly patients have an altered distribution volume because of an increased proportion of fat tissue. Protein binding is also reduced (Stefan, 2011).

The pharmacodinamics of drugs in the elderly are complex. The rate and intensity of adverse effects tend to be higher. For most of the antiepileptic drugs a reduction in dose in comparison with young adults is required to avoid adverse effects and the premise of starting low and go slow is a particularly useful advise.

Drugs interactions are very frequent and can complicate the treatment of seizures. Polypharmacy is the rule in older people and treatment adherence declines as the number of prescribed drugs rises (Brodie *et al.*, 2009).

The majority of epilepsies which appeared in the elderly can be controlled in monotherapy but in some series it has been reported a drug-resistant epilepsy in 21% of patients (Hernández-Ronquillo *et al.*, 2018).

The tendency is to treat after a first unprovoked seizure in the presence of a brain lesion or epileptiform abnormalities in the EEG. For a first seizure of unknown origin to treat should be individualized. There is also a tendency to use new antiepileptic drugs like levetiracetam, lacosamide, lamotrigine, eslicarbazepine, oxcarbazepine, zonisamide, perampanel and gabapentin due to their better tolerability in comparison with old antiepileptic drugs (carbamazepine, phenytoin, sodium valproate, phenobarbitone).

Lamotrigine obtained significantly better retention (71%) compared with carbamazepine (42%) and fewer patients dropped out because of adverse events with lamotrigine (18%) *versus* carbamazepine (42%) (Brodie *et al.*, 1999). In another comparative study lamotrigine treatment was better tolerated than carbamazepine or gabapentin (Rowan, 2005). Lamotrigine had the highest 12-month retention rate (79%) in comparison with levetiracetam (73%), gabapentin (59%), phenytoin (59%), topiramate (56%), carbamazepine (48%) and oxcarbazepine (24%). Lamotrigine had the highest 12-month seizure-freedom rate (54%) followed by levetiracetam (43%) (Arif *et al.*, 2010). Other observational studies have found effectiveness of lamotrigine monotherapy at low dose in the elderly (Mauri *et al.*, 2005). Recent studies have shown effectiveness with lacosamide, perampanel and zonisamide. The advantage of intravenous formulation of some of new antiepileptic drugs (levetiracetam, lacosamide, brivaracetam) can help to choose treatment in the elderly patients.

Surgery treatment for epilepsy is rare in elderly patients because epilepsy is easily treated with antiepileptic drugs. Nevertheless, in some series resective epilepsy surgery has been succesfully performed (Stefan, 2011).

Conclusion

Acute symptomatic seizures and epilepsy in elderly patients need to be considered a frequent medical condition with special difficulties in diagnosis and special considerations in pharmacological treatment.

There are electroclinical patterns which can be considered as special situations in the elderly. We can consider true epileptic syndromes.

– The syndrome of *transient epileptic amnesia* characterized by:
- recurrent and frequent episodes of amnesia on waking;
- brief duration (median: 30–60 minutes);
- other cognitive functions intact during the attacks;
- olfactory or gustatory hallucinations and automatisms in 40% of cases;
- common persistent memory difficulties;
- interictal focal EEG abnormalities in more tan 30% of patients;
- neuroimaging usually without specific findings;
- good response to antiepileptic drugs.

– The syndrome of *confusional status associated with PLEDs* in the EEG. It occurs not only in elderly patients but it can be considered a peculiar electroclinical syndrome characterized by:
- acute confusional status;
- EEG with periodic epileptiform discharges;
- cortical or subcortical lesions on neuroimaging in the majority of cases;
- hyperperfusion on SPECT during the ictal period;
- a clear correlation between clinical and EEG findings.

– The syndrome of *senile myoclonic epilepsy* in elderly patients with Down syndrome and Alzheimer's dementia. It is characterized by:
- myoclonic seizures predominantly on awakening followed by GTCS;
- spike-wave and polyspike-wave bilateral EEG discharges with possible photoparoxysmal response;
- progressive cognitive decline.

– *De novo absence status epilepticus* of late life. It is characterized by:
- sudden onset of confusion that can last hours or even days;
- a history of long-remitted absence epilepsy in early life in many cases;
- in most, triggered by psychotropic drug toxicity or withdrawl (particularly benzodiazepines);
- generalized spike and wave discharges;
- disappearance of clinical and EEG changes after intravenous benzodiazepine;
- no tendency to recur (long-term antiepileptic treatment usually not required.

The *de novo absence status epilepticus* can also be considered an acute symptomatic epilepsy induced by drugs, drug withdrawl or favoured by metabolic disturbances such as hypoglycemia, hypocalcemia or uremia.

– *Focal reflex seizures with nonketotic hyperglycemia.* It can be also considered an acute symptomatic epilepsy syndrome in the elderly. It is characterized by:
- focal sensitive-motor seizures induced by voluntary movements;
- hyperglycemia with no cetoacidosis;
- excellent response to metabolic disorder improvement.

REFERENCES

Abubakr A, Wambacq I (2005): Seizures in the elderly: Video/EEG monitoring analysis. *Epilepsy Behav* 7: 447–450.

Amatniek JC, Hauser WA, Del Castillo-Manzaneda C, *et al.* (2006): Incidence and predictors of seizures in patients with Alzheimer's disease. *Epilepsia* 47: 867–872.

Arif H, Buchsbaum R, Pierro J, *et al.* (2010): Comparative effectiveness of 10 antiepileptic drugs in older adults with epilepsy. *Arch Neurol* 67: 408–415.

Assal F, Papazyan JP, Slosman DO, Jallon P, Goerres GW (2001): SPECT in periodic lateralized epileptiform discharges (PLEDs): a form of partial status epilepticus? *Seizure* 10: 260–264.

Benavente LF, Salas-Puig J (2007): Pure Sleep Seizures risk of seizures while awake. *Epileptic Disord* 9: 65–70.

Bilo L, Meo R, Ruosi P, de Leva MF, Striano S (2009): Transient epileptic amnesia: an emerging late-onset epileptic syndrome. *Epilepsia* (Suppl 5): 58–61.

Brick JF, Gutrecht JA, Ringel RA (1989): Reflex epilepsy and nonketotic hyperglycemia in the elderly: a specific neuroendocrine syndrome. *Neurology* 39: 394.

Brodie MJ, Overstall PW, Giorgi L(1999): Multicentre, double-blind, randomised comparison between lamotrigine and carbamacepine in elderly patients with newly diagnosed epilepsy. *Epilepsy Res* 37: 81–87.

Brodie MJ, Elder MT, Kwan P (2009): Epilepsy in later life. *Lancet Neurol* 8: 1019–1030.

Butler CR, Graham KS, Hodges JR, Kapur N, Wardlaw JM, Zeman AZJ (2007): The syndrome of transient epileptic amnesia. *Ann Neurol* 61: 587–598.

Butler CR, Bhaduri A, Acosta-Cabronero J, *et al.* (2009): Transient epileptic amnesia: regional brain atrophy and its relationship to memory deficits. *Brain* 132: 357–368.

Cleary P, Shorvon S, Tallis R (2004): Late-onset seizures as a predictor of subsequent stroke. *Lancet* 363: 1184–1186.

D'Alessandro R, Guarino M, Greco G (2004): Risk of seizures while awake in pure sleep epilepsies: a prospective study. *Neurology* 62: 254–257.

De Simone R, Salas-Puig X, Gélisse P, Crespel A, Genton P (2010): Senile myoclonic epilepsy: Delineation of a common condition associated with Alzheimer's disease in Down syndrome. *Seizure* 19: 383–389.

Fernandez-Torre JL, Rebollo M, Gutiérrez A, López-Espadas F, Hernández-Hernández MA (2011): Nonconvulsive status epilepticus in adults: Electroclinical differences between proper and comatose forms. *Clin Neurophysiol* 123: 244–251.

García-García J, Calleja S, De la Vega V, Salas-Puig J, Lahoz CH (2004): Heraldic seizure. *Seizure* 13: 328–330.

Hernández-Ronquillo L, Adams S, Ballendine S, Téllez-Centeno JF (2018): Epilepsy in elderly population: Classification, etiology and drug resistance. *Epilepsy Res* 140: 90–94.

Hauser WA, Annegers JF, Kurland LT (1993): Incidence of epilepsy and unprovoked seizures in Rochester, Minnesota: 1935–1984 *Epilepsia* 34: 453–468.

Kalamangalam GP, Diehl B, Burgess RC (2007): Neuroimaging and Neurophysiology of Periodic Lateralized Epileptiform Discharges: Observations and Hypotheses. *Epilepsia* 48: 1396–1405.

Kawai M, Hrachovy RA, Franklin PJ, Foreman PJ (2007): Video-EEG monitoring in a geriatric veteran population. *J Clin Neurophysiol* 24: 429–432.

Kellinghaus C, Loddenkemper T, Dinner DS, Lachwani D, Lüders HO (2004): Seizure semiology in the elderly: A video analysis. *Epilepsia* 45: 263–267.

Krämer G (2001): Epilepsy in the Elderly: Some clinical and pharmacotherapeutic aspects. *Epilepsia* 42 (Suppl 3): 55–59.

Loiseau P (1997): Pathologic processes in the Elderly and their association with seizures. In: Rowan AJ, Ramsay RE (eds). *Seizures and Epilepsy in the Elderly*. pp. 63–86. Boston: Butterwoth-Heinemann.

Mauri JA, Tejero C, Mercade JM, Padro L, Salas-Puig J (2005): Lamotrigine and epilepsy in the elderly: observational study of low-dose monotherapy. *Int J Clin Pract* 59: 651–654.

Mc Bride AE, Shih TT, Hirsch LJ (2002): Video-EEG monitoring in the Elderly: A review of 94 patients. *Epilepsia* 43: 165–169.

Michel VH, Sebban C, Debray-Meignan S, *et al.* (2011): Electroclinical features of idiopathic generalized epilepsies in the elderly: a geriatric hospital-based study. *Seizure* 20: 292–298.

Mosbah A, Tramoni E, Guedj E, *et al.* (2016): Clinical, neuropsychiological and metabolic characteristics of transient epileptic amnesia syndrome. *Epilepsia* 55: 699–706.

Pitkänen A, Roivainen R, Lukasiuk K (2016): Development of epilepsy after ischemic stroke. *Lancet Neurol* 15: 185–197.

Rowan AJ, Ramsay RE, Collins JF (2005): New onset geriatric epilepsy: a randomized study of gabapentin, lamotrigine and carbamazepine. *Neurology* 64: 1868–1873.

Santamarina E, Abraira L, Toledo M, *et al.* (2018): Prognosis of post-stroke status epilepticus: Effects of time difference between the two events *Seizure* 60: 172–177.

Scaldaferri BS, Vanacore N, Trebbastoni A, Francia A, D'Amico A, Prencipe M (2010): Seizures in Alzheimer's disease: A retrospective study of a cohort of outpatients. *Epileptic Disord* 12: 16–21.

Seang Lim K, Tin Tan C (2010): Epilepsies in the Elderly. In: Panayiotopoulos CP (ed). *Atlas of Epilepsies*. pp: 1314–1320. London: Springer.

Sen A, Capelli V, Husain M (2018): Cognition and dementia in older patients with epilepsy. *Brain* 141: 1592–1608.

Sheth RD, Drazkowski MD, Sirven JI, Gidal BE, Hermann BP (2006): Protracted ictal confusion in elderly patients. *Arch Neurol* 63: 529–532.

Silveira DC, Jehi L, Chapin J, *et al.* (2011). Seizure semiology and aging. *Epilepsy Behav* 20: 375–377.

So EL, Annegers JF, Hauser WA, O'Brien PC, Whisnant JP (1996): Population based-study of seizure disorders after cerebral infarction. *Neurology* 46: 350–355.

Stefan H (2011): Epilepsy in the elderly: facts and challenges. *Acta Neurol Scand* 124: 223–237.

Suarez-Moro R, Salas-Puig J, Amorin M, Roiz C, Lahoz CH (1999): SPECT findings in reflex seizures induced by movement in non-ketotic hyperglycemia. *Epileptic Disord* 1: 199–201.

Terzano MG, Parrino L, Mazzuchi A, Moretti G (1986): Confusional states with periodic latealized epileptiform discharges (PLEDs): a peculiar epileptuc syndrome in the elderly. *Epilepsia* 27: 446–457.

Thomas P, Beaumanoir A, Genton P (1992): "*De novo*" absence status of late onset: report of 11 cases. *Neurology* 42: 104–110.

Veran O, Kahane P, Thomas P, Hamelin S, Sabourdy C, Vercueil L (2010): *De novo* epileptic confusion in the elderly: A 1-year prospective study. *Epilepsia* 51: 1030–1035.

WITH VIDEO SUPPLEMENTS

CHAPTER 24

EPILEPSY AND INBORN ERRORS OF METABOLISM

Douglas R Nordli[1], Jr, Christian Korff[2] and Thomas Bast[3]

[1] Pediatric Epilepsy, Children's Memorial Hospital, Feinberg School of Medicine, Northwestern University, Chicago, USA
[2] Pediatric Neurology, University Hospitals, Geneva, Switzerland
[3] Department of children and adolescents, Epilepsy Centre Kork, Kehl, Germany

Introduction

Epilepsies due to inborn errors of metabolism (IEM) are important to recognize for prognostic and treatment reasons. Many are inherited in an autosomal recessive fashion and therefore have strong genetic implications for other family members. An identification of the underlying disorder can also allow the clinician to provide more accurate information for the affected individual. Most importantly some conditions can be treated, and for these children early, effective treatment can have a lasting and profound impact on their lives.

IEMs also present a particular challenge to the clinician for most are not diagnosed by their clinical features alone, instead, they are suspected when routine laboratory tests reveal an abnormality, such as comprehensive newborn screening, or when the patient presents with an unexplained encephalopathy, refractory seizures, or both. This reality is a sharp contrast to the syndromes and diagnoses found in other chapters in this book. Indeed, the remarkable success of clinical epileptology is that a skilled clinician equipped with an accurate history, a thorough physical examination, and a few details of an electroencephalogram can make an accurate clinical diagnosis of an underlying epilepsy syndrome in many patients. It is therefore disappointing that the same does not apply to inborn errors of metabolism. Many of these disorders present when the patient is quite young and during this time of life there is a relatively limited repertoire of ictal expression (Nordli *et al.*, 1997). Neonates and infants display only a small variety of seizures and their electroencephalographic features are similarly constrained. As a result, the approximate 50 or so inborn errors of metabolism that present with seizures end up having many common features.

Modern technology, including the use of expanded newborn screening (NBS) with tandem mass spectrometry and next generation sequencing has completely changed the landscape. Many disorders are now identified by comprehensive screening programs or whole exome sequencing. An accurate knowledge of NBS in each of our local areas can help us to ensure that testing is not redundant or worse yet, spotty.

Considering all of this, how can we, as clinicians be most effective? As neurologists and pediatricians with a special interest in children we are accustomed to beginning our medical thought processes with the age of the patient. This is probably the single most important starting point for the differential diagnosis. Accordingly, this chapter is organized into those disorders that commonly present in newborn, infancy and childhood/adolescence. A detailed discussion of the many IEMs is beyond the scope of this chapter, and nowadays detailed and up-to-date information on each condition is readily available at online resources including Online Mendelian Inheritance in Man (www.ncbi.nlm.nih.gov/omim). Instead, we focus on when to suspect an IEM and accordingly we begin each section with a brief discussion of the prototypic epilepsy syndrome. Where possible we group disorders either by common modes of presentation, or some other common theme such as the sub-cellular organelle involved or the general class of biochemical defect (*e.g.*, defect involving amino acids). Also, salient clinical features, prominent EEG manifestations and other findings are highlighted to aid the clinician in the identification of the underlying disorder. In addition, we list key screening tests that help to identify these disorders. We also highlight those disorders that have important treatment implications. Finally, we close with an organized approach to the diagnosis of the various IEMs.

Common pathogenic mechanisms

Anyone who has gazed at a wall chart of biochemical pathways quickly realizes that the health and well-being of our cells depends upon the intricate balance of thousands of simultaneous chemical reactions involving hundreds of pathways and scores of different classes of compounds. Molecules shuttle between one pathway and the next, sometimes acting as building blocks for one pathway, and sometimes a portion of the metabolism of another. An individual compound might simultaneously modulate the speed of several enzymatic reactions, influence the bioenergetics of the cells, or act as a critical neurotransmitter. It is no surprise, therefore, that few of the IEM have only one mechanism of action responsible for the generation of seizures and neurological injury. More often, several mechanisms are operant including the imbalance of excitatory and inhibitory neurotransmission, a reduction in available fuel for normal cell processes, accumulation of toxic substances, cytotoxic cell edema with resultant poor perfusion, and interference with normal maturation of the nervous system.

Energy failure

A central and critical theme of epileptogenesis in IEM is energy failure. GLUT1DS or De Vivo disease is characteristic of this group of diseases (De Vivo *et al.*, 1991). In this condition there is a failure of adequate transport of glucose into the central nervous system because of a mutation in the glucose transporter. The body has an adequate concentration of glucose so there are no systemic symptoms and no ketosis. This deprives the brain of both of its typical energy sources resulting in both paroxysmal symptoms and continual dysfunction. De Vivo disease commonly presents within the first year of life because the energy demands of the young brain relative to the remainder of the body markedly exceed those of any other time of life. Furthermore, not all regions of the brain appear to be equally effected and, PET studies show involvement of the thalamus and other deep grey structures (Pascual *et al.*, 2002). This explains the development of generalized spike-wave discharges and refractory absence seizures, since these are known to arise from pathology in the thalamo-cortical relations. Other IEMs that deprive the brain of adequate energy including respiratory chain defects and mitochondrial disorders often involve the deep grey nuclei to an even more profound degree so that visible changes are seen on MR imaging (Lee *et al.*, 2008). Since energy is required to move ions across electrochemical gradients and regulate the production of the essential neurotransmitters, it is easy to understand how energy failure could produce refractory seizures, particularly in metabolically vulnerable regions of the brain.

Imbalance of excitation and inhibition

In other circumstances IEM can produce an imbalance in the ratio of excitatory to inhibitory neurotransmitters. A good example of this category would be pyridoxine dependent epilepsy where the pre-treatment depleted pyridoxine reserves limit the decarboxylation of glutamate to GABA (Stockler *et al.*, 2011). This results in excessive excitation, seizures, and profound EEG abnormalities including burst-suppression and hypsarrhythmia.

Accumulation of toxic substances

A build-up of toxic substances occurs in a variety of storage disorders, urea cycle defects, amino acidurias and organic acidurias Substances like ammonia may directly and severely impair neurological function resulting in encephalopathy and seizures.

Newborn

There are four well characterized epilepsy syndromes presenting in the newborn, two have largely normal EEG backgrounds and are not associated with IEMs: benign neonatal convulsions and benign familial neonatal convulsions. Two others have markedly disorganized backgrounds with burst-suppression: early myoclonic encephalopathy (EME) (Aicardi & Goutières, 1978) and Ohtahara syndrome (Ohtahara *et al.*, 1976). EME is the prototypic epilepsy syndrome in this epoch of life associated with inborn errors. There are very rare case reports of IEM in Ohtahara syndrome.

Early myoclonic encephalopathy (EME)

In the newborn the epilepsy syndrome most clearly associated with IEM is early myoclonic encephalopathy as described by Aicardi (Aicardi & Goutières, 1978). This is characterized by refractory seizures, often myoclonic, with a variable burst-suppression pattern. Published causes of EME include nonketotic hyperglycinemia, methylmalonic acidemia, propionic acidemia, D-glyceric acidemia, sulfite oxidase deficiency/molybdenum cofactor deficiency, Leigh's syndrome, carbamyl-phosphate synthetase deficiency, pyridoxine dependency, Menkes disease and peroxisomal disorders (Vigevano & Bartuli, 2002). An inspection of this list shows that the majority of these are organic and amino acidurias and the most prominent of these is non-ketotic hyperglycinemia. One could simplify this list to the following five considerations: organic/amino acidemias, urea cycle defect, disorders of the mitochondria, peroxisomal diseases, Menkes disease, and pyridoxine dependency. All disease categories are represented in this list including disorders of energy metabolism, neurotransmission and neuronal toxicity *(Table I)*.

Table I **Inborn errors of metabolism causing EME**

Nonketotic hyperglycinemia
Propionic acidemia
Methylmalonic acidemia
D-glyceric acidemia
Carbamyl-phophate synthetase deficiency
Pyridoxine dependency
Molybdenum cofactor deficiency
Menkes disease
Zellweger syndrome
Possibly mitochondrial disorders

▼ Or, simplified
Organic/amino acidurias
Urea cycle defects
Disorders of sub cellular organelles:
– peroxisomes
– mitochondria
Menkes disease
Pyridoxine dependency

▼ Important diagnostic tests for EME
Complete blood count
Chemistry profile including liver function tests
Urine organic acids
Amino acid profile in CSF, blood and urine
Lactate/pyruvate in CSF and blood
Serum ammonia
Serum ceruloplasmin and copper
Sulfite test in fresh urine
Very long chain fatty acids
Pyridoxine challenge

Early infantile epileptic encephalopathy or Ohtahara syndrome was first described in 1976 and has some similar features to EME except that in the former tonic seizures predominate, the burst-suppression pattern does not change significantly with state, and there is a higher predominance of structural abnormalities on imaging. Very rare cases of cytochrome c oxidase deficiency or Leigh encephalopathy have been reported (Tatsuno *et al.*, 1984).

Epilepsies other than EME in the newborn with IEM

The minority of patients seen in the newborn period will have a well-characterized epilepsy syndrome. Some authors have referred to patients with severe epilepsies who do not fit into either Ohtahara or EME as early-onset epileptic encephalopathy (EOEE, Deprez *et al.*, 2010). Importantly, these authors have shown that some of these patients have identifiable mutations in various genes including *STXBP1*. Still other patients may show a mixture of focal, myoclonic and tonic seizures with abnormal backgrounds but not meeting criteria for burst-suppression. Every type of seizure has been described to be associated with IEMs, so this cannot be used as a distinguishing feature. Likewise, details of EEG findings in IEMs are often lacking, and are usually described as showing excessive discontinuity to the extreme of burst-suppression, excessive multifocal sharps, or both. Therefore, any neonate with persistent seizures without a clearly identifiable cause should be evaluated for an IEM and the newly discovered channelopathies, particularly if there is accompanying encephalopathy.

IEMs that present in the newborn include: nonketotic hyperglycinemia; isovaleric, methymalonic and propionic aciduria; maple syrup urine disease; pyridoxine dependency, pyridoxal phosphate dependency; holocarboxylase deficiency; D-2-hydroxyglutaric aciduria, 3-phophoglycerate dehydrogenase deficiency; adenylsuccinate lyase deficiency; methylene tetrahydrofolate reductase deficiency (MTHFR Deficiency); GABA transaminase deficiency; congenital disorders of glycosylation; developmental delay, epilepsy and neonatal diabetes (DEND); hyperinsulinism, hyperammonemia (HiHA); neonatal ceroidlipofuscinosis with cathepsin deficiency; creatine deficiency; peroxisomal disorders, urea cycle disorders; dihydropyrimidine dehydrogenase deficiency; molybdenum cofactor deficiency; carnitine palmitoyltransferase types I and II; pyruvate carboxylase deficiency; pyruvate dehydrogenase deficiency and disorders of biotin (Cook & Walker, 2011; Prasad & Hoffmann, 2010). In short, every class of metabolic derangement may present in the very young, and most of these have few distinguishing clues *(Table II)*.

Infancy

Prototypic disorder of IEM in infancy: West syndrome

The epilepsy syndrome most closely associated with inborn errors of metabolism in infancy is West syndrome (WS). The classic triad of West syndrome is infantile spasms, developmental delay and hypsarrhythmia. A large number of IEMs have been identified, but the most commonly mentioned are: biotinidase deficiency, pyridoxine deficiency, mitochondrial disorders (Shah *et al.*, 2002; Sadleir *et al.*, 2004), Menkes Disease (Prasad *et al.*, 2011), congenital disorder of glycosylation type III (Stibler *et al.*, 1999), organic and amino acidurias including phenylketonuria (Low *et al.*, 1957) and others (Wolf *et al.*, 2009), peroxisomal disorders (Buoni *et al.*, 2007), and lysosomal disorders (Nordli & De Vivo, 2002). Incidentally, there are a growing number of important genetic causes for WS, but this is outside the scope of this chapter (Paciorkowski *et al.*, 2011). Vigevano & Bartuli (2002) make the point that even though there are a variety of IEMs associated with WS, they account for only a small fraction of the total cases *(Table III)*.

Table II **Epileptic encephalopathies in the newborn**

Nonketotic hyperglycinemia
Isovaleric, methymalonic and propionic aciduria
Maple syrup urine disease
Pyridoxine dependency, pyridoxal phosphate dependency
Holocarboxylase deficiency
D-2-hydroxyglutaric aciduria
3-phophoglycerate dehydrogenase deficiency
Adenylsuccinate lyase deficiency
Methylene tetrahydrofolate reductase deficiency (MTHFR deficiency)
GABA transaminase deficiency
Congenital disorders of glycosylation
Developmental delay, epilepsy and neonatal diabetes (DEND)
Hyperinsulinism, hyperammonemia (HiHA)
Neonatal ceroidlipofuscinosis with cathepsin deficiency
Creatine deficiency
Peroxisomal disorders
Urea cycle disorders
Dihydropyrimidine dehydrogenase deficiency
Molybdenum cofactor deficiency
Carnitine palmitoyltransferase types I and II
Pyruvate carboxylase deficiency
Pyruvate dehydrogenase deficiency
Disorders of biotin

Table III **Inborn errors of metabolism associated with West syndrome**

Biotinidase deficiency
Pyridoxine dependency
Menkes disease
Mitochondrial disorders
Organic acidurias
Amino acidopathies
Congenital disorder of glycosylation type III
Lysosomal hydrolase deficiencies

Non-syndromic infantile epilepsies with IEMs

As with neonates, some infants have forms of epilepsy that do not yet fit into one of the recognized syndromes. Those infants with unexplained, poorly controlled seizures, and encephalopathy should be evaluated for IEMs. Some additional causes of infantile seizures are: GM1 and GM2 gangliosidoses; neuronal ceroid lipofuscinosis; infantile neuroaxonal dystrophy; Glut-1 deficiency; late-onset multiple carboxylase deficiency; disorders of cerebral and peripheral folate metabolism; disorders of neurotransmitter synthesis; arginase deficiency (urea cycle defect); amino and organic acidurias; and sialidoses (Prasad & Hoffmann, 2010).

Child/adolescence

Progressive myoclonus epilepsy

Progressive myoclonus epilepsy (PME) usually begins in late childhood or adolescence. It is characterized by myoclonic seizures, tonic-clonic seizures, worsening ataxia and progressive dementia (Ramachandran *et al.*, 2009; Berkovic *et al.*, 1993). Recognized causes of PME include Unverricht-Lundborg, myoclonus epilepsy with ragged red fibers (MERRF), Lafora disease, neuronal ceroid lipofuscinoses (NCL), and sialidoses types I and II. There is considerable overlap in the clinical features for the various causes, but there are some distinguishing features including the ocular examination: optic atrophy would suggest NCL whereas a cherry red spot or lens opacity suggests a sialidosis. Myopathy, hearing loss and lipomas are seen in MERRF. All of the disorders are inherited in an autosomal recessive fashion except for MERRF, which shows maternal inheritance and Kufs disease which may rarely show a dominant inheritance. In all cases the EEGs may initially have normal backgrounds with superimposed generalized or multifocal spikes. In most cases the EEGs deteriorate over time with loss of sleep architecture and sometimes a prominent reduction in amplitude. Many have photosensitivity, and cases of late infantile NCL may show large amplitude visual evoked responses. An occipital predominance is classically seen in Lafora, but occipital spikes are also present in other conditions. Sialidoses may have runs of vertex maximal fast activity preceding massive myoclonic jerks.

Treatment

Until recently, none of the conditions had a specific treatment, but the FDA recently approved cerliponase alfa as a treatment for *CLN2*, caused by tripeptidyl peptidase-1 (TPP1) deficiency. This treatment has been approved to slow loss of walking ability in symptomatic patients three years and older. Avoidance of phenytoin is important with Unverricht-Lundborg disease and drugs useful in treatment of other forms of myoclonic epilepsies have generally been used.

Diagnosis

Previously, biopsies were very useful to secure the diagnosis, but currently, gene tests or enzyme assays are available for all of these diagnoses (www.genetests.org). There are commercially available panels that will test for Lafora, Unverricht-Lundborg, and MERRF from one sample. A careful eye examination may help to suggest either the sialidoses or NCL and sialidosis can be tested by checking the urine for sialyloligosaccharides. Most forms of NCL can now be confirmed by either enzyme assays, gene tests, or both *(Table IV)*. Finally, commercial laboratories offer NGS specific panels for progressive myoclonus epilepsy that cover most of these diseases.

Table IV Causes of PME

Unverricht-Lundborg disease
Myoclonus epilepsy with ragged red fibers (MERRF)
Lafora disease
Neuronal ceroid lipofuscinoses : Late infantile Finnish late infantile Late-infantile variant Turkish late infantile Juvenile Adult
Sialidoses types I and II

Overview of IEMs

Overview of organic and amino acidurias

Amino acidurias are so-called because of the disturbances in the concentration of amino acids normally present in the urine. Amino acids are involved in a large number of complex pathways and are particularly important because of their role in neurotransmission, and thus their relevance to epilepsy (Lee, 2011). Disorders of the amino acid metabolism may affect branched – chain amino acids, sulfur – containing amino acids and aromatic amino acids. Organic acidurias refer to similar disturbances, but involve compounds that are organic acids and lack an amino group. These present with very similar features since most organic acidurias derive from altered metabolism of amino acids. Some other organic acidurias involve defects in fatty acid oxidation and therefore may have a component of altered energy metabolism as well. The most severe cases present very early in life, shortly after feeding has commenced with altered mental status and seizures. There are few distinguishing clinical features so determination of the disorder depends upon analysis of organic acids in the urine, and amino acids in the CSF, blood and urine.

Types of organic acidemia include maple syrup urine disease (MSUD), propionic acidemia, methymalonic acidemia (MMA), methylmalonic acidurias and homocystinuria, isovaleric acidemia, biotin-unresponsive 3-methylcrotonyl-CoA carboxylase deficiency, 3-hydroxy-3-methylglutaryl-CaA (HMG-CoA) lyase deficiency, ketothiolase deficiency, and glutaricacidemia type 1 (GA 1). In most circumstances the disorder will be identified by an excess of certain compounds with the notable exception of disorders of serine which present with low serine and glycine levels either in the fasting blood or routine CSF analysis.

Maple syrup urine disease (MSUD), a classic form of organic aciduria

MSUD was described by Menkes and colleagues in 1954 and results from mutations of any of four different genes which control the branched-chain α-keto acid dehydrogenase complex (Chuang, 1998). This results in accumulations in leucine, isoleucine and valine. Testing is generally performed in most extended NBS so that asymptomatic individuals can now be identified. Otherwise, patients present with lethargy sometimes in the first few weeks of life. Intermittent increases in tone, tremor, myoclonic jerks and repeated flexion-extension movement of the limbs are seen. Focal seizures emerge and uncontrolled cerebral edema develops in untreated individuals. A characteristic odor, for which the disorder derived its name, can be detected in the urine and cerumen. The neuropathology is remarkable for diffuse myelin loss with cystic degeneration of the white matter, and sometimes associated disorders of neuronal migration. Comb-like mu rhythms with bursts of 7–9 Hz spindle-like sharp waves have been reported (Tharp, 1992).

Important diagnostic tests

Plasma, urine and CSF amino acids are diagnostic and show elevation of branched-chain amino acids. Metabolic acidosis and ketosis are also present.

Treatment

The mainstay of treatment is protein restriction, thiamine supplementation and avoidance of branched-chain amino acids from the diet (Chuang *et al.*, 2006). Liver transplantation can partially restore the enzyme function and is considered in presymptomatic individuals (Feier *et al.*, 2016).

Prototypic aminoaciduria: nonketotic hyperglycinemia or glycine encephalopathy

This autosomal recessive condition is caused by a defect in the large glycine cleavage enzyme system which is responsible for degrading glycine in all regions of the body, including the brain (Applegarth & Toone, 2004). Derangements of mitochondrial lipoate synthesis and transportation of glycine to the extracellular compartment may produce a similar phenotype (Baker *et al.*, 2014; Kurolap *et al.*, 2016). Glycine accumulates in the brain where it achieves toxic levels. The mitochondrial enzyme system is composed of four units (designated P, H, T, and L). The most common mutation involves GLDC and causes P protein dysfunction. Glycine can have an excitatory action in the brain, in contrast to its inhibitory function in the spinal cord.

Symptoms are usually expressed within the first 48 hours of life with lethargy, apnea, and seizures. Hiccoughs may be seen by day of life 4 or 5. Cortical malformations and corpus callosum defects may be present.

Important diagnostic test

Amino acids in the CSF and blood collected at the same time for the level of glycine.

Treatment

There is no long-term effective treatment for the disorder, though diazepam may help to blunt seizures and dextromethorphan, an NMDA agonist has been used to some advantage, albeit transient in some cases (Hamosh *et al.*, 1998; Zammarchi *et al.*, 1994). Treatments to normalize plasma glycine (such as benzoate) have shown some improvements in motor skills and a reduction in seizures (Bjoraker *et al.*, 2016).

Urea cycle defects

Urea cycle disorders (UCDs) are due to defects in the removal of excess nitrogen from the body. Results with tandem mass spectroscopy in newborn screening found urea cycle defects in approximately 1/70,000 live births (Couce *et al.*, 2011). These are all inherited in an autosomal recessive fashion except for the commonest condition: ornithine transcarbamylase (OTC) deficiency which is X-linked dominant. These disorders present similarly and often in the newborn. They result, at least in part, from ammonia elevations. Affected newborns feed poorly, are lethargic and begin having convulsions within 1–5 days after birth. These symptoms can progress to herniation from increased intracranial pressure as a result of diffuse cerebral edema. Milder cases can present later and some patients may be completely asymptomatic in heterozygotic females until they experience some type of stressful event.

Diagnostic tests

The diagnosis is suspected when there are elevations in serum ammonia, absence of urine ketones, and respiratory alkalosis. Plasma amino and urine organic acids can help to distinguish the various conditions. This diagnosis can be confirmed by gene sequencing.

The EEG shows a low-voltage slowed background with multifocal epileptiform discharges. Two patients studied by Verma and coworkers in 1984 demonstrated episodes of sustained monorhythmic theta activity (Verma *et al.*, 1984).

Treatment

Hemodialysis in the acute setting has been used to reduce serum ammonia and can be lifesaving. Subsequently, protein restriction and medical therapy aimed at lowering serum ammonia are also used.

Mitochondrial disorders

The young brain has such high energy demands that disorders involving the mitochondria often produce neurological symptoms. The overlap between mitochondrial disorders and epilepsy was reviewed (Rahman, 2012). Multiple organ involvement and lactic acidosis are cardinal features but these are not present in call cases. Refractory epilepsy occurs in isolation, or with other neurologic problems including retinal pigmentary changes, optic atrophy, hearing loss, developmental delays, neuropathy, and myopathy. Myoclonic epilepsy is sometimes seen with mitochondrial disease, but almost any seizure type can occur. The EEG features are variable. For example, the EEG features of mitochondrial encephalopathy with lactic acidosis and stroke-like events (MELAS) show focal slowing and interictal epileptiform discharges, but MERRF has generalized spike-wave activity. There are over 2,000 nuclear DNA genes involved in mitochondrial function and an additional 37 maternally inherited mitochondrial DNA (mtDNA) genes. About 80% of mitochondrial disorders follow autosomal recessive, the remainder shows a maternal inheritance pattern.

Diagnosis

Abnormalities in plasma amino acids, acylcarnitines, lactate, pyruvate, and urine organic acids can indicate a mitochondrial disorder. One can measure mitochondrial enzyme activity in multiple tissues and conduct specific genetic testing (Rahman, 2012).

Treatment

It is critical to minimize worsening because of metabolic or physiologic stresses. Various cofactors and supplements are often used. Ketogenic diet has been advocated in certain respiratory chain defects (Lee *et al.*, 2008). Valproate should be avoided in an uncertain diagnostic situation. Valproate is contraindicated in Alpers disease with *POLG1* mutation (Saneto *et al.*, 2010).

Pyruvate dehydrogenase deficiency

Pyruvate dehydrogenase (PDH) complex is composed of three enzymes: pyruvate decarboxylase (E1), dihydrolipoyl transacetylase (E2), and dihydrolipoyl dehydrogenase (E3). The E1 alpha -subunit is particularly important, as it contains the E1 active site, and mutations in this region are the most common cause of PDH deficiency (Chun *et al.*, 1995).

There is a wide variety of clinical expression from acute lactic acidosis in infancy with severe neurologic impairment in affected boys to a slowly progressive neurodegenerative disorder which is more commonly seen in girls. Typically, lactate and pyruvate are both elevated but the lactate to pyruvate ratio is normal. Agenesis of the corpus callosum and other structural abnormalities may be present.

Infantile spasms and myoclonic seizures are common presentations. EEG findings range from multifocal slow spike-and-wave discharges to hypsarhythmia. The ketogenic diet is, to varying degrees beneficial (Sofou *et al.*, 2017).

Pyruvate carboxylase deficiency

Pyruvate carboxylase converts pyruvate to oxaloacetate using biotin as a cofactor. Neonates can present with severe lactic acidemia and often perish within the first few months of life. Infants may have episodes of lactic acidemia precipitated by an infection, accompanied by failure to thrive and hypotonia. The lactate to pyruvate ratio is typically elevated. There are characteristic abnormalities in the plasma amino acids profile and urinary organic acids. Infantile spasms and hypsarrhythmia may develop. Seizures are related to the energy dysfunction that occurs secondary to Krebs cycle dysfunction. Treatment with the ketogenic diet or corticotropins may markedly exacerbate the disorder and should be avoided (De Vivo *et al.*, 1977; Rutledge *et al.*, 1989).

Leigh syndrome

Subacute necrotizing encephalomyelopathy is also known as Leigh syndrome. In addition to pyruvate dehydrogenase deficiency defects in nuclear and mitochondrial complexes 1 to 5 have been identified. It may be autosomal recessive or dominant, X- linked or maternally inherited (DiMauro & De Vivo, 1996).

Infants usually present with acute to subacute regression, hypotonia, lactic acidosis, and failure to thrive. As the disease progresses there is spasticity, abnormal eye movements, and central respiratory failure. Bilateral deep grey matter involvement is evident on neuroimaging and white matter lesions may also be present, although biotin and thiamine-responsive disorders as well as vigabatrin toxicity are other considerations for these imaging findings.

Disorders with potential for central replacement therapy

Glut1DS

The Glut-1 transporter deficiency syndrome was first described in 1991 by De Vivo and is the prototypic example of energy failure (De Vivo *et al.*, 1991). This autosomal dominant condition results from a loss of functional glucose transport across the blood-brain barrier. The transporter is encoded by the *SLC2A* gene. The spectrum of presentation is evolving. The classic clinical features included developmental delay, ataxia, hypotonia, infantile seizures, and acquired microcephaly. Paroxysmal eye-head movements, paroxysmal exertional dyskinesia, hemiplegic migraine and refractory absence seizures have also been reported (Pearson *et al.*, 2017).The defect reduces the CSF-to- blood glucose ratio to half of normal (typically, CSF glucose is less than 40 mg/dL). In addition, a low lactate concentration might be seen. Additional confirmation of impaired glucose transport can be performed through assays in erythrocytes and clinical genetic testing is available. Seizures are found in the majority of patients and when they begin in infancy are usual focal. As the child matures other seizure types including absence, myoclonic, astatic, and generalized tonic-clonic may be seen. The EEG is usually normal between seizures, but generalized 2.5- to 4-Hz spike-wave discharges are observed in more than one third of children older than 2 years of age (Leary *et al.*, 2003).

Diagnosis

Screening for lumbar puncture should be considered in those with refractory epilepsy. Confirmation can be obtained by analysis of erythrocyte transport and also by genetic testing.

Treatment

Early initiation of the ketogenic diet is effective in the treatment of the paroxysmal features of the illness (Wang *et al.*, 2005). More than 90% reduction in seizures has been reported as well as improvement in cognitive skills (Kass *et al.*, 2016; Ramm-Pettersen *et al.*, 2014).

Folic acid disorders

As defined by Ramaekers and Blau, cerebral folate deficiency associates neurological symptoms, a low concentration of 5-methyltetrahydrofolate (5-MTHF) in the cerebrospinal fluid, and normal peripheral folate metabolism (Ramaekers & Blau, 2004). It can result from various mechanisms, which include insufficient dietary intake, and congenital or acquired malabsorption syndromes, in which low folate concentration is also noted in the peripheral blood. In addition, isolated cerebral folate deficiency has been described in a small number of infants. These patients typically present with non-specific neurologic signs, such as irritability and sleep disturbance at around four months of life. Developmental delay, spastic diplegia, abnormal movements, ataxia, head growth deceleration, and autistic features typically occur on follow-up. Myoclonic-atonic seizures, absences, or generalized tonic-clonic seizures were also observed in a minority of the reported patients, but EEG details are lacking. Isolated cerebral folate deficiency might be explained by the presence of autoantibodies directed against folate receptors, or by mutations in *FOLR1*, the gene that encodes the FR1 folate receptor protein 1 (Ramaekers & Blau, 2004; Hyland *et al.*, 2010). Finally, cerebral folate deficiency has been reported in association with various diseases, such as Rett syndrome, Aicardi-Goutières syndrome, hypomyelination with atrophy of the basal ganglia, and dihydropteridine reductase deficiency (Hyland *et al.*, 2010). The underlying mechanisms that lead to folate depletion in these diseases are somewhat controversial and remain to be fully understood.

Diagnosis

Cerebrospinal fluid 5-MTHF screening should be considered in infants who present unexplained progressive neurological symptoms, particularly if they present with the relatively homogeneous clinical picture of the patients with the isolated form described above. Etiologies for peripheral folate metabolism disturbances should be excluded in parallel.

Treatment

Folate supplementation might be deleterious and is contraindicated. However, treatment with 0.5–1 mg/kg/day folinic acid, a stable and metabolically active folate compound, may help improving neurological symptoms, particularly in those diagnosed before 6 years (Ramaekers & Blau, 2004).

Cerebral creatine deficiency

Creatine plays an important role in energy storage and transmission, mostly in the central nervous system and the muscle. The two sources of creatine are dietary intake and endogenous anabolism. Creatine biosynthesis results from the transformation of arginine and glycine into guanidinoacetate (GAA) and ornithine by arginine:glycine amidinotransferase (AGAT). The second step, catabolized by guanidinoacetate methyltransferase (GAMT), involves the methylation of GAA into creatine. Cerebral creatine deficiency may be due to hereditary enzymatic defects of AGAT or GAMT, or to dysfunction of the protein responsible for the transport of creatine from the blood to the central nervous system. The latter may be due to a defect on the gene that encodes the creatine transporter, *SLC6A8*. The main clinical symptoms of cerebral creatine deficiency include developmental delay, autism, and epilepsy. Seizures are observed in more than 80% of GAMT-deficient and in dysfunctional *SLC6A8* patients. In GAMT deficiency, seizures may be particularly difficult to treat (Mikati *et al.*, 2013). They usually start between 10 months and 3 years, and consist of myoclonias, generalized tonic-clonic seizures, focal seizures, head nods and drop attacks (Nasrallah *et al.*, 2010). Those observed in association with *SLC6A8* defects are typically easy to treat.

Diagnosis

The measurement of urinary GAA and creatine, the calculation of GAA/creatinine and creatine/creatinine ratios, and proton magnetic resonance spectroscopy are used as powerful screening methods. Genetic analyses are available for the 3 genes described above (Nasrallah *et al.*, 2010).

Treatment

Oral supplementation with 300–400 mg/kg/day creatine monohydrate may help improve the clinical symptoms due to both enzymatic defects (Wolf *et al.*, 2009; Stockler-Ipsiroglu *et al.*, 2014). Ornithine supplementation and arginine restriction may be useful, as well. Creatine intake is not effective in the presence of an abnormal transporter, however.

Biotin disorders

Biotin is an essential vitamin that serves as a cofactor for four carboxlyases in the human body: acetyl-CoA carboxylase alpha and beta, propionyl-CoA carboxylase (PCC), 3-methylcrotonyl-CoA carboxylase (MCC), and pyruvate carboxylase (PC) (Zempleni *et al.*, 2008). Among many functions, these enzymes are active in the metabolism of fatty acids, aminoacids and glucose; they also help to regulate genes involved in carbohydrate metabolism. A stable and sufficient biotin concentration is therefore essential to maintain a normal function of vital organs, such as the heart and brain. Biotin homeostasis is regulated by 3 main proteins: biotinidase, the pancreatic enzyme responsible for releasing free biotin from digested proteins and biocytin, also involved in biotin transport to peripheral tissues, and in the recycling of holocarboxylase synthetase degradation products; the sodium-dependent multivitamin transporter, responsible of biotin uptake from various tissues, such as the intestine, the kidney, and the liver; and holocarboxylase synthetase, which catalyzes biotin attachment to the above-mentioned enzymes and to histones.

Deficiencies in the biotin cycle may lead to a severe clinical picture, that includes neurologic and cutaneous manifestations (Zempleni *et al.*, 2008). Biotinidase deficiency, also called late-onset multiple carboxylase deficiency, usually presents between the third and sixth month of life with myoclonia, developmental delay and hypotonia. Infantile spasms have been reported as well. Additional important signs include laryngeal stridor, seborrheic or atopic dermatitis, alopecia, conjunctivitis, and later autistic behavior, hearing loss and optic atrophy (Lyon *et al.*, 2006). Most patients will present with metabolic acidosis episodes, which sometimes result in coma and death. Eighty percent of the patients will have intermittent organic aciduria in the course of their disease, an important clue in the diagnosis.

Diagnosis

Organic acid profile should be analyzed in urine and cerebrospinal fluid, as screening measures in all children who present with unexplained refractory seizures and developmental delay. In biotinidase deficiency, the measurement of residual enzymatic activity can be tested in serum, leukocytes, fibroblasts or cerebrospinal fluid, and is usually very low (Lyon *et al.*, 2006a, b). Genetic sequencing is also clinically available.

Treatment

Biotin oral supplementation (10–100 mg/day) may lead to rapid seizure control and substantial clinical improvement in biotinidase deficiency and in some cases of holocarboxylase deficiency (Wolf *et al.*, 2009; Lyon *et al.*, 2006a, b).

Disorders of serine metabolism

L-serine is a non-essential amino-acid that plays an important role in central nervous system development and function. Its main sources are dietary intake and internal metabolism, via the degradation of proteins and phospholipids, or via internal synthesis, either (reversibly) from glycine by serine-hydroxymethyl transferase (SHMT), or from 3 phosphoglycerate by 3-phosphoglycerate dehydrogenase (3-PGDH), phosphoserine aminotransferase (PSAT) and phosphoserine phosphatase (PSPH). In the central nervous system, the cells in which these steps take place are the astrocytes. In addition, the astrocytic AMPA-receptors, excited by glutamate released from adjacent pre-synaptic neurons, activate the transformation by serine racemase (SR) of L-serine into D-serine, which in turn will contribute to the opening of the post-synaptic NMDA-receptor. CNS deficiency of serine may be caused by a defect in the serine transporter, ASCT1 (Damseh *et al.*, 2015).

3-PGDH deficiency is classically associated with developmental delay, congenital microcephaly, and refractory seizures of all types, including epileptic spasms. Milder phenotypes have been reported, particularly in children with later age of onset. PSAT deficiency shares some PGDH deficiency characteristics, and may provoke developmental delay, refractory seizures, hypertonia and acquired microcephaly. Seizures were not present in the only patient with PSPH reported to date (Tabatabaie *et al.*, 2010).

Diagnosis

Routine amino acid analysis will reveal low concentrations of L-serine and glycine in the plasma and in the cerebrospinal fluid, in most situations. Two exceptions exist: in the juvenile form of 3-PGDH deficiency and in PSPH deficiency, glycine concentrations are normal in both compartments (Tabatabaie *et al.*, 2010).

Treatment

L-serine oral supplementation, up to 300–500 mg/kg/day (Wolf *et al.*, 2009), may dramatically improve the clinical symptoms (Tabatabaie *et al.*, 2010; Livet *et al.*, 2005). Adding glycine, up to 300 mg/kg/day, might be of benefit if seizures are refractory.

Pyridoxine-dependent epilepsy

Pyridoxine-dependent epilepsy (PDE) is an autosomal recessive disorder caused by a deficiency of α-aminoadipic semialdehyde dehydrogenase (Stockler *et al.*, 2011). This is due to mutations in *ALDH7A1* gene which encodes antiquitin (ATQ). ATQ is an aldehyde dehydrogenase in the lysine degradation pathway. Its deficiency leads to an accumulation of α-aminoadipic semialdehyde (AASA), piperideine-6-carboxylate (P6C) and pipecolic acid, which can be used as diagnostic markers in CSF, urine, and plasma. Refractory seizures often develop in the first week of life manifested by focal seizures, myoclonia or epileptic spasms. EEG tracings may show discontinuity with bursts of diffuse high amplitude delta activity followed by periods of relative attenuation. A burst-suppression may be seen shortly after treatment, which ultimately normalizes with continued pyridoxine. Rarely, hypsarrhythmia is seen.

Folinic acid responsive condition was originally thought to be a separate condition, but subsequent work has shown that it is identical to PDE. Some individuals do not respond to pyridoxine but do respond to pyridoxal-L-phosphate (PLP). Most of these have an abnormality in the enzyme that forms PLP, but some do not. Some advocate using PLP at a dose of 30 mg/kg/day as an alternative to pyridoxine, and others reserve it for patients who fail to respond to three days of pyridoxine treatment.

Important diagnostic tests

Screening can be done in blood or urine looking for AASA and P6C concentrations and also in the blood for pipecolic acid. Confirmation can be made by mutational analysis.

Treatment

Pyridoxine at 100 mg per day or 30 mg/kg/day until biochemical tests exclude the diagnosis. PLP at doses of 30 mg/kg/day may be used if pyridoxine fails (Stockler *et al.*, 2015). Responders may experience apnea, so IV injection should not be performed without the availability of rapid respiratory support. Lysine restriction and arginine supplementation have also been recommended (Coughlin *et al.*, 2015; Al Teneiji *et al.*, 2017).

Lysosomal hydrolase deficiencies

Lysosomal storage disorders are a group of inherited diseases, mostly autosomal recessive, in which the accumulation of incompletely digested macromolecules leads to the dysfunction of various cell types and organs, such as the central nervous system (Kruer & Steiner, 2011). A deficient activity of lysosomal hydrolases, an abnormal processing of proteins involved in their synthesis or activation, or a dysfunctional transport of digested molecules from lysosomes to other cell compartments, may all provoke storage disorders. These are typically classified according to the type of accumulated substrate, and include glycogen storage disease type 2, mucopolysaccharidoses, lipidoses, sphingolipidoses, mucolipidoses, and oligosaccharidoses. Although epilepsy is not a prominent feature in most of these diseases, seizures and EEG changes may be more frequent and suggestive in some of them.

Neuronal ceroid lipofuscinoses, lysosomal storage disorders in which cortical dysfunction are prominent, are treated separately.

Tay-Sachs disease is a sphingolipidosis due to a defect of hexosaminidase A, which leads to the accumulation of a ganglioside, GM2, in neurons. Typical symptoms include excessive startle response, and progressive macrocephaly, motor and cognitive impairment. The optic fundus examination reveals a characteristic cherry-red spot. Myoclonic seizures, sometimes associated with diffuse spike-waves, may be observed. The interictal EEG is normal at onset, but voltage progressively decreases as the disease progresses (Gaitanis, 2011). Death occurs at 3–5 years. The EEG in GM1 gangliosidosis, another sphingolipidosis due to a dysfunction of beta-galactosidase, shows slow activity in the theta range, prominent in temporal regions (Gaitanis, 2011).

Mucopolysaccharidosis type III presents between 1 and 6 years with developmental delay and behavioral problems. Progressive dementia and epilepsy appear on evolution. The interictal EEG may be normal, or show diffuse slow waves or low voltage fast activity (Gaitanis, 2011).

Niemann-Pick disease is due to a defect in acid sphingomyelinase. The patients who suffer from type C usually present between 3 and 8 years with ataxia, vertical gaze palsy and hepatosplenomegaly, and may exhibit myoclonic seizures with time. The interictal EEG may reveal diffuse slowing, or high-amplitude diffuse activity in the alpha range, enhanced by photic stimulation (Gaitanis, 2011).

Gaucher disease results from a defect in glucocerebrosidase, with accumulation of glucocerebroside in the macrophage-monocyte system that leads to hepatosplenomegaly and neurological impairment, such as oculomotor apraxia and cerebral atrophy in subtype III. Seizures may be observed in type II and III, and the interictal EEG may show 6–10 Hz rhythmical sharp waves, polyspikes and spike-waves (Gaitanis, 2011). Seizures and non-specific EEG abnormalities, mainly slowing of the background activity, may be observed in the course of metachromatic leukodystrophy, a disorder in which sulfated glycolipids accumulate, due to a defect in arylsulfatase A.

Krabbe disease patients may present with tonic spasms in their first year of life. This disorder is due to a defect in galactosylceramidase.

Diagnosis

Screening tests when lysosomal storage disorders are suspected include skeletal x-rays, ophtalmological and audiological investigations, echocardiography and peripheral blood smear. Oligosaccharides and glycosaminoglycans may be elevated in urine. Enzymatic activities measured in white blood cells or fibroblasts are available. DNA analysis may be performed for confirmation of a gene defect.

Treatment

Enzyme replacement therapy is available for some lysosomal storage disorders, but seems less effective in improving the neurological manifestations. Hematopoietic stem cell transplantation may also be effective, particularly if performed early in the course of certain of these diseases. A combination of both methods might even bring better outcomes. There are two current treatments for Gaucher: enzyme replacement therapy and substrate reduction therapy.

Peroxisomal disorders

Peroxisomes disorders are due to an inability to degrade very-long-chain-fatty acids (VLCFA) and branched-chain fatty acid. They also involve defects where there is an inability to synthesize plasminogen. The epilepsy presentation is not sufficiently distinct to allow characterization by clinical features alone. Most of these disorders present with seizures either in the neonatal or infantile period. The EEG features are largely dependent upon the age and severity of the conditions. The younger and more severe patients may have multifocal seizures, infants who are a bit older may present with hypsarhythmia, and those older still may have generalized EEG features. Disorders of the peroxisome have been divided into three categories: i) disorders of peroxisomal biogenesis (Zellweger syndrome spectrum [ZSS]); (ii) disorders of a single peroxisomal enzyme (X-linked adrenoleukodystrophy [XALD], acyl-coenzyme A [acyl-CoA] oxidase deficiency); and (iii) disorders with deficiencies of multiple peroxisomal enzymes (rhizomelic chondrodysplasia punctata). These conditions can be screened by sending an assay of VLCFA. Patients with Zellweger syndrome spectrum have focal motor seizures without secondary generalization involving all parts of the body. Zellweger is the most extreme portion of this spectrum with pronounced cortical malformations. The interictal electroencephalogram of patients with ZSS shows infrequent bilateral independent multifocal spikes, predominantly in the fronto-central regions. Less frequently, hypsarhythmia has been reported (Takahashi *et al.*, 1997). Hypsarhythmia is seen with neonatal adrenoleukodystrophy and D-bifunctional protein deficiency (DBPD).

Treatment

Treatment is generally symptomatic. Gene therapy including bone marrow transplantation has been used in XALD and screening has been added to some NBS panels.

Neuronal ceroid lipofuscinoses

Neuronal ceroid lipofuscinoses (NCL) are inherited (mostly autosomal recessive) lysosomal storage disorders, in which ceroid lipofuscin, an autofluorescent degradation product, accumulates in lysosomes and provokes the degeneration of neurons (Mole &Williams, 1993). Ten subtypes have been identified (NCL1-NCL10), that share the clinical features of progressive dementia and motor signs, refractory epilepsy and early death. In addition, most patients present with intention myoclonus (or polymyoclonus), retinal degeneration and subsequent visual loss. Cerebral imaging shows progressive cortical and cerebellar atrophy. Extraneurological involvement is absent. NCLs may be classified in groups according to their age of onset.

The earliest form, a subtype of NCL10, presents as congenital microcephaly and neonatal (possibly antenatal) seizures. It is due to mutations in the *CTSD* gene that codes for cathepsin D, a lysosomal enzyme implicated in neuronal stability (Kohlschutter & Schulz, 2009).

Infantile NCL (Santavuori-Haltia-Hagberg disease), or NCL1, is due to mutations in the gene *CLN1* that results in a defect in palmitoyl-protein thioesterase (PPT1), and mostly starts between 6 and 24 months. It is characterized by its particularly rapid and extensive destruction of neurons, and frequently manifests as autistic regression initially, followed by seizures, myoclonus, ataxia, visual failure, and general health decline that rapidly leads to a vegetative state and death at around 7 years (Lyon *et al.*, 2006b). On EEG, there is an early loss of electroclinical activity, with diminution of amplitude leading to a flat trace within 2 years ("vanishing EEG"). An early feature is a lack of attenuation of the alpha rhythm with eye opening.

Late infantile NCL, or NCL2 (Jansky-Bielschowsky disease), is due to gene mutations in *CLN2* that leads to a defect in tripeptidyl-peptidase (TPP1), and usually starts between 2 and 4 years with sleep difficulties and seizures (generalized tonic-clonic seizures, atonic falls or staring spells). Polymyoclonus, ataxia and visual loss due to optic atrophy and macular degeneration appear later, as the disease progresses. On EEG, high somatosensory evoked potentials may be noted, and characteristic giant visual evoked potentials are elicited with photic stimulation at low rates (1–2 Hz), particularly in the early stages of the disease. Death usually occurs around the end of the first decade, but life expectancy may be longer (Lyon *et al.*, 2006a).

Juvenile NCL (Batten disease or Spielmeyer-Vogt disease) is the most frequently encountered NCL group, and accounts for 50% of all cases (Lyon *et al.*, 2006). In addition to the classical form, NCL3, due to *CLN3* defects, juvenile NCL includes various subtypes, such as the Finnish type, due to mutations in *CLN5*, and Northern epilepsy, due to mutations in *CLN8*. Unlike most other forms, the latter is rarely associated with loss of vision and myoclonus. NCL3 usually presents between 4 and 6 years as progressive loss of vision, with total blindness developing within 2 to 4 years, followed over years by dementia, seizures and motor disturbances. EEG findings include general disorganization and diffuse spike-and-slow-wave complexes (Gaitanis, 2011). Kuf's disease, the adult form, starts at around 30 years.

Diagnosis

Enzymatic activity assays are the initial diagnostic step, based on the age of onset, and genetic analyses may confirm the diagnosis. Cytoplasmic vacuoles in lymphocytes are characteristic of NCL3, and are detectable on a routine blood smear. Electroretinography is a useful screening test for most NCL and may detect abnormalities even before clinical evidence of visual disturbance appears. Ultrastructural analysis of skin (usually axillary) biopsies allows identification of characteristic intracellular inclusions for each age group (Lyon *et al.*, 2006a, b). Prenatal genetic screening is possible.

Treatment

Enzyme replacement (cerliponase alfa) has been approved by the FDA for CLN2 disease. Gene therapy and stem cell therapy are under evaluation for some NCLs. Supporting measures include the treatment of behavioral and psychiatric troubles, dystonia and spasticity, and antiepileptic drugs.

Congenital disorders of glycosylation

More than 100 disorders of glycosylation (CDG) have been described since their initial characterization in 1980. CDGs may result in aberrant protein folding and stability which can impact multiple systems and cause multi-organ dysfunction. Most of these diseases are protein hypoglycosylation disorders, due to a defect in the attachment of N-glycans or of O-glycans. A group of diseases in which N- and O-glycosylation defects occur in combination have been described. Lipid hypoglycosylation disorders have also been reported (Jaeken, 2010). CDG can affect all organs, including central nervous system in an important number of patients, and should be suspected in any unexplained clinical syndrome, according to certain authors. The most frequent CDG subtype is phosphomannomutase 2 deficiency (PMM2-CDG), formerly known as CDG-Ia, an autosomal recessive disorder of N-glycosylation that usually starts in infancy, but may present at any age, including in adults with a very mild phenotype. Its typical clinical characteristics are non-progressive neurological signs, such as ataxia, abnormal eye movement, hypotonia and hyporeflexia, an abnormal distribution of subcutaneous fat tissue, inverted nipples and cerebellar atrophy. Variable degrees of developmental delay, failure to thrive, and dysmorphic features may also be present, among many other possible manifestations. Stroke-like episodes and epilepsy may appear after infancy (Jaeken, 2010). Difficult-to treat seizures of all types, including epileptic spasms, may be observed in a majority of the other, apparently much rarer, CDGs (Sparks & Krasnewich, 2011). In this group, PIGM-CDG is important to recognize because treatment is available. This disorder of glycosylphosphatidylinositol(GPI)-anchor glycosylation is due to a genetic defect that causes histone hypoacetylation at the *PIGM* promoter (Jaeken, 2010). It presents in infancy with splanchnic vein thrombosis and epilepsy.

Diagnosis

Serum transferrin gylcosylation analysis is the recommended CDG screening test. Further analyses, such as enzymatic activity, glycan intermediates measurement, and molecular genetic tests may be required, based on the availability and clinical presentation, in order to precise the CDG subtype (Jaeken, 2010; Sparks & Krasnewich, 2011). Next generation sequencing panels are now available that cover the known CDGs.

Treatment

Treatment options only exist for 3 subtypes of CDG: MPI-CDG and SLC35C1-CDG, in which neurological symptoms are mostly absent; and PIGM-CDG, as mentioned before, in which butyrate, a histone deacetylase inhibitor, increases *PIGM* transcription, and is able to improve the control of seizures (Jaeken, 2010).

Protocol for evaluating IEM

Step 1. Obtain screening blood and urine samples

The goal is to rapidly determine if there are any underlying metabolic derangements needing immediate attention and start collection of data for the most common and treatable conditions. The highest priority is to exclude hypoglycemia (with or without ketosis), acidosis, hyperammonemia, or electrolyte abnormalities. In all patients we will assume that at a minimum a baseline EEG has been performed including portions recorded awake and asleep. Increasingly, continuous EEG recordings are being used in critically ill neonates and infants both to evaluate for seizures and also to important discern the impact of treatments on the background rhythms.

Step 1
Plasma glucose
Blood gases
Plasma lactate
Serum ammonia
Chemistry profile
Complete blood count
Blood and urine amino acids
Urine organic acids
Plasma and urine creatine; guanidinoacetic acid
Plasma acylcarnitine profile
Biotinidase
Urinanalysis

Step 2. Organize a MRI including spectroscopy, if available

MRI can provide valuable clues to the presence of an underlying metabolic disease by the character and distribution of abnormalities. White matter lesions might suggest a leukodystrophy whereas involvement of the deep grey structures can occur with energy failure disorders and other conditions (Rahman, 2012).

Step 3. Perform lumbar puncture to evaluate for other treatable conditions.

If the results of the initial screening tests and imaging does not strongly implicate a specific diagnosis then proceeding to a lumbar puncture to evaluate for other conditions is a reasonable next step. This should be analyzed for glucose, lactate/pyruvate, and amino acids. Samples can also be sent to evaluate for B6 dependency, folate and defects in biogenic amines. Neurotransmitter levels including biogenic amines (dopamine and serotonin metabolites), neopterin, and biopterin can also be examined.

Step 4. Initiate treatment with pyridoxine or pyridoxal phosphate

There are various protocols for proceeding with pyridoxine, although nearly all authorities recommend oral supplementation with 30 mg/kg/day for at least 3–5 days, whether or not there is an EEG response to IV infusion. Some will substitute pyridoxal 5 phophate for pyridoxine, or administer it after a trial of pyridoxine.

Step 5. Consider NGS if resources permit or perform additional studies to evaluate for other conditions as indicated

If the resources permit NGS may be the most efficient next step in the evaluation. If no other condition is suggested from the evaluation to this point that it may be reasonable to pause, and reassess the patient at a later date. If an IEM is still strongly suspected and the resources do not exist to perform NGS then further selective screening tests can be performed. Additional tests may include:

– VLCFA (very long chain fatty acids).

– Lysosomal enzyme analysis in leukocytes.

– Succinyladenosine for adenylosuccinase deficiency (a disorder of purine/pyrimidine metabolism).

– PPT1/TPP1 levels for neuronal ceroid lipofuscinosis.

– Transferrin glycosylation studies via mass spectroscopy (previously transferrin isoelectric focusing).

Serum copper/ceruloplasmin for Menkes.

If there are specific abnormalities then specific enzyme studies, genetic studies or both may help to clarify the underlying diagnosis.

REFERENCES

Aicardi J, Goutières F (1978): Encéphalopathie myoclonique néonatale. *Rev EEG Neurophysiol* 8: 99–101.

Al Teneiji A, Bruun TU, Cordeiro D, *et al.* (2017): Phenotype biochemical features, genotype and treatment outcome of pyridoxine-dependent epilepsy. *Metab Brain Dis* 32: 443–451.

Applegarth DA, Toone JR (2004): Glycine encephalopathy (nonketotic hyperglycinaemia): review and update. *J Inherit Metab Dis* 27: 417–422.

Baker PR 2nd, Friederich MW, Swanson MA, *et al.* (2014): Variant non ketotic hyperglycinemia is caused by mutations in LIAS, BOLA3 and the novel gene GLRX5. *Brain* 137: 366–379.

Berkovic SF, Cochius J, Andermann E, Andermann F (1993): Progressive myoclonus epilepsies: clinical and genetic aspects. *Epilepsia* 34 (Suppl 3): S19–30.

Bjoraker KJ, Swanson MA, Coughlin CR 2nd, *et al.* (2016): Neurodevelopmental outcome and treatment efficacy of benzoate and dextromethorphan in siblings with attenuated nonketotic hyperglycinemia. *J Pediatr* 170: 234–239.

Buoni S, Zannolli R, Waterham H, Wanders R, Fois A (2007): D-bifunctional protein deficiency associated with drug resistant infantile spasms. *Brain Dev* 29: 51–54.

Chuang DT (1998). Maple syrup urine disease: it has come a long way. *J Pediatr* 132: S17–S23.

Chuang DT, Chuang JL, Wynn RM (2006): Lessons from genetic disorders of branched-chain amino acid metabolism. *J Nutr* 136 (1 Suppl): 243S–249S.

Chun K, MacKay N, Petrova-Benedict R, *et al.* (1995): Mutations in the X-linked E1 alpha subunit of pyruvate dehydrogenase: exon skipping, insertion of duplicate sequence, and missense mutations leading to the deficiency of the pyruvate dehydrogenase complex. *Am J Hum Genet* 56: 558–569.

Cook P, Walker V (2011): Investigation of the child with an acute metabolic disorder. *J Clin Pathol* 64: 181–191.

Couce ML, Castiñeiras DE, Bóveda MD, *et al.* (2011): Evaluation and long-term follow-up of infants with inborn errors of metabolism identified in an expanded screening programme. *Mol Genet Metab* 104: 470–475.

Coughlin CR 2nd, van Karnebeek CD, Al-Hertani W, *et al.* (2015): Triple therapy with pyridoxine, arginine supplementation and dietary lysine restriction in pyridoxine-dependent epilepsy: Neurodevelopmental outcome. *Mol Genet Metab* 116: 35–43.

Damseh N, Simonin A, Jalas C, *et al.* (2015): Mutations in SLC1A4, encoding the brain serine transporter, are associated with developmental delay, microcephaly and hypomyelination. *J Med Genet* 52: 541–547.

Deprez L, Weckhuysen S, Holmgren P, *et al.* (2010): Clinical spectrum of early-onset epileptic encephalopathies associated with *STXBP1* mutations. *Neurology* 75: 1159–1165.

De Vivo DC, Trifiletti RR, Jacobson RI, Ronen GM, Behmand RA, Harik SI (1991): Defective glucose transport across the blood-brain barrier as a cause of persistent hypoglycorrhachia, seizures, and developmental delay. *N Engl J Med* 325: 703–709.

De Vivo DC, Haymond MW, Leckie MP, Bussman YL, McDougal DB Jr, Pagliara AS (1977): The clinical and biochemical implications of pyruvate carboxylase deficiency. *J Clin Endocrinol Metab* 45: 1281–1296.

DiMauro S, De Vivo DC (1996): Genetic heterogeneity in Leigh syndrome. *Ann Neurol* 40: 5–7.

Feier F, Schwartz IV, Benkert AR, *et al.* (2016): Living related versus deceased donor liver transplantation for maple syrup urine disease. *Mol Genet Metab* 117: 336–343.

Gaitanis J (2011). EEG of degenerative disorders of the central nervous system. In: Schomer D and Lopes da Silva FH (eds) *Niedermeyer's Electroencephalography: Basic Principles, Clinical Applications and Related Fields*, pp. 281–298. Philadelphia: Lippincott Williams and Wilkins.

Hamosh A, Maher JF, Bellus GA, Rasmussen SA, Johnston MV (1998): Long-term use of high-dose benzoate and dextromethorphan for the treatment of nonketotic hyperglycinemia. *J Pediatr* 132: 709–713.

Hyland K, Shoffner J, Heales SJ (2010): Cerebral folate deficiency. *J Inherit Metab Dis* 33: 563–570.

Jaeken J (2010): Congenital disorders of glycosylation. *Ann N Y Acad Sci* 1214: 190–198.

Kass HR, Winesett PT, Bessone SK, Turner Z, Kossoff EH (2016): Use of dietary therapies amongst patients with GLUT1 deficiency syndrome. *Seizure* 35: 83–87.

Kohlschutter A, Schulz A (2009). Towards understanding the neuronal ceroid lipofuscinoses. *Brain Dev* 31: 499–502.

Kruer M, Steiner R. (2011). Lysosomal storage diseases. Medscape Reference, from http://emedicine.medscape.com/article/1182830-overview#showall.

Kurolap A, Armbruster A, Hershkovitz T, *et al.* (2016): Loss of Glycine Transporter 1 Causes a Subtype of Glycine Encephalopathy with Arthrogryposis and Mildly Elevated Cerebrospinal Fluid Glycine. *Am J Hum Genet* 99: 1172–1180.

Leary LD, Wang D, Nordli DR Jr, Engelstad K, De Vivo DC (2003): Seizure characterization and electroencephalographic features in Glut-1 deficiency syndrome. *Epilepsia* 44: 701–707.

Lee W T (2011): Disorders of amino acid metabolism associated with epilepsy. *Brain Dev* 33: 745–752.

Lee YM, Kang HC, Lee JS, *et al.* (2008): Mitochondrial respiratory chain defects: underlying etiology in various epileptic conditions. *Epilepsia* 49: 685–690.

Livet MO, Aicardi J, Plouin P, Mancini J, Chabrol B (2005): Epilepsy and inborn errors of metabolism. In: Roger J, Bureau M, Dravet C, Genton P, Tassinari CA, Wolf P (eds) *Epileptic syndromes in infancy, childhood and adolescence*, pp. 423–440. Montrouge: John Libbey Eurotext.

Low NL, Bosma JF, Armstrong MD (1957): Studies on phenylketonuria. VI. EEG studies in phenylketonuria. *AMA Arch Neurol Psychiatry* 77: 359–365.

Lyon G, Kolodny EH, *et al.* (2006a): Late infantile progressive genetic encephalopathies. In: Lyon G, Kolodny EH, Pastores GM (eds) *Neurology of hereditary metabolic diseases of children*, pp. 179–242. New York: McGraw-Hill.

Lyon G, Kolodny EH, *et al.* (2006b): Early infantile progressive metabolic encephalopathies: clinical problems and diagnostic considerations. In: Lyon G, Kolodny EH, Pastores GM (eds) *Neurology of hereditary metabolic diseases of children*, pp. 65–178. New York: McGraw-Hill.

Mikati AG, Abu Gheida I, Shamseddine A, Mikati MA, Karam PE (2013): Epileptic and electroencephalographic manifestations of guanidinoacetate-methyltransferase deficiency. *Epileptic Disord* 15: 407–416.

Mole SE, Williams RE (1993): Neuronal Ceroid-Lipofuscinoses. In: Pagon A, Bird TD, Dolan CR, Stephens K (eds) GeneReviews [Internet]. Seattle (WA): University of Washington, Seattle; 1993-.2001 Oct 10 [updated 2010 Mar 02].

Nasrallah F, Feki M, Kaabachi N (2010): Creatine and creatine deficiency syndromes: biochemical and clinical aspects. *Pediatr Neurol* 42: 163–171.

Nordli DR.Jr, C W Bazil, Scheuer ML, Pedley TA (1997): Recognition and classification of seizures in infants. *Epilepsia* 38: 553–560.

Nordli DR Jr, DeVivo DC (2002): Classification of infantile seizures: implications for identification and treatment of inborn errors of metabolism. *J Child Neurol* 17 (Suppl 3): 3S3–7; discussion 3S8.

Ohtahara S, Ishida T, Oka E, *et al.* (1976): On the specific age-dependent epileptic syndromes: the early-infantile epileptic encephalopathy with suppression-burst. *No To Hattatsu* 8: 270–280.

Paciorkowski AR, Thio LL, Dobyns WB (2011): Genetic and biologic classification of infantile spasms. *Pediatr Neurol* 45: 355–367.

Pascual JM, Van Heertum RL, Wang D, Engelstad K, De Vivo DC (2002): Imaging the metabolic footprint of Glut1 deficiency on the brain. *Ann Neurol* 52: 458–464.

Pearson T S, Pons R, Engelstad K, Kane SA, Goldberg ME, De Vivo DC (2017): Paroxysmal eye-head movements in Glut1 deficiency syndrome. *Neurology* 88: 1666–1673.

Prasad AN, Hoffmann GF (2010): Early onset epilepsy and inherited metabolic disorders: diagnosis and management. *Can J Neurol Sci* 37: 350–358.

Prasad AN, Levin S, Rupar CA, Prasad C (2011). Menkes disease and infantile epilepsy. *Brain Dev* 33: 866–876.

Rahman S (2012): Mitochondrial disease and epilepsy. *Dev Med Child Neurol* 54: 397–406.

Ramachandran N, Girard JM, Turnbull J, Minassian BA (2009): The autosomal recessively inherited progressive myoclonus epilepsies and their genes. *Epilepsia* 50 (Suppl 5): 29–36.

Ramaekers VT, Blau N (2004): Cerebral folate deficiency. *Dev Med Child Neurol* 46: 843–851.

Ramm-Pettersen AK, Stabell E, Nakken KO, KK Selmer (2014): Does ketogenic diet improve cognitive function in patients with GLUT1-DS? A 6- to 17-month follow-up study. *Epilepsy Behav* 39: 111–115.

Rutledge SL, Snead OC 3rd, Kelly DR, *et al.* (1989): Pyruvate carboxylase deficiency: acute exacerbation after ACTH treatment of infantile spasms. *Pediatr Neurol* 5: 249–252.

Sadleir LG, Connolly MB, Applegarth D, *et al.* (2004): Spasms in children with definite and probable mitochondrial disease. *Eur J Neurol* 11: 103–110.

Saneto RP, Lee IC, Koenig MK, *et al.* (2010): POLG DNA testing as an emerging standard of care before instituting valproic acid therapy for pediatric seizure disorders. *Seizure* 19: 140–146.

Shah NS, Mitchell WG, Boles RG (2002): Mitochondrial disorders: a potentially under-recognized etiology of infantile spasms. *J Child Neurol* 17: 369–372.

Sofou K, Dahlin M, Hallbook T, Lindefeld M, Viggedal G, Darin N (2017): Ketogenic diet in pyruvate dehydrogenase complex deficiency: short- and long-term outcomes. *J Inherit Metab Dis* 40: 237–245.

Sparks S, Krasnewich D (2011): Congenital disorders of glycosylation Overview. In: Pagon RA, Bird TD, Dolan CR, Stephens K, editors. GeneReviews [Internet]. Seattle (WA): University of Washington, Seattle; 1993-.2005 Aug 15 [updated 2011 Aug 11].

Stibler H, Gylje H, Uller A (1999): A neurodystrophic syndrome resembling carbohydrate-deficient glycoprotein syndrome type III. *Neuropediatrics* 30: 90–92.

Stockler S, Plecko B, Gospe SM Jr *et al.* (2011): Pyridoxine dependent epilepsy and antiquitin deficiency: clinical and molecular characteristics and recommendations for diagnosis, treatment and follow-up. *Mol Genet Metab* 104: 48–60.

Stockler-Ipsiroglu S, van Karnebeek C, Longo N, *et al.* (2014): Guanidinoacetate methyltransferase (GAMT) deficiency: outcomes in 48 individuals and recommendations for diagnosis, treatment and monitoring. *Mol Genet Metab* 111: 16–25.

Tabatabaie L, Klomp LW, Berger R, de Koning TJ (2010): L-serine synthesis in the central nervous system: a review on serine deficiency disorders. *Mol Genet Metab* 99: 256–262.

Takahashi Y, Suzuki Y, Kumazaki K, *et al.* (1997): Epilepsy in peroxisomal diseases. *Epilepsia* 38: 182–188.

Tatsuno M, Hayashi M, Iwamoto H, Sasaki Y, Hara M (1984): Autopsy case of Leigh's encephalopathy with wide lesions in central nervous system and early infantile epileptic encephalopathy with burst suppression. *No To Hattatsu* 16: 68–75.

Tharp BR (1992): Unique EEG pattern (comb-like rhythm) in neonatal maple syrup urine disease. *Pediatr Neurol* 8: 65–68.

Verma NP, Hart ZH, Kooi KA (1984): Electroencephalographic findings in urea-cycle disorders. *Electroencephalogr Clin Neurophysiol* 57: 105–112.

Vigevano F, Bartuli A (2002): Infantile epileptic syndromes and metabolic etiologies. *J Child Neurol* 17 (Suppl 3): 3S9–13; discussion 13S14.

Wang D, Pascual JM, Yang H, *et al.* (2005): Glut-1 deficiency syndrome: clinical, genetic, and therapeutic aspects. *Ann Neurol* 57: 111–118.

Wolf NI, García-Cazorla A, Hoffmann GF (2009): Epilepsy and inborn errors of metabolism in children. *J Inherit Metab Dis* 32: 609–617.

Zammarchi E, Donati MA, Ciani F, Pasquini E, Pela, P Fiorini P (1994): Failure of early dextromethorphan and sodium benzoate therapy in an infant with nonketotic hyperglycinemia. *Neuropediatrics* 25: 274–276.

Zempleni J, Hassan YI, Wijeratne SS (2008): Biotin and biotinidase deficiency. *Expert Rev Endocrinol Metab* 3: 715–724.

Epileptic Syndromes in Infancy, Childhood and Adolescence (6th ed), M. Bureau, P. Genton, C. Dravet, A. V. Delgado-Escueta, R. Guerrini, C.A. Tassinari, P. Thomas & P. Wolf

WITH VIDEO SUPPLEMENTS

CHAPTER 25
GENETICALLY DETERMINED FOCAL EPILEPSIES

■ Fabienne Picard[1] and Ingrid E. Scheffer[2]

[1] Department of Neurology, University Hospital and Medical School of Geneva, Switzerland
[2] Epilepsy Research Centre, Department of Medicine, the University of Melbourne, Austin Health, Department of Paediatrics, the University of Melbourne, Royal Children's Hospital, Florey and Murdoch Children's Research Institutes, Melbourne, Australia

With the emphasis on aetiology in the new 2017 Classification of the epilepsies (Scheffer *et al.*, 2017), the genetic basis of many focal epilepsies is becoming increasingly recognized. This includes many of the focal epilepsies previously regarded as "idiopathic, symptomatic or cryptogenic" epilepsies in the old classification. Aetiology is now divided into six groups: structural, genetic, infectious, metabolic, immune and unknown. These groups are not exclusive such that a patient's aetiology may include two or more groups, as exemplified by tuberous sclerosis which has both a structural and genetic basis. A genetic etiology was historically based on clinical genetic evidence drawn from twin and family studies; however, it is increasingly based on the identification of a genetic mutation (or pathogenic variant).

The genetics of the epilepsies is a rapidly evolving field, and has depended upon clinicians for recognition of specific epilepsy syndromes. In the past, the inheritance pattern of a syndrome was the first step in uncovering its genetic basis. However, the major advances in clinical epileptology, together with the recent revolution in molecular and imaging technology, has enabled increasing sophistication in the diagnosis of epilepsy syndromes, and underpinned the remarkable progress in epilepsy genetics.

Thus, in the past twenty-four years, clinicians have identified several new focal (previously termed partial, Fisher *et al.*, 2017) epilepsy syndromes following single gene inheritance including autosomal dominant nocturnal frontal lobe epilepsy (ADNFLE), familial temporal lobe epilepsies (FTLE), familial focal epilepsy with variable foci (FFEVF) and rare familial Rolandic epilepsies. These conditions do not correspond to epilepsy syndromes of individuals but to "familial epilepsy syndromes". This means that for each affected family member, the clinical picture is not identical and is similar to a picture of focal epilepsy that may occur in a sporadic patient who does not have a family history of seizures. The rate of pharmacoresistance may be higher than in non-genetic focal epilepsies (higher than 30%), possibly depending on the underlying genetic mutation. The neurologic status and intelligence of affected individuals are typically normal and interictal EEG abnormalities are scarce in some of these syndromes. The peculiarity of these conditions is therefore the familial occurrence of specific epilepsy syndromes, related to an inherited molecular defect. In these syndromes, the penetrance is around 60–70%, such that obligate gene carriers who do not have a history of seizures often exist within a family.

It is not always possible to classify families into one of the recognized syndromes because these familial syndromes show phenotypic overlap and because it may be difficult to localize the focal epilepsy for some patients on the basis of ictal semiology and scalp EEG recordings. In addition, some families are too small for the identification of the syndrome of FFEVF as there are too few individuals to show the characteristic familial pattern of multiple foci (Dibbens *et al.*, 2013). Future molecular genetic findings may help to solve the overlap between familial focal epilepsy syndromes.

Taking a family history of seizure disorders

Understanding the genetic component to a patient's epilepsy is an important clue to the diagnosis. A careful family history should be part of a routine epilepsy evaluation. A pedigree can be constructed relatively quickly and should denote both sides of the patient's family and clearly indicate the relationship of the patient to other affected family members. Details about relatives' seizures should be obtained as this may aid in the diagnosis of a familial epilepsy syndrome. The clinician should also enquire whether family members have had any type of paroxysmal attack including febrile seizures or isolated seizures, or other paroxysmal neurological disorders such as movement disorders.

Specific questioning about consanguinity is essential as this may not be volunteered but may implicate a genetic basis. Bilineal inheritance is not uncommon, where both the maternal and paternal lines have a history of seizures, and may be a clue to complex inheritance where a patient has inherited more than one epilepsy gene.

Patients often do not know their family history and should be encouraged to talk to others in the family, particularly the elderly matriarchs who may know of early childhood attacks in other family members, long since forgotten. Thus, the patient should be encouraged to provide more significant detail about the family history at subsequent visits. The older generations may initially be reticent to discuss a family history of seizures as they feel guilty about "passing on" a disorder. But with gentle education regarding genetic issues, they may volunteer carefully guarded family secrets of major relevance.

Autosomal dominant nocturnal frontal lobe epilepsy (ADNFLE)/Sleep-related hypermotor epilepsy (SHE)

ADNFLE was first recognized as a familial focal epilepsy in 1994 in families from Australia, Canada and the United Kingdom (Scheffer *et al.*, 1994). Prior to this, ADNFLE was originally described as a movement disorder, paroxysmal nocturnal dystonia (Lugaresi & Cirignotta, 1981; Lugaresi *et al.*, 1986). This syndrome is characterized by clusters of motor seizures arising from sleep. It follows autosomal dominant inheritance with 70% penetrance. There is considerable intrafamilial variation in epilepsy severity (Scheffer *et al.*, 1995a; Picard *et al.*, 2000). This syndrome is not rare with more than one hundred and fifty ADNFLE families reported to date (Scheffer *et al.*, 1995a; Magnusson *et al.*, 1996; Oldani *et al.*, 1996, 1998; Phillips *et al.*, 1998; Khatami *et al.*, 1998; Picard *et al.*, 2000; Ito *et al.*, 2000; Combi *et al.*, 2004; Hwang *et al.*, 2011; Chen *et al.*, 2017). Sporadic cases of nocturnal frontal lobe epilepsy (NFLE), with a similar clinical picture, are even more frequent (Oldani *et al.*, 1998). Some may represent unrecognized familial cases or *de novo* mutations of genes causing ADNFLE (Phillips *et al.*, 2000; Heron *et al.*, 2012).

Recently a new term, SHE, has been proposed, as the seizures are sleep-related, rather than strictly nocturnal, and the location of the epileptic zone may not be frontal, in particular, the operculo-insular cortex may be implicated (Tinuper *et al.*, 2016). For familial cases following autosomal dominant inheritance, ADSHE has been suggested.

Clinical features

The mean age at onset of ADNFLE is between 8 and 11.5 years (Scheffer *et al.*, 1995a; Oldani *et al.*, 1998; Picard *et al.*, 2000). Age at onset is below 20 years in 85% of cases; however, it may range from 2 months to 56 years. Seizures occur from sleep, frequently in clusters, with a mean of eight seizures per night typically over a few hours (Scheffer *et al.*, 1995a). Diurnal seizures may be observed in the more severe cases, particularly when patients are going through a period of poor seizure control and seizures continue following a cluster through the night. Seizures may begin with a nonspecific aura prior to a motor seizure with hyperkinetic (frantic movements of bipedal activity, pelvic thrashing), tonic or dystonic features. In the latter case, abrupt and sudden, rapidly changing movements of the limbs and the trunk are observed, leading to various brief dystonic postures. During the seizure, a sensation of being unable to "get one's breath" has been reported by many patients and may be akin to a choking feeling. Awareness may be retained through the seizure, which has often led to misdiagnoses of parasomnias, night terrors or even hysteria (Scheffer *et al.*, 1995a).

Seizures are stereotyped and of short duration (usually less than one minute) (Scheffer *et al.*, 1995a). In Picard *et al.*'s study (2000) of 23 patients, the mean seizure duration was 30 seconds. Oldani *et al.*'s video-polysomnographic study (1998) recorded all episodes of nocturnal repetitive motor activity and classified them into four categories (minimal, minor, major and prolonged episodes) according to duration, semiology and complexity of motor behavior. Although control subjects may present nocturnal movements that resemble minimal (duration 3–10 seconds) or minor (duration 10–30 seconds) episodes, the semiology of the episodes provides a clear differentiation between the control subjects and the patients: patients' episodes were stereotyped, and always included sudden movements with dyskinetic or dystonic components (Oldani *et al.*, 1996).

The main provocative factors for seizures are sleep deprivation (30% patients) and stress (30%). Rare focal to bilateral tonic-clonic seizures (previously called secondarily generalized seizures) are observed in nearly half the patients. They may occur at the onset of epilepsy or during the course of the disease. Neurological examination is normal.

Psychiatric and neuropsychological disturbances are not infrequent; in some cases, they are subtle and require focused testing to detect features of frontal lobe dysfunction. Psychiatric disturbances have been reported in approximately 25% of the patients, particularly during the active phase of their epilepsy. Behavioral disorders including irritability, aggression and impulsive behavior, with fugue states during adolescence, were the most frequent findings (Picard *et al.*, 2000). An ADNFLE Norwegian family included one patient with schizophrenia and three others with other psychiatric problems (Magnusson *et al.*, 2003). In addition, two families with typical ADNFLE and mental retardation have been described (Khatami *et al.* 1998; Cho *et al.*, 2003), as well as two families with unusually severe ADNFLE, with associated psychiatric, behavioral, and cognitive features including neurodevelopmental regression (Derry *et al.*, 2008). In these latter families, childhood behavioural disturbance took a variety of forms, from aggressive and destructive behaviors to prominent distractibility and overactivity. In adulthood, the most frequent psychiatric diagnoses were depression, personality disorder and one patient had paranoid schizophrenia. Intellectual disability was present in a quarter of the affected family members.

A neuropsychological pilot study performed on 11 individuals from four ADNFLE families with different mutations in nicotinic receptor subunits (see below – "Molecular genetic studies") demonstrated cognitive dysfunction with a fronto-temporal pattern in most subjects (Picard *et al.*, 2009). ADNFLE patients from the original large family with the first ADNFLE mutation showed impairments on tasks requiring cognitive flexibility against a background of well-preserved intellectual abilities (Wood *et al.*, 2010).

Considerable intrafamilial and interfamilial clinical variability is observed in the severity of the epilepsy, response to antiepileptic therapy, neuropsychological and psychiatric co-morbidity. The ictal symptoms vary greatly from one individual to another within a family, with ictal video-EEG recordings and functional neuroimaging confirming different regions of onset within the frontal lobe in different family members (Hayman *et al.*, 1997).

EEG and neuroimaging studies

Interictal EEG is often normal. Studies vary with between 12 and 65% of patients showing anterior focal epileptiform abnormalities (Scheffer *et al.*, 1995a; Oldani *et al.*, 1998; Picard *et al.* 2000). These abnormalities are not specific. It is important to note that in 75% of patients, abnormalities are only visible during sleep recordings (Oldani *et al.*, 1998). Ictal EEG may also fail to show any ictal discharges with studies identifying an ictal pattern in only 40 to 88% of patients. It consists of either sharp waves/repetitive 8–11 Hz spikes, rarely in the form of a recruiting pattern, or rhythmic theta activity that may be bifrontal or unilateral frontal, or a diffuse desynchronization. Ictal recordings are often obscured by movement artifact. The lack of epileptiform activity may reflect the inaccessibility of the focus to scalp EEG recordings. The focus may only be apparent with highly specific depth electrode studies. In Oldani *et al.*'s study (1998), 26% patients had both a normal interictal and ictal scalp EEG. It is interesting to note that when unilateral interictal or ictal EEG abnormalities are identified, they remain lateralized to the same side throughout the evolution of the disorder.

The video-EEG-polysomnographic recordings show that the seizures occur during non-rapid eye movement (NREM) sleep, mainly in stage 2 sleep. Moreover, seizures apparently are initiated from sleep spindles *(Figure 1)*, which are physiological neuronal oscillations that recur periodically, usually every 5–10 seconds, during stage 2 NREM sleep, with a maximum over the frontal regions, and are generated by thalamocortical circuitry.

Intracerebral EEG recordings performed in one patient with a typical picture of ADNFLE surprisingly demonstrated that seizures originated from the left insular cortex. Ictal surface EEG showed diffuse flattening or left frontoprecentral fast activity at the onset of the seizures, and ictal SPECT using 99mTc-ethyl cysteinate dimer (ECD) showed left frontal hyperperfusion, correlating with the right-sided predominance of the ictal motor symptoms (Picard *et al.*, 2000; Ryvlin *et al.*, 2006). In this patient, the aura (tingling sensation in the back) could be reproduced only by stimulation of the insular cortex.

MRI studies were first considered normal in all patients. However, the recent identification of focal cortical dysplasia (FCD) in some patients with familial focal epilepsy, including ADSHE, and a mutation in a gene that is part of the GATOR1 complex has revolutionized the field of genetic focal epilepsies (Scheffer *et al.*, 2014). This means that both lesional (or "structural") epilepsies, and non-lesional SHE, occur in family members with ADSHE and also in families with FFEVF (Weckhuysen *et al.*, 2016).

Functional imaging studies include ictal SPECT and interictal PET using fluoro-deoxyglucose (FDG). In 1997, Hayman *et al.* reported nuclear imaging findings in two patients with ADNFLE from different families. One individual had congruent focal hypometabolism on interictal PET with focal hyperperfusion on ictal SPECT in the left frontopolar region, while the other, who had a mutation in the $\alpha 4$ subunit gene of the nicotinic acetylcholine receptor, showed right parasagittal, midfrontal hyperperfusion on ictal SPECT. Picard *et al.* (2000) performed an ictal SPECT using 99mTc- ECD in one patient showing left frontal hyperperfusion (as reported above). Ictal SPECT in other patients showed hypoperfusion in both frontal lobes in one (Ito *et al.*, 2000), and hyperperfusion in the body of the cingulate gyrus in two others (Cho *et al.*, 2008).

FDG-PET performed in six patients from a Korean family showed no clear abnormality; however, after SPM analysis, a decrease in glucose uptake was observed in the superior and middle frontal gyri, and in

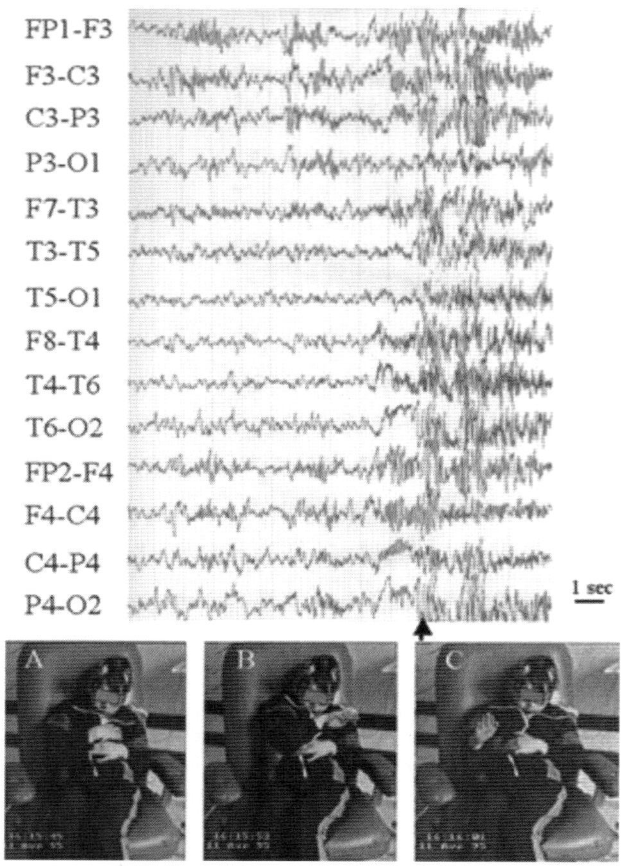

Figure 1 **Ictal EEG of a child with ADNFLE (paper speed, 15 mm/sec). The seizure occurred during stage 2 of NREM sleep, characterized by sleep spindles. A change in the EEG began 1 second before the first clinical manifestations (arrow), with a fast bifrontal rhythm of high amplitude with a frequency of 12 Hz, for which the localization and morphology were very similar to the sleep spindles observed in the preceding seconds. This was followed by muscle artefact without visible underlying EEG abnormalities. Clinical features were tachypnea related to a "feeling of being out of breath" followed by forced, abrupt and irregular movements of the extremities and the trunk (photographs A, B, C). Photograph A shows the patient 8 seconds after the arrow denoting the initial clinical manifestations.**

central and anterior parietal areas (Cho *et al.*, 2003). In our FDG-PET study of five ADNFLE patients with different nicotinic receptor mutations, we observed decreased metabolism in the right and left anterior orbitofrontal cortex, in the right and left opercular regions and in the right supramarginal gyrus (Picard *et al.*, 2006).

Dopaminergic receptor D(1) density was also analyzed using [(11)C]-SCH23390 and PET in 12 ADNFLE subjects with a nicotinic receptor mutation (Fedi *et al.*, 2008). Reduced D(1) receptor binding was observed in the right putamen and may represent increased extracellular dopamine levels or, more likely, receptor downregulation. Alterations in mesostriatal dopaminergic circuits were then proposed to contribute to nocturnal paroxysmal motor activity in ADNFLE.

Evolution and treatment

When seizures continue throughout life in a given patient, the stereotyped character of seizure semiology, without any progression, is a striking feature of ADNFLE. An exception is seen when seizures begin in early childhood, with seizures evolving from tonic attacks to classical NFLE seizures with dystonic or hyperkinetic components. Thereafter, the ictal semiology remains unchanged throughout life in the same patient, even after 30 years of evolution, although attacks may become more subtle. In a minority of cases, seizures may only occur for a few months (Scheffer *et al.*, 1995a). In many, seizures persist for years but tend to disappear with age, around the fourth or fifth decade, or sometimes even in the third decade, without relapse after cessation of drug therapy. This was observed in patients who had been refractory to antiepileptic medication over several years.

Carbamazepine is the most effective antiepileptic medication in ADNFLE, and completely suppresses seizures in about 70% of patients. Carbamazepine is indeed much more effective than valproate in this syndrome (Scheffer *et al.*, 1995a; Picard *et al.*, 2000). Low dosages of carbamazepine (around 600 mg/day in adults) are sufficient, which may give evidence of pathophysiological mechanisms that are different from those of other epilepsies. It may be noted that this high sensitivity to carbamazepine is also observed in paroxysmal neurological disorders (paroxysmal kinesigenic choreoathetosis) in which pathogenic mechanisms involve basal ganglia and related structures. According to Hirose & Kurahashi (2010), ADNFLE patients with a specific nicotinic receptor mutation (α4-S252L) (see below – "Molecular genetic studies") are more responsive to zonisamide than carbamazepine. Pharmacoresistance to carbamazepine and other antiepileptic drugs was observed in 30% of patients. Anecdotally, two pilot studies showed a possible benefit of nicotine patches in pharmacoresistant patients (Willoughby *et al.*, 2003; Brodtkorb &

Picard, 2006). Lastly, a clear improvement with vagal nerve stimulation has been reported in one patient with a severe form of ADNFLE with repeated episodes of status epilepticus (Carreno *et al.*, 2010), whereas we observed an absence of efficacy in another case with very frequent pharmacoresistant nocturnal hypermotor seizures (personal observation).

In the patients with a recognised FCD, epilepsy surgery is a good option as the outcome is excellent (Baulac *et al.*, 2015) (cf. Familial focal epilepsy with variable foci).

Many of the reported families with ADNFLE contain one pharmacoresistant individual whereas other affected family members have shown a good response to antiepileptic medication, confirming the high intra-familial variability in epilepsy severity.

Molecular genetic studies

ADNFLE was the first non-lesional "idiopathic" epilepsy for which a responsible gene was identified. Several groups of genes have now been implicated in ADNFLE including those encoding subunits of the neuronal nicotinic acetylcholine receptor (nAChR), a potassium channel subunit gene *(KCNT1)* for severe ADNFLE, and genes involved in the mTOR (mechanistic or mammalian target of rapamycin) pathway.

Mutations have been identified in three genes encoding nAChR subunits in twenty families (which corresponds to about 10% of reported ADNFLE families) and in five sporadic cases. nAChRs are pentameric ligand-gated ion channel receptors which consist of different functional subunit combinations. Twelve subunits (α2-α10 and β2-β4) have been identified (Buisson *et al.*, 1999; Sgard *et al.*, 2000). The major brain receptors in human are made from the assembly of α4 and β2 subunits (in a 2α/3β ratio), which may explain why both subunits are associated with ADNFLE. The nAChRs are excitatory receptor channels permeable to cations (Na^+, K^+, Ca^{2+}). The endogenous ligand is acetylcholine (ACh), while nicotine constitutes an exogenous ligand. There are two isoforms with different stoichiometry: $(\alpha4)3(\beta2)2$ is the low affinity subtype and $(\alpha4)2(\beta2)3$ is the high affinity subtype, with a 100-fold higher affinity to ACh and nicotine. Most of the nAChRs are presynaptic and have a neuromodulatory role consisting of an enhanced release of the neurotransmitter present in the neurons on which they are located (GABA, glutamate, dopamine, nore-pinephrine, serotonin or ACh). Other nAChRs are postsynaptic and mediate fast excitatory synaptic transmission. The nAChRs are involved in cognition and in the regulation of the sleep/wake cycle.

Mutations identified in *CHRNA4*, the gene encoding the α4 subunit of the nAChR, are: i) "S248F" (or S280F using the alternative coding system), a missense mutation replacing serine with phenylalanine in position 248 in the amino acid sequence, observed in four families, that are respectively Australian, Spanish, Norwegian and Scottish (Steinlein *et al.*, 1995, 2000; Saenz *et al.*, 1999; McLellan *et al.*, 2003); ii) "776ins3" (or L291 dup), an insertion of three nucleotides at nucleotide position 776, leading to the insertion of a leucine in the amino acid sequence, in a Norwegian family (Steinlein *et al.*, 1997); iii) "S252" (or S284L), a missense mutation replacing a serine by a leucine in position 252 in the amino-acid sequence in a Japanese family, a Polish family, a Korean family, a *de novo* mutation in a mother-son pair of Lebanese origin, and a sporadic Australian girl (Hirose *et al.*, 1999; Rozycka *et al.*, 2003; Cho *et al.*, 2003; Phillips *et al.*, 2000; unpublished data); iv) "T265I" (or T293I) in a German family (Leniger *et al.*, 2003); v) "R308H" (or R336H) amino-acid exchange outside the transmembrane domain, in the second intracellular loop between the third and fourth transmembrane domains (Chen *et al.*, 2009); and vi) *de novo* I275F in one Chinese patient (Wang *et al.*, 2014). The four first mutations are located within exon 5, coding for the second transmembrane domain (TM2) of the α4 subunit, which constitutes the wall of the ionic pore of the nicotinic receptor (Buisson *et al.*, 1999).

Six mutations (V287L, V287M, I312M, V308A, V337G and L301V) have been identified in *CHRNB2*, the gene encoding the nAChRβ2 subunit, in Italian, Scottish, English, Spanish, Chinese and Turkish families (De Fusco *et al.*, 2000; Phillips *et al.*, 2001; Bertrand *et al.*, 2005; Diaz-Otero *et al.*, 2008; Liu *et al.*, 2011; Chen *et al.*, 2015; Hoda *et al.*, 2008). These mutations are located in the second (TM2) and third (TM3) transmembrane domains of the subunit, which play an important role in channel gating, except for V337G which is located in the C2 loop between TM3 and TM4.

Lastly, two mutations (I279N and I297F) have been identified in *CHRNA2*, the gene encoding the nAChR α2 subunit (in the first and second transmembrane domain, respectively), each in one family (Aridon *et al.*, 2006; Conti *et al.*, 2015).

Thus mutations have been found not just in segments that directly contribute to the structure of the ion gate (8/14 mutations in TM2), but also close to the outer ring of TM2 or in transmembrane regions that are not part of the ion channel inner wall.

Comparison of the ADNFLE phenotype in a Scottish family with a *CHRNA4* mutation and another Scottish family with a *CHRNB2* mutation showed that the phenotypes associated with different genes were indistinguishable (McLellan *et al.*, 2003).

Functional studies

Electrophysiological studies of oocytes injected with an equivalent amount of mutant and wild type (non-mutant) *CHRNA4* alleles to reflect the dominant inheritance pattern of ADNFLE resulted in expression of mutant heterozygous receptors. The only common functional effect for different mutations was a significant increase in sensitivity to ACh of the mutant receptors (Phillips *et al.*, 2001; Moulard *et al.*, 2001; Bertrand *et al.*, 2002; Leniger *et al.*, 2003; Hoda *et al.*, 2009). Another mutation, the *CHRNB2* V287L mutation, caused retardation of channel desensitization (De Fusco *et al.*, 2000). Thus, contrary to the first conclusions obtained from the assessment of homozygous mutant receptors, recent studies suggest a gain of function of the mutant nicotinic receptor for the various mutations, despite different effects for different mutations. In contrast, another study of five mutations proposed a reduction of the Ca^{2+} dependence of the ACh response that may explain an increase of glutamate release during bouts of synchronous activity, as an alternative common mechanism (Rodrigues-Pinguet *et al.*, 2003). The study of Son *et al.* (2009) showed defective regulation of the intracellular subunit stoichiometry of nicotinic receptors carrying ADNFLE mutations that could be pathogenic, and normalization of this defective stoichiometry under nicotine, which could explain how nicotine patches may suppress seizures in ADNFLE patients (Son *et al.*, 2009). An increased ratio of high affinity receptors/low affinity receptors was shown for several mutations (Steinlein *et al.*, 2012; Nichols *et al.*, 2016).

However, the precise mechanisms leading to epileptogenesis in ADNFLE remain unresolved.

A PET-scan using [^{18}F]-F-A-85380, a ligand with a high affinity and specificity for α4β2 nAChRs, allowed the study of the nAChR cerebral distribution in a group of patients with ADNFLE carrying a nAChR mutation, in comparison with a group of control subjects (Picard *et al.*, 2006). A significant increase of nicotinic receptor density was found in the patients in the mesencephalon, suggesting a role of the brainstem ascending cholinergic system which projects to the thalamus and activates at the time of arousals during sleep. Some authors suggest a link between sleep spindles and onset of ADNFLE seizures (Picard *et al.*, 2007) while others suspect that ADNFLE seizures may be initiated by K-complexes (El Helou *et al.*, 2008).

An interesting correlation with the observation that carbamazepine is efficacious in patients with ADNFLE is the finding that mutant α4β2 nicotinic receptors are more sensitive to this drug than normal receptors, and readily inhibited at pharmacological concentrations (Picard *et al.*, 1999; Bertrand *et al.*, 2002). However, the effect varies depending on the mutations (Di Resta *et al.*, 2010), and other mutations do not change the receptor carbamazepine sensitivity or may even decrease the receptor sensitivity towards carbamazepine (Hoda *et al.*, 2009). In accordance with these experimental data, an absence of efficacy of carbamazepine is frequent in ADNFLE patients carrying these specific mutations (Hoda *et al.*, 2009). Di Resta *et al.* (2010) also showed an increased effect of oxcarbazepine on mutant receptors.

Several transgenic animal (mice and rat) models of ADNFLE have been generated (Zhu *et al.*, 2008; for a review, see Boillot & Baulac, 2016). A *CHRNA4* knockout mouse shows increased anxiety in its behavioural phenotype compared with wild type, but no spontaneous seizures (Ross *et al.*, 2000). Point mutation knock-in mice with hypersensitive α4 nicotinic receptors show increased anxiety and dopaminergic deficits (Labarca *et al.*, 2001), and increased sensitivity to agonist-induced seizures (Fonck *et al.*, 2003), supporting the possible involvement of gain-of-function α4 receptors in ADNFLE. Knock-in mice harboring a mutation that is found in human ADNFLE (α4-S248F) responded to modest nicotine injections with a behavior that closely resembled the dystonic head and limb semiology of ADNFLE attacks (Teper *et al.*, 2007). An increased sensitivity to nicotine-induced seizures was also reported in α4-L9'A and in transgenic β2-V286L rat (Fonck 2005; Shiba, 2015). *CHRNB2* knock-out mice show abnormal functional organization in the dorsal lateral geniculate nucleus (Grubb *et al.*, 2003), reduced sensitivity to nicotine-induced locomotor depression (Tritto *et al.*, 2004) and reduced fragmentation of non-REM sleep by micro-arousals (Lena *et al.*, 2004). One study suggested a potential pathogenic role of the mutant nicotinic receptors during development: in a mouse model, the mutant receptors were responsible for abnormal formation of neuronal circuits and/or long-lasting alteration of network assembly in the developing brain (Manfredi *et al.*, 2009).

Mutations in *CHRNA4* and *CHRNB2* account for only a minority (around 10%) of ADNFLE families. Linkage to α4 and β2 subunits has indeed been excluded in most families (Steinlein *et al.*, 1995; Phillips *et al.*, 1998; Picard *et al.*, 2000). Linkage to 15q24, close to the region containing α3, α5 and β4 nicotinic subunit genes, has been demonstrated in one family (Phillips *et al.*, 1998); however, the linkage seems to be actually external to the interval containing the cluster of nicotinic subunits (Bonati *et al.*, 2000). A mutation in the promoter of the corticotropin-releasing hormone (CRH) gene was reported in one family (Combi *et al.*, 2005). The pathophysiological link between CRH and nAChRs in ADNFLE is still obscure.

As orexin is the other principal substance involved in arousal induction from sleep besides ACh, we searched for mutations in the orexin system (the single preproorexin gene, *HCRT*, which encodes orexin-A and orexin-B, and the *HCRTR1* and *HCRTR2* genes, which encode the two receptors). However, the analysis of the three genes in 21 ADNFLE unrelated probands failed to identify any potentially pathological variants (Bouchardy *et al.*, 2011).

Mutations in the three genes that make up the GATOR1 complex *(DEPDC5, NPRL2, NPRL3)* have been recently identified in about 12% of ADNFLE families. As NFLE/SHE is one of the phenotypes seen in FFEVF, it is not surprising that smaller families may just have individuals with this focal seizure syndrome (see "Familial focal epilepsy with variable foci") (Scheffer *et al.*, 2014; Dibbens *et al.*, 2013; Picard *et al.*, 2014).

Familial temporal lobe epilepsy (FTLE)

FTLE can be subdivided into mesial (FMTLE) and lateral forms, the latter also known as autosomal dominant epilepsy with auditory features (Ottman *et al.*, 1995). Inheritance of seizures is clearly autosomal dominant in some families, but others show patterns more suggestive of complex inheritance (Crompton *et al.*, 2010). Both forms usually begin in adolescence or adult life, with a mean age at onset of 24 years (range: 1–63, median: 15–18.5 years depending on the study).

Familial mesial temporal lobe epilepsy (FMTLE)

Electroclinical features

In the classical form of FMTLE, there is no history of febrile seizures and no abnormalities on MRI. More than 20 families with this form (without a history of familial febrile seizures) have been reported (Berkovic *et al.*, 1996; Cendes *et al.*, 1998; Gambardella *et al.*, 2000; Regesta *et al.*, 2002). FMTLE is characterized by mesial temporal lobe auras that may have psychic, or more rarely autonomic or special sensory components (Berkovic *et al.*, 1996). *Déjà vu* constitutes the most common psychic symptom. Other common symptoms are fear, nausea, tachycardia, a sense of slow motion, and complex visual or auditory distortions. Somatosensory auras consist of diffuse numbness or tingling. Focal aware seizures (auras) occur in about 90% of patients and focal impaired awareness seizures, usually preceded by an aura in 65%. Rare focal to bilateral tonic-clonic seizures occur in about 70% of patients. There is intrafamilial variability of ictal symptoms. Some patients are not easily diagnosed, when their symptoms are mild and then ignored or regarded as normal phenomena. Interictal EEG abnormalities are rare. Evolution is usually benign. This familial mesial temporal lobe epilepsy contrasts with the frequent cases of sporadic temporal lobe epilepsies with hippocampal sclerosis in which there is often a history of febrile seizures, often prolonged, and in which the age at onset of temporal lobe seizures is around 9 years, with frequent pharmacoresistance.

Heterogeneity of FMTLE became apparent when TLE families with more severe syndromes were described, with frequent hippocampal sclerosis and a variable association with febrile seizures (Vadlamudi *et al.*, 2003; Gambardella *et al.*, 2009). In these cases, epilepsy begins in the first to third decade of life (mean age at onset around 10 years). Interictal EEGs show frequent temporal discharges. Patients are often pharmacoresistant. There is still debate as to whether hippocampal sclerosis may be the consequence of febrile seizures (in some cases), of ongoing seizures or of an early developmental lesion.

A few families with individuals with both febrile seizures and temporal lobe seizures, but without hippocampal abnormalities on MRI, have also been reported. A common genetic susceptibility to both types of seizures is likely in these families (Baulac *et al.*, 2001; Claes *et al.*, 2004).

Molecular genetic studies

No causal genes have been identified solely for the classical form of FMTLE (with no hippocampal sclerosis and no febrile convulsions) or in FMTLE with hippocampal sclerosis and febrile convulsions. There are, however, families with MTLE who have mutations of the genes in the GATOR1 complex. Smaller families may only have a FMTLE phenotype rather than the heterogeneous phenotypic picture that is typically seen in larger families with FFEVF (Dibbens *et al.*, 2013).

Autosomal dominant lateral temporal lobe epilepsy (ADLTLE) (or autosomal dominant epilepsy with auditory features ADEAF)

Electroclinical features

Autosomal dominant lateral TLE (ADLTLE) is a self-limited, pharmacoresponsive syndrome with onset in late adolescence (Ottman *et al.*, 1995; Poza *et al.*, 1999; Michelucci *et al.*, 2000). The most frequent ictal symptom consists of auditory hallucinations such as ringing or humming (36 to 55% of patients), but some patients have other symptoms, alone or in association, such as visual hallucinations, olfactory symptoms, or aphasic seizures (Winawer *et al.*, 2000; Michelucci *et al.*, 2003). Seizures are sometimes triggered by external noises (Michelucci *et al.*, 2009). Interictal EEGs are normal or show mild abnormalities. Previous reports described normal MRIs in all patients, except for abnormalities in the lateral cortex of the temporal lobe in one family (Kobayashi *et al.*, 2003). However, functional impairment in language processing was shown using auditory evoked potentials (AEP), fMRI with an auditory description decision task and a tone discrimination task, and magnetoencephalography (MEG) with auditory stimuli (Brodtkorb *et al.*, 2005; Ottman *et al.*, 2008). Response to antiepileptic treatment is usually good with an overall benign outcome (Michelucci *et al.*, 2009); apart from a family with two pharmacoresistant patients and recurrent focal status epilepticus (Di Bonaventura *et al.*, 2009).

Molecular genetic studies

About half of the ADLTLE families have mutations in *LGI1*, the leucine-rich glioma inactivated gene 1, also called epitempin, located on chromosome 10q (Kalachikov *et al.*, 2002; Michelucci *et al.*, 2003; Ottman *et al.*, 2004; Berkovic *et al.*, 2004a; Kawamata *et al.*, 2010). The estimated penetrance of *LGI1* mutations is 67% (about two-thirds of individuals who inherit a mutation in *LGI1* will develop epilepsy) (Rosanoff & Ottman, 2008).

It is interesting to note that even one family with sensory aphasic seizures without auditory symptoms had a *LGI1* mutation (Michelucci *et al.*, 2003). Pisano *et al.* (2005) reported a family in which the *LGI1* mutation might underlie both ADLTLE and a specific interictal neuropsychological deficit of abnormal phonologic processing. There are no clinical differences between *LGI1* mutated and non-mutated families. *LGI1* mutations have also been found in about 2% of sporadic cases with focal epilepsy with auditory features of unknown aetiology (Nobile *et al.*, 2009). Twenty-five *LGI1* mutations have been described in familial and sporadic lateral temporal epilepsy patients. The mutations are distributed throughout the gene and are mostly missense mutations occurring in both the N-terminal and C-terminal protein domains. No obvious genotype-phenotype correlation can be identified, the phenotype being rather homogeneous. Both truncating and missense mutations prevent secretion of mutant proteins, suggesting that *LGI1* mutations result in a loss of function (Nobile *et al.*, 2009; Striano *et al.*, 2008).

LGI1 was first thought to be a tumour suppressor gene. The function of the LGI1 protein remains unknown but sequence analysis showed that it is not an ion channel subunit. It is probably not membrane-bound and it shares the epitempin repeat with another epilepsy gene, the *MASS1/VLGR1* gene, mutated in the Frings mouse model of audiogenic seizures (Skradski *et al.*, 2001) and in one small family with febrile seizures (Nakayama *et al.*, 2002). The LGI1 protein has a role in postnatal development of glutamatergic circuits in the hippocampus of transgenic mice: the mutant protein LGI1 inhibited dendritic pruning and increased the spine density to markedly increase excitatory synaptic transmission (Zhou *et al.*, 2009). The transmembrane proteins ADAM22 and ADAM23 constitute LGI1 receptors. Owuor *et al.* (2009) demonstrated that LGI1 binding to ADAM23 is necessary to correctly pattern neuronal morphology and connectivity between neurons, while another study (Thomas *et al.*, 2010) showed that a specific Nogo receptor 1 facilitates LGI1 binding to ADAM22. A mouse model heterozygous for the *LGI1* mutation showed lowered seizure thresholds and provided evidence for how LGI1 may serve as a major determinant of brain excitation (Fukata *et al.*, 2010): "extracellularly secreted LGI1 appeared to link two epilepsy-related receptors in the brain, ADAM22 and ADAM23, and organizes a transsynaptic protein complex that includes presynaptic potassium channels and postsynaptic AMPA receptor scaffolds. A lack of LGI1 disrupts this synaptic protein connection and selectively reduces AMPA receptor-mediated synaptic transmission in the hippocampus".

Interestingly, LGI1 is also the autoantigen associated with limbic encephalitis previously attributed to voltage-gated potassium channels (Lai *et al.*, 2010). LGI1 is the major target of potassium channel antibodies (Irani *et al.*, 2010; Yates, 2010).

In addition to *LGI1*, mutations have been recently identified in *RELN*. RELN encodes *reelin*, a glycoprotein regulating neuronal migration (Hong *et al.*, 2000) and it does not interfere with channels. An Italian-American study identified 7 heterozygous missense mutations in *RELN* in 7 families with ADEAF who did not have *LGI1* mutations (Dazzo *et al.*, 2015). A study of 40 Italian families with ADLTE recently showed that 18% harbored *RELN* mutations (Michelucci *et al.*, 2017). There were no significant clinical differences between families with *LGI1* mutations and those with *RELN* mutations, except for a higher rate of left-sided EEG abnormalities in the *RELN* families.

Familial focal (partial) epilepsy with variable foci (FFEVF)

Electroclinical features

Familial focal epilepsy with variable foci is an autosomal dominant epilepsy with focal seizures emanating from different regions of cortex in different family members (Scheffer *et al.*, 1998). Thus a single family may include individuals with frontal lobe epilepsy, temporal lobe epilepsy, parietal lobe epilepsy or occipital lobe epilepsy. Seizure semiology is constant for each individual. Eleven large families were recognized prior to gene identification (Scheffer *et al.*, 1998; Xiong *et al.*, 1999; Picard *et al.*, 2000; Callenbach *et al.*, 2003; Berkovic *et al.*, 2004b; Klein *et al.*, 2012). Penetrance is incomplete (estimated at around 60%), as suggested by the absence of a history of seizures in some obligate gene carriers.

Mean age at seizure onset is 13 years (median age, 10 years), with a large range extending from 1 month to 52 years (Berkovic *et al.*, 2004b). Not all brain regions appear equally susceptible, because most of the patients have their epileptic focus in the frontal or temporal lobe, as indicated by the ictal symptoms. Focal seizures with or without awareness occur. Temporal lobe seizures may present as psychic phenomena or olfactory hallucinations. Sixty to 86% of the patients have focal to bilateral tonic-clonic seizures. Severity of the epilepsy varies markedly within a family.

Subtly different phenotypes of FFEVF occur in different families. In some families, seizures occur exclusively or predominantly during sleep with some individuals having typical nocturnal frontal lobe epilepsy (or sleep-related hypermotor epilepsy) (Xiong *et al.*, 1999; Picard *et al.*, 2000; Berkovic *et al.*, 2004b; Scheffer *et al.*, 2014); this similarity has led to some families being diagnosed as ADNFLE and showing that ADNFLE in this setting is a subset of FFEVF. In these families, interictal epileptiform features may be rare. In other families (Scheffer *et al.*, 1998; Callenbach *et al.*, 2003; Klein *et al.*, 2012), seizures occur predominantly awake and interictal EEG studies show active epileptiform abnormalities. These discharges remain constant in location in affected individuals over many years even without ongoing seizures (Scheffer *et al.*, 1998).

Seven of 8 of the original families with FFEVF had a mutation of *DEPDC5*, with many more small FFEVF families identified (Dibbens *et al.*, 2013, see below). *DEPDC5* is a gene of the GATOR1 complex in the mTOR pathway. More than 70% of patients with *DEPDC5* mutations had frontotemporal epilepsies, including NFLE. Later many further families were found to have mutations of the other members of the GATOR1 complex, *NPRL2* and *NPRL3* (see "Molecular genetic studies"). The phenotypes of *NPRL2* and *NPRL3* are most frequently NFLE (or "SHE"), followed by TLE, and then FLE (without a nocturnal predominance) (Ricos *et al.*, 2016). Drug resistance seems higher than in other familial focal epilepsies (Picard *et al.*, 2014; Tsai *et al.*, 2017), and an increased risk of SUDEP seems to emerge with these diseases (Bagnall *et al.*, 2016; Weckhuysen *et al.*, 2016).

Epileptiform abnormalities on EEG studies have also been found in some at-risk individuals who have never had seizures (16 to 18% of the studied at-risk members) (Scheffer *et al.*, 1998; Picard *et al.*, 2000), presumably representing a marker of carrier status of the FFEVF genetic mutation. Intellectual disability is seen in rare affected family members and autism spectrum disorders have also been noted (Klein *et al.*, 2012). Neurological examination is usually normal.

While MRI was first considered to be normal in all patients, a major breakthrough took place in the field of autosomal dominant non lesional focal epilepsies in 2013 with the identification of mutations in *DEPDC5*. Focal cortical dysplasia (FCD) has since been identified in more than 15 patients from families carrying a *DEPDC5* mutation (Scheffer *et al.*, 2014; Baulac *et al.*, 2015; Scerri *et al.*, 2015; D'Gama *et al.*, 2015) and in at least 4 patients with *NPRL2* or *NPRL3* mutation (Sim *et al.*, 2016; Weckhuysen *et al.*, 2016) (see below, Molecular genetic studies). The MRI aspect is usually a bottom-of-the-sulcus dysplasia (Scheffer *et al.*, 2014) with a blurring of the grey-white matter junction and a possible transmantle sign. More rarely, subtle band heterotopias, bilateral perisylvian polymicrogyria (Ricos *et al.*, 2016) and hemimegalencephaly (D'Gama *et al.*, 2015) have been reported. The localizations are most often in the frontal lobe, premotor, superior frontal gyrus, inferior frontal gyrus, mesial prefrontal, precentral, or fronto-opercular, insular or in the cingulate cortex. In the patients with FCD, drug resistance is very high (Scheffer *et al.*, 2014; Baulac *et al.*, 2015) and intellectual disability and psychiatric disorders are more frequent.

In most cases with FFEVF, a good response to therapy with antiepileptic medications is observed. In the few patients with FCD, epilepsy surgery is an excellent option, as 6/8 patients were seizure-free after surgery and one showed worthwhile improvement (Baulac *et al.*, 2015; Sim *et al.*, 2016; Scerri *et al.*, 2015). From a histological point of view, FCD type IIa (Baulac *et al.*, 2015; Scerri *et al.*, 2015) and IIb (D'Gama *et al.*, 2015) have been reported. In case of surgery contraindication, because of the localization of the FCD or other, ketogenic diet therapies may help patients with FCD and epilepsy, as shown in children (Guerrini, 2015). Everolimus, already used for tuberous sclerosis (TSC)-associated epilepsy, is a promising future option after formal trials in GATOR1 diseases.

Molecular genetic studies

Linkage studies of the original Australian family suggested linkage to chromosome 2 (Scheffer *et al.*, 1998), while seven families were mapped to chromosome 22q11-q12, including the Australian family following reanalysis (Xiong *et al.*, 1999; Callenbach *et al.*, 2003; Berkovic *et al.*, 2004b; Klein *et al.*, 2012). Mutations in *DEPDC5*, on chromosome 22, were identified in 7 out of 8 large families with FFEVF (Dibbens *et al.*, 2013) and in 10 out of 82 families with autosomal dominant focal epilepsies that were too small for a diagnosis of FFEVF. Ishida *et al.* (2013) also identified mutations in two large FFEVF families and in 4 small families. Tsai *et al.* (2017) reported a Taiwanese FFEVF family with a *DEPDC5* mutations. DEPDC5 forms the GATOR1 complex with NPRL2 and NPRL3. GATOR1 is a repressor of the mechanistic (formerly mammalian) target of rapamycin, also known as mTOR. Together with other proteins, they make up the mTORC1 complex. This complex regulates cell proliferation, motility, survival and protein synthesis. Mutations were later found in *NPRL2* and *NPRL3* in families and sporadic cases of focal epilepsy, including asymptomatic family members (Sim *et al.*, 2016; Ricos *et al.*, 2016; Weckhuysen *et al.*, 2016). About 80% of the families with a clear diagnosis of FFEVF have mutations in GATOR1 genes.

Autosomal dominant rolandic epilepsy with speech dyspraxia and the epilepsy-aphasia spectrum disorders

This rare syndrome was first described in 1995, in an Australian family with autosomal dominant inheritance (Scheffer *et al.*, 1995b). It consisted of typical Rolandic epilepsy in most family members with the proband having a developmental and epileptic encephalopathy. Affected individuals had speech dyspraxia, persisting into adult life (Turner *et al.*, 2015). The mean age of seizure onset was 5 years (median: 6 years, range: 1.5–10 years). Seizures typically occurred in the first two hours of falling asleep and included unilateral facial and upper limb tonic and clonic activity, sometimes preceded by paraesthesia. All individuals had rare focal to bilateral tonic-clonic seizures. Epilepsy and speech dyspraxia occurred in all affected individuals except one who was elderly and gave no history of childhood seizures. The speech phenotype showed both dysarthria and dyspraxia (Turner *et al.*, 2015). The dyspraxia consisted of difficulties in organizing and coordinating the high-speed movements necessary to produce fluent and/or intelligible speech. Other oral movements requiring coordination such as moving the tongue in and out or side to side were poorly performed. Cognitive difficulties were evident in younger generations.

Interictal EEGs showed frequent epileptiform activity during the active phase of the epilepsy. Focal epileptiform discharges were localized to the centro-temporal regions, either unilateral or bilateral and independent, and activated by sleep. A horizontal dipole could be seen. Neuroimaging studies (MRI or CT brain scan) were normal.

A similar family, of French origin, in which affected members had Rolandic seizures with oral and speech dyspraxia and a variable degree of mental retardation, was mapped to chromosome Xq and a variant found in the gene *SRPX2* (Roll *et al.*, 2006). SRPX2 is a secreted sushi-repeat containing protein expressed in neurons of the human adult brain, including the Rolandic area. The mutation led to a gain-of-glycosylation of the protein. Another mutation was identified in this gene in a male with Rolandic seizures and bilateral perisylvian polymicrogyria and his maternal aunts with intellectual disability who did not have epilepsy also carried the mutation. Later this family was found to have a mutation in *GRIN2A* (see below). A third family with a variant form of Rolandic epilepsy, speech impairment, oromotor apraxia and cognitive deficit was reported (Kugler *et al.*, 2008).

Molecular genetic studies

It took eight years to identify the causative gene and it turned out to be relevant to the broad group of epilepsy-aphasia spectrum disorders (Tsai *et al.*, 2013). *GRIN2A* encodes the NR2A (GluN2A) subunit of the N-methyl-D-aspartate (NMDA) receptor, a key excitatory glutamatergic receptor. Mutations in *GRIN2A* were identified in the original Australian family and the French family. Just as importantly they were found in 9–20% of probands with epilepsy-aphasia spectrum disorders such as epileptic encephalopathy with continuous spike-wave in sleep and Landau-Kleffner syndrome (Carvill *et al.*, 2013; Lesca *et al.*, 2013). Mutations were also found in about 5% of individuals with benign epilepsy with centrotemporal spikes, although the affected individuals had a more complex phenotype suggestive of the epilepsy-aphasia spectrum disorders (Lemke *et al.*, 2013). Mutations were inherited in an autosomal dominant manner or *de novo* in sporadic cases. Functional studies were consistent with loss of function of the NMDA receptor (Carvill *et al.*, 2013; Lesca *et al.*, 2013). Many patients with *GRIN2A* mutations are being identified and a distinctive speech pattern of dysarthria and dyspraxia has been observed and assists with recognition of this disorder (Turner *et al.*, 2015).

Autosomal recessive Rolandic epilepsy with paroxysmal exercise-induced dystonia and writer's cramp

A single consanguineous Italian family has been described with this rare condition in two siblings and their first cousin (Guerrini *et al.*, 1999). During childhood, all affected individuals had rare awake unilateral orofaciobrachial seizures, during which they were dysarthric but responsive. Interictal EEGs showed Rolandic spikes. Paroxysmal exercise-induced dystonia also occurred in childhood. It presented as hemidystonia, alternating between right and left sides, or involving axial muscles. Writer's cramp began in childhood and persisted into adolescence. Neurological examination between attacks or during adolescence only revealed mild horizontal nystagmus. MRI studies were normal in all three patients.

Linkage mapping assuming autosomal recessive inheritance identified a common homozygous haplotype spanning 6 cM on chromosome 16, within the region for familial infantile convulsions and paroxysmal choreoathetosis (Szepetowski *et al.*, 1997). These two disorders could therefore be caused by the same gene.

Focal (partial) epilepsy with pericentral spikes (PEPS)

Focal epilepsy with pericentral spikes was described in a single Brazilian family as a benign syndrome with: i) onset in the first to second decade of life; ii) characteristic pericentral spikes on EEG; iii) no MRI abnormalities and no febrile seizures.

The reported seizure types are: hemiclonic, hemitonic, episodes of epigastric pain and focal seizures of temporal lobe origin. A peculiarity of this syndrome is that patients may present with more than one focal seizure type. Linkage to chromosome 4p15 was demonstrated (Kinton *et al.*, 2002).

According to Limviphuvadh *et al.* (2010), arguments based on protein sequence analysis and patient-specific chromosomal deletions are provided for *LGI2* as the prime candidate gene for PEPS among the 52 genes known at the genome locus 4p15. They suggest that patients diagnosed with PEPS or similar phenotypes be screened for mutations in *LGI2* (and other shortlisted candidate genes) to test this hypothesis.

New genetic syndromes with focal and generalized seizures

Familial adult myoclonic epilepsy (FAME)

Familial adult myoclonic epilepsy (FAME) is defined by autosomal dominant inheritance, adult onset of myoclonus of the extremities, infrequent tonic-clonic seizures in some family members and a benign course (Uyama *et al.*, 2005). It overlaps with autosomal dominant cortical myoclonus and epilepsy (ADCME), benign adult familial myoclonic epilepsy (BAFME) and familial cortical myoclonic tremor associated with epilepsy (FCMTE).

Autosomal dominant cortical myoclonus and epilepsy (ADCME) with focal and generalized seizures has been described in a family with eight affected members (Guerrini *et al.*, 2001, 2005) and likely represent a variant of FAME. Age at onset was between 12 and 50 years. All patients presented predominantly distal semi-continuous rhythmic myoclonus and generalized tonic-clonic seizures, while three also had focal impaired awareness seizures. All patients had fronto-temporal and generalized interictal EEG abnormalities.

Sixty Japanese families and a Chinese family have been mapped to chromosome 8q24 (Plaster *et al.*, 1999), while many Italian families and an Australian-New Zealand family were mapped to 2p11.1-q12.2 (de Falco *et al.*, 2003; Guerrini *et al.*, 2001, 2005; Crompton *et al.*, 2012). Additional FAME loci have been mapped to chromosome 2q11 in which a mutation in *ADRA2B* has been identified; chromosome 5p15 in which a mutation in CTNND2 was described (van Rootselaar *et al.*, 2017); chromosome 3q26.32-q28 and chromosome 1q32 in which a mutation in *CNTN2* was reported.

Very recently, a novel and fascinating type of mutation has been identified in Japanese families mapping to the chromosome 2 locus. It comprises an intronic expansion of pentanucleotide repeats, TTTCA or TTTTA, in *SAMD12* (Ishiura *et al.*, 2018). Interestingly two families that did not carry either of these repeats had similar non-coding penta-repeats identified in introns of different genes, *TNRC6A* or *RAPGEF2*. It is presumed that expansions of either the TTTCA or TTTTA motifs play a role through RNA-mediated toxicity mechanisms, irrespective of the gene in which the pentanucleotide repeat is located.

Genetic epilepsy with febrile seizures plus (GEFS+)

Although GEFS+ was initially conceptualized as a generalized familial epilepsy syndrome, subsequent reports have shown that many families include some members with focal seizures (Scheffer & Berkovic, 1997; Scheffer *et al.*, 2009; Zhang *et al.*, 2017). These include temporal and frontal lobe seizure disorders and in many cases, but not all, may follow a history of classical febrile seizures or febrile seizures plus (Abou-Khalil *et al.*, 2001; Ito *et al.*, 2002; Baulac *et al.*, 2001). In some instances, temporal lobe epilepsy has been associated with hippocampal sclerosis and, in others, the absence of hippocampal sclerosis has been demonstrated pathologically with surprisingly successful surgical outcome (Scheffer *et al.*, 2007).

Molecular genetic studies have shown sodium channel subunit gene mutations in a small proportion of GEFS+ families and include the genes encoding both the alpha 1 subunit, *SCN1A*, and the beta 1 subunit, *SCN1B* (Abou-Khalil *et al.*, 2001; Ito *et al.*, 2002; Wallace *et al.*, 2002; Scheffer *et al.*, 2007; Zhang *et al.*, 2017). In addition, mutations of the $GABA_A$ receptor subunit gene, *GABRG2*, have been associated with hemiclonic seizures (Baulac *et al.*, 2001).

GLUT1 deficiency syndrome

Finally, it has been shown that families with autosomal dominant Glucose Transporter 1 syndrome, associated with mutations of the gene *SLC2A1*, may have individuals with generalized and focal epilepsies. While generalized absence epilepsies predominate, rare family members may have multifocal or temporal lobe epilepsy (Mullen *et al.*, 2010).

REFERENCES

Abou-Khalil B, Ge Q, Desai R, *et al.* (2001): Partial and generalized epilepsy with febrile seizures plus and a novel *SCN1A* mutation. *Neurology* 57: 2265–2272.

Aridon P, Marini C, Di Resta C, *et al.* (2006): Increased sensitivity of the neuronal nicotinic receptor alpha 2 subunit causes familial epilepsy with nocturnal wandering and ictal fear. *Am J Hum* Genet 79: 342–350.

Bagnall RD, Crompton DE, Petrovski S, *et al.* (2016): Exome-based analysis of cardiac arrhythmia, respiratory control, and epilepsy genes in sudden unexpected death in epilepsy. *Ann Neurol* 79: 522–534.

Baulac S, Huberfeld G, Gourfinkel-An I, *et al.* (2001): First genetic evidence of GABA(A) receptor dysfunction in epilepsy: a mutation in the gamma2-subunit gene. *Nat Genet* 28: 46–48.

Baulac S, Ishida S, Marsan E, *et al.* (2015): Familial focal epilepsy with focal cortical dysplasia due to DEPDC5 mutations. *Ann Neurol* 77: 675–683.

Berkovic SF, McIntosh A, Howell RA, Mitchell A, Sheffield LJ, Hopper JL (1996): Familial temporal lobe epilepsy: A common disorder identified in twins. *Ann Neurol* 40: 227–235.

Berkovic SF, Izzillo P, McMahon JM, *et al.* (2004a): LGI1 mutations in temporal lobe epilepsies. *Neurology* 62: 1115–1119.

Berkovic SF, Serratosa JM, Phillips HA, *et al.* (2004b): Familial partial epilepsy with variable foci: clinical features and linkage to chromosome 22q12. *Epilepsia* 45: 1054–1060.

Bertrand D, Picard F, Le Hellard S, *et al.* (2002): How mutations in the nAChRs can cause ADNFLE epilepsy. *Epilepsia* 43 (Suppl 5): 112–122.

Bertrand D, Elmslie F, Hugues E, *et al.* (2005): The CHRNB2 mutation I312M is associated with epilepsy and distinct memory deficits. *Neurobiol Dis* 20: 799–804.

Boillot M, Baulac S (2016): Genetic models of focal epilepsies. *J Neurosci Methods* 260: 132–143.

Bonati MT, Asselta R, Duga S, *et al.* (2000): Refined mapping of CHRNA3/A5/B4 gene cluster and its implications in ADNFLE. *Neuroreport* 11: 2097–2101.

Bouchardy I, Steinlein O, Combi R, *et al.* (2011): Mutations of the orexin system, a regulator of sleep arousal, are not a common cause of ADNFLE. *Neurology* 76: 1272–1273.

Brodtkorb E, Steinlein OK, Sand T (2005): Asymmetry of long-latency auditory evoked potentials in LGI1-related autosomal dominant lateral temporal lobe epilepsy. *Epilepsia* 46: 1692–1694.

Brodtkorb E, Picard F (2006): Tobacco habits modulate autosomal dominant nocturnal frontal lobe epilepsy. *Epilepsy Behav* 9: 515–520.

Buisson B, Curtis L, Bertrand D (1999): Neuronal nicotinic acetylcholine receptor and epilepsy. In: Berkovic S, Genton P, Hirsch E, Picard F (eds) *Genetics of Focal Epilepsies*, pp. 187–202. London: John Libbey.

Callenbach PM, van den Maagdenberg AM, Hottenga JJ, *et al.* (2003): Familial partial epilepsy with variable foci in a Dutch family: clinical characteristics and confirmation of linkage to chromosome 22q. *Epilepsia* 44: 1298–1305.

Carreno M, Garcia-Alvarez D, Maestro I, *et al.* (2010): Malignant autosomal dominant frontal lobe epilepsy with repeated episodes of status epilepticus: successful treatment with vagal nerve stimulation. *Epileptic Disord* 12: 155–158.

Carvill GL, Regan BM, Yendle SC, *et al.* (2013): *GRIN2A* mutations cause epilepsy-aphasia spectrum disorders. *Nat Genet* 45: 1073–1076.

Cendes F, Lopes-Cendes I, Andermann E, Andermann F (1998): Familial temporal lobe epilepsy: A clinically heterogeneous syndrome. *Neurology* 50: 554–557.

Chen Y, Wu L, Fang Y, *et al.* (2009): A novel mutation of the nicotinic acetylcholine receptor gene CHRNA4 in sporadic nocturnal frontal lobe epilepsy. *Epilepsy Res* 83: 152–156.

Chen Z, Wang L, Wang C, *et al.* (2015): Mutational analysis of CHRNB2, CHRNA2 and CHRNA4 genes in Chinese population with autosomal dominant nocturnal frontal lobe epilepsy. *Int J Clin Exp Med* 8: 9063–9070.

Cho YW, Motamedi GK, Laufenberg I, *et al.* (2003): A Korean kindred with autosomal dominant nocturnal frontal lobe epilepsy and mental retardation. *Arch Neurol* 60: 1625–1632.

Cho YW, Yi SD, Lim JG, Kim DK, Motamedi GK (2008): Autosomal dominant nocturnal frontal lobe epilepsy and mild memory impairment associated with CHRNB2 mutation I312M in the neuronal nicotinic acetylcholine receptor. *Epilepsy Behav* 13: 361–365.

Claes L, Audenaert D, Deprez L, *et al.* (2004): Novel locus on chromosome 12q22-q23.3 responsible for familial temporal lobe epilepsy associated with febrile seizures. *J Med Genet* 41: 710–714.

Combi R, Dalprà L,Tenchini ML, Ferini-Strambi L (2004): Autosomal dominant nocturnal frontal lobe epilepsy. A critical overview. *J Neurol* 251: 923–934.

Combi R, Dalpra L, Ferini-Strambi L, Tenchini ML (2005): Frontal lobe epilepsy and mutations of the corticotropin-releasing hormone gene. *Ann Neurol* 58: 899–904.

Conti V, Aracri P, Chiti L, *et al.* (2015): Nocturnal frontal lobe epilepsy with paroxysmal arousals due to CHRNA2 loss of function. *Neurology* 84: 1520–1528.

Crompton DE, Scheffer IE, Taylor I, *et al.* (2010): Familial mesial temporal lobe epilepsy: a benign epilepsy syndrome showing complex inheritance. *Brain* 133: 3221–3231.

Crompton DE, Sadleir LG, Bromhead CJ, *et al.* (2012): Familial Adult Myoclonic Epilepsy (FAME): recognition of mild phenotypes and refinement of the 2q locus. *Arch Neurol* 69: 474–481.

Dazzo E, Santulli L, Posar A, *et al.* (2015): Autosomal dominant lateral temporal epilepsy (ADLTE): novel structural and single-nucleotide LGI1 mutations in families with predominant visual auras. *Epilepsy Res* 110: 132–138.

De Falco FA, Striano P, de Falco A, *et al.* (2003): Benign adult familial myoclonic epilepsy: genetic heterogeneity and allelism with ADCME. *Neurology* 60: 1381–1385.

De Fusco M, Becchetti A, Patrignani A, *et al.* (2000): The nicotinic receptor b2 subunit is mutant in nocturnal frontal lobe epilepsy. *Nat Genet* 26: 275–276.

Derry CP, Heron SE, Phillips F, *et al.* (2008): Severe autosomal dominant nocturnal frontal lobe epilepsy associated with psychiatric disorders and intellectual disability. *Epilepsia* 49: 2125–2129.

D'Gama AM, Geng Y, Couto JA, *et al.* (2015) Mammalian target of rapamycin pathway mutations cause hemimegalencephaly and focal cortical dysplasia. *Ann Neurol* 77: 720–725.

Diaz-Otero F, Quesada M, Morales-Corraliza J, *et al.* (2008): Autosomal dominant nocturnal frontal lobe epilepsy with a mutation in the CHRNB2 gene. *Epilepsia* 49: 516–520.

Dibbens LM, de Vries B, Donatello S, *et al.* (2013): Mutations in *DEPDC5* cause Familial Focal Epilepsy with Variable Foci. *Nat Genet* 45: 546–551.

Di Bonaventura C, Carni M, Diani E, *et al.* (2009): Drug resistant ADLTE and recurrent partial status epilepticus with dysphasic features in a family with a novel LGI1mutation: electroclinical, genetic, and EEG/fMRI findings. *Epilepsia* 50: 2481–2486.

Di Resta C[1], Ambrosi P, Curia G, Becchetti A (2010): Effect of carbamazepine and oxcarbazepine on wild-type and mutant neuronal nicotinic acetylcholine receptors linked to nocturnal frontal lobe epilepsy. *Eur J Pharmacol* 643: 13–20.

El Helou J, Navarro V, Depienne C, *et al.* (2008): K-complex-induced seizures in autosomal dominant nocturnal frontal lobe epilepsy. *Clin Neurophysiol* 119: 2201–2204.

Fedi M, Berkovic SF, Scheffer IE, *et al.* (2008): Reduced striatal D1 receptor binding in autosomal dominant nocturnal frontal lobe epilepsy. *Neurology* 71: 795–798.

Fisher RS, Cross JH, French JA, *et al.* (2017): Operational classification of seizure types by the International League Against Epilepsy: Position Paper of the ILAE Commission for Classification and Terminology. *Epilepsia* 58: 522–530.

Fonck C, Nashmi R, Deshpande P, *et al.* (2003): Increased sensitivity to agonist-induced seizures, straub tail, and hippocampal theta rhythm in knock-in mice carrying hypersensitive alpha 4 nicotinic receptors. *J Neurosci* 23: 2582–2590.

Fonck C, Cohen BN, Nashmi R, *et al.* (2005): Novel seizure phenotype and sleep disruptions in knock-in mice with hypersensitive alpha 4* nicotinic receptors. *J Neurosci* 25: 11396–11411.

Fukata Y, Lovero KL, Iwanaga T, *et al.* (2010): Disruption of LGI1-linked synaptic complex causes abnormal synaptic transmission and epilepsy. *Proc Natl Acad Sci USA* 107: 3799–3804.

Gambardella A, Messina D, Le Piane E, *et al.* (2000): Familial temporal lobe epilepsy-Autosomal dominant inheritance in a large pedigree from Southern Italy. *Epilepsy Res* 38: 127–132.

Gambardella A, Labate A, Giallonardo A, Aguglia U (2009): Familial mesial temporal lobe epilepsies: clinical and genetic features. *Epilepsia* 50 (Suppl 5): 55–57.

Grubb MS, Rossi FM, Changeux JP, Thompson ID (2003): Abnormal functional organization in the dorsal lateral geniculate nucleus of mice lacking the beta 2 subunit of the nicotinic acetylcholine receptor. *Neuron* 40: 1161–1172.

Guerrini R, Bonanni P, Nardocci N, Parmeggiani L, Casari G (1999): Autosomal recessive Rolandic epilepsy with paroxysmal exercise induced dystonia and writer's cramp: delineation of the syndrome and gene mapping to chromosome 16p12–11.2. *Ann Neurol* 45: 344–352.

Guerrini R, Bonanni P, Patrignani A, *et al.* (2001): Autosomal dominant cortical myoclonus and epilepsy (ADCME) with complex partial and generalized seizures: A newly recognized epilepsy syndrome with linkage to chromosome 2p11.1-q12.2. *Brain* 124: 2459–2475.

Guerrini R, Parmeggiani L, Marini C, Brovedani P, Bonanni P (2005): Autosomal dominant cortical myoclonus and epilepsy (ADCME) with linkage to chromosome 2p11.1-q12.2. *Adv Neurol* 95: 273–279.

Guerrini R, Duchowny M, Jayakar P, *et al.* (2015): Diagnostic methods and treatment options for focal cortical dysplasia. *Epilepsia* 56: 1669–1686.

Hayman M, Scheffer IE, Chinvarun Y, Berlangieri SU, Berkovic SF (1997): Autosomal dominant nocturnal frontal lobe epilepsy: demonstration of focal frontal onset and intrafamilial variation. *Neurology* 49: 969–975.

Heron SE, Smith KR, Bahlo M, *et al.* (2012): Missense mutations in the sodium-gated potassium channel gene *KCNT1* cause severe autosomal dominant nocturnal frontal lobe epilepsy. *Nat Genet* 44: 1188–1190.

Hirose S, Iwata H, Akiyoshi H, *et al.* (1999): A novel mutation of *CHRNA4* responsible for autosomal dominant nocturnal frontal lobe epilepsy. *Neurology* 53: 1749–1753.

Hirose S, Kurahashi H (2010): Autosomal dominant nocturnal frontal lobe epilepsy. In: Pagon RA, Bird TC, Dolan CR, Stephens K (eds) *GeneReviews*, online. Seattle (WA): University of Washington.

Hoda JC, Wanischeck M, Bertrand D, Steinlein OK (2009): Pleiotropic functional effects of the first epilepsy-associated mutation in the human *CHRNA2* gene. *FEBS Lett* 583: 1599–1604.

Hwang SK, Makita Y, Kurahashi H, Cho YW, Hirose S (2011): Autosomal dominant nocturnal frontal lobe epilepsy: a genotypic comparative study of Japanese and Korean families carrying the CHRNA4 Ser284Leu mutation. *J Hum Genet* 56: 609–612.

Irani SR, Alexander S, Waters P, *et al.* (2010): Antibodies to Kv1 potassium channel-complex proteins leucine-rich, glioma inactivated 1 protein and contactin-associated protein-2 in limbicencephalitis, Morvan's syndrome and acquired neuromyotonia. *Brain* 133: 2734–2748.

Ishida S, Picard F, Rudolf G, *et al.* (2013): Mutations of DEPDC5 cause autosomal dominant focal epilepsies. *Nat Genet* 45: 552–555.

Ishiura H, Doi K, Mitsui J, *et al.* (2018): Expansions of intronic TTTCA and TTTTA repeats in benign adult familial myoclonic epilepsy. *Nat Genet* 50: 581–590.

Ito M, Kobayashi K, Fujii T, *et al.* (2000): Electroclinical picture of autosomal dominant nocturnal frontal lobe epilepsy in a Japanese family. *Epilepsia* 41: 52–58.

Ito M, Nagafuji H, Okazawa H, *et al.* (2002): Autosomal dominant epilepsy with febrile seizures plus with missense mutations of the (Na+)-channel alpha 1 subunit gene, SCN1A. *Epilepsy Res* 48: 15–23.

Kalachikov S, Evgrafov O, Ross B, *et al.* (2002): Mutations in LGI1 cause autosomal-dominant partial epilepsy with auditory features. *Nat Genet* 30: 335–341.

Kawamata J, Ikeda A, Fujita Y, Usui K, Shimohama S, Takahashi R (2010): Mutations in LGI1 gene in Japanese families with autosomal dominant lateral temporal lobe epilepsy: the first report from Asian families. *Epilepsia* 51: 690–693.

Khatami R, Neumann M, Schulz H, Kölmel HW (1998): A family with autosomal dominant nocturnal frontal lobe epilepsy and mental retardation. *J Neurol* 245: 809–810.

Kinton L, Johnson MR, Smith SJ, *et al.* (2002): Partial epilepsy with pericentral spikes: a new familial epilepsy syndrome with evidence for linkage to chromosome 4p15. *Ann Neurol* 51: 740–749.

Klein KM, O'Brien TJ, Praveen K, *et al.* (2012): Familial focal epilepsy with variable foci mapped to chromosome 22q12: expansion of the phenotypic spectrum. *Epilepsia* 53: e151–5.

Kobayashi E, Santos NF, Torres FR, *et al.* (2003): Magnetic resonance imaging abnormalities in familial temporal lobe epilepsy with auditory auras. *Arch Neurol* 60: 1546–1551.

Kugler SL, Bali B, Lieberman P, *et al.* (2008): An autosomal dominant genetically heterogeneous variant of Rolandic epilepsy and speech disorder. *Epilepsia* 49: 1086–1090.

Labarca C, Schwarz J, Deshpande P, *et al.* (2001): Point mutant mice with hypersensitive alpha 4 nicotinic receptors show dopaminergic deficits and increased anxiety. *Proc Natl Acad Sci USA* 98: 2786–2791.

Lai M, Huijbers MG, Lancaster E, *et al.* (2010): Investigation of LGI1 as the antigen in limbic encephalitis previously attributed to potassium channels: a case series. *Lancet Neurol* 9: 776–785.

Lemke JR, Lal D, Reinthaler EM, *et al.* (2013): Mutations in *GRIN2A* cause idiopathic focal epilepsy with rolandic spikes. *Nat Genet* 45: 1067–1072.

Lena C, Popa D, Grailhe R, Escourrou P, Changeux JP, Adrien J (2004): Beta2-containing nicotinic receptors contribute to the organization of sleep and regulate putative micro-arousals in mice. *J Neurosci* 24: 5711–5718.

Leniger T, Kananura C, Hufnagel A, Bertrand S, Bertrand D, Steinlein OK (2003): A new mutation with low penetrance in nocturnal frontal lobe epilepsy. *Epilepsia* 44: 981–985.

Lesca G, Rudolf G, Bruneau N, *et al.* (2013): *GRIN2A* mutations in acquired epileptic aphasia and related childhood focal epilepsies and encephalopathies with speech and language dysfunction. *Nat Genet* 45: 1061–1066.

Limviphuvadh V, Chua LL, Eisenhaber F, Adhikari S, Maurer-Stroh S (2010): Is LGI2 the candidate gene for partial epilepsy with pericentral spikes? *J Bioinform Comput Biol* 8: 117–127.

Liu H, Lu C, Li Z, *et al.* (2011): The identification of a novel mutation of nicotinic acetylcholine receptor gene CHRNB2 in a Chinese patient: Its possible implication in non-familial nocturnal frontal lobe epilepsy. *Epilepsy Res* 95: 94–99.

Lugaresi E, Cirignotta F (1981): Hypnogenic paroxysmal dystonia: epileptic seizure or a new syndrome? *Sleep* 4: 129–138.

Lugaresi E, Cirignotta F, Montagna P (1986): Nocturnal paroxysmal dystonia. *J Neurol Neurosurg Psychiatry* 49: 375–380.

Magnusson A, Nakken KO, Brubakk E (1996): Autosomal dominant frontal lobe epilepsy. *Lancet* 347: 1191–1192.

Magnusson A, Stordal E, Brodtkorb E, Steinlein O (2003): Schizophrenia, psychotic illness and other psychiatric symptoms in families with autosomal dominant nocturnal frontal lobe epilepsy caused by different mutations. *Psychiatr Genet* 13: 91–95.

Manfredi I, Zani AD, Rampoldi L, *et al.* (2009): Expression of mutant beta2 nicotinic receptors during development is crucial for epileptogenesis. *Hum Mol Genet* 18: 1075–1088.

McLellan A, Phillips HA, Rittey C, *et al.* (2003): Phenotypic comparison of two Scottish families with mutations in different genes causing autosomal dominant nocturnal frontal lobe epilepsy. *Epilepsia* 44: 613–617.

Michelucci R, Passarelli D, Pitzalis S, Dal Corso G, Tassinari CA, Nobile C (2000): Autosomal dominant partial epilepsy with auditory features: description of a new family. *Epilepsia* 41: 967–970.

Michelucci R, Poza JJ, Sofia V, *et al.* (2003): Autosomal dominant lateral lobe epilepsy: clinical spectrum, new epi-tempin mutations, and genetic heterogeneity in seven European families. *Epilepsia 44:* 1289–1297.

Michelucci R, Pasini E, Nobile C (2009): Lateral temporal lobe epilepsies: clinical and genetic features. *Epilepsia* 50 (Suppl 5): 52–54.

Michelucci R, Pulitano P, Di Bonaventura C, *et al.* (2017): The clinical phenotype of autosomal dominant lateral temporal lobe epilepsy related to reelin mutations. *Epilepsy Behav* 68: 103–107.

Moulard B, Picard F, le Hellard S, *et al.* (2001): Ion channel variation causes idiopathic epilepsies. *Brain Res Rev* 36: 275–284.

Mullen SA, Suls A, De Jonghe P, Berkovic SF, Scheffer IE (2010): Absence epilepsies with widely variable onset are a key feature of familial GLUT1 deficiency. *Neurology* 75: 432–440.

Nakayama J, Fu YH, Clark AM, *et al.* (2002): A nonsense mutation of the *MASS1* gene in a family with febrile and afebrile seizures. *Ann Neurol* 52: 654–657.

Nichols WA, Henderson BJ, Marotta CB, *et al.* (2016): Mutation Linked to Autosomal Dominant Nocturnal Frontal Lobe Epilepsy Reduces Low-Sensitivity $\alpha 4\beta 2$, and Increases $\alpha 5\alpha 4\beta 2$, Nicotinic Receptor Surface Expression. *PLoS One* 11: e0158032.

Nobile C, Michelucci R, Andreazza S, *et al.* (2009). LGI1 mutations in autosomal dominant and sporadic lateral temporal epilepsy. *Hum Mutat* 30: 530–536.

Oldani A, Zucconi M, Ferini-Strambi L, Bizzozero D, Smirne S (1996). Autosomal dominant nocturnal frontal lobe epilepsy: electroclinical picture. *Epilepsia* 37: 964–976.

Oldani A, Zucconi M, Asselta R, *et al.* (1998): Autosomal dominant nocturnal frontal lobe epilepsy. A video-polysomnographic and genetic appraisal of 40 patients and delineation of the epileptic syndrome. *Brain* 121: 205–223.

Ottman R, Risch N, Hauser WA, *et al.* (1995): Localization of a gene for partial epilepsy to chromosome 10q. *Nat Genet* 10: 56–60.

Ottman R, Winaver MR, Kalachikov S, *et al.* (2004): LGI1 mutations in autosomal dominant partial epilepsy with auditory features. *Neurology* 62: 1120–1126.

Ottman R, Rosenberger L, Bagic A, *et al.* (2008): Altered language processing in autosomal dominant partial epilepsy with auditory features. *Neurology* 71: 1973–1980.

Owuor K, Harel NY, Englot DJ, Hisama F, Blumenfeld H, Strittmatter SM (2009): LGI1-associated epilepsy through altered ADAM23-dependent neuronal morphology. *Mol Cell Neurosci* 42: 448–457.

Phillips HA, Scheffer IE, Crossland KM, *et al.* (1998): Autosomal dominant nocturnal frontal lobe epilepsy: genetic heterogeneity and a probable second locus at 15q24. *AmJ Hum Genet* 63: 1108–1116.

Phillips HA, Marini C, Scheffer IE, Sutherland GR, Mulley JC, Berkovic SF (2000): A *de novo* mutation in a family with autosomal dominant nocturnal frontal lobe epilepsy. *Ann Neurol* 48: 264–267.

Phillips HA, Favre I, Kirkpatrick M, *et al.* (2001): CHRNB2 is the second acetylcholine receptor subunit associated with autosomal dominant nocturnal frontal lobe epilepsy. *Am J Hum Genet* 68: 225–231.

Picard F, Bertrand S, Steinlein O, Bertrand D (1999): Mutated nicotinic receptors responsible for autosomal dominant nocturnal frontal lobe epilepsy are more sensitive to carbamazepine. *Epilepsia* 40: 1198–1209.

Picard F, Baulac S, Kahane P, *et al.* (2000): Dominant partial epilepsies: a clinical, electrophysiological and genetic study of 19 European families. *Brain* 123: 1247–1262.

Picard F, Bruel D, Servent D, *et al.* (2006): Alteration of the *in vivo* nicotinic receptor density in ADNFLE patients: a PET study. *Brain* 129: 2047–2060.

Picard F, Mégevand P, Minotti L, *et al.* (2007): Intracerebral recordings of nocturnal hyperkinetic seizures: demonstration of a longer duration of the pre-seizure sleep spindle. *Clin Neurophysiol* 118: 928–939.

Picard F, Pegna AJ, Arntsberg V, *et al.* (2009): Neuropsychological disturbances in frontal lobe epilepsy due to mutated nicotinic receptors. *Epilepsy Behav* 14: 354–359.

Picard F, Makrythanasis P, Navarro V, *et al.* (2014): *DEPDC5* mutations in families presenting as autosomal dominant nocturnal frontal lobe epilepsy. *Neurology* 82: 2101–2106.

Pisano T, Marini C, Brovedani P, *et al.* (2005): Abnormal phonologic processing in familial lateral temporal lobe epilepsy due to a new LGI1 mutation. *Epilepsia* 46: 118–123.

Plaster NM, Uyama E, Uchino M, *et al.* (1999): Genetic localization of the familial adult myoclonic epilepsy (FAME) gene to chromosome 8q24. *Neurology* 56: 1180–1183.

Poza JJ, Saenz A, Martinez-Gil A, *et al.* (1999): Autosomal dominant lateral temporal epilepsy: clinical and genetic study of a large basque pedigree linked to chromosome 10q. *Ann Neurol* 42: 182–188.

Regesta G, Tanganelli P (2002): Temporal lobe epilepsy of adult age of possible idiopathic nature. *Seizure* 11: 131–135.

Ricos MG, Hodgson BL, Pippucci T, *et al.* (2016): Mutations in the mammalian target of rapamycin pathway regulators NPRL2 and NPRL3 cause focal epilepsy. *Ann Neurol* 79: 120–131.

Rodrigues-Pinguet N, Jia L, Li M, *et al.* (2003): Five ADNFLE mutations reduce the Ca2+ dependence of the mammalian alpha4beta2 acetylcholine response. *J Physiol* 550: 11–26.

Roll P, Rudolf G, PereiraS, *et al.* (2006): SRPX2 mutations in disorders of language cortex and cognition. *Hum Mol Genet* 15: 1195–1207.

Rosanoff MJ, Ottman R (2008): Penetrance of LGI1 mutations in autosomal dominant partial epilepsy with auditory features. *Neurology* 71: 567–571.

Ross SA, Wong JYF, Clifford JJ, *et al.* (2000): Phenotypic characterization of an α4 neuronal nicotinic acetylcholine subunit knockout mouse. *J Neuroscience* 20: 6431–6441.

Rozycka A, Skorupska E, Kostyrko A, Wieslaw H, Trzceciak H (2003): Evidence for S284L mutation of the CHRNA4 in a white family with autosomal dominant nocturnal frontal lobe epilepsy. *Epilepsia* 44: 1113–1117.

Ryvlin P, Minotti L, Demarquay G, *et al.* (2006): Nocturnal hypermotor seizures, suggesting frontal lobe epilepsy, can originate in the insula. *Epilepsia* 47: 755–765.

Saenz A, Galan J, Caloustian C, *et al.* (1999): Autosomal dominant nocturnal frontal lobe epilepsy in a Spanish family with a ser252phe mutation in the CHRNA4 gene. *Arch Neurol* 56: 1004–1009.

Scerri T, Riseley JR, Gillies G, *et al.* (2015): Familial cortical dysplasia type IIA caused by a germline mutation in DEPDC5. *Ann Clin Transl Neurol* 2: 575–580.

Scheffer IE, Berkovic SF (1997): Generalized epilepsy with febrile seizures plus. A genetic disorder with heterogeneous clinical phenotypes. *Brain* 120: 479–490.

Scheffer IE, Bhatia KP, Lopes-Cendes I, *et al.* (1994): Autosomal dominant frontal epilepsy misdiagnosed as sleep disorder. *Lancet* 343: 515–517.

Scheffer IE, Bhatia KP, Lopes-Cendes I, *et al.* (1995a): Autosomal dominant nocturnal frontal lobe epilepsy. A distinctive clinical disorder. *Brain* 118: 61–73.

Scheffer IE, Jones L, Pozzebon M, Howell RA, Saling MM, Berkovic SF (1995b): Autosomal dominant Rolandic epilepsy and speech dyspraxia: A new syndrome with anticipation. *Ann Neurol* 38: 633–642.

Scheffer IE, Phillips HA, O'Brien CE, *et al.* (1998): Familial partial epilepsy with variable foci: A new partial epilepsy syndrome with suggestion of linkage to chromosome 2. *Ann Neurol* 44: 890–899.

Scheffer IE, Harkin LA, Grinton BE, *et al.* (2007): Temporal lobe epilepsy and GEFS+ phenotypes associated with SCN1B mutations. *Brain* 130: 100–109.

Scheffer IE, Zhang YH, Jansen FE, Dibbens L (2009): Dravet syndrome orgenetic (generalized) epilepsy with febrile seizures *plus*? *Brain Dev* 31: 394–400.

Scheffer IE, Heron SE, Regan BM, *et al.* (2014): Mutations in mammalian target of rapamycin regulator DEPDC5 cause focal epilepsy with brain malformations. *Ann Neurol* 75: 782–787.

Scheffer IE, Berkovic S, Capovilla G, *et al.* (2017): ILAE classification of the epilepsies: Position paper of the ILAE Commission for Classification and Terminology. *Epilepsia* 58: 512–521.

Sgard F, Bertrand S, Charpantier E, *et al.* (2000): Alpha10, a novel human nicotinic acetylcholine receptor subunit. XXXth Annual congress of the Society For Neurosciences. New-Orleans USA; Poster 613.5.

Shiba Y, Mori F, Yamada J, *et al.* (2015): Spontaneous epileptic seizures in transgenic rats harboring a human ADNFLE missense mutation in the β2-subunit of the nicotinic acetylcholine receptor. *Neurosci Res* 100: 46–54.

Sim JC, Scerri T, Fanjul-Fernández M, *et al.* (2016): Familial cortical dysplasia caused by mutation in the mammalian target of rapamycin regulator NPRL3. *Ann Neurol* 79: 132–137.

Skradski SL, Clark AM, Jiang H, White HS, Fu YH, Ptâcek LJ (2001): A novel gene causing a mendelian audiogenic mouse epilepsy. *Neuron* 31: 537–544.

Son CD, Moss FJ, Cohen BN, Lester HA (2009): Nicotine normalizes intracellular subunit stoichiometry of nicotinic receptors carrying mutations linked to autosomal dominant nocturnal frontal lobe epilepsy. *Mol Pharmacol* 75: 1137–1148.

Steinlein OK, Mulley JC, Propping P, *et al.* (1995): A missense mutation in the neuronal nicotinic acetylcholine receptor α4 subunit is associated with autosomal dominant nocturnal frontal lobe epilepsy. *Nat Genet* 11: 201–203.

Steinlein OK, Magnusson A, Stoodt J, *et al.* (1997): An insertion mutation of the CHRNA4gene in a family with autosomal dominant nocturnal frontal lobe epilepsy. *Hum Mol Genet* 6: 943–948.

Steinlein OK, Stoodt J, Mulley JC, Berkovic SF, Scheffer IE, Brodtkorb E (2000): Independent occurence of the CHRNA4 Ser248Phe mutation in a Norwegian family with nocturnal frontal lobe epilepsy. *Epilepsia* 41: 529–535.

Steinlein OK, Hoda JC, Bertrand S, Bertrand D (2012): Mutations in familial nocturnal frontal lobe epilepsy might be associated with distinct neurological phenotypes. *Seizure* 21: 118–123.

Striano P, de Falco A, Diani E, *et al.* (2008): A novel loss-of-function LGI1 mutation linked to autosomal dominant lateral temporal epilepsy. *Arch Neurol* 65: 939–942.

Szepetowski P, Rochette J, Berquin P, Piussan C, Lathrop GM, Monaco AP (1997): Familial infantile convulsions and paroxysmal choreoathetosis: a new neurological syndrome linked to the pericentromeric region of human chromosome 16. *Am J Hum Genet* 61: 889–898.

Teper Y, Whyte D, Cahir E, *et al.* (2007): Nicotine-induced dystonic arousal complex in a mouse line harboring a human autosomal-dominant nocturnal frontal lobe epilepsy mutation. *J Neurosci* 27: 10128–10142.

Thomas R, Favell K, Morante-Redolat J, *et al.* (2010): LGI1 is a Nogo receptor 1 ligand that antagonizes myelin-based growth inhibition. *J Neurosci* 30: 6607–6612.

Tinuper P, Bisulli F, Cross JH, *et al.* (2016): Definition and diagnostic criteria of sleep-related hypermotor epilepsy. *Neurology* 86: 1834–1842.

Tritto T, McCallum SE, Waddle SA, *et al.* (2004): Null mutant analysis of responses to nicotine: deletion of beta2 nicotinic acetylcholine receptor subunit but not alpha7 subunit reduces sensitivity to nicotine-induced locomotor depression and hypothermia. *Nicotine Tob Res* 6: 145–158.

Tsai MH, Vears DF, Turner SJ, *et al.* (2013): Clinical genetic study of the epilepsy-aphasia spectrum. *Epilepsia* 54: 280–287.

Tsai MH, Chan CK, Chang YC, *et al.* (2017): DEPDC5 mutations in familial and sporadic focal epilepsy. *Clin Genet* 92: 397–404.

Turner SJ, Mayes AK, Verhoeven A, Mandelstam SA, Morgan AT, Scheffer IE (2015): *GRIN2A*: an aptly named gene for speech dysfunction. *Neurology* 84: 586–593.

Uyama E, Fu YH, Ptacek LJ (2005): Familial adult myoclonic epilepsy (FAME). *Adv Neurol* 95: 281–288.

Vadlamudi L, Scheffer IE, Berkovic SF (2003): Genetic of temporal lobe epilepsy. *J Neurol Neurosurg Psychiatry* 74: 1359–1361.

van Rootselaar AF, Groffen AJ, de Vries B, *et al.* (2017): delta-Catenin (CTNND2) missense mutation in familial cortical myoclonic tremor and epilepsy. *Neurology* 89: 2341–2350.

Wallace RH, Scheffer IE, Parasivam G, *et al.* (2002): Generalized epilepsy with febrile seizures plus: mutation of the sodium channel subunit SCN1 B. *Neurology* 58: 1426–1429.

Wang MY, Liu XZ, Wang J, Wu LW (2014): A novel mutation of the nicotinic acetylcholine receptor gene CHRNA4 in a Chinese patient with non-familial nocturnal frontal lobe epilepsy. *Epilepsy Res* 108: 1927–1931.

Weckhuysen S, Marsan E, Lambrecq V, *et al.* (2016): Involvement of GATOR complex genes in familial focal epilepsies and focal cortical dysplasia. *Epilepsia* 57: 994–1003.

Willoughby JO, Pope KJ, Eaton V (2003): Nicotine as an antiepileptic agent in ADNFLE: an N-of-one study. *Epilepsia* 44: 1238–1240.

Winaver MR, Ottman R, Hauser WA, Pedley TA (2000): Autosomal dominant partial epilepsy with auditory features: defining the phenotype. *Neurology* 54: 2173–2176.

Wood AG, Saling MM, Fedi M, *et al.* (2010): Neuropsychological function in patients with a single gene mutation associated with autosomal dominant nocturnal frontal lobe epilepsy. *Epilepsy Behav* 17: 531–535.

Xiong L, Labuda M, Li DS, *et al.* (1999): Mapping of a gene determining familial partial epilepsy with variable foci to chromosome 22q11-q12. *Am J Hum Genet* 65: 1698–1710.

Yates D (2010): Neuroimmunology: Antibodies target LGI1 rather than potassium channels in limbic encephalitis. *Nat Rev Neurol* 6: 467.

Zhang Y-H, Burgess R, Malone JP, *et al.* (2017): Genetic Epilepsy with Febrile Seizures Plus: Refining the spectrum. *Neurology* 89: 1210–1219.

Zhou YD, Lee S, Jin Z, *et al.* (2009): Arrested maturation of excitatory synapses in autosomal dominant lateral temporal lobe epilepsy. *Nat Med* 15: 1208–1214.

Zhu G, Okada M, Yoshida S, *et al.* (2008): Rats harboring S284L Chrna4 mutation show attenuation of synaptic and extrasynaptic GABAergic transmission and exhibit the nocturnal frontal lobe epilepsy phenotype. *J Neurosci* 28: 12465–12476.

CHAPTER 26
AUTOIMMUNE EPILEPSIES AND ENCEPHALOPATHIES

Sukhvir Wright[1,2] and Angela Vincent[3]

[1] School of Life and Health Sciences, Aston University, Birmingham, United Kingdom
[2] Department of Paediatric Neurology, Birmingham Children's Hospital, Birmingham, United Kingdom
[3] Weatherall Institute of Molecular Medicine and Nuffield Department of Clinical Neurosciences, John Radcliffe University Hospital, Oxford, United Kingdom

Introduction

When antibodies were first discovered in blood by Jules Bordet at the turn of the 20th century, early researchers believed antibodies and the immune system were solely designed to protect us from disease. The concept of *autoimmune* disease, where the immune system itself becomes a destructive pathological force acting against the host's own cells, was coined "horror autotoxicus" by Paul Ehrlich, meaning the immune system could never turn on itself. This was following experiments where he failed to show the production of autoantibodies in goats who were immunized with their own red blood cells (Chang, 2014; Mackay, 2010). Ehrlich's condemnation of autoimmunity overshadowed the interpretation of important discoveries over the next 30 years including early models of experimental autoimmune encephalomyelitis relevant to multiple sclerosis (EAE) (Rivers & Schwentker, 1935). The discoveries of the Coombs test in autoimmune haemolytic anaemia, anti-nuclear antibodies in SLE, rheumatoid factor and thyroid receptor antibodies during the 1940s and 1950s heralded the beginning of the acceptance of autoimmunity as a pathological process. These discoveries were translated into animal models, and improvements in microscopy enabled detection of immunological deposits in frozen sections of tissues and detection of antibodies in serum of patients with suspected autoimmune diseases (Mackay, 2010).

In 1957, guidelines to establish whether a human disease was autoimmune in origin were published by Witebsky (Witebsky *et al.*, 1957), modelled on Koch's postulates to define microbiological pathogenicity. These defining criteria for autoantibody pathogenicity were revised in light of advances in molecular biology and require evidence from three main areas, listed in *Table I* (Rose &Bona, 1993).

In the 1970s, autoimmunity as a disease mechanism in the nervous system gained credence with the discovery of pathogenic *peripheral* nervous system autoantibodies as described in myasthenia gravis (acetylcholine receptor (AChR) antibodies) and Lambert-Eaton syndrome (pre-synaptic voltage-gated calcium channels (VGCC:P/Q type). These classical autoantibody-mediated diseases fulfil Witebsky's criteria as the autoantibodies bind to the extracellular domain of membrane proteins, can be measured easily in patient serum, cause pathologically relevant effects *in vivo* and *in vitro*, and affected patients show substantial improvements with immunotherapy (Lang *et al.*, 1984; Newsom-Davis *et al.*, 1978b; Newsom-Davis *et al.*, 1978a; Toyka *et al.*, 1977). Many of these features are also directly applicable to the now well recognised central nervous system autoantibodies (for example to the N-methyl-D-aspartate receptor (NMDAR)), that play a pathogenic role in epileptic encephalopathy in both adults and children. In this chapter, we will discuss the link between inflammation, autoimmune disease and epilepsy, the neuronal autoantibodies most relevant to paediatric encephalopathy and epilepsy, as well as review existing evidence on diagnosis, treatment and evidence of pathogenicity.

Inflammation, autoimmune disease and epilepsy

The central nervous system is no longer considered "immune-privileged", or separate, from the effects and influence of the innate and adaptive immune system both locally within the brain and

Table I Modified Witebsky's postulates of pathogenicity define an autoimmune disease

Presence of an antibody that can bind the target antigen or tissue
Reproduction of disease in a normal recipient by direct transfer of autoantibody – An example is transplacental transmission of pathogenic autoantibodies from an affected mother to foetus in utero. This also applies to direct infusion of pathogenic human autoantibodies to experimental animals.
Reproduction of autoimmune diseases in experimental animal models – Here, once the antigen is identified in the human disease, the equivalent antigen is isolated in an experimental animal and the essential features of the disease are reproduced by active immunization.
Circumstantial evidence from clinical clues – These include clinical history of other autoimmune diseases in the same individual or family members, lymphocytic infiltration of target organ, HLA association and favourable response to immunotherapy.

systemically (Kipnis, 2016; Ransohoff *et al.*, 2003; Banks & Erickson, 2010). These inflammatory processes can precipitate and sustain seizure activity through neuronal hyper-excitability and may contribute to the development of refractory epilepsy in the longer term (Vezzani *et al.*, 2011; Marchi *et al.*, 2014).

Febrile seizures and Rasmussen's encephalitis are examples of paediatric epilepsy syndromes closely linked to brain inflammation and are discussed in detail in Chapters 9 and 18 of this book. Other childhood epilepsy syndromes, although not directly thought to be "neuroimmunological" are treated with and respond well to immunotherapy. An example includes West syndrome/infantile spasms, an electroclinical infantile epileptic encephapalopathy syndrome, where hormonal treatment (adrenocorticotrophic hormone and/or prednisolone) alone or combined with vigabatrin is an effective treatment for stopping the spasms (O'Callaghan *et al.*, 2017; Hancock *et al.*, 2013). Corticosteroids and other immunotherapies including intravenous immunoglobulin (IVIG), have also been used in the treatment of patients on the epilepsy-aphasia spectrum including those with Landau-Kleffner syndrome (LKS) and continuous spike and waves during slow-wave sleep syndrome (CSWSS) (Buzatu *et al.*, 2009; Mikati *et al.*, 2002; Arts *et al.*, 2009). However, here, the evidence for efficacy is limited to case series and retrospective reports, and the relevance of autoimmunity as a disease process has not yet been proven (Granata *et al.*, 2011). Moreover, two Cochrane reviews have not found sufficient evidence for the efficacy of corticosteroids in treating childhood epilepsies, apart from epileptic spasms (Mehta *et al.*, 2015; Gayatri *et al.*, 2007).

Systemic autoimmune/inflammatory disorders that are known to be associated with an increased risk of epilepsy and other neurological symptoms include systemic lupus erythromatous (SLE) and Hashimoto's thyroiditis. In SLE, the proportion of patients with epilepsy is significantly higher than controls (Watad *et al.*, 2018), although the exact disease mechanism is not yet known (Palace & Lang, 2000). These and other similar observations have led to wider studies investigating the association of epilepsy and autoimmune disease. One such population-level study in the United States, found the risk of epilepsy was significantly heightened among patients with autoimmune diseases, and this effect was especially pronounced in children (Ong *et al.*, 2014).

The next sections and main aim of this chapter are to describe the conditions associated with specific central nervous system autoantibodies, but it is first important to mention how the antibodies are measured.

Neuronal antibody tests

Immunohistology

Many groups use immunohistology for the detection of antibodies binding to neuronal proteins. Rodent brain sections are fixed and exposed to diluted serum or CSF. IgG antibodies are then detected with a secondary anti-human IgG labelled with an enzymic or fluorescent probe. This method can detect with some confidence certain antibodies, but in most cases needs to be followed up by specific tests.

Cell-based assays

Over the last 20 years, most novel antibody detection has involved establishment of an antigen-specific cell-based assay (CBA). These are based on the binding of patient IgG antibodies to the surface of human embryonic kidney (HEK) cells which have been transfected with DNAs for the antigen (Leite *et al.*, 2010; Irani *et al.*, 2010b). There are two main versions of the CBA: transfected cells that are exposed to the patients' antibodies while still alive (*i.e.* before fixation), so as to ensure that only antibodies binding to the extracellular domains are identified, or transfected cells that are fixed and permeabilised before exposure to the antibodies. The latter are more convenient as they can be stored at 4° C, but they can show reduced sensitivity or detect antibodies that bind to intracellular, non-pathogenic epitopes.

There are now also commercial antibody kits that can be used. The main source provides chips containing a mosaic of cells with different antigens on their surface. A single dilution of serum or CSF is applied and binding to one of the different antigens (*e.g.*, NMDAR, AMPAR, GABARs) can be determined. These kits are very useful and now widely available.

When requesting antibody tests, it is important to be aware of the relevance of serum or CSF testing. Serum is always diluted for testing, whereas CSF can be applied undiluted. Ideally both should be tested (paired serum and CSF samples). The general recommendation is to test CSF for NMDAR, AMPAR and GABAR antibodies, but for LGI1 and CASPR2 (antibodies complexed to the voltage gated potassium channel), serum can be more useful as the CSF levels tend to be low.

Neuronal antibody mediated epileptic encephalopathies NMDA receptor antibody encephalitis

Presentation

Synaptic function and transmission is essential for the processing and storing of information in the central nervous system. Excitatory synaptic transmission is mediated by the neurotransmitter glutamate and glutamate receptors of both metabotropic (*e.g.*, mGluRs, G protein coupled receptors) and ionotropic class (ligand-gated ion channel). The N-methyl-D-aspartic receptor (NMDAR) is an ionotropic glutamate receptor; activation of the receptor is required for long-term potentiation and long-term depression, processes thought to underlie learning and memory (Bear & Malenka, 1994). The functional importance of NMDARs in normal brain function and neural plasticity is best illustrated by the catastrophic neuroimmunological syndrome seen in NMDAR-Ab encephalitis patients when specific circulating antibodies bind to the extracellular membrane portion of the receptor, causing defects in normal synaptic function (Dalmau *et al.*, 2008).

The first cases of NMDAR-Ab encephalitis were described in young females (age 14–44 years) presenting with a severe encephalopathy displaying psychiatric symptoms, seizures, cognitive and autonomic dysfunction, florid movement disorders, and decreased levels of consciousness, that in some cases led to hypoventilation, coma and death (Dalmau *et al.*, 2007). Interestingly in this case series, all patients had a teratoma (11 ovarian, one mature teratoma in the mediastinum), and given their positive clinical response to tumour removal and immunotherapy, NMDAR-Ab encephalitis was initially reported as a paraneoplastic encephalitis in young women. All subsequent studies have expanded the affected groups of patients and described cases in both males and females, adults and children, with and without underlying tumours (Irani *et al.*, 2010b; Armangue *et al.*, 2013; Titulaer *et al.*, 2013, Florance *et al.*, 2009, Wright *et al.*, 2015a). In children, the estimated incidence of NMDAR-Ab encephalitis is 0.85 per million children per year (from a United Kingdom Study [Wright *et al.*, 2015a]). An associated tumour with NMDAR-Ab encephalitis is predominantly found in female patients (14–45 years), and nearly all (96%) are ovarian teratomas (Titulaer *et al.*, 2013), as described in the first case series. Other malignancies have also been found in NMDAR-Ab encephalitis patients, including testicular teratomas, Hodgkin's lymphoma, small cell carcinoma, glioblastoma and neuroblastoma (Irani *et al.*, 2010b; Zandi *et al.*, 2009; Fujii *et al.*, 2013). Tumours are much less common in young children, the youngest reported patient with NMDAR-Ab encephalitis and a tumour was 7 years old (Titulaer *et al.*, 2013).

Even though the characteristic symptoms described above seen during the illness in both adults and children, there has been some debate as to the symptom presentation of disease in these two groups of patients (Rosenfeld *et al.*, 2012). In adults, the most common presenting symptoms are, on the whole, neuropsychiatric, for example delusions, hallucinations, psychosis and abnormal behaviour. Some studies have suggested that a more *neurological* phenotype including abnormal movements, seizures and focal or sensory deficits are more commonly the first symptoms in children (Armangue *et al.*, 2013; Favier *et al.*, 2018). However, even in the youngest patients, bizarre and atypical behaviour is well recognised and needs to be actively sought in the clinical history (Wright *et al.*, 2015a; Goldberg *et al.*, 2014). Speech delay and even "autistic regression" has been described in the presentation, with stereotypies, expressive dysphasia and mutism seen in both autism and NMDAR-Ab encephalitis; occurrence of these symptoms in cases of subacute neuroregression in patients < 3 years, should prompt testing of NMDAR antibodies (Hacohen *et al.*, 2016; Scott *et al.*, 2014). As in younger patients, the complex neuropsychiatric presentation of NMDAR-Ab encephalitis can lead to a delayed diagnosis in adult patients with pre-existing intellectual disability and autism, who may also have communication difficulties. Disruption in sleep, low mood, confusion, and even autonomic symptoms are commonly attributed to neuroleptic malignant syndrome or catatonia (Kiani *et al.*, 2015). Increased awareness of NMDAR-Ab encephalitis will ensure early testing for the disease and prompt therapeutic decisions to improve outcomes.

Further expansion of the NMDAR-Ab encephalitis phenotype has included patients presenting with predominance of one of the major symptoms (on occasion without co-existing encephalopathy), for example movement disorder (Hacohen *et al.*, 2014b) psychiatric features (Kayser *et al.*, 2013), and seizures (Niehusmann *et al.*, 2009).

The five cases of temporal lobe epilepsy in young women presented by Niehusmann *et al.*, all had associated features of NMDAR-Ab encephalitis, which included psychiatric disturbance, speech dysfunction, decreased level of consciousness. Four out of five patients responded to immunotherapy (Niehusmann *et al.*, 2009). An observational study describing 13 adult male patients, found 61.5% (8/13) presented initially with a seizure which was focal in five (Viaccoz *et al.*, 2014). By contrast, only 8/58 (12%) female cases presented with seizures initially, and these were mostly generalized. A similar study in a large cohort of 577 patients, found that even though seizures as an initial symptom were more common in men than women (27% *vs.* 11%); in both groups psychiatric features were still the most frequent initial symptom (Titulaer & Dalmau, 2014).

NMDAR-Ab encephalitis can also present *de novo* in the recovery period following viral mediated encephalitis as seen with Herpes simplex virus (HSV) encephalitis. Often previously misdiagnosed as a HSV relapse, recurrent failure to isolate the virus in the relapse CSF samples and the florid movement disorder on presentation (particularly in children), led to the discovery that these relapses were in fact NMDAR-Ab mediated (Hacohen *et al.*, 2014a; Mohammad *et al.*, 2014; Hoftberger *et al.*, 2013a). Patients respond to immunotherapy with no evidence of viral recurrence following use of immunomodulatory therapies (Armangue *et al.*, 2015; Armangue *et al.*, 2014).

Underlying malignancy and previous HSV infection are the main susceptibility factors for NMDAR-Ab encephalitis identified to date, as no conclusive genetic associations have yet been made. However, one paediatric case series from New Zealand found a higher incidence of NMDAR-Ab encephalitis in children with Maori or pacific Island ancestry as well as a more severe phenotype, suggesting genetic susceptibility may be a factor in some populations (Jones *et al.*, 2017).

Investigations

NMDAR-Ab antibodies are present in the CSF and serum of affected patients, with positivity confirmed by combinations of testing with immunohistology (binding of antibodies to rodent brain slices), immunocytochemistry (binding of antibodies to neuronal cultures *in vitro*), and cell based assay (CBA) techniques, as described above). For maximal sensitivity and specificity serum *and* CSF samples should be tested in all suspected cases of autoimmune encephalitis including NMDAR-Ab encephalitis (Irani *et al.*, 2014); for determination of relapse, CSF antibody titres may be more predictive (Gresa-Arribas *et al.*, 2014).

Interestingly, conventional brain MRI scans are normal in up to 79% of affected patients (Titulaer *et al.*, 2013; Wright *et al.*, 2015a; Irani *et al.*, 2010b), with abnormalities identified as being reversible, subtle, grey and white matter non-enhancing lesions. This clinic-radiological paradox has since been further explained by results of functional brain imaging studies which demonstrate alterations and impairment of functional connectivity in large scale networks (Finke *et al.*, 2013; Peer *et al.*, 2017): memory impairment correlated with hippocampal and medial temporal lobe network connectivity, and psychosis symptoms correlated with disruption to fronto-pariental networks, offering some explanation for the major clinical symptoms (Peer *et al.*, 2017).

In comparison to the low yield of diagnostic positivity in conventional MRI, the EEG in NMDAR-Ab encephalitis is abnormal in > 90% of patients (Armangue *et al.*, 2013; Titulaer *et al.*, 2013; Wright *et al.*, 2015a); most commonly reported as encephalopathic with or without epileptiform discharges. "Extreme delta brush" describes a distinct EEG waveform found in up to 30% of NMDAR-Ab encephalitis patients during the illness, and is characterised by rhythmic delta activity superimposed with beta frequency oscillations on each delta wave (Schmitt *et al.*, 2012; Kirkpatrick *et al.*, 2011; Veciana *et al.*, 2015). Previously only described in premature infants, it is most commonly seen in severely affected adult patients, perhaps reflecting prolonged illness and intensive care admission. Reports of paediatric patient EEGs suggest that early and longitudinal EEG patterns can be pathognomonic and aid in the differentiation between epileptiform and non-epileptiform movements (Gitiaux *et al.*, 2013; Nosadini *et al.*, 2014; Gataullina *et al.*, 2011). Recent studies have used EEG data from NMDAR-Ab encephalitis patients to non-invasively assess the synaptic level dysfunction using dynamic causal modelling (Symmonds *et al.*, 2018; Cooray *et al.*, 2015). These methods hold promise for future non-invasive assessment of treatment effects and prediction of prognosis in affected patients.

Table II summarises the current expert consensus opinion on the diagnostic criteria for NMDAR-Ab encephalitis in adults (Graus *et al.*, 2016). These diagnostic criteria have also been shown to have high sensitivity and specificity in paediatric patients, with all positive patients fulfilling the criteria within a median of 2 weeks (range 1–6 weeks) from first symptom onset (Ho *et al.*, 2017). The criteria can guide the prompt use of immunotherapy before antibody results are available.

Treatment and outcome

As in most autoantibody-mediated diseases, treatment of NMDAR-Ab encephalitis is aimed at removal of circulating antibodies (plasma exchange) and suppression of the immune system with steroids (often referred to as "1st line" immunotherapy) or reduced production of antibodies (using Rituximab and other immunomodulatory agents), referred to as "2nd line" treatment. The removal of an associated tumour if present, and any additional oncological therapy, is essential and correlates with improved outcome overall (Dalmau

Table II **Diagnostic criteria for NMDAR-Ab encephalitis (From Graus *et al.*, 2016)**

*Probable anti-NMDA receptor encephalitis**

Diagnosis can be made when all three of the following criteria have been met:

1. Rapid onset (less than 3 months) of at least four of the six following major groups of symptoms:
   - Abnormal (psychiatric) behaviour or cognitive dysfunction
   - Speech dysfunction (pressured speech, verbal reduction, mutism)
   - Seizures
   - Movement disorder, dyskinesias, or rigidity/abnormal postures
   - Decreased level of consciousness
   - Autonomic dysfunction or central hypoventilation

2. At least one of the following laboratory study results:
   - Abnormal EEG (focal or diffuse slow or disorganised activity, epileptic activity, or extreme delta brush)
   - CSF with pleocytosis or oligoclonal bands

3. Reasonable exclusion of other disorders

Diagnosis can also be made in the presence of three of the above groups of symptoms accompanied by a systemic teratoma

*Definite anti-NMDA receptor encephalitis**

Diagnosis can be made in the presence of one or more of the six major groups of symptoms and the presence of IgG anti-GluN1 antibodies†, after reasonable exclusion of other disorders

* Patients with a history of herpes simplex virus encephalitis in the previous weeks might have relapsing immune-mediated neurological symptoms (post-herpes simplex virus encephalitis). †Antibody testing should include testing of CSF. If only serum is available, confirmatory tests should be included (e.g., live neurons or tissue immunohistochemistry, in addition to cell-based assay).

et al., 2008). With early recognition and prompt treatment, a significant neurological improvement is seen in 81% of patients (Titulaer *et al.*, 2013). There is no controlled trial to provide high quality evidence on the optimal therapeutic strategy, however a large cohort analysis appears to suggest the additional benefits of second line therapy when first line therapy fails (Titulaer *et al.*, 2013). Relapses occur in 12–23% of patients, are often less severe than the original disease episode and respond to immunotherapy (Titulaer *et al.*, 2013; Wright *et al.*, 2015a; Irani *et al.*, 2010b).

Pathogenicity and epileptogenicity of NMDAR-Abs

Pathogenic effects of the antibodies have been studied *in vitro* and *in vivo*. On dissociated rodent hippocampal neurons, patient NMDAR-Abs (usually CSF) caused a selective reduction in surface membrane NMDARs, resulting in "NMDAR hypofunction" (Hughes *et al.*, 2010). This was reversible on removal of the NMDAR-Abs, and mediated by autoantibody cross-linking of the receptors and internalization (Moscato *et al.*, 2014). In keeping with the Witebsky's postulates of pathogenicity, *in vivo* passive transfer experiments with human NMDAR-Abs have been successful in replicating, in part, the symptoms of disease (Planaguma *et al.*, 2014; Wright *et al.*, 2015b). Cognitive and memory deficits were seen in mice after 14 days of CSF infusion with human CSF containing NMDAR antibodies (Planaguma *et al.*, 2014). Post-mortem analysis revealed a progressive decrease of total and synaptic NMDAR clusters. In another intraventricular passive transfer mouse model, lowered seizure threshold was found in NMDAR-Ab IgG injected mice implanted with wireless EEG transmitters (Wright *et al.*, 2015b) when given a sub-convulsive dose of PTZ. No spontaneous seizures or movement disorders were seen in either model, and psychosis-related phenotypes were not assessed.

Future directions

Treatment of NMDAR-Ab encephalitis has remained largely unchanged for the last 10 years and no randomised controlled trial evidence yet exists for the timing and choice of first line and second line immunotherapies. These important therapeutic decisions are made on a case by case basis relying on the experience of the physician and adherence to pragmatic principles of safe and effective immunomodulatory treatment. Future research, including long-term outcome data and audit of clinician treatment strategies, should serve to inform planning of future trials of new and existing immunotherapies (Bartolini & Muscal, 2017; Titulaer *et al.*, 2013).

Limbic encephalitis and facio-brachial dystonic seizures mediated by LGI1 antibodies

The Leucine-rich glioma inactivated 1 (LGI1) protein is complexed to the voltage gated potassium channel (VGKC-complex) which functions to control membrane excitability. LGI1 is a secreted synaptic protein that organises a trans-synaptic complex with the ADAM22/23 proteins, an important interaction that has been shown to regulate AMPAR mediated synaptic transmission (Fukata *et al.*, 2006). The LGI1 protein also prevents inactivation of the voltage-gated potassium channels (VGKCs) through the cytoplasmic regulatory protein Kvβ (Schulte *et al.*, 2006), and is recognised as an essential protein for neurodevelopment (Ribeiro *et al.*, 2008; Xie *et al.*, 2015).

LGI1 antibodies were historically identified by radioimmunoassay as "VGKC-complex antibodies" (Buckley *et al.*, 2001), until their true antigenic identity as a protein complexed with the VGKCs was revealed (Irani *et al.*, 2010a), and also identified independently (Lai *et al.*, 2010). In children, LGI1 antibodies (LGI1-Abs) are uncommon, and although VGKC-complex antibodies are found in a proportion of patients with neuroinflammatory conditions (Hacohen *et al.*, 2015) they appear to bind to intracellular epitopes and are unlikely to be pathogenic (Lang *et al.*, 2017).

In adults, LGI1-Abs are found in facio-brachial dystonic seizures (FBDS) which can evolve into or be part of the clinical presentation of a limbic encephalitis (LE) (Irani *et al.*, 2011). FBDS presents in older males most commonly, with brief repetitive dystonic seizure-like events that can occur hundreds of times a day (Irani *et al.*, 2011; Irani *et al.*, 2013; Andrade *et al.*, 2011). In the early stages of FBDS, the characteristic hyponatraemia of LE and temporal lobe changes on MRI may not be seen, and scalp EEG is normal in most patients. Immunotherapy produces a clear reduction in seizures and can prevent the development of LE, thus improving the cognitive outcome of affected patients. Often, anti-epileptic drugs are ineffective, and interestingly associated severe cutaneous reactions with these medications have been observed in up to 41% of patients (Irani *et al.*, 2011). This may be explained by recent studies reporting specific HLA subtypes in patients with LGI1 encephalitis (Mueller *et al.*, 2018; Binks *et al.*, 2018; Kim *et al.*, 2017).

The youngest patient described so far with LGI1 antibodies is a 14 year-old boy with Type 1 diabetes mellitus presenting with subacute memory dysfunction, left hippocampal swelling on imaging (*Figure 1A-D* – **scans of this boy – need to ask permission**) and positive oligoclonal bands in the cerebrospinal fluid (Schimmel *et al.*, 2018). He developed psychiatric features, but not FBDS, instead episodes of half-sided pallor and paraesthesia of the face with ptosis lasting up to 1 minute were reported. His EEG remained normal throughout, and he made good recovery with plasma exchange and immunotherapy, although some residual memory problems remain. The coexisting autoimmune disease in this patient and response to immunotherapy suggest the LGI1 antibodies were pathogenic in this case, despite the partial phenotype. Previously, testing of paediatric autoimmune encephalitis cohorts for LGI1 antibodies has failed to find positive cases compared to NMDAR-Abs (*Figure 1E*); future studies should include partial phenotypes and those with risk factors such as preexisting autoimmune disease.

Gamma-aminobutyric acid A ($GABA_A$) and gamma-aminobutyric acid B ($GABA_B$) receptor encephalitis

GABA receptors mediate inhibitory synaptic transmission throughout the central nervous system, and the GABAergic synapse is the target for anti-epileptic drugs commonly used in children, for example benzodiazepines, vigabatrin, topiramate and valproate (Rogawski & Loscher, 2004).

$GABA_A$ encephalitis

The $GABA_A$ receptor mediates the majority of fast inhibitory transmission in the brain. $GABA_A$ receptors are pentameric channels composed of different combinations of the 16 known subunits (Barnard *et al.*, 1998). A functional $GABA_A$ receptor will require at least 2 of the α and β subunit types, and an additional gamma or delta subunit to be functional (Galanopoulou, 2008). Recently, autoantibodies to the $GABA_A$ receptor have been identified in a severe form of autoimmune encephalitis with refractory seizures and extensive MRI cortical/subcortical FLAIR abnormalities (Petit-Pedrol *et al.*, 2014; Pettingill *et al.*, 2015; Ohkawa *et al.*, 2014). Most antibodies bind to the α1/β3 subunits or α1,γ2 (Pettingill *et al.*, 2015). The severity of seizures appears to be one of the hallmarks of this disease, with refractory status epilepticus and epilepsia partialis continua reported in 50% of patients (Petit-Pedrol *et al.*, 2014); all 3 paediatric patients reported in this case series developed status epilepticus as well as varying symptoms of memory, cognitive and affective problems, and movement disorder. A recent case report identified $GABA_A$ receptor antibodies in a case of Febrile Infection-related epilepsy syndrome (FIRES) (Caputo *et al.*, 2018); the patient responded to a combination of high-dose-steroids and intravenous infusion of ketamine with complete recovery of neurological function which is unusual for children with FIRES (Kramer *et al.*, 2011). Additional antibodies have been

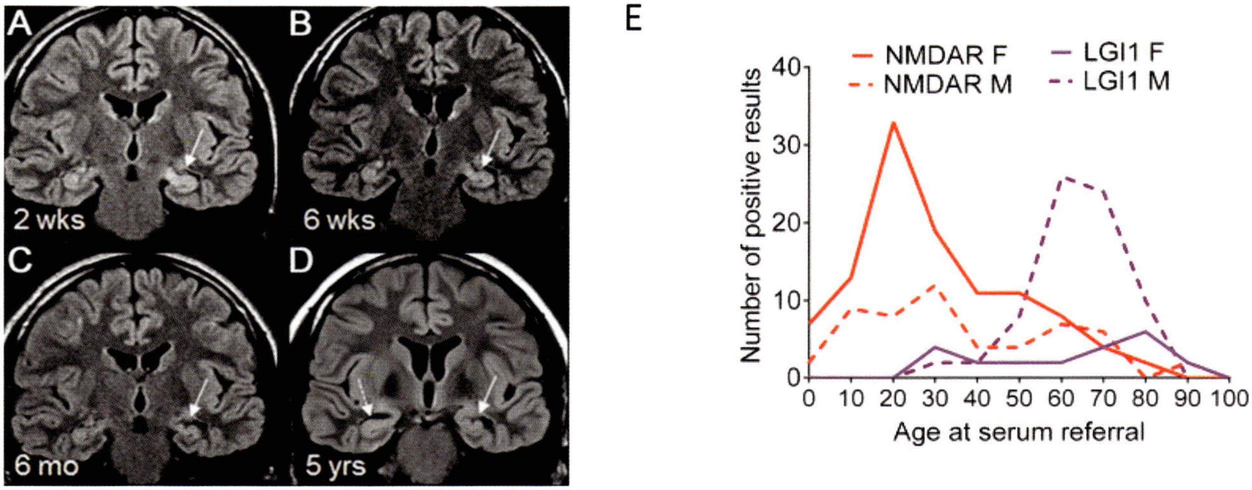

Figure 1 A-D: **MRI of 14-year-old boy with LGI-Ab encephalitis and frequency of LGI-Abs in childhood. Serial fluid-attenuated inversion recovery magnetic resonance imagingrevealing development of left sided hippocampal sclerosis (arrows). In D, the loss of the internal structure of the right hippocampus and a slightly increased signal suggests that the right hippocampus, too, has become sclerotic (dashed arrow), reproduced from Schimmel *et al.*, 2018.** E: **Age distributions of patients with different antibodies detected by cell-based assays in one year (2015) by the Oxford diagnostic service. NMDAR (red) antibodies are more common in children and younger females than males particularly below the age of 30. LGI1 (purple) antibodies, by contrast, are typically found in older males with fewer females, reproduced from Hacohen & Vincent 2018.**

reported in the $GABA_A$ receptor antibody patients (*e.g.*, $GABA_BR$, GAD65 and TPO), as well as paraneoplastic associations (*e.g.*, invasive thymoma, Hodgkins lymphoma), other autoimmune diseases (opsoclonus-myoclonus, Type 1 IDDM, stiff-person syndrome), and post viral meningitis occurrence similar to NMDAR-Ab encephalitis (Petit-Pedrol *et al.*, 2014; Pettingill *et al.*, 2015; Ohkawa *et al.*, 2014; Nikolaus *et al.*, 2018). In terms of pathogenicity, $GABA_AR$ antibodies reduce surface levels of $GABA_AR$'s (Pettingill *et al.*, 2015; Petit-Pedrol *et al.*, 2014), and selectively reduced miniature IPSC amplitude and frequency without affecting miniature EPSCs in one electrophysiological study (Ohkawa *et al.*, 2014). Loss of synaptic $GABA_A$ receptors by internalization is thought to underlie the resistance seen to benzodiazepines in refractory status epilepticus (Goodkin *et al.*, 2005) which may explain the refractory seizures in this disease.

$GABA_B$ encephalitis

The G-protein coupled $GABA_B$ receptors are composed of two subunits $GABA_B1$ and $GABA_B2$, and mediate pre- and post-synaptic inhibition. Autoantibodies to the $GABA_B$ receptor have been reported in a number of adult case series (Lancaster *et al.*, 2010; Hoftberger *et al.*, 2013b; Dogan Onugoren *et al.*, 2015); patients presenting with symptoms of LE, often with early or prominent seizures (Lancaster *et al.*, 2010). The EEG shows encephalopathy, partly with epileptiform discharges in some patients (Dogan Onugoren *et al.*, 2015). Up to 50% of all cases had an underlying small cell lung cancer (SCLC). Response to immunotherapy and oncological treatment was variable with full or partial improvement reported to be between 20–83% (Hoftberger *et al.*, 2013b; Dogan Onugoren *et al.*, 2015).

$GABA_BR$-Ab encephalitis patients who respond best to immunotherapy are those with LE in the context of SCLC (Jeffery *et al.*, 2013). Paediatric cases of $GABA_B$ encephalitis are very rare, one case report describes a presentation of encephalopathy, refractory seizures, and a mixed movement disorder (opsoclonus, ataxia and chorea) in a 3-year-old child (Kruer *et al.*, 2014). Unfortunately, this patient died of overwhelming sepsis despite treatment with intravenous corticosteroids and immunoglobulins. Unlike $GABA_AR$ antibodies, there is no reduction of $GABA_BR$ levels on *in vitro* hippocampal neurons exposed to $GABA_BR$ antibodies (Lancaster *et al.*, 2010). Limited electrophysiological studies suggest a direct inhibitory effect on the receptor causing a network effect (Nibber *et al.*, 2017).

GABA receptor antibodies in children are rare, but given the positive therapeutic responses with immunotherapy in selected cases, cases of refractory status epilepticus should be investigated.

Other neuronal surface antibodies in epileptic encephalopathy

α-amino-3-hydroxy-5-methyl-4-isoxazolepropionic acid (AMPA) receptor antibodies

The heteromeric AMPA receptor (AMPAR), composed of four subunits (GluA 1–4), is an ionotropic transmembrane glutamate receptor that mediates the majority of fast synaptic transmission throughout the CNS. Autoantibodies to this receptor are rare and found mainly in adult limbic encephalitis; often patients will also have an underlying malignancy which predicts a poor outcome (Hoftberger *et al.*, 2015; Joubert *et al.*, 2015; Lai *et al.*, 2009). In the 1990s, AMPAR antibodies were reported in paediatric patients with Rasmussen's encephalitis which is a rare, progressive disorder characterised by severe frequent unilateral seizures leading to cognitive decline and subsequent hemiparesis from the affected side (see Chapter 18) (Rogers *et al.*, 1994). These findings were not replicated in subsequent studies (Watson *et al.*, 2004), but a recent report identified antibodies to the GluA2 and GluA3 subunits when co-expressed in a cell-line in 2/52 Rasmussen's encephalitis patient sera (Nibber *et al.*, 2016). However, these antibodies were identified during the disease course rather than at onset, casting doubt on their pathogenic potential in this disease.

Glycine receptor antibodies

The glycine receptor belongs to the superfamily of ligand-gated ion channels. The main function is to mediate inhibitory neurotransmission in the spinal cord and brain stem. This pentameric receptor is composed from two α-subunits and three β-subunits. Glycine receptor antibodies were first described in adult patients with progressive encephalomyelitis with rigidity and myoclonus (PERM) and stiff person syndrome (SPS), but the phenotype has been expanded with increased identification of these antibodies in patients with LE, epileptic encephalopathy and brainstem encephalitis (Carvajal-Gonzalez *et al.*, 2014; Crisp *et al.*, 2017). Only one case of PERM in childhood has been described in a 14 months old, who responded well to immunotherapy despite the relapsing nature of her disease (Damasio *et al.*, 2013). Other rare paediatric presentations have included focal status epilepticus and progressive dyskinesia as well as encephalopathy, again responding to immunotherapy (Chan *et al.*, 2017; Carvajal-Gonzalez *et al.*, 2014).

Non-surface/intracellular neuronal antibodies

Glutamic acid D-carboxylase (GAD) is a rate-limiting cytosolic enzyme of GABA synthesis; antibodies to GAD have been predominantly associated with adult SPS (Solimena *et al.*, 1990), but are now associated with LE, focal epilepsy and cerebellar ataxia (Honnorat *et al.*, 2001; Malter *et al.*, 2010; Lilleker *et al.*, 2013). Response to immunotherapy is variable and often, affected patients, including children, have a poor outcome (Lilleker *et al.*, 2014; Haberlandt *et al.*, 2011). Controversy exists over the pathological significance of GAD-Abs, and many studies investigating GAD-Abs and their relevance in neurological disease are often testing samples and treating patients many years after disease onset (Veri *et al.*, 2013). More long-term prospective trials are needed to clarify the clinical significance of GAD antibodies in epilepsy.

Onconeural antibodies

The most common paraneoplastic antibody, anti-Hu, is still very rare in children, with a recent single centre study finding only 8 positive patients < 18 years of age. Two of these patients had neuroblastoma and opsoclonus-myoclonus, the remaining 6 had classic LE but no evidence of cancer (Honnorat *et al.*, 2013). These 6 patients were treated with anti-epileptic drugs and immunotherapy; however, the management of epilepsy was difficult in all cases.

The other onconeuronal antibodies relevant to paediatric epileptic encephalopathy are listed in *Table III*.

Antibodies in demyelinating diseases of childhood

Focal or generalised seizures can be part of the presentation of Acute Disseminated Encephalomyelitis (ADEM), a CNS inflammatory demyelinating disease of childhood, characterised by encephalopathy, polyfocal CNS deficits and multifocal brain MRI lesions (Pohl *et al.*, 2016; Pohl & Tenembaum, 2012; Dale, 2003). Response to immunotherapy is good, with generally a favourable outcome, although some patients may relapse (Pohl *et al.*, 2016). Antibodies to the myelin-oligodendrocyte protein (MOG-Abs) have been identified in ADEM patients, predicting a non-multiple sclerosis but multiphasic disease course (Baumann *et al.*, 2016; Hacohen *et al.*, 2018). MOG-ab associated disease includes adult cases of unilateral cerebral cortical encephalitis presenting with generalised epileptic seizures, with or without encephalopathy, which are responsive to anti-epileptic drugs and immunotherapy (Ogawa *et al.*, 2017). In fact, recent cohort studies in both children and adults show that MOG-Ab

Table III Neuronal targets in paediatric autoimmune epileptic encephalopathy

Neuronal target	Cell surface or intracellular	Paraneoplastic	Frequency in paediatric patients and phenotypic features
NMDAR	Cell-surface	Ovarian teratoma, neuroblastoma, testicular germinoma	Common, F > M, ~ 40% of cases Encephalopathy, neuropsychiatric features, seizures, movement disorder, dysautonomia
AMPAR	Cell-surface	Lung cancer,thymic tumour, breast cancer	Rare Encephalitis, seizures, psychiatric features
$GABA_A$	Cell-surface	Invasive thymoma	Rare, but increasing case reports Encephalitis, status epilepticus, refractory seizures, FIRES
$GABA_B$	Cell-surface	Small cell lung carcinoma	Rare LE
LGI1	Cell-surface	Thymoma, small-cell lung carcinoma, breast, prostate cancer	Rare, one case report in young male with IDDM LE, FBDS
Glycine receptor	Cell-surface	About 15%, thymoma, lymphoma	Rare,one paediatric case of PERM PERM, SPS, epileptic encephalopathy
GAD65	Intracellular	Not common but occasional thymoma; renal, breast GI tract carcinoma	Rarely reported in children, poor outcome SPS, LE, refractory seizures (temporal lobe)
Hu	Intracellular	Classically small-cell carcinoma; neuroblastoma in children	Rare overall but most common paraneoplastic antibody in children; tumour not always found in children LE, neuropathy (autonomic, peripheral, sensory), brainstem encephalitis
Ma1, Ma2	Intracellular	Testicular, breast, colon cancer	Rare, case report of 14-year-old girl with severe encephalopathy, seizures, status dystonicus, no tumour LE, polyneuropathy, encephalomyelitis
Tr (Delta/notch like epidermal growth factor- related receptor)	Intracellular	Breast cancer, small cell lung cancer, and Hodgkin's disease	Rare Reported in 12 year old girl with Hodgkin lymphoma

GI: gastrointestinal; LE: limbic encephalitis; LEMS: Lambert Eaton Myasthenic Syndrome; PERM: progressive encephalomyelitis with rigidity and myoclonus; SPS: stiff-person syndrome.

associated disease is more likely to present with seizures, and incur an increased risk of developing long-term "autoimmune epilepsy" (Hamid *et al.*, 2018; Rosser *et al.*, 2019).

A summary of all relevant neuronal targets in paediatric autoimmune epilepsy and encephalopathy is shown in *Table III*.

Paediatric epilepsy cohort studies

Given the dizzying array of antibodies that may be implicated in the aetiology of paediatric and adult epilepsy, researchers have attempted to assess systematically well-characterised epilepsy cohorts (without encephalitis) to assess their frequency and significance.

The frequency of previous cohort studies has varied between 9–13% positivity for low levels of neuronal antibodies, and were found more commonly in epilepsy of "unknown cause" and often focal epilepsy (Brenner *et al.*, 2013; Majoie *et al.*, 2006; Suleiman *et al.*, 2013). These studies also included testing for VGK-complex antibodies rather than for the specific antigens including LGI1, so may not be significant in terms of an auto-immune epilepsy diagnosis. In long term studies (up to 15 year follow-up) there was no significant difference in response to standard antiepileptic drugs or long-term outcome between antibody positive and antibody-negative patients (Wright *et al.*, 2016). In a more recent prospective multi-centre study, 101 children with new onset seizures presenting to hospital in Switzerland were tested for serum neuronal antibodies and no specific neuronal antibodies were identified using the commercial assays available (Garcia-Tarodo *et al.*, 2018).

In paediatric epilepsy and new-onset seizures without encephalitis, neuronal antibodies are rarely found and testing should be limited to those presenting with associated symptoms suggestive of an underlying autoimmune encephalopathy (*e.g.*, neuropsychiatric features, behavioural change, movement disorder, autonomic symptoms, refractory status epilepticus).

Treatment of paediatric autoimmune encephalitis and encephalopathy

In the absence of consensus guidelines on the treatment of autoimmune encephalitis and encephalopathy most clinicians in practice follow a pragmatic step-wise approach to treatment *(Figure 2)*. As with NMDA encephalitis, in autoimmune epileptic encephalopathy, "first-line" treatment will begin in the form of pulsed intravenous high dose steroids, intravenous immunoglobulin and/or plasma exchange. Escalation to "second-line immunotherapy" is often as a result of failure to respond to first line treatment, relapse, or the severity of presenting illness (Titulaer *et al.*, 2013). Options include rituximab, cyclophosphamide, azathioprine, mycophenolate mofetil and methotrexate (Ramanathan *et al.*, 2014; Lim *et al.*, 2015; Toledano & Pittock, 2015; Linnoila *et al.*, 2014). These agents are not

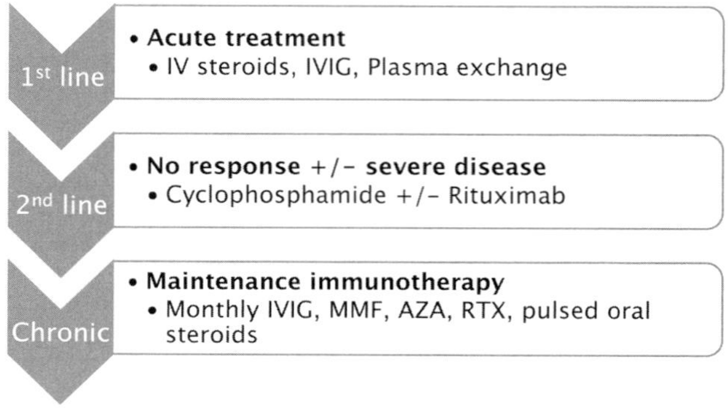

AZA Azathioprine; IVIG: Intravenous immunoglobulin; MMF: Mofetil mycophenolate; RTX: Rituximab

Figure 2 **Suggested pathway for treatment of autoimmune encephalopathies** (adapted from Dale *et al.*, 2016).

without risk and require careful consideration and monitoring for potential serious side effects (Dale *et al.*, 2014). Patients respond well to immunotherapy with the best therapeutic responses seen in those diagnosed and treated early, and with tumour removal, if applicable (Titulaer *et al.*, 2013; Wright *et al.*, 2015a; Byrne *et al.*, 2015). In reality, each individual patient will need a personalised plan of treatment depending on the antigen under attack, stage of disease and their response to treatment; all patients however need prompt recognition of disease and initiation of first-line treatment.

Conclusions

Based on the Witebsky criteria there is sufficient evidence that neuronal surface antibodies are pathogenic in paediatric autoimmune encephalitis and encephalopathy. With the combination of specific antibody detection methods, recognition of clinical phenotypes and judicious use of ancillary investigations, affected patients should now be diagnosed and treated promptly. Overwhelming evidence points to early diagnosis being a crucial factor in terms of outcome. With the developing nervous system it is even more important to preserve and support the integrity of a child's developmental trajectory. With an increased understanding of the pathogenic mechanisms of the CNS auto antibodies, the relationship to the immune system and genetic susceptibility, the time is ripe for further research into future specific and existing therapies to improve patient recovery times and eventual outcome.

REFERENCES

Andrade DM, Tai P, Dalmau J, Wennberg R (2011): Tonic seizures: a diagnostic clue of anti-LGI1 encephalitis? *Neurology* 76: 1355–1357.

Armangue T, Leypoldt F, Malaga I, *et al.* (2014): Herpes simplex virus encephalitis is a trigger of brain autoimmunity. *Ann Neurol* 75: 3173–3123.

Armangue T, Moris G, Cantarin-Extremera V, *et al.* (2015): Autoimmune post-herpes simplex encephalitis of adults and teenagers. *Neurology* 85: 1736–1743.

Armangue T, Titulaer MJ, Malaga I, *et al.* (2013): Pediatric anti-N-methyl-D-aspartate receptor encephalitis-clinical analysis and novel findings in a series of 20 patients. *J Pediatr* 162: 850–856.e2.

Arts WF, Aarsen FK, Scheltens-De Boer M, Catsman-Berrevoets CE (2009): Landau-Kleffner syndrome and CSWS syndrome: treatment with intravenous immunoglobulins. *Epilepsia* 50 (Suppl 7): 55–58.

Banks WA, Erickson MA (2010): The blood-brain barrier and immune function and dysfunction. *Neurobiol Dis* 37: 26–32.

Barnard EA, Skolnick P, Olsen RW, *et al.* (1998): International Union of Pharmacology. XV. Subtypes of gamma-aminobutyric acidA receptors: classification on the basis of subunit structure and receptor function. *Pharmacol Rev* 50: 291–313.

Bartolini L, Muscal E (2017): Differences in treatment of anti-NMDA receptor encephalitis: results of a worldwide survey. *J Neurol* 264: 647–653.

Baumann M, Hennes EM, Schanda K, *et al.* (2016): Children with multiphasic disseminated encephalomyelitis and antibodies to the myelin oligodendrocyte glycoprotein (MOG): Extending the spectrum of MOG antibody positive diseases. *Mult Scler* 22: 1821–1829.

Bear M F, Malenka R C (1994): Synaptic plasticity: LTP and LTD. *Curr Opin Neurobiol* 4: 389–399.

Binks S, Varley J, Lee W, *et al.* (2018): Distinct HLA associations of LGI1 and CASPR2-antibody diseases. *Brain* 141: 2263–2271.

Brenner T, Sills GJ, Hart Y, Howell S, Waters P, Brodie MJ, Vincent A, Lang B (2013): Prevalence of neurologic autoantibodies in cohorts of patients with new and established epilepsy. *Epilepsia* 54: 1028–1035.

Buckley C, Oger J, Clover L, *et al.* (2001): Potassium channel antibodies in two patients with reversible limbic encephalitis. *Ann Neurol* 50: 73–78.

Buzatu M, Bulteau C, Altuzarra C, Dulac O, Van Bogaert P (2009): Corticosteroids as treatment of epileptic syndromes with continuous spike-waves during slow-wave sleep. *Epilepsia* 50 (Suppl 7): 68–72.

Byrne S, Walsh C, Hacohen Y, *et al.* (2015): Earlier treatment of NMDAR antibody encephalitis in children results in a better outcome. *Neurol Neuroimmunol Neuroinflamm* 2, e130.

Caputo D, Iorio R, Vigevano F, Fusco L (2018): Febrile infection-related epilepsy syndrome (FIRES) with super-refractory status epilepticus revealing autoimmune encephalitis due to GABAAR antibodies. *Eur J Paediatr Neurol* 22: 182–185.

Carvajal-Gonzalez A Leite MI, Waters P, *et al.* (2014): Glycine receptor antibodies in PERM and related syndromes: characteristics, clinical features and outcomes. *Brain* 137: 2178–2192.

Chan DW, Thomas T, Lim M, Ling S, Woodhall M, Vincent A (2017): Focal status epilepticus and progressive dyskinesia: A novel phenotype for glycine receptor antibody-mediated neurological disease in children. *Eur J Paediatr Neurol* 21: 414–417.

Chang C (2014): Autoimmunity: from black water fever to regulatory function. *J Autoimmun* 48–49: 1–9.

Cooray GK, Sengupta B, Douglas P, Englund M, Wickstrom R, Friston K (2015): Characterising seizures in anti-NMDA-receptor encephalitis with dynamic causal modelling. *Neuroimage* 118: 508–519.

Crisp SJ, Balint B,Vincent A (2017): Redefining progressive encephalomyelitis with rigidity and myoclonus after the discovery of antibodies to glycine receptors. *Curr Opin Neurol* 30: 310–316.

Dale RC (2003): Acute disseminated encephalomyelitis. *Semin Pediatr Infect Dis* 14: 90–95.

Dale RC, Brilot F, Duffy LV, *et al.* (2014): Utility and safety of rituximab in pediatric autoimmune and inflammatory CNS disease. *Neurology* 83: 142–150.

Dale RC, Nosadini M, Lim M (2016): Therapeutic decision making in autoimmune and inflammatory disorders of the central nervous system in children. *JICNA* 16: 112.

Dalmau J, Gleichman AJ, Hughes EG, *et al.* (2008): Anti-NMDA-receptor encephalitis: case series and analysis of the effects of antibodies. *Lancet Neurol* 7: 1091–1098.

Dalmau J, Tuzun E, Wu HY, *et al.* (2007): Paraneoplastic anti-N-methyl-D-aspartate receptor encephalitis associated with ovarian teratoma. *Ann Neurol* 61: 25–36.

Damasio J, Leite MI, Coutinho E, *et al.* (2013): Progressive encephalomyelitis with rigidity and myoclonus: the first pediatric case with glycine receptor antibodies. *JAMA Neurol* 70: 498–501.

Dogan Onugoren M, Deuretzbacher D, Haensch CA, *et al.* (2015): Limbic encephalitis due to GABAB and AMPA receptor antibodies: a case series. *J Neurol Neurosurg Psychiatry* 86: 965–972.

Favier M, Joubert B, Picard G, *et al.* (2018): Initial clinical presentation of young children with N-methyl-aspartate receptor encephalitis. *European Journal of Paediatric Neurology* 22: 404–411.

Finke C, Kopp UA, Scheel M, *et al.* (2013): Functional and structural brain changes in anti-N-methyl-D-aspartate receptor encephalitis. *Ann Neurol* 74: 284–296.

Florance NR, Davis RL, Lam C, *et al.* (2009): Anti-N-methyl-D-aspartate receptor (NMDAR) encephalitis in children and adolescents. *Ann Neurol* 66: 11–18.

Fujii H, Kubo S, Yunoki T, *et al.* (2013): Glioblastoma with ovarian teratoma having N-methyl-D-aspartate receptor (NMDAR) antibody in CSF – a case report. *Rinsho Shinkeigaku* 53: 712–715.

Fukata Y, Adesnik H, Iwanaga T, Bredt DS, Nicoll RA, Fukata M (2006): Epilepsy-related ligand/receptor complex LGI1 and ADAM22 regulate synaptic transmission. *Science* 313: 1792–1795.

Galanopoulou AS (2008): GABA(A) Receptors in Normal Development and Seizures: Friends or Foes? *Curr Neuropharmacol* 6: 1–20.

Garcia-Tarodo S, Datta AN, Ramelli GP, Marechal-Rouiller F, Beni CG, Korff CM (2018): Circulating neural antibodies in unselected children with new-onset seizures. *Eur J Paediatr Neurol* 22: 396–403.

Gataullina S, Plouin P, Vincent A, Scalais E, Nuttin C, Dulac O (2011): Paroxysmal EEG pattern in a child with N-methyl-D-aspartate receptor antibody encephalitis. *Dev Med Child Neurol* 53: 764–67.

Gayatri NA, Ferrie CD, Cross H (2007): Corticosteroids including ACTH for childhood epilepsy other than epileptic spasms. *Cochrane Database Syst Rev* Cd005222.

Gitiaux C, Simonnet H, Eisermann M, *et al.* (2013): Early electro-clinical features may contribute to diagnosis of the anti-NMDA receptor encephalitis in children. *Clin Neurophysiol* 124: 2354–2361.

Goldberg EM, Titulaer M, De Blank PM, Sievert A, Ryan N (2014): Anti-N-methyl-D-aspartate receptor-mediated encephalitis in infants and toddlers: case report and review of the literature. *Pediatr Neurol* 50: 181–184.

Goodkin HP, Yeh JL, Kapur J (2005): Status epilepticus increases the intracellular accumulation of GABAA receptors. *J Neurosci* 25: 5511–5520.

Granata T, Cross H, Theodore W, Avanzini G (2011): Immune-mediated epilepsies. *Epilepsia* 52 (Suppl 3): 5–11.

Graus F, Titulaer MJ, Balu R, *et al.* (2016): A clinical approach to diagnosis of autoimmune encephalitis. *Lancet Neurol* 15: 391–404.

Gresa-Arribas N, Titulaer MJ, Torrents A, *et al.* (2014): Antibody titres at diagnosis and during follow-up of anti-NMDA receptor encephalitis: a retrospective study. *Lancet Neurol* 13: 167–177.

Haberlandt E, Bast T, Ebner A, *et al.* (2011): Limbic encephalitis in children and adolescents. *Arch Dis Child* 96: 186–191.

Hacohen Y, Deiva K, Pettingill P, *et al.* (2014a): N-methyl-D-aspartate receptor antibodies in post-herpes simplex virus encephalitis neurological relapse. *Mov Disord* 29: 90–96.

Hacohen Y, Dlamini N, Hedderly T, *et al.* (2014b): N-methyl-D-aspartate receptor antibody-associated movement disorder without encephalopathy. *Dev Med Child Neurol* 56: 190–193.

Hacohen Y, Singh R, Rossi M, *et al.* (2015): Clinical relevance of voltage-gated potassium channel-complex antibodies in children. *Neurology* 85: 967–975.

Hacohen Y, Wong YY, Lechner C, *et al.* (2018): Disease Course and Treatment Responses in Children With Relapsing Myelin Oligodendrocyte Glycoprotein Antibody-Associated Disease. *JAMA Neurol* 75: 478–487.

Hacohen Y, Wright S, Gadian J, *et al.* (2016): N-methyl-d-aspartate (NMDA) receptor antibodies encephalitis mimicking an autistic regression. *Dev Med Child Neurol* 58: 1092–1094.

Hamid SHM, Whittam D, Saviour M, *et al.* (2018): Seizures and Encephalitis in Myelin Oligodendrocyte Glycoprotein IgG Disease *vs.* Aquaporin 4 IgG Disease. *JAMA Neurol* 75: 65–71.

Hancock EC, Osborne JP, Edwards SW (2013): Treatment of infantile spasms. *Cochrane Database Syst Rev* 6: Cd001770.

Ho ACC, Mohammad SS, Pillai SC, *et al.* (2017): High sensitivity and specificity in proposed clinical diagnostic criteria for anti-N-methyl-D-aspartate receptor encephalitis. *Dev Med Child Neurol* 59: 1256–1260.

Hoftberger R, Armangue T, Leypoldt F, Graus F, Dalmau J (2013a): Clinical Neuropathology practice guide 4–2013: post-herpes simplex encephalitis: N-methyl-Daspartate receptor antibodies are part of the problem. *Clin Neuropathol* 32: 251–254.

Hoftberger R, Titulaer MJ, Sabater L, *et al.* (2013b): Encephalitis and GABAB receptor antibodies: novel findings in a new case series of 20 patients. *Neurology* 81: 1500–1506.

Hoftberger R, Van Sonderen A, Leypoldt F, *et al.* (2015): Encephalitis and AMPA receptor antibodies: Novel findings in a case series of 22 patients. *Neurology* 84: 2403–2412.

Honnorat J, Didelot A, Karantoni E, *et al.* (2013): Autoimmune limbic encephalopathy and anti-Hu antibodies in children without cancer. *Neurology* 80: 2226–2232.

Honnorat J, Saiz A, Giometto B, *et al.* (2001): Cerebellar ataxia with anti-glutamic acid decarboxylase antibodies: study of 14 patients. *Arch Neurol* 58: 225–230.

Hughes EG, Peng X, Gleichman AJ, *et al.* (2010): Cellular and synaptic mechanisms of anti-NMDA receptor encephalitis. *J Neurosci* 30: 5866–5875.

Irani SR, Alexander S, Waters P, *et al.* (2010a): Antibodies to Kv1 potassium channel-complex proteins leucine-rich, glioma inactivated 1 protein and contactin-associated protein-2 in limbic encephalitis, Morvan's syndrome and acquired neuromyotonia. *Brain* 133: 2734–2748.

Irani SR, Bera K, Waters P, *et al.* (2010b): N-methyl-D-aspartate antibody encephalitis: temporal progression of clinical and paraclinical observations in a predominantly non-paraneoplastic disorder of both sexes. *Brain* 133: 1655–1667.

Irani SR, Gelfand JM, Al-Diwani A, Vincent A (2014): Cell-surface central nervous system autoantibodies: Clinical relevance and emerging paradigms. *Ann Neurol* 76: 168–184.

Irani SR, Michell AW, Lang B, *et al.* (2011): Faciobrachial dystonic seizures precede Lgi1 antibody limbic encephalitis. *Ann Neurol* 69: 892–900.

Irani SR, Stagg CJ, Schott JM, *et al.* (2013): Faciobrachial dystonic seizures: the influence of immunotherapy on seizure control and prevention of cognitive impairment in a broadening phenotype. *Brain* 136: 3151–3162.

Jeffery OJ, Lennon VA, Pittock SJ, Gregory JK, Britton JW, Mckeon A (2013): GABAB receptor autoantibody frequency in service serologic evaluation. *Neurology* 81: 882–887.

Jones HF, Mohammad SS, Reed PW, *et al.* (2017): Anti-N-methyl-d-aspartate receptor encephalitis in Maori and Pacific Island children in New Zealand. *Dev Med Child Neurol* 59: 719–724.

Joubert B, Kerschen P, Zekeridou A, *et al.* (2015): Clinical Spectrum of Encephalitis Associated With Antibodies Against the alpha-Amino-3-Hydroxy-5-Methyl-4-Isoxazolepropionic Acid Receptor: Case Series and Review of the Literature. *JAMA Neurol* 72: 1163–1169.

Kayser MS, Titulaer MJ, Gresa-Arribas N, Dalmau J (2013): Frequency and characteristics of isolated psychiatric episodes in anti-N-methyl-d-aspartate receptor encephalitis. *JAMA Neurol* 70: 1133–1139.

Kiani R, Lawden M, Eames P, *et al.* (2015): Anti-NMDA-receptor encephalitis presenting with catatonia and neuroleptic malignant syndrome in patients with intellectual disability and autism. *BJPsych Bull* 39: 32–35.

Kim TJ, Lee ST, Moon J, *et al.* (2017): Anti-LGI1 encephalitis is associated with unique HLA subtypes. *Ann Neurol* 81: 183–192.

Kipnis J (2016): Multifaceted interactions between adaptive immunity and the central nervous system. *Science* 353: 766–771.

Kirkpatrick MP, Clarke CD, Sonmezturk HH, Abou-Khalil B (2011): Rhythmic delta activity represents a form of nonconvulsive status epilepticus in anti-NMDA receptor antibody encephalitis. *Epilepsy Behav* 20: 392–394.

Kramer U, Chi CS, Lin K L, *et al.* (2011): Febrile infection-related epilepsy syndrome (FIRES): pathogenesis, treatment, and outcome: a multicenter study on 77 children. *Epilepsia* 52: 1956–1965.

Kruer MC, Hoeftberger R, Lim KY, *et al.* (2014): Aggressive Course in Encephalitis With Opsoclonus, Ataxia, Chorea, and Seizures: The First Pediatric Case of gamma-Aminobutyric Acid Type B Receptor Autoimmunity. *JAMA Neurol* 71: 620–623.

Lai M, Hughes EG, Peng X, *et al.* (2009): AMPA receptor antibodies in limbic encephalitis alter synaptic receptor location. *Ann Neurol* 65: 424–434.

Lai M, Huijbers MG, Lancaster E, *et al.* (2010): Investigation of LGI1 as the antigen in limbic encephalitis previously attributed to potassium channels: a case series. *Lancet Neurol* 9: 776–785.

Lancaster E, Lai M, Peng X, *et al.* (2010): Antibodies to the GABA(B) receptor in limbic encephalitis with seizures: case series and characterisation of the antigen. *Lancet Neurol* 9: 67–76.

Lang B, Makuch M., Moloney T, *et al.* (2017): Intracellular and non-neuronal targets of voltage-gated potassium channel complex antibodies. *J Neurol Neurosurg Psychiatry* 88: 353–361.

Lang B, Molenaar PC, Newsom-Davis J, Vincent A (1984): Passive transfer of Lambert-Eaton myasthenic syndrome in mice: decreased rates of resting and evoked release of acetylcholine from skeletal muscle. *J Neurochem* 42: 658–662.

Leite MI, Waters P, Vincent A (2010): Diagnostic use of autoantibodies in myasthenia gravis. *Autoimmunity* 43: 371–379.

Lilleker J, Biswas V, Mohanraj R (2013): Relevance of Gad Antibodies in Adults with Epilepsy: Experience in a Tertiary Clinic. *J Neurol Neurosurg Psychiatry* 84: e2.

Lilleker JB, Biswas V, Mohanraj R (2014): Glutamic acid decarboxylase (GAD) antibodies in epilepsy: Diagnostic yield and therapeutic implications. *Seizure* 23: 598–602.

Lim M, Hacohen Y, Vincent A (2015): Autoimmune encephalopathies. *Pediatr Clin North Am* 62: 667–685.

Linnoila JJ, Rosenfeld MR, Dalmau J (2014): Neuronal surface antibody-mediated autoimmune encephalitis. *Semin Neurol* 34: 458–466.

Mackay IR (2010): Travels and travails of autoimmunity: a historical journey from discovery to rediscovery. *Autoimmun Rev* 9: A251–258.

Majoie HJ, De Baets M, Renier W, Lang B, Vincent A (2006): Antibodies to voltage-gated potassium and calcium channels in epilepsy. *Epilepsy Res* 71: 135–141.

Malter MP, Helmstaedter C, Urbach H, Vincent A, Bien CG (2010): Antibodies to glutamic acid decarboxylase define a form of limbic encephalitis. *Ann Neurol* 67: 470–478.

Marchi N, Granata T, Janigro D (2014): Inflammatory pathways of seizure disorders. *Trends Neurosci* 37: 55–65.

Mehta V, Ferrie CD, Cross JH, Vadlamani G (2015): Corticosteroids including ACTH for childhood epilepsy other than epileptic spasms. *Cochrane Database Syst Rev* Cd005222.

Mikati MA, Saab R, Fayad MN, Choueiri RN (2002): Efficacy of intravenous immunoglobulin in Landau-Kleffner syndrome. *Pediatr Neurol* 26: 298–300.

Mohammad SS, Sinclair K, Pillai S, *et al.* (2014): Herpes simplex encephalitis relapse with chorea is associated with autoantibodies to N-Methyl-D-aspartate receptor or dopamine-2 receptor. *Mov Disord* 29: 117–122.

Moscato EH, Peng X, Jain A, Parsons TD, Dalmau J, Balice-Gordon RJ (2014): Acute mechanisms underlying antibody effects in anti-N-methyl-D-aspartate receptor encephalitis. *Ann Neurol* 76: 108–119.

Mueller SH, Farber A, Pruss H, *et al.* (2018): Genetic predisposition in anti-LGI1 and anti-NMDA receptor encephalitis. *Ann Neurol* 83: 863–869.

Newsom-Davis J, Pinching AJ, Vincent A, Wilson SG (1978a): Function of circulating antibody to acetylcholine receptor in myasthenia gravis: investigation by plasma exchange. *Neurology* 28: 266–272.

Newsom-Davis J, Vincent A, Wilson SG, Ward CD, Pinching AJ, Hawkey C (1978b): Plasmapheresis for myasthenia gravis. *N Engl J Med* 298: 456–457.

Nibber A, Clover L, Pettingill P, *et al.* (2016): Antibodies to AMPA receptors in Rasmussen's encephalitis. *Eur J Paediatr Neurol* 20: 222–227.

Nibber A, Mann EO, Pettingill P, *et al.* (2017): Pathogenic potential of antibodies to the GABAB receptor. *Epilepsia Open* 2: 355–359.

Niehusmann P, Dalmau J, Rudlowski C, *et al.* (2009): Diagnostic value of N-methyl-D-aspartate receptor antibodies in women with new-onset epilepsy. *Arch Neurol* 66: 458–464.

Nikolaus M, Knierim E, Meisel C, *et al.* (2018): Severe GABAA receptor encephalitis without seizures: A paediatric case successfully treated with early immunomodulation. *Eur J Paediatr Neurol* 22: 558–562.

Nosadini M, Boniver C, Zuliani L, *et al.* (2014): Longitudinal Electroencephalographic (EEG) Findings in Pediatric Anti-N-Methyl-D-Aspartate (Anti-NMDA) Receptor Encephalitis: The Padua Experience. *J Child Neurol* 30: 238–245.

O'Callaghan FJ, Edwards SW, Alber FD, *et al.* (2017): Safety and effectiveness of hormonal treatment *versus* hormonal treatment with vigabatrin for infantile spasms (ICISS): a randomised, multicentre, open-label trial. *Lancet Neurol* 16: 33–42.

Ogawa R, Nakashima I, Takahashi T, *et al.* (2017): MOG antibody-positive, benign, unilateral, cerebral cortical encephalitis with epilepsy. *Neurol Neuroimmunol Neuroinflamm* 4: e322.

Ohkawa T, Satake S, Yokoi N, Miyazaki Y, Ohshita T (2014): Identification and characterization of GABA(A) receptor autoantibodies in autoimmune encephalitis. *J Neurosci* 34: 8151–8163.

Ong MS, Kohane IS, Cai T, Gorman MP, Mandl KD (2014): Population-level evidence for an autoimmune etiology of epilepsy. *JAMA Neurol* 71: 569–574.

Palace J, Lang B (2000): Epilepsy: an autoimmune disease? *J Neurol Neurosurg Psychiatry* 69: 711–714.

Peer M, Pruss H, Ben-Dayan I, Paul F, Arzy S, Finke C (2017): Functional connectivity of large-scale brain networks in patients with anti-NMDA receptor encephalitis: an observational study. *Lancet Psychiatry* 4: 768–774.

Petit-Pedrol M, Armangue T, Peng X, *et al.* (2014): Encephalitis with refractory seizures, status epilepticus, and antibodies to the GABAA receptor: a case series, characterisation of the antigen, and analysis of the effects of antibodies. *Lancet Neurol* 13: 276–286.

Pettingill P, Kramer HB, Coebergh JA, *et al.* (2015): Antibodies to GABAA receptor alpha1 and gamma2 subunits: clinical and serologic characterization. *Neurology* 84: 1233–1241.

Planaguma J, Leypoldt F, Mannara F, *et al.* (2014): Human N-methyl D-aspartate receptor antibodies alter memory and behaviour in mice. *Brain* 138: 94–109.

Pohl D, Alper G, Van Haren K, *et al.* (2016): Acute disseminated encephalomyelitis: Updates on an inflammatory CNS syndrome. *Neurology* 87: S38–45.

Pohl D, Tenembaum S (2012): Treatment of acute disseminated encephalomyelitis. *Curr Treat Options Neurol* 14: 264–275.

Ramanathan S, Mohammad SS, Brilot F, Dale RC (2014): Autoimmune encephalitis: recent updates and emerging challenges. *J Clin Neurosci* 21: 722–730.

Ransohoff RM, Kivisakk P, Kidd G (2003): Three or more routes for leukocyte migration into the central nervous system. *Nat Rev Immunol* 3: 569–581.

Ribeiro PA, Sbragia L, Gilioli R, Langone F, Conte FF, Lopes-Cendes I: (2008): Expression profile of Lgi1 gene in mouse brain during development. *J Mol Neurosci* 35: 323–329.

Rogawski MA, Loscher W (2004): The neurobiology of antiepileptic drugs. *Nat Rev Neurosci* 5: 5 553–64.

Rogers SW, Andrews PI, Gahring LC, *et al.* (1994): Autoantibodies to glutamate receptor GluR3 in Rasmussen's encephalitis. *Science* 265: 648–651.

Rose NR, Bona C (1993): Defining criteria for autoimmune diseases (Witebsky's postulates revisited). *Immunol Today* 14: 426–430.

Rosenfeld MR, Titulaer MJ, Dalmau J (2012): Paraneoplastic syndromes and autoimmune encephalitis: Five new things. *Neurol Clin Pract*, 2, 215–223.

Rossor T, Benetou C, Wright S, *et al.* (2019): Early predictors of epilepsy and subsequent relapse in children with acute disseminated encephalomyelitis. *Mult Scler* Feb 7: 1352458518823486 [In press].

Schimmel M, Fruhwald MC, Bien CG (2018): Limbic encephalitis with LGI1 antibodies in a 14-year-old boy. *Eur J Paediatr Neurol*, 22, 190–193.

Schmitt SE, Pargeon K, Frechette ES, Hirsch LJ, Dalmau J, Friedman D (2012): Extreme delta brush: a unique EEG pattern in adults with anti-NMDA receptor encephalitis. *Neurology* 79: 1094–1100.

Schulte U, Thumfart JO, Klocker N, *et al.* (2006): The epilepsy-linked Lgi1 protein assembles into presynaptic Kv1 channels and inhibits inactivation by Kvbeta1. *Neuron* 49: 697–706.

Scott O, Richer L, Forbes K, *et al.* (2014): Anti-N-methyl-D-aspartate (NMDA) receptor encephalitis: an unusual cause of autistic regression in a toddler. *J Child Neurol* 29: 691–694.

Solimena M, Folli F, Aparisi R, Pozza G, De Camilli P (1990): Autoantibodies to GABA-ergic neurons and pancreatic beta cells in stiff-man syndrome. *N Engl J Med* 322: 1555–1560.

Suleiman J, Wright S, Gill D, *et al.* (2013): Autoantibodies to neuronal antigens in children with new-onset seizures classified according to the revised ILAE organization of seizures and epilepsies. *Epilepsia* 54: 2091–2100.

Symmonds M, Moran CH, Leite MI, *et al.* (2018): Ion channels in EEG: isolating channel dysfunction in NMDA receptor antibody encephalitis. *Brain* 141: 1691–1702.

Titulaer MJ, Dalmau J (2014): Seizures as first symptom of anti-NMDA receptor encephalitis are more common in men. *Neurology* 82: 550–551.

TItulaer MJ, Mccracken L, Gabilondo I, *et al.* (2013): Treatment and prognostic factors for long-term outcome in patients with anti-NMDA receptor encephalitis: an observational cohort study. *Lancet Neurol* 12: 157–165.

Toledano M, Pittock SJ (2015): Autoimmune Epilepsy. *Semin Neurol* 35: 245–258.

Toyka KV, Drachman DB, Griffin DE, *et al.* (1977): Myasthenia gravis. Study of humoral immune mechanisms by passive transfer to mice. *N Engl J Med* 296: 125–131.

Veciana M, Becerra JL, Fossas P, *et al.* (2015): EEG extreme delta brush: An ictal pattern in patients with anti-NMDA receptor encephalitis. *Epilepsy Behav* 49: 280–285.

Veri K, Uibo O, Talvik T, *et al.* (2013): Newly-diagnosed pediatric epilepsy is associated with elevated autoantibodies to glutamic acid decarboxylase but not cardiolipin. *Epilepsy Res* 105: 86–91.

Vezzani A, French J, Bartfai T, Baram TZ (2011): The role of inflammation in epilepsy. *Nat Rev Neurol* 7: 31–40.

Viaccoz A, Desestret V, Ducray F, *et al.* (2014): Clinical specificities of adult male patients with NMDA receptor antibodies encephalitis. *Neurology* 82: 556–563.

Watad A, Tiosano S, Bragazzi NL, *et al.* (2018): Epilepsy among Systemic Lupus Erythematosus Patients: Insights from a Large Database Analysis. *Neuroepidemiology* 50: 1–6.

Watson R, Jiang Y, Bermudez I, *et al.* (2004): Absence of antibodies to glutamate receptor type 3 (GluR3) in Rasmussen encephalitis. *Neurology* 63: 43–50.

Witebsky E, Rose NR, Terplan K, Paine J R, Egan RW (1957): Chronic thyroiditis and autoimmunization. *J Am Med Assoc* 164: 1439–1447.

Wright S, Geerts AT, Jol-Van Der Zijde CM, *et al.* (2016): Neuronal antibodies in pediatric epilepsy: Clinical features and long-term outcomes of a historical cohort not treated with immunotherapy. *Epilepsia* 57: 823–831.

Wright S, Hacohen Y, Jacobson L, *et al.* (2015a): N-methyl-D-aspartate receptor antibody-mediated neurological disease: results of a UK-based surveillance study in children. *Arch Dis Child* 100: 521–526.

Wright S, Hashemi K, Stasiak L, *et al.* (2015b): Epileptogenic effects of NMDAR antibodies in a passive transfer mouse model. *Brain* 138: 3159–3167.

Xie YJ, Zhou L, Jiang N, *et al.* (2015): Essential roles of leucine-rich glioma inactivated 1 in the development of embryonic and postnatal cerebellum. *Sci Rep* 5: 7827.

Zandi M S, Irani S R, Follows G, Moody AM, Molyneux P, Vincent A (2009): Limbic encephalitis associated with antibodies to the NMDA receptor in Hodgkin lymphoma. *Neurology* 73: 2039–2040.

CHAPTER 27
BRAIN PARASITIC INFECTIONS

Sofia S. Sanchez[1,2], Isidro Gonzales[2], Marco T. Medina[3], Antonio Delgado-Escueta[4] and Hector H. Garcia[2,5]

[1] Universidad Peruana Cayetano Heredia, Lima, Peru
[2] Cysticercosis Unit, Instituto Nacional de Ciencias Neurologicas, Jirón Ancash 1271, Lima, Peru
[3] School of Medical Sciences, University of Honduras, Tegucigalpa, Honduras
[4] Epilepsy Genetics-Genomics Labs, Neurology and Research Services, Veterans Affairs Greater Los Angeles Healthcare System, West Los Angeles, USA
[5] Center for Global Health – Tumbes and Department of Microbiology, Universidad Peruana Cayetano Heredia

The increased prevalence of epilepsy in developing countries is the composite result of several contributing factors including infections (bacteria, parasites, virus), trauma, poor delivery conditions and genetic factors (Newton & Garcia, 2012; Gracia *et al.*, 2010) among others. Multiple parasitic infections can affect the human brain, and from them at least two (neurocisticercosis and malaria) are significant contributors to the global burden of seizures and epilepsy (Newton & Garcia, 2012; Ndimubanzi *et al.*, 2010).

From all parasites affecting humans, most of them could potentially invade the human brain. Many nematodes have a life cycle that involves access of the larvae to the circulatory system, a pass through the lungs, deglution and then establishment in the intestinal lumen. Other, including some protozoa (*E. hystolitica*), trematodes and cestodes, can also reach the nervous system *via* the circulation after they penetrate the intestinal wall and reach a small vessel, and another group can access via the olfactory epithelium. Once in the brain, parasites may cause seizures by diverse mechanisms that may involve diffuse damage and ischemia (malaria), local damage and inflammation (*Taenia solium*, *Toxoplasma*, *Gnathostoma*, *Toxocara*), mass effect (hydatid disease, cysticercosis). Brain invasion, however, does not necessarily result in evident symptoms and many (likely the vast majority) of individuals remain apparently asymptomatic. For most parasites, only small numbers of cases of symptomatic central nervous involvement can be found (Kristensson *et al.*, 2013). Recently, an indirect effect damaging the neural cells by a cross-reactive immune reaction to antigens of the river blindness causative agent *Onchocerca volvulus* has been demonstrated in head nodding syndrome, a particular type of epilepsy described in several African settings (Johnson *et al.*, 2017).

Significant causes of epilepsy: malaria and neurocysticercosis

Malaria (*Plasmodium falciparum*)

Malaria is the most frequent neurological disease of parasitic origin worldwide. From the four species of *Plasmodium* affecting humans, only *P. falciparum* causes cerebral malaria (CM) according to the World Health Organization (WHO, 2018). Cerebral malaria is defined as an unexplained coma in a patient with malarial parasitemia. Approximately 10% of the cases result in chronic epilepsy (Postels & Birbeck, 2013). In sub-Saharan Africa, it is common and severe in children between 6 months and 5 years old, while in Southeast Asia (area of lower transmission) it is more common in older children and adults (Newton & Warrell, 1998).

Life cycle

Plasmodium is transmitted by the bite of the malaria-infected female *Anopheles* mosquito, inoculating sporozoites to the human host, which infects liver cells and mature into schizonts. After that, merozoites are released from the liver into the blood stream, where they invade the erythrocytes. Then, the parasites undergo asexual multiplication inside the erythrocytes. The ring stage trophozoites mature into schizonts, which rupture releasing merozoites (Marsh *et al.*, 1996; Newton & Krishna, 1998; Newton *et al.*, 1998; Postels & Birbeck, 2013).

After that, during a blood meal, the gametocytes are ingested by an *Anopheles* mosquito and inside the mosquito's stomach; they penetrate the macrogametes generating zygotes, which invade the midgut wall of the mosquito where they develop into oocysts. They grow, rupture, and release sporozoites, which make their way to the mosquito's salivary glands (Marsh *et al.*, 1996; Newton & Krishna, 1998; Newton *et al.*, 1998; Postels & Birbeck, 2013).

Clinical presentation

Almost half of the infected population is asymptomatic (O'Meara *et al.*, 2008). Prodromal symptoms are common and may take the form of fever, anorexia, cough, or vomiting. This period usually last less than 1 day. After that, the child falls into a coma or has a seizure before. Usually, African children only have "cerebral" disease, with rapid onset of coma, seizures, and compromise of the nervous system at multiple levels. In adults, central nervous system compromise occurs together with failure of other organ systems, mostly renal and respiratory *(Figure 1)* (Birbeck *et al.*, 2010; Idro *et al.*, 2005; Molyneux *et al.*, 1989).

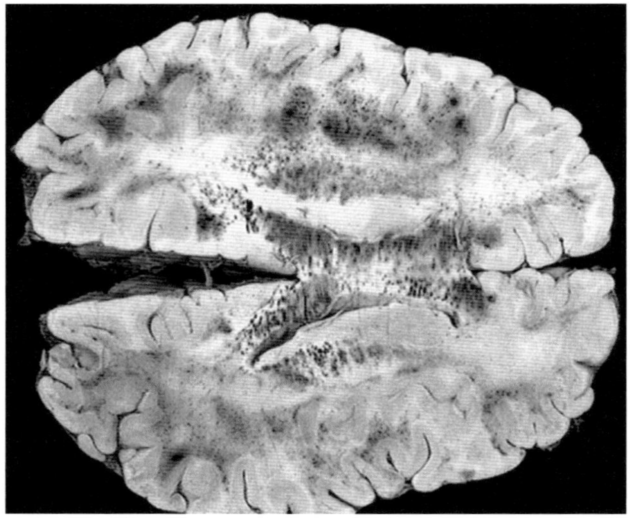

Figure 1 **Macroscopical pathology of cerebral malaria showing numerous petechial hemorrhages. (From Chimelli. A morphological approach to the diagnosis of protozoal infections of the central nervous system. *Pathol Res Int*, 2011, with permission.)**

From 40 to 80% of patients present generalized or partial seizures (Birbeck *et al.*, 2010b; Crawley *et al.*, 1996). Nystagmoid movements, conjugate eye deviation, breathing alterations, and other autonomic phenomena have all been correlated with epileptiform electroencephalogram pattern, suggesting these clinical manifestations may be ictal (Birbeck *et al.*, 2010b; Holding *et al.*, 1999). For those who survive CM, neurological sequelae are common, such as: epilepsy, cognitive impairment, behavioral disorders, and neurological deficits which include motor, sensory, and language disorders (Birbeck *et al.*, 2010a).

Malarial retinopathy can be detected by indirect ophthalmoscopy. This finding is 95% sensitive and 90% specific in identifying parasitemic children whose comas are caused by the malaria parasite. There are four main findings of malaria retinopathy: retinal whitening, retinal hemorrhages, papilledema, and changes in the appearance of retinal vessels (Beare *et al.*, 2006). The severity of this entity is positively correlated with the risk of death (Beare *et al.*, 2004).

Laboratory and radiological findings

Findings can include hypoglycemia, metabolic acidosis, hyponatremia and thrombocytopenia (Enwere *et al.*, 1998). After the onset of coma, generalized (symmetrical or asymmetrical), or focal slowing is frequently seen in the EEG (Crawley *et al.*, 2001). Seizures are often partial with or without secondary generalization, but can be primarily generalized (Postels & Birbeck, 2013). Twenty percent of children without history of seizures after their coma have subclinical seizures on examination. (Birbeck *et al.*, 2010a). Approximately 28% of patients had status epilepticus (overt or electrographic) (Idro *et al.*, 2005). Children with prolonged coma and retinopathy can show computed tomography (CT) scan abnormalities such as large vessel infarction and edema, both supratentorial and brainstem, while in adults, magnetic resonance imaging (MRI) findings include: cortical and subcortical infarcts, diffuse cerebral edema, gray and white matter abnormalities of the thalamus and cerebellum, and brainstem demyelination (Postels & Birbeck, 2013; Potchen *et al.*, 2010; Vyas *et al.*, 2012).

Cerebral malaria and epilepsy

Either electrographic or clinical seizures are predictors for death and long-term neurological disability, and the late development of epilepsy. This highlights the importance of increasing research in the long-term consequences of infectious diseases such as malaria (Birbeck *et al.*, 2010; Christensen & Eslick, 2015; Holding *et al.*, 1999). Seizures can occur in the later part of the acute course of the illness, and an important proportion of acute seizures are complex, prolonged and recurrent, comparing with simple febrile seizures (Christensen & Eslick,

2015). The mechanisms of neurological impairment in CM are not clear; studies suggest that brain injury is occasioned by sequestration of infected erythrocytes in the cerebral vasculature, which leads to hypoxia and subsequent ischemia (Idro *et al.*, 2010; Postels & Birbeck, 2013).

Treatment

Untreated CM is probably fatal, and with antimalarials therapy (derivatives of artemisinin and cinchona alkaloids) and supportive care, 15 to 30% still die (Newton & Krishna, 1998). In successfully treated patients, coma resolves within 24 hours. Longer coma duration could be because of non-convulsive seizures, metabolic abnormalities, concomitant bacterial infections or other conditions. Initial treatment of clinical seizures should be with benzodiazepines, with longer acting antiepileptic drugs given as needed (Christensen & Eslick, 2015; Ngoungou & Preux, 2008; Postels & Birbeck, 2013).

Neurocysticercosis (*Taenia solium*)

Infection of the human brain by the cystic larvae of the pork tapeworm *Taenia solium* is a very frequent condition in developing countries with exception of Muslim societies. In endemic regions NCC consistently accounts for approximately 30% of cases of epilepsy, becoming the most frequent cause of acquired epilepsy in adults (Garcia *et al.*, 1993; Ndimubanzi *et al.*, 2010; Medina *et al.*, 1990).

Life cycle

The co-existence of poor sanitary conditions and domestic pig raising allows pigs to have contact with and ingest human stools containing tapeworm eggs. The embryos contained in the eggs are released in the small intestine, attach to the intestinal mucosa and actively cross the intestinal wall to reach the circulatory system and are thus disseminated to most tissues of the intermediate host where they develop into mature, viable cystic larvae (cysticerci). When poorly cooked infected pork containing cysticerci is ingested by a human (the only definitive host), the larvae evaginate in the intestine and grows as an adult tapeworm, usually 2 to 4 meters long. The distal tapeworm segments or proglottids are filled with mature eggs that are then released into the environment to infect another intermediate host and continue the cycle. Unfortunately humans can also become infected with eggs and develop cysticercosis, *via* fecal oral contamination (Flisser, 1994). Larvae reaching the nervous system or the eye would survive preferentially because of the protection conferred by the blood brain and the hemato-ocular barriers, and become mature cysts.

Clinical features and diagnosis

While cysts may locate in almost any brain region and can produce diverse neurological symptoms, seizures, headache and intracranial hypertension are the most frequent manifestations. Seizures result from parenchymal brain cysts (parenchymal NCC), and intracranial hypertension and hydrocephalus commonly originate from invasion of the ventricles or the subarachnoid space, particularly the Sylvian fissure and the basal cisterns (extraparenchymal NCC) (Garcia *et al.*, 2014a). NCC symptoms usually initiate in the second and third decades of life. This has been attributed to the long pre-patent survival time of the parasites, in which the cysts successfully evade the immune surveillance of the host. At some point, inflammation launches around one or more of the cysts and the host's immune reaction ends up destroying the parasite, in a process that involves local inflammation and edema. In approximately 30% of cases, a residual calcification develops after a few months. Diagnosis rests on neuroimaging techniques (computed tomography and magnetic resonance imaging) (Del Brutto *et al.*, 2017b) and is supported by specific serology, either EITB using LLGP for antibody detection or monoclonal antibody-based ELISA for antigen detection (Rodriguez *et al.*, 2012). The use of ELISA for antibody detection is suboptimal and should not be recommended (Garcia *et al.*, 2018).

Treatment

The relation between cyst degeneration and onset of symptoms led some clinicians to assume that the use of antiparasitic drugs to destroy brain cysts was unnecessary. However, viable lesions do not begin to degenerate in the short term, (Garcia *et al.*, 2014b) and moreover, the onset of cyst degeneration do not imply that all cysts will resolve in the short term, since patients may have other surviving parasites for many years. Current guidelines recommend treatment with albendazole or praziquantel plus concomitant steroid coverage (White *et al.*, 2018). More than one course of antiparasitic treatment may be required to resolve all viable lesions. Cyst resolution is associated with fewer seizure relapses in the follow up (Garcia *et al.*, 2004; Garcia *et al.*, 2014b).

Cysticercosis and epilepsy

When comparable populations are studied either by serology or neuroimaging, cysticercosis infection is strongly associated with a 2 to 3-fold higher risk of seizures and epilepsy (Garcia *et al.*, 1993; Ndimubanzi *et al.*, 2010). A proportion of cases, particularly individuals with a single degenerating brain cyst, may present seizures for a short period of time after the cyst begins to degenerate, with a good prognosis and low relapse rate (under 30%) (Rajshekhar & Jeyaseelan, 2004). This is not the case for individuals with multiple cysts or those who initiate their symptoms with already calcified disease, in whom seizures are repetitive and who also carry a sizable risk of seizure relapse after AED tapering. (Del Brutto, 1994) *(Figure 2)*.

An interesting recent finding is the association between calcified NCC (outside the hippocampal region) and hippocampal sclerosis, both in clinical epilepsy cases as well as in apparently asymptomatic general population. It suggests that NCC acts as a causative factor either by chronic inflammation or by subclinical seizure discharges (Bianchin *et al.*, 2017; Del Brutto *et al.*, 2017a).

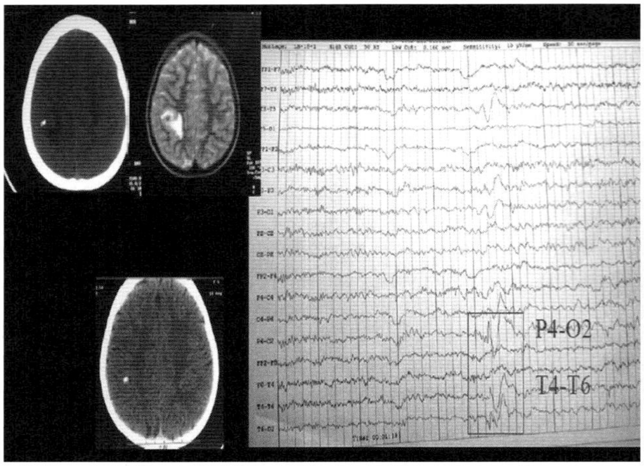

Figure 2 **Calcified neurocysticercosis with perilesional edema in a 6-year-old child with focal seizures.** **Upper left: CT and MRI demonstrating the calcified lesion with perilesional edema.** **Lower left: follow up CT demonstrating resolution of edema.** **Right: EEG demonstrating focal right parieto-temporal spike and wave complexes.**

NCC in pediatrics

Most cases of NCC in the pediatric population present as a single degenerating lesion, opening the differential with other causes of focal, contrast enhancing parenchymal brain lesions. Calcified NCC is occasionally seen. Established infections with multiple viable cysts are infrequent, and subarachnoid disease is seldom seen (Singhi & Saini, 2017). The search for a tapeworm carrier in all household members should be stressed when pediatric NCC is suspected, both to support the diagnosis as well as to eliminate the source of infection. The frequency of epilepsy associated to NCC can be reduced by community interventions (Medina *et al.*, 2011; Garcia *et al.*, 2016).

Other parasitic infections of the central nervous system

Toxocariasis (*T. canis, T. cati*)

Toxocariasis is one of the most prevalent helminth infections worldwide. In industrialized countries its prevalence ranges from 2 to 5% in urban areas, up to 37% in rural settings. In tropical regions the seroprevalence ranges from 39 to 93% (Bachli *et al.*, 2004; Fan *et al.*, 2015; Finsterer & Auer, 2007; Kazek, 2006; Magnaval *et al.*, 2001; Moiyadi *et al.*, 2007). The most common species are *T. canis* and *T. cati*, infecting dogs and cats respectively.

Life cycle

About 200,000 eggs are produced per day by an adult female *Toxocara canis*, and are released to the environment with the feces of the infected dog. Once in the soil, they require an incubation period of 1–2 weeks to become infectious (Glickman & Schantz, 1981). Embrionated *Toxocara* eggs can remain infective in the environment for several years. These are ingested by dogs or cats. Larvae can migrate to the fetus *via* placenta in pregnant dogs. In both dogs and cats the highest prevalence is found at 24 weeks of age (O'Lorcain, 1994). Humans get infected by ingestion of food contaminated with embrionated eggs. When ingested the larva is released and hatches the intestine wall to migrate to the liver and the lungs. When it reaches the systemic circulation it can migrate to any organ (Nichols, 1956; Nicoletti, 2013; Sprent, 1952).

Clinical features and diagnosis

The most common clinical manifestations are visceral larva migrans (VLM) and ocular larva migrans. Covert toxocariasis and common toxocariasis were described recently as mild *Toxocara* infection and characterized by less severe systemic manifestations. The first is more common in children while the latter is frequently found in adults (Taylor *et al.*, 1987).

Asymptomatic CNS infection is probably common. Clinically apparent neurotoxocariasis has a wide spectrum of neurological manifestations from meningitis, encephalitis and myelitis, to cerebral vasculitis (Fan *et al.*, 2015). There are few reports of peripheral nervous system manifestations like radiculitis, cranial nerves or musculo-skeletal compromise. Around 100 cases of neurotoxocariasis have been reported in the literature since 1956 (Finsterer & Auer, 2007).

The diagnosis of neurotoxocariasis is based on the presence of a high titer of anti-*Toxocara* antibody in the CSF or in the serum, presence of eosinophilia in the serum or CSF, and clinical and radiological improvement after anthelmintic therapy (Finsterer & Auer, 2007; Nicoletti, 2013; Sanchez *et al.*, 2018).

Isolated myelitis represents the most commonly reported presentation. Clinical manifestations include sensory and motor disturbances, predominantly involving the lower limbs accompanied by autonomic dysfunction (Ota, 2010; Lee, 2009). Encephalic/meningeal toxocariasis involvement is associated with a wide range of clinical manifestations including headache, seizures, focal deficits, confusional state, and cognitive impairment, with or without fever. CNS vasculitis is a rare and severe presentation presenting with headache, cognitive impairment, and acute ischemic events (Fellrath & Magnaval, 2014; Feske *et al.*, 2015).

The standard serological test is an ELISA for secretory-excretory antigens (TES) from *Toxocara canis* larvae at the second stage. ELISA for the detection of specific IgG antibodies to TES in serum has a sensitivity of 78% and a specificity of 92% for the diagnosis of VLM, although cross-reactions with other nematode infections reduce its specificity, particularly in tropical areas (Fillaux & Magnaval, 2013; Ma *et al.*, 2018). Screening with the indirect TES-IgG-ELISA, followed by confirmation with the TES-Western Blot (TES-WB), is considered an effective approach (Ma *et al.*, 2018; Rubinsky-Elefant *et al.*, 2010).

Treatment

If well there is no controlled data, the usual treatment is albendazole at 800 mg/day or 15 mg/kg/day, and the duration of treatment is variable, between 2 weeks and 3 months. Most clinicians also use steroids, and there are reports of improvement with steroid treatment only (Jabbour *et al.*, 2011).

Toxocariasis and epilepsy

A possible association between *T. canis* and epilepsy at the population level has been suggested by several case-control studies. A meta-analysis that included seven case-control studies showed a common odds ratio (OR) of 1.92 [95% confidence interval (CI) 1.50–2.44, $p < 0.001$], supporting the existence of a positive association (Deshayes *et al.*, 2016; Quattrocchi *et al.*, 2012). Seroprevalence rate of anti-*Toxocara spp.* antibodies was higher among people with epilepsy than control subjects in all the seven studies; however, these studies were retrospective, and we cannot establish a causal association (Akyol *et al.*, 2007; Arpino *et al.*, 1990; Glickman & Schantz, 1981; Nicoletti, 2013; Nicoletti *et al.*, 2002, 2007, 2008; Quattrocchi *et al.*, 2012).

A population-based survey in India demonstrated a similar prevalence of antibodies to *T. canis* in people with active epilepsy (4.7%; 5 of 106 people) compared to controls (5.7%; 6 of 106 people) (Singh *et al.*, 2012). Conversely, data from rural-community studies in Bolivia and Burundi and a hospital-based study from Italy suggests an association between *T. canis* exposure and epilepsy (Nicoletti *et al.*, 2002, 2007, 2008). In the Bolivian study, the adjusted OR was 2.70 (95% CI 1.4–5.2), while in the Burundi study it was 2.1 (95% CI 1.2–3.8), and in the Italian study it was 3.9 (95% CI, 1.9–8.0).

Toxoplasmosis (*T. gondii*)

Toxoplasmosis is likely the most common infection of the human nervous system. The parasite is present worldwide, and human exposure to the parasite is a very frequent event. In tropical countries the majority of the population demonstrates specific antibodies, and it varies between 10 and 50% in industrialized countries (Pappas *et al.*, 2009; Torgerson & Mastroiacovo, 2013).

Life cycle

In the usual cycle of the infection, *Toxoplasma gondii* (an obligate intracellular protozoa) are ingested by cats. Sexual reproduction occurs in the cat's intestines and large numbers of oocysts are shed to the environment. After a few days these oocysts become infective and are ingested by an intermediate host (usually rodents or birds). Occysts mature to tachyzoites that can infect the intermediate host's tissues and establish as tissue cysts (full of bradyzoites) in muscles or in the nervous system. The cycle is closed when cats get infected by ingesting the cysts in the meat of an infected intermediate host, or by ingesting infective oocysts. Human infection also occurs by ingesting infected meat with tissue cysts or by ingesting infective oocysts in soil, by mother-to-fetus transplacental infection, by organ transplant or blood transfusion (Soldati & Meissner, 2004; Tenter *et al.*, 2000).

Clinical features and diagnosis

Human disease depends on whether it occurred during pregnancy (characterized by congenital abnormalities and parenchymal brain calcifications), early in childhood (retinal scars), or later (silent tissue cysts that may reactivate in case of immunosuppression such as HIV infection; toxoplasmosis is still a frequent cause of neurological disease in AIDS patients in regions where highly active antiretroviral therapy is not easily accessible). More rarely, neurotoxoplasmosis may occur in immunocompetent hosts during acute *Toxoplasma* infection. Patients present with fever, headache, focal signs, seizures, altered mental status, or intracranial hypertension.

Brain *Toxoplasma* lesions frequently locate in the basal ganglia or subcortical white matter and demonstrate ring enhancing lesions with significant perilesional edema on CT or MRI. On histology the lesions may show parasites in the bradyzoite or tachyzoite stages, with central necrosis.

Diagnosis is usually achieved by serology, although tissue cysts may be observed in stained biopsy specimens. A positive IgG assay is poorly predictive in endemic regions because of the high seroprevalence of *T. gondii* infection in both the general population and in HIV patients in developing countries. Raising titers or a positive IgM test are thus required to indicate acute infection, although most disease in adults results from reactivation of old infections. PCR in amniotic fluid can be used to demonstrate congenital infections, and PCR in CSF appears useful in neurological compromise. Blood PCR is poorly sensitive but a positive finding provides a reliable diagnosis (Kotresha & Noordin, 2010; Luft & Remington, 1992; Montoya & Rosso, 2005; Remington *et al.*, 2004; Swisher *et al.*, 1994; Dard *et al.*, 2016; Villard *et al.*, 2016).

Treatment

The clinical response rate in *Toxoplasma* encephalitis is very high if it is diagnosed and treated early. Treatment is based on the combination of pyrimethamine and sulfadiazine for six weeks or more, and aims to destroy the tachyzoite forms. Leucovorin is used concomitantly with pyrimethamine to decrease hematological toxicity. Clindamycin is used as a replacement for sulfadiazine when it is not a feasible option. Imaging follow up is required to assess treatment efficacy.

Toxoplasmosis and epilepsy

Unlike NCC, malaria or possibly toxocariasis, neurotoxoplasmosis is mostly a cause of acute seizure episodes, particularly in patients with HIV, and rarely a cause of chronic epilepsy.

Free-living ameba (*Acanthamoeba spp, Balamuthia mandrillaris, Naegleria fowleri, Sappinia pedata*)

Free living ameba of the generes *Acanthamoeba, Balamuthia, Naegleria*, and more rarely *Sappinia*, can cause central nervous system infections in the human host (Visvesvara, 2013; Gelman *et al.*, 2001; Qvarnstrom *et al.*, 2009). *Naegleria* infections produce a very acute disease (primary amebic meningoencephalitis, PAM), while *Acanthamoeba* and *Balamuthia* course with a more chronic presentation, granulomatosis amebic encephalitis. Both types of presentation are highly lethal with rare survivor cases.

Life cycle

The life cycle of amebas includes a cyst stage, very resistant to adverse environmental conditions, and an active form or trophozoite, which multiplies by binary fusion. Humans get infected by the trophozites through the olfactory pathway or skin lesions.

Clinical manifestations

PAM presents very acutely with headache, fever, stiff neck, ataxia, photophobia, seizures, intracranial hypertension, lethargia, confusion, coma and death. It clinically resembles acute bacterial meningitis, and this may distract clinicians from considering *Naegleria* in the differential diagnosis and work up. Frequently the diagnosis is only determined post-mortem by immunohistochemistry or DNA assays (Carter, 1972; Martinez, 1985; Marciano-Cabral, 1988; Martinez & Visvesvara, 1997; Schuster & Visvesvara, 2004; Visvesvara & Maguire, 2006; Visvesvara, 2007; Visvesvara *et al.*, 2007b; Qvarnstrom *et al.*, 2006; Guarner *et al.*, 2007). Neuroimages in PAM demonstrate diffuse inflammation and edema, with occasional areas of infarction (Razek, 2011).

Acanthamoeba GAE is more frequent in immunosuppressed or debilitated hosts. The presentation is less abrupt and the course is chronic, with altered mental status, headache, neurologic deficits, and seizures (Martinez, 1985; Martinez & Visvesvara, 1997; Marciano-Cabral & Cabral, 2003; Schuster & Visvesvara, 2004; Khan, 2006; Visvesvara & Maguire, 2006; Visvesvara, 2007; Visvesvara *et al.*, 2007b). In the case of GAE by Balamuthia, cutaneous lesions in the face, thorax or limbs precede the neurological compromise (Bravo *et al.*, 2006; Bravo *et al.*, 2011). Neuroimages in GAE show space-occupying lesions, granulomatous or cystic in appearance, with variable degrees of perilesional edema. The differential neuroimaging diagnosis involves multiple bacterial abscesses, neurotuberculosis or neurocysticercosis (Martinez & Visvesvara, 1997; Schuster & Visvesvara, 2004; Visvesvara, 2007; Visvesvara *et al.*, 2007b). The only case caused by *Sappinia pedata* presented with loss of consciousness, headache, vomiting, and visual alterations. A temporal mass was surgically excised, the patient received a course of antibiotics, and recovered (Qvarnstrom *et al.*, 2009).

Treatment

Combined use of antibiotics (pentamidine, sulfadiazine, clarithromycin, fluconazol, and flucitosine) has resulted in several therapeutical successes in Balamuthia GAE (Deetz *et al.*, 2003; Jung *et al.*, 2004; Cary *et al.*, 2010; Doyle *et al.*, 2011). In addition, two cases in Peru responded to combined albendazole plus itraconazole plus surgical excision of skin lesions (Bravo *et al.*, 2006) and miltefosine also useful. Only a few cases have survived from PAM, usually with combined therapies including amphotericin B, miconazole and rifampicine. Miltefosine also seems to offer a promising alternative.

Amebiasis and epilepsy

As in neurotoxoplasmosis, amebic CNS infections are mostly a cause of acute seizure episodes and rarely a cause of chronic epilepsy.

Concluding remarks

Parasitic invasion of the human CNS is not a rare event, and likely (as in most infectious diseases) the majority of infected individuals remain apparently asymptomatic. The proportion of symptomatic individuals, however, would still result in a sizable number of cases of seizures and epilepsy. In particular, NCC and malaria are responsible for large numbers of PWE worldwide. Immigration and travel now make these pathologies more frequent in industrialized countries, so they should be borne in mind in differential diagnosis.

REFERENCES ▶

Abdel Razek AA, Watcharakorn A, Castillo M (2011): Parasitic diseases of the central nervous system. *Neuroimaging Clin N Am* 21: 815–841.

Akyol A, Bicerol B, Ertug S, Ertabaklar H, Kiylioglu N (2007): Epilepsy and seropositivity rates of *Toxocara Canis* and *Toxoplasma Gondii*. *Seizure* 16: 233–237.

Arpino C, Gattinara GC, Piergili D, Curatolo P (1990): Toxocara infection and epilepsy in children: a case-control study. *Epilepsia* 31: 33–36.

Bachli H, Minet JC, Gratzl O (2004): Cerebral toxocariasis: a possible cause of epileptic seizure in children. *Childs Nerv Syst* 20: 468–472.

Beare NA, Riva CE, Taylor TE, *et al.* (2006): Changes in optic nerve head blood flow in children with cerebral malaria and acute papilloedema. *J Neurol Neurosurg Psychiatry* 77: 1288–1290.

Beare NA, Southern C, Chalira C, Taylor TE, Molyneux ME, Harding SP (2004): Prognostic significance and course of retinopathy in children with severe malaria. *Arch Ophthalmol* 122: 1141–1147.

Bianchin MM, Velasco TR, Wichert-Ana L, Dos Santos AC, Sakamoto AC (2017): Understanding the association of neurocysticercosis and mesial temporal lobe epilepsy and its impact on the surgical treatment of patients with drug-resistant epilepsy. *Epilepsy Behav* 76: 168–177.

Birbeck GL, Beare N, Lewallen S, *et al.* (2010a): Identification of malaria retinopathy improves the specificity of the clinical diagnosis of cerebral malaria: findings from a prospective cohort study. *Am J Trop Med Hyg* 82: 231–234.

Birbeck GL, Molyneux ME, Kaplan PW, *et al.* (2010b): Blantyre Malaria Project Epilepsy Study (BMPES) of neurological outcomes in retinopathy-positive paediatric cerebral malaria survivors: a prospective cohort study. *Lancet Neurol* 9: 1173–1181.

Bravo F G, Cabrera J, Gotuzzo E (2006): Cutaneous manifestations of infection by free-living amebas. In: Tyring SK, Lupi O, Hengge UR (eds.). *Tropical Dermatology*. Edinburgh, New York: Elsevier Churchill Livingstone, pp. 49–55.

Bravo F G, Alvarez P J, Gotuzzo E (2011): *Balamuthia mandrillaris* infection of the skin and central nervous system: an emerging disease of concern to many specialties in medicine. *Curr Opin Infect Dis* 24: 112–117.

Carter RF (1972): Primary amoebic meningo-encephalitis. An appraisal of present knowledge. *Trans. Roy Soc Trop Med Hyg* 66: 193–208.

Cary LC, Maul E, Potter C, Wong P, Nelson PT, Given C II, Robertson W Jr (2010): *Balamuthia mandrillaris* meningoencephalitis: survival of a pediatric patient. *Pediatrics* 125: 699–703.

Christensen SS, Eslick GD (2015): Cerebral malaria as a risk factor for the development of epilepsy and other long-term neurological conditions: a meta-analysis. *Trans R Soc Trop Med Hyg* 109: 233–238.

Crawley J, Smith S, Kirkham F, Muthinji P, Waruiru C, Marsh K (1996): Seizures and status epilepticus in childhood cerebral malaria. *QJM* 89: 591–597.

Crawley J, Smith S, Muthinji P, Marsh K, Kirkham F (2001): Electroencephalographic and clinical features of cerebral malaria. *Arch Dis Child* 84: 247–253.

Dard C, Fricker-Hidalgo H, Brenier-Pinchart MP, Pelloux H (2016): Relevance of and new developments in serology for toxoplasmosis. *Trends Parasitol* 32: 492–506.

Deetz TR, Sawyer MH, Billman G, Schuster FL, Visvesvara GS (2003): Successful treatment of *Balamuthia* amoebic encephalitis: presentation of 2 cases. *Clinical Infectious Diseases* 37: 1304–1312.

Del Brutto OH (1994): Prognostic factors for seizure recurrence after withdrawal of antiepileptic drugs in patients with neurocysticercosis. *Neurology* 44: 1706–1709.

Del Brutto OH, Issa NP, Salgado P, *et al.* (2017a): The association between neurocysticercosis and hippocampal atrophy is related to age. *Am J Trop Med Hyg* 96: 243–248.

Del Brutto OH, Nash TE, White AC Jr, *et al.* (2017b): Revised diagnostic criteria for neurocysticercosis. *J Neurol Sci* 372: 202–210.

Deshayes S, Bonhomme J, De La Blanchardiere A (2016): Neurotoxocariasis: a systematic literature review. *Infection* 44: 565–574.

Doyle JS, Campbell E, Fuller A, *et al.* (2011): *Balamuthia mandrillaris* brain abscess successfully treated with complete surgical excision and prolonged combination antimicrobial therapy. *J Neurosurg* 114: 458–462.

Dubey JP (1998): Re-examination of resistance of *Toxoplasma gondii* tachyzoites and bradyzoites to pepsin and trypsin digestion. *Parasitology* 116: 43–50.

Enwere G, Van Hensbroek MB, Adegbola R, *et al.* (1998): Bacteraemia in cerebral malaria. *Ann Trop Paediatr* 18: 275–278.

Fan CK, Holland CV, Loxton K, Barghouth U (2015): Cerebral toxocariasis: silent progression to neurodegenerative disorders? *Clin Microbiol Rev* 28: 663–686.

Fellrath JM, Magnaval JF (2014): Toxocariasis after slug ingestion characterized by severe neurologic, ocular, and pulmonary involvement. *Open Forum Infect Dis* 1. doi: 10.1093/ofid/ofu063.

Feske SK, Goldberg M, Dudzinski DM, Gonzalez RG, Kovach AE (2015): Case records of the Massachusetts general hospital. Case 29–2015. A 38-year-old pregnant woman with headache and visual symptoms. *N Engl J Med* 373: 1154–1164.

Fillaux J, Magnaval JF (2013): Laboratory diagnosis of human toxocariasis. *Vet Parasitol* 193: 327–336.

Finsterer J and Auer H (2007): Neurotoxocarosis. *Rev Inst Med Trop Sao Paulo* 49: 279–287.

Flisser A (1994): Taeniasis and cysticercosis due to *Taenia solium*. *Prog Clin Parasitol* 4: 77–116.

Garcia HH, Castillo Y, Gonzales I, *et al.* (2018): Low sensitivity and frequent cross-reactions in commercially available antibody detection ELISA assays for taenia solium cysticercosis. *Trop Med Int Health* 23: 101–105.

Garcia HH, Gilman R, Martinez M, *et al.* (1993): Cysticercosis as a major cause of epilepsy in Peru. *Lancet* 341: 197–200.

Garcia HH, Gonzales I, Lescano AG, *et al.* (1981): Epidemiology and pathogenesis of zoonotic toxocariasis. *Epidemiol Rev* 3: 230–250.

Garcia HH, Nash TE, Del Brutto OH (2014b): Clinical symptoms, diagnosis, and treatment of neurocysticercosis. *Lancet Neurol* 13: 1202–1125.

Garcia HH, Pretell EJ, Gilman RH, *et al.* (2004): A trial of antiparasitic treatment to reduce the rate of seizures due to cerebral cysticercosis. *N Engl J Med* 350: 249–258.

Gavidia M, Rodriguez L, Najar E, Umeres H, Pretell EJ (2014a): Efficacy of combined antiparasitic therapy with praziquantel and albendazole for neurocysticercosis: a double-blind, randomised controlled trial. *Lancet Infect Dis* 14: 687–695.

Gelman BB, Rauf SJ, Nader R, *et al.* (2001): Amoebic encephalitis due to *Sappinia Diploidea*. *JAMA* 285: 2450–2451.

Goswick SM, Brenner GM (2003): Activities of therapeutic agents against *Naegleria Fowleri* and in a mouse model of primary amebic meningoencephalitis. *J Parasitol* 89: 837–842.

Gracia F, de Lao SL, Castillo L, *et al.* (1990). Epidemiology of epilepsy in Guaymi Indians from Bocas del Toro Province, Republic of Panama. *Epilepsia* 31: 718–23.

Guarner J, Bartlett J, Shieh WJ, Paddock CD, Visvesvara GS, Zaki SR (2007): Histopathologic spectrum and immunohistochemical diagnosis of amebic meningoencephalitis. *Mod Pathol* 20: 1230–1237.

Holding PA, Stevenson J, Peshu N, Marsh K (1999): Cognitive sequelae of severe malaria with impaired consciousness. *Trans R Soc Trop Med Hyg* 93: 529–534.

Idro R, Jenkins NE, Newton CR (2005): Pathogenesis, clinical features, and neurological outcome of cerebral malaria. *Lancet Neurol* 4: 827–840.

Idro R, Marsh K, John CC, Newton CR (2010): Cerebral malaria: mechanisms of brain injury and strategies for improved neurocognitive outcome. *Pediatr Res* 68: 267–274.

Jabbour RA, Kanj SS, Sawaya RA, Awar GN, Hourani MH, Atweh SF (2011): *Toxocara canis* myelitis: clinical features, magnetic resonance imaging (MRI) findings, and treatment outcome in 17 patients. *Medicine (Baltimore)* 90: 337–343.

Johnson TP, Tyagi R, Lee PR, *et al.* (2017): Nodding syndrome may be an autoimmune reaction to the parasitic worm *Onchocerca volvulus*. *Sci Transl Med* 9: 377.

Jung S, Schelper RL, Visvesvara GS, Chang HT (2004): *Balamuthia mandrillaris* meningoencephalitis in an immunocompetent patient: an unusual clinical course and a favorable outcome. *Arch Pathol Lab Med* 128: 466–468.

Kazek B, Jamroz E, Mandera M, Bierzyńska-Macyszyn G, Kluczewska E, Marszał E (2006): The cerebral form of toxocarosis in a seven-year-old patient. *Folia Neuropathol* 44: 72–76.

Khan Na (2006): *Acanthamoeba*: biology and increasing importance in human health. *FEMS Microbiol Rev* 30: 564–595.

Kotresha D and Noordin R (2010): Recombinant proteins in the diagnosis of toxoplasmosis. *APMIS* 118: 529–542.

Kristensson K, Masocha W, Bentivoglio M (2013): Mechanisms of CNS invasion and damage by parasites. In: Garcia HH, Tanowitz HB, Del Brutto OH (eds) *Neuroparasitology and Tropical Neurology*. Amsterdam: Elsevier. Vol 114. pp. 11–22.

Luft BJ and Remington JS (1992): Toxoplasmic encephalitis in AIDS. *Clin Infect Dis* 15: 211–222.

Ma G, Holland CV, Wang T, *et al.* (2018): Human toxocariasis. *Lancet Infect Dis* 18: E14–E24.

Magnaval JF, Glickman LT, Dorchies P, Morassin B (2001): Highlights of human toxocariasis. *Korean J Parasitol* 39: 1–11.

Marciano-Cabral F (1988): Biology of *Naegleria spp*. *Microbiol Rev* 52: 114–133.

Marciano-Cabral F and Cabral G (2003): *Acanthamoeba spp*. as agents of disease in humans. *Clin Microbiol Rev* 16: 273–307.

Marsh K, English M, Crawley J, Peshu N (1996): The pathogenesis of severe malaria in african children. *Ann Trop Med Parasitol* 90: 395–402.

Martinez AJ (1985): Free-living amebas: natural history, prevention, diagnosis, pathology, and treatment of disease. CRC Press. Boca Raton, Florida. pp: 156.

Martinez AJ, Visvesvara GS (1997): Free-living, amphizoic and opportunistic amebas. *Brain Pathol* 7: 583–598.

Medina MT, Rosas E, Rubio-Donnadieu F, Sotelo J (1990): Neurocysticercosis as the main cause of late-onset epilepsy in Mexico. *Arch Intern Med* 150: 325–327.

Medina MT, Aguilar-Estrada RL, Alvarez A, *et al.* (2011): Reduction in rate of epilepsy from neurocysticercosis by community interventions: the Salama, Honduras study. *Epilepsia* 52: 1177–1185.

Moiyadi A, Mahadevan A, Anandh B, Shivashankar RS, Chickabasavaiah YT, Shankar SK (2007): Visceral larva migrans presenting as multiple intracranial and intraspinal abscesses. *Neuropathology* 27: 371–374.

Molyneux, ME, Taylor, TE, Wirima, JJ, Borgstein A (1989): Clinical features and prognostic indicators in paediatric cerebral malaria: a study of 131 comatose malawian children. *Q J Med* 71: 441–459.

Montoya JG, Rosso F (2005): Diagnosis and management of toxoplasmosis. *Clin Perinatol* 32: 705–726.

Ndimubanzi PC, Carabin H, Budke CM, *et al.* (2010): A systematic review of the frequency of neurocysticercosis with a focus on people with epilepsy. *Plos Negl Trop Dis* 4: E870.

Newton CR, Garcia HH (2012): Epilepsy in poor regions of the world. *The Lancet* 380: 1193–1201.

Newton CR, Krishna S (1998): Severe falciparum malaria in children: current understanding of pathophysiology and supportive treatment. *Pharmacol Ther* 79: 1–53.

Newton CR, Taylor TE, Whitten RO (1998): Pathophysiology of fatal falciparum malaria in african children. *Am J Trop Med Hyg* 58: 673–683.

Newton CR, Warrell DA (1998): Neurological manifestations of falciparum malaria. *Ann Neurol* 43: 695–702.

Ngoungou EB and Preux PM (2008): Cerebral malaria and epilepsy. *Epilepsia* 49: 19–24.

Nichols (1956): The etiology of visceral larva migrans: I. diagnostic morphology of infective second-stage *Toxocara* larvae. *J Parasitol* 42: 349–362.

Nicoletti A (2013): Toxocariasis. In: Garcia HH, Tanowitz HB, Del Brutto OH (eds.), *Neuroparasitology and tropical neurology*. Handbook of clinical neurology, vol. 114, pp. 217–228.

Nicoletti A, Bartoloni A, Reggio A, *et al.* (2002): Epilepsy, cysticercosis, and toxocariasis: a population-based case-control study in rural Bolivia. *Neurology* 58: 1256–1261.

Nicoletti, A, Bartoloni A, Sofia V, *et al.* (2007): Epilepsy and toxocariasis: a case-control study in Burundi. *Epilepsia* 48: 894–899.

Nicoletti A, Sofia V, Mantella A, *et al.* (2008): Epilepsy and toxocariasis: a case-control study in Italy. *Epilepsia* 49: 594–599.

O'lorcain P (1994): Epidemiology of *Toxocara spp*. in stray dogs and cats in Dublin, Ireland. *J Helminthol* 68: 331–336.

O'meara WP, Bejon P, Mwangi TW, *et al.* (2008): Effect of a fall in malaria transmission on morbidity and mortality in Kilifi, Kenya. *Lancet* 372: 1555–1562.

Page FC (1967): Re-definition of the genus *Acanthamoeba* with descriptions of three species. *J Protozool* 14: 709–724.

Page FC (1988): *A New Key to Freshwater and Soil Gymnamoebae: with Instruction for Culture*. Ambleside. Cumbria: Freshwater Biological Association, p. 122.

Pappas G, Roussos N, Falagas ME (2009): Toxoplasmosis snapshots: global status of *Toxoplasma gondii* seroprevalence and implications for pregnancy and congenital toxoplasmosis. *Int J Parasitol* 39: 1385–1394.

Postels DG and Birbeck GL (2013): Cerebral Malaria. In: Garcia HH, Tanowitz HB, Del Brutto OH (eds.), *Neuroparasitology and Tropical Neurology*. Handbook of clinical neurology, vol. 114, pp. 91–102.

Potchen MJ, Birbeck GL, Demarco JK., *et al.* (2010): Neuroimaging findings in children with retinopathy-confirmed cerebral malaria. *Eur J Radiol* 74: 262–268.

Quattrocchi G, Nicoletti A, Marin B, Bruno E, Druet-Cabanac M, Preux PM (2012): Toxocariasis and epilepsy: systematic review and meta-analysis. *Plos Negl Trop Dis* 6: E1775.

Qvarnstrom Y, Visvesvara GS, Sriram R, Da Silva AJ (2006): Multiplex real-time PCR assay for simultaneous detection of *Acanthamoeba spp.*, *Balamuthia mandrillaris*, and *Naegleria fowleri*. *J Clin Microbiol* 44: 3589–3595.

Qvarnstrom Y, Da Silva AJ, Schuster FL, Gelman BB, Visvesvara GS (2009): Molecular confirmation of *Sappinia pedata* as a causative agent of amoebic encephalitis. *J Infect Dis* 199: 1139–1142.

Rajshekhar V, Jeyaseelan L (2004): Seizure outcome in patients with a solitary cerebral cysticercus granuloma. *Neurology* 62: 2236–2240.

Remington JS, Thulliez P, Montoya JG (2004): Recent developments for diagnosis of toxoplasmosis. *J Clin Microbiol* 42: 941–945.

Rodriguez S, Wilkins P, Dorny P (2012): Immunological and molecular diagnosis of cysticercosis. *Pathog and Glob Health* 106: 286–298.

Rubinsky-Elefant G, Hirata CE, Yamamoto JH, Ferreira MU (2010): Human toxocariasis: diagnosis, worldwide seroprevalences and clinical expression of the systemic and ocular forms. *Ann Trop Med Parasitol* 104: 3–23.

Sanchez SS, Garcia HH, Nicoletti A (2018): Clinical and magnetic resonance imaging findings of neurotoxocariasis. *Front Neurol* 9: 53.

Schuster FL, Visvesvara GS (2004): Free-living amoebae as opportunistic and non-opportunistic pathogens of humans and animals. *Int J Parasitol* 34: 1001–1027.

Schuster FL, Guglielmo BJ, Visvesvara GS (2006a): *In vitro* activity of miltefosine and voriconazole on clinical isolates of free-living amebas: *Balamuthia mandrillaris, Acanthamoeba spp., and Naegleria fowleri*. *J Eukaryot Microbiol* 53: 121–126.

Singh G, Bawa J, Chinna D, *et al.* (2012): Association between epilepsy and cysticercosis and toxocariasis: a population-based case-control study in a slum in india. *Epilepsia* 53: 2203–2208.

Singhi P, Saini AG (2019): Pediatric neurocysticercosis. *Indian J Pediatr* 86: 76–82.

Soldati D, Meissner M (2004): Toxoplasma as a novel system for motility. *Curr Opin Cell Biol* 16: 32–40.

Sprent JF (1952): On the migratory behavior of the larvae of various *Ascaris* species in white mice. Distribution of larvae in tissues. *J Infect Dis* 90: 165–176.

Swisher CN, Boyer K, Mcleod R (1994): Congenital toxoplasmosis, the toxoplasmosis study group. *Semin Pediatr Neurol* 1: 4–25.

Taylor MR, Keane CT, O'connor P, Girdwood RW, Smith H (1987): Clinical features of covert toxocariasis. *Scand J Infect Dis* 19: 693–696.

Tenter AM, Heckeroth AR, Weiss LM (2000): *Toxoplasma gondii*: from animals to humans. *Int J Parasitol* 30: 1217–1258.

Torgerson PR, Mastroiacovo P (2013): The global burden of congenital toxoplasmosis: a systematic review. *Bull World Health Organ* 91: 501–508.

Villard O, Cimon B, L'Ollivier C, *et al.* (2016): Serological diagnosis of *Toxoplasma gondii* infection: recommendations from the french national reference center for toxoplasmosis. *Diagn Microbiol Infect Dis* 84: 22–33.

Visvesvara GS (2007): Pathogenic and opportunistic free-living amebae. In: Murray PR, Baron EJ (eds.), *Manual of clinical microbiology*. Washington DC: ASM Press, pp. 2082–2091.

Visvesvara GS, Moura H, Schuster FL (2007b): Pathogenic and opportunistic free-living amoebae: *Acanthamoeba spp., Balamuthia mandrillaris, Naegleria fowleri*, and *Sappinia diploidea*. *FEMS Immunol Med Microbiol* 50: 1–26.

Visvesvara GS, Maguire JH (2006): Pathogenic and opportunistic free-living amebas: *Acanthamoeba spp. Balamuthia mandrillaris, Naegleria fowleri*, and *Sappinia diploidea*. In: Guerrant RL, Walker DH, Weller PF (eds.), *Tropical Infectious Disease: Principles, Pathogens and Practice*, vol. 2. Philadelphia: Churchill Livingstone (Elsevier), pp. 1114–1125.

Visvesvara GS, Schuster FL, Martinez AJ (1993): *Balamuthia mandrillaris*, N. G., N. Sp, agent of amebic meningoencephalitis in humans and other animals. *J Eukaryot Microbiol* 40: 504–514.

Visvesvara GS, Stehr-Green JK (1990): Epidemiology of free-living ameba infection. *J Protozool* 37: 25s–33s.

Visvesvara GS (2013): Infections with free-living amebae. In: Garcia HH, Tanowitz HB, Del Brutto OH (eds.) *Neuroparasitology and Tropical Neurology*. Handbook of clinical neurology, vol. 114. pp. 153–168.

Vyas S, Gupta V, Hondappanavar A, *et al.* (2012): Magnetic resonance imaging of cerebral malaria. *J Emerg Med* 42: E117–E119.

World Health Organization (2018). Malaria Fact Sheet No. 94 Retrieved 11 April 2018, From: http://www.who.int/mediacentre/factsheets/fs094/en/

WITH VIDEO SUPPLEMENTS

CHAPTER 28
COMPLEX REFLEX EPILEPSIES

Yushi Inoue[1] and Peter Wolf[2]

[1] National Epilepsy Centre, Shizuoka Institute of Epilepsy and Neurological Disorders, Japan
[2] Danish Epilepsy Centre Filadelfia, Dianalund, Denmark

Introduction

The precipitation of seizures by specific sensory or cognitive stimuli, often referred to as "reflex epilepsy", is found in many epilepsy syndromes, both idiopathic and symptomatic. Some of these conditions such as photosensitivity and eye closure sensitivity seem to be genetic traits, which can be found across syndromes although they may cluster with certain clinical entities. They would only be considered a syndrome of its own if a patient had only (or almost only) precipitated seizures, which is rare. Thus, photosensitivity is a trait, which is mostly but not exclusively found with idiopathic generalized epilepsies (IGE) where it is most frequent in juvenile myoclonic epilepsy (JME). There are some cases with reflex seizures only, and this condition has been called photosensitive epilepsy. This has, however, not become a recognized syndrome of its own because the trait is found much more frequently with IGE than standing alone.

According to the provocation mechanism, "reflex" seizures can be divided into a simple and a complex group. The former comprises seizure precipitation by simple sensory stimuli and by movements, the second precipitation by complex mental and emotional processes, although the distinction is somewhat arbitrary. Latency from stimulus onset to the clinical or EEG event is usually longer in the complex than in the simple group.

This chapter deals with three types of complex precipitating mechanisms: i) hearing music and voices: ii) language, including reading; and iii) other complex cognitive tasks.

Induction by hearing music and voices

Listening to music "sounds in melodic or harmonic combination" (Zifkin & Zatorre, 1998), particularly to pieces of music with emotional effect, may elicit seizures (Critchley, 1937).

Demographics and description

Wieser *et al.* (1997, 2004) reviewed 83 cases of musicogenic epilepsy, and Avanzini (2003) 88 cases. The age of onset of epilepsy was at 27.7 years (± 12.5) and the first musically provoked seizure at 28.1 years (± 9.8). An exceptional case of a 6-month-old boy was reported (Lin *et al.*, 2003). Only 14 patients had exclusively musically triggered seizures and 48 patients had both musicogenic seizures and spontaneous seizures. In half of the patients with sufficient information, the provoking music was specific, *i.e.*, music of a certain style or a certain composer, or even only a certain musical piece triggered the seizures. Sometimes, even thinking or dreaming about music can induce seizures (Jallon *et al.*, 1989). In others, music of any type may be sufficient (Vizioli, 1989). In some cases, seizures may initially occur exclusively in response to music and subsequently generalize to other auditory stimuli, such as voice or nonmusical sound (Genc *et al.*, 2001; Gélisse *et al.*, 2003), while in some others, there were initially non-musicogenic, but thereafter exclusively musicogenic seizures. More than 70% of the patients with available information were interested or talented in music. Such interest in the provoking activities is also observed in other types of seizures induced by higher brain function.

In one-third, familiarity and/or affective content were reported as a very important aspect of the triggering mechanism. The importance of music-associated emotion was often indicated, as the information conveyed by music is primarily emotional, in contrast to propositional language.

The induced seizures were complex partial seizures (with or without secondary generalization) often preceded by an aura: auditory hallucinations of simple (sound) or complex character (tune, rhythm, voice), epigastric discomfort, smell, experiential phenomena, and emotion such as anxiety and fear. A complex focal seizure induced by listening to a song that triggered a seizure in real life is shown on *Figure 1*. The feeling preceding the seizures was more often unpleasant (76%) than pleasant (Pittau *et al.*, 2008). There was often a latency of several minutes during which the patient must be continually exposed to the stimulus for the seizure to occur, and autonomic symptoms and signs may be noted before overt ictal behaviour begins.

In some, playing instruments or singing a song were even more provocative than simple listening (Tayah *et al.*, 2006; Duanyu *et al.*, 2010).

EEG and imaging studies

In 63%, a seizure focus was localized to the temporal lobe, more often on the right side. There were several reports indicating temporal onset of the ictal EEG discharges: among 60 patients with ictal EEG findings, the focus was right temporal in 48%, left temporal in 32%, and bitemporal in 8%; the remaining 12% had generalized or nonfocal alterations on their EEGs (Pittau *et al.*, 2008). Equivalent current dipoles using interictal EEG were located in the right posterior transverse temporal gyrus (Shibata *et al.*, 2006).

Usually no structural brain lesion can be found (Kaplan, 2003), except some cases. According to the literature review of Pittau *et al.* (2008), the MRI (available in 14 cases) was normal in eleven patients; unspecified right-sided lesions were reported in two patients and a left-sided astrocytoma was described in one (Anneken *et al.*, 2006). Ictal SPECT studies (available in six cases) demonstrated abnormality on the right in four patients and on the left in two. A PET study performed on four patients was normal in three and revealed right-sided abnormality in one. An ictal PET revealed increased metabolism in the right anterio-mesial temporal lobe (Mehta *et al.*, 2009). fMRI signal increase was found in the left anterior temporal lobe and the right gyrus rectus at an early phase (Morocz *et al.*, 2003), and over the right fronto-temporo-occipital area before the seizure onset (Pittau *et al.*, 2008), or also in other areas in addition to the epileptogenic area (Marrosu *et al.*, 2009; Diekmann *et al.*, 2014).

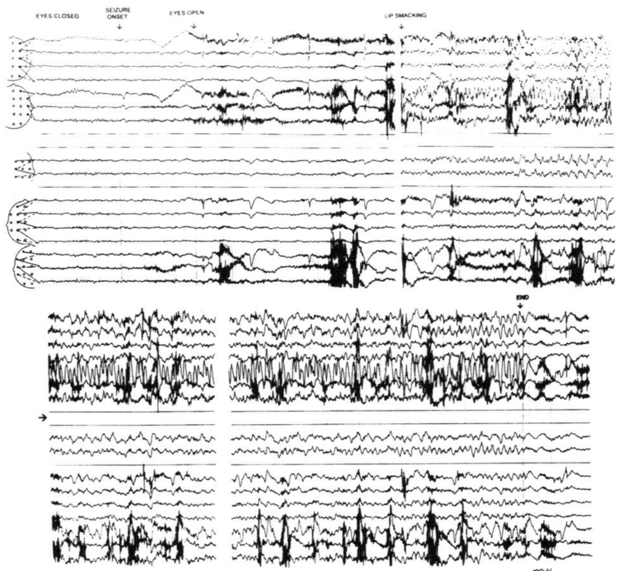

Centre Saint-Paul

Figure 1 **Musicogenic epilepsy, ictal recording, abstracts from a seizure that lasted 1 minute and 48 seconds in a 45-yr old woman. Seizure provoked by listening to the tune that triggered her first seizure two years earlier. The clinical onset is marked by a feeling of anxiety and uneasiness without EEG changes; later apperance of rhythmic theta activity over the right temporal leads. The clinical and EEG seizure stops as soon as the music stops. The patient never experienced secondary generalization. She later developed seizures also triggered by music or specific sounds that originated also in the left temporal lobe. The epilepsy was drug-resistant.**

Tayah *et al.* (2006) reported 3 patients with musicogenic epilepsy who underwent intracranial EEG investigation. The seizures started in the right lateral temporal lobe, right medial temporal lobe and independently from both medial temporal lobes in each patient. The first patient had a right anterior temporal lobe resection that spared the hippocampus. This patient remained seizure free for 12 years. The second patient underwent resection of the right medial temporal lobe and was free from seizures for 3 years. The authors concluded that musicogenic seizures could arise from multiple temporal lobe foci, although there was a right side preponderance as well as relationship to emotion. Mehta *et al.* (2009) revealed an ictal intracranial EEG onset in the right hippocampus and amygdala, followed by early spread into the parahippocampal gyrus and the lateral temporal lobe, then Heschl's gyrus and the right frontal lobe, in a 24-year-old MRI negative woman who subsequently underwent right temporal lobectomy and became seizure free. Duanyu *et al.* (2010) also performed intracranial EEG in a 14-year-old boy and found the epileptogenic focus localized to the middle part of the lateral temporal lobe on the left side. Resection of the temporal neocortex rendered the patient seizure free. The morphological diagnosis was focal cortical dysplasia type 1b. Wang *et al.* (2012) studied a 42-year-old professional composer with aura consisting of buzzing or muffled sounds consistently triggered by songs with familiar melody and lyrics by invasive EEG recording. All the electrophysiological data including MEG pinpointed seizure onset at planum temporale on the left side. A limited resection of left superior temporal gyrus sparing eloquent cortex made the seizures disappear. The pathology was focal cortical dysplasia type 1. Tezer *et al.* (2014) reported a female patient in whom the seizures precipitated by listening to affective music in her native language originated from the right hippocampus, while spontaneous seizures came from the left hippocampus. They speculated that emotions and memory related to past worries triggered by music were responsible for seizure precipitation on the right side. Diekmann *et al.* (2014) studied a 32-year-old male patient with seizures induced by a specific piece of Russian music accompanied by a certain pleasant feeling by using fMRI-EEG where BOLD signal alterations were not only found in the left temporo-frontal epileptogenic focus determined by ictal EEG, but also in areas known for their role in the processing of emotion. They speculated that dysfunction of the regulation processes of musically-induced emotions, and not the musical stimulus itself, led to the seizures.

Mechanism of music induction

The mechanism of music induction is not well understood. Sparr, (2003) mentioned a variety of components of musical perception (pitch, melody, rhythm and emotional response), variety of musical abilities in humans, and difference of the location of music in brain by gender and experience. Therefore, music as stimulus is very complex in the brain as well as in individuals. It appeared that, rather than the tone or timbre of the sound stimulus, more complex or interacting factors operate as a precipitant (Kaplan, 2003). Musical stimuli may have widespread effects on neural activity in human temporal lobes extending well beyond the restricted primary auditory area. A neural system that is dedicated to processing musically relevant auditory features involving bilateral cortical and subcortical territories, with right hemisphere dominance, may be activated. There must be also a strong contribution of emotion to the music induction.

Treatment

Joynt *et al.* (1966) reported on a patient treated with sensory extinction, *i.e.*, playing either innocuous music or short passages of unpleasant music prior to playing the seizure-producing music. Although the results of conventional treatment using antiepileptic medication have not been pooled, some patients were apparently very intractable and considered for epilepsy surgery. Although the reported outcome after surgery was good, the presurgical evaluation may be challenging, because neuroimaging often revealed no structural abnormality.

Complex auditory induction other than by music

Other related complex trigger mechanisms seem to be extremely rare. There is one report where singing and recitation, but not listening to music, induced seizures with head turning in a very young boy with temporo-central spikes (Herskowitz *et al.*, 1984).

Forster *et al.* (1969) reported a 53-year-old female who had post-traumatic epilepsy with focal seizures with aphasia. These were precipitated by hearing the voices of three particular radio announcers, independently of the texts. No other voices could provoke a seizure. The authors suggested that an element of prosody may have played a significant role in seizure provocation, and there may have been an emotional factor. Ramani, (1991) published a similar case of a 45-year-old woman with cryptogenic right temporal lobe seizures triggered by a particular female co-host in a popular TV entertainment program. Systematic testing revealed that the patient was sensitive to the performer's voice and not to visual stimulation, emotional anticipation or background music, nor to other programs or other female voices. Another case of voice-induced seizure was reported by Tsuzuki & Kasuga (1978). It was a woman who had EEG discharges triggered by verbal stimulation, particularly if someone spoke to the patient directly. These cases share some similarities to the language-induced epilepsy to be discussed in the next section.

Nosological place

The cases of musicogenic epilepsy were characterized by rather late onset, temporal lobe seizure semiology, often unrevealing imaging findings, and epileptiform EEG discharges in the temporal region, more often on the right side. The medial temporal lobe may not be the initial seizure onset zone, but becomes necessarily involved in the seizure development as indicated by the seizure semiology and ictal intracranial EEG. A neural system dedicated to processing musically relevant auditory features with involvement of limbic system for emotion may trigger the seizure. According to Mameniskiene and Wolf (2018), the fact that of the many patients with TLE, only very few have musicogenic seizures, and that unusually many of these have above average musical abilities, indicates that the seizures are generated in an enriched pre-existing functional-anatomical network. Therefore, their ictogenic mechanisms seem to have an intermediate place between the reflex mechanisms in system epilepsies which use physiological functional-anatomic networks (see below), and other focal reflex seizures that originate in pathological ad hoc networks related to the epileptogenic lesion.

The epilepsy is symptomatic or cryptogenic focal without exception.

Language-related induction

Certain modalities of language may trigger seizures in rare instances. Michelucci *et al.* (2004) reported a case of telephone-induced temporal lobe epilepsy. The patient's seizures consisted of dizziness, distortion and attenuation of sound, inability to understand language, slowing or arrest of speech. Only answering telephone induced the seizures. Ictal EEG started in the probably language dominant temporal lobe. The same authors (2007) reported another patient with similar symptomatology. The seizures were evoked almost exclusively by answering the telephone, and consisted of subjective feeling of distortion or attenuation of environmental sounds, inability to understand the language and to speak appropriately, loss of contact, and inconsistent secondary generalization. Sometimes the patient reported complex auditory hallucinations such as music or voices at the onset of seizures. The patient harboured a *de novo* mutation of leucine-rich, glioma-inactivated 1 *(LGI1)/Epitempin* gene.

Brodtkorb *et al.* (2005) also described a patient whose seizures were triggered by unexpected interruption by verbal command. During seizures, voices became distorted. The patient had difficulty understanding conversations and to trace the spatial direction of sounds. The syllables floated together with an echoing character. He could not understand the words and express himself. Other auditory stimuli did not provoke seizures. This patient belongs to a family with autosomal dominant lateral temporal lobe epilepsy (ADLTE) with mutations in *LGI1* gene.

The prominent feature of aphasia and the auditory precipitant of seizure may help to identify the *LGI1* gene-related syndrome. Usui *et al.* (2009) confirmed significantly large N100m signals (a magnetic counterpart of N1/N100 in EEG) in patients with ADLTE.

Similar cases were also reported. Inoue *et al.* (1999) suggested a group of patients whose seizures often occurred when using language such as conversing or reading. The seizures consisted of fluent paraphasia, paragraphia and comprehension deficit. The syllables uttered during seizures contained many neologisms and the same syllables were often repeated and tended to rhyme. Seizure focus was on the left side.

Lee *et al.* (1980) described a 48-year-old man who had recurrent seizures after an anastomosis of the left superficial temporal to the left middle cerebral artery. Speaking induced jaw jerking; silent reading induced jerking of right face, jaw and neck; reading aloud induced stuttering and writing induced dysgraphia. Canevini *et al.* (2001) reported a 57-year-old patient with a left frontal traumatic lesion who presented with facial myoclonic jerks triggered by speaking and listening to spoken language.

There was also a report of Rasmussen encephalitis with aphasic seizures precipitated by listening to speech and conversation or reading but not by own speech in its early phase (El Tawil *et al.*, 2016).

In contrast to these apparently focal epilepsy cases, Geschwind & Sherwin, (1967) reported a case where seizures were triggered by three modalities of language, *i.e.*, reading, writing and speaking, and the ictal EEG showed bilaterally symmetrical spike and polyspike and wave complexes. They assumed that an electrical focus resided in some portion of the so-called centrencephalic system. They used the term "language-induced epilepsy" and drew attention to a close link to the cases designated as primary reading epilepsy or graphogenic epilepsy described below.

Orofacial reflex myocloni (ORM)

This is the most common type of language-related seizure consisting of single or very brief volleys of small, lightning-like myocloni in the lips, tongue, throat or jaw triggered by reading and talking. They occur primarily in two syndromes, Primary Reading Epilepsy and Juvenile Myoclonic Epilepsy.

Primary reading epilepsy (PRE)

Of two types of seizure precipitation by reading originally described by Bickford *et al.* (1956) and termed primary and secondary reading epilepsy (RE), the "primary" variant has received much more attention. A comprehensive review of the literature was written for the second edition of this book (Wolf, 1992) and included 111 cases published in 60 papers. Metaanalysis of this literature led to the conclusion that RE is a benign idiopathic epilepsy syndrome preferentially related to the temporo-parietal region of the language dominant hemisphere but also to other regions functionally involved in reading. Later reports have added several details but not fundamentally changed this conclusion.

Description of seizures and findings of functional investigations

The clinical hallmark are abnormal sensations or movements (tonic or myoclonic) which develop in clear consciousness after a certain amount of reading, in the musculature which is involved in reading and talking: tongue, jaw, lips, face and throat. This seizure type was reported for all but four of the 111 patients (Wolf, 1992). Language suspension during the seizure may mimic stuttering (Michel *et al.*, 2004).

These motor seizures may sooner or (mostly) later be followed by a generalized tonic-clonic (GTC) seizure when the patients continue to read. Nineteen patients of the review had, either along with the motor phenomena, or independent from them, or alone, some kind of ocular and visual seizures, and these had no uniform semiology. The symptoms were clearly dyslexic in six patients, and probably dyslexic in three; four reported phosphenes or other simple visual hallucinations; three had oculomotor manifestations, and three were unclassifiable.

A singular case of a Saudi girl who had typical absences with 3 Hz generalized spike-and-wave (SW) since age 10 which were precipitated by reading the Koran in Arabic as well as by hyperventilation (Singh *et al.*, 1995) was investigated too superficially to confirm the precipitation by reading as such rather than, *e.g.*, emotional involvement (Ribble, 1936), *e.g.*, with hyperventilation. The authors of another report of absences precipitated by reading, television and checkerboard pattern (Matricardi *et al.*, 1991) did not consider this a case of primary RE.

Whereas the above-mentioned visual and ocular seizure types are undoubtedly focal, and related to the occipital and angular regions, the classification of the more common motor ictal phenomena of PRE is less obvious. In most reports, there is no comment as to whether they were unilateral or bilateral, and it seems that, often, it was even not attempted to clarify this. Both varieties, however, have been reported, and our own material, which is included in the review, comprises video documentations of both unilateral facial myocloni with bilateral EEG discharges, and bilateral myoclonus with unilateral discharge. As much of the musculature involved receives bihemispheric innervations, the observation of bilateral motor patterns from focal epileptic activity is not unexpected. On the other hand, one-sided local motor symptoms would be a very unusual expression of truly generalized seizure activity.

While the interictal EEGs in these patients were normal in 80%, reading provocation in the EEG resulted in the registration of paroxysmal activity in 73 (77%) of the 95 patients who were thus investigated. This may consist of sharp waves or single, rarely repetitive SW complexes. In 23 (32% of positive EEGs), this activity was bilateral and symmetric whereas an equal number of patients (22 or 30%) had unilateral or focal epileptiform discharges, and in the remaining 28 (38%) the findings were bilateral but not symmetric. The lateralization in 39 cases was to the left hemisphere, in five to the right, and in six, shifting between both sides. In one exceptional patient (Gastaut & Tassinari, 1966), two seizures were recorded (one prolonged partial and the other, GTC) of which one began focally at electrode P3 and the other, at P4. Maillard *et al.* (2010) also reported 2 patients where reading induced independent bilateral temporal lobe seizures. A regional distribution of the epileptiform discharge could be defined in 55 cases and was parieto-temporal (sometimes extending to the central or occipital regions) in 44, and frontal (with possible extension to central or anterior temporal channels) in the remaining 11.

Vaudano *et al.* (2012) analyzed ictal MEG in a patient and found activity extending precentrally into Brodmann area 6. Anzellotti *et al.* (2013) also performed an EEG/MEG study in a patient and found a right and left middle frontal gyrus hyperactivation in the early event with a bilateral to left and anterior to posterior cortical recruitment.

Other functional investigations than the EEG/MEG with specific provocation have added important information. An ictal HMPAO SPECT in one patient showed focal hyperperfusion of both frontal lobes, and the left temporal area in a right-handed subject (Miyamoto *et al.*, 1995). In another right-handed patient the same investigation revealed ictal hyperperfusion in the right superior temporal region (Kücük *et al.*, 1999). Koepp *et al.* (1998a) studied five RE patients with [11C] Diprenorphine (Dpn) PET scans at rest and with reading-induced seizures. The Dpn volume of distribution was decreased in the thalamus, left frontal lobe, right posterior temporal and left inferior parietal lobes after seizures. This finding suggests release of endogenous opioids at these sites after reading-induced seizures. Koepp *et al.* (1998b) performed a comparison of EEG, MRI and PET in one patient and found the assumption confirmed that RE is due to abnormal activity in the complex bilateral network subserving reading.

Gavaret *et al.* (2009) reported a right-handed patient whose ictal semiology was characterized by palinopsia and dyslexia. Ictal high resolution EEG showed rhythmic discharges in left temporo-parieto-occipital junction channels, with left occipito-temporal predominance. MRI fusion of the co-registered subtraction between ictal and interictal 99mTc-ECD SPECT individualized relative hyperperfusion affecting the left occipito-parietal junction area, the left lateral middle and inferior temporal gyri and the left inferior frontal area. They suggest that besides reading-induced myoclonic jerks of the jaw, a second variant of reading epilepsy may exist with seizures manifested by visual symptoms and/or dyslexia that originate from the occipito-temporal region of the dominant hemisphere, corresponding to the posterior part of the neural network that underlies the function of reading. Olberg *et al.* (2016) also reported spells with letters dancing before the eyes and those with jaw jerking in a same patient who showed reduced PET metabolism both in the left temporooccipital cortex and frontal/orbitofrontal locations. However, as reported above, there is too much overlap between these two presentations to support an independent variant.

Archer *et al.* (2003) studied patients with RE using spike-triggered fMRI and found the spike activity overlapped with reading activity in the left middle frontal gyrus, a structure recruited during working memory cognitive tasks, in addition to the finding of an unusual gyrus branching anteriorly off the left central sulcus. They therefore postulated that the spikes of RE spread from working memory areas into adjacent motor cortex, activating a cortical-subcortical circuit. In a series of fMRI studies in nine patients with PRE (Salek-Haddadi *et al.*, 2009), ictal fMRI revealed activations within cortical (right medial frontal gyrus) and subcortical (left putamen) areas during reading induced seizures. Whilst there were no gross abnormalities in cognitive or motor organization, most of the cortical areas were either in close proximity or directly overlapping with the areas activated by cognitive and motor functions. These subcortical areas may be closely linked to areas of hyperexcitable cortex, which constitute part of the normal reading network or physiological motor function. Another EEG- fMRI study (Vaudano *et al.*, 2012) found that BOLD signal changes in the left deep piriform cortex (PFC) and left Brodmann area (BA) 6 preceded seizures and occurred before BOLD changes were observed in thalamus and right inferior frontal gyrus (BA44). They suggest an important role of deep cortical and subcortical structures, in particular the frontal PFC, as key regions in initiating and modulating seizure activity. Fumuro *et al.* (2015) conducted a multimodal (MEG, EEG, diffusion tractography, fMRI) study in a patient with Katakana (Japanese syllabogram comparable with the alphabets in European language)-induced reading epilepsy and found activation of both the left posterior basal temporal area and left lateral frontal area by reading. They suggest that the selective subsystems including articulation and morphological processing served as the seizure onset and symptomatogenic zones and network hyperexcitability within the left hemisphere contributed to the development of clinical seizures.

Thus, the clinical findings and the data of functional ancillary studies converge to suggest that the generation of seizures in RE is neither focal nor bilateral synchronous, *i.e.* "generalized", but related to a set of functionally interactive anatomical sites with clustering at the motor and language areas of the dominant hemisphere in some patients but probably other clusters in others. This will be further discussed below.

Syndromatic features, treatment and course

There is a high degree of heredity, which is often specific. Of 75 patients of the meta-analysis of Wolf, (1992) with information on the family, 34 (46%) had affected relatives. Of a total of 47 reported affected relatives, reasonably detailed information was available in 20, and of these, 11 had PRE.

PRE is a syndrome of male preponderance. In 104 cases with this information, the ratio was 67:37, or 1.8. The onset is in adolescence with a mean of 17–18 years, with only three cases below 12, and only five beyond 25 years of age. This indicates that the pathomechanism is not primarily related to reading which is learned much earlier, but to the biological maturation of a subsystem, which becomes epileptogenic and happens to be involved in reading.

All patients have seizures provoked by reading of linguistic material in some form of script. This may include nonsense texts, unknown and known foreign languages, various alphabets, shorthand, unusual directions of presentation, and even Braille (Forster & Daly, 1973). It includes arithmetic material when it is lettered out, but may exclude it when presented in figures (Wolf, 1992; Meyer & Wolf, 1973). Understanding of the material read is not required. Reading aloud is more provocative than silent reading, and the precipitating effect increases with increasing difficulties at reading the material (Yalçin *et al.*, 1998). The precipitating mechanisms may include some related activities such as talking (in 27%), writing (in 11%), or reading of musical scores (three observations). Single spontaneous seizures were reported in only four cases. They should not exclude the diagnosis when all typical features are present.

RE may be treated by partial stimulus avoidance. This is especially possible in the cases with little or delayed propensity to develop GTCS. These patients may learn to carefully dose their reading, stop if necessary, and thus avoid convulsive seizures. If this is not possible, the drug of first choice is valproic acid, but also clonazepam and levetiracetam seem to be effective (Haykal *et al.*, 2012). Oxcarbazepine was reported to be effective in one report (Gregory *et al.*, 2013) but not in another (Mayer *et al.*, 2006).

Follow-up of more than 10 years in 29 patients of the literature (Wolf, 1992) indicated a good prognosis, and this was confirmed in a report of 18 patients of the Mayo Clinic (Radhakrishnan *et al.*, 1995) who have been followed for periods of 4 to 40 years. Complete remission, however, seems rarely to occur.

Nosological place

RE is, in the International Classification of Epilepsies and Epileptic Syndromes (Commission, 1989) included in the idiopathic localization-related epilepsies. It clearly fulfills the criteria of an idiopathic disorder as it is not caused or occasioned by any definable injury to the brain, and has a frequent, often specific genetic background. The seizure patterns and ancillary findings that suggest seizure generation in a functionally interactive subsystem of the central nervous system were discussed above. They justify inclusion in the class of "localization-related epilepsies". These are being integrated in the concept of system epilepsies (Avanzini *et al.*, 2012) whereas the 2017 position paper of the ILAE Commission on Classification (Scheffer *et al.*, 2017) considers them as "self-limited focal epilepsies" which is misleading as they have no local causes. The prototype of these is idiopathic childhood epilepsy with centro-temporal spikes, and there is one report of a 30-year-old patient who had the latter syndrome with typical nocturnal focal motor seizures from age 8 with spontaneous remission at age 12, and developed typical reading epilepsy at age 17 (Valenti *et al.*, 1999).

ORM in juvenile myoclonic epilepsy (JME)

Radhakrishnan *et al.* (1995) have proposed to consider RE a generalized epilepsy because they were impressed by its conjunction with JME. This occurred in four of their patients. Compared with the whole literature, this seems to be a rather unusual cluster as the combination had otherwise only been seen in two of our own patients. In all six cases, the myoclonic jerks of the upper limbs typical for JME were not precipitated by reading but occurred spontaneously, mostly in the morning hours and after sleep deprivation. Radhakrishnan *et al.* therefore talked about "co-occurrence" rather than identity of RE and JME which left the nosological question open.

New light was shed on this question by Mayer (Mayer & Wolf, 1997) who routinely questioned a series of newly admitted patients with JME about perioral myocloni during reading, and investigated many of them with video EEG. As a preliminary result it appears that about one quarter of patients with JME may have this trait. In addition, and without systematic investigation, it was found in twelve other patients of this hospital, ten with symptomatic or cryptogenic localization-related epilepsy and two with epilepsy with grand mal on awaking (Wolf & Mayer, 2000). In these non-RE cases, however, the perioral myocloni were precipitated by talking much more often than by reading. Subsequently, Da Silva Sousa *et al.* (2005) described 4 patients with JME in whom coexistence of praxis- and language (reading, speaking)-induced jerks was documented. Mayer *et al.* (2006) observed ORM in 9 of 25 JME patients (36%) tested in a video-EEG neuropsychological protocol.

Guaranha *et al.* (2011) in a systematic video-EEG investigation of 65 JME patients including a cognitive test battery found ORM in 26%. Thus it appeared that these were not particular to PRE but also quite common in JME. Here, however, they are precipitated in the first place by talking, especially emotional talking, and only in about 40% of cases also by reading.

In addition, the prognostic significance in both syndromes is different. Whereas PRE not necessarily requires pharmacotherapy, ORM in JME indicate a less benign course since Guaranha *et al.* (2011) found that of the JME patients who at follow-up had persistent seizures 53.8% were language-sensitive and 16,7% were not.

Other conditions

As already mentioned, systematic questioning about ORM revealed their existence also in some cases of symptomatic and cryptogenic focal epilepsies (Wolf & Mayer, 2000). Valenti *et al.* (2006) reported a large family where stuttering was induced by speaking, reading, and calculation. The stuttering was due to positive focal myoclonus of the jaw. Some of the family members also had myoclonus of the arms. A similar but slightly different family was reported by Kasteleijn-Nolst Trenité *et al.* (2015) where talking-induced jaw jerks appeared around age 50 years in addition to photosensitive limb jerks in 4 (spontaneous in 3) of 18 family members without provocation by reading or writing. There was a mutation of *SCNM1* gene.

The conclusion of these new findings was that ORM are not a specific finding in PRE but a more common trait, easily escaping attention and requiring systematic search to be diagnosed (Yacubian *et al.*, 2015). This reflex epileptic trait is the presenting symptom of PRE and frequent in JME but can also be observed in conjunction with other epilepsy syndromes, both generalized and focal.

The mechanism of precipitation of ORM

Many theories about the responsible mechanism(s) of precipitation have been proposed, especially in the early history of PRE. Often, these were much influenced by observations with single, and sometimes exceptional, patients. The increasing numbers of observations, many of them including sophisticated investigations have, however, resulted in a much clearer picture.

The only feature of the precipitating mechanism, which is common to all patients, is the formal act of transforming linguistic material displayed in some graphic system into phonetic speech (audible or internal), which needs not to be semantically understood. The more difficult this formal task, the more it becomes provocative. Reading aloud is more provocative than silent reading, and turbulences (*e.g.*, graphic, phonetic or semantic difficulties and anomalies), which disturb a smooth performance, often have a significant influence.

Modern concepts of the neurophysiology of reading are in accord with, and can help to understand the clinical and EEG findings in RE (Ritaccio *et al.*, 1992; Wolf, 1994; Koutroumanidis *et al.*, 1998; Pegna *et al.*, 1999). Reading is considered to be a bihemispheric cooperative performance (Taylor, 1988), where the phonological representation is more on the left and the semantic representation more on the right side. Involvement of the phonological track is indispensable for the mechanism of reading epilepsy but semantics may become involved through the constant interhemispheric exchange in the reading process. Pegna *et al.* (1999) experimentally investigating one patient along these lines concluded that there may be two forms of PRE, lexical and non-lexical (the latter triggered by non-word reading).

Primarily semantic reading as it occurs in logographic script systems would be expected to be less provocative, and indeed RE seems to be very rare in Japan. The Japanese patient reported by Miyamoto *et al.* (1995) had seizures when reading an English textbook.

The pathophysiology of RE involves multiple sensorimotor, cognitive and integrative cortical processes whose complexity seems to remove them from reflex theories. Interestingly, however, the pathological system seems to respond, at its periphery, in simple veritably reflex-like ways (Wolf, 1994) where the "proprioceptive bombardment" from the speech musculature results in "reflex firing through the same motor segment" (Bickford *et al.*, 1956). In the case of seizures precipitated by reading Braille, the myoclonic response was in the right hand (Forster & Daly, 1973).

ORM in JME appear less specific as their generation seems not necessarily to comprise reading but otherwise involve the functional-anatomic network for linguistic communication (Wolf, 2017).

Praxis-induced seizures

The observations which some authors (Goossens *et al.*, 1990; Inoue *et al.*, 1994) have started to lump together have appeared under a variety of names, including Epilepsia arithmetices, drawing-induced seizures, chess and card epilepsy, seizures during card games and draughts, reflex epilepsy evoked by decision making or by specific psychic activity, seizures evoked by Rubik's cube, seizures induced by thinking, reflex epilepsy with response to games of chance, calculations and spatial decisions, and writing-induced (graphogenic) epilepsy. The term praxis-induced (PI) seizures was proposed after (Inoue *et al.*, 1994).

In this section, clinical, EEG, and some other features are described for 92 patients who were aware that their seizures were induced by higher mental activity as mentioned above, and who were reported in the available publications before 2004 (references in Wolf & Inoue, 2012). Thereafter, results of more recent publications are added (see also Yacubian & Wolf, 2014).

Description

There are 31 female patients (33.7%) and 61 male patients (66.3%). Seizures usually started during adolescence (range 11 months to 67 years with a mean of 15.0 and a median of 14 years). Sixteen patients had a history of febrile seizures, eight with minor head injuries, three patients with meningitis/encephalopathy, and two with perinatal hypoxia. Two patients suffered from migraine as well. The personal history of 57 out of 84 patients with relevant information shows no notable events. One patient had Horner's syndrome of undetermined cause, otherwise there was no neurological impairment in 83 of 84 patients. Intellectual function was described in 60 patients, often average or above average, but two patients were described as below average intelligence, and the mean IQ of 22 patients examined was 92.6 (74–121).

Seizure type

The seizures of these patients consisted of myoclonias (78 patients, 84.8%), absences (34 patients, 37%), episodes of impairment of consciousness (complex partial seizures? two patients), spells with falling (one patient), visual and Jacksonian motor seizures (one patient), and GTCS (80 patients, 87%). The latter started suddenly or were preceded by a series of myoclonic jerks of increasing frequency. In 25 patients (27%), asymmetrical or focal features of the seizure were described: myoclonias predominantly occurring in one hand in 18 patients (left side in four), versive movements at the onset of the seizure in eight, and focal seizure onset in two patients. Almost all patients (57 among 69 patients) had spontaneous seizures in addition to induced seizures.

Electroencephalography

The interictal EEG presented bilateral spike, spike-wave or poly-spike-wave discharges during baseline or hyperventilation in 54 (74%) of the 73 patients where information is available, with focal accentuation in seven, and additional focal spikes or slow waves in eight. Only one patient with visual and Jacksonian seizures had exclusively focal spikes (Maruko *et al.*, 1974). Eighteen patients had no interictal paroxysmal activity. Twelve of 62 patients (19.4%) showed a photoparoxysmal response. However, the mean age at examination was 26.2 years (84 patients, 13–67 years), so that in some patients earlier photosensitivity might have been missed.

Precipitation

In the clinical history, the most frequently reported stimuli which evoked seizures were calculation in 42 patients (45.7%), writing in 34 (37%), playing cards in 31 (33.7%), playing chess or similar games in 27 (29.3%), other games such as punchi or videogames in

15 (16.3%), constructive activity in twelve (13%), drawing in eleven (12%), thinking, especially spatial one in ten (10.9%), decision making in two, with additional complex finger manipulation in 19 (20.7%). In seven patients, playing musical instruments was also the trigger. There were two patients whose seizures were also triggered by talking, two by reading and another two by eating. The seizures induced by talking and reading did not involve the arms but perioral muscles. In 58 patients (63%) there was more than one effective trigger. It has often been suggested to specifically inquire about reflex activation since the patients rarely reported it spontaneously. Concentration of attention and stress, or fatigue and strong motivation (Striano *et al.*, 1993) may be important additional contributors to the precipitation of seizures.

Reflex EEG activation

Reflex activation of the paroxysmal EEG discharges by various neuropsychological tasks was confirmed in 82 patients, of whom 15 had not shown epileptiform discharge in the routine EEG. There are two reports in which the patients never had provoked seizures but the EEG was easily activated by mathematical or spatial stimuli (Wiebers *et al.*, 1979; Anderson & Wallis, 1986). These two patients are included in the analysis. The evoked paroxysmal EEG discharges were almost the same as in the interictal state: bilateral spike, spike-wave or poly-spike-wave discharges in 57 of the 60 patients described, with focal accentuation in 14, and additional focal spikes in one. Three patients showed only focal spikes. Paroxysmal EEG activity could be induced by mental activity which was previously not noticed by every patient: constructive activity in 31 patients, calculation in 21, drawing in 13, writing in 10, chess in seven, cards in four, spatial thinking in two, and reading in four. It has often been suggested that the reproduction of the situation of seizure induction in real life, which often includes emotional involvement and stress, is difficult in the EEG laboratory where many patients also have an increased level of awareness.

Matsuoka *et al.* (2000) reported the results of the inclusion in standard EEG investigation of cognitive tasks (neuropsychological EEG activation: NPA) comprising reading, speaking, writing, written and arithmetic calculation, and spatial construction in 480 Japanese patients with epilepsy. These tasks provoked epileptic discharges in 38 patients (7.9%) and were accompanied by myoclonic seizures in 15 patients, absence seizures in 8, and simple partial seizures in one They found that NPA was effective in 36 (24.7%) of 146 idiopathic generalized epilepsy patients, especially in JME (22 of 45 patients, 49%). The most effective trigger was writing (26 out of 38 patients, 68.4%), followed by spatial construction (63.2%), written calculation (55.3%), mental calculation (7.9%) and reading (5.3%). The discharges evoked were quite similar to those that appeared spontaneously. They consisted of diffuse and symmetric spike-wave or polyspike-wave complexes, but were sometimes accompanied by both symmetric and asymmetric bilateral spike-wave complexes that predominated over the central derivations.

Hasegawa *et al.* (1981) reported one left-handed patient whose paroxysms were often observed in the right hemisphere in response to writing and calculation, and in the left hemisphere, to constructive activity.

It seems that absences and other non-convulsive seizures were more often induced by abstract thinking such as spatial tasks or mental calculation, and myoclonias more often by activities involving hand or finger movements (Ohtaka *et al.*, 1977; Yamamoto *et al.*, 1990).

Neuroimaging

Lateral ventricle asymmetry was observed in two patients, and slight cortical atrophy in one of 45 patients where neuroradiological finding were mentioned. Yamamoto *et al.* (1992) conducted a SPECT study in twelve patients with JME and EEG discharges induced by higher mental activity, and found abnormalities in eight: an increase of rCBF on the anterior half of unilateral cortex, a decrease of rCBF of unilateral thalamus, or both.

Genetics

The family history was described in 84 patients, of which 60 were negative. Eighteen patients (21%) had family members affected by epilepsy, and six patients by occasional seizures. However, the type of epilepsy in most of these cases could not be established. Apart from one pair of siblings (Goossens *et al.*, 1990), no familial cases homologous as to seizure precipitation seem to have been reported, but this may very well have to do with insufficient questioning.

Therapy

Most patients present spontaneous as well as evoked seizures, but in some cases all seizures are provoked. In these cases avoiding the trigger stimulus may be sufficient to control seizures.

Three of the 25 patients in Goossens *et al.* (1990) were seizure-free without medication by avoiding specific activating stimuli. Of the various drug treatments reported, valproic acid and benzodiazepines (clonazepam and clobazam) seemed to have been most frequently used and reasonably effective.

It is interesting to note that, of the patients with JME in Shizuoka, those with PI seizures obtained complete seizure control in only 31% against 69% in the non-provoked group. Almost all these patients could recognize the likelihood of seizures occurring and tried to avoid the precipitating factors in their daily lives. The most effective drugs, here, were valproate, clonazepam or zonisamide (Inoue *et al.*, 1994). Matsuoka *et al.* (2002) investigated the long-term course of seizure susceptibility in two patients with JME and found them to remain sensitive to neuropsychological provocative tasks for more than 20 years.

Findings from more recent publications

The number of the patients where computer games could induce seizures has increased (Chuang, 2006a). Chuang *et al.* (2006b) investigated cases with seizures induced by various games or game-related materials, especially by playing or watching mah-jong, a complicated game requiring thinking, memory, decision-making and manual handling (Kwan *et al.*, 2000; Wan *et al.*, 2005; Chang *et al.*, 2007), and divided into two groups. Group 1 (10 patients) was attributed to certain focal/diffuse pathologic changes of cortex with higher age at onset, whereas, group 2 (12 patients) had both game-induced seizures and spontaneous ones: absence, myoclonus or GTCs. The onset ages were during adolescence and the seizures were therapy responsive. These latter cases were regarded as praxis-induced seizures in the context of idiopathic generalized epilepsy. The clinical characteristics of group 1 was further studied in 56 patients (An *et al.*, 2015): male predominance, seizure onset in adulthood (mean 35.1 ± 16.3 years: 17–70), focal seizures (simple focal seizures or secondarily GTCS), and mean seizure latency after playing mah-jong of 6.1 hours (1–15). Wu *et al.* (2010) reported that five cases with mah-jong-induced epilepsy had nonketotic hyperglycemia at the occurrence of seizure. Lee *et al.* (2006) investigated 17 patients with seizures induced by playing oriental card or board games (Go Stop or baduk) and found male preponderance, higher age at seizure onset (ranging from 18 to 66 years, mean 42.3 years), family history of epilepsy in 24%, normal MRI in 76%, no generalized discharges in EEG, latency to occurrence of actual seizure (GTC or absence-like) of 2–20 hours and after lack of sleep in 82%. These cases may involve both group 1 and group 2.

Another report (Lee *et al.*, 2012) with 11 patients with seizures induced by playing Go Stop or baduk games came to the similar results and suggested that aging may be an important factor in generation of this type of reflex epilepsy with adult onset cognitive task-induced seizures.

Fukuma *et al.* (2016) recorded an ictal EEG in a patient who had attacks induced by playing mah-jong first at age 62 years and frequently after age 81 years. The ictal EEG demonstrated a clear right parietal lobe origin, with postictal hypoperfusion in the right parietal area in SPECT.

Feddersen *et al.* (2015) reported a patient with postanoxic intention myoclonus and focal motor seizures triggered by Sudoku puzzles. EEG onset was right centro-parietal, ictal fMRI showed maximal right central activation and ictal/interictal SPECT hyperperfusion of the posterior cingulate gyrus.

A case with praxis-induced seizures with successful surgery outcome was described by Racicot *et al.* (2016). A 23-year-old left-handed woman with medically intractable praxis-induced reflex seizures starting at age 10 years, mainly precipitated by writing, underwent selective resection of subtle end-of-sulcus cortical dysplasia in the right inferior parietal lobule resulting in freedom from seizures. Oshima *et al.* (2003) described a patient with arrest of motion and speech accompanied by a jerking sensation in the right hand, with or without actual jerks, exclusively induced by writing. They argued that their nonlesional case with ictal theta activity belongs to the graphogenic epilepsy as a variant of language-induced epilepsy. This case may represent reflex writing seizures in the context of symptomatic focal epilepsy.

The following reported cases were considered as idiopathic epilepsy with praxis-induced seizures. Abreu *et al.* (2005) described a right-handed patient with seizures induced in the right hand by writing in whom ictal EEG showed generalized polyspike-waves maximum over the right parieto-central area, ictal SPECT showed hyperperfusion over the right parieto-frontal region, and fMRI showed left frontal activation. They hypothesized the mechanism underlying writing-triggered seizures may be a generalized seizure process with a focal cortical trigger. Kho *et al.* (2006) reported a similar case where, however, only drawing induced myoclonus of the both arms. Mikati & Shamseddine (2005) reported a case with calculation-induced myoclonus. Tatsuzawa *et al.* (2010) reported a right-handed patient in whom generalized epileptiform discharges occurred during the Shogi, a Japanese chess, Wisconsin card sorting test, and block design test. There was a report of 13-year-old boy who had myoclonias and GTC while playing with Lego® bricks (Zylicz *et al.*, 2013). EEG showed generalized polyspike waves. Glenn *et al.* (2012) reported a case with myoclonic seizures induced by performing manual tasks starting at age 39 years. Building a bird house induced myoclonia during Video-EEG with bilateral discharges. They suggest that praxis-induced seizure may appear in the IGE subgroup of adult myoclonic epilepsy.

Mann *et al.* (2004) studied EEG back-averaging of the myoclonus registered during a chess match and during neuropsychological testing with Kohs cubes, which were the main triggers in a JME patient. The back-averaging showed bilateral spikes in the fronto-central cortical area. Tanaka *et al.* (2006) performed a MEG study during writing activation in two right-handed patients with graphogenic epilepsy, and found equivalent current dipoles clustered in the left centro-parietal area. de León *et al.* (2016) also performed an MEG study and the source reconstruction localized the epileptogenic area to the right premotor frontal cortex. Vidal-Dourado *et al.* (2016) showed enhanced excitability in the somatosensory cortex of JME patients through somatosensory evoked potentials study.

Karachristianou (2005) studied the effects of higher mental activity on the EEG in 30 JME patients; 76.6% showed EEG activation to at least one neuropsychological task and 4 tasks, two involving the use of the hands and two without manual involvement like mental calculation and mental spatial manipulation, were associated with a high frequency of EEG activation (43–60%).

Guaranha *et al.* (2009) performed a comprehensive neuropsychological activation study comprising 76 JME patients under video-EEG. Twenty-nine of 76 patients (38.2%) presented provocative effect. Action-programming tasks (reading aloud, speaking, writing, written calculation, drawing and spatial construction) were more effective than thinking (reading silently and mental calculation) in provoking epileptiform discharges (23.7% *vs.* 11%). They also found inhibitory effects by these tasks in 28 of 31 (90.3%), which supports the possibility of nonpharmacologic therapeutic interventions in JME.

Beniczky *et al.* (2012) studied 60 JME patients and found cognitive activation in 18% (task-specific), while inhibition in 29% (non-specific), when the spontaneous fluctuations of epileptiform discharges were accounted for.

Concerning the reflexogenic mechanism, Ferlazzo *et al.* (2005) summarized the previous notion that the hyperexcitable regions and systems activated by stimuli, that can be diffuse but not necessarily uniform and differ in degree and extent, are suspected to produce epileptic activity that involves the cortico-reticular or cortico-cortical pathways, with the result of generalized or bilateral epileptic events. Vollmar *et al.* (2011) examined 30 JME patients and 26 healthy controls using fMRI paradigm of visuomotor coordination and working memory. They reported, with increasing cognitive demand, increasing co-activation of the primary motor cortex and supplementary motor area, and increased functional connectivity between the motor system and fronto-parietal cognitive networks. Furthermore, the concomitant physiological deactivation of the default mode network during the cognitive tasks was impaired. These findings may provide an explanation of praxis-induction in JME.

Concerning treatment and outcomes, Guaranha *et al.* (2011) followed 65 JME patients and found sensitivity to praxis as one of the factors significantly suggesting moderate or poor seizure control. Uchida *et al.* (2015) indicated that praxis-induction traits in JME patients is related to seizures without preferential circadian occurrence and reduced response to antiepileptic drugs. In JME patients with praxis-induction, relative risk of stress as a precipitant of seizures increased 3.82 times as compared with JME without any reflex epileptic traits.

Mental processes involved in PI

Several attempts were made to clarify the mental processes involved in PI. Ingvar & Nyman (1962) emphasized the role of focusing attention. Forster (1977) reported that the three factors of complex decision-making, sequential decision-making and stress might play a deterministic role in seizure induction. Cirignotta *et al.* (1980) argued the importance of foreseeing the consequence of decision and introduced the term "strategic thinking", *i.e.*, considering a sequence of moves based on evaluating the consequences of previous moves (Siegel *et al.*, 1992). Wilkins *et al.* (1982) stressed the involvement of spatial processes in seizures induced by thinking. These findings led to the authors to conclude that photosensitivity and praxis sensitivity reflect an increased, but spatially different excitability of the cortex.

In the review of 92 patients described above, there were 48 patients from Japan. This uneven distribution may be of interest if taken into consideration together with the rarity of reading epilepsy in Japan. However, the high prevalence of PI as a triggering factor among JME patients became noted also in other countries. Thus, Wolf & Mayer, (2000) found in a questionnaire survey that 19 out of 62 responding patients with JME (31%) referred to praxis induction. The responses comprised stimuli such as writing (7), decision-making (4), computer tasks and video games (6), calculations (6), thinking (8), and playing the piano (1).

Chifari *et al.* (2004) reported two siblings in whom myoclonic jerks of the right arm and hand were triggered exclusively by writing that required a higher degree of concentration. The complexity and length of writing tasks played a major role in triggering myoclonic jerks which were readily elicited by writing philosophical texts in mother tongue or copying, and above all taking dictation of texts in a foreign language, while reading, thinking, calculation, drawing or typing never elicited epileptic myoclonus. This report is of interest in two ways: first, it identified a gradient of effectiveness in eliciting reflex writing seizures that is directly proportional to the difficulty of writing tests, similarly to that described in RE, and secondly, it further supports the notion that writing-induced seizures, like other praxis-induced seizures, represent an inherited trait of seizures precipitated by specific mode of activation occurring mainly within idiopathic generalized epilepsies.

Comparison of seizure precipitation by reading and praxis

There is a certain extent of overlap between the two conditions, reading epilepsy and praxis induction, as writing is an occasional precipitating factor in the first, and a frequent one in the second.

Exceptionally, patients having one of the two conditions also respond to the typical stimulus of the other. They have similar ages of onset, are usually idiopathic, and always (RE) or most frequently (PI) benign with a good response to similar drugs. The rates of photosensitive subjects are similar (9 *vs.* 19%). The precipitating stimuli in both most frequently need some time to become noxious, and the mechanisms of action are highly complex; they involve both higher cortical, and motor performances together, and the ictal motor symptoms start in that motor segment where the precipitating motor activity takes place.

But, in addition to the different modes of precipitation, the two conditions also differ in a variety of other significant respects, which are listed below:

– seizure types: perioral reflex myoclonias and unique types of focal visual seizures in RE; typical seizures of juvenile idiopathic generalized epilepsies in PI;
– unprovoked seizures: very rare in RE; common in PI;
– clinical response to stimulus: confined to a restricted functional cortical system unless secondary generalization occurs in RE; rapidly generalizing, first to non-convulsive, and eventually later to convulsive seizures in PI;
– interictal EEG: mostly negative in RE; mostly positive in PI;
– ictal EEG: bilateral symmetric, bilateral asymmetric, and unilateral/focal discharges about equally frequent, single sharp waves or brief SW volleys in RE; nearly always bilateral, mostly symmetric, runs of SW in PI;
– genetics: strongly suggestive of specific gene in RE; part of the polygenic setting of JME in PI;
– nosology: RE is a syndrome of its own; PI is a subgroup across juvenile idiopathic generalized epilepsy syndromes, similar in this respect to photosensitivity.

Considering the relation of RE and PI to JME, the important difference is that, although perioral reflex myoclonias are most common in these two of all epilepsy syndromes, true co-occurrence of RE and JME is rare, and reading in these cases has never been reported to provoke the myoclonic jerks typical for JME. In contradistinction, praxis-induction may provoke the classical seizures of juvenile idiopathic generalized epilepsies, though often with an otherwise unusual local onset.

REFERENCES

Abreu P, Ribeiro M, Forni A, Pires I, Sousa G (2005): Writing epilepsy: a neurophysiological, neuropsychological and neuroimaging study. *Epilepsy Behav* 6: 463–466.

An D, Zou X, Chen T, Yan B, Liu L, Zhou D (2015): Clinical characteristics and prognosis of mah-jong-induced epilepsy: A cohort review of 56 patients. *Epilepsy Behav* 53: 117–119.

Anderson NE, Wallis WE (1986): Activation of epileptiform activity by mental arithmetic. *Arch Neurol* 43: 624–626.

Anneken K, Fischera M, Kolska S, Evers S (2006): An unusual case of musicogenic epilepsy in a patient with a left fronto-temporal tumour. *J Neurol* 253: 1502–1504.

Anzellotti F, Franciotti R, Onofrj M (2013): Temporal recruitment of cortical network involved in reading epilepsy with paroxysmal alexia: a combined EEG/MEG study. *Seizure* 22: 156–158.

Archer JS, Briellmann RS, Syngeniotis A, Abbott DF, Jackson GD (2003): Spike-triggered fMRI in reading epilepsy: involvement of left frontal cortex working memory area. *Neurology* 60: 415–421.

Avanzini G (2003): Musicogenic seizures. *Ann NY Acad Sci* 999: 95–102.

Avanzini G, Manganotti P, Meletti S, *et al.* (2012). The system epilepsies: A pathophysiological hypothesis. *Epilepsia* 53: 771–778.

Beniczky S, Guaranha MS, Conradsen I, *et al.* (2012): Modulation of epileptiform EEG discharges in juvenile myoclonic epilepsy: an investigation of reflex epileptic traits. *Epilepsia* 53: 832–839.

Bickford RG, Whelan JL, Klass DW, Corbin KB (1956): Reading epilepsy: clinical and electroencephalographic studies of a new syndrome. *Trans Amer Neurol Assoc* 81: 100–102.

Brodtkorb E, Michler RP, Gu W, Steinlein OK (2005): Speech-induced aphasic seizures in epilepsy caused by *LGI1* mutation. *Epilepsia* 46: 963–966.

Canevini MP, Vignoli A, Sgro V, *et al.* (2001): Symptomatic epilepsy with facial myoclonus triggered by language. *Epileptic Disord* 3: 143–146.

Chang RS, Cheung RT, Ho SL, Mak W (2007): Mah-jong-induced seizures: case reports and review of twenty-three patients. *Hong Kong Med* J 13: 314–318.

Chifari R, Piazzini A, Turner K, Canger R, Canevini MP, Wolf P (2004): Reflex writing seizures in two siblings with juvenile myoclonic epilepsy. *Acta Neurol Scand* 109: 232–235.

Chuang YC (2006a): Massively multiplayer online role-playing game-induced seizures: a neglected health problem in Internet addiction. *Cyberpsychol Behav* 9: 451–456.

Chuang YC, Chang WN, Lin TK, Lu CH, Chen SD, Huang CR (2006b): Game-related seizures presenting with two types of clinical features. *Seizure* 15: 98–105.

Cirignotta R, Cicogna P, Lugaresi E (1980): Epileptic seizures during card games and draughts. *Epilepsia* 21: 137–140.

Commission on Classification and Terminology of the ILAE (1989): Proposal for revised classification of epilepsies and epileptic syndromes. *Epilepsia* 30: 389–399.

Critchley M (1937): Musicogenic epilepsy. *Brain* 60: 13–27.

da Silva Sousa P, Lin K, Garzon E, Ceiki Sakamoto A, Yacubian EM (2005): Language- and praxis-induced jerks in patients with juvenile myoclonic epilepsy. *Epileptic Disord* 7: 115–121.

de León SC, Niso G, Canuet L, *et al.* (2015): Praxis-induced seizures in a patient with juvenile myoclonic epilepsy: MEG-EEG coregistration study. *Epilepsy Behav* 5: 1–5.

Diekmann V, Hoppner AC (2014): Cortical network dysfunction in musicogenic epilepsy reflecting the role of snowballing emotional processes in seizure generation: an fMRI-EEG study. *Epileptic Disord* 16: 31–44.

Duanyu N, Yongjie L, Guojun Z, Lixin C, Liang Q (2010): Surgical treatment for musicogenic epilepsy. *J Clin Neurosci* 17: 127–129.

El Tawil S, Morris R, Mullatti N, Nashef L, Rajakulendran S (2016): Adult onset Rasmussen's encephalitis associated with reflex language induced seizures responsive to Rituximab therapy. *Seizure* 42: 60–62.

Feddersen B, Vollmar C, Rémi J, Stephan T, Flanagin VL, Noachtar S (2015): Seizures from solving Sudoku puzzles. *JAMA Neurology* 72: 1524–1526.

Ferlazzo E, Zifkin BG, Andermann E, Andermann F (2005): Cortical triggers in generalized reflex seizures and epilepsies. *Brain* 128: 700–710.

Forster FM, Hansotia P, Cleeland CS, Ludwig A (1969): A case of voice-induced epilepsy treated by conditioning. *Neurology* 19: 325–331.

Forster FM, Daly RF (1973): Reading epilepsy in identical twins. *Trans Amer Neurol Ass* 98: 186–188.

Forster FM (1977): *Reflex Epilepsy, Behavioral Therapy and Conditional Reflexes*, pp. 94–134. Springfield: Thomas.

Fukuma K, Ihara M, Miyashita K, *et al.* (2016): Right parietal source in Mahjong-induced seizure: a system epilepsy of focal origin. *Clin Case Rep* 4: 948–951.

Fumuro T, Matsumoto R, Shimotake A, *et al.* (2015): Network hyperexcitability in a patient with partial reading epilepsy: converging evidence from magnetoencephalography, diffusion tractography, and functional magnetic resonance imaging. *Clin Neurophysiol* 126: 675–681.

Gastaut H, Tassinari CA (1966): Triggering mechanisms in epilepsy: the electroclinical point of view. *Epilepsia* 7: 85–138.

Gavaret M, Guedj E, Koessler L, *et al.* (2010): Reading epilepsy from the dominant temporo-occipital region. *J Neurol Neurosurg Psychiatry* 81: 710–715.

Gelisse P, Thomas P, Padovani R, Hassan-Sebbag N, Pasquier J, Genton P (2003): Ictal SPECT in a case of pure musicogenic epilepsy. *Epileptic Disord* 5: 133–137.

Genc BO, Genc E, Tastekin G, Iihan N (2001): Musicogenic epilepsy with ictal single photon emission computed tomography (SPECT): could these cases contribute to our knowledge of music processing? *Eur J Neurol* 8: 191–194.

Geschwind N, Sherwin I (1967): Language-induced epilepsy. *Arch Neurol* 16: 25–31.

Glenn M, Carrazana EJ, Lopez MR, Wallace DM (2012): Late-onset, praxis-induced myoclonic epilepsy. *Epileptic Disord* 14: 167–171.

Goossens L, Andermann F, Andermann E, Remillard GM (1990): Reflex seizures induced by calculation, card or board games, and spatial tasks: a review of 25 patients and delineation of the epileptic syndromes. *Neurology* 40: 1171–1176.

Gregory LK, Broomail EM (2013): Teaching Video NeuroImages: Reading epilepsy: A seizure in a thousand words (or less). *Neurology* 81: e100.

Guaranha MS, da Silva Sousa P, de Araujo-Filho GM, *et al.* (2009): Provocative and inhibitory effects of a video-EEG neuropsychologic protocol in juvenile myoclonic epilepsy. *Epilepsia* 50: 2446–2455.

Guaranha MS, Filho GM, Lin K, Guilhoto LM, Caboclo LO, Yacubian EM (2011): Prognosis of juvenile myoclonic epilepsy is related to endophenotypes. *Seizure* 20: 42–48.

Hasegawa T, Matsuoka H, Takahashi T, Okuma T (1981): Myoclonic seizures induced by writing, calculation with figures and constructive acts – with special reference to neuropsychological EEG activation. *Psychiatry Neurol Japan* 83: 199–210.

Haykal MA, El-Feki A, Sonmezturk HH, Abou-Khalil BW (2012): New observations in primary and secondary reading epilepsy: excellent response to levetiracetam and early spontaneous remission. *Epilepsy Behav* 23: 466–470.

Herskowitz J, Rosman NP, Geschwind N (1984): Seizures induced by singing and recitation: a unique form of reflex epilepsy in childhood. *Arch Neurol* 41: 1102–1103.

Ingvar DH, Nyman GE (1962): Epilepsia arithmetices: a new psychologic trigger mechanism in a case of epilepsy. *Neurology* 12: 282–287.

Inoue Y, Seino M, Tanaka M, Kubota H, Yamakaku K, Yagi, K (1994): Epilepsy with praxis-induced seizures. In: Wolf P (ed) *Epileptic Seizures and Syndromes*, pp. 81–91. London: John Libbey.

Inoue Y, Mihara T, Fukao K, Kudo T, Watanabe Y, Yagi K (1999): Ictal paraphasia induced by language activity. *Epilepsy Res* 35: 69–79.

Jallon P, Heraut LA, Vanelle JM (1989): Musicogenic epilepsy. In: Beaumanoir A, Gastaut H, Naquet R (eds) *Reflex Seizures and Reflex Epilepsies*, pp. 269–274. Geneva: Éditions Médecine & Hygiène.

Joynt RJ, Green D, Green R (1966): Musicogenic epilepsy. *JAMA* 179: 501–504.

Kaplan PW (2003): Musicogenic epilepsy and epileptic music: a seizure's song. *Epilepsy Behav* 4: 464–473.

Karachristianou S, Bostantjopoulou S, Katsarou Z, Kazis A (2005): Neuropsychological EEG activation in patients with juvenile myoclonic epilepsy. *Functional Neurology* 19: 185–189.

Kasteleijn-Nolst Trenité DG, Volkers L, Strengman E, *et al.* (2015): Clinical and genetic analysis of a family with two rare reflex epilepsies. *Seizure* 29: 90–96.

Kho KH, van den Bergh WM, Spetgens WP, Leijten FS (2006): Figuring out drawing-induced epilepsy. *Neurology* 66: 723–726.

Koepp MJ, Richardson MP, Brooks DJ, Duncan JS (1998a): Focal cortical release of endogenous opioids during reading-induced seizures. *Lancet* 352: 952–955.

Koepp MJ, Hansen ML, Pressler RM, *et al.* (1998b): Comparison of EEG, MRI and PET in reading epilepsy: a case report. *Epilepsy Res* 29: 251–257.

Koepp MJ, Caciagli L, Pressler RM, Lehnertz K, Beniczky S (2016): Reflex seizures, traits, and epilepsies: from physiology to pathology. *Lancet Neurol* 15: 92–105.

Koutroumanidis M, Koepp MJ, Richardson MP, *et al.* (1998): The variants of reading epilepsy. A clinical and video-EEG study of 17 patients with reading-induced seizures. *Brain* 121: 1409–1427.

Kücük NÖ, Yigit A, Ibis E, Aras G, Sener HÖ, Mutluer N (1999): Functional imaging in reading epilepsy: A case report. *Ann Nucl Med* 13: 355–356.

Kwan SY, Su MS (2000): Mah-jong epilepsy: a new reflex epilepsy. *Zhonghua Yi Xue Za Zhi (Taipei)* 63: 316–321.

Lee SI, Sutherling WW, Persing JA, Butler AB (1980): Language-induced seizure: a case of cortical origin. *Arch Neurol* 37: 433–436.

Lee SA, Choi EJ, Kang JK (2006): Reflex epilepsy induced by playing oriental card or board games. *J Clin Neurol* 2: 262–267.

Lee MK, Yoo JS, Cho YJ, Lee BI, Heo K (2012): Reflex epilepsy induced by playing Go-stop or Baduk games. *Seizure* 21: 770–774.

Lin KL, Wang HS, Kao PF (2003): A young infant with musicogenic epilepsy. *Pediatr Neurol* 28: 379–381.

Maillard L, Vignal JP, Raffo E, Vespignani H (2009): Bitemporal form of partial reading epilepsy: Further evidence for an idiopathic localization-related syndrome. *Epilepsia* 51: 165–169.

Mameniskiene R, Wolf P (2018): Precipitation and inhibition of seizures in focal epilepsies. *Expert Rev Neurother* [Epub ahead of print].

Mann MW, Gueguen B, Guillou S, Debrand E, Soufflet C (2004): Chess-playing epilepsy: a case report with video-EEG and back averaging. *Epileptic Disord* 6: 293–296.

Marrosu F, Barberini L, Puligheddu M, *et al.* (2009): Combined EEG/fMRI recording in musicogenic epilepsy. *Epilepsy Res* 84: 77–81.

Maruko K, Ono T, Ishige K, Takaya Y, Yashima Y (1975): A case of Mah-jong induced epilepsy. *Psychiatry* (Japan) 17: 709–715.

Matricardi M, Brinciotti M, Paciello F (1991): Reading epilepsy with absences, television-induced seizures, and pattern sensitivity. *Epilepsy Res* 9: 145–147.

Matsuoka H, Takahashi T, Sasaki M, *et al.* (2000): Neuropsychological EEG activation in patients with epilepsy. *Brain* 123: 318–330.

Matsuoka H, Takahashi T, Sasaki M, Yoshida S, Numachi Y, Sato M (2002): The long-term course of seizure susceptibility in two patients with juvenile myoclonic epilepsy. *Seizure* 11: 126–130.

Mayer T, Wolf P (1997): Reading epilepsy: related to juvenile myoclonic epilepsy? *Epilepsia* 38 (Suppl 3): 18–19.

Mayer TA, Schroeder F, May TW, Wolf P (2006): Perioral reflex myoclonias: a controlled study in patients with JME and focal epilepsies. *Epilepsia* 47: 1059–1067.

Mehta AD, Ettinger AB, Perrine K, *et al.* (2009): Seizure propagation in a patient with musicogenic epilepsy. *Epilepsy Behav* 14: 421–424.

Meyer J, Wolf P (1973): Über primäre Leseepilepsie. Mit einem kasuistischen Beitrag. *Nervenarzt* 44: 155–160.

Michel V, Burbaud P, Taillard J, *et al.* (2004): Stuttering or reflex seizure? A case report. *Epileptic Disord* 6: 181–185.

Michelucci R, Gardella E, de Haan GJ, *et al.* (2004): Telephone-induced seizures: a new type of reflex epilepsy. *Epilepsia* 45: 280–283.

Michelucci R, Mecarelli O, Bovo G, *et al.* (2007): A *de novo* LGI1 mutation causing idiopathic partial epilepsy with telephone-induced seizures. *Neurology* 68: 2150–2151.

Mikati MA, Shamseddine AN (2005): Refractory calculation-induced idiopathic generalized epilepsy: a case report and review of the literature. *Epilepsia* 46 (Suppl 10): 48–50.

Miyamoto A, Takahashi S, Tokumitsu A, Oki J (1995): Ictal HMPAO-single photon emission computed tomography findings in reading epilepsy in a Japanese boy. *Epilepsia* 36: 1161–1163.

Morocz IA, Karni A, Haut S, Lantos G, Liu G (2003): fMRI of triggerable aurae in musicogenic epilepsy. *Neurology* 60: 705–709.

Ohtaka T, Miyasaka M (1977): A case of language-induced epilepsy precipitated mainly by writing. *Psychiatry Neurol Japan* 79: 587–601.

Olberg HK, Eichele T, Schwarzlmüller T, Lind J, Hjelland IE, Engelsen BA (2016): Combined variants in reading epilepsy; coexisting anterior and posterior variants camouflaged as heat cramps where the patient finds his own diagnosis searching the internet. *Epilepsy Behav Case Rep* 5: 75–77.

Oshima T, Hirose K, Murakami H, Suzuki S, Kanemoto K (2003): Graphogenic epilepsy: a variant of language-induced epilepsy distinguished from reading- and praxis-induced epilepsy. *Seizure* 12: 56–59.

Pegna AJ, Picard F, Martory MD, *et al.* (1999): Semantically-triggered reading epilepsy: An experimental case study. *Cortex* 35: 355–356.

Pittau F, Tinuper P, Bisulli F, *et al.* (2008): Videopolygraphic and functional MRI study of musicogenic epilepsy. A case report and literature review. *Epilepsy Behav* 13: 685–692.

Racicot F, Obaid S, Bouthillier A, *et al.* (2016): Praxis-induced reflex seizures mainly precipitated by writing due to a parietal focal cortical dysplasia. *Epilepsy Behav Case Rep* 6: 52–54.

Radhakrishnan K, Silbert PL, Klass DW (1995): Reading epilepsy. An appraisal of 20 patients diagnosed at the Mayo Clinic, Rochester, Minnesota, between 1949 and 1989, and delineation of the epileptic syndrome. *Brain* 118: 75–89.

Ramani V (1991): Audiogenic epilepsy induced by a specific television performer. *N Engl J Med* 325: 134–135.

Ribble M (1936): Ego dangers and epilepsy. *Psychoanal Quart* 5: 71–86.

Ritaccio AL, Hickling EJ, Ramani V (1992): The role of dominant premotor cortex and grapheme to phoneme transformation in reading epilepsy. *Arch Neurol* 49: 933–939.

Salek-Haddadi A, Mayer T, Hamandi K, *et al.* (2009): Imaging seizure activity: a combined EEG/EMG-fMRI study in reading epilepsy. *Epilepsia* 50: 256–264.

Shibata N, Kubota F, Kikuchi S (2006): The origin of the focal spike in musicogenic epilepsy. *Epileptic Disord* 8: 131–135.

Siegel M, Kurzrok N, Barr WB, Rowan AJ (1992): Game-playing epilepsy. *Epilepsia* 33: 93–97.

Striano S, Orsini A, Vitolo S (1983): Epilepsia arithmetices: clinical and EEG study of a case and characteristics of precipitating factors. *Acta Neurol* (Napoli) 38: 14–19.

Singh B, Anderson L, Al Gashlan M, Al-Shahwan SA, Riela AR (1995): Reading-induced absence seizures. *Neurology* 45: 1623–1624.

Sparr SA (2003): Amusia and musicogenic epilepsy. *Curr Neurol Neurosci Rep* 3: 502–507.

Tanaka N, Sakurai K, Kamada K, Takeuchi F, Takeda Y, Koyama T (2006): Neuromagnetic source localization of epileptiform activity in patients with graphogenic epilepsy. *Epilepsia* 47: 1963–1967.

Tatsuzawa Y, Yoshino A, Nomura S (2010): A case of seizures induced by abstract reasoning. *Epilepsy Behav* 17: 552–554.

Tayah TF, Abou-Khalil B, Gilliam FG, Knowlton RC, Wushensky CA, Gallagher MJ (2006): Musicogenic seizures can arise from multiple temporal lobe foci: intracranialEEG analyses of three patients. *Epilepsia* 47: 1402–1406.

Taylor MM (1988): The bilateral cooperative model of reading. In: De Kerckhove D, Lumsden CJ (eds) *The Alphabet and the Brain*, pp. 322–361. Berlin, Heidelberg: Springer.

Tezer FI, Bilginer B, Oguz KK, Saygi S (2014): Musicogenic and spontaneous seizures: EEG analyses with hippocampal depth electrodes. *Epileptic Disord* 16: 500–505.

Tsuzuki H, Kasuga I (1978): Paroxysmal discharges triggered by hearing spoken language. *Epilepsia* 19: 147–154.

Uchida CG, de Carvalho KC, Guaranha MS, G *et al.* (2015): Phenotyping juvenile myoclonic epilepsy. Praxis induction as a biomarker of unfavorable prognosis. *Seizure* 32: 62–68.

Usui K, Ikeda A, Nagamine T, *et al.* (2009): Abnormal auditory cortex with giant N100m signal in patients with autosomal dominant lateral temporal lobe epilepsy. *Clin Neurophysiol* 120: 1923–1926.

Valenti MP, Tinuper P, Cerullo A, Carcangiu R, Marini C (1999): Reading epilepsy in a patient with previous idiopathic focal epilepsy with centro-temporal spikes. *Epileptic Disord* 1: 167–171.

Valenti MP, Rudolf G, Carre S, *et al.* (2006): Language-induced epilepsy, acquired stuttering, and idiopathic generalized epilepsy: phenotypic study of one family. Epilepsia 47: 766–772.

Vaudano AE, Carmichael DW, Salek-Haddadi A, *et al.* (2012): Networks involved in seizure initiation A reading epilepsy case studied with EEG-fMRI and MEG. *Neurology* 79: 249–253.

Vidal-Dourado M, Nunes KF, Guaranha MS, Giuliano LM, Yacubian EM, Manzano GM (2016): Expression of praxis induction on cortical excitability in juvenile myoclonic epilepsy. *Clin Neurophysiol* 127: 2551–2560.

Vizioli R (1989): Musicogenic epilepsy. *Int J Neurosci* 47: 159–164.

Vollmar C, O'Muircheartaigh J, Barker GJ, *et al.* (2011): Motor system hyperconnectivity in juvenile myoclonic epilepsy: a cognitive functional magnetic resonance imaging study. *Brain* 134: 1710–1719.

Wan CL, Lin TK, Lu CH, Chang CS, Chen SD, Chuan YC (2005): Mah-Jong-induced epilepsy: a special reflex epilepsy in Chinese society. *Seizure* 14: 19–22.

Wang ZI, Jin K, Kakisaka Y, Burgess RC, *et al.* (2012): Interconnections in superior temporal cortex revealed by musicogenic seizure propagation. *J Neurol* 259: 2251–2254.

Wiebers DO, Westmoreland BF, Klass DW (1979): EEG activation and mathematical calculation. *Neurology* 29: 1499–1503.

Wieser HG, Hungerbühler H, Siegel AM, Buck A (1997): Musicogenic epilepsy: review of the literature and case report with ictal single photon emission computed tomography. *Epilepsia* 38: 200–207.

Wieser HG (2004): Musicogenic seizures and findings on the anatomy of musical perception. In: Wolf P, Inoue Y, Zifkin B (eds) *Reflex Epilepsies-Progress in Understanding*, pp. 79–91. Montrouge: John Libbey.

Wilkins A, Zifkin B, Andermann F, McGovern E (1982): Seizures induced by thinking. *Ann Neurol* 11: 608–612.

Wolf P (1992): Reading epilepsy. In: Roger J, Bureau M, Dravet C, Dreifuss FE, Perret A, Wolf P (eds) *Epileptic Syndromes in Infancy, Childhood and Adolescence*, 2nd ed, pp. 281–298. London: John Libbey.

Wolf P (1994): Reading epilepsy. In: Wolf P (ed) Epileptic Seizures and Syndromes, pp. 67–73. London: John Libbey.

Wolf P (2017): Reflex epileptic mechanisms in humans: Lessons about natural ictogenesis. *Epilepsy Behav* 71: 118–123.

Wolf P, Mayer T (2000): Juvenile myoclonic epilepsy: a syndrome challenging syndromic concepts? In: Schmitz B, Sander T (eds): *Juvenile Myoclonic Epilepsy. The Janz Syndrome*, pp. 33–39. Petersfield: Wrightson Biomedical.

Wolf P, Inoue Y (2012): Complex reflex epilepsies. In: Bureau M, Genton P, Dravet C, Delgado-Escueta A, Tassinari CA, Thomas P, Wolf P (eds). *Epileptic syndromes in infancy, childhood and adolescence* (5th ed), pp. 529–543. Montrouge: John Libbey Eurotext.

Wu YJ, Tsai JJ, Huang CW (2010): Nonketotic hyperglycemia-related reflex epileptic seizures induced by mah-jong playing. *Epilepsy Behav* 19: 533–535.

Yacubian EM, Wolf P (2014): Praxis induction. Definition, relation to epilepsy syndromes, nosological and prognostic significance. A focused review. *Seizure* 23: 247–251.

Yacubian EM, Wolf P (2015): Orofacial reflex myocloni. Definition, relation to epilepsy syndromes, nosological and prognosis significance. A focused review. *Seizure* 30: 1–5.

Yamamoto S, Yamamoto J, Kawasaki T, *et al.* (1992): A pathophysiological consideration of 21 cases of reflex epilepsy induced by higher mental activity. *Jpn J Psychiat Neurol* 46: 440–443.

Yalçin AD, Forta H (1998): Primary reading epilepsy. *Seizure* 7: 325–327.

Yamamoto S, Egawa I, Yamamoto J, *et al.* (1990): A case of reflex epilepsy induced by higher mental activities, mainly by arithmetices. *J Jpn Epil Soc* 8: 22–28.

Zifkin BG, Zatorre RJ (1998): Musicogenic epilepsy. In: Zifkin BG, Andermann F, Beaumanoir A, Rowan AJ (eds) Reflex Epilepsies and Reflex Seizures: *Advances in Neurology*, vol. 75, pp. 273–281. Philadelphia: Lippincott-Raven.

Zylicz SA, Schippers HM, Tromp SC (2013): Lego®-induced seizures: from an exceptional case towards the building blocks of generalised epilepsy. *Seizure* 22: 326–327.

WITH VIDEO SUPPLEMENTS

CHAPTER 29

EPILEPSIES AND CHROMOSOMAL DISORDERS

Pierre Genton[1], Carla Marini[2], Nadia Bahi Buisson[3], Anna Kaminska[3], Maurizio Elia[4] and Giuseppe Gobbi[5]

[1] Centre Saint-Paul, Henri-Gastaut Hospital, Marseille, France
[2] Children's Hospital A. Meyer and University of Florence, Florence, Italy
[3] Pediatric Neurology, Hôpital Necker Enfants-Malades, Paris, France
[4] IRCCS Oasi Maria SS, Troina (EN), Italy
[5] Child Neurology and Psychiatry Unit, Maggiore "C.A. Pizzardi" Hospital, Bologna, Italy

Introduction

Chromosomal abnormalities do not represent a frequent cause of seizure disorders (Jennings & Bird, 1981), but they carry a high risk for seizures (Holmes, 1987). Many chromosomal abnormalities are associated with central nervous system malformations and other neurological alterations resulting in mental retardation and seizures that are more frequent than in the general population (Kumada *et al.*, 2005). Certain chromosomal syndromes are specifically associated with epilepsy and show a particular clinical and EEG pattern: 1p36 monosomy, Wolf-Hirschhorn syndrome, Angelman syndrome, ring chromosome 20 syndrome, Miller-Dieker syndrome, 18q- syndrome, and Down syndrome (Pollack *et al.*, 1978; Boyd *et al.*, 1988; Musumeci *et al.*, 1988; Guerrini *et al.*, 1989, 1990a, b; Sgrò *et al.*, 1995; Viani *et al.*, 1995; Guerrini *et al.*, 1997; Bahi-Buisson *et al.*, 2005; Sorge & Sorge, 2010). Other chromosomal anomalies associated with epilepsy have no specific patterns of seizures, *e.g.*, the 14r syndrome, the Klinefelter syndrome, the fragile-X syndrome.

A detailed analysis of electroclinical patterns of the epilepsies associated with a chromosomal disorder may be useful in clinical practice. Chromosomal abnormalities are responsible for approximately 6% of central nervous system malformations (Carter, 1977), and it may be important to establish whether epilepsy is due to the seizure susceptibility due to abnormal gene function or results from structural central nervous system abnormalities.

Major progress in our understanding of epilepsy resulted from the development of new genetic technologies, such as high-resolution chromosome banding, fluorescent in situ hybridization (FISH), and molecular biology. Oligonucleotide array comparative genome hybridization (array CGH) and SNP (single nucleotide polymorphisms) array are well established for genome-wide exploration of microchromosomal variation. A more detailed analysis of electroclinical patterns of the epilepsies may help detect specific genes affecting seizure susceptibility (Anderson & Hauser, 1990). We may quote an example provided by the clinical picture associated with a unique chromosomal rearrangement at 2q24: the epilepsy phenotype is dependent on the extent of a deletion, with widely different phenotypes associated with minimally different deletions, the difference depending on the inclusion of neuronal receptor genes (Pereira *et al.*, 2006).

Only those chromosomal abnormalities that are highly associated with epilepsy are considered in this chapter, and we will especially focus on the specific epileptic syndromes that may contribute to the diagnosis of the chromosomopathy. The role of copy number variants (CNVs) in the pathogeny of epilepsies will also be discussed.

Wolf-Hirschhorn syndrome (WHS, 4p- syndrome, monosomy 4p; including Pitt-Rogers-Danks syndrome)

WHS is a contiguous gene syndrome resulting from terminal deletion of the short arm of chromosome 4. The frequency of WHS is estimated at 1/50,000-1/20,000 births, with a female preponderance of 2:1. No single gene deletion or intragenic mutation have been shown to confer the full WHS phenotype (Battaglia *et al.*, 2008a).

WHS is characterized by low birth weight, severe growth retardation with delayed bone age, severe mental defect, microcephaly, "Greek helmet" profile, closure defects (cleft lip or palate, coloboma of the eye, cardiac septal defects) and high prevalence of seizures (80–90%). Other clinical features include hemangioma of the forehead, prominent glabella, beaked nose, short phyltrum, micrognathia, carp-shaped mouth, low-set simple ears, hypertelorism, wide and downward slanting palpebral fissures, epicanthus, renal hypoplasia, hypospadias, pulmonary isomerism, common mesentery, abnormal dermal ridges, sacral dimple, and diaphragmatic hernia. Microencephaly, abnormal gyral pattern, grey matter heterotopias, dysplasia of nuclear structures (especially lateral geniculate bodies and dentate nuclei), and hypoplasia of the corpus callosum have been reported (Guthrie *et al.*,1971; Lazjuk *et al.*, 1980; Gottfried *et al.*, 1981; Battaglia *et al.*, 2008a). In at least one-third of cases, death occurs during the first year of life because of severe systemic malformations, cardiac failure, or pulmonary infection (Wolf *et al.*, 1965; Hirschhorn *et al.*, 1965; Fujimoto & Wilson, 1990). Hepatic (and other) neoplasms seem to occur with increased frequency (Battaglia *et al.*, 2018).

It appears that deletion of band 4p16 is necessary for full expression of the phenotype (Buli *et al.*, 1990). *De novo* deletions have been reported by Quarrell *et al.* (1991) and by Thies *et al.* (1992). Molecular studies indicated that the deleted segment might be of paternal or maternal origin (Thies *et al.*, 1992). Wright *et al.* (1998) came to a similar conclusion from analysis of a patient with WHS and two patients with Pitt-Rogers-Danks syndrome (PRDS). They found that the two conditions result from the absence of identical genetic segments and suggested that the clinical differences observed between them are likely the result of allelic variation in the remaining homolog. Therefore, the two conditions can be lumped under the same genetic entity. About 85% of 4p- cases are sporadic events, whereas the remaining 15% result from the unbalanced segregation of a parental reciprocal translocation (Lurie *et al.*, 1980; Stengel-Rutkowski *et al.*, 1984), most frequently occurring between chromosomes 4 and 8, 4 and 19 (Quarrel *et al.*, 1991) or 4 and 12 (McKeown *et al.*, 1987).

The shortest region of overlap of the deletions observed in WHS patients, the WHS critical region, has been confined to a region of 165 kb (Wright *et al.*, 1997), located between loci D4S166 and D4S3327. This region was sequenced during the search for the Huntington disease gene (Baxendale *et al.*, 1993) and a number of candidate genes for WHS have been identified. However, it is unclear whether a single gene or more are involved in the WHS phenotype. One of these genes is *WHSC1* (Stec *et al.*, 1998; Zollino & Doronzio, 2018), and another one is *LETM1*; but *FGFRL1* is considered the best candidate that accounts for the typical facial appearance (Yamamoto-Shimoyima *et al.*, 2018).

Epilepsy and EEG

Epileptic seizures constitute a major medical concern during the first years of life, occurring in 50 to 100% of patients (Guthrie *et al.*, 1971; Centerwall *et al.*, 1975; Jennings & Bird, 1981; De Grouchy & Turleau,1984; Stengel-Rutkowski *et al.*, 1984; Kagitani-Shimono *et al.*, 2005; Battaglia *et al.*, 2008). Seizures usually begin with a peak incidence at around 9–10 months. They may be clonic or tonic, unilateral with or without secondary generalization, or tonic-clonic from the onset (Estabrooks *et al.*, 1994; Reid *et al.*, 1996; Ogle *et al.*, 1996; Battaglia, 1997; Battaglia *et al.*, 1999a, b; Battaglia & Carey 1999, 2000; Battaglia *et al.*, 2008a). They are frequently triggered by fever, may last 15 minutes or longer, and often occur in clusters (Sgrò *et al.*, 1995; Zankl *et al.*, 2001; Battaglia *et al.*, 2008a). In over 50% unilateral or generalized clonic or tonic-clonic status epilepticus occurs during the early years, despite adequate antiepileptic treatment (Battaglia *et al.*, 2008a). Between 1 and 5 years of age, almost two thirds of the patients develop atypical absences, often with a mild myoclonic component, mainly involving the eyelids and axial and limbs muscles (Sgrò *et al.*, 1995; Battaglia, 1997; Battaglia *et al.*, 1999, 2004, 2008a). Other seizure types associated with WHS include migrating partial seizures, epileptic spasms, myoclonic seizures, tonic seizures, and complex focal seizures (CFS) (Kanazawa *et al.*, 1991; Zankl *et al.*, 2001; Motoi *et al.*, 2016; Itakura *et al.*, 2016).

Distinctive EEG patterns are observed in about 70% of patients. These patterns are essentially of two types: i) frequent, diffuse, atypical slow sharp element, spike and wave complexes often occurring in long bursts activated by slow wave sleep, with paroxysmal activity associated with atypical absences, not unlike the Angelman syndrome (Matsumoto *et al.*, 1992; Sugimoto *et al.*, 1992; Mizuguchi *et al.*, 1994); ii) frequent high amplitude, fast spike-polyspike and wave complexes over the posterior third, triggered by eye closure (Parmeggiani *et al.*, 1993; Sgrò *et al.*, 1995; Battaglia *et al.*, 2003). These abnormalities may be present in patients who have not experienced seizures (Bahi-Buisson *et al.*, 2005).

With regard to pathogenesis of the epilepsy, it has been demonstrated that genes encoding the $\alpha2$,$\alpha4$, $\beta1$, and $\gamma1$ GABAA subunit receptors are clustered on chromosome 4p13-4q11 (McKeman & Whiting, 1996). Molecular studies have identified that the critical region in 4p- syndrome is located within 4p16.3 (Anvret *et al.*, 1991) and that the genes encoding the GABAA-receptor subunits $\alpha2$ and $\beta1$ are both located on chromosome 4 in bands p12-p13 and may be adjacent (Buckle *et al.*, 1989). Although the deletion does not encompass the 4p12-p13 region, reduction of gene product in an adjacent band could contribute to the high epileptogenicity. The presence of generalized spike-and-wave discharges in patients with WHS is in keeping with the models of epileptogenesis resulting from reduced GABAergic inhibition and with the hypothesized role of GABAA-receptor function defect in producing the electroclinical pattern in Angelman syndrome (AS). The electroclinical similarities that exist between WHS and AS suggest that this peculiar electroclinical pattern of epilepsy has a common pathogenesis.

Diagnosis

Standard chromosome analysis detects large deletions involving the 4p16.3 band in approximately 50%–60% of individuals with WHS who have a deletion with no other cytogenetic abnormality ("pure deletion"); however, G-banded cytogenetic studies or fluorescently labelled probes (FISH) alone may not reveal other complex genomic alterations that help determine the type of rearrangement leading to the 4p16.3 deletion. About 40%–50% of affected individuals have an unbalanced translocation with both a deletion of 4p and a partial trisomy of a different chromosome arm. These unbalanced translocations may be *de novo* or inherited from a parent with a balanced rearrangement. The remaining individuals have other complex rearrangements leading to a 4p16.3 deletion (*e.g.*, ring 4) (South *et al.*, 2008). Prenatal diagnosis can be suspected, *e.g.*, on intrauterine growth retardation and the typical facial appearance and/or cleft palate and confirmed by karyotyping and/or SNP array (Xing *et al.*, 2018).

Treatment

Epilepsy is usually effectively controlled by valproate (VPA) alone or associated with ethosuximide (ESM). In a minority of patients there may be a need to add a benzodiazepine (BZD). Bromides have been recommended as the initial treatment, especially for the prevention of status epilepticus (Kagitani-Shimono *et al.*, 2005). A large retrospective survey showed that clobazam, lamotrigine and levetiracetam were useful, while carbamazepine, oxcarbazepine or phenytoin were not or even aggravated seizures (Ho *et al.*, 2018). Despite early severity, the long-term outcome of epilepsy seems to be good, as seizures tend to disappear with age (Battaglia, 2005 b; Battaglia & Carey, 2005).

Angelman syndrome (partial monosomy 15q)

Angelman syndrome (AS) is a severe neurodevelopmental disorder with a heterogenous genetic aetiology always related to absence of a maternal contribution to chromosome 15q11-q13 (Knoll *et al.*, 1990). AS was firstly reported by Angelman (1965) in 3 patients with severe mental retardation and he called them "puppet children". Bower and Jeavons (1967) coined the name "happy puppet syndrome". The eponym "Angelman syndrome" was suggested by Williams and Frias (1982) because the term "happy puppet" may appear derisive. A consensus for diagnostic criteria was established (Williams *et al.*, 1995). Consistent characteristics (100%) are: severe developmental delay, speech impairment with no or minimal use of words, better receptive and nonverbal communication, ataxia and tremulous movements of limbs, behavioural uniqueness such as hyperactivity, hand flapping, frequent and inappropriate laughter. Frequent characteristics (more than 80%) are: postnatal microcephaly, seizures, onset usually before age 3 years, abnormal characteristic EEG pattern with large amplitude slow spike-waves (2–3 Hz) facilitated by eye closure. Associated characteristics (20–80%) are: flat occiput, occipital groove, protruding tongue, wide mouth, hypopigmentation (similar to that found in Prader-Willi syndrome and found only in cases with deletion), sleep disturbances.

Most of the cases are not diagnosed during infancy as typical behavioural features are overlooked, and dysmosphism is discrete. With time however, delayed milestones, lack of appropriate language development, deceleration of head growth, epilepsy, the appearance of jerky movements and sleep disorders, they become evident.

Genetics and physiopathology

The chromosomal origin of AS was first recognized by the finding of a 15q11-q13 deletion using high resolution chromosomal analysis and, later on, the deletion was found to be of maternal origin (conversely, the same deletion is paternal in Prader-Willi syndrome [Kapian *et al.*, 1987; Buxton *et al.*, 1994; Magenis *et al.*,1990]). These findings suggest that the 15q11-q13 genomic region is subjected to genomic imprinting, an epigenetic modification that allows differential expression of genes depending on their parental origin (Knoll *et al.*, 1989; Williams *et al.*, 1990). There are four classes of AS, according to the different genetic etiologies: i) *de novo* deletion of 15q11-q13 (70% of cases); ii) paternal uniparental disomy (5%) (Freeman *et al.*, 1993; Malcolm *et al.*, 1991); iii) defect of imprinting (5%); and iv) mutation of the maternal copy of the ubiquitin-protein ligase gene (*UBE3A*) (Matsuura *et al.*, 1997). In a small percentage of cases, no genetic anomaly can be identified (Fiumara *et al.*, 2010).

Recurrence risk differs according to the genetic type (Stalker & Williams,1998). Most cases due to a large *de novo* deletion have a low (< 1%) risk of recurrence, the same is true for AS due to uniparental disomy (in the absence of a parental translocation) (Antonarakis *et al.*, 1993; Greger *et al.*, 1997; Robinson *et al.*, 1993a). In other cases, with mutations of the imprinting center or UBE3A gene mutations, the risk of recurrence may be as high as 50% (Moncla *et al.*, 1999).

The presence in the commonly deleted region, 15q 11 -q 13, of a cluster of genes coding for 3 subunits of the GABAa receptor complex ($\beta3$, $\alpha5$, $\gamma3$) may indicate that GABA neurotransmission is involved in AS. It has been suggested that cortical hyperexcitability might result from reduced GABAergic inhibition (Guerrini *et al.*, 1996). Neurochemical study of the cerebellar cortex demonstrated markedly reduced GABA contents possibly related to failure to develop or loss of Purkinje cells and inhibitory GABAergic interneurons (Jay *et al.*, 1991). Morecver, a 60–80% reduction in BDZ binding has been shown in most brain regions of a mutant mouse exhibiting a deletion involving a chromosomal region homologous to the one associated with AS in humans (Nakatsu *et al.*, 1993).

In mouse models, the defect of the imprinting center in deleted cases decreases the expression of maternal *UBE3A* (Lewis *et al.*, 2019). The *UBE3A* mutation was reproduced in mice and induced a pro-epileptic phenotype that was rescued by postnatal reinstatement of *UBE3A* (Gu *et al.*, 2019). In humans, some variants of *UBE3A* mutations are associated w th a mild type of AS (Sadhwani *et al.*, 2018).

Epilepsy and EEG

The onset of epilepsy is often before 3 years: the incidence is around 25% during the first year, vs close to 90% within 3 years (Guerrini *et al.*, 1993; Matsumoto *et al.*, 1992; Sugimoto *et al.*, 1994; Viani *et al.*, 1995; Zori *et al.*, 1992; Clayton-Smith, 1993; Saitoh *et al.* 1994; Fiumara *et al.*, 2010). In infants, seizures tend to occur in a febrile context. The onset of epilepsy usually precedes the diagnosis of AS (Valente *et al.*, 2006). Atypical absences, myoclonic seizures, generalized tonic clonic seizures (GTCS), and clonic unilateral seizures are among the main ictal patterns (Guerrini *et al.*, 1996; Matsumoto *et al.*, 1992; Sugimoto *et al.*, 1994; Viani *et al.*, 1995). CFS with eye deviation and vomiting, possibly indicating occipital lobe origin, are quite frequent (Viani *et al.*, 1995). On the contrary, infantile spasms with hypsarrhythmia are exceptional. Non-convulsive status epilepticus has been reported in more than half (Matsumoto *et al.*, 1992; Sugimoto *et al.*, 1994). They are responsible for episodes of regression with worsening of ataxia and myoclonic jerks. Viani *et al.* (1995) found EEG evidence of transient myoclonic status epilepticus in 9 of 18 AS patients. These myoclonic statuses were described as "myoclonic epilepsy ("myoclonic status") in non-progressive encephalothies" by Dalla Bernardina *et al.* (1985), later renamed as "myoclonic encephalopathy in non-progressive disorders" (Berg *et al.*, 2010). This syndrome is also observed in other genetic encephalopathies such as Wolf-Hirschhorn and Willi-Prader syndromes (Darra *et al.*, 2017).

EEG patterns in AS are quite characteristic. According to Boyd *et al.* (1988), there are three typical patterns: i) generalized rhythmic 4–6 Hz activity not influenced by eye closure *(Figure 1)*; ii) rhythmic delta activity at 2–3 Hz over the anterior regions (confirmed by Laam *et al.*, 1996); iii) spikes and sharp waves mixed with 3–4 Hz components of amplitude higher than 200 μV, mainly posterior and triggered by eye closure.

During episodes of non-convulsive status, high amplitude spike and waves become subcontinuous during wakeness and sleep *(Figure 2a)*. These abnormalies dramatically improve after treatment with a concomittant clincal improvement.

Polygraphic recordings during myoclonic status or shorter myoclonic episodes reveal that each spike is accompanied by a myoclonic potential (Guerrini *et al.*, 1996), and is therefore a fast-bursting cortical myoclonus (Goto *et al.*, 2015). There is inter-hemispheric latency between the cortical spikes, and a corresponding latency from one side to the other, consistent with transcallosal spread. Myoclonus shows a rostrocaudal pattern, indicating cortical rather than brainstem origin (Guerrini *et al.*, 1996). However, Elia *et al.* (2009) showed that in some cases, myoclonic jerks are not correlated with EEG paroxysmal abnormalities; massive myoclonic jerks may also be recorded *(Figure 2b)*. In other patients, myoclonus may remain erratic, showing no apparent relation with EEG abnormalities (Viani *et al.*, 1995). Myoclonus typically ceases during sleep (Viani *et al.*, 1995; Guerrini *et al.*, 1996) whereas the continuous EEG anomalies can persist (Dalla Bernardina *et al.*, 1985). In addition, AS patients may exhibit a quasi-continuous focal or multifocal rhythmic myoclonus at about 11 Hz, mainly involving hands and face, producing a mild jerking or twitching *(Figure 3)*.

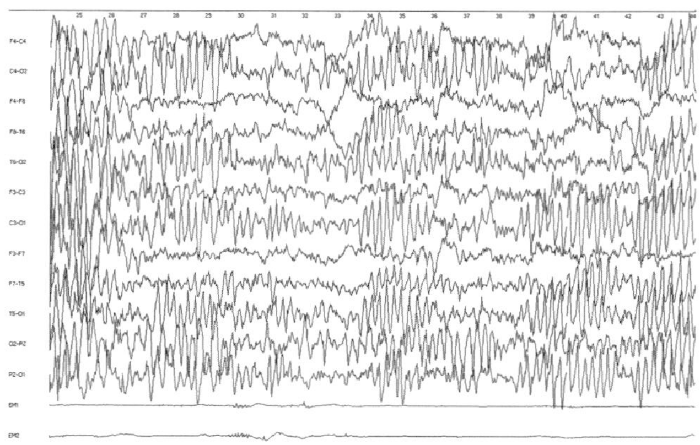

Figure 1 **Angelman syndrome in a 3-year-old patient. Waking EEG: typical background activity composed by high amplitude, diffuse monorythmic theta waves (5–6 Hz), most prominent in posterior regions (amplitude: 150 μV/cm).**

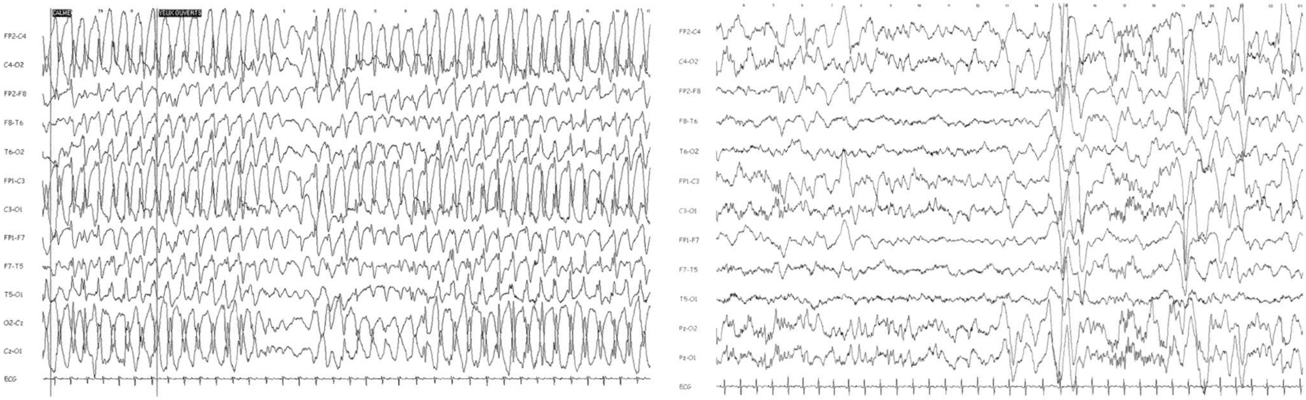

Figure 2

Angelman syndrome: Left. **Waking EEG in a 2-year-old patient: status of epileptic absences with high amplitude spike and waves, maximal in both frontal regions, subcontinuous at 2 Hz.** Right. **Waking EEG in a 3-year-old patient: massive myoclonia on EMG on deltoids, at the same time burst of spikes (amplitude: 100 μV/cm).**

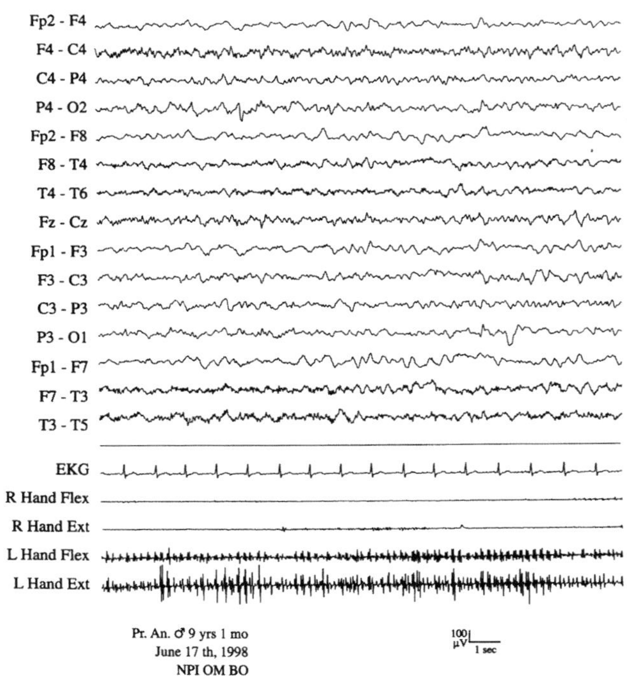

Figure 3 **Angelman syndrome: 9-year old patient. Quasi-continuous rhythmic myoclonus at about 11 Hz in the left hand, mimicking tremor.**

These patterns appear early in life, from the 4th month, and represent a precious tool for the early diagnosis. With time EEG abnormalities change and Buoni *et al.* (1999) and Laan *et al.* (2005) describe high voltage slow burst activity of 1–3 Hz mixed with high amplitude 4–6 Hz activity in children younger than 4 years, evolving to 4–6 Hz activity from posterior regions mixed with spike and waves in following years until puberty. The long-term evolution of the characteristic EEG and seizure patterns has been evaluated (Uemura *et al.*, 2005): most patients enter longlasting seizure remission after the age of 20, but some isolated seizures can occur even after the age of 30; EEG changes decrease with age and epileptiform anomalies tend to disappear after age 20. Other authors have stressed the abatement of EEG changes and seizures, that may occur as soon as 8 years after the onset (Galvan-Manso *et al.*, 2005). However, adult patients may show a very slow background rhythm, at times mixed with focal or multifocal spikes, and may still exhibit bursts of slow activity intermixed with spikes, often associated with jerking, and longlasting episodes of myoclonic status *(Figure 4)*. In their analysis of

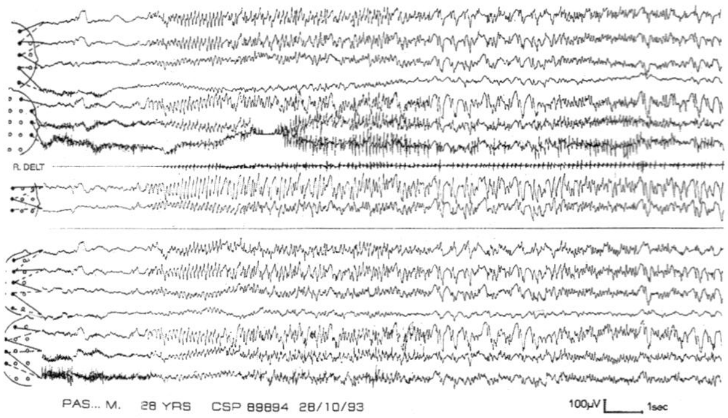

Figure 4 **Angelman syndrome: 28-year-old female patient with myoclonic status. Fluctuating fast and slow activities on the EEG. Note the fast-bursting myoclonus recorded on the right deltoid muscle.**

53 adolescent and adult cases, Prasad *et al.* (2018) confirm the relative abatement of epilepsy but show that tremor and myoclonus may increase with age, together with anxiety and behavioral disturbances. Pollack *et al.* (2018) have also stressed the fact that nonepileptic myoclonus may predominate after childhood.

Diagnosis

The presentation of AS is fairly characteristic, and the diagnosis relies mostly on the constant clinical criteria. However, in infants, the presence of nonepileptic abnormal movements due to the underlying encephalopathy, often prevents from recognizing the myoclonus (Dalla Bernardina *et al.*, 1985). The diagnosis may be hampered in young children.

It may be hampered in young children because of the absence of some typical manifestations and in older patients because of the changing behavioural characteristics. The EEG is useful for diagnosis at any age. The clinical diagnosis is confirmed by high-resolution chromosome analysis (Saitoh *et al.*, 1994) or, when this is negative, by the mutation analysis of *UBE3A* gene. Patients tested negative could bear a not yet identified genetic anomaly involving *UBE3A* activity. FISH analysis performed on metaphase chromosomes identifies deletions and subtle translocations. The analysis is carried out through commercially available probes mapping to the common deletion interval, which are used in combination with an alpha satellite probe and an additional single-copy control probe (Delach *et al.*, 1994). Microsatellite analysis by PCR can be employed to detect both deletions and uniparental disomies. Such analysis can demonstrate the lack of maternal genetic contribution resulting from either paternal uniparental disomy or deletion of the maternal 15q11-q13 region (Mutirangura *et al.*, 1993). The methylation test is based on a Southern blot analysis performed with probes that detect parental origin of alleles on the basis of their methylation status. In the case of AS, this analysis demonstrates only paternal contribution (Giliessen-Kaesbach *et al.*, 1995). When the clinical diagnosis is suggestive, cases without the classical molecular anomalies may be proposed for the search of *UBE3A* mutations. The remaining AS cases without identifiable molecular abnormalities account for about 5%.

The deletion phenotype is generally linked to a more severe clinical picture (Minassian *et al.*, 1998). Patients with UPD are less severely affected, with only 20% having epileptic seizures (Lossie *et al.*, 2001). Patients with imprinting anomalies have an even milder course with better communication skills (Nicholls *et al.*, 1998). *UBE3A* mutation patients are similar to deletion patients as far as concerns seizures, microcephaly and absence of speech.

Treatment

While seizures tend to be drug resistant in infancy and early childhood, the severity of epilepsy may show attenuation from later childhood onwards (Zori *et al.*, 1992). In contrast to previous reports, Laan *et al.* (1996, 1997) found that 92% of AS adult patients continue to have epileptic seizures. Status myoclonicus or non-convulsive status epilepticus is usually stopped with BZD (Viani *et al.*, 1995; Guerrini *et al.*, 1996), although they may become intractable, such as in two patients of our series (Viani *et al.*, 1995). Particularly effective is the association of BZD with VPA for long-term treatment of epilepsy (Viani *et al.*, 1995). VPA and ESM in association are also effective in patients presenting recurrent status myoclonicus. CBZ may cause myoclonus and worsening of the absence seizures (Viani *et al.*, 1995). Topiramate (TPM) has been found effective in five children with AS, possibly because of its GABAergic properties (Franz *et al.*, 2000). A survey, conducted in the US by Internet questionnaires addressed to lay AS organizations confirmed the widespread use of the VPA-clonazepam combination, and the positive effect of TPM and ESM (Nolt *et al.*, 2003); however, this study also mentions the use of phenytoin (PHT) and CBZ, which points to insufficient information of some families. Cortical myoclonus in AS patients may be treated with good results with high doses of piracetam (140 mg/kg/day or more) (Guerrini *et al.*, 1996).

Among the newer anticonvulsants, lamotrigine (LTG) was evaluated in 5 patients with positive results in three (Dion *et al.*, 2007). Levetiracetam (LEV) has been reported as successful in a child with non-convulsive status (Weber, 2010), and has also been suggested as a primary treatment option (together with LTG) by a questionnaire survey among AS lay organizations (Thibert *et al.*, 2009). The ketogenic diet gave good results in recent retrospective studies with most of the patients showing a more than 50% seizure reduction (Caraballo *et al.*, 2017). Other means, like steroids or vagal nerve stimulation, await further trials.

Disturbance of normal sleep patterns are frequent and pervasive problems in children and adolescents with AS have been confirmed by polygraphic studies (Miano *et al.*, 2004). Such disturbances may require specific management.

Ring chromosome 20 syndrome

The ring chromosome 20 syndrome (r20S) was first suggested by Borgaonkar *et al.* in 1976, and is characterized by mild to moderate mental deficiency, behavioural disorders and epilepsy (Jalbert *et al.*, 1977; Herva *et al.*, 1977; Porfirio *et al.*, 1987). It stands out among chromosomal disorders associated with epilepsy because no dysmorphism is apparent, thus often delaying genetic evaluation; the electroclinical syndrome is characteristic in most patients with a triad associating recurrent nonconvulsive status, drug-resistant frontal lobe seizures and a characteristic EEG; however, this triad is not fully specific (Gago-Veiga *et al.*, 2018). The onset is in childhood with frequent daytime atypical absences and an EEG with long-lasting bilateral slow activity intermixed with spikes (Inoue *et al.*, 1997; Canevini *et al.*, 1998; Roubertie *et al.*, 2000; Petit *et al.*, 2000). Seizures are refractory to treatment and a range of comorbidities such as intellectual disability, regression, behavioural disorders and even dysmorphism may occur. Some patients may have normal intelligence and performance: among 4 patients, mental retardation was only apparent in one (Biraben *et al.*, 2001). The aetiology of the seizures and the other less penetrant comorbidities characteristic of r20S remain unknown. Most cases are sporadic and involve true mosaicism for the ring chromosome, but familial cases have been reported (Back *et al.*, 1989; Canevini *et al.*, 1998; Unterberger *et al.*, 2018).

Epilepsy and EEG

Seizures usually begin in childhood, and are reported as loss of contact, lasting from seconds to minutes, or even hours, in the form of nonconvulsive status: these episodes are sometimes not clearly distinguished from the patient's baseline behaviour, and may precede other seizure types for years before being recognized as seizures. They may be associated with automatic behaviour, wandering, and a mimic of fear. Myoclonias, particularly perioral myoclonias, but also eyelid myoclonias, may be present during part or all of the nonconvulsive seizures (Petit *et al.*, 1999; Biraben *et al.*, 2001; Vignoli *et al.*, 2016). Nonconvulsive seizures or status occur frequently, sometimes several times per week, and may be triggered by particular factors or situations: Takahashi *et al.* (1995) reported a boy in whom seizures were triggered by videogames; in general, adverse psychological events (such as quarrels) are the most common factor in other patients (Roubertie *et al.*, 2000). Such triggering factors, and the particular behaviour associated with nonconvulsive episodes, may lead to the diagnosis of nonepileptic seizures. Other types of seizures are: short lasting focal motor seizures, CFS with fear and in some cases hallucinations; in CFS a secondary generalization can occur. Frequent sleep-related subtle frontal lobe seizures have also been described as a characteristic trait (Augustijn *et al.*, 2001). Gelastic seizures have been seen (Dimova *et al.*, 2012). Refractory status epilepticus has also been reported (Hirano *et al.*, 2016).

Epilepsy does not remit in adults and is usually drug-resistant. Although most patients experience a stable, chronic condition, some may deteriorate mentally and behaviourally (Augustijn *et al.*, 2001). Neuroimaging studies have been normal in most cases, but one case has been reported with a frontal cortical dysplasia (Takahashi *et al.*, 1995; Inoue *et al.*, 1997); in this patient, the removal of this lesion did not improve epilepsy. Severe, intractable nonconvulsive status epilepticus has been reported, with prolonged coma and lethal outcome (Jacobs *et al.*, 2008).

The interictal EEG may be normal or may show uni- or bilateral sharp or slow changes without specific features, sometimes in the form of longlasting theta slowing without associated clinical symptoms (Biraben *et al.*, 2001). During nonconvulsive status, the EEG shows high-amplitude rhythmic slow activity at 2–3 Hz, with superimposed spikes or slow waves that predominate over the frontal regions *(Figure 5)* (Inoue *et al.*, 1997; Canevini *et al.*, 1998). The onset and offset of such states are usually sudden. Some patients may exhibit rhythmic, high-amplitude slow waves discharge during such states, or only comparatively low-voltage rhythmic slow activity. Compared with other types of epilepsies associated with recurrent episodes of absence status, the EEG changes found in r20S appear less ample and less "spiky" (Inoue *et al.*, 1997), with a frequently typical aspect of diffuse theta slowing (*Figure 6*). Other seizures, such as generalized tonic clonic or motor seizures that may resemble tonic seizures, are usually associated with diffuse changes from the onset. The existence of focal EEG changes is debatable. Biraben *et al.* (2001) recorded several brief motor seizures that were all associated with diffuse fast activities; such seizures occurred during a long nonconvulsive state, which they did not interrupt. Magnetoencephalography localized the typical slow ictal discharges to the medial frontal lobe regions, with possible bilateral spread to temporal lobes (Tanaka *et al.*, 2004).

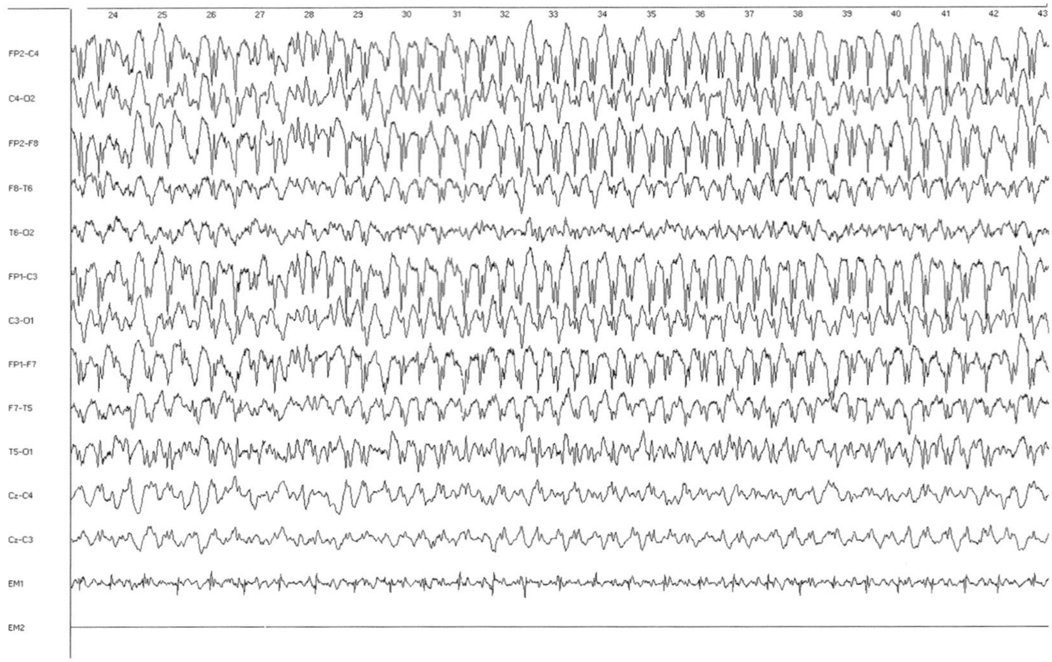

Figure 5

Ring chromosome 20 syndrome in a 12-year-old patient. Waking EEG during an episode of fluctuating consciousness and mutism. Continuous diffuse slow spike and waves at 2–3 Hz, rhythmic and synchronous, maximal over both frontal regions (amplitude: 100 μV/cm).

Genetics and diagnosis

Reported cases tend to be sporadic: a familial case has been reported (Back *et al.*, 1989). In this family, there were three carriers of the ring anomaly, and two of them were affected and had the typical clinical features including epilepsy. The "silent" forms prevalence of the r20 anomaly is unknown. The mosaicism is usually postzygotic. The formation of the ring is associated with loss of telomeric material on both arms of chromosome 20. These terminal deletions can be demonstrated by molecular cytogenetic techniques (Brandt *et al.*, 1993). The severity of mental retardation appears to correlate with the percentage of abnormal lymphocytes, while the epilepsy does not (Inoue *et al.*, 1997). Although this hypothesis has been challenged by the observation of some patients with severe mental retardation and epilepsy who have a very low percentage of abnormal lymphocytes, while others have normal intelligence in spite of a high percentage of positive mitoses. When the probability of the r20S is high, at least 100 mitoses should be examined, as only a very small percentage of peripheral cells may exhibit the characteristic ring formation. These terminal deletions can be demonstrated by molecular cytogenetic techniques (Brandt *et al.*, 1993) or FISH analysis. Review of case reports has shown that the onset of seizures is inversely correlated with the degree of mosaicism in blood, with earlier seizure onset associated with a higher loading for the ring chromosome (Nishiwaki *et al.*, 2005; Herrgard *et al.*, 2007).

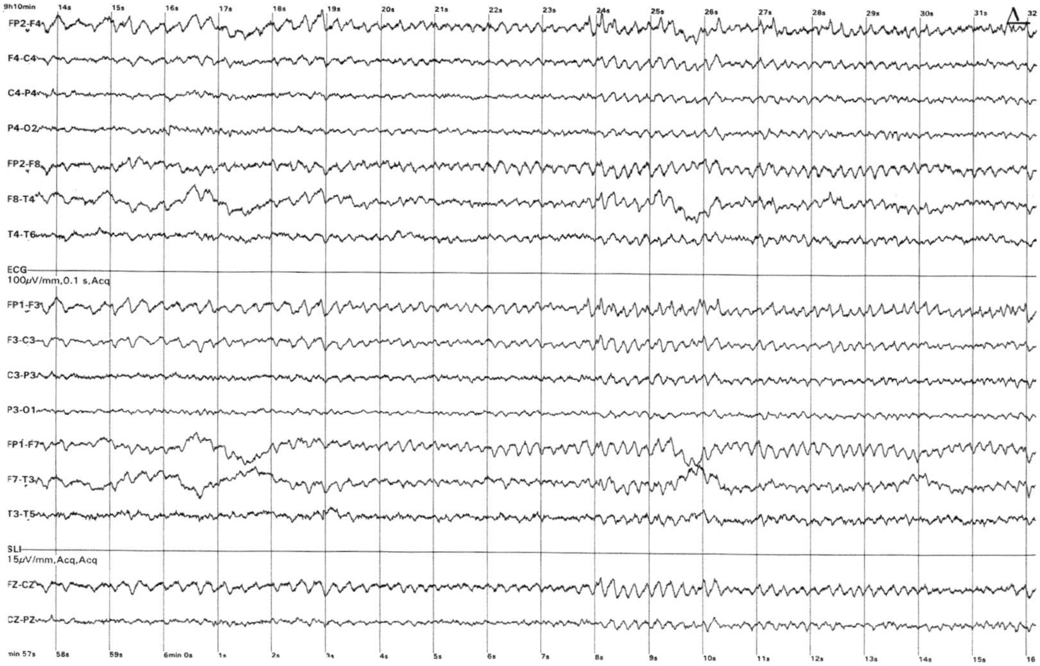

Figure 6

Ring chromosome 20 syndrome in a 20-year-old patient. Waking EEG during an episode of atypical absence. Continuous diffuse theta activity at 3–4 Hz, predominating frontally. This episode lasted 15 minutes. Amplitude: 100 µV/cm.

Data demonstrates that the r20S is heterogeneous with both mosaic and nonmosaic rings (Conlin *et al.*, 2011). The mosaic group represents the majority of patients. Deletions are only detected in patients with nonmosaic rings, indicating that the mechanism of formation is very different between the 2 groups of patients. In the mosaic group, the ring is formed postzygotically by telomere-telomere fusion, while the non-mosaic rings may have formed during meiosis. There is a phenotype-genotype correlation with mosaic patients having later seizure onset and a lower likelihood of additional findings such as intellectual disability or dysmorphic features. According to Corbin *et al.* (2011), several theories may explain the r20S phenotype including: i) candidate gene deletion; ii) silencing of gene expression through telomere position effect; and iii) the deleterious effect of ring instability on cell viability and function. The telomeric regions of chromosome 20 contain two genes that have been implied in the genesis of dominantly transmitted epilepsies, *i.e.*, benign neonatal familial convulsions *(KCNQ2)* (Singh *et al.*, 1998) and autosomal dominant frontal lobe nocturnal seizures *(CHRNA4)* (Steinlein *et al.*, 1995); however, there is very little overlap of these conditions with the r20S. The majority of r20 patients do not have any detectable deletions and those deleted have heterogeneous deletions with no genes that were uniformly deleted in all patients (Conlin *et al.*, 2011). However, alteration of gene expression due to a telomere position effect is possible. This may explain why patients with non-ring deletions of the chromosome 20 do not present the same r20S phenotype.

Subcortical mechanisms appear to be prominent, as shown by the diffuse and partly subcortical ictal changes found in SPECT studies (Biraben *et al.*, 2001). However, some authors stress the focal nature of the epilepsy on clinical and EEG grounds (Holopainen *et al.*, 1994; Yamadera *et al.*, 1998). A deficit in the expression of the gene encoding human carboxypeptidase L was found in one patient (Halal *et al.*,1992).

Clinically, the r20S can be distinguished from other epilepsies characterized by recurrent nonconvulsive status epilepticus, either as a complication of childhood or juvenile-onset idiopathic generalized epilepsy in adolescents or young adults, or as situation-related seizures in the elderly (Thomas *et al.*, 1992). Two further epileptic syndromes may be discussed in this context. The first is a syndrome of "phantom absences" associated with recurrent episodes of absence status, and rare GTCS (Panayiotopoulos et al., 1995a), and the second is "absence status epilepsy" (Genton *et al.*, 2008). They concern adults with normal IQ, no behavioural disturbances, and who belong to the idiopathic generalized epilepsies; this is also the case for some children with recurrent episodes of absence status (Santucci *et al.*, 1985). The second concerns the syndrome of perioral myoclonias with absences (Panayiotopoulos *et al.*, 1995b): patients with this apparently idiopathic form of absence epilepsy seem to have mild to moderate mental retardation, and some may indeed have the r20S. A phenotype similar to the r20S has been reported in the ring chromosome 17 (Ricard-Mousnier *et al.*, 2007).

Treatment

All reports have stressed the drug-resistance of epilepsy in the r20S and there is no report on a clear aggravating effect of any drug. Lacosamide (Onder & Tezer, 2016), retigabine (Walleigh *et al.*, 2013) showed efficacy in single cases, while the VPA-LTG combination was helpful in two patients who had experienced non-convulsive status (Vignoli *et al.*, 2009). A possible involvement of basal ganglia in the genesis of the seizures, with decreased DOPA uptake, has been demonstrated by a PET study (Biraben *et al.*, 2004; Del Sole *et al.*, 2010) and may open new therapeutic possibilities. One patient was operated for frontal lobe cortical dysplasia without success (Inoue *et al.*, 1997). A 6-year old girl benefited from vagal nerve stimulation (Chawla *et al.*, 2002), but this positive effect has not been confirmed. Given the possibility of significant triggering factors or circumstances, patients with the r20S may benefit from psychological help. It may be noted here that paroxetine given at 20 mg/d because of associated anxiety decreased markedly the frequence of seizures in 3 out of 6 of our patients (unpublished).

Trisomy 21 (Down syndrome)

Down syndrome (DS) is one of the commonest chromosomal disorders and aetiologies of congenital mental retardation, with an incidence estimated at 1/800 births. It is significantly associated with epilepsy. DS is usually diagnosed at birth or even prenatally and is associated with well-known dysmorphic features: growth retardation, hypotonia, flat faces with brachycephaly and upward-slanted eyes, epicanthal folds, small ears, simian crease, hypogonadism and congenital heart malformations. In DS, there is a higher risk of leukemia and there is a significant increase, in patients aged 35 or more, of Alzheimer-like dementia. The prevalence of epilepsy increases with age in DS: this prevalence is not much higher than in the general population in infants and children, at 1.4% (Tatsuno *et al.*, 1984), but reaches 12.2% in patients aged 35 or more (Veall, 1974). A bimodal distribution of epilepsy, with early onset in the first year of life in 40% and late onset after the age of 30 in another 40% was also noted (Pueschel *et al.*, 1991). In DS, seizures occur in various settings and a clear relationship between age and type of seizures or epilepsy is present.

Genetics and physiopathology

The additional copy of chromosome 21 combined with imbalance in expression of chromosome 21 and non-chromosome 21 genes are proposed to result in the many phenotypes that characterize DS (Wiseman *et al.*, 2009). Trisomy of chromosome 21 genes has a significant impact on the development of multiple tissues. Of these, the upregulation dual-specificity tyrosine-(Y)-phosphorylation-regulated kinase 1A (*DYRK1A*) and regulator of calcineurin 1 (*RCAN1*), may lead to a disregulation of neuronal differentiation, and several alterations of the development of many cell types, leading to heart defects and abnormal learning and memory (Arron *et al.*, 2006).

The critical region for DS has been mapped to 21q22.3. Brain size and weight are usually within the low normal ranges for age, but significant changes are present. The gyral pattern of the brain surface is simplified, and there are cytoarchitectonic changes such as decreased small granular cells, which play a role in GABAergic inhibition, lower neuronal density, retarded myelination and dysgenesis of dendritic spines (Becker *et al.*, 1986; Ross *et al.*, 1984; Wisniewski & Schmidt-Sidor, 1989). The changes might paradoxically result in overinhibition, accounting for the high prevalence of epilepsy in DS (Araujo *et al.*, 2015). These changes have been implicated in both the delayed onset of age-related epilepsies such as infantile spasms and Lennox-Gastaut syndrome, and in the occurrence of reflex seizures (Guerrini *et al.*, 1990a). Alzheimer-like neuropathological changes have been demonstrated in both demented and non-demented ageing DS patients. Dementia is more frequent (prevalence: 13.3%), occurs at an earlier age (mean: 54,7 years), and is significantly associated with late-onset epilepsy (Tyrrell *et al.*, 2001 review in Menendez, 2005). Acquired factors, such as hypoxic brain damage, in some cases as the consequence of congenital heart disease, have also been considered to play a significant role in the occurrence of epileptic seizures (Stafstrom *et al.*, 1991; Stafstrom, 1993).

Epilepsy and EEG

In patients with DS, seizures can be ascribed to a variety of causes, including cardiac dysfunction and hypoxia. However, specific epilepsy types can be found, and we will limit ourselves here to both the epilepsies found in the younger age classes and to those that appear as significantly related to DS.

Infantile spasms (IS) are particularly frequent (Tatsuno *et al.*, 1984; Stafstrom *et al.*, 1991). Their incidence is increased at 2 to 5% in DS *vs.* 0.3 to 0.5 per 1,000 births in the general population (Pueschel *et al.*, 1991). Under certain circumstances, the Ts65Dn mouse model of DS may exhibit extensor spasms (Cortez *et al.*, 2009). In DS, the EEG may show the features of "idiopathic" West syndrome, *i.e.*, symmetric hypsarrhythmia, which reappears between spasms during a cluster (Silva *et al.*, 1996). IS remain often unrecognized by carers and are diagnosed late, which may cause a poorer response to therapy (Eisermann *et al.*, 2003). However, the overall prognosis is somewhat better than average for IS, with a lower incidence of chronic epilepsy and of increased developmental delay (Beatty *et al.*, 2017), and a good response to vigabatrin (VGB) in 4 out of 5 cases (Nabbout *et al.*, 2001), or to ACTH, in a series of 37 cases in which it was also noted that children with DS and heart malformations were more likely to have infantile spasms (Daniels *et al.*, 2011).

In children, there is a lower incidence of febrile seizures (0.9%) compared with the overall prevalence of around 3% in the general population (Stafstrom *et al.*, 1991). A retrospective study showed that 6% (15/252) pediatric and adolescent patients with DS had seizures: 8 had focal seizures, 1 had infantile spasms, 1 had Lennox-Gastaut syndrome, and 5 had GTCS (Smigielska-Kuzia *et al.*, 2009). However, children with DS and epilepsy may exhibit specific traits:

– The most characteristic trait is the high prevalence of reflex seizures (Guerrini *et al.*, 1990a; Pueschel & Louis, 1993), which may present as generalized or as focal epilepsies *(Figure 7)*. Many types of seizures can be found, including massive myoclonias, falls, tonic spasms.

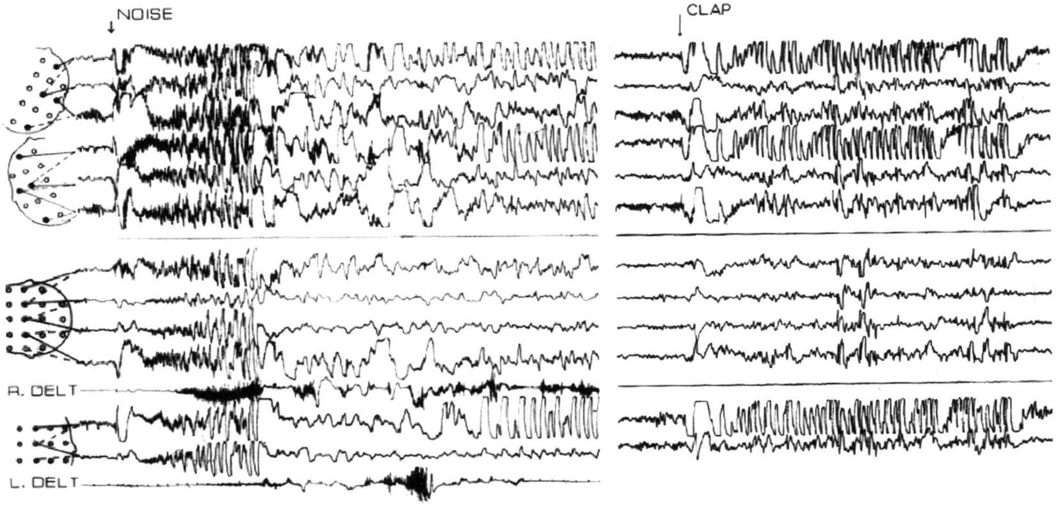

Figure 7

Down syndrome in a 12-year-old female. She developed reflex absences triggered by surprise or sudden noises at age 9 years, and soon after reflex tonic seizures with the same precipitants. A full-blown Lennox-Gastaut syndrome became apparent soon after. The EEG polygraphic recording shows: (left) a short tonic seizure triggered by a sudden noise and (right) an atypical absence triggered by an unexpected clap. Amplitude: 100 µV/cm.

Various stimuli may be involved, including light, noise, contact, and self-stimulation may also occur.

– The Lennox-Gastaut syndrome (LGS) may occur in patients with DS but remains uncommon. However, among six cases with reflex seizures, 3 had LGS (Guerrini *et al.*, 1989). In two cases, the onset of LGS coincided with the onset of reflex seizures *(Figure 7)*, while in the last case the reflex seizures began one year after onset of the LGS. In some cases, with the onset of purely reflex seizures, the sensitivity to external stimuli abates and the clinical and EEG features evocative of LGS appear thereafter (Lugo *et al.*, 1999; Ferlazzo *et al.*, 2009). The onset of LGS in patients with DS is late, around age 10. The course is usually severe.

– A number of middle-aged patients with DS, with, or usually without prior epilepsy, exhibit epileptic seizures that accompany or follow the onset of mental deterioration, mostly in the form of a myoclonic epilepsy, labeled "senile myoclonic epilepsy" (Genton & Paglia, 1994; De Simone *et al.*, 2010; d'Orsi *et al.*, 2014) or "late onset myoclonic epilepsy in DS" (LOMEDS) (Moller *et al.*, 2002). Alzheimer-type degeneration was found in autopsied cases (Wisniewski *et al.*, 1985; Pueschel *et al.*, 1991; Pueschel & Louis, 1993; Stafstrom, 1993). Senile myoclonic epilepsy, with a characteristic flow of events starting with awakening massive myoclonic jerks associated with SW discharges, followed by GTCS and by erratic myoclonus with concomittent slowing of the EEG background, occurs in practically all DS patients who exhibit Alzheimer-like dementia. It is increasingly recognized and may be the most common type of progressive myoclonic epilepsy (De Simone *et al.*, 2010; d'Orsi *et al.*, 2014) *(Figure 8)*. Its prevalence is indeed high: among 60 DS patients with dementia, 26 developed seizures (16 had prominent myoclonus) within 2 years (Gholipour *et al.*, 2017).

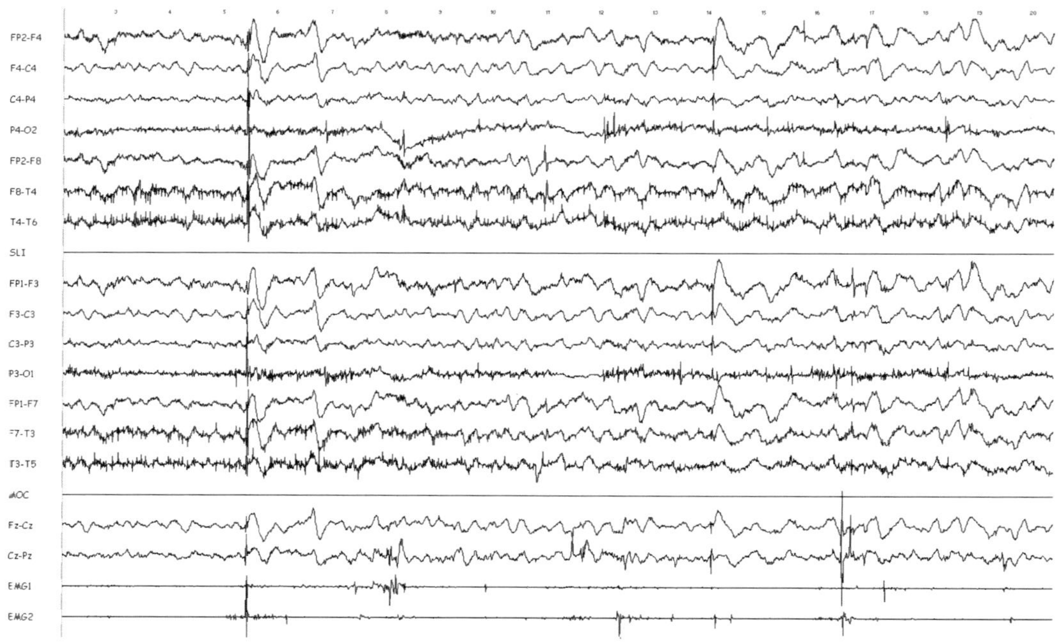

Figure 8

Down syndrome: 55-year-old female patient. Onset of Alzheimer-like dementia at age 51, occurrence of myoclonias soon after, and of GTCS within 2 years. Note diffuse slowing and the coexistence of generalized spike-wave discharges (associated with bilateral myoclonic jerks) and of erratic myoclonus, not clearly associated with EEG changes. EMG1 and 2 are right and left deltoid muscles. Recording speed 15 mm/s; 100 mV/10mm.

– Epilepsies that mimic idiopathic generalized forms, with a benign course and a good response to therapy, may occur in DS patients (Guerrini *et al.*, 1990b, case 1), and it is not well understood whether such cases are coincidental or not. It must be noted that they may exhibit special features, like photosensitivity, which may be related to the apparently higher prevalence of reflex epilepsies in DS.

In adolescents, as well as in older children and in young adults, the prevalence of various forms of focal or generalized epilepsies appears to be only slightly above average, and no specific features have been reported.

Thus, epilepsy presents itself with higher prevalence and in a large variety of forms in DS at all ages. Prognosis of epilepsy, and therapeutic response may vary according to the form of epilepsy, from benign, easily treatable forms to severe and intractable symptomatic generalized epilepsies. Treatment should thus be based on a syndromic approach of epilepsy: probably, the most common type of epilepsy in DS, the senile myoclonic form, responds to VPA and LEV initially, but progresses towards drug resistance; patients usually decease 4–8 years after seizure onset (De Simone *et al.*, 2010).

Monosomy 1 p36 (1p36 deletion syndrome)

Monosomy 1p36 (1p36 deletion syndrome) is the most common terminal deletion syndrome seen in humans, occurring in approximately 1 in 5,000 live births (Jordan *et al.*, 2015). The affected patients show a recognizable phenotype: microcephaly, brachycephaly, large and late-closing anterior fontanels, prominent forehead, straight eyebrows, short palpebral fissures, deep-set eyes, flat nasal bridge, midface hypoplasia, elongated philtrum, pointed chin, hypotonic face, low-set malformed and posterior rotated ears are found in > 75% of subjects. Also found in > 75% is intellectual disability, poor or absent speech, muscle hypotonia, brachycampodactyly, short feet, and brain anomalies. Less frequently found: congenital heart defects, visual problems including visual inattention, hearing loss mostly of the sensorineural type, skeletal anomalies, gastrointestinal and urogenital anomalies, cardiomyopathy, congenital hypothyroidism and behavioural disorders (Battaglia *et al.*, 2008 b; Battaglia & Shaffer, 2008).

Seizures occur in 44% to 58% of affected individuals. Structural brain abnormalities are present in 88% of affected individuals and include dilatation of the lateral ventricles and subarachnoid spaces, cortical atrophy and hypoplasia, thinning, and total or partial broadness of the corpus callosum. Less common anomalies are delay in myelination, multifocal hyperintensities in the white matter and periventricular nodular heterotopia (Neal *et al.*, 2006).

Epilepsy and EEG

The epilepsy phenotype is highly variable (Bahi-Buisson *et al.*, 2008). Seizures generally start in infancy or childhood from 4 days to 2 years 8 months (Heilstedt *et al.*, 2001, 2003; Bahi-Buisson *et al.*, 2008; Battaglia *et al.*, 2008b). The seizure types include infantile spasms, GTCS, complex or simple focal seizures, myoclonic seizures and absences. Their control with current antiepileptic drugs is quite good. The spectrum of EEG abnormalities includes hypsarrhythmia, focal and multifocal spikes and asymmetry of slow wave activity (*Figure 9*). First seizures are either generalized or focal. Infantile spasms are the most frequent type of seizures (36.4% of 22 cases according to Verrotti *et al.*, 2018), and are associated with hypsarrhythmia. IS may either be the presenting seizure type or may follow other seizure types. All kind of seizures seem to improve with time and only a few cases of intractable epilepsy are reported, especially among patients with structural brain abnormalities. When detected in adolescents or adults, the phenotype appears somewhat milder, as a majority of patients are able to walk and have gained some language skills (Brazil *et al.*, 2014).

Diagnosis/testing

The clinical suspicion of 1p36 deletion syndrome is confirmed by detection of a deletion of the most distal band of the short arm of chromosome 1 (1p36). Conventional G-banded cytogenetic analysis, FISH, or array GH can all be used to detect deletions, the latter being necessary for the more complex rearrangements. Four classes of rearrangements can be identified in individuals (Battaglia & Shaffer, 2008): an apparently "pure" *de novo* terminal deletion (52%), interstitial deletion (29%), more complex rearrangements including more than one deletion or deletions with duplications, triplications, insertions, and/or inversions (12%), and derivative chromosome 1 resulting from an unbalanced translocation (7%).

Investigators have searched for correlations between size of the 1p deletion and severity of clinical manifestations. Wu *et al.* (1999) and Heilstedt *et al.* (2003b) suggested a complete genotype-phenotype correlation, identifying the critical regions for certain features and considering 1p36 deletion syndrome as a contiguous gene deletion syndrome. Deletions above 6.2 Mb are associated with the most severe neurological handicap (Shimada *et al.*, 2015). However, Gajecka *et al.* (2007) found no correlation between deletion size and number of observed clinical features in a large cohort; even individuals with small (< 3 Mb) deletions of 1p36 presented with most of the features commonly associated with the syndrome. Redon *et al.* (2005) hypothesized that the features associated with 1p36 deletion syndrome may result from a position effect rather than a contiguous gene deletion syndrome.

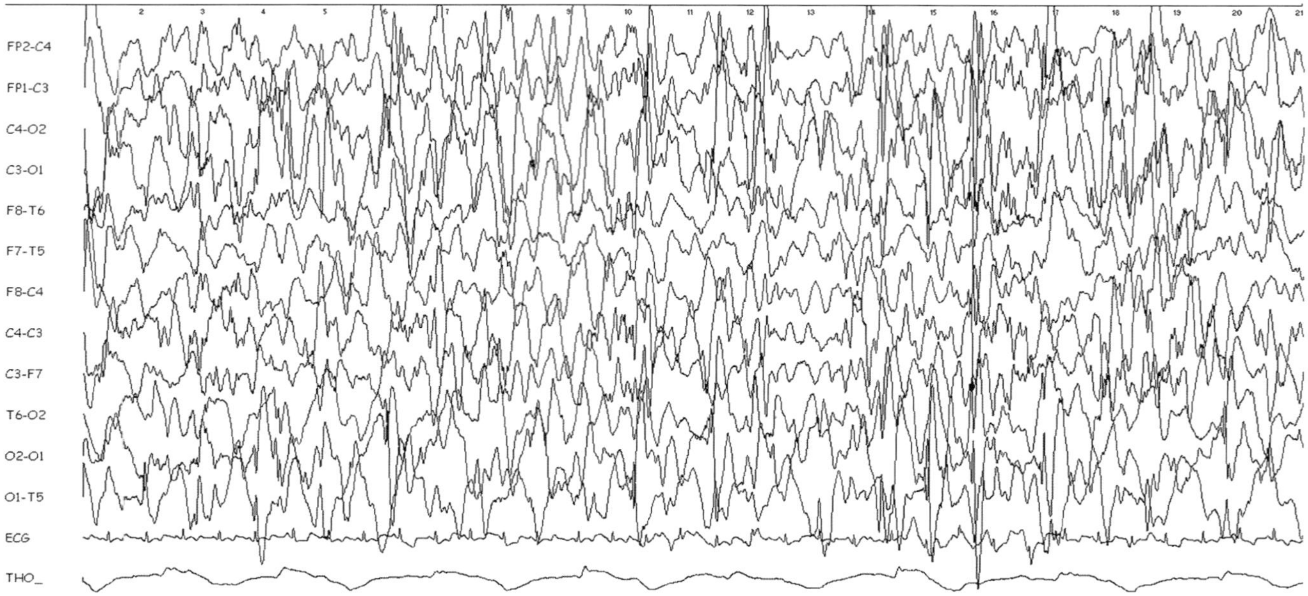

Figure 9

Monosomy 1p36 in a 12-month-old patient, sleep EEG: high amplitude delta slow waves intermixed with theta activity and multifocal spikes with an hypsarrhythmic pattern (amplitude: 100 µV/cm).

Rosenfeld *et al.* (2010) reported on five individuals with 200–823 kb overlapping deletions of proximal 1p36.33, four of which apparently *de novo*. The smallest region of deletion overlap is 174 Kb and contains five genes; these genes are likely candidates for some of the phenotypic features in monosomy 1p36. The RERE gene, located in the proximal part of the deleted region, may be causative of laryngo-oesophagal malformations (Pelizzo *et al.*, 2019), and *de novo* mutations may cause a phenotype with many of the 1p36 deletion syndrome (Fregeau *et al.*, 2016). Other genes deleted in a subset of the patients likely play a contributory role in the phenotypes, including GABRD and seizures, PRKCZ and neurologic features, and SKI and dysmorphic and neurologic features. Prenatal diagnosis, triggered by the US detection of multiple malformation, has been reported using SNP array (Ji *et al.*, 2017).

Fragile-X syndrome (Martin Bell syndrome)

Fragile-X syndrome (FraXS) is another one of the common causes of inherited mental retardation, with a severity that may range from mild to profound. Both males and females may be affected, but in agreement with X-linked inheritance, the phenotype is more severe in males. However, some boys present only learning disabilities. Associated clinical features include delayed speech, muscular hypotonia, joint hyperlaxity, macro-orchidism in postpuberal males, and facial dysmorphism consisting in a long narrow face, prominent forehead, large ears, small mandible, and a high-arched palate. Hyperactive or autistic behaviour, independent of the degree of mental retardation, may occur. Only recently was a high incidence of epilepsy recognized in FraXS. There is no correlation between the occurrence of seizures and the degree of mental retardation.

Fragile-X syndrome has a prevalence of 1/1,000 to 1/2,610 males (Webb *et al.*, 1986; Turner *et al.*, 1986) according to classical studies, based on induction of the Xq27.3 fragile site as a cytogenetic marker for the disorder. After the discovery of the FMR1 gene and the molecular diagnostic test for FXS, these prevalence estimates were revised to approximately 1/4,000 males (Turner *et al.*, 1996). Subsequent studies have estimated the prevalence to range from 1/3,717 to 1/8,918 in the general population of European descent (De Vries *et al.*, 1997; Crawford *et al.*, 2001). By means of an assay of 36,124 newborn males, an incidence in males of 1/5,161 was found (Coffee *et al.*, 2009). It is estimated that 1 in 1,000 females are carriers (Blomquist *et al.*, 1983).

Genetics and pathophysiology

The X-chromosome shows a fragile site at Xq27.3 (FraXA), when cells are grown in a folic-deprived medium. Recent molecular genetic studies showed that FraXS results from a dynamic mutation of the *FMR1* gene due to the expansion of a CGG-trinucleotide sequence located in exon 1. As a consequence, the gene is transcriptionally silenced. A molecular genetic analysis, mostly performed by Southern blot analysis, allows the detection of carriers and affected individuals.

The normal FMR-1 alleles contain 6-52 copies of the CGG repeat, whereas males with more than 200 copies are affected with the disease (full mutation). Nonaffected transmitting males have a premutation with 50-200 copies. Females bearing the premutation are phenotypically normal and usually do not express the fragile site. Premutation expansions are frequent in the general population, with estimates of 1/113-259 females and 1/260-800 males (Bourgeois *et al.*, 2009). However, recent studies have changed the view that there are no clinical manifestations associated with the premutation condition. Individuals with the premutation can present a late-onset neurodegenerative disorder, fragile X-associated tremor/ataxia syndrome (FXTAS), which affects nearly 40% of premutated males and 8% of premutated females over 50 years (Jacquemont *et al.*, 2004). In addition, primary ovarian insufficiency (POI) affects approximately 16–25% of premutated females. Comorbid psychiatric illness is also seen in a subgroup of premutation carriers, both males and females, children and adults (Bourgeois *et al.*, 2009).

Females with more than 200 copies (full mutation) may be normal or mentally affected (about 30%) and can show mild facial features of FraXS. Premutations tend to expand when transmitted to offspring through female carriers, and the risk of expansion to a full mutation correlates with the size of the premutation (Heitz *et al.*, 1992). In association with the full mutation, the promoter region of the FMR1 gene is hypermethylated and the transcription of the gene is repressed (Pieretti *et al.*, 1991). Two additional fragile sites reside in the distal Xq, FraXE and FraXF. FraXF is not clearly associated with a specific phenotype, but FraXE may cause mental impairment, usually milder than that observed for patients bearing a mutation at the FraXA locus. This information is important in order to understand the true predisposition.

In postmortem studies, long, thin, dysmorphic, or increased cortical dendrites have been found; brain MRI has also shown an increase in hippocampal volume. A transgenic mouse with FraXS is available. The knockout mice bearing the full mutation of *FMR1* gene are substantially more susceptible to audiogenic-induced seizures than the wild-type mice. This finding seems to confirm the role of cortical hyperexcitability in causing epilepsy in FraXS (Musumeci *et al.*, 2000, 2007).

FMRP may play a role in the regulation of mRNA in the cortical dendrites. The dendritic spines are longer and frequently immature in shape in the pyramidal cells of the V layer of the visual cortex in FMR1 knockout mice. In the same animal model, the mossy fibres of the dentate gyrus of the hippocampus have an abnormal distribution. The cortical expression of the GluR1 receptors is depressed postsynaptically, and long-term potentiation is reduced (Musumeci *et al.*, 2000). A reduced number of mGlu5 receptors have been linked to the constitutive forms of Homer proteins, with possible consequent alterations in synaptic plasticity (Giuffrida *et al.*, 2005).

There is now a great amount of evidence that the consequences of group 1 metabotropic glutamate receptor (Gp1 mGluR) activation are exaggerated in the absence of the FMRP, probably reflecting altered dendritic protein synthesis. Abnormal mGluR signaling could be responsible for the remarkably diverse neurological and psychiatric symptoms in FraXS, including seizures, delayed cognitive development, anxiety, and movement disorders (Bear, 2005). A FMR-1 knockout mouse model has been developed, but its phenotype significantly differs from the human (review in Telias, 2019). The dFMR1 mutant Drosophilia melanogaster is also considered a model of the human FraXS and exhibits similar reduction of synaptic activities (review in Specchia *et al.*, 2019).

Epilepsy and EEG

Premutation (55-200 repeats) carriers do not exhibit increased prevalence of epilepsy, but a variety of neuropsychiatric disorders including in children: anxiety, AHDH, or autism spectrum disorders, and in adults: anxiety, depression and obsessive-compulsive disorder (Hagerman *et al.*, 2018). The prevalence of epilepsy in patients with FraXS is 10 to 20% (Wisniewski *et al.*, 1985; Musumeci *et al.*, 1999; Incorpora *et al.*, 2002; Berry-Kravis, 2002). Age at onset of epilepsy is in the first 15 years of life and ranges between 2 and 12 years in most patients (Wisniewski *et al.*, 1985; Guerrini *et al.*, 1993, Musumeci *et al.*, 1999; Berry-Kravis, 2002).

There is a clear polymorphism in epilepsy. Complex focal seizures (CFS) occurred in 89.3% and simple focal seizures in 25% of patients with epilepsy (Musumeci *et al.*, 1999). In the same study, GTCS were present in 46.4% and were rare in about half of them, whereas in other studies they were the most frequently mentioned seizure type (Finelli *et al.*, 1985; Wisniewski *et al.*, 1985; Guerrini *et al.*, 1993). One individual with West syndrome followed by Lennox-Gastaut syndrome has been reported (Musumeci *et al.*, 1988). Febrile seizures were reported in only two out of the 28 patients with epileptic seizures. In one case, status epilepticus occurred when drug therapy with PB and PHT was discontinued (Musumeci *et al.*, 1999). In another series (Berry-Kravis, 2002), 12 patients (75%) had focal epilepsy and four males (25%) had generalized seizures only. Four of the 12 individuals with focal seizures had focal motor attacks with speech arrest and onset in sleep only. Four individuals had CFS occurring in wakefulness and sleep, and four had both focal and GTCS. All four individuals with generalized seizures had GTCS. Epilepsy is usually not severe; seizures have a low frequency of recurrence and are usually responsive to anticonvulsants. Two patients had experienced an isolated seizure (Guerrini *et al.*, 1993). The age at the last seizure is between 2 and 47 years. Three patients had a phenotype mimicking Panayiotopoulos syndrome, with seizure onset between ages 4 and 7 reported and with remission of seizures before age 14 (Bonnani *et al.*, 2017).

According to Musumeci *et al.* (1999), an age-related cortical hyperexcitability in FraXS seems to be demonstrated by the presence of spikes in the EEGs of patients without seizures, by the presence of spikes evoked by finger tapping and by the presence of giant somatosensory evoked potentials. In fact, a characteristic EEG pattern has been described in young FraXS males (Musumeci *et al.*, 1988, 1999; Kluger *et al.*, 1996) and has been considered as a "marker" for the condition: bi- or triphasic spikes of medium or high amplitude, usually over the central or centrotemporal regions but sometimes over the posterior regions, or multifocal, isolated or in brief sequences, rarely associated with spike and wave complexes, and dramatically activated by sleep, similar to those of benign childhood epilepsy with centrotemporal spikes (BECTS) (*Figure 10*). This pattern was found in about 50% of patients younger than 12 years, with or without seizures, by Musumeci *et al.* (1988) and was confirmed by others (Wisniewski *et al.*, 1991; Berry-Kravis, 2002), while other investigators found Rolandic spikes in only 9 and 10% of 33 and 30 patients in the same age class, respectively (Guerrini *et al.*, 1993; Incorpora *et al.*, 2002). Spikes tend to disappear in adulthood, and when present

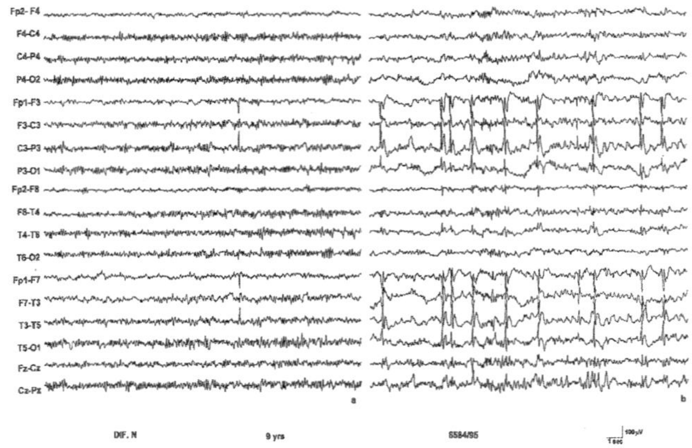

Figure 10 **9-year-old male with FraXS. Waking EEG showing a single spike localized over the central-temporal regions of the right hemisphere** (a)**; during sleep, paroxysmal abnormalities are markedly activated over the same regions** (b)**.**

at that age they are usually non-specific, rare and limited to only one location. No other types of EEG abnormalities have been observed in prepubertal children. In 6 out of 8 patients with a full mutation in exon 1 of the FraXS mental retardation-1 gene, focal seizures occurred during sleep. The relation between FMR-1 protein and cortical hyperexcitability in FraXS is not yet explained.

The apparent relationship with BECTS has been excluded by linkage analysis, which excluded the fragile-X locus as candidate gene for BECTS (Rees *et al.*, 1993, in Musumeci *et al.*, 1999). Moreover, children with BECTS were molecularly studied by Kluger *et al.* (1996) for FraXS and only one case carried a fragile-X premutation (with an intermediate range of repeats of 50-200).

Diagnosis

All mentally retarded males must be investigated for FraXS. Clinical and EEG findings may be suggestive. Molecular genetic analysis of the FMR-1 gene is mandatory. Epileptic seizures, including focal motor or CFS with or without secondary generalization and focal EEG abnormalities are only rarely reported in fragile-X female carriers. However, it has been suggested that screening for fragile-X would be appropriate for all females with mental retardation but also for mentally normal females with focal seizures (Singh *et al.*, 1999).

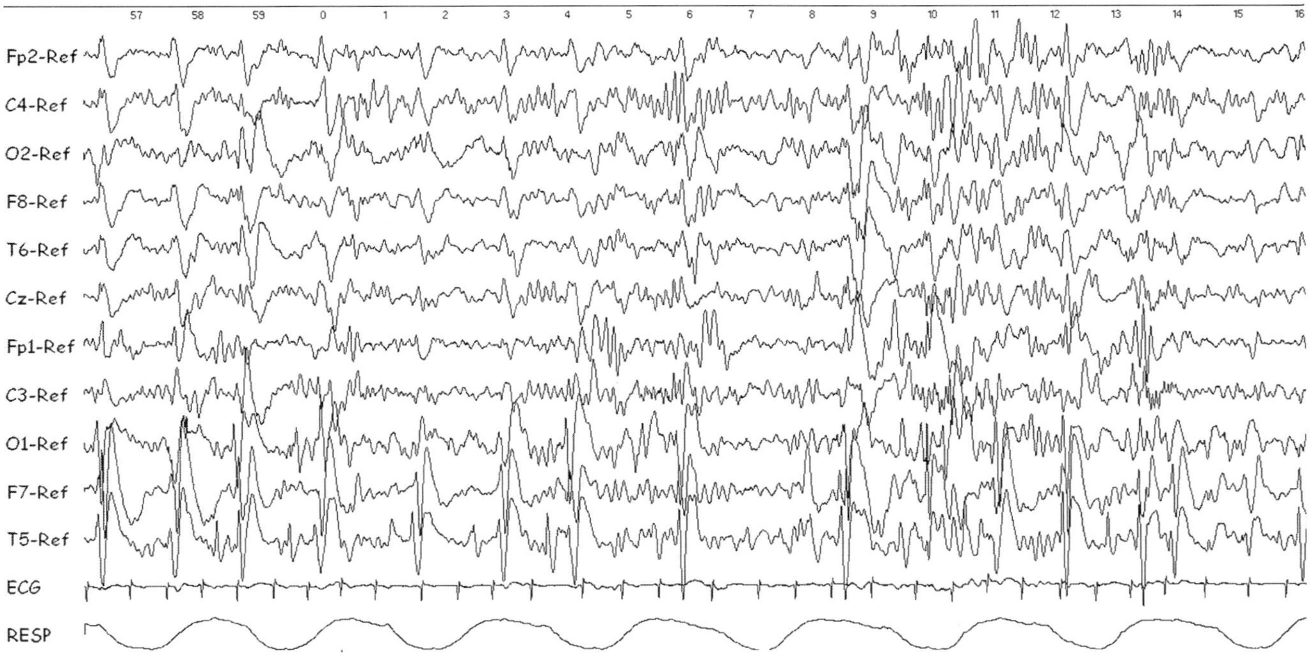

Figure 11

Lissencephaly in a 9-month-old patient, sleep EEG: "alpha like" activity with high amplitude maximal in both central regions and polyphasic spikes maximal in right frontal and temporo-occipital areas (amplitude: 200 µV/cm).

Treatment

Seizures are controlled in most, usually in monotherapy (Wisniewski *et al.*, 1985). Seizures persisted into adulthood in 25% FraXS patients (Musumeci *et al.*, 1999). AEDs which produced complete or good control in the well-controlled individuals include VPA, CBZ, PHT, ESM (Berry-Kravis, 2002). A patient with drug-resistant temporal lobe epilepsy and hippocampal sclerosis has been successfully operated (Kenmuir *et al.*, 2015). Beyond the scope of this chapter, breakthrough, genetic-based therapeutic advances are using viral-mediated gene therapy or targeting reactivation of the silenced *FMR1* gene (Kumari *et al.*, 2019).

Lissencephalies: Miller-Dieker syndrome and isolated lissencephaly

The Miller-Dieker Lissencephaly Syndrome (MDS) is characterized by lissencephaly type 1, or classical lissencephaly, with characteristic dysmorphic facial features and large 17p13-3 deletions. Classical lissencephaly is a human brain malformation characterized by a "four-layered" cortex composed of a molecular layer, an outer cellular layer (true cortex), a cell-sparse layer, and a deep cellular layer composed of heterotopic incompletely migrated neurons

(Barkowich, 1991). Classical lissencephaly may be complete or incomplete with both agyric and pachygyric regions. The origin of lissencephaly appears to be an arrest of the normal migration process at about the fourth month of gestation when the normal foetal cortex looks like a lissencephalic cortex.

Children with classical lissencephaly have a rather homogeneous neurological presentation, with severe mental retardation, severe motor disabilities with profound hypotonia and spastic tetraplegia, feeding problems and epilepsy; this is referred to as Isolated Lissencephaly Sequence (ILS). In MDS, the following characteristic facial changes are associated: bitemporal narrowing, prominent forehead, short nose with upturned nares, a long thin upper lip and small jaw. Associated abnormalities include low-set and posteriorly rotated ears, mild congenital heart malformations, clinodactyly, camptodactyly, cryptorchidism, and sacral dimples.

Genetics and physiopathology

Two genes associated with classical lissencephaly have been cloned (review by Dobyns *et al.*, 1999): *LIS1* located on chromosome 17p13.3, and *XLIS* (DCX) from Xq22.3-q23. Large deletions of 200kb or more extending from LIS1 toward the 17p telomere cause MDS whereas smaller deletions or point mutations of *LIS1* and mutations of *XLIS* (DCX) in affected males result in ILS (named ILS17 and ILSX respectively). Mutations of *XLIS* (DCX) cause subcortical band heterotopia (also called "double cortex") in affected females (Dobyns *et al.*, 1999). As for ILS17, boys with ILSX may have either a completely normal facial appearance or subtle abnormalities such as wide nasal bridge and epicanthal folds, which do not resemble MDS (Dobyns *et al.*, 1999).

Neuroimaging studies showed consistent differences in the gyral patterns. The malformation is more severe posteriorly in individuals with LIS1, either with MDS or ILS17, and more severe anteriorly in individuals with XLIS (DCX) mutations (Dobyns *et al.*, 1999). There are also differences in severity of the gyral malformation between MDS and ILS17, being greater in MDS. Hypoplasia of the cerebellar vermis proved to be more common with *XLIS* (DCX) mutations. Neurological abnormalities differ slightly between patients with MDS, ILS17 or ILSX. In general, this seems to be correlated with the lissencephaly grade, type of mutation detected and severity of epilepsy (Dobyns *et al.*, 1999). Most children with MDS have a shorter lifespan.

In patients with no FISH abnormalities and no mutations on gene sequencing, multiplex ligation-dependent probe amplification (MLPA) has increased the detection of genomic deletions/duplication in the encompassing the LIS1 region. *LIS1* gene abnormalities are frequently associated with a posterior-anterior gradient (Dobyns *et al.*, 1999; Mei *et al.*, 2008).

A smaller number of patients with lissencephaly present mutations in the *TUBA1A* gene associated with a posterior-anterior gradient (Poirier *et al.*, 2007). *DCX*, *LIS1* and *TUBA1A* genes regulate microtubule and cytoplasmicdyne in function interfering with neuronal migration *LIS1* is also required for cellular proliferation and intracellular transport (Leventer *et al.*, 2001). A small percentage of patients have mutations in the reelin (*RELN*) gene, which is thought to be associated with arresting neuronal migration and promoting normal cortical lamination (Dulabon *et al.*, 2000). RELN mutations are associated with an autosomal recessive lissencephaly with cerebellar hypoplasia (Hong *et al.*, 2000).

Children with submicroscopic duplications at 17p13.3 and a milder phenotype were recently described: they had cognitive, neurobehavioural symptoms and structural brain abnormalities (dysgenesis of the corpus callosum, mild volume loss in the cerebellum, occipital cortex and cerebrum).

The children did not have seizures, although one carrier mother did. Mutant mice with increased LIS1 expression had smaller brains and with a disorganized ventricular zone although cortical layer identity was preserved and radial glia scaffold was aligned in a normal fashion (Bi *et al.*, 2009). Another rare form of lissencephaly associated with abnormal genitalia (with or without corpus callosum abnormalities) is found in children with *ARX* mutations (Kato *et al.*, 2004). Interestingly, mutations in this gene are also present in patients with West syndrome without a visible abnormality of cortical migration. *ARX* gene is expressed in the forebrain and regulates non-radial migration of interneurons (Kitamura *et al.*, 2002).

Epilepsy and EEG

Early onset epilepsy (usually before 8 weeks of age; in 82% within the first six months of life according to Herbst *et al.*, [2016]) with refractory seizures are the main clinical features in both patients with facial dysmorphisms of classical lissencephaly and those with lissencephaly (Daube & Chou, 1966; Garcia *et al.*, 1978; Jones *et al.*, 1980). Dulac *et al.* (1983), Gastaut *et al.* (1987) and Mori *et al.* (1994) have described in details the characteristic EEG findings of classical lissencephaly (agyria-pachygyria).

Typically, seizures begin in the first months of life with massive bilateral myoclonus or epileptic spasms without typical hypsarrythmia (Gastaut *et al.*, 1987), or with focal motor seizures. Spasms may be preceded by apnoeic spells or tonic seizures (Miller, 1963; Mori *et al.*, 1994). Although epileptic spasms and massive bilateral myoclonus are frequent, they were not invariably present in the Gastaut's series (Gastaut *et al.*, 1987). Periodic spasms are a seizure type extremely suggestive and frequent in patients with classical lissencephaly, including those with MDS (Gobbi *et al.*, 1987, 1996). Periodic spasms may persist after the first year of life. Tonic seizures are common by the end of the second year and usually represent, in older patients, the main seizure type together with focal seizures with secondary generalization. Tonic seizures are never associated with the typical interictal slow spike and wave pattern of the Lennox-Gastaut syndrome (Gastaut *et al.*, 1987).

The main interictal EEG finding is represented by abnormal high-amplitude fast activity, predominantly in the alpha and beta frequency bands, at all ages studied. The amount of fast activity is quite variable in the first six to eight months. In some cases, beta activity is already prominent at five months, with very little slower rhythms, while in other cases delta and theta activities are clearly preponderant. When fast and slow activity are combined, the slower waves may appear notched, at times resembling spike-wave complexes. In accordance with Gastaut *et al.* (1987), we believe that it has been erroneously interpreted as hypsarrhythmia. The fast activity persists on eyes opening and is little modified by sleep. Vertex sharp waves, sleep spindles and theta activity of deeper sleep are absent, but 14 Hz sleep spindles have been found in early infancy. Usually, a FISH analysis with a specific LIS1 probe, which is commercially available, is necessary to confirm MDS. In addition, a mutational analysis of DCX or LIS1 is necessary to detect point mutations in non-deleted patients. In patients who are negative for deletions/mutations of LIS1 or for mutations of *DCX* gene, MLPA analysis of *LIS1* gene and research for mutations of *TUBA1A*, *RELN*, and *ARX* genes should be performed.

Epileptic seizures in MDS and other lissencephalies are refractory to treatment. Some improvement may be achieved with steroids or benzodiazepines, and patients often respond to phanobarbital or vigabatrin (Herbst *et al.*, 2016). Perampanel has brought relief, especially against myoclonic seizures, in 4/5 patients (Ikemoto *et al.*, 2019).

Other chromosomal disorders associated with seizures

Trisomy 12p

Trisomy of the short arm of chromosome 12 represents a rare multiple congenital craniofacial anomalies/mental retardation syndrome. It occurs approximatively in 1/50,000 births (Stengel-Rutkowski *et al.*, 1981), and is considered to result in abortions in most cases, newborns exhibiting often mosaicism (Roberts *et al.*, 2016). Neurological findings consist of severe mental retardation without language development and generalized hypotonia. Dysmorphic features include a round face with a short neck, high and prominent forehead, flat/undeveloped occiput, hypertelorism, bilateral epicanthus, broad nasal bridge, long phyltrum, prominent lower lip, low-set ears, and micrognatia. Life expectancy in pure cases of trisomy 12p does not appear particularly impaired; mosaic patients fare better than those with complete 12p trisomy. Neuropathological investigations showed non-homogeneous findings ranging from normal results to several cortical dysplastic lesions (Fryns *et al.*, 1974; Nielsen *et al.*, 1977). Neuroimaging may also disclose basal ganglia calcifications, cortical-subcortical atrophy, "cisterna magna" and abnormal white matter signals (Guerrini *et al.*, 1990b; Elia *et al.*, 1995a).

This chromosomal disease may be caused either by a malsegregation of a balanced parental chromosomal rearrangement or by a *de novo* occurrence in a mosaic or regular fashion (McKusick, 1994). In most patients the breakpoint is at band 12p11. Allen *et al.* (1996) suggest that there is some variability in the phenotypic expression, in relation to the breakpoint, and, following the extent of the 12p trisomy and the presence of other chromosomal aneusomies, 12p trisomy may be subdivided into five categories:

- partial pure trisomy 12p with duplication point distal to 12p11 without involvement of other chromosomes (Tayei *et al.*, 1989);
- 12p trisomy associated with cell line mosaicism (Karki & Walters, 1990);
- pure 12p trisomy with an additional trisomy or monosomy of the short arm of an acrocentric chromosome;
- complete 12p trisomy with monosomy or trisomy of nonacrocentric chromosomes other than 12p;
- complete 12p trisomy with trisomic involvement of 12q.

Epileptic seizures have been reported in all five categories with the exception of the first, which is also characterized by a more benign presentation of the syndrome; seizures occur in most patients after the age of 7 years (Segel *et al.*, 2006). The susceptibility to develop epilepsy is variably influenced by severity and distribution of brain anomalies and by the occurrence of perinatal respiratory problems. Most seizures reported are generalized convulsive, either febrile or not, or myoclonic in infancy or childhood. Exhaustive description of the electroclinical findings has been reported by Guerrini *et al.* (1990b). Myoclonic absences with onset after the age of three years associated with an ictal and interictal 3-Hz spikes and polyspike waves EEG seem to represent a common seizure and EEG pattern (Guerrini *et al.*, 1990b; Elia *et al.*, 1995a), and such unusual EEG changes have also been reported in two patients with pericentric inversion of chromosome 12 (Grosso *et al.*, 2004a). Three voltage-gated K-channel genes are clustered together in the 12p13 band (McKusick, 1994, pp. 176–260). Seizures appear well controlled by AEDs.

Ring chromosome 14

Ring chromosome 14 (r14) is a rare chromosomal anomaly with a fairly specific clinical presentation that includes epilepsy as a major trait. The genetic anomaly occurs as a mosaicism, but homogenous r14 cases have been reported, who do not differ from other patients (Raoul *et al.*, 1984). There is no clear phenotypic difference between patients with the r14 anomaly and other patients with deletions of chromosomal material in the same region without ring formation, but there may be marked differences in the amount and nature of deleted material, as assessed by molecular markers (Wintle *et al.*, 1995): the r14 apparently represents the smallest form of 14q monosomy. The terminal q region of chromosome 14 is known to carry the genes of the immunoglobulin heavy chain gene cluster, but no major changes in immunoglobulins have been found in r14, and the deletion appears to occur distally (Krawczun *et al.*, 1984). Dysregulation of *FOXG1* has been reported (Alosi *et al.*, 2015).

The phenotype of patients with the r14 syndrome was defined some years ago and updated (Réthoré *et al.*, 1984; Zollino *et al.*, 2009): there is a quite evocative association of short stature, early-onset epilepsy, mental retardation (marked to profound in most patients), speech impairment, microcephaly, and facial dymorphisms with a narrow, elongated face, arched palate, short palpebral fissures, flat nasal bridge and retrognathia. Ocular anomalies include cortical cataract, yellow-white spots on mid-peripheral retina and refractive errors (Hisatomi *et al.*, 2000). No specific neuroanatomic changes have been reported, with the exception of a slight hypoplasia of the corpus callosum on MRI in one case (Ono *et al.*, 1999), and a left temporal hypodensity on CT scan in another case (Shirasaka *et al.*, 1992). Some patients may exhibit only discrete dysmorphisms, as a patient who had only "almond shaped eyes" in association with epilepsy, mental retardation and macular spots (de Blois *et al.*, 1990).

Epilepsy begins early in life, usually during the first year (Ville *et al.*, 2009), and the incidence is 100% (Giovannini *et al.*, 2013). The patients have mostly a generalized symptomatic form of epilepsy, but may also exhibit CFS, which may occur in clusters, and a fronto-central origin of seizures has been evidenced in some patients (Ono *et al.*, 1999). The epilepsy is reported as drug-resistant in most cases, status epilepticus is frequent, and the severity of epilepsy is negatively correlated to the mental development (Giovannini *et al.*, 2013). A milder epileptic, mental and dysmorphic phenotype has been associated with r14 mosaicism in a boy otherwise characterized by growth retardation and blepharophimosis (Hou, 2004), or in three other patients with mosaicism or monosomy, with evidence of focal epilepsy in the latter (Morimoto *et al.*, 2003).

Inv-dup(15) syndrome

The inv-dup(15) or idic(15) syndrome (inverted duplication of proximal chromosome or isodicentric 15 chromosome) is the most common genetic disorder of a heterogeneous group of the extra structurally abnormal chromosomes (ESACs) whose presence results in tetrasomy 15p and partial tetrasomy 15q. Although poorly known, prevalence at birth of inv-dup(15) is estimated to be 1 in 30,000 with a sex ratio of almost 1 (Schinzel & Niedrist, 2001; Battaglia, 2008). However, a higher incidence is possible due to underascertainment.

The typical phenotype of the inv-dup(15) syndrome, containing the Prader-Willi/Angelman syndrome (PWS/AS) region, is characterized by mental retardation ranging from medium to severe, severe language delay and deficit, hypotonia, ataxia, autistic or autistic-like behaviour, and epilepsy. Mild dysmorphic features can be occasionally found such as microcephaly, frontal bossing, oedematous palpebrae, micropenis and hypospadias. All patients present with highly variable in severity behavioural problems classifiable as pervasive developmental disorders (PDD) or autism (Battaglia *et al.*, 1997; Cabrera *et al.*, 1998; Takeda *et al.*, 2000; Buoni *et al.*, 2000; Borgatti *et al.*, 2001; Battaglia, 2008). Survival is not markedly affected.

In their review of 45 cases, Matricardi *et al.* (2018) found at onset epileptic spasms in 51%, focal seizures in 26%, atypical absences in 11% and falls in 9%. The most common type of epilepsy is symptomatic generalized epilepsy of the Lennox-Gastaut type with intractable seizures and severe evolution (Battaglia *et al.*, 1997; Borgatti *et al.*, 2001; Takeda *et al.*, 2000; Takeda *et al.*, 2000; Torrisi *et al.*, 2001; Battaglia, 2008; Battaglia *et al.*, 2016). West syndrome later followed by drug-resistant cryptogenic myoclonic epilepsy has also been described (Cabrera *et al.*, 1998); Aguglia *et al.* (1999) described reflex seizures beginning 5–20 seconds after the onset of repeated cheek-kissing from the mother or after viewing of pleasant or funny events. They were characterized by bilateral discharges involving mainly the temporal regions and evolving into myoclonic absence-like seizures. Non-emotional stimuli, such as a pinch, sucking or rubbing cheeks, or the sound of the kiss alone, failed to provoke seizures. The seizures were drug-resistant. Focal symptomatic epilepsy has been reported in one case by Borgatti *et al.* (2001), but may be more frequent, and some of Lennox-Gastaut type epilepsies may have evolved from focal epilepsies. We nevertheless observed a patient with inv-dup(15) syndrome who had a benign epilepsy with centro-temporal spikes, with a benign evolution. The EEG pattern was typical for BECTS (*Figure 12*). Two further cases with large deletions and mild phenotypes were also reported (Chifari *et al.*, 2002).

In 1997, Battaglia *et al.* reported in detail the EEG abnormalities observed in four patients with inv-dup(15). All EEGs were abnormal, showing: i) slow background activity; ii) absence or poverty of the

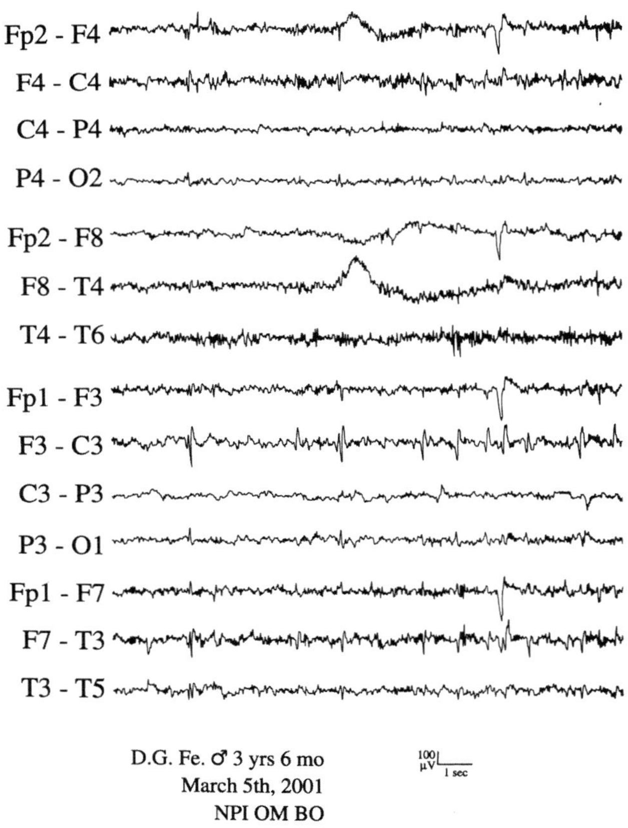

Figure 12 **Patient with 47,xy,inv-dup 15 syndrome. Brief sequence of medium or high amplitude bi-triphasic spikes localized over the left centro-temporal region.**

rhythmic activities usually elicited over the posterior third of the brain on eye closure; iii) multifocal discharges with variable hemispheric predominance; iv) frequent, large amplitude, generalized paroxysms, lasting 2 to 20 seconds, characterized by slow sharp element-spike/wave complexes, mostly accompanied by atypical absences; v) frequent generalized bursts of fast rhythms during slow wave sleep in 2 of the 4 patients, accompanied by tachypnea and/or by an upward rolling of the eyes, and/or by tonic fits; and vi) disruption of the usual sleep structure. Other EEG findings include generalized rhythmic 3.5–4 Hz spike-and-wave discharges, lasting 4–6 seconds (Chifari *et al.*, 2002), diffuse spikes, polyspikes, and ill-defined polyspike/wave complexes, with variable hemispheric predominance (Battaglia, 2008).

In cytogenetic investigation it is fairly frequent to find supernumerary marker chromosomes, which are defined as extrastructurally abnormal chromosomes (ESAC) (Hook & Cross, 1987). *In situ* hybridization demonstrated that 50% of them is derived from pericentromeric region of chromosome 15 and these ESAC have been defined inv-dup(15) (Schreck *et al.*, 1977). Extrachromosomes derived from chromosome 15 and containing the Prader-Willi/Angelman syndrome region are the cause of the inv-dup(15) (ESAC-15) syndrome (Leana-Coxetal, 1994). Robinson *et al.* (1993b) demonstrated that presumably the inv-dup(15) syndrome resulted from an illegitimate recombination event between two different chromosomes 15, and that all patients showed a maternal origin of the duplicated chromosome. The clinical severity appears to be associated with dosage of the PWS/AS region rather than with differences in the extent of the duplicated segment. Wandstrat *et al.* (1998) delineated the breakpoints of a large inv-dup(15), that includes the PWS/AS chromosomal region (15q 11 -q 13). They described two types of inv-dup(15): those that break between D15S12 and D15S24, near the distal boundary of the PWS/AS chromosomal region, and those that share a breakpoint immediately proximal to D15S1010. At least two additional breakpoints have been identified that account for the formation of small and medium inv-dup(15). These four breakpoints represent hotspots for rearrangement because they contain repeated sequences. Parent-of-origin studies revealed that, in all the analysed cases, the inv-dup(15) was maternal in origin. In the patient reported by Aguglia *et al.* (1999), molecular genetic investigations revealed a correct methylation pattern of the chromosomes 15, and three copies (two maternal and one paternal) of the segment 15q11-q13, including the *GABRB3* gene. The authors hypothesize that an overexpression of cerebral gamma-aminobutyric acid (GABA)-mediated inhibition accounts for the severe epilepsy that they observed in their patient. Actually, the PWS/AS region includes genes for these two syndromes, the gene for G ABRB3 and GABRA5, and the gene P. Gene P seems to be important since a deletion of P alleles in mice causes a re-arrangement of GABRB3 and GABRA5 receptors producing a phenotype consisting of ataxia and epileptic seizures (Nakatasu *et al.*, 1993). Similarly, it could be hypothesized that a tetrasomy of these genes, such as the one observed in large inv-dup(15), may alterate GABA receptor activity (Battaglia *et al.*, 1997). Nevertheless, the influence of gene content of the marker chromosome, particularly the three gamma-aminobutyric acid-A receptor subunit genes, may represent the link between epilepsy, mental retardation, and PDD (Borgatti *et al.*, 2001).

An additional gene located more distally in the region SLC12A6 (solute carrier, family 12, member 6), coding for a cation chloride cotransporter and expressed in the brain, heart, skeletal muscle, and kidney, could also be implicated in the pathogenesis of seizures (Caron *et al.*, 2000). A study performed on post-mortem brain tissue from two individuals with 15q11-13 hexasomy and 15q11-13 tetrasomy respectively, has suggested that genetic copy number variation, combined with additional genetic or environmental influences on epigenetic mechanisms, impact clinical heterogeneity and the outcome of inv-dup(15) (Hogart *et al.*, 2009).

Klinefelter (XXY) syndrome

The Klinefelter syndrome (KS) (Klinefelter *et al.*, 1942) is a frequent condition that is usually recognized only in post-pubertal males, in the context of infertility, or, earlier in life, in the context of mild to moderate mental retardation and/or behavioural or psychiatric disorders. The overall prevalence is around 1.7/1,000 male births (Court Brown, 1969). Epilepsy is rarely the presenting symptom, and the prevalence of seizures ranges between 2 and 10% (Becker *et al.*, 1966; Zuppinger *et al.*, 1967; Nielsen & Pedersen, 1969; Genton *et al.*, 1992). Although it appears to exceed the prevalence found in the general population, it is apparently close to the overall prevalence of seizures in psychiatric or mentally retarded populations (Boltshauser *et al.*, 1978). The genetic anomaly is represented by the presence of one or more extra X chromosomes, mostly as a consequence of no disjunction during meiosis. Around 80% of patients have only one extra X chromosome. Mosaicism with coexistence or normal (46, XY) and abnormal (46, XXY) populations is common, while mixo-ploidy is present in a minority of cases. The severity of symptoms is usually higher in patients with multiple X chromosomes.

The clinical presentation may be very evocative in some patients, while others have no clear dysmorphism or dysfunction and present only in the context of male infertility (usually with azoospermia without marked peripheral hypogonadism) or mild mental retardation. Testicular atrophy (with or without ectopy) is constant in post-pubertal patients but may escape a neurologist's attention. The characteristic, but inconstant dysmorphic features include markers of male hypogonadism ("eunuchoidism") in adolescents or adults: gynecomasty, increased body height, long limbs, narrow shoulders and broad hips, decreased body hair. Many patients have normal mental performance, but the IQ is in average 10 to 15 points below that of the normal population, and only 15–20% can be considered mentally impaired (English *et al.*, 1989). Psychiatric problems may be the obvious presenting symptoms in some patients, ranging from high anxiety to psychotic-like behaviour (Yeragani & Hopkinson, 1981; Miyamoto *et al.*, 1992). Tremor may also be present (Boltshauser *et al.*, 1978). Neuropathology changes appear as non-specific, although polymicrogyria and megalencephaly was described in one case (Budka, 1978).

EEG changes may be present, even in patients who do not experience seizures, but are often nonspecific: slight background slowing, with or without focal sharp anomalies (Nielsen & Pedersen, 1969; Nielsen & Tsuboi, 1974). Patients with epilepsy may exhibit various clinical and EEG changes. A case with infantile spasms has been reported (Inoue *et al.*, 2012). Tatum *et al.* reported in 1998 the largest known series of patients with KS and epilepsy: interestingly, most of their patients have a generalized form of epilepsy, including typical absences and generalized tonic-clonic seizures, with typical generalized discharges on the EEG (Genton *et al.*, 1992; Tatum *et al.*, 1998). However, other patients clearly have focal types of seizures and EEG changes. In agreement with Elia *et al.* (1995b), the epilepsy is usually mild, and seizures are easily controlled by medication, but is considered nevertheless a significant contributor to the increased mortality found in KS (Swerdlow *et al.*, 2005). Overall, epilepsy associated with the KS does not have a homogenous presentation, different from the syndrome associated with another X-chromosome anomaly, the triple X syndrome, with posterior EEG changes and treatable epilepsy (Grosso *et al.*, 2004b).

18q-syndrome

The 18q- deletion syndrome is due to a terminal deletion in the long arm of chromosome 18 with variable breakpoints. It is associated with various dysmorphism with microcephaly, turricephaly, deep-set eyes, carp shaped mouth, broad nasal bridge, high arched or cleft palate, small hands and feet, frequent cardiac anomalies. Patients show moderate to severe mental retardation, aggressive behaviour, ataxia, dysmetria, and hypotonia. Additionnally, it is associated with disturbed myelination thought to be due to haploinsufficiency of the gene for myelin basic protein and frequent cardiac anomalies. MRI hypersignals found in the white matter are not related to dysmyelination, as usually stated (the myelin basic protein gene is on 18q23), but rather to gliosis (Tanaka *et al.*, 2011).

Several reports suggest the association of epilepsy and 18q- syndrome (Sturm *et al.*, 2000; Grosso *et al.*, 2005; Stephenson, 2005). Early epilepsy can be a feature of the syndrome. The reported seizures are frequently autonomic epileptic seizures with cardiac arrhythmia and apnoea simulating nonepileptic syncope.

6q Terminal deletion syndrome

The 6q terminal deletion syndrome is a rare form of contiguous gene defects with mental retardation, facial dysmorphism, genital hypoplasia, and structural anomalies of the CNS, including periventricular heterotopia corpus callosum dysgenesis, polymicrogyria (Conti *et al.*, 2013). Five patients with 6q terminal deletion (ranging between 9 and 16 Mb) associated with a specific clinical and EEG pattern were described (Elia *et al.*, 2006). In all cases, seizures were characterized by vomiting, cyanosis, head and eye version, with or without loss of consciousness. In four cases, the interictal EEG showed posterior spike-and-wave complexes, which were activated by sleep (*Figure 13*). No patient had status epilepticus or prolonged seizures. The MRI revealed colpocephaly and dysgenesis of the corpus callosum and brainstem in four patients; three of them also had hypertrophic massa intermedia. Seizure outcome was rather good in all patients.

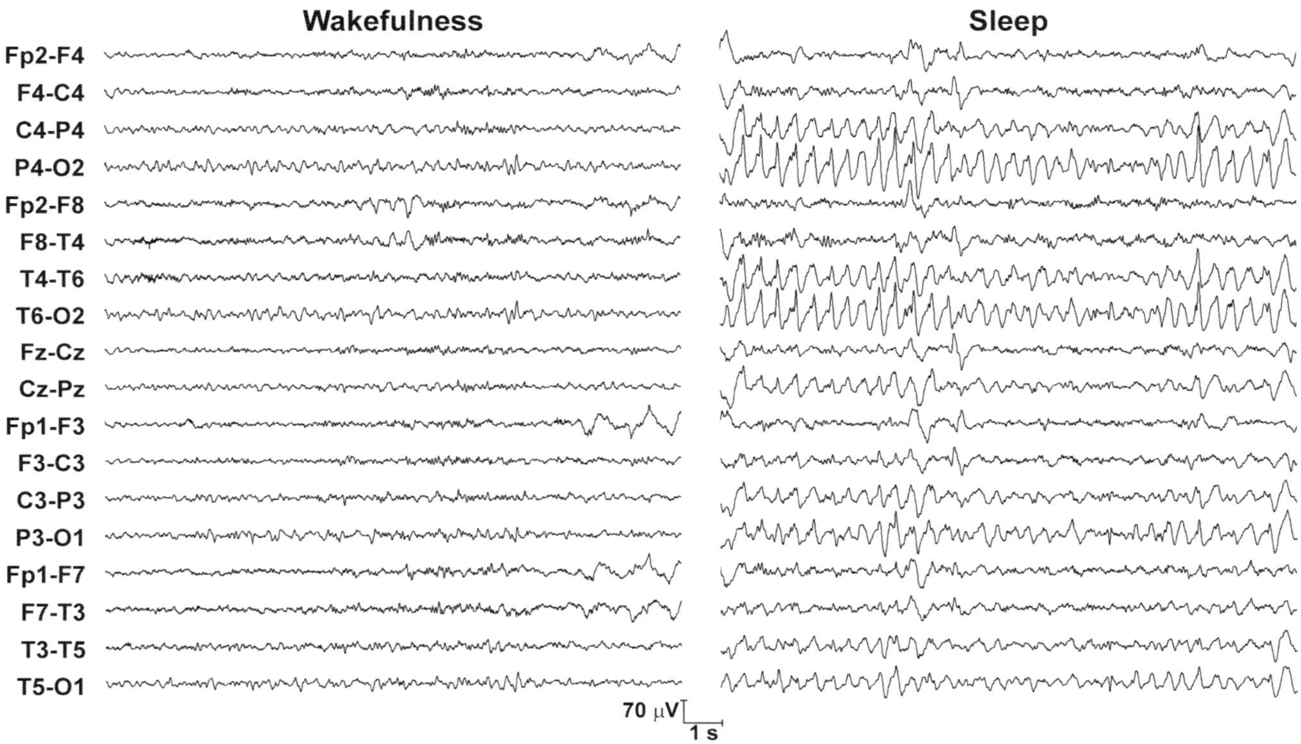

Figure 13

Waking EEG of a male subject with 6q terminal deletion syndrome.
Left: **Note the presence of sharp waves over the posterior regions of the right hemisphere.**
Right: **During sleep, very long sequences of slow waves or spike-and-wave complexes are present over the posterior regions.**

Rare, non-recurrent, copy number variants (CNVs) and epilepsy

Deletions and duplications which affect DNA copy number, are collectively known as copy number variants (CNVs). Rare CNVs - less than 1% - (Valsesia *et al.*, 2013) have been established as important risk factors for epilepsies, both in children and in adults (Meffor, 2014; Kessi *et al.*, 2018; Borlot *et al.*, 2017; Coppola *et al.*, 2019). Recurrent CNV "hotspots" predispose to different types of epilepsies including focal and generalized seizures (Heinzen *et al.*, 2010; Olson *et al.*, 2014), epileptic encephalopathies (Mefford *et al.*, 2011) genetic generalized epilepsy with intellectual disability (ID) (De Kovel *et al.*, 2010, Mullen *et al.*, 2013), atypical Rolandic epilepsy (Reinthaler *et al.*, 2016), fever-associated syndromes (Hartmann *et al.*, 2015) and absence epilepsy (Addis *et al.*, 2016).

The percentages of patients with epilepsy carrying pathogenic CNVs varies between 5 to 12% of patients according to inclusion criteria and methodology used (Mefford *et al.*, 2010; Olson *et al.*, 2014; Borlot *et al.*, 2017; Kessi *et al.*, 2018; Coppola *et al.*, 2019). When seizures comorbid with a wide range of neurodevelopmental and neuropsychiatric conditions the percentage of patients with pathogenic CNVs increases considerably (Coppola *et al.*, 2019, in press). Although a search for CNV is undoubtedly worthwhile in people with epilepsy, it may not be that such CNVs drive only epilepsy, indeed, for patients ascertained through their epilepsy, the presence of additional features including neurodevelopmental disorders or non-neurological co-morbidities, points to an elevated likelihood of finding an underlying pathogenic CNV (Coppola *et al.*, 2019, in press).

Up until 5 years ago, CNVs were mostly detected through array-based comparative genomic hybridization (aCGH) and then single nucleotide polymorphism (SNP) arrays. These technologies allowed the detection of submicroscopic CNVs that were too small to be recognized by routine karyotype analysis. Thanks to array-based technologies, surveys of large CNVs (> 50 Kbp) first associated CNVs in genomic hotspots such as 15q11.2 and 16p13.11 with generalized epilepsy (Helbig *et al.*, 2009; De Kovel *et al.*, 2010). Other studies have further shown the importance of large and *de novo* CNVs as well as identified a few associations with specific genes (Saitsu *et al.*, 2008). Rare genic CNVs were typically found in around 10% of epilepsy patients (Mefford *et al.*, 2010; Mefford *et al.*, 2011; Adis *et al.*, 2018) and CNVs larger than 1 Mbp were significantly enriched in patients compared to controls (Lal *et al.*, 2015). Unfortunately, small CNVs and other types of SVs could not be efficiently or consistently detected using these technologies.

More recent technological advances including next-generation sequencing (CNV seq) and Whole Genome Sequencing (WGS), both holding the potential to identify pathogenic CNVs, provide the possibility of a more comprehensive characterization of the role of CNVs in epilepsy (Carvill & Mefford, 2015; Monlong *et al.*, 2018; Coppola *et al.*, 2019, in press). Investigating the occurrence of pathogenic CNVs through genomic-based methodologies has further improved the diagnostic yield in allowing the evaluation of a greater number of patients, the detection of smaller CNVs compared to microarrays (Gilissen *et al.*, 2014), and the detecting of balanced structural variation as well (Redin *et al.*, 2017). Also, regions of Uniparental Disomy (UPD), that can be associated with disorders of genomic imprinting, can be identified. The detection of CNVs from WGS requires the appropriate CNV detection algorithm (Monlong *et al.*, 2018).

The detection of CNVs using NGS or WGS methodologies will inevitably produce a very large amount of genetic data and, the navigation through such vast data requires some rules and regulations, to establish the possible pathogenicity of a "suspected culprit" CNVs. Indeed, international guidelines emphasize the importance to consider the occurrence of the CNVs in the general population, the recurrence associated to a similar phenotype, the parental inheritance, the CNVs size and the gene content (review and summary in Nowakowska, 2017). Thus, WGS has high diagnostic yield and decreasing costs and might be destined to replace arrayCGH studies in some patients.

Conclusion

Chromosomal abnormalities do not represent a frequent cause of seizure disorders, but chromosomal syndromes carry a higher risk for seizures, and seizures are part of the clinical phenotype in some of the chromosomal disorders. Some chromosomal abnormalities result in intractable seizures, while epilepsy in others it has a more favourable prognosis.

Seizure susceptibility may correlate with the severity of structural brain abnormalities or with the extent of the chromosomal derangement. Seizure susceptibility may also be related to factors that alter cortical excitability, such as changes in neurotransmitters, probably depending on the specific involved genes. This seems to be the case of several conditions such as Angelman, 4p- syndrome, trisomy 12p, fragile-X syndrome, and inv-dup(15) syndrome, and it seems to depend on the extension of gene derangement. This probably may also explain the similarity of EEG pattern in Angelman and 4p-syndromes.

A more detailed analysis of electroclinical patterns of the epilepsy associated with chromosomopathy, especially when seizures present with specific interictal and ictal EEG patterns, may help to detect specific genes affecting seizure susceptibility (Anderson & Hauser, 1990). The awareness of the associations between syndromes due to chromosomal abnormalities and epilepsy, together with knowledge of their response to treatment and the expected outcome, should be of help in planning rational treatment and counselling of the families.

REFERENCES ▶

Addis L, Rosch RE, Valentin A, *et al.* (2016): Analysis of rare copy number variation in absence epilepsies. *Neurol Genet* 2(2): e56.

Aguglia U, Le Piane E, Gambardella A, *et al.* (1999): Emotion-induced myoclonic absence-like seizures in a patient with inv-dup (15): syndrome: a clinical, EEG, and molecular genetic study. *Epilepsia* 40: 1316–1319.

Allen TL, Brothman AR, Carey JC, Chance PF (1996): Cytogenetic and molecular analysis in trysomy 12p. *Am J Med Genet* 63: 250–256.

Alosi D, Klitten LL, Bak M, et al. (2015): Dysregulation of FOXG1 by ring chromosome 14. *Mol Cytogenet* 8: 24.

Anderson EV, Hauser WA (1990): Genetics. In: Dam M, Gram M, eds. *Comprehensive Epileptology*, pp. 57–74. New York: Raven Press.

Angelman H (1965): "Puppet" children: a report on three cases. *Dev Med Child Neurol* 7: 681–683.

Antonarakis SE, Avramopoulos D, Blouin JL, Talbot CC Jr, Schinzel AA (1993): Mitotic errors in somatic cells cause trisomy 21 in about 4.5% of cases and are not associated with advanced maternal age. *Nat Genet* 3: 146–150.

Anvret M, Nordenskjold M, Stolpe L, Johansson L, Brondum-Nielsen K (1991): Molecular analysis of 4p deletion associated with the Wolf-Hirschhorn syndrome moving the critical segment towards the telomere. *Hum Genet* 86: 481–483.

Araujo BH, Torres LB, Guilhoto LM (2015): Cerebal overinhibition could be the basis for the high prevalence of epilepsy in persons with Down syndrome. *Epilepsy Behav* 53: 120–125.

Arron JR, Winslow MM, Polleri A, *et al.* (2006): NFAT dysregulation by increased dosage of DSCR1 and DYRK1A on chromosome 21. *Nature* 441: 595–600.

Augustijn PB, Parra J, Wouters CH, Joosten P, Lindhout D, van Emde Boas W (2001): Ring chromosome 20 epilepsy syndrome in children: electro-clinical features. *Neurology* 57: 1108–1111.

Back E, Voiculescu I, BrÂnger M, Wolff G (1989): Familial ring (20) chromosomal mosaicism. *Hum Genet* 83: 148–154.

Bahi-Buisson N, Ville D, Eisermann M, Plouin P, Kaminska A, Chiron C (2005): Epilepsy in chromosome aberrations. *Arch Pediatr* 12: 449–458.

Bahi-Buisson N, Guttierrez-Delicado E, Soufflet C, *et al.* (2008): Spectrum of epilepsy in terminal 1p36 deletion syndrome. *Epilepsia* 49: 509–515.

Barkovich AJ, Koch TK, Carrol CL (1991): The spectrum of lissencephaly: report of ten patients analyzed by magnetic resonance imaging. *Ann Neurol* 30: 139–146.

Battaglia A (2005): Del 1p36 syndrome: a newly emerging clinical entity. *Brain Dev* 27: 358–361.

Battaglia A (2008): The inv dup (15) or idic (15) syndrome (Tetrasomy 15q). *Orphanet J Rare Dis* 19: 3–30.

Battaglia A, Shaffer LG (2008): 1p36 deletion syndrome. In: Pagon RA, Bird TD, Dolan CR, Stephens K (eds) *Source Gene Reviews* [Internet].

Battaglia A, Gurrieri F, Bertini E, et al. (1997): The inv-dup(15) syndrome: a clinically recognizable syndrome with altered behavior, mental retardation, and epilepsy. *Neurology* 48: 1081–1086.

Battaglia D, Zampino G, Zollino M, *et al.* (2003): Electroclinical patterns and evolution of epilepsy in the 4p- syndrome. *Epilepsia* 44: 1183–1190.

Battaglia A, Filippi T, Carey JC (2008a): Update on the clinical features and natural history of Wolf-Hirschhorn (4p-) syndrome: experience with 87 patients and recommendations for routine health supervision. *Am J Med Genet C Semin Med Genet* 148C (4): 246–251.

Battaglia A, Hoyme HE, Dallapiccola B, *et al.* (2008b): Further delineation of deletion 1p36 syndrome in 60 patients: a recognizable phenotype and common cause of developmental delay and mental retardation. *Pediatrics* 121: 404–410.

Battaglia A, Bernardini L, Torrente I, Novelli A, Scarselli G (2016): Spectrum of epilepsy and electroencephalogram patterns in idic (15) syndrome. *Am J Med Genet* 170: 2531–2539.

Battaglia A, Calhoun ARUL, Lortz A, Carey JC (2018): Risk of hepatic neoplasms in Wolf-Hirschhorn syndrome (4p-): Four new cases and review of the literature. *Am J Med Genet* 176: 2389–2394.

Baxendale S, MacDonald ME, Mott R, *et al.* (1993): A cosmid contig and high resolution restriction map of the 2 megabase region containing the Huntington's disease gene. *Nat Genet* 4: 181–186.

Bear MF (2005): Therapeutic implications of the mGluR theory of fragile X mental retardation. *Genes Brain Behav* 4: 393–398.

Beatty CW, Wrede JE, Blume HK (2017): Diagnosis, treatment, and outcomes of infantile spasms in the Trisomy 21 population. *Seizure* 45: 184–188.

Becker KL, Hoffman DL, Albert A, Underdahl LO, Mason HL (1966): Klinefelter syndrome: clinical and laboratory findings in 50 patients. *Arch Intern Med* 118: 314–321.

Becker KL, Armstrong DL, Chan F (1986): Dendritic atrophy in children with Down's syndrome. *Ann Neurol* 20: 520–526.

Berg AT, Berkovic SF, Brodie MJ et al. (2010): Revised terminology and concepts for organization of seizures and epilepsies: report of the ILAE Commission on Classification & Terminology, 2005-2009. *Epilepsia* 51: 676–685.

Berry-Kravis E (2002): Epilepsy in fragile X syndrome. *Dev Med Child Neurol* 44: 724–728.

Bi W, SapirT, Shchelochkov OA, *et al.* (2009): Increased LIS1 expression affects human and mouse brain development. *Nat Genet* 41: 168–177.

Biraben A. Odent S, Lucas J, *et al.* (2001): Chromosome 20 en anneau et épilepsie: diversité des crises étudiées en vidéo-EEG. Un mécanisme sous-cortical d'épileptogénèse est-il au premier plan ? *Épilepsies* 13: 9–15.

Biraben A, Semah F, Ribeiro MJ, Douaud G, Remy P, Depaulis A (2004): PET evidence for a role of the basal ganglia in patients with ring chromosome 20 epilepsy. *Neurology* 63: 73–77.

Blomquist HK, Gustavson KH, Hoimgren G, Nordenson 1, Palsson-Strae U (1983): Fragile X syndrome in mildly retarded children in a northern Swedish country. *Clin Genet* 24: 393–398.

Boltshauser E, Meyer M, Deonna T (1978): Klinefelter syndrome and neurological disease. *J Neurol* 219: 253–259.

Bonanni P, Casellato S, Fabbro F, Negrin S (2017): Epilepsy in fragile-X-syndrome mimicking panayiotopoulos syndrome: Description of three patients. *Am J Med Genet A* 173: 2753–2757.

Borgaonkar DS, Lacassie YE, Stoll C (1976): Usefulness of chromosome catalog in delineating new syndromes. *Birth Defect* 12: 87–95.

Borlot F, Regan BM, Bassett AS, Stavropoulos DJ, Andrade DM (2017): Prevalence of Pathogenic Copy Number Variation in Adults With Pediatric-Onset Epilepsy and Intellectual Disability. *JAMA Neurol* 74: 1301–1311.

Borgatti R, Piccinelli P, Passoni D, *et al.* (2001): Relationship between clinical and genetic features in "inverted duplicated chromosome 15" patients. *Pediatr Neurol* 24: 111–116.

Bourgeois JA, Coffey SM, Rivera SM, *et al.* (2009): A review of fragile X premutation disorders: expanding the psychiatric perspective. *J Clin Psychiatry* 70: 852–862.

Bower BD, Jeavons PM (1967): The "happy puppet" syndrome. *Arch Dis Child* 42: 298–302.

Boyd SG, Harden A, Patton MA (1988): The EEG in early diagnosis of Angelman's (happy puppet) syndrome. *Eur J Pediatr* 147: 508–513.

Brandt CA, Kierkegaard O, Hindkjaer J, Jensen PKA, Pedersen S, Therkelsen AJ (1993): Ring chromosome 20 with loss of telomeric sequences detected by multicolour PRINS. *Clin Genet* 44: 26–31.

Brazil A, Stanford K, Smolarek T, Hopkin R (2014): Delineating the phenotype of 1p36 deletion in adolescents and adults. *Am J Med Genet* 164 A: 2496–2503.

Buckle VJ, Fujita N, Ryder-Cook AS, *et al.* (1989): Chromosomal localization of GABA(A) receptor subunit genes: relationship to human genetic disease. *Neuron* 3: 647–654.

Budka H (1978): Megalencephaly and chromosomal anomaly. *Acta Neuropathol* 43: 263–266.

Buli M, Warburton D (1990): Monosomy 4p. In: Buyse ML (ed) *Birth Defect Encyclopedia*, pp. 334–335. Cambridge, MA: Blackwell Scientific Publications.

Buoni S, Sorrentino L, Farnetani MA, Pucci L, Fois A (2000): The syndrome of inv-dup (15) clinical, electroencephalographic, and imaging findings. *J Child Neurol* 15: 380–385.

Buoni S, Grosso S, Pucci L, Fois A (1999): Diagnosis of Angelman syndrome: clinical and EEG criteria. *Brain Dev* 21: 296–302.

Buxton JL, Chan CJ, Gilbert H, *et al.* (1994): Angelman syndrome associated with a maternal 15q11-13 deletion of less than 200 kb. *Hum Molec Genet* 3: 1409–1413.

Cabrera JC, Marti M, Toledo L, Gine R, Vazquez C (1998): West's syndrome associated with inversion duplication of chromosome 15. *Rev Neurol* 26: 77–79.

Canevini MP, Sgro V, Zuffardi O, *et al.* (1998): Chromosome 20 ring: a chromosomal disorder associated with a particular electroclinical pattern. *Epilepsia* 39: 942–951.

Caraballo R, Darra F, Reyes G, Armeno M, Cresta A, Mestre G, Bernardina BD (2017): The ketogenic diet in patients with myoclonic status in nonprogressive encephalopathy. *Seizure* 51: 1–5.

Caron L, Rousseau F, Gagnon E, Isenring P (2000): Cloning and functional characterization of a cation-Cl- cotransporter-interacting protein. *J Biol Chem* 13: 32027–32036.

Carter CO (1977): Genetics of common singie malformations. *Br Med Bull* 32: 21–28.

Centerwall WR, Thompson WP, Allen IE, Fobes CD (1975): Translocation 4p- syndrome. *Am J Dis Child* 122: 366–370.

Chawla J, Sucholeiki R, Jones C, Silver K (2002): Intractable epilepsy with ring chromosome 20 syndrome treated with vagal nerve stimulation: case report and review of the literature. *J Child Neurol* 17: 778–780.

Chifari R, Guerrini R, Pierluigi M, et al. (2002): Mild generalized epilepsy and developmental disorder associated with large inv dup(15). *Epilepsia* 43: 1096–1100.

Clayton-Smith J (1993): Clinical research on Angelman syndrome in the United Kingdom: observations on 82 affected individuals. *Am J Med Genet* 46: 12–15.

Coffee B, Keith K, Albizua I, *et al.* (2009): Incidence of fragile X syndrome by newborn screening for methylated FMR1 DNA. *Am J Hum Genet* 85: 503–514.

Conlin LK, Kramer W, Hutchinson AL, *et al.* (2011): Molecular analysis of ring chromosome 20 syndrome reveals two distinct groups of patients. *J Med Genet* 48: 1–9.

Conti V1, Carabalona A, Pallesi-Pocachard E, *et al.* (2013): Periventricular heterotopia in 6q terminal deletion syndrome: role of the C6orf70 gene. *Brain* 136: 3378–3394.

Coppola A, Cellini E, Stamberger H, *et al.* (2019): Diagnostic implications of genetic copy number variation in epilepsy plus. *Epilepsia* 2019, in press

Cortez MA, Shen L, Wu Y, *et al.* (2009): Infantile spasms and Down syndrome: a new animal model. *Pediatr Res* 65: 499–503.

Court Brown WM (1969): Sex chromosome aneuploidy in man and its frequency, with special reference to mental subnormality and criminal behavior. *Int Rev Exp Pathol* 7: 31–38.

Crawford DC, Acuna JM, Sherman SL (2001): FMR1 and the fragile X syndrome: human genome epidemiology review. *Genet Med* 3: 359–371.

Dalla Bernardina B, Trevisan E, Colamaria V, Magaudda A (1985): Myoclonic epilepsy ("myoclonic status") in non-progressive encephalothies. In: Roger J, Dravet C, Bureau M, Dreifuss FE, Wolf P (eds) *Epileptic Syndromes in Infancy, Childhood and Adolescence*, pp 68–72. London: John Libbey

Darra F, Fontana E, Dalla Bernardina B (2017): Myoclonic Status in nonprogressive Encephalopathies. In: Pellock JM, Nordli DR Jr, Sankar R, Wheless JW (eds) *Pellock's Pedaitric Epilepsy Diagnosis and Therapy*, pp. 373–382. New York: Demos Medical Publishing.

Daube JR, Chou SM (1966): Lissencephaly: two cases. *Neurology* 16: 179–191.

d'Orsi G, Specchio LM; Apulian Study Group on Senile Myoclonic Epilepsy (2014): Progressive myoclonus epilepsy in Down syndrome patients with dementia. *J Neurol* 261: 1584–1597.

De Blois MC, Caille B, Rethore MO, Dufier JL, Lejeune J (1990): r14 syndrome without major dysmorphism. *Ann Genet* 33: 155–158.

De Grouchy J, Turleau C (1984): Clinical Atlas of Human Chromosomes, 2nd ed. New York: John Wiley.

de Kovel CG, Trucks H, Helbig I, *et al.* (2010): Recurrent microdeletions at 15q11.2 and 16p13.11 predispose to idiopathic generalized epilepsies. *Brain* 133: 23–32.

De Simone R, Puig XS, Gélisse P, Crespel A, Genton P (2010): Senile myoclonic epilepsy: delineation of a common condition associated with Alzheimer's disease in Down syndrome. *Seizure* 19: 383–389.

De Vries BB, van der Ouweland AM, Duivenvoorden HJ and the collaborative fragile X study group (1997): Screening and diagnosis for the fragile X syndrome among the mentally retarded: an epidemiological and psychological survey. *Am J Hum Genet* 61: 660–667.

Delach JA, Rosengren SS, Kaplan L, *et al.* (1994): Comparison of high resolution chromosome banding and fluorescent in situ hybridization (FISH) for the laboratory evaluation of Prader-Willi syndrome and Angelman syndrome. *Am J Med Genet* 52: 85–91.

Del Sole A, Chiesa V, Lucignani G, *et al.* (2010): Exploring dopaminergic activity in ring chromosome 20 syndrome: a SPECT study. QJ Nucl Med Mol Imaging 54: 564–569.

Dimova P1, Boneva I, Todorova A, Minotti L, Kahane P (2012): Gelastic seizures in ring chromosome 20 syndrome: a case report with video illustration. *Epileptic Disord* 14: 181–186.

Dion MH, Novotny EJ Jr, Carmant L, Cossette P, Nguyen DK (2007): Lamotri-gine therapy of epilepsy with Angelman's syndrome. *Epilepsia* 48: 593–596.

Dobyns WB, Truwit CL, Ross ME, *et al.* (1999): Differences in the gyral pattern distinguish chromosome 17-linked and X-linked lissencephaly. *Neurology* 53: 270–277.

Dulabon L, Olson EC, Taglienti MG, *et al.* (2000): Reelin binds alpha3beta1 integrin and inhibits neuronal migration. *Neuron* 27: 33–44.

Eisermann MM, De La Raillere A, Dellatolas G, *et al.* (2003): Infantile spasms in Down syndrome-effects of delayed anticonvulsive treatment. *Epilepsy Res* 55: 21–27.

Elia M (2009): Myoclonic status in nonprogressive encephalopathies: an update. *Epilepsia* 50 (Suppl 5): 41–44.

Elia M, Musumeci SA, Ferri R, *et al.* (1995a): Trisomy 12p and epilepsy with myoclonic absences: a new case. *Epilepsia* 36 (Suppl. 3): S2.

Elia M, Musumeci SA, Ferri R, Scuderi C, Del Gracco S, Stefanini MC (1995b): Seizures in Klinefelter's syndrome: a clinical and EEG study of five patients. *Ital J Neurol Sci* 16: 231–238.

Elia M, Striano P, Fichera M, *et al.* (2006): 6q terminal deletion syndrome is associated with a distinctive EEG and clinical pattern. A report of five cases. *Epilepsia* 47: 830–838.

English CJ, Davison EV, Bhatei MS, Barrett L (1989): Chromosome studies of males in an institution for the mentally handicapped. *J Med Genetics* 26: 379–381.

Ferlazzo E, Adjien CK, Guerrini R, *et al.* (2009): Lennox-Gastaut syndrome with late-onset and prominent reflex seizures in trisomy 21 patients. *Epilepsia* 50: 1587–1594.

Finelli PF, Pueschei SM, Padre-Mendoza T, O Brien MM (1985): Neurological findings in patients with fragile-X syndrome. *J Neurol Neurosurg Psychiatry* 48: 150–153.

Fiumara A, Pittalà A, Cocuzza M, Sorge G (2010): Epilepsy in patients with Angelman syndrome. *Italian Journal of Pediatrics* 36: 31.

Franz DN, Glauser TA, Tudor C, Williams S (2000): Topiramate therapy of epilepsy associated with Angelman's syndrome. *Neurology* 54: 1185–1188.

Freeman SB, May KM, Pettay D, Fernhoff PM, Hassold TJ (1993): Paternal uniparental disomy in a child with a balanced 15;15 translocation and Angelman syndrome. *Am J Med Genet* 45: 625–630.

Fregeau B, Kim BJ, Hernández-García A, *et al.* (2016): *De novo* Mutations of RERE Cause a Genetic Syndrome with Features that Overlap Those Associated with Proximal 1p36 Deletions. *Am J Hum Genet* 98: 963–970.

Fryns JP, Van den Berge H, Van Herck G, Cassimpan JJ (1974): Trisomy 12p due to familial t (2p-; 6q+) translocation. *Hum Genet* 24: 247–252.

Fujimoto A, Wilson MG (1990): Growth retardation in Wolf-Hirschhorn syndrome. *Hum Genet* 84: 296–297.

Gago-Veiga AB, Toledano R, García-Morales I, *et al.* (2018): Specificity of electroclinical features in the diagnosis of ring chromosome 20. *Epilepsy Behav* 80: 215–220.

Gajecka M, Mackay KL, Shaffer LG (2007): Monosomy 1p36 deletion syndrome. *Am J Med Genet C Semin Med Genet* 145: 346–356.

Galvan-Manso M, Campistol J, Conill J, Sanmarti FX (2005): Analysis of the characteristics of epilepsy in 37 patients with the molecular diagnosis of Angelman syndrome. *Epileptic Disord* 7: 19–25.

Garcia CA, Dunn D, Trevor R (1978): The lissencephaly (Agyria): syndrome in siblings. Computerized tomographic and neuropathologic findings. *Arch Neurol* 35: 608–611.

Gastaut H, Pinsard N, Raybaud C, Aicardi J, Zifkin B (1987): Lissencephaly (Agyria-Pachygyria) clinical findings and serial EEG studies. *Dev Med Child Neurol* 29: 167–180.

Genton P, Medina MT, Roger J, Murcia de Medina M, Mattei MG, Guerrini R (1992): Syndrome de Klinefelter (dysgénésie gonadique avec caryo-type 47, XXY) et épilepsie: 5 observations. *Boll Lega It Epil* 79/80: 69–70.

Genton P, Paglia G (1994): Épilepsie myoclonique sénile? Myoclonies épileptiques d'apparition tardive dans le syndrome de Down. *Epilepsies* 6: 5–11.

Genton P, Ferlazzo E, Thomas P (2008): Absence status epilepsy: delineation of a distinct idiopathic generalized epilepsy syndrome. *Epilepsia* 49: 642–649.

Gholipour T, Mitchell S2 Sarkis RA, Chemali Z (2017): The clinical and neurobehavioral course of Down syndrome and dementia with or without new-onset epilepsy. *Epilepsy Behav* 68: 11–16.

Giliessen-Kaesbach G, Cross S, Kaya-Westerloh S, Passarge E, Horsthernke B (1995): DNA methylation based testing of 450 patients suspected of having Prader-Willy syndrome. *J Med Genet* 32: 88–92.

Gilissen G, Hehir-Kwa JY, Thung DT, *et al.* (2014): Genome sequencing identifies major causes of severe intellectual disability. *Nature* 511: 344–347.

Giovannini S1, Marangio L, Fusco C *et al.* (2013): Epilepsy in ring 14 syndrome: a clinical and EEG study of 22 patients. *Epilepsia* 54: 2204–2213.

Giuffrida R, Musumeci S, D'Antoni S, *et al.* (2005): A reduced number of metabotropic glutamate subtype 5 receptors are associated with constitutive homer proteins in a mouse model of fragile X syndrome. *J Neurosci* 25: 8908–8916.

Gobbi G, Bruno L, Pini A, Giovanardi Rossi P, Tassinari CA (1987): Periodic spasms: an unclassified type of epileptic seizure in childhood. *Dev Med Child Neurol* 29: 766–775.

Gobbi G, Pini A, Parmeggiani A, *et al.* (1996): Periodic spasms in Cortical dysplasia. In: Guerrini R, Andermann F, Canapicchi R, Roger J, Zifkin BJ, Pfanner P (eds), *Dysplasias of Cerebral Cortex and Epilepsy*, pp. 311–321. Philadelphia: Lippincott-Raven Publishers.

Goto M, Saito Y, Honda R *et al.* (2015): Episodic tremors representing cortical myoclonus are characteristic in Angelman syndrome due to UBE3A mutations. *Brain Dev* 37:,216–222.

Gottfried M, Lavine L, Roessmann U (1981): Neuropathological findings in Wolf-Hirschhorn (4p-) syndrome. *Acta Neuropathol* (Berl) 55: 163–165.

Greger V, Knoll JHM, Wagstaff J, *et al.* (1997): Angelman syndrome associated with an inversion of chromosome 15q11.2q24.3. *Am J Hum Genet* 60: 574–580.

Grosso S, Pucci L, Farnetani M, *et al.* (2004a): Epilepsy and electroencephalographic findings in pericentric inversion of chromosome 12. *J Child Neurol* 19: 604–608.

Grosso S, Farnetani MA, Di Bartolo RM, *et al.* (2004b): Electroencephalographic and epileptic patterns in X chromosome anomalies. *J Clin Neurophysiol* 21: 249–253.

Grosso S, Pucci L, Di Bartolo RM, *et al.* (2005): Chromosome 18 aberrations and epilepsy: a review. *Am J Med Genet* 134: 88–94.

Gu B, Carstens KE, Judson MC *et al.* (2019): Ube3a reinstatement mitigates epileptogenesis in Angelman syndrome model mice. *J Clin Invest* 129:,163–168.

Guerrini R, Battaglia A, Stagi P, *et al.* (1989): Caratteristiche elettrocliniche dell'epilessia nella Sindrome di Down. *Boll Lega It Epil* 66/67: 317–319.

Guerrini R, Bureau M, Mattei MG, Battaglia A, Galland MC, Roger J (1990): Trisomy 12p syndrome: a chromosomal disorder associated with generalized 3-Hz spike and wave discharges. *Epilepsia* 31: 557–566.

Guerrini R, Genton P, Bureau M, Dravet C, Roger J (1990): Reflex seizures are frequent in patients with Down syndrome and epilepsy. *Epilepsia* 31: 406–417.

Guerrini R, Dravet C, Ferrari AR, *et al.* (1993): Evoluzione dell'epilessia nelle più frequenti forme genetiche con ritardo mentale (sindrome di Down e sindrome dell'X fragile). *Ped Med Chir* 15: 19–22.

Guerrini R, De Lorey TM, Bonanni P, *et al.* (1996): Cortical myoclonus in Angelman syndrome. *Ann Neurol* 40: 39–48.

Guthrie RD, Aase JM, Asper AC, *et al.* (1971): The 4p-syndrome: a clinically recognizable chromosomal deletion syndrome. *Am J Dis Child* 122: 421–425.

Hagerman RJ, Protic D, Rajaratnam A *et al.* (2018): Fragile X-Associated Neuropsychiatric Disorders (FXAND). *Front Psychiatry* 9: 564. eCollection 2018.

Halal F, Chitayat D, Parikh H, *et al.* (1992): Ring chromosome 20 and possible assignment of the structural gene encoding human carboxypeptidase-L to the distal segment of the long arm of chromosome 20. *Am J Med Genet* 43: 576–579.

Hartmann C, von Spiczak S, Suls A, *et al.* (2015): Investigating the genetic basis of fever-associated syndromic epilepsies using copy number variation analysis. *Epilepsia* 56: e26–e32

Heilstedt HA, Burgess DL, Anderson AE, *et al.* (2001): Loss of the potassium channel beta-subunit gene, KCNAB2, is associated with epilepsy in patients with 1p36 deletion syndrome. *Epilepsia* 42: 1103–1111.

Heilstedt HA, Ballif BC, Howard LA, *et al.* (2003): Physical map of 1p36, placement of breakpoints in monosomy 1p36, and clinical characterization of the syndrome. *Am J Hum Genet* 72: 1200–1212.

Heinzen EL, Radtke RA, Urban TJ, *et al.* (2010): Rare deletions at 16p13.11 predispose to a diverse spectrum of sporadic epilepsy syndromes. *Am J Hum Genet* 86: 707–718.

Helbig I, Mefford HC, Sharp AJ, *al.* (2009): 15q13.3 microdeletions increase risk of idiopathic generalized epilepsy. *Nat genet* 41: 160–172

Heitz D, Devys D, Imbert G, Kretz C, Manciel JL (1992): Inheritance of the fragile X permutation is a major determinant of the transition to full mutation. *J Med Genet* 29: 794–801.

Herbst SM, Proepper CR, Geis T, *et al.* (2016): LIS1-associated classic lissencephaly: A retrospective, multicenter survey of the epileptogenic phenotype and response to antiepileptic drugs. *Brain Dev* 38: 399–406.

Herrgard E, Mononen T, Mervaala E, *et al.* (2007): More severe epilepsy and cognitive impairment in the offspring of a mother with mosaicism for the ring 20 chromosome. *Epilepsy Res* 73: 122–128.

Herva R, Saarinen I, Leikkonen L (1977): The r (20) syndrome. *J Med Genet* 14: 281–283.

Hirano Y, Oguni H, Nagata S (2016): Refractory and severe status epilepticus in a patient with ring chromosome 20 syndrome. *Brain Dev* 38: 746–749.

Hirschhorn K, Cooper HL, Firschein IL (1965): Deletion of short arms of chromosome 4-5 in a child with defects of midline fusion. *Humancenetik* 1: 479–482.

Hisatomi T, Kira R, Sakamoto T, Inomata H (2000): A case of ring 14 chromosome with ocular manifestations. *Nippon Ganka Gakkai Zasshi* 104: 121–124.

Ho KS, Markham LM, Twede H, *et al.* (2018): A survey of antiepileptic drug responses identifies drugs with potential efficacy for seizure control in Wolf-Hirschhorn syndrome. *Epilepsy Behav* 81: 55–61.

Hogart A, Leung KN, Wang NJ, *et al.* (2009): Chromosome 15q11-13 duplication syndrome brain reveals epigenetic alterations in gene expression not predicted from copy number. *J Med Genet* 46: 86–93.

Holmes GL (1987): *Diagnosis and Management of Seizures in Children*. Philadelphia: W. B. Saunders, pp. 56–71.

Holopainen I, Penttinen M, Lakkala T, Aarimaa T (1994): Ring chromosome 20 mosaicism in a girl with complex partial seizures. *Dev Med Child Neurol* 36: 70–73.

Hong SE, Shugart YY, Huang DT, *et al.* (2000): Autosomal recessive lissencephaly with cerebellar hypoplasia is associated with human RELN mutations. *Nat Genet* 26: 93–96.

Hook EB, Cross K (1987): Extra structurally abnormal chromosomes (ESAC): detected at amniocentesis: frequency in approximately 75,000prenatal cytogenic diagnoses and associations with maternal and paternalage. *Am J Hum Genet* 54: 748–756.

Hou JW (2004): Mosaic ring chromosome 14 and monosomy 14 presenting with growth retardation, epilepsy, and blepharophimosis. *Chang Gung Med J* 27: 373–378.

Ikemoto S, Hamano SI, Hirata Y, Matsuura R, Koichihara R (2019): Perampanel in lissencephaly-associated epilepsy. *Epilepsy Behav* Case Rep 11: 67–69.

Incorpora G, Sorge G, Sorge A, Pavone L (2002): Epilepsy in fragile X syndrome. *Brain Dev* 24: 766–769.

Inoue Y, Fujiwara T, Matsuda K, *et al.* (1997): Ring chromosome 20 and non convulsive status epilepticus. A new epileptic syndrome. *Brain* 120: 939–953.

Inoue H, Orita T, Matsushige T, Hasegawa S, Ichiyama T (2012): Klinefelter's syndrome complicated with West syndrome in a 4-month-old boy. *Brain Dev* 34: 148–150.

Itakura A, Saito Y, Nishimura Y, *et al.* (2016): Successful treatment of migrating partial seizures in Wolf-Hirschhorn syndrome with bromide. *Brain Dev* 38: 658–662.

Jacobs J, Bernard G, Andermann E, Dubeau F, Andermann F (2008): Refractory and lethal status epilepticus in a patient with ring chromosome 20 syndrome. *Epileptic Disord* 10: 254–259.

Jacquemont S, Hagerman RJ, Leehey MA, *et al.* (2004): Penetrance of the fragile X-associated tremor/ataxia syndrome in a premutation carrier population. *JAMA* 291: 460–469.

Jalbert P, Jalbert H, Sele B, *et al.* (1977): Chromosome 20 en anneau: un nouveau syndrome. *Ann Genet* 20: 258–262.

Jay V, Becker LE, Chan F-W, Perry TL (1991): Puppet-like syndrome of Angelman: a pathologic and neurochemical study. *Neurology* 41: 416–422.

Jennings MT, BirdTD (1981): Genetic influences in the epilepsies. *Am J Dis Child* 135: 450–457.

Ji X, Hu H, Wang Y, *et al.* (2017): Prenatal diagnosis of two fetuses with chromosome 1p36 deletion syndrome. *Zhonghua Yi Xue Yi Chuan Xue Za Zhi* 34: 853–856.

Jones KL, Gilbert EF, Kaveggia EG, Opitz JM (1980): The Miller-Dieker syndrome. *Pediatrics* 66: 277–281.

Jordan VK, Zaveri HP, Scott DA (2015): 1p36 deletion syndrome: an update. *Appl Clin Genet* 8: 189–200.

Kagitani-Shimono K, Imai K, Otani K, *et al.* (2005): Epilepsy in Wolf-Hirschhorn syndrome (4p-). *Epilepsia* 46: 150–155.

Kanazawa O, Irie N, Kawai I (1991): Epileptic seizures in the 4p syndrome. Report of 2 cases. *Jpn J Psychiatry Neurol* 45: 653–659.

Kapian LC, Wharton R, Elias E, *et al.* (1987): Clinical heterogenicity associated with deletions in the long ann of chromosorne I 5: report of 3 new cases and their possible genetic significance. *Am J Med Genet* 28: 45–53.

Karki CB, Walters RM (1990): Trisomy 12p mosaicism syndrome. *J Ment Def Res* 34: 75–80.

Kato M, Das S, Petras K, *et al.* (2004): Mutations of ARX are associated with striking pleiotropy and consistent genotype-phenotype correlation. *Hum Mutat* 23: 147–159.

Kenmuir C, Richardson M, Ghearing G (2015): Surgical treatment for medically refractory focal epilepsy in a patient with fragile X syndrome. *Brain Dev* 37: 916–918.

Kessi M, Xiong J, Wu L *et al.* (2018): Copy Number Variations and predictors in children with intellectual disability and epilepsy. *Front Neurol* 9: 947.

Kitamura K, Yanazawa M, Sugiyama N, *et al.* (2002): Mutation of ARX causes abnormal development of forebrain and testes in mice and X-linked lissencephaly with abnormal genitalia in humans. *Nat Genet* 32: 359–369.

Klinefelter HF Jr, Reifenstein EC Jr, Albright F (1942): Syndrome characterized by gynecomastia, aspermatogenesis without aleydigism and increased secretion of follicle-stimulating hormone. *J Clin Endocrinol* 2: 615–627.

Kluger G, Bohm I, Laub MC, Waldenmaier C (1996): Epilepsy and fragile X gene mutations. *Pediatric Neurology* 15: 358–360.

Knoll JHM, Nicholls RD, Magenis R, *et al.* (1990): Angelman syndrome: three molecular classes identified with chromosome 15q11q13-specific DNA markers. *Am J Hum Genet* 47: 149–155.

Krawczun M, Melink G, Cervenka J (1984): Ring chromosome 14 and immunoglobulin locus. *Am J Med Genet* 17: 465–469.

Kumada T, Ito M, Miyajima T (2005): Multi-institutional study on the correlation between chromosomal abnormalities and epilepsy. *Brain Dev* 2: 127–134.

Kumari D, Gazy I, Usdin K (2019): Pharmacological Reactivation of the Silenced FMR1 Gene as a Targeted Therapeutic Approach for Fragile X Syndrome. *Brain Sci* 9(2). E39.

Laan LA, Den Boer AT, Hennekam RC, Renier WO, Brouwer OF (1996): Angelman syndrome in adulthood. *Am J Med Genet* 66: 356–360.

Laan LA, Renier WO, Arts LFM, Buntinx IM, *et al.* (1997): Evolution of epilepsy and EEG findings in Angelman syndrome. *Epilepsia* 38: 195–199.

Laan LA, Vein AA (2005): Angelman syndrome: is there a characteristic EEG? *Brain Dev* 27: 80–87.

Lal D, Ruppert AK, Trucks H, *et al.* (2015): Burden Analysis of Rare Microdeletions Suggests a Strong Impact of Neurodevelopmental Genes in Genetic Generalised Epilepsies. *PLOS Genetics* 11:e1005226.

Leana-Cox J, Jenkis L, Palmer CG, *et al.* (1994): Molecular cytogenetic analysis of inv dup (15) chromosomes, using probes specific for Prader-Willi/Angelman syndrome region: clinical implications. *Am J Hum Genet* 54: 748–756.

Leventer RJ, Cardoso C, Ledbetter DH, Dobyns WB (2001): LIS1: from cortical malformation to essential protein of cellular dynamics. *Trends Neurosci* 24: 489–492.

Lewis MW, Vargas-Franco D, Morse DA, Resnick JL (2019): A mouse model of Angelman syndrome imprinting defects. *Hum Mol Genet* 28: 220–229.

Lossie AC, Whitney MM, Amidon D, *et al.* (2001): Distinct phenotypes distinguish the molecular classes of Angelman syndrome. *J Med Genet* 12: 834–845.

Lugo R, Bureau M, Dravet C, Viallat D, Genton P (1999): Particularités du syndrome de Lennox-Gastaut dans la trisomie 21. *Épilepsies* 11: 213.

Lurie IW, Lazjuk GI, Ussova YI, *et al.* (1980): The Wolf-Hirschhorn syndrome. *Clin Genet* 17: 375–385.

Magenis RE, Toth-Fejel S, Allen LJ, *et al.* (1990): Comparison of the 15q deletions in Prader-Willi and Angelman syndromes: specific regions, extent of deletions, parental origin, and clinical consequences. *Am J Med Genet* 35: 333–349.

Malcolm S, Clayton-Smith J, Nichols M, *et al.* (1991): Uniparental paternal disomy in Angelman's syndrome. *Lancet* 337: 694–697.

Matricardi S, Darra F, Spalice A, *et al.* (2018): Electroclinical findings and long-term outcomes in epileptic patients with inv dup (15). *Acta Neurol Scand* 137: 575–581.

Matsumoto A, Kumagai T, Miura K, Miyazaki S, Hayakawa C, Yamanaka T (1992): Epilepsy in Angelman syndrome associated with chromosome 15q deletion. *Epilepsia* 33: 1083–1090.

Matsuura T, Sutcliffe JS, Fang P, *et al.* (1997): *De novo* truncating mutations in E6-AP ubiquitin-protein ligase gene (UBE3A) in Angelman syndrome. *Nat Genet* 15: 74–77.

McKeown C, Read AP, Dodge A, Stecko O, Mercer A, Harris R (1987): Wolf-Hirschhorn locus is distal to D4S10 on short arm of chromosome 4. *J Med Genet* 24: 410–412.

McKeman RM, Whiting PJ (1996): Which GABAA-receptor subtypes really occur in the brain? 19: 139–143.

McKusick VA (1994): *Mendelian Inheritance in Man. A Catalog of Human Genes and Genetic Disorders,* 11th ed. Baltimore: John Hopkins University Press.

Mei D, Lewis R, Parrini E, Lazarou LP, Marini C, Pilz DT, Guerrini R (2008): High frequency of genomic deletions-and a duplication-in the LIS1 gene in lissencephaly: implications for molecular diagnosis. *J Med Genet* 45: 355–361.

Mefford HC (2014): CNVs in epilepsy. *Curr Genet Med Rep* 2: 162–167.

Mefford HC, Muhle H, Ostertag P, *et al.* (2010): Genome-Wide Copy Number Variation in Epilepsy: Novel Susceptibility Loci in Idiopathic Generalized and Focal Epilepsies. *PLoS Genetics* 6 (5): e1000962.

Mefford HC, Yendle SC, Hsu C, *et al.* (2011): Rare copy number variants are an important cause of epileptic encephalopathies. *Ann Neurol* 70: 974–985.

Menendez M (2005): Down syndrome, Alzheimer's disease and seizures. *Brain Dev* 27: 246–252.

Miano S, Bruni O, Leuzzi V, Elia M, Verrillo E, Ferri R (2004): Sleep polygraphy in Angelman syndrome. *Clin Neurophysiol* 115: 938–945.

Minassian BA, DeLorey TM, Olsen RW, *et al.* (1998): Angelman syndrome: correlations between epilepsy phenotypes and genotypes. *Ann Neurol* 43: 485–493.

Miyamoto A, Kitawaki K, Koida H, Nagao K (1992): Klinefelter's syndrome and epileptic psychosis: a case report. *Jpn J Psychiatry Neurol* 46: 61–65.

Miller JQ (1963): Lissencephaly in two siblings. *Neurology* 13: 841–850.

Mizuguchi M, Tsukamoto K, Suzuki Y, *et al.* (1994): Myoclonic epilepsy and a maternally derived deletion of 15pter? q 13. *Clin Genet* 45: 44–47.

Moller JC, Hamer HM, Oertel WH, Rosenow F (2002): Late-onset myoclonic epilepsy in Down's syndrome (LOMEDS). *Seizure* (Suppl. A): 303–305.

Moncla A, Malzac P, Voelckel MA, Auquier P, Girardot L, Mattei MG, *et al.* (1999): Phenotype-genotype correlation in 20 deletion and 20 non-deletion Angelman syndrome patients. *EurJ Hum Gen* 7: 131–139.

Monlong J, Girard SL, Meloche C (2018): Global characterization of copy number variants in epilepsy patients from whole genome sequencing. *PLoS Genet* 14: e1007285.

Mori K, Hashimoto T, Tayama M, *et al.* (1994): Serial EEG and sleep plygraphic studies on lissencephaly (agyria-pachygyria). *Brain Dev* 16: 365–373.

Morimoto M, Usuku T, Tanaka M, *et al.* (2003): Ring chromosome 14 with localization-related epilepsy: three cases. *Epilepsia* 44: 1245–1249.

Motoi H, Okanishi T, Kanai S, *et al.* (2016): Wolf-Hirschhorn (4p-) syndrome with West syndrome. *Epilepsy Behav* Case Rep 6: 39–41.

Mullen SA, Carvill GL, Bellows S, *et al.* (2013): Copy number variants are frequent in genetic generalized epilepsy with intellectual disability. *Neurology* 81: 1507–1515.

Mutirangura A, Greenberg F, Butier MG, *et al.* (1993): Multiplex PCR of three dinucleotide repeats in the Prader-Willi/Angelman critical region (15q11-q13): molecular diagnosis and mechanism of uniparental disomy. *Hum Mol Genet* 2: 143–151.

Musumeci SA, Colognola RM, Ferri R, *et al.* (1988): Fragile X syndrome: a particular epileptogenic EEG pattern. *Epilepsia* 29: 41–47.

Musumeci SA, Hagerman RJ, Ferri R, *et al.* (1999): Epilepsy and EEG findings in males with fragile X syndrome. *Epilepsia* 40: 1092–1099.

Musumeci SA, Bosco P, Calabrese G, *et al.* (2000): Audiogenic seizures susceptibility in transgenic mice with fragile X syndrome. *Epilepsia* 41: 19–23.

Musumeci SA, Calabrese G, Bonaccorso CM, *et al.* (2007): Audiogenic seizure susceptibility is reduced in fragile X knockout mice after introduction of FMR1 transgenes. *Exp Neurol* 203: 233–240.

Nabbout R, Melki I, Gerbaka B, Dulac O, Akatcherian C (2001): Infantile spasms in Down syndrome: good response to a short course of vigabatrin. *Epilepsia* 42: 1580–1583.

Nakatsu Y, Tyndale RF, DeLorey TM, *et al.* (1993): A cluster of three GABAA receptor subunit genes is deleted in a neurological mutant of the mouse p locus. *Nature* 364: 448–450.

Neal J, Apse K, Sahin M, Walsh CA, Sheen VL (2006): Deletion of chromosome 1p36 is associated with periventricular nodular heterotopia. *Am J Med Genet A* 140: 1692–1695.

Nicholls RD, Saitoh S, Horsthemke B (1998): Imprinting in Prader-Willi and Angelman syndromes. *Trends Genet* 14: 194–200.

Nielsen J, Pedersen E (1969): Electro-encephalographic findings in patients with Klinefelter's syndrome and the XYY syndrome. *Acta Neurol Scand* 45: 87–94.

Nielsen J, Tsuboi T (1974): Electroencephalographic examination in the XYY syndrome and in Klinefelter's syndrome. *Br J Psychiatry* 125: 236–237.

Nielsen J, Venter M, Holm V, Askjaer SA, Reske-Nielsen E (1977): A newborn child with karyotype 47,XX, + der(12) (12pter?12q12: 8q24?8qter),t(8;12) (q24;q12) pat. *Hum Genet* 35: 357–362.

Nolt DH, Mott JM, Lopez WL (2003): Assessment of anticonvulsant effectiveness and safety in patients with Angelman's syndrome using an Internet questionnaire. *Am J Health Syst Pharm* 60: 2583–2587.

Nowakowska B (2017): Clinical interpretation of copy number variants in the human genome. *J Appl Genet* 58: 449–457.

Onder H, Tezer FI (2016): Significant Improvements of EEG and Clinical Findings With Oral Lacosamide in a Patient With Ring Chromosome 20. *Clin EEG Neurosci* 47: 330–332. Epub 2015 Aug 2.

Ono J, Nishiike K, Imai K, Otani K, Okada S (1999): Ring chromosome 14 complicated with complex partial seizures and hypoplastic corpus callosum. *Pediatr Neurol* 20: 70–72.

Panayiotopoulos CP, Giannakodimos S, Chroni E (1995a): Typical absences in adults. In: Duncan JS, Panayiotopoulos CP (eds) *Typical Absences and Related Epileptic Syndromes,* pp. 289–297. London: Churchill Livingstone.

Panayiotopoulos CP, Ferrie CD, Giannakodimos S, Robinson RO (1995b): Perioral myoclonia with absences. In: Duncan JS, Panayiotopoulos CP (eds) *Typical Absences and Related Epileptic Syndromes,* pp. 221–230. London: Churchill Livingstone.

Parmeggiani A, Gobbi G, Guerrini R, Poggioli D, Giovanardi Rossi P (1993): Epileptic seizures in patients with 4p- syndrome. *Epilepsia* 34 (Suppl. 2): 177.

Pelizzo G, Puglisi A, Lapi M, *et al.* (2018): Type IV Laryngotracheoesophageal Cleft Associated with Type III Esophageal Atresia in 1p36 Deletions Containing the RERE Gene: Is There a Causal Role for the Genetic Alteration? *Pediatr Case Rep* 4060527.

Pereira S, Vieira JP, Cau P, Genton P, Szepetowski P (2006): Epilepsy and deletions at chromosome 2q24. *Am J Med Genet* 140: 1354–1355.

Petit J, Roubertie A, Inoue Y, Genton P (1999): Non-convulsive status in the ring chromosome 20 syndrome: a video illustration of 3 cases. *Epileptic Disorders* 1: 237–241.

Pieretti M, Zhang FP, Fu YH, *et al.* (1991): Absence of expression of the FMR-1 gene in fragile X syndrome. *Cell* 66: 817–822.

Poirier K, Keays DA, Francis F, *et al.* (2007): Large spectrum of lissencephaly and pachygyria phenotypes resulting from *de novo* missense mutations in tubulin alpha 1A (TUBA1A). *Hum Mutat* 28: 1055–1064

Pollack MA, Golden GS, Schnlidt R, *et al.* (1978): Infantile spasms in Down syndrome: a report of 5 cases and review of the literature. *Ann Neurol* 3: 406–408.

Pollack SF, Grocott OR, Parkin KA, *et al.* (2018): Myoclonus in Angelman syndrome. *Epilepsy Behav* 82: 170–174.

Porfirio B, Valorani MG, Giannotti A, Sabetta G, Dalla Piccola B (1987): Ring chromosome 20 phenotype. *J Med Genet* 24: 375–377.

Prasad A, Grocott O, Parkin K, Larson A, Thibert RL (2018): Angelman syndrome in adolescence and adulthood: A retrospective chart review of 53 cases. *Am J Med Genet* 176: 1327–1334.

Pueschel SM, Louis S, McKnight P (1991): Seizure disorders in Down syndrome. *Arch Neurol* 48: 318–320.

Pueschel SM, Louis S (1993): Reflex seizures in Down syndrome. *Child's Nerv Syst* 9: 23–24.

Quarrell OWJ, Snell RG, Curtis MA, Roberts SH, Harper PS, Shaw DJ (1991): Paternal origin of the chromosomal deletion resulting in Wolf-Hirschhorn syndrome. *J Med Genet* 28: 256–259.

Olson H, Shen Y, Avallone J, *et al.* (2014): Copy number variation plays an important role in clinical epilepsy. *Ann Neurol* 75: 943–958.

Raoul O, Razavi F, Lescs MC, Bouhanna A (1984): Ring chromosome 14. I. A case report on homogeneous r(14). *Ann Genet* 27: 88–90.

Redin C, Brand H, Collins RL, *et al.* (2017): The genomic landscape of balanced cytogenetic abnormalities associated with human congenital anomalies. *Nat Genet* 49: 36–45

Redon R, Rio M, Gregory SG, *et al.* (2005): Tiling path resolution mapping of constitutional 1p36 deletions by array-CGH: contiguous gene deletion or "deletion with positional effect" syndrome. *J Med Genet.* 42: 166–171.

Reinthaler EM, Lal D, Lebon S, *et al.* (2014): Duplications confer risk for typical and atypical Rolandic epilepsy. *Hum Mol Genet* 23: 6069–6080.

Rethore MO, Caille B, Huet de Barochez Y, de Blois MC, Ravel A, Lejeune J (1984): Ring chromosome 14. II. A case report of r(14) mosaicism. The r(14) phenotype. *Ann Genet* 27: 91–95.

Ricard-Mousnier B, N'Guyen S, Dubas F, Pouplard F, Guichet A (2007): Ring chromosome 17 epilepsy may resemble that of ring chromosome 20 syndrome. *Epileptic Disord* 9: 327–331.

Roberts W, Zurada A, Zurada-Zielinska A, *et al.* (2016): Anatomy of trisomy 12. *Clin Anat* 29: 633–637.

Robinson WP, Binkert F, Gine R, *et al.* (1993): Clinical and molecular analysis of five inv dup(15) patients. *Eur J Hum Genet* 1: 37–50.

Robinson WP, Bernasconi F, Mutirangura A, et al. (1993): Nondisjunction of chromosome 15: origin and recombination. *Am J Hum Genet* 53: 740–751.

Rosenfeld JA, Crolla JA, Tomkins S, *et al.* (2010): Refinement of causative genes in monosomy 1p36 through clinical and molecular cytogenetic characterization of small interstitial deletions. *Am J Med Genet A* 152: 1951–1959.

Ross MH, Galaburda AM, Kemper TL (1984): Down's syndrome: is there a decreased population on neurons? *Neurology* 34: 909–916.

Roubertie A, Petit J, Genton P (2000): Chromosome 20 en anneau: un syndrome épileptique identifiable. *Rev Neurol* 156: 149–153.

Sadhwani A1, Sanjana NE2, Willen JM *et al.* (2018): Two Angelman families with unusually advanced neurodevelopment carry a start codon variant in the most highly expressed UBE3A isoform. *Am J Med Genet* 176: 1641–1647.

Saitoh S, Harada N, Jinno Y, *et al.* (1994): Molecular and clinical study of 61 Angelman syndrome patients. *Am J Med Genet* 52: 158–163.

Saitsu H, Kato M, Mizuguchi T, *et al.* (2008): *De novo* mutations in the gene encoding STXBP1 (MUNC18-1) cause early infantile epileptic encephalopathy. *Nat Genet* 40: 782–788.

Santucci M, Giovanardi Rossi P, Salvi F, Ambrosetto G (1985): Stato di assenza isolato nel bambino. *Boll Lega It Epil* 49/50: 143–144.

Schinzel A, Niedrist D (2001): Chromosome imbalances associated with epilepsy. *Am J Med Genet* (Semin Med Genet). 106: 119–124.

Schreck RR, Breg WR, Erlanger BF, *et al.* (1977): Preferential derivation of abnormal human G-Group-like chromosomes from chromosome 15. *Hum Genet* 36: 1–12.

Segel R, Peter I, Demmer LA, *et al.* (2006): The natural history of trisomy 12p. *Am J Med Genet* 140: 695–703.

Sgro V, Riva E, Canevini MP, *et al.* (1995): 4p(-) syndrome: a chromosomal disorder associated with a particular EEG pattern. *Epilepsia* 36: 1206–1214.

Shimada S, Shimojima K, Okamoto N *et al.* (2015): Microarray analysis of 50 patients reveals the critical chromosomal regions responsible for 1p36 deletion syndrome-related complications. *Brain Dev* 37: 515–526.

Shirasaka Y, Ito M, Okuno T, Fujii T, Nozaki K, Mikawa H (1992): Ring 14 chromosome with complex partial seizures: a case report. *Brain Dev* 14: 257–260.

Silva ML, Cieuta C, Guerrini R, Plouin P, Livet MO, Dulac O (1996): Early clinical and EEG features of infantile spasms in Down syndrome. *Epilepsia* 37: 977–982.

Smigielska-Kuzia J, Sobaniec W, Kulak W, Bockowski L (2009): Clinical and EEG features of epilepsy in children and adolescents in Down syndrome. *J Child Neurol* 24: 416–420.

Singh N.A, Charlier C, Stauffer D, *et al.* (1998): A novel potassium channel gene, KCNQ2, is mutated in an inherited epilepsy of newborns. *Nat Genet* 18: 25–29.

Singh R, Sutherland G, Manson J (1999): Partial seizures with focal epileptogenic electroencephalographic patterns in three related female patients with fragile-X syndrome. *J Child Neurol* 14: 108–112.

Sorge G, Sorge A (2010): Epilepsy and chromosomal abnormalities. *Ital J Pediatr* 3: 36: 36????????????. **ATTENTION À REVOIR**

South ST, Hannes F, Fisch GS, Vermeesch JR, Zollino M (2008): Pathogenic significance of deletions distal to the currently described Wolf-Hirschhorn syndrome critical regions on 4p16.3. *AmJ Med Genet C Semin Med Genet* 148 C: 270–274.

Specchia V, Puricella A, D'Attis S *et al.* (2019): Drosophilia melanogaster as a Model to Study the Multiple Phenotypes, Related to Genome Stability of the Fragile-X Syndrome. *Front Genet* 10: 10.

Stafstrom CE, Patxot OF, Gilmore HE, Wisniewski KE (1991): Seizures in children with Down syndrome: etiology, characteristics and outcome. *Dev Med Child Neurol* 33: 191–200.

Stafstrom CE (1993): Epilepsy in Down syndrome: clinical aspects and possible mechanisms. *Am J Ment Retard* 98 (Suppl.): 12–26.

Stalker HJ, Williams CA (1998): Genetic counseling in Angelman syndrome: the challenges of multiple causes. *Am J Med Genet* 77: 54–59.

Stec I, Wright TJ, Van Ommen G-JB, De Boer PAJ, *et al.* (1998): WHSC1, a 90 kb SET domain-containing gene, expressed in early development and homologous to a Drosophila dysmorphy gene maps in the Wolf-Hirschhorn syndrome critical region and is fused to IgH in t(4;14) multiple myeloma. *Hum Molec Genet* 7: 1071–1082.

Stengel-Rutkowski S, Warkotsch A, Schimanek P, *et al.* (1984): Familial Wolf's syndrome with a hidden 4p deletion by translocation of an 8p segment. Unbalanced inheritance from a maternal translocation (4;8) (p15.3;p22). Case report, review and risk estimates. *Clin Genet* 25: 500–521.

Stengel-Rutkowski S, Alber A, Manken JD, *et al.* (1981): New chromosomal dysmorphic syndromes. *Eur J Pediatr* 136: 249–262.

Steinlein OK, Mulley JC, Propping P, Wallace RH, Phillips HA, Sutherland GR (1995): A missense mutation in the neuronal nicotinic acetylcholine receptor a-4 subunit is associated with autosomal dominant nocturnal frontal lobe epilepsy. *Nat Genet* 11: 201–203.

Stephenson JB (2005): Autonomic seizures in 18q- syndrome. *Brain Dev* 2: 125–126.

Sturm K, Knake S, Schomburg U, *et al.* (2000): Autonomic seizures versus syncope in 18q- deletion syndrome: a case report. *Epilepsia* 8: 1039–1043.

Sugimoto T, Yasubara A, Ohta T, *et al.* (1992): Angelman syndrome in three siblings: characteristic epileptic seizures and EEG abnormalities. *Epilepsia* 33: 1078–1082.

Sugimoto T, Araki A, Yasuhara A, Woo M, Nishida N, Sasaki T (1994): Angelman syndrome in three siblings: genetic model of epilepsy associated with chromosomal DNA deletion of the GABAA receptor. *Jpn J Psychiatry Neurol* 42: 271–273.

Swerdlow AJ, Higgins CD, Schoemaker MJ, *et al.* (2005): Mortality in patients with Klinefelter syndrome in Britain: a cohort study. *J Clin Endocrinol Metab* 90: 6516–6522.

Takahashi Y, Shigematsu H, Kubota H, Inoue Y, Fujiwara T, Yagi K, Seino M (1995): Non photosensitive video game-induced partial seizures. *Epilepsia* 36: 837–841.

Takeda Y, Baba A, Nakamura F, *et al.* (2000): Symptomatic generalized epilepsy associated with an inverted duplication of chromosome 15. *Seizure* 9: 145–150.

Tanaka N, Kamada K, Takeuchi F (2004): Ictal magnetoencephalographic study in a patient with ring 20 syndrome. *J Neurol Neurosurg Psychiatry* 75: 488–490.

Tanaka R, Iwasaki N, Hayashi M, *et al.* (2012): Abnormal brain MRI signal in 18q-syndrome not due to dysmyelination. *Brain Dev* 34: 234–237.

Tatsuno M, Hayashi M, Iwamoto H, Suzuki Y, Kuroki Y (1984): Epilepsy in childhood Down syndrome. *Brain Dev* 6: 37–44.

Tatum WO, Passaro EA, Elia M, Guerrini R, Gieron M, Genton P (1998): Seizures in Klinefelter's syndrome. *Pediatr Neurol* 19: 275–278.

Tayei S, McCorquodale MM, Rutherford, *et al.* (1989): A case of *de novo* trisomy 12p syndrome. *Clin Genet* 35: 382–386.

Telias M (2019): Fragile X Syndrome Pre-Clinical Research: Comparing Mouse- and Human-Based Models. *Methods Mol Biol* 1942: 155–162.

Thibert RL, Conant KD, Braun EK, Bruno P, Said RR, Nespeca MP, Thiele EA (2009): Epilepsy in Angelman syndrome: a questionnaire-based assessment of the natural history and current treatment options. *Epilepsia* 50: 2369–2376.

Thies U, Back E, Wolff G, Schroeder-Kurth T, Hager H-D, Schroder K (1992): Clinical, cytogenetic and molecular investigations in three patients with Wolf-Hirschhorn syndrome. *Clin Genet* 42: 201–205.

Thomas P, Beaumanoir A, Genton P, Dolisi C, Chatel M (1992): *De novo* Absence Status of Late Onset. Report of 11 cases. *Neurology* 42: 104–110.

Torrisi L, Sangiorgi E, Russo L, Gurrieri F (2001): Rearrangements of chromosome 15 in epilepsy. *Am J Med Genet, Seminars in Medical Genetics* 106: 125–128.

Turner G, Robinson H, Laing S, Purvis-Smith S (1986): Preventive screening for the fragile X syndrome. *N Engl J Med* 315: 607–609.

Turner G., Webb T, Wake S, Robinson H (1996): Prevalence of fragile X syndrome. *Am J Med Genet* 64: 196–197.

Uemura N, Matsumoto A, Nakamura M, *et al.* (2005): Evolution of seizures and electroencephalographical findings in 23 cases of deletion type Angelman syndrome. *Brain Dev* 27: 383–388.

Unterberger I, Dobesberger J, Schober H, *et al.* (2018): A further case of familial ring chromosome 20 mosaicism - molecular characterization of the ring and review of the literature. *Eur J Med Genet* S1769-7212(18)30256-8.

Valente KD, Koiffmann CP, Fridman C, *et al.* (2006): Epilepsy in patients with Angelman syndrome caused by deletion of the chromosome 15q11-13. *Arch Neurol* 63: 122–128.

Veall RM (1974): The prevalence of epilepsy among mongols related to age. *J Ment Defic Res* 18: 99–106.

Verrotti A1, Greco M1, Varriale G *et al.* (2018): Electroclinical features of epilepsy monosomy 1p36 syndrome and their implications. *Acta Neurol Scand* 138: 523–530.

Viani F, Romeo A, Viri M, *et al.* (1995): Seizure and EEG Patterns in Angelman Syndrome. *J Child Neurol* 10: 467–471.

Vignoli A, Canevini MP, Darra F, *et al.* (2009): Ring chromosome 20 syndrome: a link between epilepsy onset and neuropsychological impairment in three children. *Epilepsia* 50: 2420–2427.

Vignoli A, Bisulli F, Darra F, *et al.* (2016): Epilepsy in ring chromosome 20 syndrome. *Epilepsy Res* 128: 83–93.

Ville D, De Bellescize J, Nguyen MA, *et al.* (2009): Ring 14 chromosome presenting as early-onset isolated partial epilepsy. *Dev Med Child Neurol* 11: 917–922.

Walleigh DJ, Legido A, Valencia I (2013): Ring chromosome 20: a pediatric potassium channelopathy responsive to treatment with ezogabine. *Pediatr Neurol* 49: 368–369.

Wandstrat AE, Leana-Cox J, Jenkins L, Schwartz S (1998): Molecular cytogenetic evidence for a common breakpoint in the largest inverted duplications of chromosome 15. *Am J Hum Genet* 62: 925–936.

Webb TP, Bundey SE, Thacke Al, Todd I (1986): Population incidence and segregation ratios in the Martin-Bell syndrome. *Am J Med Genet* 23: 573–580.

Weber P (2010): Levetiracetam in non-convulsive status epilepticus in a child with Angelman syndrome. *J Child Neurol* 25: 393–396.

Williams CA, Frias JL (1982): The Angelman ("happy puppet"): syndrome. *Am J Med Genet* 11: 463–460.

Williams CA, Zori RT, Stone JW, *et al.* (1990): Maternal origin of 15q11-13 deletions in Angelman syndrome suggests a role forgenomic imprinting. *Am J Med Genet* 35: 350–353.

Williams CA, Angelman H, Clayton-Smith J, *et al.* (1995): Angelman syndrome: consensus for diagnostic criteria. *Am J Med Genet* 56: 237–238.

Wintle RF, Costa T, Haslam RH, Teshima IE, Cox DW (1995): Molecular analysis redefines three human chromosome 14 deletions. *Hum Genet* 95: 495–500.

Wiseman FK, Alford KA, Tybulewicz VLJ, Elizabeth MC, Fisher EMC (2009): Down syndrome-recent progress and future prospects. *Hum Mol Genet*: 18, Review Issue R75–R83.

Wisniewski KE, French JH, Fernando S, *et al.* (1985): Fragile X syndrome: associated neurological abnormalities and developmental disabilities. *Ann Neurol* 18: 665–669.

Wisniewski KE, Dalton AJ, McLachlan DRC, Wen G, Wisniewsky HM (1985): Alzheimer's disease in Down syndrome: clinicopathologic studies. *Neurology* 35: 957–961.

Wisniewski KE, Schmidt-Sidor B (1989): Postnatal delay of myelin formation in brains from Down syndrome infants and children. *Clin Neuropathol* 8: 55–62.

Wisniewski KE, Segan SM, Miczejesji EA, Sersen EA, Rudelli RD (1991): The Fra (X): syndrome: neurological, electrophysiological, and neuropathological abnormalities. *Am J Med Genet* 38: 47–80.

Wolf U, Reinwein H, Porsch R, *et al.* (1965): Defizienz an den kurzen Armen eines Chromosoms Nr. 4. *Humancenetik* 1: 397–413.

Wright TJ, Ricke DO, Denison K, *et al.* (1997): A transcript map of the newly defined 165 kb Wolf-Hirschhorn syndrome critical region. *Hum Molec Genet* 6: 317–324.

Wright TJ, Clemens M, Quarrell O, Altherr MR (1998): Wolf-Hirschhorn and Pitt-Rogers-Danks syndromes caused by overlapping 4p deletions. *Am J Med Genet* 75: 345–350.

Wu YQ, Heilstedt HA, Bedell JA, *et al.* (1999): Molecular refinement of the 1p36 deletion syndrome reveals size diversity and a preponderance of maternally derived deletions. *Hum Mol Genet* 8: 313–321.

Xing Y, Holder JL Jr, Liu Y *et al.* (2018): Prenatal diagnosis of Wolf-Hirschhorn syndrome: from ultrasound findings, diagnostic technology to genetic counseling. *Arch Gynecol Obstet* 298: 289–295.

Yamadera H, Kobayashi K, Sugai K, Suda H, Kaneko S (1998): A study of ring 20 chromosome karyotype with epilepsy. *Psychiatry Clin Neurosci* 52: 63–68.

Yamamoto-Shimojima K, Kouwaki M, Kawashima Y *et al.* (2018): Natural histories of patients with Wolf-Hirschhorn syndrome derived from variable chromosomal abnormalities *Congenit Anom* (Kyoto), *in press*.

Yeragani VK, Hopkinson G (1981): Klinefelter's syndrome with atypical presenting features. *Can J Psychiatry* 26: 567–568.

Zollino M, Doronzio PN (2018): Dissecting the Wolf-Hirschhorn syndrome phenotype: WHSC1 is a neurodevelopmental gene. *J Hum Genet* 63: 859–861.

Zollino M, Seminara L, Orteschi D, *et al.* (2009): The ring 14 syndrome: clinical and molecular definition. *Am J Med Genet* 149: 1116–1124.

Zuppinger K, Engel E, Forbes AP, Mentooth L, Claffey J (1967): Klinefelter's syndrome: a clinical and cytogenetic study in 24 cases. *Acta Endocrinol* 54: 5–48.

WITH VIDEO SUPPLEMENTS

CHAPTER 30

PROGRESSIVE MYOCLONUS EPILEPSIES

Roberto Michelucci[1], Jose Maria Serratosa[2], Antonio V. Delgado Escueta[3], Pierre Genton[4], Patrizia Riguzzi[1], Carlo Alberto Tassinari[1] and Michelle Bureau[4]

[1] IRCCS Istituto delle Scienze Neurologiche di Bologna, Bologna, Italy
[2] Neurology Service, Hospital Universitario Fundacion Jiménez Diaz, Universidad Autonoma de Madrid and Ciberer, Madrid, Spain
[3] Department of Neurology, David Geffen School of Medicine, University of California, Los Angeles, USA
[4] Centre Saint-Paul, Hospital Henri Gastaut, Marseille, France

Introduction and historical overview

Progressive myoclonus epilepsies (PMEs) constitute a heterogenous group of rare specific genetic diseases that share a common phenotype characterized by the association of epileptic seizures, prominent myoclonus, and a progressive neurologic deterioration. The concept of PME was established in 1903 by H. Lundborg, who was referring to the description published by H. Unverricht in 1891 of a familial condition characterized by "myoclonia". This was a disease beginning with epileptic seizures of the clonic or clonic-tonic-clonic type, which were followed by action myoclonus and ataxia. This condition became known as Unverricht-Lundborg disease (ULD), and other conditions were gradually added to this category, sometimes identified with eponymous names (such as Ramsay-Hunt syndrome). A great deal of controversy started with Lafora's discovery of PAS+ neuronal inclusion bodies in 1911, and continued through the discovery of specific pathologic inclusions in neuronal ceroidlipofuscinoses (NCL) and identification of MERRF (myoclonic epilepsy with ragged-red fibres) (Fukuhara *et al.*, 1980).

Efforts to clarify the field (Roger, 1985; Berkovic & Andermann, 1986; Berkovic *et al.*, 1986; Tassinari *et al.*, 1989; Roger *et al.*, 1990; Genton *et al.*, 1990) culminated in an international workshop in Marseille in 1989, which led to the revision of the nosology of PMEs (Marseille Consensus Group, 1990). With improved nosology came significant progress in the elucidation of their clinical picture and the discovery of their genetic defects.

Definitions and classification

The full-blown PME syndrome is characterized by the following:

- *myoclonus* involving a combination of parcellar or segmental, arrhythmic, asynchronous, asymmetrical myoclonias, and massive myoclonias;
- *epilepsy* usually with generalized tonic-clonic, clonic-tonic-clonic or clonic seizures, although other types of seizures, *e.g.*, absences and focal seizures, may also occur (Michelucci *et al.*, 2002);
- *mental deterioration* culminating in dementia, and neurological symptoms which nearly always include cerebellar manifestations;
- and variable genetic transmission, autosomal recessive in most.

The intensity of the various clinical features varies depending on the aetiology. In ULD, for instance, the intellectual deficit, if present at all, develops very late, whereas Lafora disease (LD) causes rapidly evolving dementia and neurologic deterioration, and most forms of NCL have slowly progressing dementia. A wide range of neurological and of sensory symptoms may be encountered: *e.g.*, blindness due to retinal impairment in the case of juvenile NCL, and deafness or optical atrophy in MERRF. The general progression of the disease also varies considerably from one aetiology to another, with ULD showing a less severe and slower course than LD or NCL. However, even within the same disease and the same family (*e.g.* ULD), significant differences may be encountered in terms of severity and progression of symptoms.

The overall prognosis has relatively improved in ULD thanks to early diagnosis by genetic testing and progress in the management of patients with this type of PME: drugs such as phenytoin are now being avoided, since they have been found to have aggravating side effects on the associated neurological symptoms (Elridge *et al.*, 1983); the rational use of agents such as valproate, benzodiazepines, piracetam and recently zonisamide, topiramate and levetiracetam has had a major impact on the control of epilepsy and myoclonus in ULD. However, etiologically oriented therapies remain scarce. Measures such as providing social and educational structures for patients have also contributed towards slowing down the progression of the disease. However, none of our attempts to slow, modify or cure the rapidly progressing and fatal syndromes of the infantile and late infantile forms of NCL and the invariably fatal Lafora type of PME have been succesful until recently. With the success attained in trials of nusinersen (Spinraza) for spinal muscular atrophy (SMA), cerliponase alfa (brineura) for late infantile NCL or Batten disease, eteplirsen (Exondys51) for Duchenne muscular dystrophy, and Edaravone for Amiotrophic Lateral Sclerosis and self-complementary adeno-associated viral serotype 9 (scAAV9) delivered gene replacement therapy in SMN1 related SMA, there is now hope for many of the various PMEs.

In the 1989 International Classification of Epilepsy and Epileptic Syndromes (Commission on Classification and Terminology of the ILAE, 1989), PMEs were included in the category of symptomatic generalized epilepsies. In the 2010's proposal for the establishment of a new classification, PMEs have been listed separately as a group among the various genetic epileptic syndromes (Berg *et al.*, 2010). In the recent position paper of the ILAE Commission for Classification and Terminology (Scheffer *et al.*, 2017), PMEs have not been specifically addressed although they can be included in the "epilepsy syndromes" category within the combined focal and generalized epilepsies or developmental and/or epileptic encephalopathies.

It is difficult to propose a classification of the PMEs: in this chapter, we have chosen to list them in order of approximate frequency, and will emphasize the most relatively common types among these rare conditions.

Frequency and distribution

PMEs are rare conditions and much of the former nosographic controversies were due to the low incidence of the PMEs in developed Western countries and to differences between the experiences of various centres. The prevalence of the various forms of PME varies from one country, and even from one region, to another. PMEs inherited by autosomal recessive transmission may have a relatively higher prevalence in geographic isolates with a marked founder effect (*e.g.*, NCL in Scandinavia, ULD in La Réunion Island), or in cultures that favour consanguinous marriages, *e.g.*, for ULD in Northern Africa or LD in the Karnakata state of Southern India (Acharya *et al.*, 1993). Some etiologies seem to be focused on a single ethnic group or place: dentato-rubral-pallido-luysian atrophy (DRPLA) (Naito & Oyanagi, 1982) and galactosialidosis have been observed mostly in Japan and Asian countries, although these conditions have now been diagnosed elsewhere. Other seemingly rare forms have been reported in a wide range of populations: Gaucher's disease, for instance, or mitochondrial encephalomyopathy with myoclonus epilepsy (of the MERRF type). The juvenile form of NCL is frequent in Scandinavia, while the late infantile form is found in other regions. It must also be noted that some "genetically negative" patients who had been ascribed to classical conditions, like ULD, have led to the discovery of new, rare forms of PME; single families with a particular type of PME have also been described, and await replication. Even today, some isolated or familial cases of PME remain unexplained and cannot be categorized among the known types. The true frequency of PMEs has not yet been definitely established, especially in developing Third World countries, where they are not accurately diagnosed.

Patients' geographical and ethnic background should therefore be taken into account in making diagnoses. In the large population followed at the Centre Saint-Paul in Marseille, PMEs account for less than 1% of all epilepsy cases and consist of 154 cases followed between 1960 and 2011: the PME series includes in the vast majority of cases ULD (70 patients, 45%) and LD (45 patients, 29%), while there is a low prevalence of NCL (18 patients, 12%) and of other aetiologies or unsolved cases (21 patients, 14%). Similarly, in a large study involving 25 epilepsy centres in Italy, 204 PME cases were identified over a 15–year period, spanning between January 1998 and December 2012: in this series ULD and LD accounted for 37.7% and 18.1% of the cases, respectively, while another 15% had a variety of rare genetic disorders (including NCL – 6% –, MERRF, Gaucher disease, sialidosis and others) and almost 28% of cases were undiagnosed (Franceschetti *et al.*, 2014). Only recently, after publication, genetic advances have reduced the amount of the undiagnosed patients, some of them showing new conditions, such as MEAK (myoclonus epilepsy and ataxia due to potassium channel mutation). Therefore, the French and Italian series are quite similar and reflect the Mediterranean pool of PMEs. In Finland, there are many cases of NCL and ULD, but LD is hardly seen. At the Neurological Institute in Montreal, numerous cases of NCL have been treated, mainly due to the existence of a NCL "focus" in Newfoundland.

Diagnosis

The clinical characteristics of the major types of PME have been summarized on *Table I* and will be further detailed below. The diagnosis of a specific form of PME can often be suspected clinically on the basis of:

i) anamnestic data (familial, ethnic and geographic background, age at onset and order of progression of symptoms);

ii) a precise clinical assessment looking for myoclonus, seizures, and associated symptoms, especially cognitive decline, sensory and cerebellar signs;
iii) EEG and video/polygraphic recordings at wakeful and in sleep states.

The diagnostic hypotheses usually result from a confrontation of all these elements. For many of these diseases, a molecular genetic test that confirms diagnosis is now available in clinical practice, but the classic biochemical and pathological procedures used in the diagnosis of PMEs should still be kept in mind. Genetic panels including *EPM1*, *EPM2A*, *EPM2B*, mitochondrial and NCL genes of PME are now available commercially and newer, more recently discovered ULD-like PME genes are being incorporated and developed into the PME panels. Because there is now FDA approved treatment in Batten disease, and trials in more forms of NCL and LD are beginning, genotyping of PMEs should be done in most cases where a treatment is being offered. Useful diagnostic procedures for the various forms of PME have been listed on *Table II*. Thus, in clinical practice, the diagnosis of PME can now be made early and the best possible treatment offered.

In infants and younger children, the diagnosis can now be made at the early stage, and distinguished from inborn errors of metabolism (this group of diseases clearly overlaps with PMEs (see chapter 23) or various epileptic encephalopathies, including Dravet and Lennox-Gastaut syndromes (see chapters 9 and 11). In older children and adolescents both ULD and LD can mimic, for several weeks to months or even years, the much more common juvenile myoclonic epilepsy (JME) or other forms of idiopathic generalized epilepsy (IGE), as seizures and myoclonias are prominent after awakening in all. However, discrete clinical signs such as interictal myoclonias, erratic myoclonias or mild cognitive changes, especially in LD, or abnormal background activity on the EEG, and especially drug resistance should prompt genetic testing which leads to the correct diagnosis. Some cases of JME treated with inadequate drugs may experience severe exacerbation of myoclonus and mimic PME (Genton *et al.*, 2000).

At the borderline of PMEs are some conditions that should be briefly discussed:

- *progressive myoclonus ataxia (PMA)* is a still useful clinical entity (Marsden *et al.*, 1990). It covers a clinical picture characterized by myoclonus associated with ataxia; epileptic seizures, if they occur at all, are rare. The aetiologies of PMA overlap to a large extent with those of PMEs, but some cases do not fit into any of the known PME categories;
- *Northern epilepsy* is a syndrome reported from Finland, which is characterized by childhood-onset generalized epileptic seizures with dementia occurring later in life, and a protracted course, without myoclonus (review in Ranta & Lehesjoki, 2000). This condition, shown to be related to the CLN8 gene mutations, was subsequently found outside Finland and named "variant late-infantile" NCL (Mitchell *et al.*, 2001);
- a comparatively benign syndrome with onset in adulthood, of generalized seizures and cortical myoclonus has been reported from Japan as *familial benign myoclonus epilepsy of adult onset* (or familial adult myoclonic epilepsy, FAME) (Okino, 1997), and linked to chromosome 8q24 (Mikami *et al.*, 1999). However, in several Italian families fulfilling the diagnostic criteria of FAME, a different locus on chromosome 2p has been discovered, suggesting genetic heterogeneity (Guerrini *et al.*, 2001). In two unrelated italian families with linkage to chromosome 2p, an in-frame insertion/deletion of the ADRAB gene encoding the alpha2 adrenergic receptor subtype b, has been reported (De Fusco *et al.*, 2014). Finally, two further loci (5p and 3q) have been reported in families with comparable non-progressive clinical features (Depienne *et al.*, 2010, Yeetong *et al.*, 2013).

Unverricht-Lundborg disease (ULD or EPM1)

This condition was described repeatedly under many different names from two main sources, *i.e.*, the Baltic region and Scandinavia (Unverricht, 1891; Koskiniemi *et al.*, 1974; Koskiniemi, 1986), Southern Europe and the Mediterranean region (Roger *et al.*, 1968; Tassinari *et al.*, 1989; Genton *et al.*, 1990). It was thought that "Baltic myoclonus" and "Mediterranean myoclonus" (formerly referred to as Ramsay Hunt syndrome) were different entities, Baltic myoclonus being more severe. This apparent difference was mainly due to the widespread use of phenytoin in Northern Europe and phenobarbital and valproate in Southern Europe. Phenytoin has an aggravating effect on ULD; phenobarbital does not, while valproate may improve myoclonus. Clinicians finally agreed that these disorders were but one (Marseille Consensus Group, 1990) before genetic studies confirmed the identity and relative homogeneity of cystatin B (CSTB) mutations in chromosome 21q as the cause of ULD (Lehesjoki *et al.*, 1991; Malafosse *et al.*, 1992). Mutations in three other genes, *PRICKLE1, SCARB2, and KCN1* have been reported in *CSTB* mutation negative patients, presenting with symptoms resembling ULD (Bassuk *et al.*, 2008; Berkovic *et al.*, 2008; Dibbens *et al.*, 2009; Muona *et al.*, 2015). Following identification of the underlying genes, these disorders are now collectively classified as ULD-like PMEs. The classical form of ULD, related to the CSTB mutation, will be described here.

ULD is the most common cause of PME worldwide. ULD is also the most common type of PME around the Mediterranean and is enriched in Scandinavia especially Finland. Its prevalence is very low in countries like Japan (Kagitani-Shimono *et al.*, 2002). Interestingly, in

Table I Summary of clinical features in the main types of progressive myoclonus epilepsies (PME)

Type of PME	Specific clinical signs and symptoms	Age at onset (years)	Evolution/prognosis
Unverricht-Lundborg type (EPM1)	No associated symptoms Cognitive impairment: nil to moderate Some cases with myoclonus only Renal failure/nephritic syndrome in some Ataxia prominent at onset	7–16 (86%: 9–13)	Severe in a minority of cases Usually mild/chronic Some patients with minimal impairment Stabilizes in adulthood
Scarb2/LIMP2 variant	Renal failure/nephritic syndrome in some	15–25	Severe in most
PRICKLE variant	Ataxia prominent at onset	5–10	Preservation of intellect
MEAK (myoclonus epilepsy and ataxia due to potassium channel mutation)	Early onset, prominent myoclonus, *de novo* mutations, improvement with fever	3–15	Preservation of intellect, wheelchair bound since late teen age
North Sea PME	Early onset ataxia, multiple seizure types, areflexia, scoliosis	2–5	Preservation of intellect, wheelchair bound since adolescence, death in adult age
Lafora disease (EPM2)	Depression, rapid course of dementia Visual symptoms (ictal) Rapid progression	6–19 (typically 14–15)	Very severe Death within 2–10 years Some slowly progressive cases
Ceroid lipofuscinoses (Batten)			
Late infantile (Jansky-Bielschowsky)	Impaired vision leading to blindness	1–4	Severe in all forms
Juvenile (Spielmeyer-Vogt)	Cognitive impairment with variable course	4–14	Severe in all forms
Adult (Kufs)	Variable; visual impairment in some	11–50	Usually severe
Myoclonic epilepsy with ragged-red fibres (MERRF)	Maternal inheritance pattern, associated neurological, muscular and sensory deficits (deafness most common), variability of clinical presentation	3–65	Variable, from very mild to very severe; severity may be due to varying levels of abnormal mitochondrial DNA
Sialidosis (type 1)	Prominent facial myoclonus Burning hands and feet, cherry-red spot	8–25	Variable, sometimes benign Preserved intellect in most
Sialidosis (type 2)	Skeletal changes, coarse facies Congenital, infantile, juvenile	Earlier than type 1	Very severe in most Developmental delay
Galactosialidosis, late infantile type Galactosialidosis, juvenile type	Dysomorphia, mental retardation, ataxia, vision loss, angiokeratomas	Early childhood Adolescence or later	Severe (but rarely in PME) Usually severe (Often PME)
Dentato-rubro-pallido-luysian atrophy (DRPLA)	Chorea, dementia variable	Childhood – adolescence	Variable, often severe
Gaucher's disease (type III)	Saccadic eye movements, gaze palsy, hearing loss, splenomegaly possible	Variable	Variable, severe in most cases
Juvenile form of Huntington's chorea	GTCS, dementia, later myoclonus	Childhood	Very severe
Senile myoclonic epilepsy	Dementia followed by myoclonic seizures, GTCS and erratic myoclonus	Adult/middle age	Seen in early-onset Alzheimer's disease, especially in Down syndrome

Table II Confirmation of diagnosis in progressive myoclonus epilepsies (PME)

Type of PME	Procedure	Biology and/or pathology	Genetics Molecular biology
Unverricht-Lundborg type (EPM1)	Molecular biology	None	EPM1 (cystatin B) – 21q22.3 Expansion of CCCCGCCCCGCG dodecamer or point mutations
Scarb2/LIMP2 variant	Molecular biology	*Renal biopsy*	*Scarb2/LIMP2* gene – 4q13–21
PRICKLE variant	Molecular biology	None	*PRICKLE1* gene – 12q12
MEAK (myoclonus epilepsy and ataxia due to potassium channel mutation)	Molecular biology	None	kCN1 c.959G>A *de novo* mutations
North Sea PME	Molecular biology	None	GOSR2 mutations
Lafora disease (EPM2)	Biopsy: skin (armpit, sweat glands), liver, muscle, brain Molecular biology	Lafora bodies (polyglycosans), most prominent in sweat duct cells	*EMP2A* (laforin) – 6q23-q25 *EMP2B* (malin) – 6p22 Other
Ceroid lipofuscinoses (Batten):		Storage of lipopigment in lysosomes	
Late infantile (Jansky-Bielschowsky)	Biopsy (electron microscopy) skin, rectal mucosa, brain...	Curvilinear granular inclusions	CLN2 – 11p15.5 CLN5 (Finnish variant) – 13q21.1-q32 CLN6 (Gypsy variant) – 15q21-q23 CLN7, CLN8
Juvenile (Spielmeyer-Vogt)	Idem	Fingerprint profiles (FPP)	CLN3 (16S298) – CLN9
Adult (Kufs)	Brain biopsy	FPP and osmiophilic granular profiles	CLN6 in most
Myoclonic epilepsy with ragged-red fibers (MERRF)	Muscle biopsy Molecular biology	Ragged-red fibers on light microscopy, respiratory metabolic chain deficit	Mitochondrial DNA mutations A8344G and multiple other Mixed/overlap forms (MELAS...)
	Urine	Increased urinary oligosaccharides	α-neuraminidase – 6p21.3
Sialidosis (types 1 and 2)	Lymphocytes, fibroblasts Molecular biology	Assessment of neuraminidase	
Galactosialidosis	Lymphocytes, fibroblasts Molecular biology	Associated β-galactosidase deficit	Protein/cathepsin A – 20q13
Dentato-rubro-pallido-luysian atrophy (DRPLA)	Molecular biology	None	Atrophin, CAG expansion on 12p13
Gaucher's disease (type III)	Serum lymphocytes, fibroblasts bone marrow, liver...	Increased acid phosphatase β-glucocerebrosidase deficit glucocerebroside storage	Glucosidase beta acid (GBA) on 1q21 Leu444Pro most common
Juvenile form of Huntington's chorea	Molecular biology	None	Huntington, CAG expansion on 4p16.3
Early-onset PME (Van Bogaert)	Molecular biology	None	Potassium channel tetramerization domain (KCTD7) on 7q11.2

La Réunion island in the Indian Ocean, high prevalence, marked consanguinity and a founder effect was traced to a single immigrant common ancestor from mainland France who settled there around 1750 (Moulard *et al.*, 2003).

The age at onset of ULD is consistently 6 to 18 years, and 86% of all the cases begin between 9 and 13 years of age. A late onset at age 18 years was found in a girl who had delayed puberty with her first menses at age 18 years. On the other hand an onset around 3 years was reported in an Emirati family with genetically confirmed EPM1 (Saadah *et al.*, 2014). The disease begins either insidiously with action activated, stimulus sensitive myoclonus which is noticeable in the morning upon wakening, or more suddenly with nocturnal clonic or clonic-tonic-clonic seizures. Myoclonus gradually becomes invalidating and is particularly accentuated upon wakening and when moving. Very few spontaneous jerks occur. Myoclonus makes some movements difficult to perform, such as standing up from a sitting or reclining position, or changing direction while walking. These movements require motor preparation, and can be executed only after a period of latency. Eating becomes difficult, and drinking even more so. Some myoclonic fits are triggered by performing difficult movements and develop into full-scale clonic seizures or clonic-tonic-clonic seizures with variable durations, often involving a semi-loss of consciousness. Absences have been much less frequently reported, usually in compound heterozygotes. Patients showing only myoclonus without clear epileptic seizures or very mild myoclonus non interfering with daily activities may be encountered and may represent minor forms of ULD without the full symptomatology. In this context patients with so-called "progressive myoclonic ataxia" may indeed have ULD, as suspected by Marsden *et al.* (1990).

Ataxia, dysarthria and poor coordination are generally present, to a degree which is variable but difficult to assess because of the jerks. Other neurological signs are few such as pes cavus (in three patients in our series) – a slight and stable symptom – and abolition of the tendon reflexes (in two patients). We have never observed any optic atrophy, sensory disorders, pyramidal or extrapyramidal impairments, or amyotrophy. Cognitive abilities may not be significantly affected; often cognitive changes are subtle. Some even teach that ULD is the prototype of PMEs without dementia: however, some degree of subtle mental impairment may be seen at the onset or over the course of the disease when formal neuropsychological tests are performed (Lehesjoki *et al.*, 2009). In addition, reactional psychological disorders were both pronounced and frequent. In their systematic study of 20 CSTB genetically confirmed patients, compared with a control group, Ferlazzo *et al.* (2009a) found lower scores on all short-term memory and executive function tasks, and the severity of cognitive impairment was related to duration of the disease and to the severity of myoclonus. Similarly, Giovagnoli *et al.* (2009) compared 21 ULD patients with healthy controls and cryptogenic temporal lobe epilepsy cases: abstract reasoning, attention, planning, word fluency, constructive praxis, and visuospatial memory and learning were significantly impaired in ULD patients.

Within a few years, myoclonus, ataxia, dysarthria and poor coordination slowly but steadily worsen. Epileptic seizures which can be controlled by medication seem to lessen with time. One unusual and very typical feature of ULD is the sharp fluctuation of the patients' condition between "good periods", during which they are only slightly handicapped, and "bad periods" when the myoclonus becomes more pronounced, sometimes ending in a seizure or series of seizures. The periods of remission can last from one day to several weeks, and they tend to shorten progressively during the evolutive phase of the disease. Generally speaking, depending on the speed at which the disease has progressed, ULD tends to stabilize in adulthood, and the debilitating effects of the myoclonus may also subsequently subside. Among patients followed for at least 20 years, we found that convulsive seizures tended to subside after the first 5 years, and that myoclonus stabilized or progressed only minimally after the first ten years (Magaudda *et al.*, 2006).

Canafoglia *et al.* (2017) studied retrospectively 59 Italian patients carrying the *CSTB* expansion mutation in order to investigate the time course of symptoms and prognostic factors already detectable near to disease onset. They found that disabling myoclonus occurred an average of 32 years after disease onset, whereas cognitive impairment occurred a little later. Furthermore, an age at onset of less than 12 years, the severity of myoclonus at the time of first assessment, and seizure persistence more than 10 years after onset affected the timing of disabling myoclonus and cognitive decline and were therefore predictors of a more severe outcome.

The MRI is usually normal early in the course of ULD. At later stages, atrophy in cortical motor areas, and in pons, medulla, and cerebellar hemispheres has been reported (Koskenkorva *et al.*, 2009; Mascalchi *et al.*, 2002). Internal frontal hyperosteosis has been reported (Korja *et al.*, 2007a). Thalamic and putaminal involvement have been shown by using nonconventional MRI methods of 3 D textural analysis (Suoranta *et al.*, 2016). In the few histopathological studies of the brain available, widespread degenerative changes with no evidence for storage material have been observed.

In the early stages of the disease, the EEG shows normal background activity, with a few slow discharges which become more frequent as the disease progresses (*Figure 1*). Short, subclinical generalized fast varieties (4 to 6 Hz) of spike waves (SWs) or polyspike waves (PSWs) are recorded, sometimes associated with massive myoclonias, whereas the action myoclonus is not accompanied by any changes in the EEG. Clinical and EEG sensitivity to photostimulation is observed in

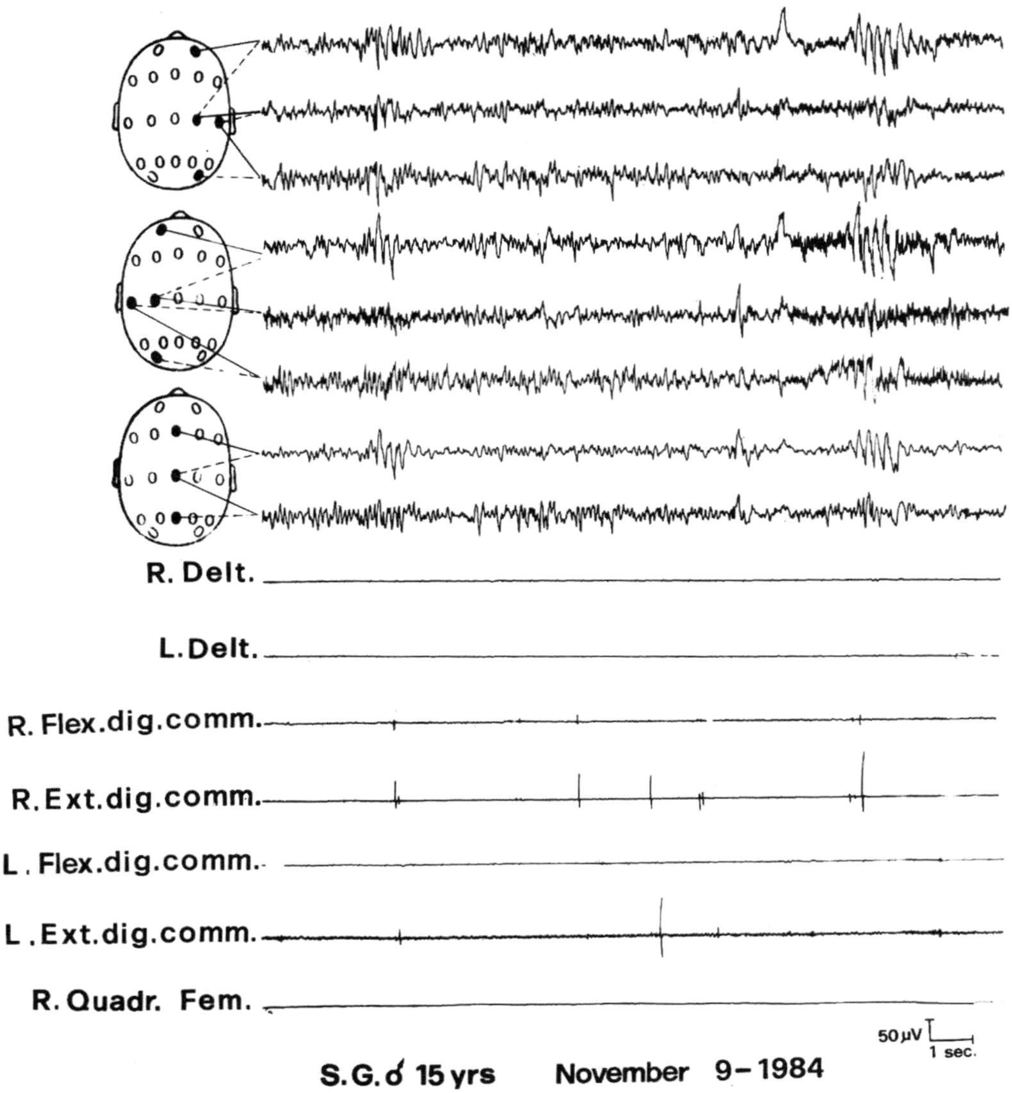

Figure 1

15-year old male patient with a 2-year history of myoclonic jerks and tonic-clonic seizures on awakening with positive genetic test for ULD. Note the normal background activity, the presence of SW discharges and erratic myoclonic jerks inconstantly correlated with the spikes.

almost 90% of all cases. The physiological sleep patterns are maintained: the paroxysmal anomalies are not noticeably aggravated during slow wave sleep, whereas during REM sleep, fast spike and polyspike discharges occur around the vertex in 83% all cases (Tassinari *et al.*, 1974) *(Figure 2)*. The amplitude of the somatosensory evoked potentials (EPs) was found to be abnormally high (Mauguière *et al.*, 1981; Tassinari *et al.*, 1989), suggesting increased cortical motor excitability. Transcranial magnetic stimulation may also show impaired motor cortical plasticity (Danner *et al.*, 2011) and abnormalities of motor cortical excitability paralleling structural alterations as demonstrated by MRI cortical thickness analysis (Danner *et al.*, 2013). The anomalies (spontaneous SW discharges, photosensitivity, polyspike discharges during REM sleep) tend to diminish with time, and are more obvious during the initial phases of the disease, when the patients are subject to frequent epileptic seizures. In the most long-established cases, a moderate slowing of the background activity and a slight attenuation of the physiological sleep patterns during the phases of slow wave sleep are mainly observed. In patients followed over more than 15 years, we found a consistent abatement of photosensitivity *(Figure 3)* and a near-disappearance of spontaneous SW discharges (Ferlazzo *et al.*, 2007). Other studies have shown the long-term abatement of cortical excitability in ULD patients (Kobayashi *et al.*, 2011). Other functional studies have pointed to a DOPAminergic deficit in ULD (Korja *et al.*, 2007b).

Cystatin B deficiency

The ULD gene was originally mapped on the distal part of chromosome 21q22.3 in families of patients with ULD evaluated in Finland (Lehesjoki *et al.*, 1991). This linkage was confirmed in Mediterranean patients (Malafosse *et al.*, 1992) and labelled EPM1, as the first gene chromosomally located in the PME group. Using positional cloning strategy, Pennacchio *et al.* (1996) identified a previously described protein, cystatin B (CSTB, also known as stefin B) as the deficient gene product. CSTB is a ubiquitously expressed 98 amino acid protein comprising a molecular weight of approximately 11 kDa. CSTB is a protease inhibitor that inhibits *in vitro* several lysosomal cysteine proteases, called cathepsins, by tight, reversible binding. Cathepsins non-selectively degrade intracellular proteins and participate in apoptosis.

Pennacchio *et al.* (1996) observed two heterozygous point mutations in CSTB. Since ULD is an autosomal recessive disease, this observation was unexplained until Lalioti *et al.* (1997a) showed that the most common mutation is an unstable expansion of a 12–nucleotide, dodecamer, repeat (5'-CCCCGCCCCGCG-3'), in the promoter region of CSTB (Lalioti *et al.*, 1997b; Virtaneva *et al.*, 1997). This is normally polymorphic with two or three copies present. EPM1-associated alleles have been reported to contain at least 30 repeat copies. The expansion mutation is found in approximately 90% of the disease alleles worldwide and in homozygous form in the majority of the patients, especially in populations with a founder effect. No significant correlation between the length of the expanded repeats and the age of onset or disease severity or anticipation has been reported in early studies (Lalioti *et al.*, 1998); only recently, however, with more detailed phenotyping of the patients, it has been shown that the actual size of the longer CSTB expansion mutation allele is likely to have a modulating effect on the age at disease onset, myoclonus severity, and cortical neurophysiology (Hypponen *et al.*, 2015). EPM1-related homozygous point mutations in CSTB have been rarely reported (Lalioti *et al.*, 1997b; Pinto *et al.*, 2012). All other point mutations identified in EPM1 patients have been found as compound heterozygotes with the expansion allele (Lalioti *et al.*, 1997a). These point mutations change single amino acids, affect splice sites or predict truncated proteins. The reported missense mutations are likely to affect the interaction of the CSTB protein with its target cysteine proteases. These compound heterozygotes with the expansion and missense point mutations, which account for almost 11% of EPM1 patients, usually show a more severe phenotype with frequent refractory seizures and a more severe cognitive impairment and EEG picture *(Figure 4)* (Koskenkorva *et al.*, 2011; Canafoglia *et al.*, 2012), with a possible gender difference (Assenza *et al.*, 2017).

Most functional changes associated with the mutations described in ULD appear to alter the lysosome-associated functions of cystatin B (Alakurtti *et al.*, 2005). Reduced CSTB expression, increased cathepsin B activities, impaired redox homeostasis and more apoptotic cell death are the primary pathological consequence of repeat expansion mutations in the majority of EPM1 mutations. Repeat expansion mutations reduce CSTB mRNA expression with less than 10% of expression in cells compared to controls (Joensuu *et al.*, 2007). Consequently, CSTB protein expression and its inhibition of cathepsins are also significantly reduced in cells of EPM1 patients. Decreased inhibitory activity of CSTB correlates with enhanced activity of cathepsins B, L, and S and implies more cell death (Rinne *et al.*, 2002). As for point mutations in ULD, these missense mutant proteins fail to associate with lysosomes, when transiently over-expressed in cells, implying an essential role of lysosomal localization for the physiological function of CSTB (Lalioti *et al.*, 1997a; Joensuu *et al.*, 2007).

A mouse model for EPM1 provides evidence that cystatin B deficient ULD is a primary neurodegenerative disorder with apoptotic cell death affecting specific neuronal populations. The *Cstb-/-* mice develop myoclonic seizures by one month of age and progressive ataxia by six months of age and thus replicate two clinical features of EPM1. In transgenic mice, it has been shown that cystatin B deficiency causes abnormal activation of cathepsin S, C1q B-chain of complement

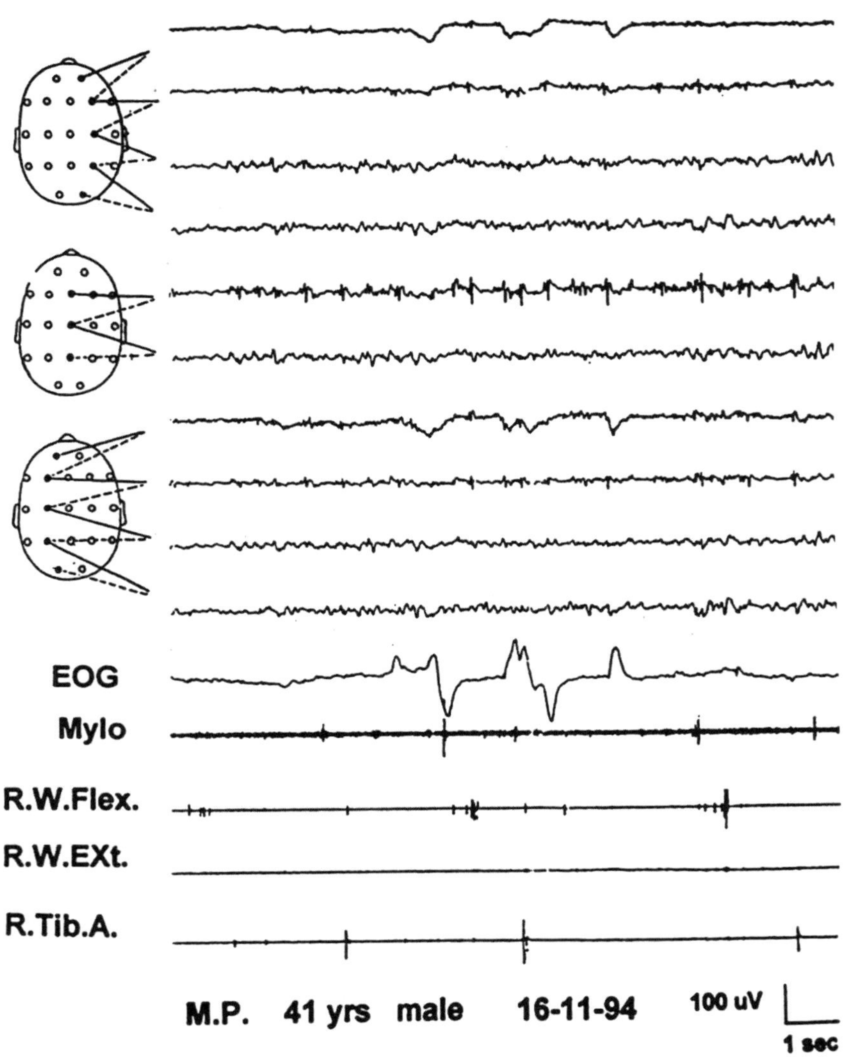

Figure 2

41-year-old male patient with a 25-year history of myoclonus, rare generalized motor seizures and cerebellar disturbance. Molecular genetic analysis led to the diagnosis of ULD. On polygraphic recording during REM sleep one can observe the occurrence of fast spikes over the vertex and the central areas and erratic myoclonic jerks.
EOG: elecro-oculogram; Mylo: mylohyoideus muscle; R.W. Flex: right wrist flexor muscles; RW Ext: right wrist extensor muscles; R Tib A: right tibialis anterior muscle.

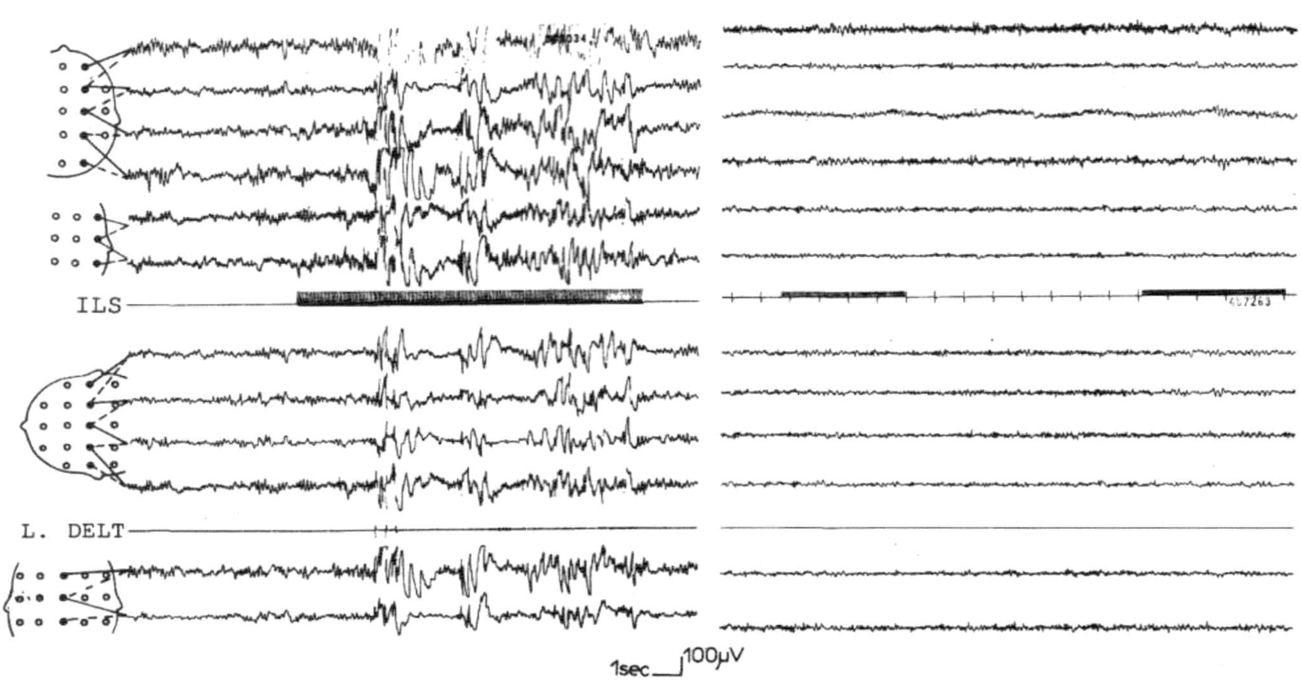

Figure 3

Male patient with ULD, onset at age 13. Evolution of photosensitivity. Left: **ILS performed at age 14, bursts of fast diffuse polyspike-waves provoking slight myoclonic jerks (L DELT).** Right: **at age 28, normal background activity and absence of photoparoxysmal response.**

(C1qB), beta2-microglobulin, glial fibrillary acidic protein (Gfap), apolipoprotein D, fibronectin 1 and metallothionein II, which are factors involved in proteolysis, apoptosis and glial activation (Lieuallen *et al.*, 2001). The neuropathological hallmark in the *Cstb-/-* mice is progressive apoptotic loss of cerebellar granule neurons, less marked neuronal apoptosis in the hippocampal formation entorhinal cortex and prosubiculum. Hyperexcitability in hippocampal slices of CSTB-/- mice was proven by responses of multiple population spikes during afferent stimuli in the CA1 region and the appearance of epileptic-like activity earlier in *Cstb-/-* mice than in wild-type mice during kainate perfusion (Francheschetti *et al.*, 2007). Impaired redox homeostasis as a key mechanism by which CSTB deficiency triggers neurodegeneration has been observed in cerebellar neurons. Both CSTB knockdown in rats and knockout in mice sensitize granule neurons to oxidative stress-induced cell death mediated by the lysosomal protease cathepsin B. CSTB deficiency triggers oxidative injury specifically in the cerebellum, leading to diminished anti-oxidant capacity and elevated lipid peroxidation (Lehtinen *et al.*, 2009). Consistent with these findings, cerebellar granule neuron degeneration is reduced in mice deficient for both CSTB and cathepsin B compared to mice deficient for CSTB only (Houseweart *et al.*, 2003). The double-knockout mice retain myoclonic seizures and ataxia suggesting that oxidative stress and CSTB may regulate neuronal excitability in EPM1 independently of deregulated cathepsin B activity. Recent experiments in the CSTB deficient mice show that inflammatory changes including microglial activation and higher serum concentrations of chemokines and proinflammatory cytokines may contribute to the disease pathology of EPM1 (Okuneva *et al.*, 2016), possibly opening

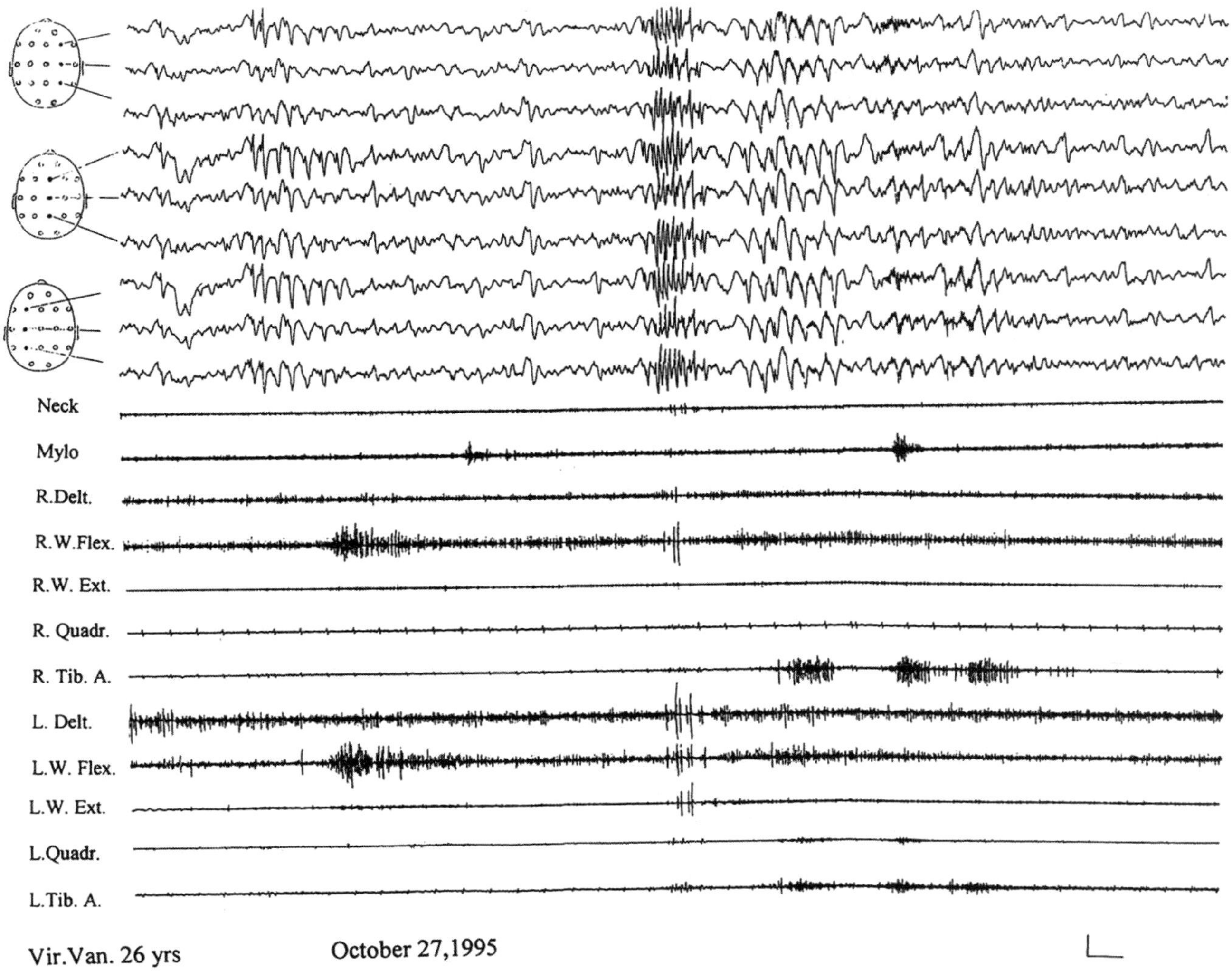

Figure 4

ULD: 26-year-old male patient showing a severe evolution of the disease with uncontrolled motor seizures and disabling myoclonus. Note the presence of slow background activity, frequent slow and fast diffuse SW and PSW discharges and abundant myoclonic jerks, related and unrelated with the paroxysmal abnormalities. This patient was a compound heterozygote for ULD CSTB mutations.

new perspectives of therapy. Indeed recent approaches using MRI and diffusion tensor imaging have uncovered early and progressive white matter tracts degeneration both in mice models (Manninen *et al.*, 2014) as well as in patients (Manninen *et al.*, 2015), which likely occurs secondary to glial activation and neuronal death.

Impairment of gabaergic inhibitory neurotransmission with loss of cortical GABA terminals has been demonstrated in the Cstb knockout mice (Buzzi *et al.*, 2012), probably contributing to both hyperexcitability of cortical neuronal networks and disruption of serotoninergic neurotransmission.

ULD-like PMEs (*PRIKLE1*, *SCARB2*, *KCNC1* and *GOSR2* related PMEs)

In recent years previously cryptogenic conditions mimicking the ULD electro-clinical phentotype and showing relative preservation of cognitive functions have been identified.

In a Palestinian Arab consanguineous family, a linkage to chr12 was found suggesting a putative *EPM1b* gene (Berkovic *et al.*, 2005). In this and two other possible related families a p.Arg104Gln mutation in the *PRICKLE1* gene encoding a protein in the non-canonical WNT signaling pathway was subsequently discovered by Bassuk *et al.* (2008). Onset was slightly younger than EPM1, between five and ten years of age with ataxia as presenting symptom followed later by action myoclonus and seizures. Intellect is generally preserved. In another consanguineous Palestinian Arab family segregating an autosomal recessive PME with early ataxia Mutation of the nuclear lamin gene *LMNB2* was found (Damiano *et al.*, 2015).

Mutations in *SCARB2* (scavenger receptor class B), or *LIMP2* (lysosomal membrane protein2), which encodes a lysosomal membrane protein, were described by Berkovic *et al.* (2008) in patients with the action myoclonus-renal failure syndrome (AMRF), and nearly simultaneously reported from Portugal in two siblings with nephrotic syndrome and PME (Balreira *et al.*, 2008). Such AMRF patients usually start at 15–25 years of age with tremor, action myoclonus, seizures, and ataxia, or with proteinuria that progresses to renal failure. Dibbens *et al.* (2009) also reported five Italian patients harboring novel mutations in *SCARB2* who showed no evidence of renal failure during up to 15 years of follow-up. Four were homozygotes, two of which were from known consanguineous unions, and one was a compound heterozygote, with mutations predicting either aberrant splicing or a truncated protein due to a frameshift alteration. Rubboli *et al.* (2011) precised the clinical and neurophysiologic phenotype in these five patients; the condition begins like classical ULD electro-clinical phenotype *(Figure 5)*, but has (in the absence of renal insufficiency) a very severe course, since four patients died around age 30 years of complications (status or pneumonia). Wider phenotypes, including demyelinating polyneuropathy and dilated cardiomyopathy were identified in a German AMRF family (Hopfner *et al.*, 2011). Neuropathological correlates of *SCARB2* associated PME were described in 2 Japanese patients and consisted of both extraneuronal brown pigment deposition especially in the cerebellar and cerebral cortices and system neurodegeneration (with diffuse neuronal loss and gliosis in the brain including the pallidoluysian and cerebello-olivary system) (Fu *et al.*, 2014).

By sequencing the exomes of 84 unrelated individuals with PME of unknown cause, a recurrent *de novo* mutation, c.959G>A (p.Arg320His), in *KCNC1* was identified as a new major cause for PME (Muona *et al.*, 2015). This gene, not previously associated with human disease, encodes KV3.1, a subunit of the KV3 voltage-gated potassium ion channels, which are major determinants of high-frequency neuronal firing. The mutation was shown to have a dominant-negative loss-of-function effect when the KV3.1 channel was analyzed *in vitro*. This novel PME, also known as MEAK, is characterized by onset between 3 and 15 years of progressively severe myoclonus and rare tonic-clonic seizures. Half of the patients were wheelchair-bound by their late teenage years and showed mild cognitive decline. Early death was not observed. EEGs showed generalized SW and PSW discharges, with documented photosensitivity in most. Interestingly transient clinical improvement with fever was noted in 6 patients likely to be related to increased channel availability at elevated temperatures, as shown by high-temperature *in vitro* recordings (Oliver *et al.*, 2017).

Another autosomal recessive and homogeneous phenotype with early-onset ataxia (average 2 years of age), areflexia, action myoclonus (starting at the mean age of 6.5 years) and seizures, scoliosis, elevated creatine kinase levels, and relative preservation of cognitive function until the late stages of the disease was ascribed to a mutation in the Golgi Qb-SNARE gene *GOSR2* (Corbett *et al.*, 2011). These patients show multiple seizure types (including tonic-clonic seizures, absence seizures and drop attacks) and typical EEG findings with generalized SW discharges with a posterior predominance and photosensitivity. This condition was rebaptized "North Sea" PME since the cases all came from countries bounding the North Sea, extending to the coastal region of Northern Norway (Boissé Lomax *et al.*, 2013).

Lafora's disease (*EPM2A* and *EPM2B*)

In 1911, Gonzalo Rodriguez Lafora described the "amyloid" bodies (intracellular deposits of poorly branched, glucose polymer or "polyglucosans") in the central nervous system of an 18-year-old

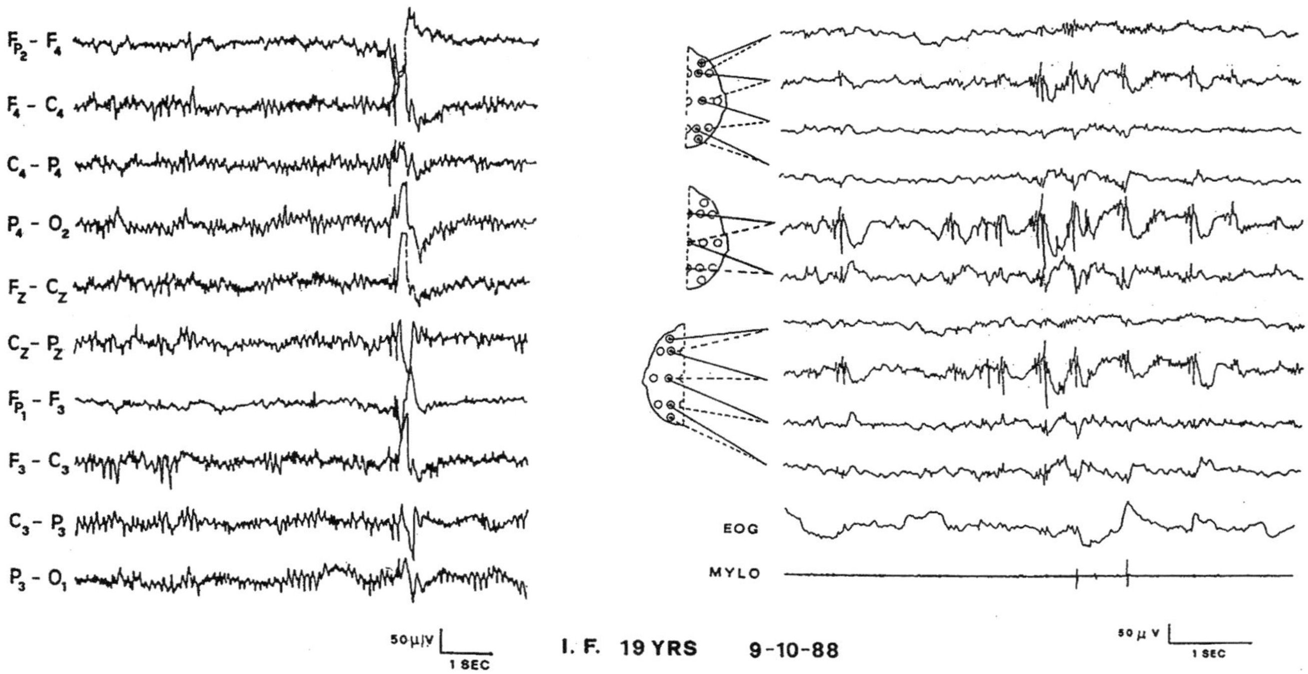

Figure 5

This male patient, aged 19, had an EEG typical for ULD. Left: **During the awake state one can observe a normal background activity with a generalized fast SW discharge.** Right: **During REM sleep, vertex and central fast spikes are particularly evident. However he had a very severe course of the disease with death occurring in the third decade; only several years later he was shown to carry SCARB2 mutation.**

male with stimulus-sensitive resting and action myoclonus, epilepsy and progressive intellectual, cerebellar and neurological deterioration. Since then, "Lafora inclusion bodies" (LBs) have been considered characteristic of this disease. In 1963, its diagnostic criteria were established: an autosomal recessive, fatal generalized multisystem disease with LBs, EEG diffuse 4–6 Hz PSWs and a rapidly PME syndrome with death within 5–10 years (Van Heycop Ten Ham & De Jager, 1963). Frequent visual auras in the clinical setting of PME, the rapid course of the illness with death occurring 10 years after onset of epilepsy, and the excessive accumulation of polyglucosan inclusion bodies in brain, muscles, liver, heart, retina, peripheral nerves and skin, separate Lafora's disease (LD) from other PMEs and make it easily recognizable. LD is more frequently found in the Mediterranean countries of Southern Europe, Northern Africa and the Middle East. It is also found in Central and Southern Asian countries, and in other countries where consanguinity occurs. The largest reported series of cases have occurred in Southern Europe, Turkey and Northern Africa, and there is also a fairly high incidence in the state of Karnataka, in Southern India (Acharya *et al.*, 1989).

The onset of the disease occurs between the ages of 6 and 19 years, most typically at 14–15 years. The age of onset and the course of the disease itself can be variable even between siblings (Tassinari *et al.*, 1978). The first symptoms are generalized tonic-clonic seizures, clonic seizures, myoclonic seizures, and absences, making it hard to separate from the idiopathic generalized epilepsies. When associated with focal visual seizures involving simple or more complex hallucinations or scotomas, LD should be suspected. Visual seizures are particularly characteristic of LD and have been reported in around 50% of the patients in the early stage (Roger *et al.*, 1983; Tinuper *et al.*, 1983). A severe resting and action myoclonus then progresses rapidly. Serious cognitive impairment with school failure usually associated with deep depression, subsequently come to the forefront, one to two years from onset of seizures and sometimes even at an earlier stage (Genton *et al.*, 1989; Ganesh *et al.*, 2000). Ataxia is sometimes difficult to assess because it is masked by the intense myoclonus. All these symptoms add up to a typical PME picture. Optic atrophy was reported in the case of a South African native with otherwise typical symptoms of Lafora's disease (De Graaf *et al.*, 1989) and personally observed in two Serbian brothers. Retinitis pigmentosa has also been described in a single LD patient (Pinto *et al.*, 2015).

Family studies have shown that EEG changes can precede the onset of clinical symptoms (Van Heycop Ten Ham & De Jager, 1963), but at the onset, the EEG is often not unlike that of idiopathic generalized epilepsy, showing a normal background activity with isolated SW and diffuse 4–6 Hz PSW discharges *(Figure 6A)*. Photosensitivity is usually present *(Figure 7)*. The paroxysmal abnormalities are not increased during sleep in LD as they are in IGE. At this stage, polygraphic recordings sometimes show the existence of sub-clinical or discrete erratic myoclonus which is not associated with the paroxysmal EEG anomalies. The EEG pattern quickly (usually within a few months, sometimes only after several years) becomes much more typical *(Figures 6B, 8, 9)*: the background activity slows down, the paroxysmal bursts begin to look more like fast SWs and PSWs and focal, particularly occipital epileptiform anomalies begin to show up. The physiological sleep patterns tend to disappear. Erratic myoclonus is liable to be recorded at this stage. Photosensitivity can persist throughout the course of the disease. The somatosensory EPs are of increased amplitude during the early stages of the disease and brainstem EPs tend to show longer latencies than in normal subjects.

In the course of LD, the myoclonus worsens and the frequency of the epileptic seizures increases, alternating with periods of apparent remission; episodes of cortical blindness may occur. In fact, the intellectual deficits increase steadily, ending in dementia, and the patients will inevitably become bedridden. Death occurs within a few years (usually 5 to 15 years) but long surviving cases, though bedridden, are increasingly observed due to improvement of long-term care. Antiepileptic and antimyoclonic drugs can nevertheless be of some help in controlling the seizures, at least during the early stages of the disease.

In most cases, it is possible to suspect the diagnosis based on the clinical signs together with the EEG data. However, since the prognosis is so poor, diagnosis should be done early both by genetic testing for *EPM2A* and *EPM2B* mutations and an axillary skin biopsy searching for PAS+ LBs in the cells of sweat gland ducts (Carpenter & Karpati, 1981). During autopsies, LBs are found in the cerebral and cerebellar cortex, hippocampus and amygdala, midbrain, hepatic parenchyma, striated and cardiac muscles. LBs are densely packed and heavily phosphorylated glycosans, with some similarities to normal corpora amylacea found in the brain of the elderly, but also sometimes in the young (Cavanagh, 1999). The location of LBs in the perikaryon and dendrites is characteristic of LD, as physiological polyglucosans are mostly found in axons and in glial cells. Their presence in the sweat glands of axillar skin biopsy material is pathognomonic for LD.

Genetic studies have pointed to the existence of clinical variants of LD, the spectrum of which is likely to increase with further progress in the elucidation of molecular mechanisms involved. Mutations within exon 1 of the *EPM2A* gene may produce a different phenotype, with childhood-onset learning difficulties and only later the more classical course (Ganesh *et al.*, 2002). Patients with *EMP2B* mutations are reported to have a slightly milder clinical course and slower progression (Gomez-Abad *et al.*, 2005). Patients with either heterozygous or homozygous D146N mutation in *EPM2B* have an atypical milder LD consisting of a later onset of symptoms, longer disease course and extended preservation of daily living activities (Baykan *et al.*, 2005; Franceschetti *et al.*, 2006; Singh *et al.*, 2006; Ferlazzo *et al.*, 2014). Interestingly these "mild" cases had also a less severe seizure phenotype (sometimes with some degree of fluctuation from one day to another), and a lower probability to show both photoparoxysmal response and giant somatosensory evoked potentials as compared to typical LD patients (Ferlazzo *et al.*, 2014).

Sixty to seventy percent of LD are due to mutations in Laforin/dual specificity phosphatase (DSP) or *EPM2A* while 30–40% are due to mutations in Malin/E3 Ubiquitin ligase or *EPM2B*.

Serratosa *et al.* (1995) used linkage analysis and homozygosity mapping to assign a gene for Lafora's disease *(EMP2A)* to 6q23–q25. Minassian *et al.* (1998) and Serratosa *et al.* (1999) reported mutations in *EPM2A* that encodes a protein called laforin, originally thought to be a protein tyrosine phosphatase and subsequently proven to be an atypical dual specificity phosphatase (Ganesh *et al.*, 2000). Mutation analysis revealed marked allelic heterogeneity in *EPM2A* (Gomez-Garre *et al.*, 2000).

However, one mutation, R241stop, was found in approximately 40% of Lafora disease patients from Spain, suggesting both founder effect and recurrence contributed to the relatively high prevalence of R241stop mutation in Spain. Laforin/DSP is associated with the plasma membrane and the rough endoplasmic reticulum, which is probably responsible for the elimination of intracellular glucosans, but might also have a direct effect on membrane excitability (Minassian *et al.*, 2001).

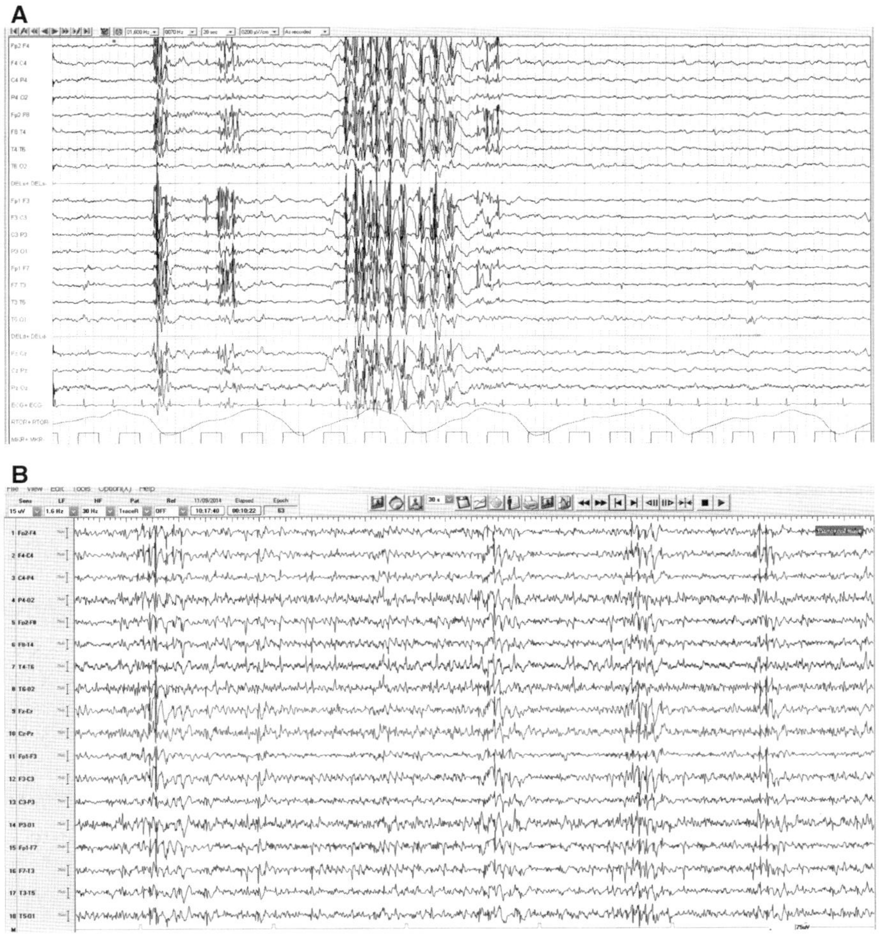

Figure 6

A: A 12-year-old girl with one year history of rare prolonged seizures with multiple coloured spots followed by loss of contact, nausea, vomitig and left upper arm jerks. There were also rare brief simple coloured spots and sporadic tonic-clonic seizures. At that time the diagnosis was benign occipital epilepsy of infancy. The EEG is characterized by normal background activity with superimposed generalized PSW discharges and left posterior focal spikes.
B: 2 years later the patient had developed myoclonic jerks in association with occipital seizures and had initial cognitive impairment. Note the slowing of the background activity and diffuse SWs associated with multiple focal spikes involving the posterior regions bilaterally. The patient was diagnosed as affected by LD by means of genetic testing analysis (homozygous mutation – c.323G>T- of the EPM2A gene).

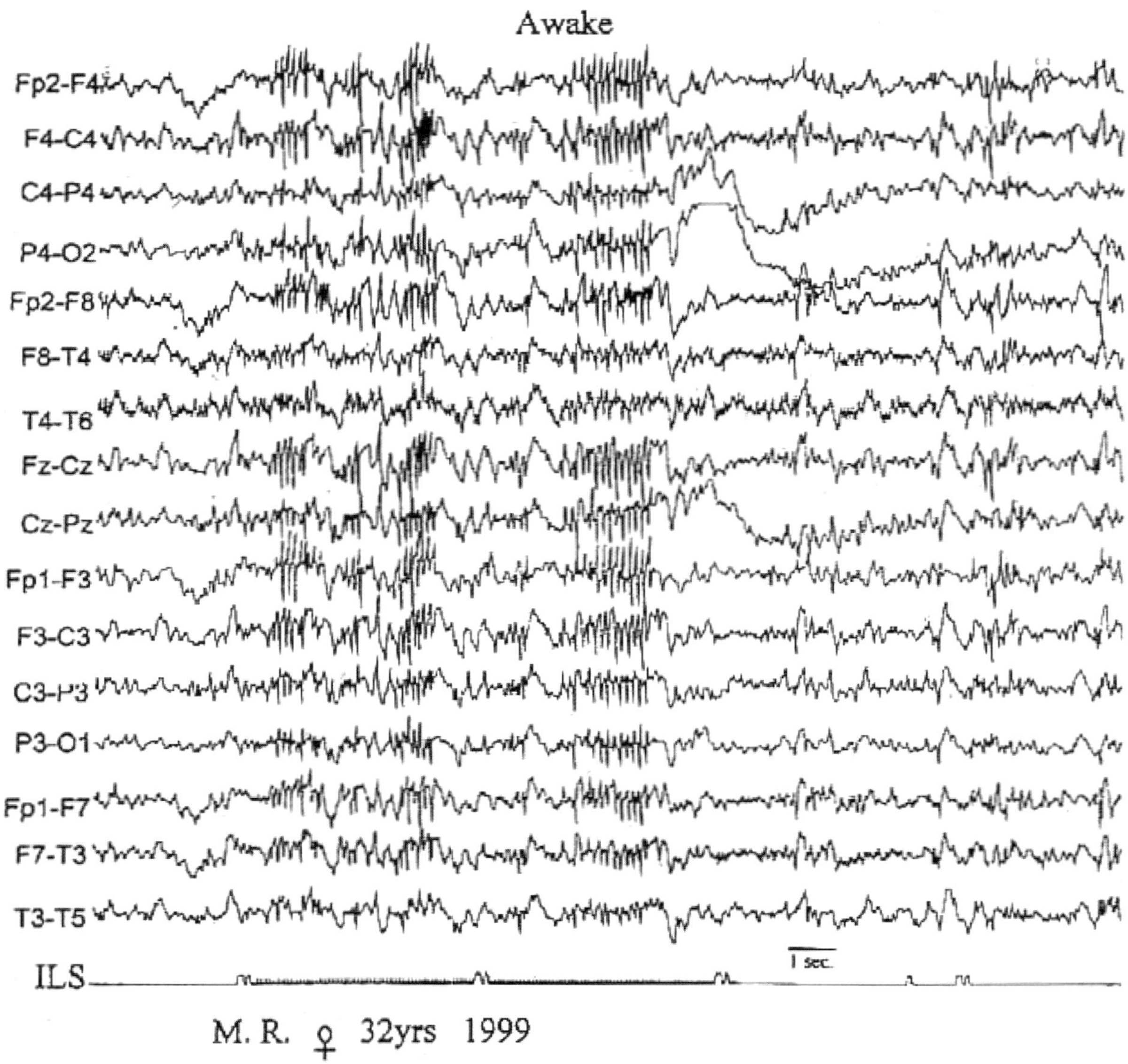

Figure 7

32-year-old LD female patient with a mild course of the disease. Note marked photosensitivity in association with a slow background activity with superimposed diffuse and multifocal spikes.

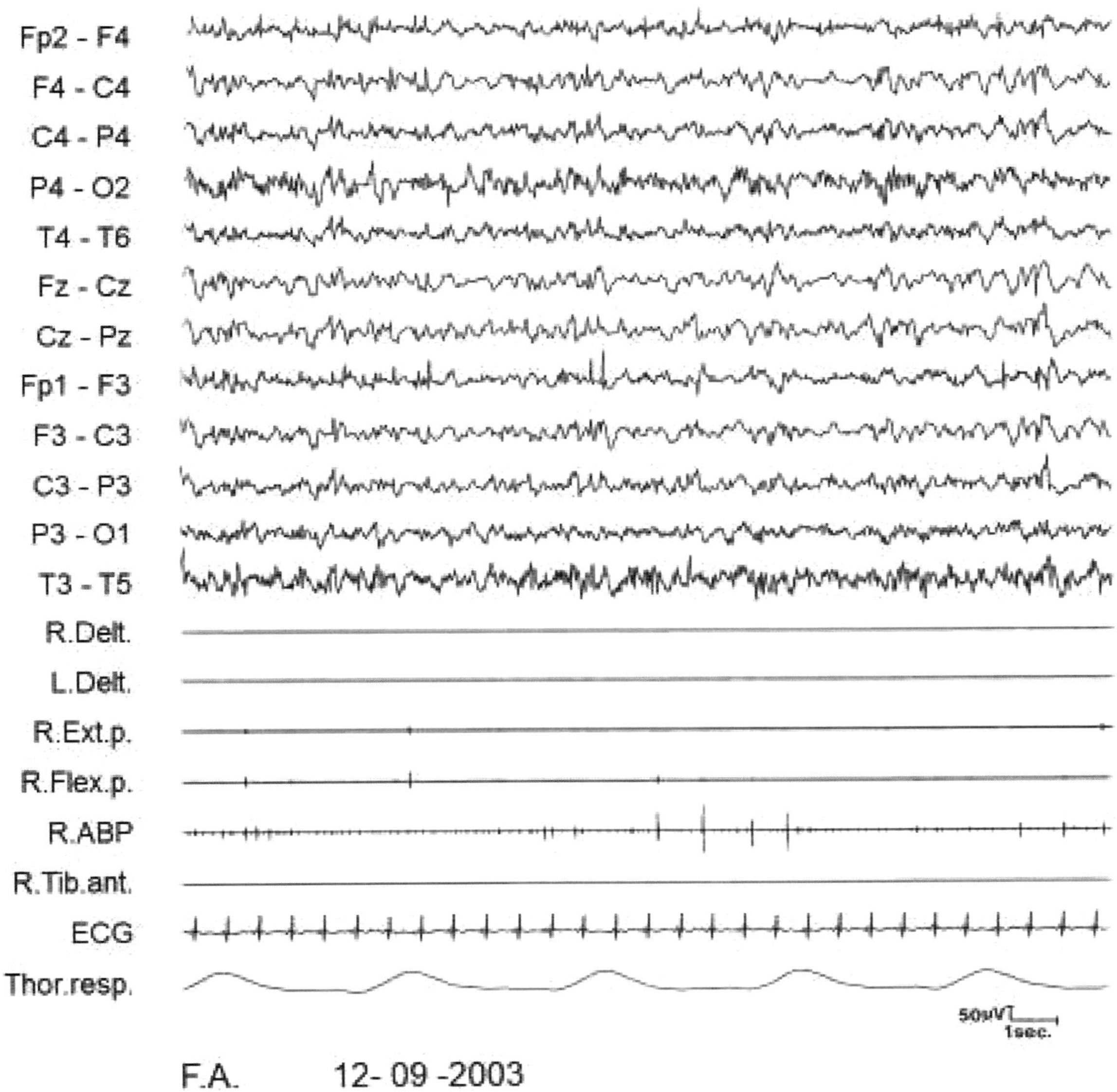

Figure 8

17-year-old male patient with LD. One can recognize marked slowing of the tracing, non modulated background activity and multiple focal spikes predominant over the central and posterior regions. Note the presence of erratic myoclonic jerks.

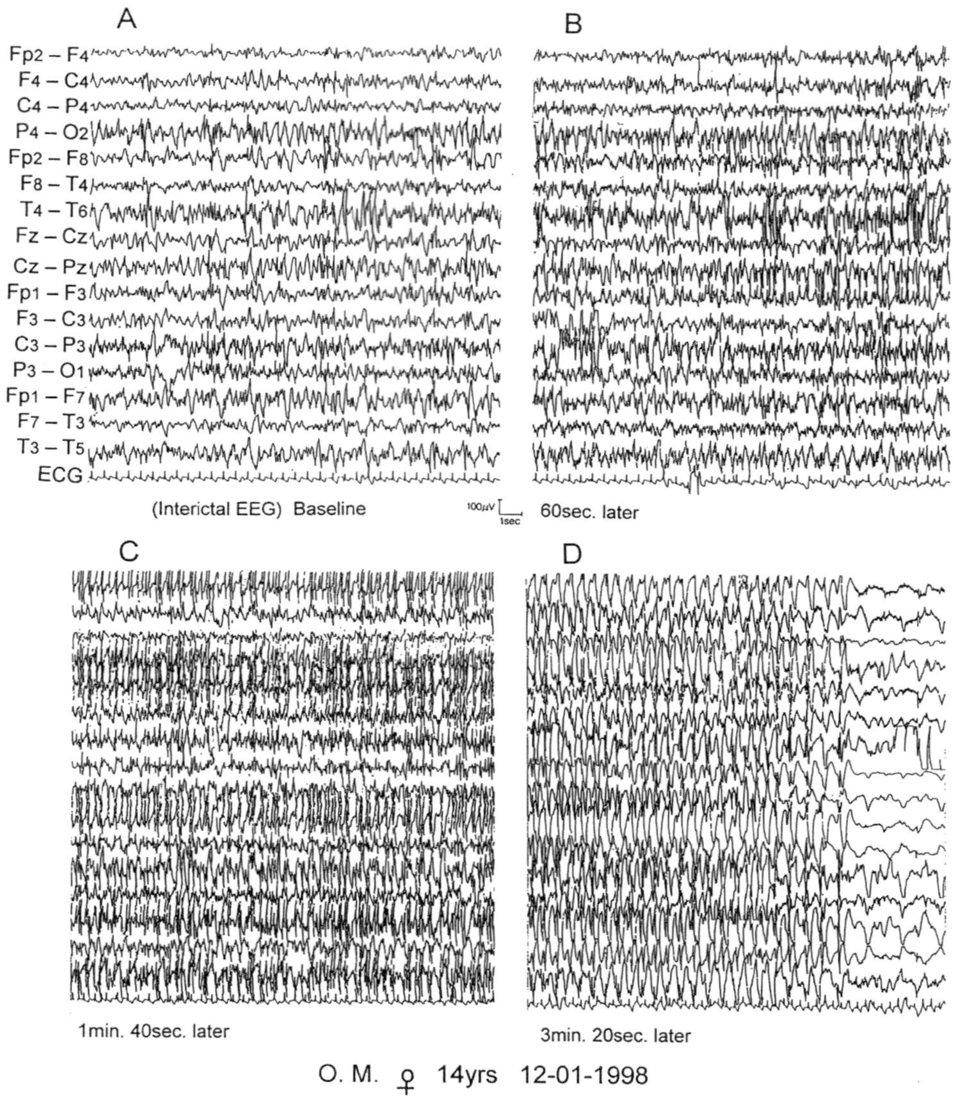

Figure 9

Appearently generalized motor seizure in a young female patient with Lafora disease. The seizure begins gradually, merging with the "interictal" background activity (a). The recruiting rhythm mainly involves the posterior regions (b) before diffusing to the whole hemispheres (c). Generalized slow SWs appear during the last stage of the seizure (d).

A second gene labelled *EPM2B* or *NHLRC1*, was mapped to 6p22 (Chan *et al.*, 2003a, 2003b). EPM2B encodes malin, a putative E3 ubiquitin ligase with a RING finger domain and six NHL motifs. Malin was found to colocalize with laforin and it was suggested that the malin-laforin interplay protected against polyglucosan body formation and epilepsy (Chan *et al.*, 2003b).

Overall the proportion of patients with *EPM2A* and *EPM2B* mutations varies among countries. In Spain *EPM2A* mutations are more common. In contrast, in Italy and France, *EPM2B* mutations predominate (Lesca *et al.*, 2010). In India and in Arabic countries, mutations are distributed evenly between *EPM2A* and *EPM2B*.

Two main mouse models of Lafora disease have been generated: the *epm2a-/-* knock-out mice *and* the *epm2b-/-* knock-out mice.

These models brought about explanations for two of the disease processes responsible for cell death in LD, accumulation of intracellular polyglucosan inclusion bodies and neurodegeneration (Ganesh *et al.*, 2002).

It was hypothesized that decreased Laforin phosphatase activities caused by EPM2a mutations result in hyperphosphorylated glycogen that forms poorly branched water-insoluble inclusions called LBs (Delgado-Escueta, 2007). LBs induce neuronal apoptosis and are the causative agent of LD. In this hypothesis of a secondarily flawed glycogen synthesis, there would be an imbalance between branching enzymes and glycogen synthase activities, glycogen synthase being favoured to go into overphosphorylated drive. The similarities between LBs and the accumulations seen in glycogen-branching enzyme deficiency, as well as data showing that overexpression of glycogen synthase can also cause plyglucosan accumulation (Raben *et al.*, 2001), support this hypothesis.

A variant of PTG, a protein that acts by activating glycogen synthase and inhibitory phosphorylase may reduce glycogen synthesis and explain a milder course of LD in some individuals (Guerrero *et al.*, 2011).

Recent hypotheses suggest that if laforin is missing phosphate accumulates and causes glycogen to become structurally abnormal an precipitate. If malin is missing reduced levels of laforin would again disturb the glycogen structure and favour its precipitation (Tiberia *et al.*, 2012). Updated reviews on the pathogenesis of LD are now available (Turnbull *et al.*, 2016; Gentry *et al.*, 2018).

Neuronal ceroid-lipofuscinoses

The neuronal ceroid-lipofuscinoses (NCL), also known as Batten Disease, are a group of neurodegenerative disorders characterized by the accumulation of autofluorescent storage positive material in the cytoplasm of neurons (Mole *et al.*, 2011). NCL are autosomal recessive conditions, classified as lysosomal storage disorders with enzymatic deficiency and structural protein dysfunction, and their clinical presentation involves major neurological symptoms (Mole *et al.*, 2005). They often but not always present as a PME, with major associated neurological and sensory (especially visual) symptoms, severe cognitive decline and motor impairment, and reduced life expectancy. NCL are rare disorders and are unequally distributed around the world, with "pockets" of higher prevalence where they are fairly common, as in Scandinavia. Classically, NCL-affected individuals have been classified into six categories (congenital, infantile, late infantile, variant late infantile, juvenile and adult) which have been mainly defined regarding the clinical onset of symptoms. However, some patients cannot be easily included in a specific group because of significant variation in the age, of onset and disease progression. Moreover, the infantile type (Santavuori *et al.*, 1974) and Northern epilepsy are not PMEs. Molecular genetics has emerged as a useful tool for enhancing subtype classification of NCL. There are 14 genetic forms (*CLN1* to *CLN14*) described to date and 360 etiological mutations, most of which have been included in the neuronal ceroid lipofuscinoses mutation database (www.ucl.ac.uk/ncl/mutation) (Kuosi *et al.*, 2012b). However, NCL are heterogeneous (Wisniewski, 2001) and most but not all of the patients with NCL can be categorized into one of the conditions recently confirmed by genetic studies, or in their variants, and further subtypes or variants are likely to exist. Despite genetic advances, for clinical purposes the classical forms of NCL will be listed according to age at onset of symptoms.

Late infantile ceroidlipofuscinosis (Jansky-Bielschowsky disease)

The late infantile NCL has been reported in various ethnic groups (Zeman *et al.*, 1970; Warburg, 1982), and is the form with the highest incidence outside Scandinavia. It begins between 1 and 4 years of age with locomotor impairment and ataxia, speech disorders and psychomotor regression; tonic-clonic seizures and myoclonus soon develop. Gradual blindness with optic atrophy generally begins before age 5, although the patients' vision usually remains fairly satisfactory for several years. The electroretinogram (ERG) is low in amplitude and later extinguished. The disease progresses rapidly and the patients are usually bedridden by the age of 5. Death occurs at the age of 3 to 10.

The EEG shows a slowing down of the background activity, slow, irregular bursts of spikes and PSW discharges. Characteristic very broad posterior polyphasic spikes are elicited by low-frequency flash stimuli *(Figure 10)*. The visual EPs are also broad, and these abnormal responses persist throughout the course of the disease (Pampiglione & Harden, 1977).

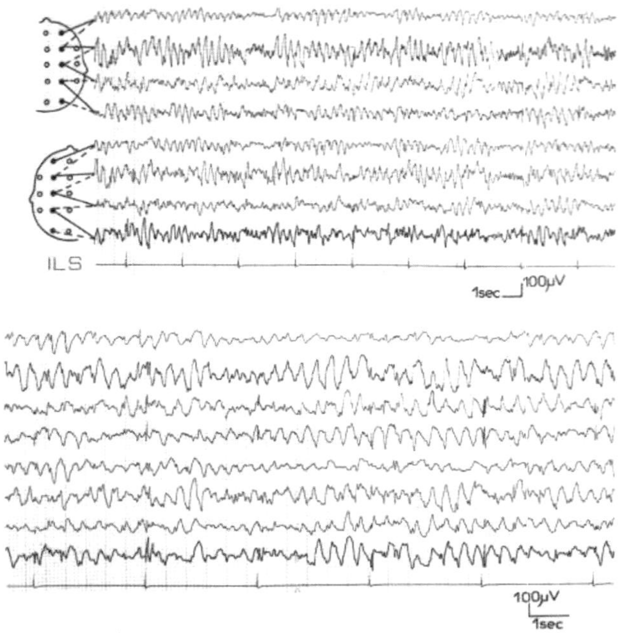

Figure 10 **5 years and 10 months old girl with late infantile NCL. Top: marked global slowing, subcontinuous slowing over the central regions and fast occipital spikes triggered by ILS flashes at 0.5 Hz. Bottom: At a slower recording speed, the time-relationship between the posterior spikes and the ILS flashes become more apparent.**

The diagnosis can be confirmed on the basis of electron microscopy showing curvilinear granular inclusions in skin, peripheral nerve or rectal mucous biopsy. The early or intermediate juvenile type described by Lake & Cavanagh (1978) on the basis of five cases has an intermediate onset, at the age of 5 to 8, and is also characterized by the fact that under electron microscopy both the curvilinear inclusions typical of the late infantile form, and the "fingerprint" profiles associated with the juvenile form are present.

The gene for the classical late infantile type of NCL *(CLN2)* maps to 11p15.5 (Sleat *et al.*, 1997; Haines *et al.*, 1998). It codes for a pepstatin-insensitive lysosomal peptidase. For prenatal diagnosis, the choice is between mutation analysis and electron microscopic examination of uncultured amniocytes for typical curvilinear bodies. A variant *(CLN5)* was identified in Finnish families and mapped to 13q21.1–q32 (Savukoski *et al.*, 1994), and the gene was shown to encode a putative transmembrane protein (Savukoski *et al.*, 1998). Another variant *(CLN6)* was reported in two consanguineous families originating from India (Sharp *et al.*, 1997) and mapped to 15q21–q23 (Gao *et al.*, 2002), at the same position where Haines *et al.* (1998) localized the gene underlying another variant found among the descendants of Spanish settlers in a small geographic area in Costa Rica. Further mutations of the *CLN6* gene were found in families from Pakistan, Roma Gypsies from Central Europe (Sharp *et al.*, 2003), Turkish (Siintola *et al.*, 2005) and Italian families (Canafoglia *et al.*, 2015). The *CLN6* gene was cloned and encodes linelin, a putative membrane-spanning protein (Gao *et al.*, 2002; Wheeler *et al.*, 2002) and has also been implicated in the adult form of NCL (see below). Interestingly only the *CLN6* patients with a teenage or adult onset presented with a classic PME phenotype before the onset of motor or cognitive impairment (Canafoglia *et al.*, 2015). The *CLN7* variant has been described in Turkish families and has distinct clinical and genetic features. Another variant, *CLN8*, also found in a subset of Turkish families, shares its locus with Northern Epilepsy (Ranta *et al.*, 2004).

Juvenile ceroidlipofuscinosis (Spielmeyer-Vogt-Sjögren disease)

The juvenile form of CLF was first described by Stengel in Norway in 1826, and later by Sjögren (1931) and by Zeman *et al.* (1970) in great detail. The gene seems to be present in nearly 1 per cent of Swedes, and the disease is particularly widespread in all the Scandinavian countries but remains uncommon elsewhere. It begins between the age of 4 and 14 (in 70% of all cases between the age of 6 and 10), and takes a fairly stereotyped course. The first symptom is a drop in visual acuity due to retinitis pigmentosa. Impairment of mental functions soon becomes evident and progresses gradually and steadily. The first neurological symptoms with onset only 2 to 3 years after the first visual symptoms are extrapyramidal signs followed by ataxia and then by pyramidal symptoms. Absence seizures or more commonly tonic-clonic seizures, begin one to four years after the onset. Segmental myoclonias begin to appear at this stage, affecting the muscles of the face in particular, and sustained myoclonic seizures eventually develop. Myoclonus is aggravated by passive movements. Massive myoclonias can proceed to clonic seizures, and clonic status is common at the terminal stage. These symptoms, however, can occur in a different sequence in about 40% of the cases, which can blur the diagnosis in the early stages, with seizures and myoclonus occurring before the characteristic visual decline (Berkovic & Andermann, 1986).

Schooling can generally be continued up to age of 10 years. At this age, the patients begin to adopt a characteristic stooping posture and articulate with difficulty due to dysarthria. They are confined to a wheelchair because of myoclonus and motor dyspraxia. Psychotic episodes can further complicate the issue, and patients used to die around age 20 years. However, improved social and educational amenities which have become available to these patients over the last years, together with improved medical care, have resulted in an increase in the life expectancy of those suffering from this disease.

In the early stages, the EEG shows a slowing of the background activity and sometimes sustained paroxysmal bursts; the changes are increased during sleep. Photic stimulation does not affect the EEG or the clinical symptoms as it does in the case of the late infantile form. The visual EPs gradually disappear, whereas the amplitude of the somatosensory EPs increases.

The diagnosis can be confirmed by evidence of vacuolated lymphocytes in peripheral blood and characteristic fingerprint profiles in the ultrastructural study of skin biopsy or lymphocytes; curvilinear inclusions can also be encountered (Goebel *et al.*, 1979). None of the various subtypes of storage material is really specific for one of the clinical forms of NCL (Carpenter *et al.*, 1977). Prenatal diagnosis can be based on electron microscopy of chorionic villi (Uvebrandt *et al.*, 1987).

The juvenile NCL was linked to chromosome 16 (Gardiner *et al.*, 1990), and a deletion has been reported on the 16S298 locus (Taschner *et al.*, 1995). The *CLN3* gene encodes for a 438-amino acid protein (International Batten disease consortium, 1995), which is a likely resident of the lysosomal/endosomal membrane, and although its function is still elusive, significant dysfunction of the lysosomal membrane is probably the major feature of this condition (Phillips *et al.*, 2005). Antenatal diagnosis is possible on amniocentesis or on chorionic biopsy material (McLeod *et al.*, 1988; Conradi *et al.*, 1989). A novel genetic variant, *CLN9*, has been described in two Serbian and German families, with extensive cellular metabolic changes, but an overall clinical presentation very similar to *CLN3* (Schulz *et al.*, 2004).

The adult form of CLF: Kufs' disease

Described by Hugo Friedrich Kufs in 1925, the adult form of NCL has a much lower incidence, appears mostly as a sporadic condition, and may be heterogenous. Type A patients present with PME, type B patients with dementia and a variety of associated movement disorders. The age at which the onset of this late form occurs ranges from 11 to 50 years (Berkovic *et al.*, 1988). As the disease develops, the symptoms are dementia accompanied by a whole range of motor deficits (ataxia, dyskinesia, athetosis), as well as convulsive seizures and myoclonias at the terminal stage, which can also take the form of epilepsy with myoclonus and gradual dementia where the neurological symptoms are more variable and inconsistent. The prognosis is very poor, since the outcome is usually fatal 10 years on average after the onset.

On EEG recordings, the background activity is slow, and generalized spike-wave discharges can be observed. One particularly noteworthy feature, however, is the high EEG and clinical sensitivity to low frequency photostimulation, which is extremely rare in adults. Visual and auditory EPs are normal, whereas giant somatosensory EPs are sometimes recorded. Histological analysis of hepatic and cutaneous biopsy samples can be difficult because of the physiological deposits of lipofuscin which accumulate with age. Typical alterations can often only be observed in brain biopsy samples, where "fingerprint" deposits and osmiophilic granular profiles can be observed under electron microscopy. Brain biopsy, which is rarely justified in the diagnosis of other types of PME, may remain a useful diagnostic tool in patients with Kuf's disease.

Most cases appear as sporadic, but a sibling pair has been reported from Ireland (Callagy *et al.*, 2000). A novel, autosomal dominant adult-onset NCL has been reported from the Netherlands (Nijssen *et al.*, 2003) in 3 affected members of a family, with ultrastructural changes not unlike those found in *CLN1*. A genetic study of sporadic and familial cases showed that *CLN6*, previously associated with late infantile NCL, was the major gene responsible for the late-onset, type A PME phenotype (Arsov *et al.*, 2011), but there is no explanation for the important differences in phenotypes between the late infantile and adult NCL. On the other hand mutations of *STSF* gene, encoding cathepsin F, a lysosomal cysteine protease, have been identified in Kuf's type B (Smith *et al.*, 2013).

Berkovic *et al.* (2016), by reevaluating the diagnosis in 47 unsolved patients collected worldwide and referred for possible Kuf's disease, confirmed the diagnosis by expert pathologic analysis and recent molecular genetic advances in only 1/3 of cases. Therefore, the diagnosis remains challenging.

Myoclonic epilepsy with "ragged-red fibres"

Myoclonic epilepsy associated with ragged-red muscular fibres (MERRF) was described by Fukuhara *et al.* in 1980, subsequent to a few preliminary reports (Tsairis *et al.*, 1973; Shapira *et al.*, 1975), and ascribed to the growing category of mitochondrial encephalomyopathies (ME). The number of patients presenting with MERRF amounts to only a very small percentage of all the cases of mitochondrial encephalomyopathy. The disease is transmitted with the mitochondrial genetic material along the maternal line in most cases (Rosing *et al.*, 1985; Harding & Holt, 1988). Pathological antecedents are often to be found among previous generations. The clinical symptoms are variable from one case to another, even among family members. Although initially described in Japan, MERRF appears to have a worldwide distribution, but remains very uncommon.

The age of onset varies between 3 and 65 years of age (Roger *et al.*, 1991). The full PME picture can occur, sometimes with focal seizures or more typically with generalized seizures. Scotogenic myoclonic seizures have been reported (Koubeissi *et al.*, 2009). A wide range of associated neurological symptoms differentiates MERRF from the other forms of PME: in a review covering 48 cases of MERRF (Roger *et al.*, 1991), there were 25 cases of deafness, 14 cases with clinical signs of myopathy, 11 cases of lactic acidosis, 11 cases of optic atrophy, 9 cases of nanism, 9 of sensory disorders, 8 cases of spasticity, 6 cases with clinical or electromyographic signs of peripheral neuropathy, 5 cases with loss of tendon reflexes, 3 cases with focal neurological symptoms, and 1 case with lipomas. The cases described by May & White (1968), involving myoclonus, ataxia and deafness and those reported by Ekbom in 1985, involving ataxia, photomyoclonus, skeletal anomalies and lipomas, probably come under the heading of MERRF. There are furthermore numerous cases in which the symptomatology of MERRF overlaps with symptoms of other ME.

The order in which the various symptoms of MERRF occur with time varies from one case to another, the onset of neurological, sensory or mental symptoms can occur several years before that of epileptic seizures, myoclonus and ataxia. Electrophysiological studies (So *et al.*, 1989; Roger *et al.*, 1991) have shown the existence of background activity anomalies (in 80% of all cases), SW discharges and generalized PSWs (73%), diffuse slow delta bursts (33%), focal anomalies (40%) and photosensitivity (26%). The normal physiological sleep patterns were either attenuated or abolished. In two cases spikes were recorded in the central regions and the vertex during REM sleep (*Figure 11*) (Roger *et al.*, 1991). Giant visual EPs were recorded in all these cases. In patients with MERRF, signs of diffuse cerebral atrophy, white matter lesions of various sizes, hypodensities or calcifications of the basal ganglia, and focal cortical hypodensities can be observed using CT scan or MRI.

The course and prognosis of MERRF vary greatly. Death can occur anytime between 3 and 30 years after the onset (Roger *et al.*, 1991). Some cases were described where the disease developed over a long period on similar lines to MERRF before complications arose, consisting of acute stroke-like episodes reminiscent of MELAS (mitochondrial encephalomyopathy with lactic acidosis and stroke-like episodes) (Byrne *et al.*, 1988; Fukuhara, 1991), and such overlap forms are not uncommon (Mongini *et al.*, 2002). Indeed, there is a spectrum of neurological symptoms in patients presenting with the three classical forms of ME, *i.e.*, MERRF, MELAS and Leigh syndrome: among 31 patients with ME, most (43% of adults, 70% of children) had an atypical clinical presentation, epilepsy was the first presenting symptoms in 53% of all cases, and even photosensitivity, which is common in MERRF, was found in one patient with MELAS and one with Leigh syndrome (Canafoglia *et al.*, 2001). Indeed, in a five-generation Belgian family with 12 affected members, a m14487T>C missense mutation affecting complex I of the mitochondrial respiratory chain, previously reported in sporadic pediatric cases with Leigh syndrome, was responsible for various phenotypes depending on the mutation load, with adult-onset PME as one of the options (Dermaut *et al.*, 2010).

MERRF can be diagnosed on the basis of the typical "ragged red fibres" observed in muscle biopsy samples. When the results are negative, it is sometimes necessary to repeat the tests on a different group of muscles; in some patients, mitochondrial abnormalities can be observed in skin tissue (Berkovic *et al.*, 1989). Even in cases with normal pathological muscular findings, it is sometimes possible to locate the seat of the deficit by performing biochemical analysis of the mitochondrial respiratory chain (Bindoff *et al.*, 1991). This however involves the use of a complex, difficult technique which cannot be applied routinely. Non-invasive techniques, such as nuclear magnetic resonance or the 2-keto[1-(13)C]isocaproicacid breath test can also be applied in screening for mitochondrial disorders (review in Parra *et al.*, 2001). However, strictly negative pathological and biochemical studies cannot exclude the diagnosis of MERRF, which relies on genetic testing for the most common mitochondrial mutation (Mancuso *et al.*, 2007).

The above mentioned procedures, starting with muscle biopsy, should be performed in clinically unclear cases, but typical forms of MERRF (as other mitochondrial disorders) are now diagnosed primarily using molecular biology and the detection of mitochondrial DNA (mDNA) mutations. The first description was reported by Shoffner *et al.* in 1990. This mutation was also present in several relatives of one of the MERRF patients who presented with other clinical forms of mitochondrial encephalomyopathy involving no myoclonus epilepsy. This mutation can also be found, albeit rarely, in families with very different phenotypes, including ophtalmoplegia and reversible respiratory failure (Wiedermann *et al.*, 2008). After this initial description, other studies have shown that the A8344G mutation is responsible for most cases of MERRF (Hammans *et al.*, 1991). In the years following the discovery of the A8344G mutation, three additional point mutations have also been found in patients with MERRF in the tRNALys gene of mtDNA as follows: T8356C, G8361A and G8363A (Rossmanith *et al.*, 2003; Santorelli *et al.*, 1996; Silvestri *et al.*, 1992). The T8356C point mutation was found in patients with MERRF who also had stroke-like episodes, suggesting an overlap between MERRF and mitochondrial encephalomyopathy with lactic acidosis and stroke-like episodes (MELAS) (Silvestri *et al.*, 1992; Nakamura *et al.*, 2010). The A8361G point mutation was described in patients associated with MERRF manifesting with deafness and dementia (Rossmanith *et al.*, 2003). The G8363A point mutation appears to be related to the presence of cardiomyopathy and deafness in patients with MERRF,

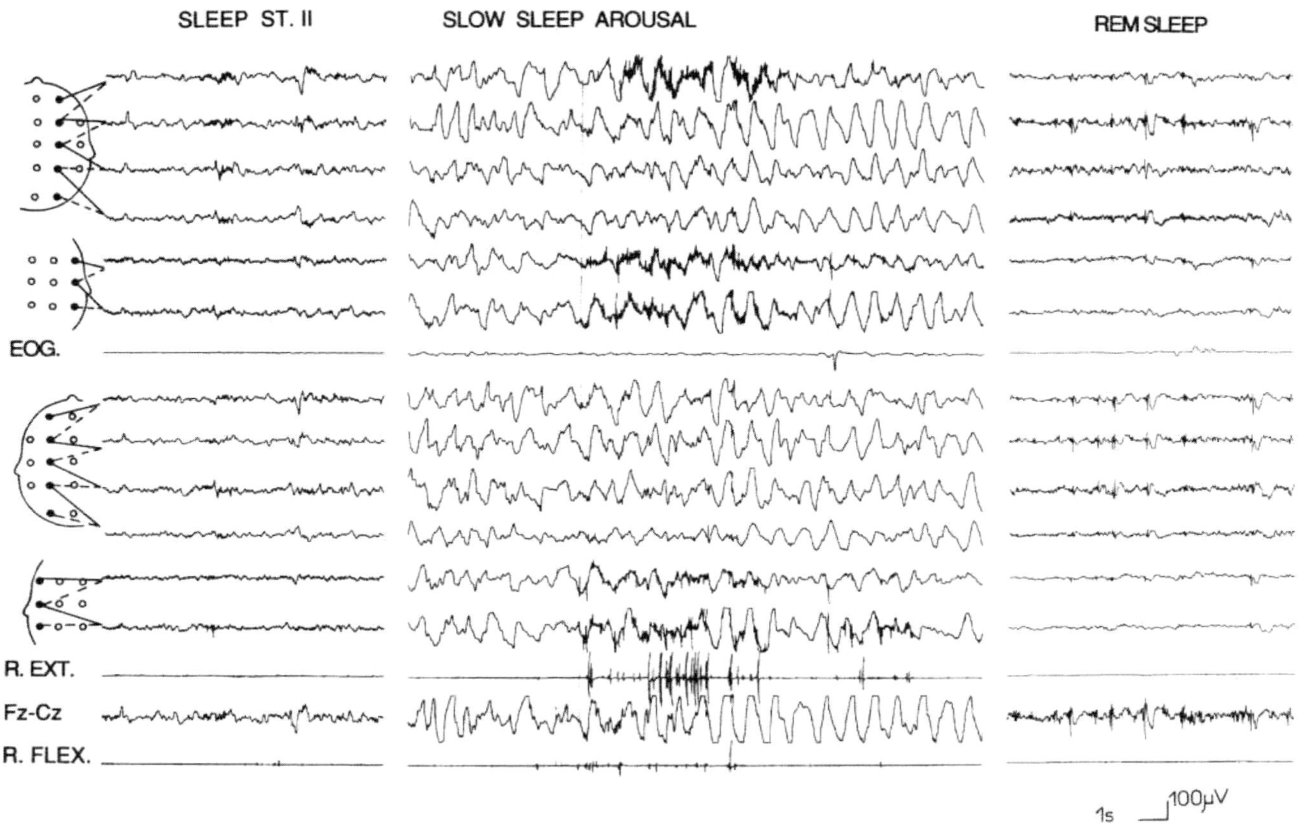

Figure 11

17-year-old male patient with MERRF. Left: **Light NREM sleep with sleep spindles and low-voltage spikes over the central areas. Middle: occurrence of myoclonic jerks during an arousal from NREM sleep.** Right: **During REM sleep, fast spikes and polyspikes over the vertex and central regions.**

and, in some cases, it overlaps with Leigh syndrome (Santorelli *et al.*, 1996). It is estimated that the A8344G mutation remains responsible for over 80% of MERRF patients: mutations T8356C, G8361A and G8363A account for approximately 10%. The remaining mutations account for less than 5% of cases, but up to 10% of MERRF patients have still no identifiable mutations in mtDNA (Hammans *et al.*, 1991; Fukuhara, 1995). The A8344G mutation appears to be specific to patients with MERRF, because this mutation has rarely been described in other mitochondrial diseases (Zeviani *et al.*, 1991). Additionally, MERRF patients who present with other mutations in mtDNA have usually been reported to present with another mitochondrial disease, such as MELAS, Leigh syndrome, Kearns-Sayre syndrome, NARP, neuropathy, deafness or pigmentary retinopathy. A MELAS/MERRF phenotype was reported in patients with a G12147A mutation (Melone *et al.*, 2004) or with a 5521G>A mutation (Herrero-Martin *et al.*, 2010).

An association with the Kearns-Sayre syndrome was described in a family with a *G3255A* mutation (Nishigaki *et al.*, 2003). A case was reported with a typical MERRF phenotype and a mutation typical for the MELAS phenotype (Brackmann *et al.*, 2012). The polymorphism of the phenotype might be due to the fact that the levels of mutant DNA vary from one subject to another (and from one tissue to another). Although the mitochondrial diseases caused by point mutations of mtDNA have heterogeneous phenotypes, the phenotype of patients with the A8344G point mutation usually results in MERRF. In rare cases, the presence of rearrangement type deletion in mtDNA or the presence of recessive missense mutations in polymerase gamma (*POLG*) gene in nuclear DNA has been associated with MERRF (Van Goethem *et al.*, 2003). Interestingly, mitochondrial dysfunction is also implied in the pathogenesis of abnormal, epileptic brain activity in seizure foci and in experimental epileptogenesis (review in Kunz, 2002). One of the mechanisms by which mitochondrial diseases, including MERRF, may cause neurological symptoms is an increased susceptibility of humans cells to apoptosis (Liu *et al.*, 2004).

Dentato-rubral-pallido-luysian atrophy

This disease with autosomal dominant transmission has been described in Japan (Naito & Oyanagi, 1982) and involves neuropathological degeneration of both the dentato-rubral and the pallido-luysian systems (Iizuka *et al.*, 1984). Although the prevalence of dentato-rubral-pallido-luysian atrophy (DRPLA) remains higher in Japan, it has now been recognized as a very uncommon disorder in other parts of the world, including the USA (where it was called the Haw River syndrome, due to a "pocket" of prevalence in African-Americans in a region of North Carolina) (Burke *et al.*, 1994) and various European countries with the inclusion of France (Destee *et al.*, 2000; Le Ber *et al.*, 2003), Turkey (Yis *et al.*, 2009) and Taiwan (Lee *et al.*, 2001). DRPLA patients in four Portuguese families apparently share a common Japanese ancestor, as shown by the fact that they have common allele that is also prevalent in Japan (Martins *et al.*, 2003). In another case, affected by mental retardation and epilepsy, DRPLA was diagnosed only when it became known the existence of a maternal aunt with a more typical form of the condition (Casseron *et al.*, 2004).

Diverse clinical pictures have been described and the onset has been reported to occur between 6 and 69 years of age. Nearly half of the cases where the onset occurs between childhood and adulthood present with PME symptoms sometimes associated with other neurological disorders, such as choreoathetosis, rapidly developing dementia or psychosis, and ataxia. Individuals with onset before age 20 years usually have a PME phenotype characterized by myoclonus, seizures, ataxia, and progressive intellectual deterioration (Naito & Oyanagi, 1982; Ikeuchi *et al.*, 1995; Tsuji, 2012). Various forms of generalized seizures (including tonic, atonic, clonic, or tonic-clonic seizures) are also observed (Tsuji, 2012). Mental deterioration is found in most cases. The EEG shows slow bursts and generalized SW discharges; no consistent pattern of photosensitivity has been observed. Patients with later onset present with various movement disorders, and choreoathetosis is also a frequent symptom in the "myoclonic" patients when they grow older. Atrophic changes in the cerebellum and brain stem, in particular the pontine tegmentum, are the typical MRI findings of DRPLA.

The genetic anomaly responsible for DRPLA was characterized as an unstable CAG triplet expansion in the exon 5 of the *atrophin* gene on chromosome 14 (Koide *et al.*, 1994). In general, an inverse correlation exists between the age at onset and the size of the expanded *ATN1* CAG repeat (Koide *et al.*, 1994; Ikeuchi *et al.*, 1995). As in other genetically transmitted diseases with unstable expansions, a genetic anticipation is possible, the most severe cases, with the earliest onset being usually related to paternal transmission. Some of the gene carriers, especially in older generations, may be nearly asymptomatic. The prevalence of the condition is probably correlated to the prevalence, in the general population, of intermediate-sized alleles containing more than 30 CAG repeats: this prevalence was 1% in the Chinese population, compared to 3% in the Japanese, which might account for the comparativeley lower prevalence of DRPLA in ethnic Chinese (Lee *et al.*, 2001). Interestingly, as in other triplet repeat diseases, there is marked somatic mosaicism concerning the size of the expansion, and in DRPLA, the largest expansions were shown to be present in glial and Pukinje cells of the cerebellum, compared with the granular cells in an early-onset patient, but they were greatest in glial cells and less in Purkinje cells in a late-onset form (Hashida *et al.*, 2001). The abnormal gene products are mutant proteins, atrophin-1, containing expanded polyglutamine stretches; the formation of intranuclear aggregates may play a part in the neuronal degeneration seen in DRPLA (Tsuji, 2000; Yamada *et al.*, 2002), but the main pathogenic factor appears to be the diffuse accumulation of the mutant atrophin-1 in nuclei. A Drosophilia model of DRPLA has been produced, in which the pathogenetic mechanism of the disease, differing from the human condition, apparently rests on severe lysosomal dysfunction (Charroux & Fanto, 2010). A mouse model with 129 CAG repeats, on the other hand, had a devastating progressive neurological condition associated with intranuclear inclusions but without evident neuronal deaths (Sato *et al.*, 2008).

Dementias and PME: neuroserpinosis, Azheimer's disease and senile myoclonic epilepsy in Down syndrome

Neuroserpin, a member of the serine proteinase inhibitor (serpin) superfamily, plays a major role in synaptogenesis and provides neuronal protection. Point mutations in neuroserpin cause aberrant conformational transitions and the formation of polymers that form inclusion bodies in the endoplasmic reticulum (Miranda & Lomas, 2006). Familial encephalopathy with neuroserpin inclusion bodies (FENIB) is an autosomal dominant form of presenile dementia (Bradshaw *et al.*, 2001) that may present with a PME phenotype. In a French family, a S52R mutation was associated with a severe PME and a frontal syndrome (Gourfinkel-An *et al.*, 2007). Sporadic non familial cases may also occur (Hagen *et al.*, 2011) and *SERPINI1* mutations are an emerging cause of childhood onset PMEs (Ranza *et al.*, 2017).

Myoclonus may be a minor feature in many of the known dementia syndromes, including multiple system atrophy, corticobasal degeneration, progressive supranuclear palsy, frontotemporal dementia, Alzheimer's disease (AD), Parkinson's disease, and other Lewy body disorders (review in Caviness, 2003). The common forms of Alzheimer's disease may be associated with myoclonus in the very late stages of their evolution. However, both the rapidly progressive forms of AD (Schmidt *et al.*, 2010) and the early-onset, familial types of AD (review in Bird, 2010) can present with a phenotype of PME, with massive and erratic jerks, in association with the disease-specific cognitive disturbances that always precede the onset of epilepsy and myoclonus. A striking PME phenotype closely following the onset of memory disorder and disorientation, around age 50, was reported in a Japanese family (Furuya *et al.*, 2003). Thus some patients, with a primary dementing disorder, may present, at some stage, with a PME phenotype. Mutation of C9orf72 was found in patient with a teen-age onset of PME followed by psychiatric disorders and dementia (van den Ameele *et al.*, 2018).

Middle-aged and elderly Down syndrome patients very commonly present a recognizable condition, called senile myoclonic epilepsy (Genton & Paglia, 1994; De Simone *et al.*, 2010) or late-onset myoclonic epilepsy in Down syndrome (Möller *et al.*, 2002) with a very reproducible sequence of events. The first symptoms of cognitive deterioration precede by 1–2 years the onset of massive myoclonic jerks, followed by GTCS and erratic myoclonus, with a fast evolution within a few years to severe dementia, full dependency and death. The patients have the neuropathologic markers of AD. This condition, which has been detailed in chapter 29, occurs in most ageing Down syndrome patients, and may well be the most common of all PMEs.

Sialidosis

The "cherry-red spot myoclonus" described in 1978 (Rapin *et al.*) is the normosomatic type 1 sialidosis, as opposed to type 2, or galactosialidosis, which is associated with dysmorphia. The biochemical impairment affects neuraminidase (α-2,6, sialidase), that is the key enzyme for the intralysosomal catabolism of sialylated glycoconjugates by removing their terminal sialic acid residues. It is inherited by recessive autosomal transmission and occurs in children of both sexes. These patients are often of Italian origin (Lowden & O'Brien, 1979), but this disease is also relatively common in Japan. Molecular studies have shed some light on the phenotypic variations. There are two main phenotypes, type I and type II sialidosis (Lowden & O'Brien, 1979), and both may present as a PME: in type I, there are no bone changes and the patients have normal intellect; type II (which has been divided into congenital, infantile and juvenile) is more severe, with earlier onset, dysostosis, coarse facies, possible optic atrophy and developmental delay.

In type I, which often presents as a typical PME, onset of the disease is characterized by moderate visual deficit, myoclonus and generalized epileptic seizures between the ages of 8 and 25, and much later onset, in middle age, has been reported (Sakazume *et al.*, 2004). Accompanying symptoms are pains of the "burning hands and feet" type, which are aggravated by exposure to heat, and ataxia. The fundus shows a cherry-red spot, which is sometimes associated with opaque, punctiform spots on the vitreous body (Durand *et al.*, 1977). In a study from Taiwan (Lai *et al.*, 2009), only 17.6% of patients had the cherry-red spot, but 82.3% developed the typical PME within five years. The myoclonias are spontaneous, and enhanced by voluntary movements and movement programming, as well as by contact. Bilateral jerks can be induced by sensory stimuli. One of the most characteristic features is the occurrence of facial myoclonias, which are spontanenous, irregular, occur predominantly around the mouth, and are insensitive to stimuli. Unlike myoclonias of the limbs, they persist during sleep.

Recently 6 adult patients belonging to 2 families have been described showing high-frequency myoclonus but no seizures and without the cardinal signs suggesting sialidosis, such as typical ocular signs and significant urinary sialic acid excretion (Canafoglia *et al.*, 2014). The EEG shows a normal to fast, low-voltage background activity, which tends to slow down as the signs of dementia appear. No photosensivity is observed. Massive myoclonias are associated with generalized SW discharges. The amplitude of the visual evoked potentials (VEP) is decreased, but that of the somatosensory EP is enlarged. Neurophysiological studies have underlined the severity of myoclonus, *e.g.*, compared to ULD (Canafoglia *et al.*, 2011). The prognosis is poor in most cases, since the myoclonus rapidly becomes severe and incapacitating. The seizures usually respond to treatment, but there exists no efficient treatment for the myoclonus. Cases have nevertheless been reported where the disease has followed a long-term course.

The biological deficit can be observed *in vitro* in lymphocytes and fibroblasts. The urinary elimination of oligosaccharides is increased. In heterozygous parents, an intermediate deficit can be observed in the neuraminidase levels. Prenatal diagnosis is possible on amniotic cell cultures (Johnson *et al.*, 1980).

The gene coding for the α-neuraminidase is located on 6p21.3 Numerous mutations have been described, and there may be a correlation between the type of mutation and the functional consequences (Bonten *et al.*, 2000; Itoh *et al.*, 2002). There is a high inverse correlation between the amount of residual enzyme activity and the severity of the condition. A study of two patients with different mutations confirmed that a V217M mutation had less consequences (with late onset and mild course) than a G243R mutation (with completely absent lysosomal neuraminidase activity) (Naganawa *et al.*, 2000). Nullizygous transgenic mice models at the Neu1 locus develop the clinical abnormalities found in early-onset sialidosis in children, including severe nephropathy, progressive oedema, splenomegaly, kyphosis and urinary excretion of sialylated oligosaccharides (De Geest *et al.*, 2002).

Galactosialidosis is characterized by deficient protein/cathepsin A (PPCA), leading to neuraminidalse and β-galactosidase inactivation by lysosomes. The infantile type is not a PME, and presents with ascites, oedema, skeletal changes in the spine, cardiomegaly, with death usually before age one year due to cardiac and renal failure.

The late infantile type is characterized by ataxia, coarse facial features, bone changes, mild mental retardation and hearing loss, but seizures are rare. The juvenile/adult type of galactosialidosis, however, often presents as a PME, with onset in adolescence, or later, into the fourth decade. Cherry red spot, corneal clouding, vision loss are present, as are chondrodystrophy short stature and quite characteristically angiokeratomas. In heterozygous parents, an intermediate neuraminidase deficit is sometimes observed, while the β-galactosidase deficit is not detectable. Prenatal diagnosis is possible by chorionic villus sampling (Kleijer *et al.*, 1979) or amniocentesis.

Less common forms of progressive myoclonus epilepsy

Gaucher's disease

Type III Gaucher's disease, which can present as PME, occurs more rarely than types I and II, and overlap with type II has been reported (Goker-Alpan *et al.*, 2003). Gaucher's disease is more prevalent among Ashkenazy Jews, and type III represents a comparatively mild form. The condition involves a storage of glucocerebroside in various organs. The age of onset varies greatly between childhood and early adulthood. The first symptoms are often saccadic horizontal eye movements and supranuclear gaze paralysis, which can be associated with strabismus, along with generalized or focal seizures. Ataxia, moderate intellectual impairment and low oculo-manual dexterity are also generally observed (Benko *et al.*, 2011). The patients are sometimes found to have hepatosplenomegaly. The typical PME phenotype is present in only a minority of cases (Kraoua *et al.*, 2010). The EEG shows a normal to slow background activity and bursts of predominantly posterior or multifocal spikes or PSW waves (Nishimura *et al.*, 1980) *(Figure 12)*. The patients are sensitive to photic stimulation, which elicits a myoclonic response. The visual EPs are normal but the somatosensory EP are abnormally enlarged in some patients (Halliday & Halliday, 1980). There are hearing abnormalities, including poor brainstem auditory EPs (Bamiou *et al.*, 2001). Specific MRI studies may show extensive white matter changes (Davies *et al.*, 2011).

The disease can be diagnosed from evidence that glucocerebroside has been stored in various organs, circulating lymphocytes and bone marrow cells, and neuronal storage can be detected in material from appendectomy or rectal biopsy. There are increased levels of chitotriosidase in plasma. The enzyme deficit can be determined from lymphocyte or fibroblast cultures (Wenger, 1978). The disease is due to a mutation in the GBA (glucosidase beta acid) gene on chromosome 1q21, with a L444P substitution most common in type III. The prognosis varies considerably from one case to another, but a life expectancy of more than 10 years can usually be predicted. There is in Sweden a particular form of this disease, which is called the Norbottinian type, from the place where it occurs. The symptoms typical of this form are fairly homogeneous, and it was probably transmitted from a single source (Svennerholm *et al.*, 1982).

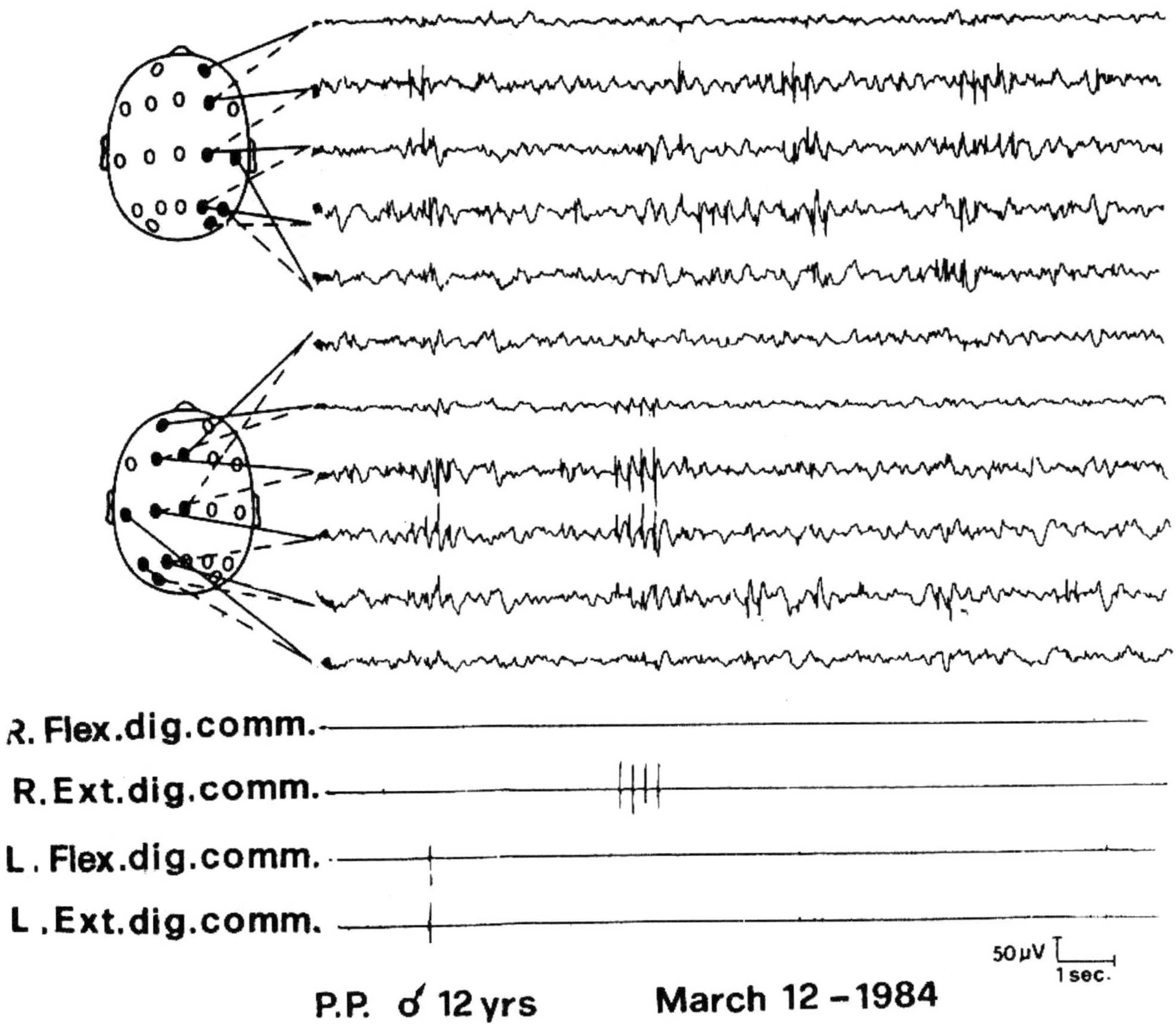

Figure 12

12-year-old boy with Gaucher's disease. One can observe the slowing of the posterior activity and the multiple and multifocal spikes involving the central and occipital regions in both hemispheres. Note that the 4 spikes on the left central region are strictly linked with 4 jerks on the right extensor *digitorum communis* muscle.

Juvenile myoclonic form of Huntington's chorea

The juvenile onset form of Huntington's chorea (HC) is rare, representing ten to 17% of all HC cases, with less than 10% having childhood onset (Gatto *et al.*, 2012). Onset is after age 3, with loss of acquired psychomotor skills, attention-deficit hyperactive disorder, cerebellar impairment, rigidity with loss of affect and dystonic posturing, or even excessive blinking (Xing *et al.*, 2008; review in Gonzalez-Alegre & Afifi, 2006). Choreic movements are not found. Epilepsy appears in general 2 years after the onset, as tonic-clonic seizures, atypical absences and massive myoclonias; erratic, asymmetric, spontaneous or action myoclonus is present in some cases and coincides mostly with worsening of epilepsy which may culminate in myoclonic or tonic-clonic status (Jervis, 1963; Garrel *et al.*, 1978). The EEG may show clinical photosensitivity even before the onset of seizures; it is later characterized by spontaneous bursts of SWs and PSWs, and a more specific finding may be represented by the occurrence of focal posterior epileptiform discharges and intermittent diffuse delta activity (Ullrich *et al.*, 2004). The prognosis is very poor, death occurring at an average of 4 to 6 years after the onset. The transmission is AD, paternal, in these myoclonic forms. HC has been mapped to 4p16.3. The abnormality is an expansion of CAG (cytosine-adenine-guanosine) triplets, equal or superior to 37 in the distal part of the gene, with early onset correlated to the number of repeats: a case with mental retardation, tremor, ataxia and cerebellar atrophy was diagnosed as early as at age 18 months, with 210–250 CAG repeats (Nicolas *et al.*, 2011). Preclinical and prenatal diagnosis raises difficult ethical problems.

Other PMEs

In spite of the recent advances in the elucidation of genetic mechanisms underlying the PMEs, there remain several conditions for which the known diagnostic categories have been excluded, either on clinical or on genetic (or on both) grounds, and there remain PME patients and families that have not been precisely categorized or receive a definite diagnosis only after many years. For example, a family with an apparently novel PME characterized by marked mental impairment, slow progression, and drug-resistant myoclonus and GTCS, with apparent onset in early adolescence but preexisting cognitive impairment (Ferlazzo *et al.*, 2009b) *(Figure 11)* only recently was shown to be caused by mutations of *CERS1*, a gene encoding for ceramide synthase 1 (Vanni *et al.*, 2014).

Van Bogaert *et al.* (2007) reported a Moroccan family with an autosomal recessive condition with onset in infancy, multifocal myoclonus, tonic-clonic seizures in some, and a mutation in the potassium channel tetramerization domain containing 7 *(KCTD7)* gene on 7q11.2, which regulates the neuronal membrane resting potential (Azizieh *et al.*, 2011). Since then mutations in *KCTD7* have been found in other cases with infantile-onset, severe PMEs including a large Turkish cohort covering 9 new cases, which confirms this gene as implicated in these conditions (Kousi *et al.*, 2012a; Krabichler *et al.*, 2012; Farhan *et al.*, 2014). In this condition the mean age of presentation of symptoms (myoclonic or tonic-clonic seizures) was 19 months and psychomotor decline became evident 0–22 months after onset of seizures and resulted in severe motor and mental retardation in all patients. Therefore, *KCTD7* mutation screening should be considered in PME patients with onset around 2 years of age followed by rapid mental and motor deterioration.

An early onset, severe PME phenotype associated with dystonia and death within the first decade was reported in a consanguineous Turkish family and mapped to 16p, but awaits elucidation (Duru *et al.*, 2010).

Coeliac disease, which may be complicated by various neurological problems, may present as a PME (Javed *et al.*, 2012). A PME-like phenotype associated with choreic movements was described in an infant with a folate transport deficiency due to a homozygous p.Cys105Arg mutation in the *LOLR1* gene (Perez-Duenas *et al.*, 2010).

Treatment

The comprehensive treatment of patients with PME should not only focus on the symptomatic therapy of myoclonus and epileptic seizures, but also take into account the specific handicaps encountered by these patients (Genton & Dravet, 1996).

An etiologically oriented treatment approach is sometimes possible. There are no reports yet of effective gene or stem cell therapy in PMEs. Enzyme replacement therapy is available in Gaucher's disease but its impact on the neurological form of the disease is moderate, as it does not markedly reverse the neurological symptoms (reviews in Germain, 2004; Davies *et al.*, 2007). In patients with MERRF, addition of coenzyme Q has not proven very efficient, and in some cases high doses have even be associated with increased severity of symptoms (Wallace *et al.*, 1991). Another etiologically oriented approach resulted in the use of an anti-oxydant, N-acetylcysteine, as a long-term treatment in patients with ULD, apparently with promising results (Hurd *et al.*, 1996). Antioxydants have been used for many years in juvenile NCL, with interesting results (Santavuori *et al.*,1988).

Metformin has been shown to ameliorate the neurological symptoms of Lafora's disease in the mice models (Berthier *et al.*, 2016; Sánchez-Elexpuru *et al.*, 2017) and has been designated as orphan drug for LD by the EMA and the FDA. However, there are no studies in human patients with LD proving an effect of this antidiabetic drug.

Development of new treatments that block the formation of lafora bodies or reduce their number are now underway, either by blocking glycogen synthase (by antisense oligonucleotides) or by enzymatically acting on LBs.

Social and psychological help is of utmost importance, and has contributed to a major progress in the field of PME care. Patients with PME are usually entitled to full benefits, but their situation may vary according to the various health systems. Patients with the most severe conditions often experience early episodes of severe depression, and patients with milder forms of PME, *e.g.*, ULD, have to cope with a lifelong problem and its consequences. Physical therapy, and education of carers and patients, may bring further improvement.

Medical treatment of PME is mainly directed against epileptic seizures and myoclonus *(Table III)* (for review, Michelucci *et al.*, 2016). Much progress has been due to the fact that some of the major antiepileptic drugs (AEDs) have been recognized as having potentially aggravating effects, either short-term (such as carbamazepine, gabapentin or vigabatrin) or long-term, such as phenytoin (Elridge *et al.*, 1983). Lamotrigine may also aggravate myoclonus in PME, as demonstrated in patients with ULD (Genton *et al.*, 2006).

Treatment will rely on a combination valproate and benzodiazepines, usually clonazepam (Iivanainen & Himberg, 1983; Roger *et al.*, 1992). Older drugs like phenobarbital and especially primidone may be useful, and ethosuximide is active against negative myoclonias, which are often found in PMEs in association with positive myoclonias (Oguni *et al.*, 1998; Wallace, 1998).

Several among the newer AEDs have been shown to have marked efficacy in the treatment of PMEs, by decreasing their generalized seizures and, to a lesser extent, their myoclonic jerks. Zonisamide has been used in LD (Yoshimura *et al.*, 2001) as well as in ULD (2 patients, Henry *et al.*, 1988; 7 patients, Kyllerman & Ben Menachem, 1998; 4 patients, Tassinari *et al.*, 1999), and has recently been evaluated, in an open-label trial, in ULD (Italiano *et al.*, 2011), showing great efficacy in the control of myoclonus. Vossler *et al.* (2008) used add on zonisamide in 30 patients with a variety of PMEs refractory to common AEDs. Topiramate also seems to have a specific antimyoclonic effect, and its efficacy has been demonstrated in a few patients with LD (Aykutlu *et al.*, 2005) and ULD (Topiramate YTC/YTCE Study Group, 2000).

In patients with debilitating myoclonus, piracetam may bring significant relief. In a controlled study, it was shown that high doses at 16 g/d were needed to have a significant effect (Koskiniemi *et al.*, 1998), and the long-term effect can be maintained over 10 years or more at doses as high as 37.5 g/d without major side-effects, although some abatement of efficacy may appear after several weeks of use (Genton *et al.*, 1999). Such high-dose treatment is not practical, although patients with PME usually accept it. The racetam family has provided another agent with very promising effect on myoclonus, levetiracetam, which has proven efficacy on photosensitive seizures (Kasteleijn-Nolst Trénité *et al.*, 1996). However, levetiracetam is not simply a more potent form of piracetam and has a distinctly different profile (Genton & vanVleymen, 2000). It was shown to be effective in the short term in ULD (Genton & Gélisse, 2000; Kinrions *et al.*, 2003; Crest *et al.*, 2004; Papacostas *et al.*, 2007). More extensive experience with levetiracetam has taught us that it cannot replace

Table III **Therapy of PMEs^**

First line AEDs	Second line AEDs	Third line strategies	Emergency treatment
Valproate	Zonisamide	5-hydroxy-L-tryptophan	Benzodiazepines i.v.*
Clonazepam	Levetiracetam	Lamotrigine	Levetiracetam i.v.
	Topiramate	N-acetylcystein	Valproate i.v.
	Piracetam	VNS or DBS	Phenytoin i.v.°
	Phenobarbital	Experimental drugs	
		Brivaracetam	
		Perampanel§	

^ Combination of multiple drugs is commonly needed.
* diazepam, lorazepam, clonazepam, midazolam
° Phenytoin may be used with success in the treatment of motor status epilepticus in late stage PMEs (Miyahara et al., 2009)
§ So far used in Lafora disease

piracetam in some patients whose myoclonus deteriorates after substitution of piracetam by levetiracetam. A combination of levetiracetam at 2,000–3,000 mg/d with a lower dose of piracetam, around 10–15 g/d, is a useful solution in such cases (Magaudda *et al.*, 2004). Levetiracetam has been increasingly used in a variety of PMEs, including Gaucher's disease for status epilepticus (Vaca *et al.*, 2012), MERRF (Mancuso *et al.*, 2006), DRPLA (Kobayashi *et al.*, 2012) and Down syndrome and senile myoclonic epilepsy (Sangani *et al.*, 2010). Thus levetiracetam is now considered a very early pharmacological treatment option in PMEs. Brivaracetam, a levetiracetam analogue, was proposed as a drug with a high potential efficacy for myoclonus as suggested in preclinical studies in a model of post-hypoxic myoclonus (Tai & Truong, 2007) and in phase II trial in photosensitive epilepsy (Kasteleijn-Nolst Trenitè *et al.*, 2007). Two prospective, multicentre, randomized, double-blind, placebo controlled, parallel-group, studies of add-on brivaracetam at doses of 5, 50 and 150 mg in a total of 106 genetically proven ULD have been recently completed (Kalviainen *et al.*, 2016). Both studies failed to reach the primary goal of redicing the severity of action myoclonus but a favorable trend was observed with brivaracetam at a dose of 50 mg/day and 87% of patients entered the long-term follow-up study. Perampanel, a selective noncompetitive antagonist of AMPA-type glutamate receptors, has an important antimycoclonic effect in LD and ULD. Goldsmith and Minassian reported 10 patients with LD whose myoclonus (in 7) and seizures (in 4) were greatly improved by perampanel at a mean dose of 6,7 mg/day. Similarly, Crespel *et al.* 2017 reported marked improvement of seizures (in all those who still had seizures) and myoclonus in 10 of 12 patients with ULD at a dose of 6 mg/day.

Less conventional drugs used as antimyoclonic agents in PME include baclofen (Awaad & Fish, 1995) and chloral hydrate (Pranzatelli & Tate, 2001). A dopaminergic agent, ropironole, has been shown to improve movement control in a patient with ULD (Karvonen *et al.*, 2010). Alcohol has also a marked antimyoclonic effect in alcohol-naïve patients that may last several hours and can be used (carefully) on social occasions (Genton & Guerrini, 1990).

New directions for a nonpharmacological treatment of myoclonus and seizures in PME can be inferred from the positive results (in a single case, with a short follow-up) of vagus nerve stimulation (VNS) in ULD (single case, Smith *et al.*, 2000), LD (two cases, Hajnsek *et al.*, 2013; Mikati & Tabbara, 2017), MERRF and Gaucher's disease (two cases, Fujimoto *et al.*, 2012): the procedure resulted in a major abatement of seizures and a decrease of cerebellar symptoms in all cases. Deep brain stimulation (DBS) has been used in a patient with PME, presumably of the ULD type, who has no benefit from VNS and a multiple drug regimen: bilateral high-frequency stimulation of the subthalamic nucleus resulted in 50% decrease of seizures (Vesper *et al.*, 2007). The same group reported on 4 further patients, stimulated in the subthalamic nucleus and additionally in the ventral intermediate nucleus, with a 30–100% reduction of myoclonic seizures, the best results occurring in the least affected cases (Wille *et al.*, 2011).

Conclusions

Our understanding of PMEs has considerably progressed and molecular genetics have shed a new light on the nosology and pathophysiology of these conditions.

PMEs are rare diseases, not all of which have a hopeless prognosis. It is now possible, in nearly all cases, to accurately diagnose these diseases using non-aggressive procedures, before they have reached the full-blown clinical stage. Treatment involves the judicious use of antiepileptic and antimyoclonic agents, but these patients' other requirements, such as the need for social and professional integration, should also be fully attended to. Genetic counselling is already possible in most cases, and some of these diseases can be diagnosed *in utero*. The next leap will concern the new therapeutic possibilities that are bound to emerge from the large body of knowledge gathered in the past years. The post-genetic era will focus on biochemistry and pharmacology and bring progress to the patient with new therapeutic approaches, hopefully with the same success attained with anti-disease treatments in other genetic neurological conditions, such as SMA and Duchenne muscular dystrophy.

REFERENCES ▶

Acharya NJ, Satishchandra P, Asha T, Shankar SK (1993): Lafora disease in South India: a clinical, electrophysiological, and pathologic study. *Epilepsia* 34: 476–487.

Aykutlu E, Baykan B, Gurses C, Bebek N, Buyukbabani N, Gokyigit A (2005): Add-on therapy with topiramate in progressive myoclonic epilepsy. *Epilepsy Behav* 6: 260–263.

Alakurtti K, Weber E, Rinne R, *et al.* (2005): Loss of lysosomal association of cystatin B proteins representing progressive myoclonus epilepsy, EPM1, mutations. *Eur J Hum Genet* 13: 208–215.

Arsov T, Smith KR, Damiano J, *et al.* (2011): Kufs disease, the major adult form of neuronal ceroid lipofuscinosis, caused by mutations in CLN6. *Am J Hum Genet* 88: 566–573.

Assenza G, Benvenga A, Gennaro E, *et al.* (2017): A novel c132–134del mutation in Unverricht-Lundborg disease and the review of literature of heterozygous compound patients. *Epilepsia* 58: e31–e35.

Awaad Y, Fish I (1995): Baclofen in the treatment of polymyoclonus in a patient with Unverricht-Lundborg disease. *J Child Neurol* 10: 68–70.

Azizieh R, Orduz D, Van Bogaert P, *et al.* (2011): Progressive myoclonic epilepsy-associated gene KCTD7 is a regulator of potassium conductance in neurons. *Mol Neurobiol* 44: 111–121.

Balreira A, Gaspar P, Caiola D, *et al.* (2008): A nonsense mutation in the LIMP-2 gene associated with progressive myoclonic epilepsy and nephrotic syndrome. *Hum Mol Genet* 17: 2238–2243.

Bamiou DE, Campbell P, Liasis A, *et al.* (2001): Audiometric abnormalities in children with Gaucher disease type 3. *Neuropediatrics* 32: 136–141.

Bassuk AG, Wallace RH, Buhr A, *et al.* (2008): A homozygous mutation in human PRICKLE1 causes an autosomal-recessive progressive myoclonus epilepsy-ataxia syndrome. *Am J Hum Genet* 83: 572–581.

Baykan B, Striano P, Gianotti S, Bebek N, Gennaro E, Gurses C, Zara F (2005): Late-onset and slow-progressing Lafora disease in four siblings with EPM2B mutation. *Epilepsia* 46: 1695–1697.

Benko W, Ries M, Wiggs EA, Brady RO, Schiffmann R, Fitzgibbon EJ (2011): The saccadic and neurological deficits in type 3 Gaucher disease. *PLoS One* 6: e22410.

Berg AT, Berkovic SF, Brodie MJ, *et al.* (2010): Revised terminology and concepts for organization of seizures and epilepsies: report of the ILAE Commission on Classification and Terminology, 2005–2009. *Epilepsia* 51: 676–685.

Berkovic SF, Andermann F (1986): The progressive myoclonus epilepsies. In: Pedley TA, Meldrum BS (eds) *Recent Advances in Epilepsy*, vol. 3, pp. 157–187. Edinburgh: Churchill Livingston.

Berkovic S. Andermann F, Carpenter S. Andermann E, Wolfe LS (1986): Progressive myoclonus epilepsies: specific causes and diagnosis. *N Engl J Med* 315: 296–305.

Berkovic SF, Andermann F. Carpenter S, Andermann E, Wolfe LS (1988): Kufs' disease. A critical reappraisal. *Brain* 111: 27–62.

Berkovic SF, Carpenter S, Evans A, *et al.* (1989): Myoclonus epilepsy and ragged-red fibres. I. A clinical, pathological, biochemical, magnetic resonance spectrographic and positron emission tomographic study. *Brain* 112: 1231–1260.

Berkovic SF, Mazarib A, Walid S, *et al.* (2005): A new clinical and molecular form of Unverricht-Lundborg disease localized by homozygosity mapping. *Brain* 128: 652–658.

Berkovic SF, Dibbens LM, Oshlack A, *et al.* (2008): Array-based gene discovery with three unrelated subjects shows SCARB2/LIMP-2 deficiency causes myoclonus epilepsy and glomerulosclerosis. *AmJ Hum Genet* 82: 673–684.

Berkovic SF, Staropoli JF, Carpenter S, *et al.* (2016): Diagnosis and misdiagnosis of adult neuronal ceroid lipofuscinosis (Kufs disease). *Neurology* 87: 579–584.

Berthier A, Payá M, García-Cabrero AM, *et al.* (2016): Pharmacological Interventions to Ameliorate Neuropathological Symptoms in a Mouse Model of Lafora Disease. *Mol Neurobiol* 53: 1296–309.

Bindoff LA, Desnuelle C, Birch-Machin MA, *et al.* (1991): Multilple defects of the mitochondrial respiratory chain in mitochondrial encephalopathy (MERRF): a clinical, biochemical and molecular *study.J Neurol Sci* 102: 17–24.

Bird TD (2010): Early-Onset Familial Alzheimer Disease. In: Pagon RA, Bird TD, Dolan CR, Stephens K, Adam MP (eds) *GeneReviews* [Internet]. Seattle (WA): University of Washington, Seattle; 1993–2010.

Boissè Lomax L, Bayly MA, Hjalgrim H, *et al.* (2013): "North Sea" progressive myoclonus epilepsy: phenotype of subjects with GOSR2 mutation. Brain 136: 1146–1154.

Bonten EJ, Arts WF, Beck M, *et al.* (2000): Novel mutations in lysosomal neuraminidase identify functional domains and determine clinical severity in sialidosis. *Hum Mol Genet* 9: 2715–2725.

Brackmann F, Abicht A, Ahting U, Schröder R, Trollmann R (2012): Classical MERRF phenotype associated with mitochondrial tRNA(Leu) (m.3243A>G) mutation. *Eur J Pediatr* 171: 859–862.

Bradshaw CB, Davis RL, Shrimpton A, *et al.* (2001): Cognitive deficits associated with a recently reported familial neurodegenerative disease: familial encephalopathy with neuroserpin inclusion bodies. *Arch Neurol* 58: 1429–1434.

Burke JR, Winfield MS, Lewis KE, *et al.* (1994): The Haw River syndrome: dentatorubropallidoluysian atrophy (DRPLA) in an African family. *Nat Genet* 7: 521–524.

Buzzi A, Chikhladze M, Falcicchia C, *et al.* (2012): Loss of cortical GABA terminals in Unverricht-Lundborg disease. *Neurobiol Dis* 47: 216–24.

Byrne E, Trounce I, Dennett X, Gligaw B, Morley JB, Marzuki S (1988): Progress from MERRF to MELAS phenotype in a patient with respiratory complex I and IV deficiency. *J Neurol Sci* 88: 327–337.

Callagy C, O'Neill G, Murphy SF, Farrell MA (2000): Adult neuronal ceroid lipofuscinosis (Kufs' disease) in two siblings of an Irish family. *Clin Neuropathol* 19: 109–118.

Canafoglia L, Franceschetti S, Antozzi C, *et al.* (2001): Epileptic phenotypes associated with mitochondrial disorders. *Neurology* 56: 1340–1346.

Canafoglia L, Franceschetti S, Uziel G, *et al.* (2011): Characterization of severe action myoclonus in sialidoses. *Epilepsy Res* 94: 86–93.

Canafoglia L, Gennaro E, Capovilla G, *et al.* (2012): Electroclinical presentation and genotype-phenotype relationships in patients with Unverricht-Lundborg disease carrying compound heterozygous CSTB point and indel mutations. *Epilepsia* 53: 2120–2127.

Canafoglia L, Robbiano A, Pareyson D, *et al.* (2014): Expanding sialidosis spectrum by genome-wide screening: NEU1 mutations in adult-onset myoclonus. *Neurology* 82: 2003–2006.

Canafoglia L, Gilioli I, Invernizzi F, *et al.* (2015): Electroclinical spectrum of the neuronal ceroid lipofuscinoses associated with CLN6 mutations. *Neurology* 85: 316–332.

Canafoglia L, Ferlazzo E, Michelucci R, *et al.* (2017): Variable course of Unverricht-Lundborg disease: Early prognostic factors. *Neurology* 89: 1691–1697.

Carpenter S, Karpati G, Andermann F, *et al.* (1977): The ultrastructural characteristics of the abnormal cytosomes in Batten-Kuf's disease. *Brain* 100: 137–156.

Carpenter S, Karpati G (1981): Sweat gland duct cells in Lafora disease: diagnosis by skin biopsy. *Neurology* 31: 1564–1568.

Casseron W, Azulay JP, Broglin D, *et al.* (2004): Phenotype variability in a caucasian family with dentatorubral-pallidoluysian atrophy. *Eur Neurol* 52: 175–176.

Cavanagh JB (1999): Corpora amylacea and the family of polyglucosan diseases. *Brain Res Rev* 29: 265–295.

Caviness JN (2003): Myoclonus and neurodegenerative disease-what's in a name? *Parkinsonism Relat Disord* 9: 185–192.

Chan EM, Bulman DE, Paterson AD, *et al.* (2003a): Genetic mapping of a new Lafora progressive myoclonus epilepsy locus (EPM2B) on 6p22. *J Med Genet* 40: 671–675.

Chan EM, Young EJ, Ianzano L, *et al.* (2003b): Mutations on *NHLRC1* cause progressive myoclonus epilepsy. *Nat Genet* 35: 125–127.

Charroux B, Fanto M (2010): The fine line between waste disposal and recycling: DRPLA fly models illustrate the importance of completing the autophagy cycle for rescuing neurodegeneration. *Autophagy* 6.6 (5).

Commission on Classification and Terminology of the International League Against Epilepsy (1989): Proposal for revised classification of epilepsies and epileptic syndromes. *Epilepsia* 30: 389–399.

Conradi G, Uvebrant P, Hökegärd KH, *et al.* (1989): First trimester diagnosis of juvenile neuronal ceroid lipofuscinosis by demonstration of fingerprint inclusion in chorionic villi. *Prenatal Diagnosis* 9: 283–287.

Corbett MA, Schwake M, Bahlo M, *et al.* (2011): A mutation in the Golgi Qb-SNARE gene GOSR2 causes progressive myoclonus epilepsy with early ataxia. *Am J Hum Genet* 88: 657–663.

Crest C, Dupont S, Leguern E., Adam C, Baulac M (2004): Levetiracetam in progressive myoclonic epilepsy: an exploratory study in 9 patients. *Neurology* 62: 640–643.

Damiano JA, Afawi Z, Bahlo M, *et al.* (2015): Mutation of the nuclear lamin gene LMNB2 in progressive myoclonus epilepsy with early ataxia. *Hum Mol Genet* 24: 4483–4490.

Danner N, Säisänen L, Määttä S, *et al.* (2011): Motor cortical plasticity is impaired in Unverricht-Lundborg disease. *Mov Disord* 26: 2095–2100.

Danner N, Julkunen P, Hyppönen J, *et al.* (2013): Alterations of motor cortical excitability and anatomy in Unverricht-Lundborg disease. *Mov Disord* 28: 1860–1867.

Davies EH, Erikson A, Collin-Histed T, Mengel E, Tylki-Szymanska A, Vellodi A (2007): Outcome of type III Gaucher disease on enzyme replacement therapy: review of 55 cases. *J Inherit Metab Dis* 30: 935–942.

Davies EH, Seunarine KK, Banks T, Clark CA, Vellodi A (2011): Brain white matter abnormalities in paediatric Gaucher Type I and Type III using diffusion tensor imaging. *J Inherit Metab Dis* 34: 549–553.

De Fusco M, Vago R, Striano P, *et al.* (2014): The $\alpha 2$ B adrenergic receptor is mutant in cortical myoclonus and epilepsy. *Ann Neurol* 75: 77–87.

De Geest N, Bonten E, Mann L, De Sousa-Hitzler J, Hahn C, D'Azzo A (2002): Systemic and neurologic abnormalities distinguish the lysosomal disorders sialidosis and galactosialidosis in mice. *Hum Mol Genet* 11: 1455–1464.

De Graaf AS, Ancker E, Rutherfoord GS. Van der Walt JJ, Rossouw DJ (1989): Lafora body disease with optic atrophy, macular degeneration and cardiac failure. *J Neurol Sci* 93: 69–84.

De Simone R, Puig XS, Gélisse P, Crespel A, Genton P (2010): Senile myoclonic epilepsy: delineation of a common condition associated with Alzheimer's disease in Down syndrome. *Seizure* 19: 383–389.

Delgado-Escueta AV (2007): Advances in lafora progressive myoclonus epilepsy. *Epilepsy Curr 7:* 61–67.

Depienne C, Magnin E, Bouteiller D, *et al.* (2010): Familial cortical myoclonic tremor with epilepsy: the third locus (FCMTE3) maps to 5p. *Neurology* 74: 2000–2003.

Dermaut B, Seneca S, Dom L, *et al.* (2010): Progressive myoclonic epilepsy as an adult-onset manifestation of Leigh syndrome due to m.14487T>C. *J Neurol Neurosurg Psychiatry* 81: 90–93.

Destee A, Delalande I, Vuillaume I, Schraen-Maschke S, Defebvre L, Sablonniere B (2000): The first identified French family with dentatorubral-pallidoluysian atrophy. *Mov Disord* 15: 996–999.

Dibbens LM, Michelucci R, Gambardella A, *et al.* (2009): SCARB2 mutations in progressive myoclonus epilepsy without renal failure. *Ann Neurol* 66: 532–536.

Durand P, Gatti R, Cavalieri S, Borrone C, Tondeur M. Michalski JC, Stercker G (1977): Sialidosis (mucolipidosis I). *Helv Paediat Acta* 32: 391–400.

Duru N, Iseri SA, Selçuk N, Tolun A (2010): Early-onset progressive myoclonic epilepsy with dystonia mapping to 16pter-p13.3. *J Neurogenet* 24: 207–215.

Ekbom K (1985): Hereditary ataxia, photomyoclonus, skeletal deformities and lipomas. *Acta Neurol Scand* 51: 393–404.

Elridge R, Iivanainen M, Stern R, Koerber I, Wilder BJ (1983): "Baltic" myoclonus epilepsy: hereditary disorder of childhood made worse by phenytoin. *Lancet* ii: 838–842.

Farhan SM, Murphy LM, Robinson JF, *et al.* (2014): Linkage analysis and exome sequencing identify a novel mutation in KCTD7 in patients with progressive myoclonus epilepsy with ataxia. *Epilepsia* 55: 106–111.

Ferlazzo E, Magaudda A, Striano P, Vi-Hong N, Serra S, Genton P (2007): Long-term evolution of EEG in Unverricht-Lundborg disease. *Epilepsy Res* 73: 219–227.

Ferlazzo E, Gagliano A, Calarese T, *et al.* (2009a): Neuropsychological findings in patients with Unverricht-Lundborg disease. *Epilepsy Behav* 14: 545–549.

Ferlazzo E, Italiano D, An I, *et al.* (2009b): Description of a family with a novel progressive myoclonus epilepsy and cognitive impairment. *Mov Disord* 24: 1016–1022.

Ferlazzo E, Canafoglia L, Michelucci R, *et al.* (2014): Mild Lafora disease: clinical, neurophysiological and genetic findings. *Epilepsia* 55: e129–e133.

Franceschetti S, Gambardella A, Canafoglia L, *et al.* (2006): Clinical and genetic findings in 26 italian patients with Lafora disease. *Epilepsia* 47: 640–643.

Franceschetti S, Sancini G, Buzzi A, *et al.* (2007): A pathogenetic hypothesis of Unverricht-Lundborg disease onset and progression. *Neurobiol Dis* 25: 675–685.

Franceschetti S, Michelucci R, Canafoglia L, *et al.* (2014): Progressive myoclonic epilepsies: definitive and still undetermined causes. *Neurology* 82: 405–411.

Fu YJ, Aida I, Tada M, *et al.* (2014): Progressive myoclonus epilepsy: extraneuronal brown pigment deposition and system neiurodegeneration in the brains of japamese patients with novel SCARB2 mutations. *Neuropathol Appl Neurobiol* 40: 551–563.

Fujimoto A, Yamazoe T, Yokota T, *et al.* (2012): Clinical utility of vagus nerve stimulation for progressive myoclonic epilepsy. *Seizure* 21: 810–812.

Fukuhara N (1991): MERRF: a clinicopathological study. Relationships between myoclonus epilepsies and mitochondrial myopathies. *Rev Neurol* 147: 476–479.

Fukuhara N (1995): Clinicopathological features of MERRF. *Muscle Nerve* 18 (Suppl 14): S90–4.

Fukuhara N, Tokiguchi S, Shirakawa K, Tsubaki T (1980): Myoclonus epilepsy asociated with ragged-red fibers (mitochondrial abnormalities). Disease entity or a syndrome? *J Neurol Sci* 47: 117–133.

Furuya H, Yasuda M, Terasawa KJ, *et al.* (2003): A novel mutation (L250V) in the presenilin 1 gene in a Japanese familial Alzheimer's disease with myoclonus and generalized convulsion. *J Neurol Sci* 209: 75–77.

Ganesh S, Agarwala KL, Ueda K, *et al.* (2000): Laforin, defective in the progressive myoclonus epilepsy of Lafora type, is a dual-specificity phosphatase associated with polyribosomes. *Hum Mol Genet* 9: 2251–2261.

Ganesh S, Delgado-Escueta AV, Sakamoto T, *et al.* (2002): Targeted disruption of the Epm2a gene causes formation of Lafora inclusion bodies, neurodegeneration, ataxia, myoclonus epilepsy and impaired behavioral response in mice. *Hum Mol Genet* 11: 1251–1262.

Gao H, Boustany RMN, Alroy J (2002): Mutations in a novel CLN6-encoded transmembrane protein cause variant neuronal ceroid lipofuscinosis in man and mouse. *Am J Hum Genet* 70: 324–335.

Gardiner M, Sandford A, Deadman M, *et al.* (1990): Batten disease (Spielmeyer-Vogt disease, juvenile onset neuronal ceroid lipofuscinosis) gene (CLN3) maps to chromosome 16. *Genomics* 8: 387–390.

Garrel S, Joannard A, Feuerstein C, Serre F (1978): Myoclonic type of Hun-tington's chorea. *Rev Electroencephalogr Neurophysiol Clin* 8: 123–128.

Gatto E, Parisi V, Persi G, *et al.* (2012): Clinical and genetic characteristics in patients with Huntington's Disease from Argentina. *Parkinsonism Relat Disord* 18: 166–169.

Genton P, Guerrini R (1990): Antimyoclonic effects of alcohol in progressive myoclonus epilepsy. *Neurology* 40: 1412–1416.

Genton P, Paglia G (1994): Épilepsie myoclonique sénile ? Myoclonies d'apparition tardive dans le syndrome de Down. *Épilepsies* 1: 5–11.

Genton P, Dravet C (1996): Treatment of epilepsies with myoclonias. In: Shorvon S, Dreifuss FE, Fish D, Thomas D (eds) *The Treatment of Epilepsy,* London: Blackwell Science, pp. 247–257.

Genton P, Gélisse P (2000): Antimyoclonic effect of levetiracetam. *Epileptic Disorders* 2: 209–212.

Genton P, van Vleymen B (2000): Piracetam and levetiracetam: close structural similarities but different phamacological profiles. *Epileptic Disorders* 2: 99–105.

Genton P, Borg M, Vigliano P, Pellissier JF, Roger J (1989): Semi-late onset and rapidly progressive case of Lafora's disease with predominant cognitive symptoms. *Europ Neurol* 29: 333–338.

Genton P, Michelucci R, Tassinari CA, Roger J (1990): The Ramsay Hunt Syndrome revisited: Mediterranean Myoclonus *versus* mitochondrialencephalomyopathy with ragged red fibers and Baltic Myoclonus. *Acta Neurol Scand* 81: 8–15.

Genton P, Guerrini R, Remy P (1999): Piracetam in the treatment of cortical myoclonus. *Pharmacopsychiatry* 32 (Suppl 1): 49–53.

Genton P, Gélisse P, Thomas P, Dravet C (2000): Do carbamazepine and phenytoin aggravate juvenile myoclonic epilepsy? *Neurology* 55: 1106–1109.

Genton P, Gélisse P, Crespel A (2006): Lack of efficacy and potential aggravation of myoclonus with lamotrigine in Unverricht-Lundborg disease. *Epilepsia* 47: 2083–2085.

Gentry MS, Guinovart JJ, Minassian, Roach PJ, Serratosa JM (2018): Lafora disease offers a unique window in neuronal glycogen metabolism. *J Biol Chem* 293: 7117–7125.

Germain DP (2004): Gaucher disease: clinical, genetic and therapeutic aspects. *Pathol Biol* (Paris) 52: 343–350.

Giovagnoli AR, Canafoglia L, Reati F, Raviglione F, Franceschetti S (2009): The neuropsychological pattern of Unverricht-Lundborg disease. *Epilepsy Res* 84: 217–223.

Goebel HH. Zeman W, Patel VK, Pullarkat RK, Lenard HG (1979): On the ultrastructural diversity and essence of residual bodies in neuronal ceroid lipofuscinosis. *Mech Aging Dev* 10: 53–70.

Goker-Alpan O, Schiffmann R, Park JK, *et al.* (2003): Phenotypic continuum in neuronopathic Gaucher disease: an intermediate phenotype between type 2 and type 3. *J Pediatr* 143: 273–276.

Gomez-Abad C, Gomez-Garre P, Gutierrez-Delicado E, *et al.* (2005): Lafora disease due to EPM2B mutations: a clinical and genetic study. *Neurology* 64: 982–986.

Gomez-Garre P, Sanz Y, Rodriguez de Cordoba SR, Serratosa JM (2000): Mutational spectrum of the EPM2A gene in progressive myoclonus epilepsy of Lafora: high degree of allelic heterogeneity and prevalence of deletions. *Eur J Hum Genet* 12: 946–954.

Gonzalez-Alegre P, Afifi AK (2006): Clinical characteristics of childhood-onset (juvenile) Huntington disease: report of 12 patients and review of the literature. *J Child Neurol* 21: 223–229.

Gourfinkel-An I, Duyckaerts C, Camuzat A, *et al.* (2007): Clinical and neuropathologic study of a French family with a mutation in the neuro-serpin gene. *Neurology* 69: 79–83.

Guerrero R, Vernia S, Sanz R, *et al.* (2011): A PTG variant contributes to a milder phenotype in Lafora disease. *PLoS One* 6: e21294.

Guerrini R, Bonanni P, Patrignani A, *et al.* (2001): Autosomal dominant cortical myoclonus and epilepsy (ADCME) with complex partial seizures and generalized seizures. A newly recognized epilepsy syndrome with linkage to chromosome 2p11–q12.2. *Brain* 124: 2459–2475.

Hagen MC, Murrell JR, Delisle MB, *et al.* (2011): Encephalopathy with neuroserpin inclusion bodies presenting as progressive myoclonus epilepsy and associated with a novel mutation in the Proteinase Inhibitor 12 gene. *Brain Pathol* 21: 575–582.

Haines JL, Boustany RMN, AlroyJ, *et al.* (1998): Chromosomal localization of two genes underlying late-infantile neuronal ceroid lipofuscinosis. *Neurogenetics* 1: 217–222.

Hajnsek S, Petelin Gadze Z, Borovecki F, *et al.* (2013): Vagus nerve stimulation in Lafora body disease. *Epilepsy Behav Case Rep* 1: 150–152.

Halliday AM, Halliday E (1980): Cerebro-somatosensory and visual evoked potentials in different clinical forms of myoclonus. In: Desmedt JE (ed) *Clinical Uses of Cerebral, Brainstem and Spinal Somatosensory Potentials*, vol. 7, Basel: Karger, pp. 292–310.

Hammans SR, Sweeney MG, Brockington M, Morgan-Hughes JA, Harding AE (1991): Mitochondrial encephalopathies: molecular genetic diagnosis from blood samples. *Lancet* 337 (8753): 1311–1313.

Harding AE, Holt IJ (1988): Mitochondrial genes and neurological disease. In: Rosenberg RN, Harding AE (eds) *The Molecular Biology of Neurological Disease*, London: Butterworths, pp. 199–210.

Hashida H, Goto J, Suzuki T, *et al.* (2001): Single cell analysis of CAG repeat in brains of dentatorubral-pallidoluysian atrophy (DRPLA). *J Neurol Sci* 190: 87–93.

Henry TR, Leppik IE, Gumnit RJ, Jacobs M (1988): Progressive myoclonus epilepsy treated with zonisamide. *Neurology* 38: 928–931.

Herrero-Martin MD, Ayuso T, Tunon MT, Martin MA, Ruiz-Pesini E, Montoya J (2010): A MELAS/MERRF phenotype associated with the mitochondrial DNA 5521G>A *mutation. J Neurol Neurosurg Psychiatry* 81: 471–472.

Hopfner F, Schormair B, Knauf F, *et al.* (2011): Novel SCARB2 mutation in action myoclonus-renal failure syndrome and evaluation of SCARB2 mutations in isolated AMRF features. *BMC Neurol* 11: 134.

Houseweart MK, Pennacchio LA, Vilaythong A, Peters C, NoebelsJL, Myers RM (2003): Cathepsin B but not cathepsins L or S contributes to the pathogenesis of Unverricht-Lundborg progressive myoclonus epilepsy (EPM 1). *J Neurobiol* 56: 315–327.

Hurd RW, Wilder BJ, Helveston WR, Uthman BM (1996): Treatment of foursiblings with progressive myoclonus epilepsy of the Unverricht-Lundborg type with N-acetylcysteine. *Neurology* 47: 1264–1268.

Hyppönen J, Äikiä M, Joensuu T, *et al.* (2015): Refining the phenotype of Unverricht-Lundborg disease (EPM1): A population-wide Finnish study. *Neurology* 84: 1529–1536.

Iivanainen M, Himberg JJ (1982): Valproate and clonazepam in the treatment of severe progressive myoclonus epilepsy. *Arch Neurol* 39: 236–238.

Iizuka R, Hirayama K, Maehara K (1984): Dentato-rubro-pallido-luysian atrophy: a clinicopathological study. *J Neurol Neurosurg Psychiatr* 47: 1288–1298.

Ikeuchi T, Koide R, Tanaka H, *et al.* (1995): Dentatorubral-pallidoluysian atrophy: clinical features are closely related to unstable expansions of trinucleotide (CAG) repeat. *Ann Neurol* 37: 769–775.

International Batten Disease Consortium (1995): Isolation of a novel gene underlying Batten disease, VLN3. *Cell* 82: 949–957. Italiano D, Pezzella M, Coppola, *et al.* (2011): A pilot open-label trial of zonisamide in Unverricht-Lundborg disease. *Mov Disord* 26: 341–343.

Italiano D, Pezzella M, Coppola A, *et al.* (2011): A pilot open-label trial of zonisamide in Unverricht-Lundborg disease. *Mov Disord* 26: 341–343.

Itoh K, Naganawa Y, Matsuzawa F, *et al.* (2002): Novel missense mutations in the human lysosomal sialidase gene in sialidosis patients and prediction of structural alterations of mutant enzymes. *J Hum* Genet 47: 29–37.

Javed S, Safdar A, Forster A, *et al.* (2012): Refractory coeliac disease associated with late onset epilepsy, ataxia, tremor and progressive myoclonus with giant cortical evoked potentials-A case report and review of literature. *Seizure* 21: 482–485.

Jervis GA (1963): Huntington's chorea in childhood. *Arch Neurol* 9: 244–257.

Joensuu T, Kuronen M, Alakurtti K, *et al.* (2007): Cystatin B: mutation detection, alternative splicing and expression in progressive myclonus epilepsy of Unverricht-Lundborg type (EPM 1) patients. *EurJ Hum Genet* 15: 185–193.

Johnson WG, Thomas GH, Miranda AF, *et al.* (1980): Congenital sialidosis: biochemical studies: clinical spectrum in 4 sibs; two successful prenatal diagnoses. *Am J Hum Genet* 32: 43A.

Kagitani-Shimono K, Imai K, Okamoto N, Ono J, Okada S (2002): Unverricht-Lundborg disease with cystatin B gene abnormalities. *Pediatr Neurol* 26: 55–60.

Kälviäinen R, Genton P, Andermann E, *et al.* (2016): Brivaracetam in Unverricht-Lundborg disease (EPM1): Results from two randomized, double-blind, placebo-controlled studies. *Epilepsia* 57: 210–221.

Karvonen MK, Kaasinen V, Korja M, Marttila RJ (2010): Ropinirole diminishes myoclonus and improves writing and postural balance in an ULD patient. *Mov Disord* 25: 520–521.

Kasteleijn-Nolst Trénité DGA, Marescaux C, Stodieck S, Edelbroek PM, Oosting J (1996): Photosensitive epilepsy: a model to study the effects of antiepileptic drugs. Evaluation of the piracetam analogue, levetiracetam. *Epilepsy Res* 25: 225–230.

Kasteleijn-Nolst Trenité, D.G., Genton, P., Parain, D., *et al.* (2007): Evaluation of brivaracetam, a novel SV2 A ligand, in the photosensitivity model. *Neurology* 69: 1027–1034.

Kinrions P, Ibrahim N, Murphy K, Lehesjoki AE, Jarvela I, Delanty N (2003): Efficacy of levetiracetam in a patient with Unverricht-Lundborg progressive myoclonus epilepsy. *Neurology* 60: 1934–1935.

Kleijer WJ, Hoogeveen A, Verheyen FW, *et al.* (1979): Prenatal diagnosis of sialidosis with combined neura-minidase and b-galactosidase deficiency. *Clin Genet* 16: 60.

Kobayashi K, Matsumoto R, Kondo T, *et al.* (2011): Decreased cortical excitability in Unverricht-Lundborg disease in the long-term follow-up: a consecutive SEP study. *Clin Neurophysiol* 122: 1617–1621.

Kobayashi K, Takeuchi A, Oka M, Akiyama M, Ohtsuka Y (2012): Amelioration of disabling myoclonus in a case of DRPLA by levetiracetam. *Brain Dev* 34: 368–371.

Koide R, Ikruchi T, Onodesa O, *et al.* (1994): Unstable expansion of CAG repeat in hereditary dentatorubral-pallidoluysian atrophy (DRPLA). *Nat Genet* 6: 9–12.

Korja M, Kaasinen V, Lamusuo S, Marttila RJ, Parkkola R (2007a): Hyperostosis frontalis interna as a novel finding in Unverricht-Lundborg disease. *Neurology* 68: 1077–1078.

Korja M, Kaasinen V, Lamusuo S, Parkkola R, Nâgren K, Marttila RJ (2007b): Substantial thalamostriatal dopaminergic defect in Unverricht-Lundborg disease. *Epilepsia* 48: 1768–1773.

Koskenkorva P, Khyuppenen J, Niskanen E, *et al.* (2009): Bilateral atrophy of the motor cortex and thalami in Unverricht-Lundborg disease: A voxel-based morphometric study. *Neurology* 73: 606–611.

Koskenkorva P, Hyppönen J, Aikiä M, *et al.* (2011): Severe phenotype in Unverricht-Lundborg disease (EPM1) patients compound heterozygous for the dodecamer repeat expansion and the c.202C>T mutation in the CSTB gene. *Neurodegener Dis* 8: 515–522.

Koskiniemi ML (1986): Baltic myoclonus. In: Fahn S, Marsden CD, Van Woert M (eds) *Myoclonus. Advances in neurology*, vol. 43, New York: Raven Press, pp. 57–64.

Koskiniemi M, Donner M, Majuri H, Haltia M, Norio R (1974): Progressive myoclonus epilepsy: a clinical and histopathological study. *Acta Neurol Scand* 50: 307–332.

Koskiniemi M, van Vleymen B, Hakamies L, Lamusuo S, Taalas J (1998): Piracetam relieves symptoms in progressive myoclonus epilepsy: a multicentre, randomised, double blind, crossover study comparing the efficacy and safety of three dosages of oral piracetam with placebo. *J Neurol Neurosurg Psychiatry* 64: 334–348.

Koubeissi MZ, Khongkhatithum C, Janus AI, Lüders H (2009): Scotosensitive myoclonic seizures in MERRF. *Neurology* 72: 858.

Kousi M, Anttila V, Schulz A, *et al.* (2012a): Novel mutations consolidate KCTD7 as a progressive myoclonus epilepsy gene. *J Med* Genet 49: 391–399.

Kousi M, Lehesjoki AE, Mole SE (2012b): Update of the mutation spectrum and clinical correlations of over 360 mutations in eight genes that underlie the neuronal ceroid lipofuscinoses. *Hum Mutat* 33: 42–63.

Krabichler B, Rostasy K, Baumann M, *et al.* (2012): Novel Mutation in Potassium Channel related Gene KCTD7 and Progressive Myoclonic Epilepsy. *Ann Hum* Genet 76: 326–331.

Kraoua I, Sedel F, Caillaud C, *et al.* (2010): A French experience of type 3 Gaucher disease: Phenotypic diversity and neurological outcome of 10 patients. *Brain Dev* 33: 131–139.

Kufs HF (1925): Über eine Spätform der amaurotischen Idiotie und ihre heredofamiliären Grundlagen. *Z ges Neurol Psychiatr* 95: 169–188.

Kunz WS (2002): The role of mitochondria in epileptogenesis. *Curr Opin Neurol* 15: 179–184.

Kyllerman M, Ben-Menachem E (1998): Zonisamide for progressive myoclonus epilepsy: long-term observations in seven patients. *Epilepsy Res* 29: 109–114.

Labauge P, Amer LO, Simonetta-Moreau M, *et al.* (2002): Absence of linkage to 8q24 in a European family with familial adult myoclonic epilepsy (FAME). *Neurology* 26: 941–944.

Lafora GR (1911): Über das Vorkommen amyloider Körperchen im Innerender Ganglienzellen. *Virchows Arch* 205: 295–303.

Lai SC, Chen RS, Wu Chou YH, *et al.* (2009): A longitudinal study of Taiwanese sialidosis type 1: an insight into the concept of cherry-red spot myoclonus syndrome. *Eur J Neurol* 16: 912–919.

Lake BD, Cavanagh NPC (1978): Early juvenile Batten's disease. A comparative subgroup distinct from other forms of Batten's disease. *J Neurol Sci* 36: 265–271.

Lalioti M, Scott HS, Buresi C, *et al.* (1997a): Dodecamer repeat in Cystatin B in progressive myoclonus epilepsy (EPM1). *Nature* 386: 847–851.

Lalioti M, Mirotsou M, Buresi C, *et al.* (1997b): Identification of mutations in Cystatin B, the gene responisble for the Unverricht-Lundborg type of progressive epilepsy (EPM1). *Am J Hum* Genet 60: 342–352.

Lalioti MD, Scott HS, Genton P, *et al.* (1998): A PCR amplification method reveals instability of the dodecamer repeat in progressive myoclonus epilepsy (EPM1) and no correlation between the size of the repeat and age at onset. *Am J Hum Genet* 62: 842–847.

Le Ber I, Camuzat A, Castelnovo G, *et al.* (2003): Prevalence of dentatorubral-pallidoluysian atrophy in a large series of white patients with cerebellar ataxia. *Arch Neurol* 60: 1097–1099.

Lee IH, Soong BW, Lu YC, Chang YC (2001): Dentatorubropallidoluysian atrophy in Chinese. *Arch Neurol* 58: 1905–1908.

Lehesjoki AE, Koskiniemi M, Sistonen P, *et al.* (1991): Localization of a gene for progressive myoclonus epilepsy to chromosome 21q22. *Proc Natl Acad Sci USA* 88: 3606–3699.

Lehesjoki AE, Kälviäinen R (2009): Unverricht-Lundborg Disease. In: Pagon RA, Bird TD, Dolan CR, Stephens K, Adam MP (eds) *Gene Reviews* [Internet]. Seattle (WA): University of Washington, Seattle; 1993–2004 [updated 2009 Jun 18].

Lehtinen MK, Tegelberg S, Schipper H, *et al.* (2009): Cystatin B deficiency sensitizes neurons to oxidative stress in progressive myoclonus epilepsy, EPM1. *J Neurosci* 29: 5910–5915.

Lesca G, Boutry-Kryza N, de Toffol B, *et al.* (2010): Novel mutations in EPM2A and NHLRC1 widen the spectrum of Lafora disease. *Epilepsia* 51: 1691–1698.

Lieuallen K, Pennacchio LA, Park M, Myers RM, Lennon GG (2001): Cystatin B-deficient mice have increased expression of apoptosis and glial activation genes. *Hum Mol Genet* 10: 1867–1871.

Liu CY, Lee CF, Hong CH, Wei YH (2004): Mitochondrial DNA mutation and depletion increase the susceptibility of human cells to apoptosis. *Ann N Y Acad Sci* 1011: 133–145.

Lowden JA, O'Brien JS (1979): Sialidosis: a review of human neuraminidase deficiency. *Am J Hum Genet* 31: 1–18.

Lundborg H (1903): *Die progressive Myoclonusepilepsie (Unverricht's Myoklonie)*. Uppsala: Almqvist and Wiskell.

Magaudda A, Gélisse P, Genton P (2004): Antimyoclonic effect of levetiracetam in 13 patients with Unverricht-Lundborg disease: clinical observations. *Epilepsia* 45: 678–681.

Magaudda A, Ferlazzo E, Nguyen VH, Genton P (2006): Unverricht-Lundborg disease, a condition with self-limited progression: long-term follow-up of 20 patients. *Epilepsia* 47: 860–866.

Malafosse A, Lehesjoki AE, Genton P, *et al.* (1992): Identical genetic locus for Baltic and Mediterranean myoclonus. *Lancet* 339 (8801): 1080–1081.

Mancuso M, Galli R, Pizzanelli C, Filosto M, Siciliano G, Murri L (2006): Antimyoclonic effect of levetiracetam in MERRF syndrome. *J Neurol Sci* 243: 97–99.

Mancuso M, Petrozzi L, Filosto M, *et al.* (2007): MERRF syndrome without ragged-red fibers: the need for molecular diagnosis. *Biochem Biophys Res Commun* 354: 1058–1060.

Manninen O, Laitinen T, Lehtimaki KK, *et al.* (2014): Progressive volume loss and white matter degeneration in cstb-deficient mice: a diffusion tensor and longitudinal volumetry MRI study. *PLoS One* 9: e90709.

Manninen O, Kostenkorva P, Lehtimaki KK, *et al.* (2015): White matter degeneration with Unverricht-Lundborg progressive myoclonus epilepsy: a translational diffusion-tensor imaging sstudy in pastients and in cystatin B deficien t mice. *Radiology* 269: 232–239.

Marsden CD, Harding AE, Obeso JA, Lu CS (1990): Progressive myoclonic ataxia (the Ramsay Hunt syndrome). *Arch Neurol* 47: 1121–1125.

Marseille Consensus Group (1990): Classification of progressive myoclonus epilepsies and related diseases. *Ann Neurol* 28: 113–116.

Martins S, Matama T, Guimaraes L, *et al.* (2003): Portuguese families with dentatorubropallidoluysian atrophy (DRPLA) share a common haplotype of Asian origin. *EurJ Hum* Genet 11: 808–811.

Mascalchi M, Michelucci R, Cosottini M, *et al.* (2002): Brainstem involvement in Unverricht-Lundborg disease (EPM1): An MRI and (1)H MRS study. *Neurology* 58: 1686–1689.

Mauguière F, Bard J, Courjon J (1981): Les potentiels évoqués somesthésiques précoces dans la dyssynergie cérébelleuse myoclonique progressive. *Rev EEG Neurophysiol* 11: 174–182.

May DL, White III (1968): Familial myoclonus, cerebellar ataxia and deafness. *Arch Neurol* 19: 331–338.

McLeod PM, Nag S, Berry G (1988): Ultrastructural studies as a method of prenatal diagnosis of neuronal ceroi lipofuscinosis. *Am J Med Genet* 5 (Suppl): 93–97.

Melone MA, Tessa A, Petrini S, *et al.* (2004): Revelation of a new mitochondrial DNA mutation (G12147A) in a MELAS/MERFF phenotype. *Arch Neurol* 61: 269–272.

Michelucci R, Serratosa J M, Genton P, Tassinari CA (2002): Seizures, myoclonus and cerebellar dysfunction in progressive myoclonus epilepsies. In: Guerrini R, Aicardi J, Andermann F, Hallett M (eds) *Epilepsy and Movement Disorders*. Cambridge: Cambridge University Press, pp. 227–249.

Michelucci R, Pasini E, Riguzzi P, Andermann E, Kalviainen R, Genton P (2016): Myoclonus and seizures in progressive myoclonus epilepsies: pharmacology and therapeutic trials. *Epileptic Disord* 18 (S2): 145–153.

Mikami M, Yasuda T, Terao A, *et al.* (1999): Localization of a gene for benign adult familial myoclonic epilepsy to chromosome 8q23.3–q24.1. *AmJ Hum Genet* 65: 745–751.

Mikati MA, Tabbara F (2017): Managing Lafora body disease with vagal nerve stimulation. *Epileptic Disord* 19: 82–86.

Minassian BA, Lee JR, Herbrick JA, *et al.* (1998): Mutations in a gene encoding a novel protein tyrosine phosphatase cause progressive myoclonus epilepsy. *Nat Genet* 2: 171–174.

Minassian BA, Andrade DM, Ianzano L, *et al.* (2001): Laforin is a cell membrane and endoplasmic reticulum-associated protein tyrosine phosphatase. *Ann Neurol* 49: 271–275.

Miranda E, Lomas DA (2006): Neuroserpin: a serpin to think about. *Cell Mol Life Sci* 63: 709–722.

Mitchell WA, Wheeler RB, Sharp JD, *et al.* (2001): Turkish variant late infantile neuronal ceroid lipofuscinosis (CLN7) may be allelic to CLN8. *Europ J Paediatr Neurol* 5 (Suppl A): 21–27.

Mittal S, Dubey D, Yamakawa K, Ganesh S (2007): Lafora disease proteins malin and laforin are recruited to aggresomes in response to proteasomal impairment. *Hum Mol Genet* 16: 753–762.

Miyahara A, Saito GY, Sugai K, *et al.* (2009): Reassessment of phenytoin for treatment of late stages progressive myoclonus epilepsy complicated with status epilepticus. *Epilepsy Res* 84: 801–809.

Mole SE, Williams RE, Goebel HH (2005): Correlations between genotype, ultrastructural morphology and clinical phenotype in the neuronal ceroid lipofuscinosis. *Neurogenetics* 6: 107–126.

Mole SE, Williams RE, Goebel HH (2011): The Neuronal Ceroid Lipofuscinoses (Batten Disease). 2nd ed. Oxford: Oxford University Press.

MöllerJC, Hamer HM, Oertel WH, Rosenow F (2002): Late-onset myoclonic epilepsy in Down's syndrome (LOMEDS). *Seizure* 11 (Suppl A): 303–305.

Mongini T, Doriguzzi C, Chiado-Piat L, Silvestri G, Servidei S, Palmucci L (2002): MERRF/MELAS overlap syndrome in a family with A3243G mtDNA mutation. *Clin Neuropathol* 21: 72–76.

Moulard B, Darcel F, Mignard D, *et al.* (2003): Founder effect in patients with Unverricht-Lundborg disease on reunion island. *Epilepsia* 44: 1357–1360.

Muona M, Berkovic SF, Dibbens LM, *et al.* (2015): A recurrent *de novo* mutation in KCNC1 causes progressive myoclonus epilepsy. *Nat Genet* 47: 39–46.

Naganawa Y, Itoh K, Shimmoto M, *et al.* (2000): Molecular and structural studies of Japanese patients with sialidosis type 1. *J Hum Genet* 45: 241–249.

Nakamura M, Yabe I, Sudo A, Hosoki K, Yaguchi H, Saitoh S, Sasaki H (2010): MERRF/MELAS overlap syndrome: a double pathogenic mutation in mitochondrial tRNA genes. *J Med Genet* 47: 659–664.

Naito H, Oyanagi S (1982): Familial myoclonus epilepsy and choreoathetosis: hereditary dentatorubral- pallidoluysian atrophy. *Neurology* 32: 798–807.

Nicolas G, Devys D, Goldenberg A, *et al.* (2011): Juvenile Huntington disease in an 18-month-old boy revealed by global developmental delay and reduced cerebellar volume. *Am J Med Genet* 155: 815–818.

Nijssen PC, Ceuterick C, van Diggelen OP, *et al.* (2003): Autosomal dominant adult neuronal ceroid lipofuscinosis: a novel form of NCL with granular osmiophilic deposits without palmitoyl protein thioesterase 1 deficiency. *Brain Pathol* 13: 574–581.

Nishigaki Y, Tadesse S, Bonilla E, *et al.* (2003): A novel mitochondrial tRNA(Leu(UUR)) mutation in a patient with features of MERRF and Kearns-Sayre syndrome. *Neuromuscul Disord* 13: 334–340.

Nishimura R, Omos-Lau N, Ajmone-Marsan C, Baranger JA (1980): Electroencephalographic findings in Gaucher Disease. *Neurology* 30: 152–159.

Oguni H, Uehara T, Tanaka T, Sunahara M, Hara M, Osawa M (1998): Dramatic effect of ethosuximide on epileptic negative myoclonus: implications forthe neurophysiological mechanism. *Neuropediatrics* 29: 29–34.

Okino S (1997): Familial benign myoclonus epilepsy of adult onset: a previously unrecognized myoclonic disorder. *J Neurol Sci* 145: 113–118.

Okuneva O, Li Z, Korber I, *et al.* (2016): Brain inflammation is accompanied by peripheral inflammation in Cstb-/- mice, a model for progressive myoclonus epilepsy. *J Neuroinflammation* 13: 298

Oliver KL, Franceschetti S, Milligan CJ, *et al.* (2017): Myoclonus Epilepsy and Ataxia due to KCNC1 Mutation: Analysis of 20 Cases and K1 Channel Properties. *Ann Neurol* 81: 677–689.

Pampiglione G, Harden A (1977): Neurophysiological identification of a late infantile form of "neuronal lipidosis". *J Neurol Neurosurg Psychiatr* 36: 323–330.

Papacostas S, Kkolou E, Papathanasiou E (2007): Levetiracetam in three cases of progressive myoclonus epilepsy. *Pharm World Sci* 29: 164–166.

Parra D, Gonzalez A, Mugueta C, Martinez A, Monreal I (2001): Laboratory approach to mitochondrial diseases. *J Physiol Biochem* 57: 267–284.

Pennacchio LA, Lehesjoki AE, Stone NE, *et al.* (1996): Mutations in the gene encoding cystatin B in progressive myoclonus epilepsy (EPM1). *Science* 271: 1731–1734.

Pérez-Duenas B, Toma C, Ormazâbal A, *et al.* (2010): Progressive ataxia and myoclonic epilepsy in a patient with a homozygous mutation in the FOLR1 gene. *J Inherit Metab Dis* 33: 795–802.

Phillips SN, Benedict JW, Weimer JM, Pearce DA (2005): CLN3, the protein associated with batten disease: structure, function and localization. *J Neurosci Res* 79: 573–583.

Pinto E, Freitas J, Duarte AJ, *et al.* (2012): Unverricht-Lundborg disease: homozygosity for a new splicing mutation in the cystatin B gene. *Epilepsy Res* 99: 187–190.

Pinto WB, de Souza PV, Pinheiro JR, *et al.* (2015): Retinitis pigmentosa in Lafora disease: expanding findings of progressivemyoclonic epilepsy. *Neurology* 85: 1087.

Pranzatelli MR, Tate ED (2001): Chloral hydrate for progressive myoclonus epilepsy: a new look at an old drug. *Pediatr Neurol* 25: 385–389.

Raben N, Lu N, Nagaraju K, *et al.* (2001): Conditional tissue-specific expression of the acid alpha-glucosidase (GAA) gene in the GAA knockout mice: implications for therapy. *Hum Mol* Genet 10: 2039–2047.

Ranta S, Lehesjoki AE (2000): Northern epilepsy, a new member of the NCL family. *Neurol Sci* 21 (Suppl 3): S43–S47.

Ranta S, Topcu M, Tegelberg S, *et al.* (2004): Variant late infantile neuronal ceroid lipofuscinosis in a subset of Turkish patients is allelic to Northern epilepsy. *Hum Mutat* 23: 300–305.

Ranza E, Garcia-Tarodo S, Varvagiannis K (2017): SERPINI1 pathogenic variants: An emerging cause of childhood-onset progressive myoclonic epilepsy. *Am J Med Genet* 173: 2456–2460.

Rapin I, Goldfisher S, Katzman R., Engel J, O'Brien JS (1978): The cherry-red spot myoclonus syndrome. *Ann Neurol* 3: 234–342.

Rinne R, Saukko P, Jarvinen M, Lehesjoki AE (2002): Reduced cystatin B activity correlates with enhanced cathepsin activity in progressive myoclonus epilepsy. *Ann Med* 34: 380–385.

Roger J (1985): Progressive myoclonic epilepsy in childhood and adolescence. In: Roger J, Dravet C, Bureau M, Dreifuss FE, Wolf P (eds). *Epileptic Syndromes in Infancy, Childhood and Adolescence*, 1st ed, pp. 302–310. London, Paris: John Libbey.

Roger J, Soulayrol R, Hassoun J (1968): La dyssynergie cérébelleuse myoclonique (syndrome de Ramsay-Hunt). *Rev Neurol* 119: 85–106.

Roger J, Pellissier JF, Bureau M, Dravet C, Revol M, Tinuper P (1983): Le diagnostic précoce de la maladie de Lafora. Importance des manifestations paroxystiques visuelles et intérêt de la biopsie cutanée. *Rev Neurol* 139: 115–124.

Roger J, Genton P, Bureau M (1990): Progressive myoclonus epilepsies. In: Dam M, Gram L (eds) *Comprehensive Epileptology*, New York: Raven Press, pp. 215–231.

Roger J, Bureau M, Dravet C, Genton P, Tassinari CA, Michelucci R (1991): La place des encéphalopathies mitochondriales dans les epilepsies-myoclonies progressives. *Rev Neurol* 147: 480–490.

Roger J, Genton P, Bureau M, Dravet C (1992): Progressive myoclonus epilepsies in childhood and adolescence. In: Roger J, Bureau M, Dravet C, Dreifuss FE, Perret A, Wolf P (eds) *Epileptic Syndromes in Infancy, Childhood and Adolescence*, 2nd ed, London: John Libbey, pp. 381–400.

Rosing HS, Hopkins LC, Wallace DC, Epstein CM, Weidenheim K (1985): Maternally inherited mitochondrial myopathy and myoclonic epilepsy. *Ann Neurol* 17: 228–237.

Rossmanith W, Raffelsberger T, Roka J, Kornek B, Feucht M, Bittner RE (2003): The expanding mutational spectrum of MERRF substitution G8361A in the mitochondrial tRNALys gene. *Ann Neurol* 54: 820–823.

Rubboli G, Franceschetti S, Berkovic SF, *et al.* (2011): Clinical and neurophysiologic features of progressive myoclonus epilepsy without renal failure caused by SCARB2 mutations. *Epilepsia* 52: 2356–2363.

Saadah M, El Beshari M, Saadah L, *et al.* (2014): progressive myoclonic epilepsy type 1: report of an Emirati family and literature review. *Epilepsy & Behavior Case Reports* 2: 112–117.

Sakazume Y, Tanaka M, Isobe I, *et al.* (2004): A case of middle-aged onset sialidosis type I. *Rinsho Shinkeigaku* 44: 541–544.

Sánchez-Elexpuru G, Serratosa JM, Sanz P, Sánchez MP (2017): 4-Phenylbutyric acid and metformin decrease sensitivity to pentylenetetrazol-induced seizures in a malin knockout model of Lafora disease. *Neuroreport* 28: 268–271.

Sangani M, Shahid A, Amina S, Koubeissi M (2010): Improvement of myoclonic epilepsy in Down syndrome treated with levetiracetam. *Epileptic Disord* 12: 151–154.

Santavuori P, Haltia M, Rapola J (1974): Infantile type of so-called neuronal ceroid lipofuscinosis. *Neuropaediatrie* 4: 375–387.

Santavuori P, Heiskala H, Westermarck T, Sainio K, Moren R (1988): Experience over 17 years with antioxidant treatment in Spielmeyer-Sjögren disease. *Am J Med* Genet (Suppl) 5: 265–274.

Santorelli FM, Mak SC, El-Schahawi M, *et al.* (1996): Maternally inherited cardiomyopathy and hearing loss associated with a novel mutation in the mitochondrial tRNA(lys) gene (G8363A). *Am J Hum Genet* 58: 933–939.

Sato T, Miura M, Yamada M, *et al.* (2008): Severe neurological phenotypes of Q129 DRPLA transgenic mice serendipitously created by en masse expansion of CAG repeats in Q76 DRPLA mice. *Hum Mol* Genet 18: 723–736.

Savukoski M, Kestila M, Williams R, *et al.* (1994): Defined chromosomal assignment of CLN5 demonstrates that at least four loci are involved in the pathogenesis of human ceroid lipofuscinosis. *Am J Hum* Genet 55: 695–701.

Savukoski M, Klockars T, Holmberg V, Santavuori P, Lander ES, Peltonen I (1998): *CLN5*, a novel gene encoding a putative transmembrane protein mutated in Finnish variant late infantile neuronal ceroid lipofuscinosis. *Nat Genet* 19: 286–288.

Schmidt C, Redyk K, Meissner B, *et al.* (2010): Clinical features of rapidly progressive Alzheimer's disease. *Dement Geriatr Cogn Disord* 29: 371–378.

Schulz A, Dhar S, Rylova S, *et al.* (2004): Impaired cell adhesion and apoptosis in a novel CLN9 Batten disease variant. *Ann Neurol* 5: 342–350.

Serratosa JM, Delgado-Escueta AV, Posada I, *et al.* (1995): The gene for progressive myoclonus epilepsy of the Lafora type maps to chromosome 6q. *Hum Mol Genet* 9: 1657–1663.

Serratosa JM, Gomez-Garre P, Gallardo ME, *et al.* (1999): A novel protein tyrosine phosphatase gene is mutated in progressive myoclonus epilepsy of the Lafora type (EPM2). *Hum Mol Genet* 8: 345–352.

Shapira Y, Cederbaum SD, Cancilla PA, Nielsen D, Lippe BM (1975): Familial poliodystrophy, mitochondrial myopathy and lactate acidemia. *Neurology* 25: 614–621.

Sharp JD, Wheeler RB, Lake BD, *et al.* (1997): Loci for classical and variant late infantile neuronal ceroid lipofuscinosis map to chromosome 11p15 and 15q21–23. *Hum Mol Genet* 6: 591–595.

Sharp JD, Wheeler RB, Parker KA, *et al.* (2003): Spectrum of CLN6 mutations in variant late infantile neuronal ceroid lipofuscinosis. *Hum Mutat* 22: 35–42.

Sheffer IE, Berkovic S, Capovilla G, *et al.* (2017): ILAE classification of the epilepsies: Position paper of the ILAE Commission for Classification and Terminology. *Epilepsia* 58: 512–521

Shoffner JM, Lott MT, Lezza AM, Seibel P, Ballinger SW, Wallace DC (1990): Myoclonic epilepsy and ragged-red fiber disease (MERRF) is associated with a mitochondrial DNA tRNA(Lys) mutation. *Cell* 61: 931–937.

Siintola E, Topcu M, Kohlschutter A, *et al.* (2005): Two novel CLN6 mutations in variant late-infantile neuronal ceroid lipofuscinosis patients of Turkish origin. *Clin Genet* 68: 167–173.

Silvestri G, Moraes CT, Shanske S, Oh SJ, DiMauro S (1992): A new mtDNA mutation in the tRNA-lys gene associated with myoclonic epilepsy and ragged-red fibers (MERRF). *Am J Hum Genet* 51: 1213–1217.

Singh S, Sethi I, Francheschetti S, *et al.* (2006): Novel NHLRC1 mutations and genotype-phenotype correlations in patients with Lafora's progressive myoclonic epilepsy. *J Med Genet* 43: e48.

Sjögren T (1931): Die amaurotische Idiotie. Klinische Beschreibung und Erblichkeit, medizinische Untersuchungen. *Lund: Hereditas* 14: 197–426.

Sleat DE, Donnelly RJ, Lackland H, *et al.* (1997): Association of mutations in a lysosomal protein with classical late-infantile neuronal ceroidlipofuscinosis. *Science* 277: 1802–1805.

Smith B, Shatz R, Elisevich K, Bespalova IN, Burmeister M (2000): Effects of vagus nerve stimulation on progressive myoclonus epilepsy of Unverricht-Lundborg type. *Epilepsia* 41: 1046–1048.

Smith KR, Dahl HHM, Canafoglia L, *et al.* (2013): Cathepsin F mutations cause Type B Kufs disease, an adult-onset neuronal ceroid lipofuscinosis. *Hum Molec Genetics* 22: 1417–1423.

So N, Berkovic S, Andermann F, Kuziecky R, Gendron D, Quesney LF (1989): Myoclonus epilepsy and ragged-red fibres (MERRF). 2. Electrophysiological studies and comparison with other progressive myoclonus epilepsy. *Brain* 112: 1261–1276.

Stengel E (1826): Account of a singular illness among four siblings in the vicinity of Reraas. Eyr (Christiana) 1: 347–352. English translation, 1982. In: Armstrong D, Koopand N, Rider JA (eds) *Ceroid lipofuscinosis (Batten's disease)*, Amsterdam, NewYork, Oxford: Elsevier Biomedical Press, pp. 17–19.

Suoranta S, Holli-Helenius K, Koskenkorva P, *et al.* (2013): 3D Texture Analysis Reveals Imperceptible MRI Textural Alterations in the Thalamus and Putamen in Progressive Myoclonic Epilepsy Type 1, EPM1.PlosOne 8: e69.

Svennerholm L, Dreborg S, Erikson A, *et al.* (1982): Gaucher disease of the Norbottinian type (type III). Phenotypic manifestation. In: Desnick RJ, Gan S, Grabowski GA (eds) *Gaucher disease: a century of delineation and research*, New York: Alan R. Liss, pp. 62–70.

Tai KK & Truong DD (2007): Brivaracetam is superior to levetiracetam in a rat model of post-hypoxic myoclonus. *J. Neural Transm* 114, 1547–1551.

Taschner PEM, de Vos N, Thompson AD, *et al.* (1995): Chromosome 16 microdeletion in a patient with juvenile neuronal ceroid lipofuscinosis (Batten disease). *Am J Hum* Genet 55: 695–701.

Tassinari CA, Bureau-Paillas M, Dalla Bernardina B, Grasso E, Roger J (1974): Etude électroencéphalographique de la dyssynergie cérébelleuse myoclonique avec épilepsie (syndrome de Ramsay-Hunt). *Rev EEG Neurophysiol* 4: 407–428.

Tassinari CA, Bureau-Paillas M, Dalla Bernardina B, *et al.* (1978): La maladie de Lafora. *Rev EEG Neurophysiol* 8: 107–122.

Tassinari CA, Michelucci R, Genton P, Pellissier JF, RogerJ (1989): Dyssynergia cerebellaris myoclonica (Ramsay Hunt syndrome): an autonomous condition unrelated to mitochondrial encephalomyopathies. *J Neurol Neurosurg Psychiatr* 52: 262–265.

Tassinari CA, Riguzzi P, Volpi L, *et al.* (1999): Zonisamide in the treatment of action myoclonus in progressive myoclonus epilepsies. Epilepsia 40: 242.

Tiberia E, Turnbull J, Wang T, *et al.* (2012): Increased laforin and laforin binding to glycogen underlie Lafora body formation in malin-deficient Lafora disease. *J Biol Chem* 287: 25650–25659.

Tinuper P, Aguglia U, Pellissier JF, Gastaut H (1983): Visual ictal phenomena in a case of Lafora disease proven by skin biopsy. *Epilepsia* 24: 214–218.

Topiramate YTC/YTCE Study Group. (2000): Nonfocal generalized tonic-clonic seizures: response during long-term topiramate treatment. *Epilepsia* 41 (Suppl 1): S77–81.

Tsairis P, Engel WK, Kark F (1973): Familial myoclonic epilepsy syndrome associated with skeletal muscle mitochondrial abnormalities. *Neurology* 23: 408.

Tsuji S (2000): Dentatorubral-pallidoluysian atrophy. *J Neural Transm* 58 (Suppl): 167–180.

Tsuji S (2012): Dentatorubral-pallidoluysian atrophy. *Handb Clin Neurol* 103: 587–594.

Turnbull J, Tiberia E, Striano P, *et al.* (2016): Lafora disease. *Epileptic Disord* 18 (52): 38–62.

Ullrich NJ, Riviello JJ Jr, Darras BT, Donner EJ (2004): Electroencephalographic correlate of juvenile Huntington's disease. *J Child Neurol* 19: 541–543.

Unverricht H (1891): Die Myoclonie, Leipzig, Wien: Franz Deuticke.

Uvebrant P, Conradi NG, Hokegard KH, Wahlstrom J, Mellqvist L (1987): First trimester diagnosis of neuronal ceroid-lipofuscinosis on chorionic villi. *Neuropediatrics* 18: 117.

Vaca GF, Lenz T, Knight EM, Tuxhorn I (2012): Gaucher disease: successful treatment of myoclonic status epilepticus with levetiracetam. *Epileptic Disord* 14: 155–158.

Van Bogaert P, Azizieh R, Désir J, *et al.* (2007): Mutation of a potassium channel-related gene in progressive myoclonic epilepsy. *Ann Neurol* 61: 579–586.

van den Ameele J, Jedlickova I, Pristoupilova A, *et al.* (2018): Teenage-onset progressive myoclonic epilepsy due to a familial C9orf72 repeat expansion. *Neurology* 90: e658–e663.

Van Goethem G, Mercelis R, Löfgren A, *et al.* (2003): Patient homozygous for a recessive POLG mutation presents with features of MERRF. *Neurology* 61: 1811–1813.

Van Heycop Ten Ham MW, De Jager H (1963): Progressive myoclonus epilepsy with Lafora bodies. Clinical-pathological features. *Epilepsia* 4: 95–119.

Vanni N, Fruscione F, Ferlazzo E, *et al.* (2014): Impairment of ceramide synthesis causes a novel progressive myoclonus epilepsy. *Ann Neurol* 76: 2016–2012.

Vesper J, Steinhoff B, Rona S, *et al.* (2007): Chronic high-frequency deep brain stimulation of the STN/SNr for progressive myoclonic epilepsy. *Epilepsia* 48: 1984–1989.

Virtaneva K, D'Amato E, Miao J, *et al.* (1997): Unstable minisatellite expansion causing recessively inherited myoclonus epilepsy, EPM1. *Nat Genet* 15: 393–396.

Vossler DG, Conry JA, Murphy JV, the ZNS-502/505 PME Study Group (2008): Zonisamide for the treatment of myoclonic seizures in progressive myoclonus epilepsy: an open label study. *Epileptic Disord* 10: 31–34.

Wallace DC, Shoffner JM, Lott MT, Hopkins LC (1991): Myoclonic epilepsy and ragged-red fiber disease (MERRF): a mitochondrial tRNALys mutation responsive to coenzyme Q10 (CoQ) therapy. *Neurology* 41 (Suppl 1): 586, S280.

Wallace SJ (1998): Myoclonus and epilepsy in childhood: a review of treatment with valproate, ethosuximide, lamotrigine and zonisamide. *Epilepsy Res* 29: 147–154.

Warburg M (1982): The natural history of Jansky-Bielschowsky's and Batten's diseases. In: Armstrong D, Koopand N, Rider JA (eds) *Ceroid Lipofuscinosis (Batten's disease)*, Amsterdam, New York, Oxford: Elsevier Biomedical Press, pp. 35–42.

Welch EM, Barton ER, Zhuo J, *et al.* (2007): PTC 124 targets genetic disorders caused by nonsense mutations. *Nature* 447: 88–93.

Wenger DA (1978): Assay of beta-glucosidase and sphingomyelinase for identification of patients and carriers of Gaucher's and Niemann-Pick eases. *Adv Exp Med Biol* 101: 707–717.

Wheeler RB, Sharp JD, Schultz RA, Joslin JM, Williams RE, Mole SE (2002): The gene mutated in variant late-infantile neuronal ceroid lipofuscinosis (CLN6) and in nclf mutant mice encodes a novel predicted transmembrane protein. *Am J Hum Genet* 70: 537–542.

Wiedemann FR, Bartels C, Kirches E, Mawrin C, Wallesch CW (2008): Unusual presentations of patients with the mitochondrial MERRF mutation A8344G. *Clin Neurol Neurosurg* 110: 859–863.

Wille C, Steinhoff BJ, Altenmüller DM, *et al.* (2011): Chronic high-frequency deep-brain stimulation in progressive myoclonic epilepsy in adulthood-report of five cases. *Epilepsia* 52: 489–496.

Wisniewski KE, Zhong N, Phillipart M (2001): Pheno/genotypic correlations of neuronal ceroid liposcinoses. *Neurology* 57: 576–581.

Xing S, Chen L, Chen X, Pei Z, Zeng J, Li J (2008): Excessive blinking as an initial manifestation of juvenile Huntington's disease. *Neurol Sci* 29: 275–277.

Yamada M, Tsuji S, Takahashi H (2002): Genotype-phenotype correlation in CAG-repeat diseases. *Neuropathology* 22: 317–322.

Yeetong P, Ausavarat S, Bhidayasiri R, *et al.* (2013): A newly identified locus for benign adult myoclonic epilepsy on chromosome 3 q26.32–3. *Eur J Hum Genet* 21: 225–228.

Yoshimura I, Kaneko S, Yoshimura N, Murakami T (2001): Long-term observations of two siblings with Lafora disease treated with zonisamide. *Epilepsy Res* 46: 283–287.

Yis U, Dirik E, Gündogdu-Eken A, Basak AN (2009): Dentatorubral pallidoluysian atrophy in a Turkish family. *TurkJ Pediatr* 51: 610–612.

Zeman W, Donahue S, Dyken P, Green J (1970): The neuronal ceroid-lipofuscinoses (Batten-Vogt syndrome). In: Vinken PS, Bruyn G (eds) *Handbook of Clinical Neurology*, vol. 10, Amsterdam: Else-vier North-Holland, pp. 588–679.

Zeviani M, Amati P, Bresolin N, *et al.* (1991): Rapid detection of the A-to-G(8344) mutation of mtDNA in Italian families with myoclonus epilepsy and ragged-red fibers (MERRF). *Am J Hum Genet* 48: 203–211.

CHAPTER 31
EPILEPSY AND MALFORMATIONS OF THE CEREBRAL CORTEX

Renzo Guerrini and Elena Parrini

Pediatric Neurology Unit and Laboratories, Children's Hospital A. Meyer, University of Florence, Firenze, Italy

Abnormal cortical development is a frequent cause of developmental disabilities and epilepsy. Improved magnetic resonance imaging (MRI) resolution makes it possible to assess the distribution and depth of cortical sulci, cortical thickness, the boundaries between grey and white matter, and variations in signal intensity. Abnormalities of any or all of these features may be observed in different malformations of cortical development (MCD), which may be restricted to discrete cortical areas or may, alternatively, be diffuse (Guerrini *et al.*, 2008; Guerrini & Dobyns, 2014). A classification scheme has been developed categorizing MCD into 3 major groups that recapitulate the main developmental steps as malformations of cell proliferation, neuronal migration, or postmigrational cortical organization and connectivity. Although the classification of MCD has advanced substantially during the past decade, in practice only a few categories are used, including lissencephaly (LIS), polymicrogyria, schizencephaly, focal cortical dysplasia (FCD), and periventricular nodular heterotopia (PNH). Emerging evidence suggests that MCD are far more heterogeneous than this classification suggests and should ideally be based on knowledge of neurobiological pathways (Guerrini & Dobyns, 2014), which is however still too incomplete to underpin a new classification proposal.

Some cortical malformations seem to be directly associated with particular epilepsy syndromes of epilepsy phenotypes. In the following sections, we will review several of the most common malformations of the cerebral cortex or of cortical elements and the types of epilepsy they are associated with.

Malformations related to abnormal proliferation of neurons and glia

Megalencephaly

The term megalencephaly refers to an abnormally large brain that exceeds the mean for age and gender by 2 SD (DeMyer, 1986). Megalencephaly has most often been classified as a disorder of brain size, but more recent studies indicate that megalencephaly with normal cortex by imaging, megalencephaly with polymicrogyria, and dysplastic megalencephaly (including classic hemimegalencephaly) as well as focal cortical dysplasia (FCD) can all result from mutations in genes in the PI3K-AKT-mTOR pathway (Lee *et al.*, 2012; Poduri *et al.*, 2012; Rivière *et al.*, 2012b; Mirzaa *et al.*, 2015).

The most common cortical malformation in megalencephaly is perisylvian polymicrogyria that looks very similar to perisylvian polymicrogyria in patients with normal or small head size. The developmental and health complications of megalencephaly differ widely. The most common problems include developmental delay, intellectual disability, and seizures that can start early in life and be intractable. Children with diffuse symmetrical or mildly asymmetrical megalencephaly, with or without associated polymicrogyria, have a large head size at birth that soon exceeds +3 SD (Mirzaa *et al.*, 2012). Their early development is delayed, and later cognitive development varies from normal to severe intellectual disability.

Megalencephaly without cortical malformations occurs in benign autosomal dominant macrocephaly, a poorly defined disorder. Several syndromes have been associated with megalencephaly and include neurofibromatosis type 1 due to NF1 microdeletions that also involve the *RNF135* gene and Sotos syndrome (with *NSD1* mutations), Weaver syndrome (with *EZH2* mutations), in addition to Bannayan-Riley-Ruvalcaba syndrome, Cowden syndrome, and severe megalencephaly with autism (all 3 with *PTEN* mutations) (Mirzaa *et al.*, 2012). Megalencephaly with polymicrogyria occurs in megalencephaly-capillary malformation syndrome (with mutations of *PIK3CA*) and megalencephaly-polymicrogyria-polydactyly-hydrocephalus syndrome (with mutations of *PIK3R2* or *AKT3*) (Mirzaa *et al.*, 2012, 2015).

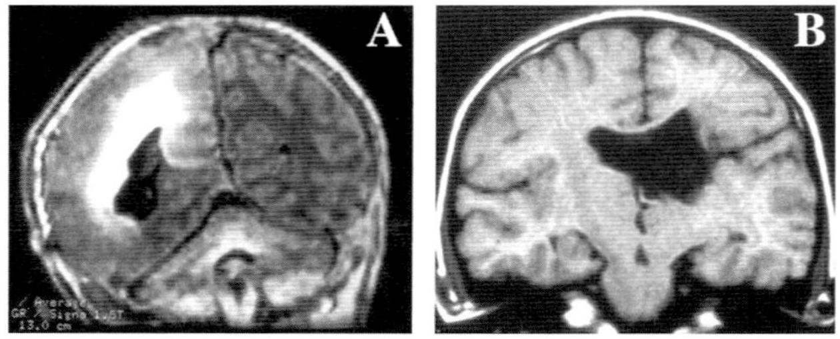

Figure 1 A. **Hemimegalencephaly in a 3-month-old boy with intractable seizures. MRI, SE, coronal section. The right hemisphere is enlarged, with thickened cortex and smooth surface. There are no digitations between the grey and white matter. High signal intensity in the white matter throughout the right hemisphere.** B. **Unilateral closed lip schizencephaly in a boy with complex partial seizures and mild hemiparesis. MRI spin-echo T1 weighted slice. The parenchymal cleft involves the left hemisphere and spans from the subarachnoid to the lateral ventricle.**

Hemimegalencephaly and focal cortical dysplasia

Hemimegalencephaly (HME) and focal cortical dysplasia (FCD) constitute a spectrum of malformations of cortical development with shared neuropathological features. In hemimegalencephaly one cerebral hemisphere is enlarged and structurally abnormal, with a thick cortex, wide convolutions and reduced sulci *(Figure 1A)*. The cortical changes in hemimegalencephaly are severe with no consistent preference for which lobes of the brain are enlarged (Salamon *et al.*, 2006). Although classical pathological studies (Robain & Gelot, 1996) had suggested that the structural abnormality is strictly unilateral, very large dysplastic megalencephalic brains have been described whose characteristics suggest a sort of bilateral asymmetric hemimegalencephaly (Guerini & Dobyns, 2014), which indicates that the distorted developmental dynamics may allow the seemingly normal hemisphere to harbour structural abnormalities in some patients. This point should prompt careful investigation of surgical candidates. Laminar organization is absent in the cortex, and the demarcation between grey and white matter is poor. There are dysmorphic neurons (up to 80 mμ in diameter) in the cortex and white matter. In about 50% of cases "balloon cells" are also observed. Hemimegalencephaly is a heterogeneous condition and its nosography is still uncertain. It has been associated with different disorders including Epidermal nevus syndrome (Zaremba *et al.*, 1978; Vigevano *et al.*, 1984; Choi & Kudo, 1981; Sakuta *et al.*, 1989; Pavone *et al.*, 1991; Dodge & Dobyns, 1995); Klippel-Trenaunay-Weber syndrome (Cheruy & Heller, 1987); Proteus syndrome (Griffiths *et al.*, 1994); Neurofibromatosis (Cusmai *et al.*, 1990); Focal alopecia (Pelayo *et al.*, 1994); Tuberous sclerosis (Maloof *et al.*, 1994), Dysembryoplastic neuroepithelial tumor (Guerrini *et al.*, 1996a); but it can also occur in isolation. In spite of these heterogeneous associations, hemimegalencephaly most often occurs without syndromic features and has been associated with mosaic mutations of *PIK3CA*, *AKT3*, and *MTOR* (Lee *et al.*, 2012). Hemimegalencephaly has also been associated with the linear nevus sebaceous syndrome (also known as Schimmelpenning syndrome) and, rarely, with CLOVES syndrome (congenital lipomatous overgrowth with vascular, epidermal, and skeletal anomalies), hemihypertrophy, and hypomelanosis of Ito (Peserico *et al.*, 1988; Williams & Elster, 1990; D'Agostino *et al.*, 2004; Tinkle *et al.*, 2005).

The clinical spectrum of hemimegalencephaly is wide, ranging from severe neonatal onset epileptic encephalopathy to individuals with normal cognitive level and late onset focal seizures. Typically, affected children have asymmetry of the skull with macrocrania, hemiparesis, hemianopia, intellectual disability and intractable seizures. Infantile spasms and a suppression burst pattern on sleep EEG have been reported (Paladin *et al.*,1989). An indication for large resections or hemispherotomy can be established within the first year of life. Hemispherectomy controls seizures in about 31% of children but seems to have a modest impact on cognitive outcome (Pulsifer *et al.*, 2004).

Histological abnormalities similar to those encountered in hemimegalencephaly may be restricted to one cerebral lobe or involve a segment measuring only a few centimeters and had originally be designated as focal cortical dysplasia (FCD) (Taylor *et al.*, 1971). This term is now used to include a spectrum of abnormalities of the laminar structure of the cortex, variably associated with cytopathological features including giant (or cytomegalic) neurons, dysmorphic neurons and balloon cells *(Figures 2 and 3B)* (Blumcke *et al.*, 2011). Balloon cells are of uncertain lineage, exhibit an abundant pale-staining cytoplasm, peripherally positioned nuclei, no cellular processes and cell-surface markers for pluripotent stem cells (Ying *et al.*, 2005). The dysplastic area is not usually sharply defined from the adjacent tissue.

A refined classification system for FCD has been proposed based on the evaluation of the clinical presentation, imaging findings, and histopathologic features of distinct clinicopathological FCD variants (Blumcke *et al.*, 2011). FCD Type I refers to isolated lesions, which present either as radial (FCD Type Ia) or tangential (FCD Type Ib) dyslamination of the neocortex, microscopically identified in one or multiple lobes. FCD Type II is an isolated lesion characterized by cortical dyslamination and dysmorphic neurons without (Type IIa) or with balloon cells (Type IIb). FCD Type III, which occurs in combination with hippocampal sclerosis (FCD Type IIIa), or with epilepsy-associated tumours (FCD Type IIIb). FCD Type IIIc is found adjacent to vascular malformations, whereas FCD Type IIId can be diagnosed in association with epileptogenic lesions acquired in early life (*i.e.*, traumatic injury, ischemic injury or encephalitis).

According to the prevailing hypothesis, FCD Type II, the form which is by far more frequent, originates from abnormal migration, maturation and cell death during ontogenesis (Ying *et al.*, 2005; Najm *et al.*, 2007). While the origin of FCD Type I remains obscure, single

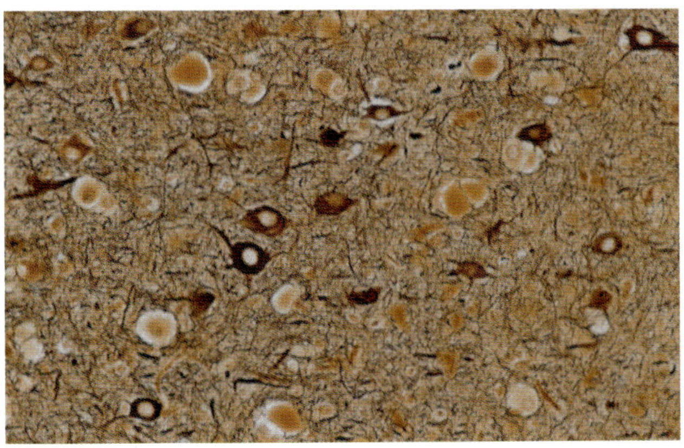

Figure 2 **Cortical dysplasia. Silver-stained section showing irregular arrangement of big neurones and pale brown "balloon-cells".**

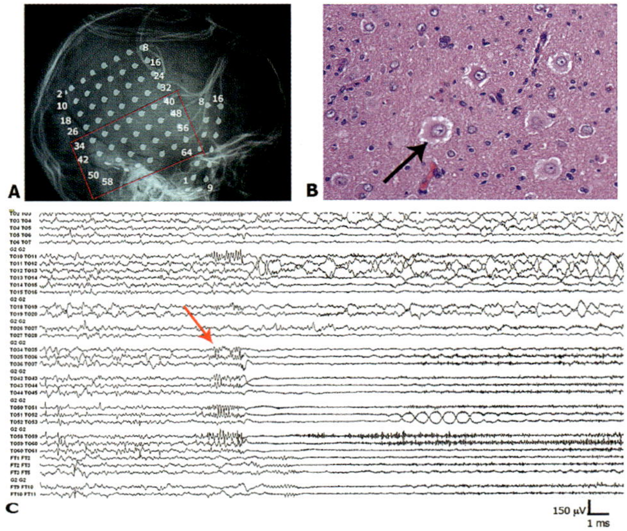

Figure 3 **A. X-ray performed after grid implantation exploring the right frontotemporal and parieto-occipital areas. Subdural electrodes indicate that the epileptogenic zone is located within the red rectangle. Grid contacts were numbered consecutively. B. Neuropathology showed Taylor-type dysplasia: hematoxylin-eosin staining. The black arrow indicates a balloon cell. C. Grid recordings showing interictal bursts of rhythmic spikes (red arrow). At seizure onset, the bursts stop and low-voltage fast discharge occurs at the same contacts.**

cell next generation sequencing studies have provided evidence that histologically similar lesions classifiable as FCD Type II are caused by somatic activating mutations in *AKT3*, *MTOR*, and *PIK3CA* and germline loss-of-function mutations in *DEPDC5*, *NPRL2*, and *TSC1/2*. These observations suggest that mutations in the same gene cause a disease continuum from FCD to hemimegalencephaly to bilateral brain overgrowth, reflecting the progenitor cell and developmental time when the mutation occurred. This hypothesis is substantiated by numerous studies that have documented pathogenic germline and mosaic mutations in genes belonging to the PI3K-AKT-mTOR pathway in the dysplasic tissue of FCD Type IIa and IIb (D'Gama *et al.*, 2015; Lim *et al.*, 2015; Sim *et al.*, 2016) *(Figure 4A, B)*. In addition, somatic duplications in the 1q chromosomal region encompassing

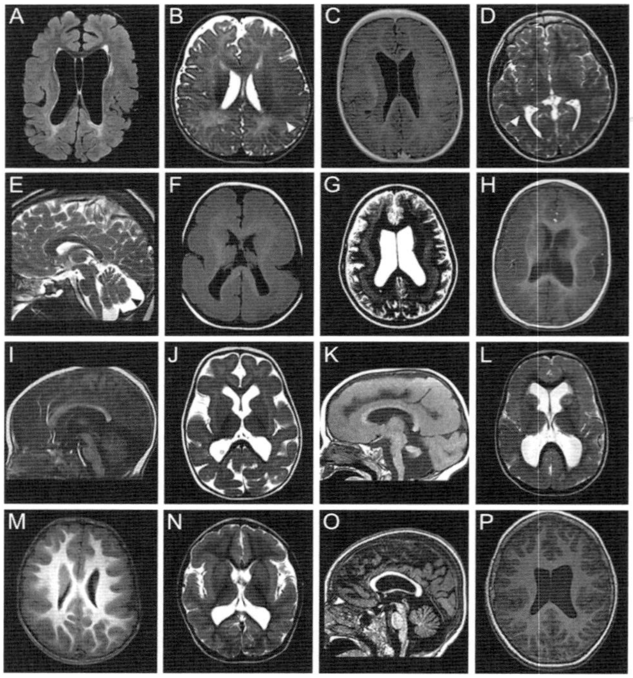

Figure 4 **Brain MRI of patients with different malformations of the cerebral cortex.**
A, B. **T1-weighted and T2-weighted axial images form patients carrying mosaic mutations in the *MTOR* gene with different percentages of mosaicism [**A: **p.Thr1977Ile, 20% of mosaicism in blood,** B: **p.Ser2215Phe, 5.5% of mosaicism in dysplastic brain tissue) showing bilateral cortical dysgyria (**A**) and focal cortical dysplasia (**B**, white arrowhead)].** C. **T1-weighted axial section. Typical, classical bilateral PNH in a girl with a *FLNA* mutation. Bilateral nodules of subependymal heterotopia are contiguous and rather symmetric, extensively lining the ventricular walls.** D, E. **T2-weighted axial section showing mild colpocephaly with unilateral PNH (white arrowhead) and T2-weighted sagittal section through the midline, showing cerebellar vermis hypoplasia (black arrowhead) with mega cisterna magna in a patient carrying a deletion in the 6q27 chromosomal region.** F. **T1-weighted axial section. Posterior to anterior pachygyria in a boy with asn *LIS1* mutation.** G. **T2-weighted axial section. Diffuse SBH in a girl with a *DCX* mutation.** H, I. **T1-weighted axial section and T1-weighted sagittal section. Thickened cortex with simplified gyral pattern and cerebellar hypoplasia in a girl with a *TUBA1A* mutation.** J, K. **T2-weighted, axial section and T1-weighted sagittal section. Lissencephaly and cerebellar hypoplasia in a girl with *RELN* mutation.** L. **T2-weighted axial section. Bilateral frontoparietal polymicrogyria in a boy with *GPR56* mutation.** M. **T1-weighted axial section. Diffuse simplified gyral pattern with prominent thickening and infolding of the sylvian fissures in a boy with *TUBB2B* mutation.** N, O. **T2-weighted axial section and T1-weighted coronal section. Pachygyria and perisylvian polymicrogyria in a girl with *DYNC1H1* mutation.** P. **Axial T1-weighted section in a patient with a mosaic *PIK3R2* mutation.**

the *AKT3* gene have been associated with megalencephaly, hemimegalencephaly, and FCD Type Ib (Poduri *et al.*, 2012; Wang *et al.*, 2013; Conti *et al.*, 2015). When performing genetic testing for disorders possibly caused by mosaic mutations, the screening of multiple tissues (*e.g.*, blood, saliva, and skin fibroblasts) is advisable. Although testing DNA extracted from blood is the gold standard for identifying *de novo* constitutive mutations, the analysis of different tissues may help in identifying mutations that are only present in a subset of somatic cells (Nellist *et al.*, 2015).

However, FCD may also derive from nongenetic causes. A link has also been postulated between FCD and perinatal or early postnatal brain injury, with subsequent cell "dedifferentiation" in the scared area (Golden & Harding, 2004; Marìn-Padilla *et al.*, 2002).

On MRI imaging, patients with FCD usually have enlarged gyri with either smooth or irregular cortical surface and increased cortical-subcortical signal intensity. Some individuals with FCD Type IIb have migration tracts underlined by hyperintense radially oriented white matter bands that extend from the dysplastic cortex to the periventricular region, an imaging feature that has been termed transmantle dysplasia (Barkovich *et al.*, 1997).

Virtually in all patients with FCD, the lesion is detected after onset of focal epilepsy, although very early seizure onset has been associated with infantile spasms with focal features (Guerrini & Filippi, 2005). FCD is a frequent cause of focal status epilepticus and is the most common pathological substrate in epilepsy surgery series, reaching up to 40% (Golden & Harding, 2004). Recordings with intracranial electrodes have demonstrated that the epileptogenic zone often extends beyond the lesion identifiable by MRI (Tassi *et al.*, 2002; Najm *et al.*, 2007). Complex seizure propagation patterns with unexpected interactions between noncontiguous sites have been documented (Duchowny *et al.*, 2000). Duchowny (2009) defined FCD as a functionally, electrophysiologically, and ultimately clinically integrated neural network disorder. As a consequence, to increase the chances of surgical success, it has been suggested that FCD should be operationally defined as a network dysfunction disorder with multifocal features rather than a localized process (Duchowny, 2009). "Intra-ictally" activated regions, capable of generating self-sustaining epileptogenesis in contiguity or at a distance from the primary zone of ictal activation, have been repeatedly documented. It is unclear to what extent seizure spread occurs through pathways that are integrated into the abnormal functional networks or if relentless epileptic discharges contribute to additional postnatal reorganization (Duchowny, 2009). Surface and intracranial EEG recordings reveal focal positive spike discharges or fast EEG frequencies, and ablation of tissue exhibiting these electrographic patterns correlates with outcome *(Figure 3A, C)* (Palmini *et al.*, 1995; Widdess-Walsh *et al.*, 2007).

Numerous studies on surgically resected human dysplastic tissue have focused on the mechanisms of epileptogenicity. Correlative light and electron microscopic methods indicate that balloon cells do not receive synaptic contacts, whereas abnormally large ectopic neurons are surrounded by hypertrophic basket formations (Alonso-Nanclares *et al.*, 2005). The density of excitatory and inhibitory synapses differs from that in the adjacent normal cortex, exhibiting increases and decreases in synaptic density as well as changes in the proportion of excitatory and inhibitory synapses; these might result in multiple changes in excitatory and inhibitory circuits (Alonso-Nanclares *et al.*, 2005).

Electrical stimulation studies have shown that the dysplastic neocortex may conserve temporal and frontal language sites (Duchowny *et al.*, 1996), but atypical motor homunculi have been revealed (Duchowny *et al.*, 2000). Magnetic source imaging suggests that, when FCD involves the sensorimotor cortex, reorganization of sensory function can be observed outside the malformed area (Burneo *et al.*, 2004). Correlative cortical stimulation and histopathologic studies suggest absence of language or motor functions in the epileptogenic perirolandic and Broca's areas that exhibit histopathological evidence of FCD with balloon cells and preservation of motor functions when no balloon cells are present (Marusic *et al.*, 2002). Although one might argue that the higher the disruption of cortical lamination the lower the ability of the cortex to subserve function, individual variability is probably very high (Guerrini *et al.*, 2015).

The most frequent clinical presentation in focal cortical dysplasia is that of a child or adolescent who develops intractable focal epilepsy. However, infantile spasms may be the first manifestation *(Figure 5A-C)*. There is no elective type of focal seizure. Focal status epilepticus is frequent (Desbiens *et al.*, 1993; Guerrini *et al.*, 1992a; Palmini *et al.*, 1995) and epilepsia partialis continua has been reported with dysplasia involving the precentral gyrus (Ferrer *et al.*, 1992; Kuzniecky *et al.*, 1988; Kuzniecky & Powers, 1993). Unless the dysplastic area is large, patients do not suffer from severe neurological deficits.

The interictal EEG shows focal, often rhythmic epileptiform discharges in about half patients (Gambardella *et al.*, 1996). These EEG abnormalities are highly specific of this type of lesion, are located over the epileptogenic area and are related to the continuous epileptiform discharges recorded during electrocorticography (EcoG) (Palmini *et al.*, 1995, 1996).

Malformations due to abnormal neuronal migration

Grey matter heterotopia

Heterotopia are agglomerates of neurons in an abnormal site. These neurons are normal in morphology and may assemble in a pattern suggestive of laminar organization, (Harding, 1996). Heterotopia can be diffuse or localized. Diffuse forms include subcortical band (or laminar) heterotopia (Barkovich *et al.*, 1994) and periventricular nodular heterotopia (PNH). Localized forms can be subependymal, unilateral or bilateral, subcortical (nodular, laminar), unilateral, or may extend from the subependymal region to the subcortex unilaterally.

Heterotopia can readily be diagnosed with MRI, showing the same signal as the normal cortex at every impulse sequence used. Heterotopic cortex may be functionally active but the surrounding cortex is often reorganized (Richardson *et al.*, 1998; Preul *et al.*, 1997; Muller *et al.*, 1998). Depth electrodes implanted in deeply located nodules and demonstrated that seizure activity usually originates both within the heterotopic cortex and the overlying cerebral cortex (Tassi *et al.*, 2005; Mirandola *et al.*, 2017; Pizzo *et al.*, 2017) or, rarely, just within the nodule (Scherer *et al.*, 2005).

Periventricular nodular heterotopia

Periventricular nodular heterotopia (PNH) consists of confluent nodules of grey matter located along the lateral ventricles (Barkovich *et al.*, 2012; Guerrini & Dobyns, 2014) *(Figure 4C)*; it ranges from isolated, single, to confluent bilateral nodules. Patients with the classic X-linked PNH typically have bilateral contiguous nodules that spare the temporal horns and mild cerebellar vermis hypoplasia with mega cisterna magna (Parrini *et al.*, 2006). Patients with rare autosomal recessive bilateral PNH may have severe

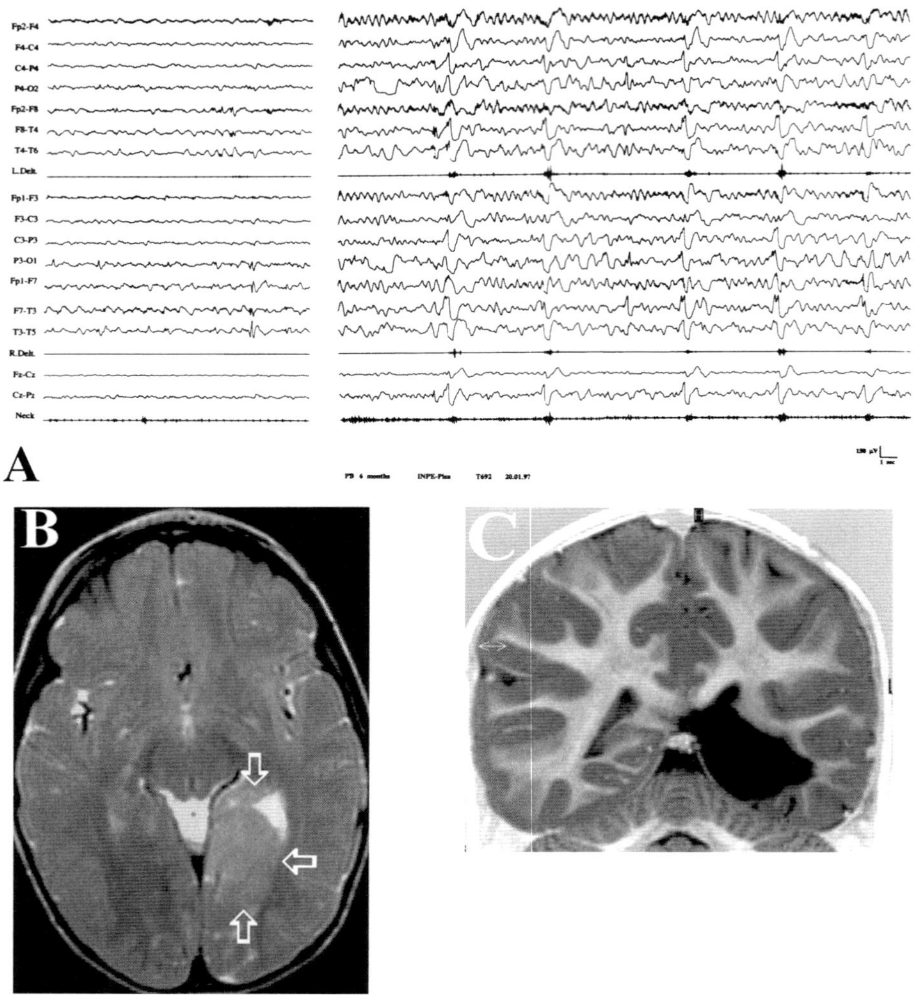

Figure 5 A. 6-month-old girl coming to our attention because of the appearance of infantile spasms. The interictal EEG (left), shows slow wave activity over both temporal regions, much more prominent on the left, where isolated spike and waves are superimposed with anterior temporal predominance. Independent sharp waves are seen over the left occipital area. Ictal recording during a series of spasms (right) shows slowing of EEG activity and captures five spasms in about 25 seconds. Spasms are accompanied by rightward eye deviation. B. Same patient as in A. MRI scan showed an area of cortical dysplasia involving the left mesiobasal part of the temporal lobe, the hippocampal region and extending back to the temporo-occipital junction (arrows). C. Same patient as in A and B. Resection of most of the abnormality, performed after intracranial recordings at age 1 year (Prof. Claudio Munari and coworkers), led to complete remission of spasms and developmental recovery. No relapse had occurred after 15 years of follow-up.

congenital microcephaly and thin overlying cortex with abnormal gyri (Sheen *et al.*, 2004a). In the fairly common posterior predominant syndromes, PNH is limited to the trigones, temporal and occipital horns, and can be associated with overlying polymicrogyria, hippocampal and cerebellar hypoplasia, or hydrocephalus (Pisano *et al.*, 2012).

The most common syndromic form of PNH (X-linked PNH) consists of bilateral contiguous or near contiguous nodules and is most often caused by *FLNA* mutations, high rates of prenatal lethality in male foetuses, and 50% recurrence risk in female offspring. All other PNH syndromes are rare. Almost 100% of families and 20% of sporadic patients harbour mutations or deletions/duplications of the *FLNA* gene (Parrini *et al.*, 2006; Clapham *et al.*, 2012). Alterations of this gene also cause coagulopathy and cardiovascular abnormalities in some patients. Only a few living male patients with periventricular nodular heterotopia owing to *FLNA* mutations have been reported (Sheen *et al.*, 2001; Guerrini *et al.*, 2004; Parrini *et al.*, 2011). Mild missense mutations or mosaic mutations account for survival of affected males who can, in turn, pass their genetic defect to their daughters. *FLNA* maps to chromosome Xq28, is composed of 48 exons, spans a 26 kb genomic region, and codes for filamin A, a 280 kDa protein with three major functional domains, allowing homodimerization and binding to actin and a wide range of cytoplasmic signaling proteins (Fox *et al.*, 1998). *FLNA* probably influences neuroblast migration during cortical development in vertebrates, and periventricular heterotopia in humans is likely to result from disruption of this process. *FLNA* also promotes orthogonal branching of actin filaments and is important for coagulation and vascular development. *FLNA* related coagulation and vascular functions, as well as gut malformations, seem to account for the prenatal or early male lethality observed in most pedigrees (Guerrini *et al.*, 2004).

Other genes cause bilateral periventricular nodular heterotopia in both genders. A rare recessive form of periventricular nodular heterotopia owing to mutations of the adenosine diphosphate-ribosylation factor guanine nucleotide exchange factor 2 (*ARFGEF2*) has been reported (Sheen *et al.*, 2004a). This gene encodes for the protein brefeldin A-inhibited GEF2 (BIG2), which is required for vesicle and membrane trafficking from the trans-Golgi network. Affected children have microcephaly, severe developmental delay, and early-onset seizures, including infantile spasms.

Other genetic forms of PNH have been associated with a few additional causative genes (*EML1, FAT4, DCHS1, NEDD4L, MAP1B*) (Cappello *et al.*, 2013; Kielar *et al.*, 2014; Broix *et al.*, 2016; Heinzen *et al.*, 2018) as well as chromosomal rearrangements, in particular 6q27 deletion including C6orf70 (also known as ERMARD) (Conti *et al.*, 2013) *(Figure 4D, E)*. Genetic heterogeneity of periventricular heterotopias is substantiated by its frequent, although inconstant, association with 30 distinct copy number variants (Cellini *et al.*, 2019). Complex phenotypes have been reported, in which periventricular heterotopia is associated with syndactyly (Dobyns *et al.*, 1997; Fink *et al.*, 1997), frontonasal dysplasia (Guerrini & Dobyns, 1998), hydrocephalus (Sheen *et al.*, 2004b), polymicrogyria (Wieck *et al.*, 2005) and severe cerebellar hypoplasia (Pisano *et al.*, 2012).

Classic periventricular nodular heterotopia with no dysmorphic features is much more frequent in women and more likely to be due to *FLNA* mutations than in atypical cases. Among carrier women, about half have *de novo* mutations of *FLNA*, whereas the remaining half have inherited mutations. Although maternal transmission is much more likely, father-to-daughter transmission is possible (Guerrini *et al.*, 2004), implying that either parent can transmit the mutation to a female proband. An affected man with periventricular nodular heterotopia caused by the *FLNA* mutation would be expected to transmit the mutation to all of his daughters, unless somatic mosaicism is present. If none of the parents has epilepsy or cognitive impairment, the proband's mother should be studied first to confirm the mutation or the brain abnormality. If the mother is mutation-negative and the proband is a female, the father should also be studied. Given that germline mosaicism of *FLNA* has never been reported in periventricular nodular heterotopia, the recurrence risk (for other children) seems to be very low when a mutation is found in the proband but when none of the parent is a carrier.

Although most patients with PNH come to medical attention because they have focal epilepsy of variable severity, there is a wide spectrum of clinical presentations, including several syndromes with intellectual disability and dysmorphic facial features. There is some correlation between the size of PNH and the likelihood of concomitant structural abnormality of the cortex and clinical severity (Parrini *et al.*, 2006), but there seems to be no correlation between the size and number of heterotopic nodules and cognitive outcome or epilepsy severity. Approximately 90% of patients with PNH have epilepsy, which can begin at any age. Dubeau *et al.* studied 33 patients with periventricular and subcortical nodular heterotopia, 29 (88%) of whom had seizures, mainly partial attacks with temporoparieto-occipital auras (Dubeau *et al.*, 1995). Seizures began between the age of 2 months and 33 years and were intractable in 27 patients (82%). The surgical approach to nodular heterotopia related epilepsy is complex and requires the use of depth electrodes in most cases (Mirandola *et al.*, 2017; Pizzo *et al.*, 2017).

Lissencephaly and subcortical band heterotopia (agyria-pachygyria-band spectrum)

Classical lissencephaly (LIS) is a severe abnormality of neuronal migration characterized by absent (agyria) or decreased (pachygyria) surface convolutions, producing a smooth cerebral surface *(Figure 4F)*. Subcortical band heterotopia (SBH) *(Figure 4G)* comprises the mild end of the same group of malformations, which may accordingly be called the agyria-pachygyria-band spectrum. In SBH, the gyral pattern may be normal or simplified with broad convolutions. Just beneath the cortical ribbon, a thin band of white matter separates the cortex from the heterotopic band of grey matter.

Different subtypes of LIS are identified based on the number of cortical layers and include 2-layered, 3-layered, and 4-layered forms (Forman *et al.*, 2005). The most common, classical LIS (4-layered form), features a very thick cortex (10–20 mm *vs.* the normal 4 mm) and no other major brain malformations. The cytoarchitecture consists of 4 primitive layers, including an outer marginal layer, which contains Cajal-Retzius neurons (layer 1); a superficial cellular layer, which contains numerous large and disorganized pyramidal neurons (layer 2) corresponding to the true cortex, a variable cell-sparse layer (layer 3), and a deep cellular layer (composed of medium and small neurons), which extends more than half the width of the mantle (layer 4) (Golden & Harding, 2004). SBH is a related disorder in which bands of grey matter are interposed in the white matter between the cortex and the lateral ventricles. Histopathology demonstrates that heterotopic neurons settle close to the cortex in a pattern suggestive of laminar organization.

Lissencephaly, subcortical band heterotopia, and lissencephaly with cerebellar hypoplasia are always genetic. Studies to date have identified 19 lissencephaly genes, which account for roughly 90% of patients (Parrini *et al.*, 2016; Di Donato *et al.*, 2017; Di Donato *et al.*, 2018). However, two major genes have been associated with classical LIS and SBH. The *LIS1* gene on chromosome 17p13.3 causes the autosomal form of LIS (Reiner *et al.*, 1993), while the doublecortin gene (*DCX* or *XLIS*) is X-linked (des Portes *et al.*, 1998; Gleeson *et al.*, 1998). Although either gene can result in either LIS or SBH, most cases of classical LIS are due to deletions or mutations of *LIS1* (Mei *et al.*, 2008), whereas most cases of SBH are due to mutations of *DCX* (Matsumoto *et al.*, 2001). *LIS1*-related LIS is more severe in the posterior brain regions (p > a gradient), whereas *DCX*-related LIS is more severe in the anterior brain (a > p gradient).

The *LIS1* gene is closely related to p > a isolated LIS syndrome (ILS). The type and position of mutations of *LIS1* do not appear to correlate with the phenotype (Uyanik *et al.*, 2007). A simplified gyral pattern in the posterior brain, with underlying SBH, has been associated with mosaic mutations of *LIS1* (Sicca *et al.*, 2003). Miller-Dieker syndrome is characterized by severe 4-layered LIS with diffuse agyria and no clear gradient, a typical facial appearance (prominent forehead, bitemporal hollowing, short nose with upturned nares, protuberant upper lip and a small jaw), and other birth defects (*e.g.*, heart malformations) (Cardoso *et al.*, 2003). Miller-Dieker syndrome (MDS) is caused by deletion of *LIS1*, however, deletion of two additional genes, *CRK* and *YWHAE*, telomeric to *LIS1*, may contribute to the most severe LIS grade and dysmorphic features (Cardoso *et al.*, 2003).

Most *DCX* mutations classically cause anterior > posterior SBH/pachygyria in females and X-linked lissencephaly (XLIS) in males. Females with *DCX* mutations have anteriorly-predominant band/pachygyria of variable severity. Favourable X-inactivation skewing or mutations with mild functional consequences are likely to explain milder phenotypes. Mutations of *DCX* have been found in all reported pedigrees, including families in which females have SBH and males have LIS, and in approximately 80% of sporadic females and 25% of sporadic males with SBH (Matsumoto *et al.*, 2001). Genomic deletions of the *DCX* gene have been identified in females with sporadic SBH and in males with X-linked lissencephaly (Mei *et al.*, 2007). Maternal germline or mosaic DCX mutations may occur in about 10% of cases of either SBH or XLIS (Gleeson *et al.*, 2000a). Hemizygous males with *DCX* mutations have classical LIS, but rare boys with missense mutations and anteriorly predominant SBH and rare females with *DCX* mutations and normal brain MRI have been described (Guerrini *et al.*, 2003; Pilz *et al.*, 1999). When a mutation in the *DCX* gene is found in a boy with LIS, mutation analysis of *DCX* should be extended to the proband's mother, even if her brain MRI is normal. If the mother is a mutation carrier, the mutation will be transmitted according to Mendelian inheritance. If the mother is not a carrier, she can still be at risk of germline mosaicism; the risk of transmitting the mutation might roughly be estimated at around 5% (Gleeson *et al.*, 2000b). For this reason, a prenatal diagnosis is indicated in every pregnancy of a woman who has a child with features of XLIS with a *DCX* mutation.

LIS1 encodes a 45 kDa protein (PAFAH1B1), which functions as a regulatory subunit of platelet-activating factor acetylhydrolase (PAF-AH) (Hirotsune *et al.*, 1998). *DCX* encodes a 40 kDa microtubule-associated protein (DCX) that is expressed in migrating neuroblasts (Gleeson *et al.*, 2000b). The DCX protein contains two tandem conserved repeats. Each of the repeats binds to tubulin and both repeats are necessary for microtubule polymerization and stabilization.

Children with the most common types of LIS (or SBH) typically appear normal as newborns. Most affected children come to medical attention during the first months of life due to neurological deficits

(Barkovich *et al.*, 2012). The major medical problems encountered are ongoing feeding problems and epilepsy of many different types. Patients with severe LIS have early developmental delay, early diffuse hypotonia, later spastic quadriplegia, and eventual profound or severe mental retardation. Rare patients with pachygyria may have moderate mental retardation. Lifespan varies in relation to different factors, including the severity of associated epilepsy. Seizures occur in over 90% of children, with onset before 6 months in about 75% of the cases (Guerrini & Filippi, 2005). Between 35 and 85% of children with classic LIS develop infantile spasms, often without classic hypsarrhythmia. Most LIS children will subsequently continue to have epileptic spasms in association with other seizure types including persisting spasms, focal and generalized tonic seizures, atypical absences, atonic and myoclonic seizures (Guerrini *et al.*, 1996a). Many children with lissencephaly have characteristic EEG changes, including diffuse fast rhythms which do not react to eye opening (Hakamada *et al.*, 1979) and high amplitude rhythmic activity, which has high specificity (< 50%) (Quirk *et al.*, 1993).

As most clinical and neurophysiological studies on children with lissencephaly were conducted before genetic distinction between XLIS and LIS1 was made, it is unknown whether these two forms have distinctive electroclinical patterns.

Subcortical band heterotopia – The main clinical manifestations of SBH are cognitive impairment and epilepsy (Barkovich *et al.*, 1994). The more severe the pachygyria and the thicker the heterotopic band, the higher are the chances of developing Lennox-Gastaut syndrome or some other generalized symptomatic epilepsy form (Barkovich *et al.*, 1994). Very early seizure onset is uncommon. Epilepsy is present in almost all patients and is intractable in about 65% of the cases. About 50% of these epilepsy patients have focal seizures, and the remaining 50% have generalized epilepsy, often within the spectrum of Lennox-Gastaut syndrome. Those with more severe MRI abnormalities have significantly earlier seizure onset and are more likely to develop Lennox-Gastaut syndrome (Barkovich *et al.*, 1994).

In SBH, depth electrode studies have demonstrated that epileptiform activity can originate directly from the heterotopic neurons, with nearly constant simultaneous involvement of the "true" cortex (Mai *et al.*, 2003). Callosotomy has been associated with worthwhile improvement in drop attacks in a few patients (Landy *et al.*, 2003; Palmini *et al.*, 1991). Epilepsy surgery for focal seizures yields poor results in most patients (Bernasconi *et al.*, 2001). Functional impairment of the cortex overlying the heterotopia is variable. Positron emission tomography (PET) studies suggest that the laminar heterotopia has the same metabolic activity as normal cortex (Lee *et al.*, 1994) and that cerebral cortex overlying the heterotopia can either retain its expected map of functional activation or show extensive reorganization (Richardson *et al.*, 1998). Extensive reorganization is also suggested by cortical stimulation studies (Little *et al.*, 2007).

Children with some LIS syndromes (especially Miller-Dieker syndrome, and severe forms of LIS with cerebellar hypoplasia or the X-linked syndrome of LIS with abnormal genitalia) have a severe course, and the most severe forms have high mortality rates. However, these data do not apply to children with less severe forms of LIS, SBH, or LIS with cerebellar hypoplasia, as all of these disorders are associated with better motor and cognitive function and longer survival (Dobyns *et al.*, 2012).

Other genes have been associated with lissencephaly or subcortical band heterotopia in rare cases. Mutations in the *ACTB* and *ACTG1* genes are associated with Baraitser-Winter cerebrofrontofacial syndrome which is characterized by the combination of hypertelorism, a broad nose with a large tip and prominent root, congenital non-myopathic ptosis, ridged metopic suture, arched eyebrows, iris or retinal coloboma, sensorineural deafness, shoulder girdle muscle bulk, and progressive joint stiffness (Rivière *et al.*, 2012a; Di Donato *et al.*, 2014; Verloes *et al.*, 2015). Many patients with *ACTB* and *ACTG1* mutations have pachygyria with an anterior-to-posterior severity gradient, similar to that observed in males with *DCX* mutations (Rivière *et al.*, 2012a; Verloes *et al.*, 2015).

Tubulinopathies and related disorders

Mutations of tubulin genes were first reported as causing LIS (for *TUBA1A*) (Keays *et al.*, 2007) or polymicrogyria (for *TUBB2B*) (Jaglin *et al.*, 2009). However, the cortical malformations seen in most individuals with mutations of tubulin or tubulin motor genes comprise a widespectrum of morphological abnormalities whose characteristics are at times distinctive but can also overlap with those of LIS and polymicrogyria by brain imaging and neuropathology (Cushion *et al.*, 2013; Poirier *et al.*, 2013). The whole malformation spectrum ranges from extreme LIS with completely absent gyri, agenesis of the corpus callosum, and severe cerebellar hypoplasia; to less severe LIS with moderate-to-severe cerebellar hypoplasia; to classic LIS, and to an atypical polymicrogyria-like cortical malformation with cerebellar hypoplasia (Cushion *et al.*, 2013; Poirier *et al.*, 2013). Cortical thickness is variable. Most children with mutations in the tubulin genes have severe intellectual disability and intractable seizures. Nine genes (*KIF2A, KIF5C, TUBA1A, TUBA8, TUBB, TUBB2B, TUBB3, TUBG1*, and *DYNC1H1*) associated with tubulinopathies have been identified. Functional studies suggest that abnormal brain development in tubulinopathies results from a dominant negative effect of heterozygous missense mutations (in the absence of loss-of-function mutations) on the regulation of microtubule-dependent mitotic processes in progenitor cells, and on the trafficking activities of the microtubule-dependent molecular motors *KIF2A, KIF5C*, and *DYNC1H1* in postmitotic neuronal cells (Poirier *et al.*, 2013). The most severe phenotype of tubulinopathies consists of LIS with cerebellar and brainstem hypoplasia. These children have profound deficits, intractable epilepsy and the most severely affected a short lifespan. Heterozygous missense mutations in the *TUBA1A* gene have been found in 30% of the patients with tubulinopathies *(Figure 4H, I)* (Kumar *et al.*, 2010; Cushion *et al.*, 2013). A less severe phenotype consists of moderate LIS with cerebellar hypoplasia with pachygyria, with callosal defects and moderate hypoplasia of the brainstem and cerebellum (Morris-Rosendahl *et al.*, 2008; Kumar *et al.*, 2010). A third phenotype has isolated LIS sequence with posterior predominant LIS matching the LIS1 pattern (Kumar *et al.*, 2010). Finally, some patients exhibit polymicrogyria plus variable agenesis of the corpus callosum as well as constant hypoplasia of the brainstem and cerebellum (Kumar *et al.*, 2010).

X-linked lissencephaly with corpus callosum agenesis and ambiguous genitalia

X-linked lissencephaly with absent corpus callosum and ambiguous genitalia (XLAG) is a severe malformation only observed in boys. The anatomoclinical spectrum includes lissencephaly with a posterior > anterior gradient and only moderate cortical thicknening (only 6 to 7 mm in X-linked lissencephaly with corpus callosum agenesis *versus* 15 to 20 mm seen in lissencephaly associated with mutations of *LIS1* or *DCX*), ambiguous genitalia, absent corpus callosum, poorly delineated and cavitated basal ganglia, postnatal microcephaly, neonatal-onset epilepsy, hypothalamic dysfunction including deficient temperature regulation, chronic diarrhea, and ambiguous genitalia with micropenis and cryptorchidism (Dobyns *et al.*, 1999; Bonneau *et al.*, 2002). Early death is not uncommon (Kato *et al.*, 2004). Brain neuropathology reveals an abnormally laminated cortex, exclusively containing pyramidal neurons, with a pattern suggesting disruption of both tangential and radial migration, dysplastic basal ganglia, hypoplastic olfactory bulbs and optic nerves, abnormal gliotic white matter containing numerous heterotopic neurons, and complete agenesis of the corpus callosum without Probst bundles (Bonneau *et al.*, 2002).

Mutations of the X-linked aristaless-related homeobox gene (*ARX*) were identified in individuals with X-linked lissencephaly with corpus callosum agenesis and ambiguous genitalia and in some female relatives (Kitamura *et al.*, 2002). Females carrying *ARX* mutations usually have normal cognitive level and normal brain MRI or callosum agenesis. Mild intellectual disability and epilepsy have been reported in rare female carriers.

The ARX protein is expressed in the ganglionic eminence and subventricular zone during early development. Its major functions are thought to be the regulation of proliferation and tangential migration of GABAergic interneurons and of radial migration of pyramidal neurons (Friocourt *et al.*, 2008). Earlier studies have indicated that the murine *Arx* gene is specifically expressed in the GABAergic neural lineages, where it controls both the specification and migration of these neurons (Colombo *et al.*, 2004). However, subsequent studies evidenced that the *Arx*-null mice show deficient tangential migration and abnormal differentiation of GABAergic interneurons in the ganglionic eminence and neocortex, as well as misplacement of radially migrating pyramidal cells, which normally do not express *Arx*.

The *ARX* gene product has two functional domains, an *aristaless* domain and a *prd*-like homeodomain. Mutations affecting these domains lead to XLAG. Non-conservative missense mutations near the c-terminal *aristaless* domain usually cause severe XLAG with microcephaly and mild cerebellar hypoplasia. Mutations in the homeodomain are in prevalence premature termination mutations; missense mutations are usually less common. Among these, non-conservative missense mutations are associated with less severe XLAG, while conservative substitutions caused Proud syndrome (ACC with abnormal genitalia). *ARX* mutations are also associated with non-malformative phenotypes including X-linked infantile spasms, Partington syndrome, dyskinetic quadriparesis with status dystonicus (Guerrini *et al.*, 2007) and X-linked nonsyndromic mental retardation (Gécz *et al.*, 2006).

Autosomal recessive lissencephaly with cerebellar hypoplasia

This form of lissencephaly, associated with severe abnormalities of the cerebellum, hippocampus and brainstem, was mapped to 7q22, and mutations were identified in the *RELN* gene (Hong *et al.*, 2000; Ross *et al.*, 2001) *(Figure 4J, K)*. Patients exhibit dysmorphic facial features and generalized seizures. *RELN* encodes a large (388 kDa) extracellular matrix protein that acts on migrating cortical neurons by binding to the very low density lipoprotein receptor (VLDLR), the apolipoprotein E receptor 2, alpha3-beta1 integrin and cadherins-related receptors (CNRs) (Hiesberger *et al.*, 1999). In mice, *Reln* mutations cause cerebellar hypoplasia, abnormal cerebral cortical neuronal migration and abnormal axonal connectivity. Neurons in affected mice fail to reach their correct location in the developing brain, disrupting the organization of the cerebellar and cerebral cortices and other laminated regions. In this animal model the cortical layering appears inverted (D'Arcangelo, 2006). Thus, Reln is thought to control cell-cell interactions critical for cell positioning in the brain.

Clinical information on patients with *RELN*-related lissencephaly is limited and insufficient to delineate a consistent spectrum of presentations.

A mutation in the *CDK5* gene has been identified in 4 individuals with LIS and cerebellar hypoplasia born from a highly consanguineous family (Magen *et al.*, 2015).

Aicardi syndrome (Aicardi *et al.*, 1969) is exclusively observed in females, with the exception of a few reported males with two X chromosomes and is thought to be caused by an X-linked gene with lethality in the hemizygous male. The very genetic cause of Aicardi syndrome remains a mystery as next generation sequencing studies have failed to uncover potential causative genes (Lund *et al.*, 2016). Genetic heterogeneity or somatic mosaicism might both explain why no genetic cause has been identified so far. The incidence rates per live births for the United States and The Netherlands are 1 per 105 000 and 1 per 93 000, respectively (Kroner *et al.*, 2008). In a large US study, the probability of survival at 27 years of age was 0.62 (95% CI, 0.47–0.77) (Kroner *et al.*, 2008). Clinical and neuroimaging features include severe intellectual disability, infantile spasms, chorioretinal lacunae and agenesis of the corpus callosum. In one study, the estimated survival rate was 75% at 6 years and 40% at 15 years (MacGregor *et al.*, 1993). It is likely that milder cases, with incomplete malformative features escape recognition. Neuropathological findings include: i) a thin unlayered cortex; ii) diffuse unlayered polymicrogyria with fused molecular layers; iii) periventricular and subcortical nodular heterotopia (Billette de Villemeur *et al.*, 1992; Ferrer *et al.*, 1986). As a result of the fusion of the molecular layers the microgyri are packed and may escape MRI recognition.

Specific electroclinical features of the syndrome include early onset infantile spasms and focal seizures. Spasms were the only seizure type in 47% of reported patients (Chevrie & Aicardi, 1986). Focal seizures often begin in the first days of life and precede the onset of spasms. Hypsarrhythmia is observed in a minority of children (Aicardi, 1996). Interictal EEG abnormalities are typically asymmetric and asynchronous (split brain EEG). Suppression bursts are at times observed. Seizures and EEG patterns change little, if at all, over time and epilepsy is often resistant. There is a low tendency to develop seizure types typical of the older child.

Malformations related to abnormal cortical organization

Most disorders of cortical organization are represented by polymicrogyria, a term designating an excessive number of small and prominent convolutions spaced out by shallow and enlarged sulci, giving the cortical surface a lumpy aspect (Friede, 1989; Barkovich *et al.*, 2012). Polymicrogyria can be localized to a single gyrus, involve portions of a hemisphere, be bilateral and asymmetric, bilateral and symmetrical, or diffuse. Sometimes, it is associated with deep clefts that may extend through the entire cerebral mantle to communicate with the lateral ventricle (schizencephaly) (Barkovich & Kjos, 1992). On MRI, it may be difficult to recognize polymicrogyria or to distinguish it from pachygyria, since the microconvolutions are often packed and merged. Cortical infolding and secondary, irregular, thickening due to packing of microgyri are quite distinctive MRI characteristics. Ultra-high field (7 Tesla) MRI reveals areas of polymicrogyria that are missed by lower field MRI investigations and confirms that larger areas of more subtle cortical abnormality are often associated to the more visible zones of disorganised cortical architecture (De Ciantis *et al.*, 2015). Macroscopically, polymicrogyria appears as an irregular or pebbled cortical surface. The perisylvian cortex is the most frequently affected. The cortex often appears thickened to 8–12 mm, but when viewed microscopically, it is overfolded and not necessarily thick. While polymicrogyria most often occurs as an isolated malformation, it can co-occur with several other brain malformations, including microcephaly, megalencephaly, grey matter heterotopia, ventriculomegaly as well as abnormalities of the septum pellucidum, corpus callosum, brainstem and cerebellum. When schizencephaly is present, the cortex edges can seem to fuse (closed lips) or stay at distance (open lips). The clefts of schizencephaly can be unilateral or bilateral. An area of polymicrogyria can occur in the cortex contralateral to a unilateral cleft (Yakovlev & Wadsworth, 1946).

In *unlayered* polymicrogyria, the external molecular layer is continuous and does not follow the profile of the convolutions, and the underlying neurons have radial (or vertical) distribution but no laminar organization (Ferrer *et al.*, 1986). Unlayered polymicrogyria is found in the border of schizencephalic clefts or in the cortex of Aicardi syndrome. It may be focal (Becker *et al.*, 1989; Galaburda *et al.*, 1985), multilobar, or diffuse (Billette de Villemeur, 1992). Its aspect suggests an early disruption of normal neuronal migration with subsequent disordered cortical organization. By contrast, four-layered polymicrogyria is characterised by primary damage to intermediate cortical layers, which would then produce a difference in growth rate between outer and inner cortical layers, with consequent excessive folding of the cortical surface (Richman *et al.*, 1974). It is not infrequent to find a combination of these two histological appearances, with areas of abnormal development or loss of neurons in middle and deep cortical layers, variably associated with an unlayered cortical structure (Harding & Copp, 1997). The pathogenesis of polymicrogyria is poorly understood.

Using CT and low-field strength MRI, polymicrogyria is difficult to discern and may only appear as a mildly thickened, irregular cortex. For this reason, polymicrogyria is frequently misdiagnosed as pachygyria. With use of high-field or ultra-high-field strength MRI with appropriate age-specific protocols, polymicrogyria can be reliably differentiated – especially the classic form of polymicrogyria with perisylvian location, schizencephaly, and several other forms – from other cortical malformations and its extent better recognized (De Ciantis *et al.*, 2015). The imaging appearance of polymicrogyria varies with the patient's age. In newborns and young infants, the malformed cortex is very thin with multiple, very small undulations. After myelination, polymicrogyria appears as thickened cortex (usually 6–10 mm) with irregular cortex-white matter junction. In schizencephaly, the grey matter lining the cleft has the imaging appearance of polymicrogyria with an irregular surface, deep infolding (the cleft), mildly thick cortex, and stippling of the interface between grey and white matter.

Polymicrogyria has been associated with a wide number of patterns and syndromes and with mutations in several genes (Guerrini & Parrini, 2010). The clinical manifestations of polymicrogyria vary widely and depend on several factors. The most severe outcomes occur in children with severe microcephaly (–3 SD or smaller), abnormal neurological examination, widespread anatomic abnormality, and additional brain malformations such as heterotopia or cerebellar hypoplasia. The best outcomes are in individuals who have localized unilateral polymicrogyria without other malformations (Guerrini & Dobyns, 2014). Polymicrogyria can affect eloquent cortical areas representing language or primary motor functions, yet if cortical gyrification and thickness are relatively spared these functions can be retained with little or no disability (Guerrini & Barba, 2010; Lenge *et al.*, 2018).

Although the topographic location of polymicrogyria is extremely variable (Leventer *et al.*, 2010), various recurrent and relatively homogeneous anatomoclinical polymicrogyria syndromes are recognized, including bilateral perisylvian (Kuzniecky *et al.*, 1993), bilateral parasagittal parieto-occipital (Guerrini *et al.*, 1997), bilateral frontal (Guerrini *et al.*, 2000), bilateral frontoparietal (Piao *et al.*, 2004), unilateral perisylvian or multilobar (Guerrini *et al.*, 1998) and generalized polymicrogyria.

Bilateral perisylvian polymicrogyria

This malformation involves the gray matter bordering the sylvian fissure on both sides. In typical cases this is almost vertical and in continuity with the central or postcentral sulcus. Neuropathological studies have been performed in a few cases before evidence for genetic heterogeneity was gathered (Kuzniecky *et al.*, 1993; Ruton *et al.*, 1994; Becker *et al.*, 1989). It is therefore unclear whether these pathologically documented cases reflect a single malformation spectrum with a homogeneous aetiology or different aetiologies with converging topography.

Patients have facio-pharingo-glosso-masticatory diplegia with dissociation of automatic (preserved) and voluntary (impaired) facial motility (Guerrini *et al.*, 1992b; Kuzniecky *et al.*, 1993). Language impairment ranges from mild dysarthria to absence of speech. Almost all patients have intellectual disability and most have epilepsy. Seizures usually begin between age 4 and 12 years and are poorly controlled in about 65% of patients. Atypical absences, tonic or atonic drop attacks and tonic-clonic seizures are the most frequent types, often occurring as Lennox-Gastaut-like syndromes *(Figure 6)*. A minority of patients (26%) have partial seizures, predominantly involving the perioral or facial muscles. Patients with drop attack seizures may benefit from anterior callosotomy (Kuzniecky *et al.*, 1994; Guerrini *et al.*, 1992b).

Bilateral parasagittal parieto-occipital polymicrogyria

This malformation was detected using MRI in a series of patients with focal epilepsy (Guerrini *et al.*, 1997). The abnormal cortex extended posteriorly to involve the occipital lobe just below the parieto-occipital sulcus and anteriorly to immediately behind the

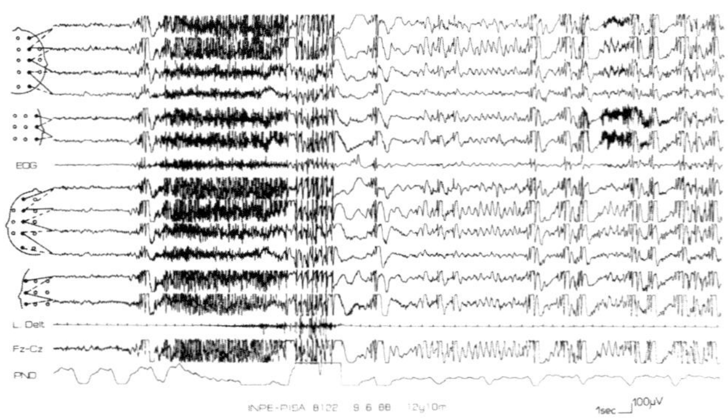

Figure 6 **12-year-old girl with bilateral perisylvian polymicrogyria and Lennox-Gastaut syndrome. Tonic seizure recorded during sleep. A generalized polyspike and slow wave discharge is followed by high amplitude fast rhythm during which a progressive tonic contraction becomes apparent on the recorded muscle (Left deltoid). The end of the tonic seizure is characterized electrically by a discharge of polyspike and wave complexes and by a suppression burst and clinically by a series of myoclonic jerks.**

precuneus and superior parietal lobule. IQs ranged from average to mild impairment. Seizures had started between ages 20 months and 15 years (mean 9 years) and were intractable in 7. Most patients had complex partial seizures, which were preceded in some by sensory symptoms. Seizure symptomatology remained constant during follow-up in all patients. A few similar isolated patients have been reported since the first series was published.

Bilateral perisylvian and parietooccipital polymicrogyria

Some patients have bilateral perisylvian polymicrogyria extending posteriorly, with the sylvian fissure prolonged across the entire hemispheric convexity up to the mesial surface. The posterior portion of this malformation therefore bears strong similarity to parasagittal parieto-occipital polymicrogyria and the anterior portion to perisylvian polymicrogyria. Most patients have severe epilepsies (Pupillo *et al.*, 1996) whose characteristics are similar to the bilateral perisylvian syndrome or may have partial epilepsies with seizure onset in the occipital or parietal lobes.

Bilateral frontal and frontoparietal polymicrogyria

Bilateral frontal polymicrogyria was described in children with developmental delay, mild spastic quadriparesis, and epilepsy (Guerrini *et al.*, 2000).

Epilepsy, seen in the majority of patients was of variable severity. Most patients were reported to have atypical absences and a full blown pattern of Lennox-Gastaut syndrome has also been described (Parrini *et al.*, 2009).

Unilateral polymicrogyria or multilobar polymicrogyria

Unilateral polymicrogyria may affect the whole hemisphere or part of it. Hypoplasia of the affected hemisphere is frequent. Unilateral on MRI may be turn out to be bilateral and extensive on microscopic examination of the brain (Guerrini *et al.*, 1992a).

Clinical characteristics of lateralized polymicrogyria have been studied in a series of 20 patients (Guerrini *et al.*, 1996b): 75% had seizures and mild to moderate hemiparesis, 70% had mild to moderate intellectual disability. Hemiparesis was typically associated with prominent mirror movements of the affected upper limb. This feature has been attributed to ipsilateral cortical representation of the sensorimotor hand area (Maegaki *et al.*, 1995). Age at seizure onset and epilepsy severity were quite variable (Guerrini *et al.*, 1996a). The most commonly reported seizure types are focal motor seizures (73%), atypical absences (47%), generalized tonic-clonic seizures (27%) and complex partial (20%). Epilepsy could be classified as focal in 80% of patients and generalized in 20%. Interictal EEG findings in most patients suggested greater cortical involvement than expected from MRI. Coexistence of multiple seizure types, inclusion of the motor cortex in the epileptogenic zone, poor delimitation of the abnormal cortex make most patients with intractable seizures and polymicrogyria unlikely candidates for epilepsy surgery.

Multilobar polymicrogyria has been observed in children with epilepsy with electrical status epilepticus during sleep (ESES, or continuous spike and waves during slow sleep – CSWS) (Guerrini *et al.*, 1998; Caraballo *et al.*, 1999; Bartolini *et al.*, 2016). Patients with this syndrome have both focal motor and atypical absence seizures and both focal and generalized interictal discharges. Sleep recordings show continuous generalized SW complexes during slow-wave phases. The condition is usually detected between ages 2 and 10 years and may last for months to years (*Figure 7A-C*). Seizures remit completely before adolescence. Although epilepsy with CSWS is infrequent, its occurrence in patients with localized polymicrogyria is not (Guerrini *et al.*, 1998, Caraballo *et al.*, 1999) and suggests that sleep EEG should be systematically performed in children with this malformative pattern. In a series of 27 patients whose follow-up extended beyond cessation of ESES, seizure outcome was consistently good (Bartolini *et al.*, 2016) and cognitive deterioration could not be clearly demonstrated after CSWS. In the same series, CSWS peaked between 5 and 7 years (mean age at onset 4.7 years) and remission of CSWS and epilepsy occurred within 2 years from onset in 21%, within 4 years in 50%, and by age 13 years in 100%. Comparative volumetric analysis of the polymicrogyric hemispheres and ipsilateral thalami *vs.* 3 subgroups featuring polymicrogyria without CSWS, benign rolandic epilepsy (BRE), and headache identified smaller thalamic and hemispheric volumes in polymicrogyria/CSWS with respect to polymicrogyria without CSWS, BRE, and controls with headache. Volumes of the malformed hemispheres and ipsilateral thalami reliably identified the risk of incurring CSWS, with a 68-fold increased risk for values lower than optimal diagnostic cut-offs. This study concluded that the polymicrogyria/CSWS syndrome is likely caused by a cortico-thalamic malformation complex and is invariably characterized by remission of epilepsy within early adolescence and that early assessment of hemispheric and thalamic volumes in children with polymicrogyria and epilepsy can reliably predict CSWS.

Although the role of resective surgery in epilepsy with ESES has not been specifically addressed, it has been hypothesized that surgery may be effective when a focal abnormality is identified (Park *et al.*, 1994). However, the good prognosis of associated epilepsy and the time limited expression of the disorder should discourage early surgical procedures in patients with CSWS.

A

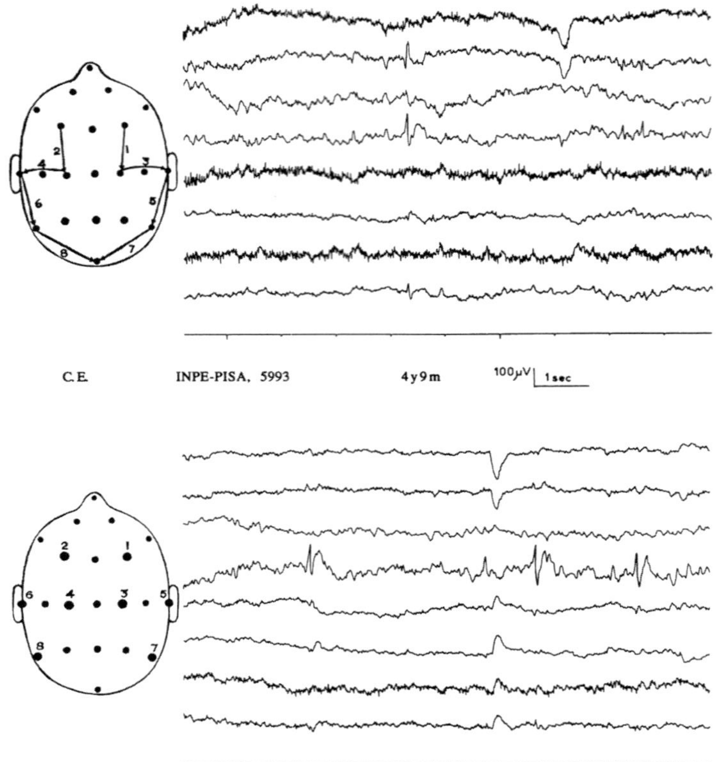
C.E.
INPE-PISA, 5993
4y9m
100µV
1 sec

B

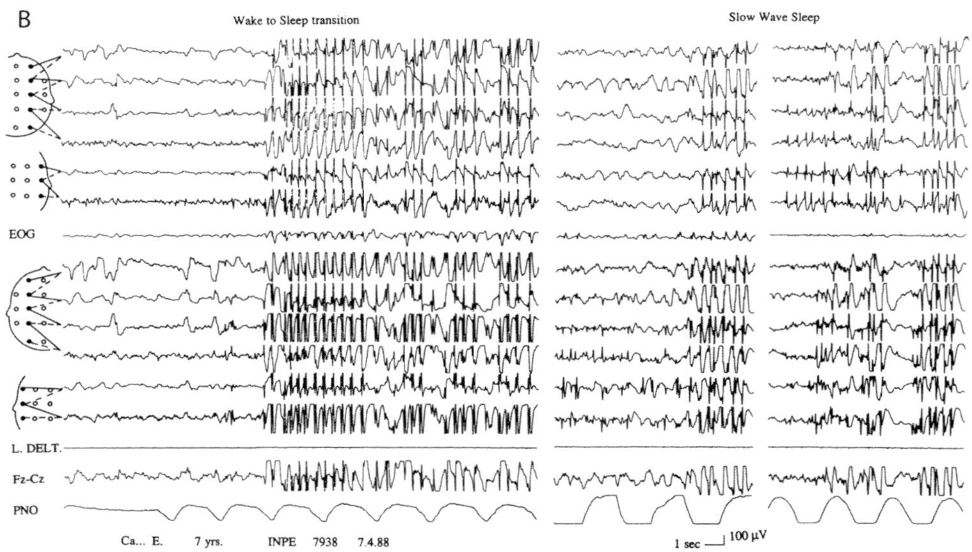
Wake to Sleep transition
Slow Wave Sleep
EOG
L. DELT.
Fz-Cz
PNO
Ca... E.
7 yrs.
INPE 7938 7.4.88
1 sec
100 µV

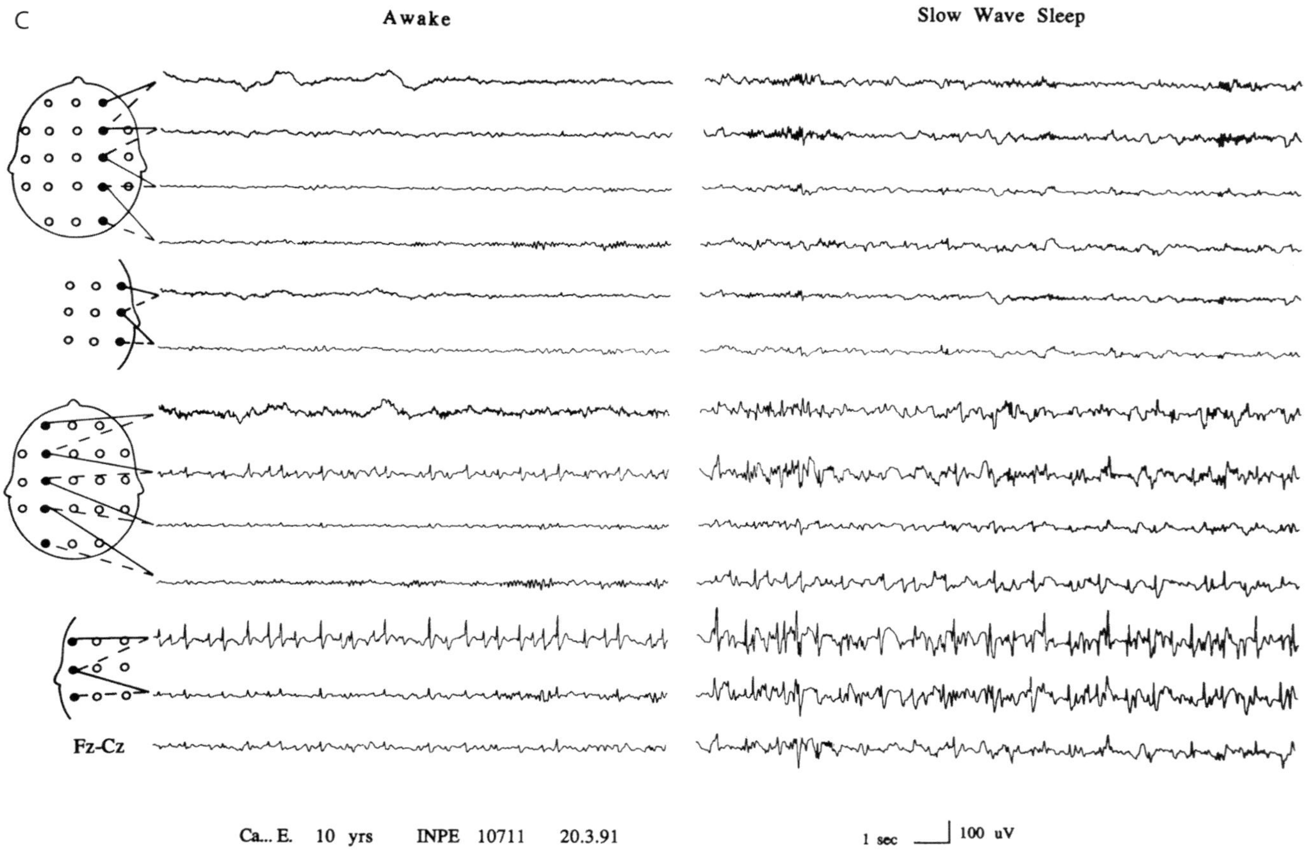

Figure 7

A. 4-year-9-month-old boy with bilateral perisylvian polymicrogyria who came to our attention because of developmental delay and anarthria. EEG showed left central spike and wave discharges. B. Since age 6 years the child started to suffer from rare sleep-related partial motor seizures involving the right arm and from multiple per day atonic absences. Sleep EEG recording showed ESES and bilateral independent spikes over the temporal areas. C. Remission of seizures and reversal of EEG abnormalities to pre ESES period were seen since age 8 years. The patient is now aged 20. No relapse of seizures has occurred.

Generalized polymicrogyria

Generalized polymicrogyria is often accompanied by microcephaly and severe-profound cognitive and motor delay, as well as epilepsy. Rather than a distinct syndrome, generalized polymicrogyria, whether symmetric or asymmetric, is the expression of a variety of partly known and largely unknown genetic and environmental factors.

Polymicrogyria involving a discrete region of one hemisphere is often detected after brain MRI, prompted by onset of focal seizures. Diffuse epileptogenesis is frequently encountered, even with seemingly limited abnormalities. Intracranial recordings suggest large epileptogenic networks, which extend well beyond the limits of the visible abnormality (Chassoux *et al.*, 2008). Consequently, surgical treatment of epilepsy is applicable to a limited number of patients in whom remission of epilepsy is not expected and large resections are feasible (Chassoux *et al.*, 2008; Ramantani *et al.*, 2013). In a large collaborative study that retrospectively analyzed 58 cases (49 SEEG and 39 corticectomy or hemispherotomies), mean age at SEEG or surgery was 28.3 years (range, 2–50) (Maillard *et al.*, 2017). Polymicrogyria was bilateral in 9 (16%) patients and unilateral in 49; 28 (48%) patients additionally had schizencephaly, heterotopia, or focal cortical dysplasia. The SEEG-determined EZ was fully concordant with polymicrogyria in only 8 (16%) cases, partially concordant in 74%, and discordant in 10%. The epileptiogenic zone included remote cortical areas in 21 (43%) cases and was primarily localized in those in 5 (10%), all related to the mesial temporal structures. At last follow-up (mean, 4.6 years; range, 1–16), 28 (72%) patients remained seizure free and shorter epilepsy duration to surgery was an independent predictor of seizure freedom. The authors confirmed that although polymicrogyria-related drug-resistant epilepsy warrants comprehensive presurgical investigations, often including SEEG, seizure freedom is feasible in a large proportion of patients and that lesion extent should not deter from exploring the possibility of epilepsy surgery.

The main problem to be faced when planning surgery is that the polymicrogyric cortex is not totally disrupted and often maintains an intrinsic functionality (Barba *et al.*, 2010; Lenge *et al.*, 2018) *(Figure 8)*.

Combined fMRI and transcranial magnetic stimulation studies in patients with polymicrogyria and hemiparesis suggest that ipsilateral corticospinal projections from the contralesional hemisphere to the paretic hand, corticospinal projections to the paretic hand originating in the polymicrogyric cortex, and bilateral motor representation are all possible (Guzzetta *et al.*, 2007; Staudt *et al.*, 2004).

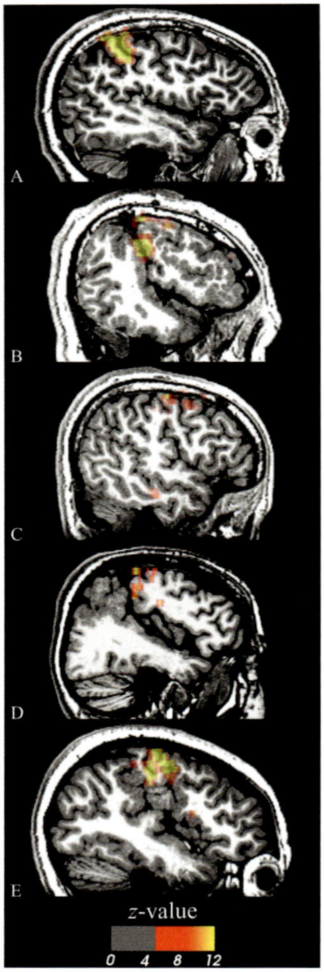

Figure 8 **Sagittal 3T MR images of a patient with seemingly cryptogenic epilepsy (A) and of four patients with perisylvian polymicrogyria (B-E). The red-yellow colormap superimposed on MRI shows fMRI activation during a hand-motor task. The patient with cryptogenic epilepsy shows a normal Sylvian fissure; those with perisylvian polymicrogyria show an abnormally vertical orientation of the Sylvian fissure which appears to be fused with the Rolandic fissure.**

Genetic bases

Numerous causes, both genetic and nongenetic, have been associated with polymicrogyria. Nongenetic causes other than hypoxia or hypoperfusion relate mainly to congenital infections, primarily cytomegalovirus (Evrard *et al.*, 1989; Barkovich & Lindan, 1994). Although the number of cases of polymicrogyria secondary to cytomegalovirus is not known, the real magnitude of the problem is probably underestimated, and an analysis for cytomegalovirus infections of dry blood spot should be performed in newborns with this malformation. Polymicrogyria is associated with a wide number of patterns and syndromes as well as mutations in several genes (Parrini *et al.*, 2016). Various types of single-gene inheritance have been hypothesized for polymicrogyria, based on observations of families with X-linked (Guerreiro *et al.*, 2000; Villard *et al.*, 2002; Santos *et al.*, 2008), autosomal dominant (Guerreiro *et al.*, 2000; Chang *et al.*, 2006), and autosomal recessive forms (Guerreiro *et al.*, 2000). Bilateral frontoparietal polymicrogyria has been associated with mutations in the *GPR56* gene in families with recessive pedigrees (Piao *et al.*, 2004) *(Figure 4L)*. However, this malformation exhibits anatomic characteristics that are more appropriately consistent with the cobblestone malformation spectrum (muscle-eye-brain disease and Fukuyama congenital muscular dystrophy) (Guerrini & Dobyns, 2014). Polymicrogyria occurs with a few types of severe congenital microcephaly, such as autosomal recessive syndromes associated with mutations in the *WDR62*, (Bilgüvar *et al.*, 2010), *NDE1* (Alkuraya *et al.*, 2011), or *KATNB1* (Mishra-Gorur *et al.*, 2014) genes. Polymicrogyria with microcephaly or normal head size has been reported with several tubulin and tubulin motor genes, especially *TUBB2B (Figure 4M)* (Jaglin *et al.*, 2009; Guerrini *et al.*, 2012) and *DYNC1H1 (Figure 4N, O)* (Poirier *et al.*, 2013). Autosomal recessive forms of polymicrogyria have been linked to mutations of *RTTN* (Kheradmand Kia *et al.*, 2012). Also, polymicrogyria has now been reported in several megalencephaly syndromes. Mutations in *PIK3R2*, a pivotal gene of the PI3K-AKT-mTOR pathway, may account for up to 15% of all patients with bilateral perisylvian polymicrogyria with or without megalencephaly (Mirzaa *et al.*, 2015) *(Figure 4P)*. In this association, patients with associated megalencephaly have more widespread polymicrogyria, more severe clinical impairment and germline mutations while those with normal head size usually have perisylvian only polymicrogyria, are less severely impaired and exhibit somatic mosaicism. Some copy-number variants have been associated with polymicrogyria (Parrini *et al.*, 2016), but only deletions in 1p36.3 and 22q11.2 have been consistently (Robin *et al.*, 2006; Dobyns *et al.*, 2008).

Schizencephaly

Schizencephaly is characterized by clefts in the cerebral mantle, surrounded by polymicrogyric cortex (Ferrer, 1984) and often co-occur with polymicrogyria in the same individual or in individuals of the same family (Muntaner, 1997) and both may occur with prenatal cytomegalovirus infection (Barkovich & Lindan, 1994) or with vascular problems related to twinning (Barth & van der Harten, 1985) or to mutations in the *COL4A1* gene (Yoneda *et al.*, 2013; Khalid *et al.*, 2018; Sato *et al.*, 2018), which tend to be also associated with porencephaly. This latter association confirms the vascular origin of schizencephaly. Schizencephaly has also been associated with environmental factors including maternal trauma, substance abuse (Barkovich & Kjos, 1992; Curry *et al.*, 2005) but these factors may also act through a vascular mechanism. Other genetic causes include chromosome aneuploidy and some rare syndromes (Curry *et al.*, 2005).

It has been suggested that considering their frequent association and shared causative factors, polymicrogyria and schizencephaly should be classified together (Barkovich *et al.*, 2005). The schizencephalic fissures are unilateral or bilateral and produce an abnormal full thickness communication between the ventricle(s) and pericerebral subarachnoid space(s). The walls of the clefts may be widely separated (open-lip schizencephaly), or closely apposed (closed-lip schizencephaly) *(Figure 1B)* and may be located in any region of the hemispheres, but are by far most frequent in the central and perisylvian area (Friede, 1989; Barkovich & Kjos, 1992). Bilateral clefts are usually symmetric in location, but not necessarily in size. Unilateral clefts, especially if large, may be associated with a localized focus of polymicrogyria in the contralateral cortex (Friede, 1989). Schizencephaly is associated with agenesis of septum pellucidum in about 30% of cases and agenesis or hypoplasia of corpus callosum in about 70% of cases. An association between unilateral or bilateral clefts, agenesis of septum pellucidum and optic nerve atrophy (so called septo-optic dysplasia) may be observed in 6 to 25% of patients (Barkovich & Kjos, 1992; Granata *et al.*, 1999; Denis *et al.*, 2000). Several sporadic patients and two siblings of both sexes harbouring germline mutations in the homeobox gene *EMX2* have been described but involvement of this gene has not been confirmed in large series (Merello *et al.*, 2008).

It is difficult to establish at which time during embryonic development schizencephaly originates. There is no agreement as to whether it should be classified as a defect originating early, with localized fault in neuronal proliferation. The presence of polymicrogyric cortex, however, is the hallmark of a disorder of cortical layering that extends through late cortical organization.

Clinical findings include focal seizures in most patients (81% of cases in one large review), usually beginning before age 3 years if bilateral clefts are present. Bilateral clefts are usually associated with severe neurological abnormalities whereas unilateral schizencephaly is usually accompanied by hemiparesis or at times detected after seizure onset in otherwise neurologically normal individuals. Patients with bilateral schizencephaly usually exhibit spastic quadriparesis, often associated with apraxia, pseudobulbar paralysis, and microcephaly (Granata *et al.*, 2005). Cognitive level is normal in 30% to 80% of patients with a unilateral cleft, whereas it is moderately to severely impaired in most patients with bilateral clefts (Barkovich & Kjos, 1992; Denis *et al.*, 2000).

Epilepsy is present in 36 to 65% of patients with schizencephaly and is refractory to antiepileptic drugs in 9% to 38% of them (Barkovich & Kjos, 1992; Packard *et al.*, 1997; Denis *et al.*, 2000). In two series (Granata *et al.*, 1999; Denis *et al.*, 2000), epilepsy was more frequently associated with unilateral schizencephaly, in comparison with bilateral cases, in which seizure intractability was less frequent. Other authors (Packard *et al.*, 1997; Barkovich & Kjos, 1992) have pointed out that bilateral open-lip schizencephaly implies an earlier age at seizure onset and more frequent drug-resistance. Severity and type of seizures does not seem to correlate with the topography of the schizencephalic cleft (Leventer *et al.*, 2008).

Selected patients with schizencephaly have been treated with surgery for epilepsy (Lee *et al.*, 1999; Maillard *et al.*, 2017). In planning surgical treatment, careful clinical, neurophysiological (including SEEG) and functional imaging studies are necessary.

REFERENCES

Aicardi J (1996): Aicardi syndrome. In: Guerrini R, Andermann F, Canapicchi R, Roger J, Zifkin BG, Pfanner P (eds). *Dysplasias of Cerebral Cortex and Epilepsy*. Philadelphia-New York: Lippincott-Raven, pp. 211–216.

Aicardi J, Chevrie JJ, Rousselie F (1969): Le syndrome agénésie calleuse, spasmes en flexion, lacunes choriorétiniennes. *Arch Franc Pédiatr* 26: 1103–1120.

Alkuraya FS, Cai X, Emery C, *et al.* (2011): Human mutations in *NDE1* cause extreme microcephaly with lissencephaly [corrected]. *Am J Hum Genet* 88: 536–547.

Alonso-Nanclares L, Garbelli R, Sola RG, *et al.* (2005): Microanatomy of the dysplastic neocortex from epileptic patients. *Brain* 128: 158–173.

Barba C, Montanaro D, Cincotta M, Giovannelli F, Guerrini R (2010): An integrated fMRI, SEPs and MEPs approach for assessing functional organization in the malformed sensorimotor cortex. *Epilepsy Res* 89: 66–71.

Barkovich AJ, Kjos BO (1992): Schizencephaly: correlation of clinical findings with MR character istics. *AJNR Am J Neuroradiol* 13: 85–94.

Barkovich AJ, Lindan CE (1994): Congenital cytomegalovirus infection of the brain: imaging analysis and embryologic considerations. *AJNR Am J Neuroradiol* 15: 703–715.

Barkovich AJ, Guerrini R, Battaglia G, *et al.* (1994): Band heterotopia: correlation of outcome with magnetic resonance imaging parameters. *Ann Neurol* 36: 609–617.

Barkovich AJ, Kuzniecky RI, Bollen AW, Grant PE (1997): Focal transmantle dysplasia: a specific malformation of cortical development. *Neurology* 49: 1148–1152.

Barkovich AJ, Kuzniecky RI, Jackson GD, Guerrini R, Dobyns WB (2005): A developmental and genetic classification for malformations of cortical development. *Neurology* 65: 1873–1887.

Barkovich AJ, Guerrini R, Kuzniecky RI, Jackson GD, Dobyns WB (2012): A developmental and genetic classification for malformations of cortical development: update 2012. *Brain* 135: 1348–1369.

Barth PG, van der Harten JJ (1985): Parabiotic twin syndrome with topicalisocortical disruption and gastroschisis. *Acta Neuropathol* 67: 345–349.

Bartolini E, Falchi M, Zellini F, *et al.* (2016): The syndrome of polymicrogyria, thalamic hypoplasia, and epilepsy with CSWS. *Neurology* 86: 1250–1259.

Becker PS, Dixon AM, Troncoso JC (1989): Bilateral opercular polymicrogyria. *Ann Neurol* 25: 90–92.

Bernasconi A, Martinez V, Rosa-Neto P, *et al.* (2001): Surgical resection for intractable epilepsy in "double cortex" syndrome yields inadequate results. *Epilepsia* 42: 1124–1129.

Bilgüvar K, Oztürk AK, Louvi A, *et al.* (2010): Whole-exome sequencing identifies recessive WDR62 mutations in severe brain malformations. *Nature* 467: 207–210.

Billette de Villemeur T, Chiron C, Robain O (1992): Unlayered polymicrogyria and agenesis of the corpus callosum: a relevant association? *Acta Neuropathol* 83: 265–270.

Blümcke I, Thom M, Aronica E, *et al.* (2011): The clinicopathologic spectrum of focal cortical dysplasias: a consensus classification proposed by an ad hoc Task Force of the ILAE Diagnostic Methods Commission. *Epilepsia* 52: 158–174.

Bonneau D, Toutain A, Laquerriere A, *et al.* (2002): X-linked lissencephaly with absent corpus callosum and ambiguous genitalia (XLAG): Clinical, magnetic resonance imaging, and neuropathological findings. *Ann Neurol* 51: 340–349.

Broix L, Jagline H, Ivanova E, *et al.* (2016): Mutations in the HECT domain of NEDD4L lead to AKT-mTOR pathway deregulation and cause periventricular nodular heterotopia. *Nat Genet* 48: 1349–1358.

Burneo JC, Bebin M, Kuzniecky RI, Knowlton RC (2004): Cortical reorganization in malformations of cortical development: a magnetoencephalographic study. *Neurology* 63: 1818–1824.

Cappello S, Gray MJ, Badouel C, *et al.* (2013): Mutations in genes encoding the cadherin receptor-ligand pair DCHS1 and FAT4 disrupt cerebral cortical development. *Nat Genet* 45: 1300–1308.

Caraballo R, Cersosimo R, Fejerman N (1999): A particular type of epilepsy in children with congenital hemiparesis associated with unilateral polymicrogyria. *Epilepsia* 40: 865–871.

Cardoso C, Leventer RJ, Ward HL, *et al.* (2003): Refinement of a 400-kb critical region allows genotypic differentiation between isolated lissencephaly, Miller-Dieker syndrome, and other phenotypes secondary to deletions of 17p13.3. *Am J Hum Genet* 72: 918–930.

Cellini E, Vetro A, Conti V, *et al.* (2019): Multiple genomic copy number variants associated with periventricular nodular heterotopia indicate extreme genetic heterogeneity. *Eur J Hum Genet* Jan 25. doi: 10.1007/s13258-019-00788-9

Chassoux F, Landre E, Rodrigo S, *et al.* (2008): Intralesional recordings and epileptogenic zone in focal polymicrogyria. *Epilepsia* 49: 51–64.

Chang BS, Apse KA, Caraballo R, *et al.* (2006): A familial syndrome of unilateral polymicrogyria affecting the right hemisphere. *Neurology* 66: 133–135.

Cheruy M, Heller FR (1987): An unusual variant of Klippel Trenaunay syndrome. *Acta Chir Belg* 87: 73–76.

Chevrie JJ, Aicardi J (1986): The Aicardi syndrome. In: Pedley TA, Meldrum BS (eds). *Recent advances in epilepsy*. Edinburgh: Churchill Livingston. pp. 189–210.

Choi BH, Kudo M (1981): Abnormal neuronal migration and gliomatosis cerebri in epidermal naevus syndrome. *Acta Neuropatho.* 53: 319–325.

Clapham KR, Yu TW, Ganesh VS, *et al.* (2012): FLNA genomic rearrangements cause periventricular nodular heterotopia. *Neurology* 78: 269–278.

Colombo E, Galli R, Cossu G, Gécz J, Broccoli V (2004): Mouse orthologue of *ARX*, a gene mutated in several X-linked forms of mental retardation and epilepsy, is a marker of adult neural stem cells and forebrain GABAergic neurons. *Dev Dyn* 231: 631–639.

Conti V, Carabalona A, Pallesi-Pocachard E, *et al.* (2013): Periventricular heterotopia in 6q terminal deletion syndrome: role of the *C6orf70* gene. *Brain* 136: 3378–3394.

Conti V, Pantaleo M, Barba C, *et al.* (2015): Focal dysplasia of the cerebral cortex and infantile spasms associated with somatic 1q21.1-q44 duplication including the AKT3 gene. *Clin Genet* 88: 241–247.

Curry CJ, Lammer EJ, Nelson V, Shaw GM (2005): Schizencephaly: heterogeneous etiologies in a population of 4 million California births. *Am J Med Genet A* 137: 181–189.

Cushion TD, Dobyns WB, Mullins JG, *et al.* (2013): Overlapping cortical malformations and mutations in TUBB2B and TUBA1A. *Brain* 136: 536–548.

Cusmai R, Curatolo P, Mangano S, Cheminal R, Echenne B (1990): Hemimegalencephaly and neurofibromatosis. *Neuropediatrics* 21: 179–182.

D'Agostino MD, Bastos A, Piras C, *et al.* (2004): Posterior quadrantic dysplasia or hemi-hemimegalencephaly: a characteristic brain malformation. *Neurology* 62: 2214–2220.

D'Arcangelo G (2006): Reelin mouse mutants as models of cortical development disorders. *Epilepsy Behav* 8: 81–90.

D'Gama AM, Geng Y, Couto JA, Martin B, Boyle EA, LaCoursiere CM, *et al.* (2015): Mammalian target of rapamycin pathway mutations cause hemimegalencephaly and focal cortical dysplasia. *Ann Neurol* 77: 720–725.

Denis D, Chateil JF, Brun M, *et al.* (2000): Schizencephaly: Clinical and imaging features in 30 infantile cases. *Brain Dev* 22: 475–483.

De Ciantis A, Barkovich AJ, Cosottini M, *et al.* (2015): Ultra-high-field MR imaging in polymicrogyria and epilepsy. *AJNR Am J Neuroradiol* 36: 309–316.

DeMyer W (1986): Megalencephaly: types, clinical syndromes, and management. *Pediatr Neurol* 2: 321–328.

Des Portes V, Pinard JM, Billuart P, *et al.* (1998): Identification of a novel CNS gene required for neuronal migration and involved in X-linked subcortical laminar heterotopia and lissencephaly syndrome. *Cell* 92: 51–61.

Desbiens R, Berkovic SF, Dubeau F, *et al.* (1993): Life-threatening focal status epilepticus due to occult cortical dysplasia. *Arch Neurol* 50: 695–700.

Di Donato N, Rump A, Koenig R, *et al.* (2014): Severe forms of Baraitser-Winter syndrome are caused by ACTB mutations rather than ACTG1 mutations. *Eur J Hum Genet* 22: 179–183.

Di Donato N, Chiari S, Mirzaa GM, *et al.* (2017): Lissencephaly: Expanded imaging and clinical classification. *Am J Med Genet A* 173: 1473–1488.

Di Donato N, Timms AE, Aldinger, *et al.* (2018): Analysis of 17 genes detects mutations in 81% of 811 patients with lissencephaly. *Genet Med* 20: 1354–1364.

Dobyns WB, Guerrini R, Czapansky-Beilman DK, *et al.* (1997): Bilateral periventricular nodular heterotopia (BPNH) with mental retardation and syndactyly in boys: a new X-linked mental retardation syndrome. *Neurology* 49: 1042–1047.

Dobyns WB, Truwit CL, Ross ME, *et al.* (1999): Difference in the gyral pattern distinguish chromose 17-linked and X-linked lissencephaly. *Neurology* 53: 270–277.

Dobyns WB, Mirzaa G, Christian SL, *et al.* (2008): Consistent chromosome abnormalities identify novel polymicrogyria loci in 1p36.3, 2p16.1-p23.1, 4q21.21-q22.1, 6q26-q27, and 21q2. *Am J Med Genet A* 146A: 1637–1654.

Dobyns WB, Guerrini R, Leventer RL (2012): Malformations of cortical development, in Swaiman KF, Ashwal S, Ferriero DM, Schor NF (eds). *Swaiman's Pediatric Neurology: Principles and Practice* (ed 5), Edinburgh: Elsevier Saunders, pp. 202–231.

Dodge NN, Dobyns WB (1995): Agenesis of the corpus callosum and Dandy-Walker malformation associated with hemimegalencephaly in the sebaceous nevus syndrome. *Am J Med Genet* 56: 147–150.

Dubeau F, Tampieri D, Lee N, *et al.* (1995): Periventricular and subcortical nodular heterotopia. A study of 33 patients. *Brain* 118: 1273–1287.

Duchowny M (2009): Clinical, functional, and neurophysiologic assessment of dysplastic cortical networks: implications for cortical functioning and surgical management. *Epilepsia* 50: 19–27.

Duchowny M, Jayakar P, Harvey AS, *et al.* (1996): Language cortex representation: effects of developmental *versus* acquired pathology. *Ann Neurol* 40: 31–38.

Duchowny M, Jayakar P, Levin B. Neurology (2000): Aberrant neural circuits in malformations of cortical development and focal epilepsy. *Neurology* 55: 423–428.

Evrard P, de Saint-Georges P, Kadhim HJ, Gadisseux JF (1989): Pathology of prenatal encephalopathies. In: French JH, De Vivo DC, Rapin I, *et al.* (eds): *Child Neurology and Developmental Disabilities*, Baltimore: Paul H. Brookes, pp. 153–176.

Ferrer I (1984): A Golgi analysis of unlayered polymicrogyria. *Acta Neuropathol* 65: 69–76.

Ferrer I, Cusi MV, Liarte A, Campistol J (1986): A Golgi study of the polymicrogyric cortex in Aicardi syndrome. *Brain Dev* 8: 518–525.

Ferrer I, Pineda M, Tallada M, *et al.* (1992): Abnormal local circuit neurons in epilepsia partialis continua associated with focal cortical dysplasia. *Acta Neuropathol* 83: 647–652.

Fink JM, Dobyns WB, Guerrini R, Hirsch BA (1997): Identification of a duplication of Xq28 associated with bilateral periventricular nodular heterotopia. *Am J Hum Genet* 61: 379–387.

Forman MS, Squier W, Dobyns WB, Golden JA (2005): Genotypically defined lissencephalies show distinct pathologies. *J Neuropathol Exp Neurol* 64: 847–857.

Fox JW, Lamperti ED, Eksioglu YZ, *et al.* (1998): Mutations in filamin 1 prevent migration of cerebral cortical ceurons in human periventricular heterotopia. *Neuron* 21: 1315–1325.

Friede RL (1989): *Developmental neuropathology* (2nd ed). New York: Springer-Verlag, p. 577.

Friocourt G, Kanatani S, Tabata H, *et al.* (2008): Cell-autonomous roles of ARX in cell proliferation and neuronal migration during corticogenesis. *J Neurosci* 28: 5794–5805.

Galaburda AM, Sherman GF, Rosen GD, Aboitiz F, Geschwind N (1985): Developmental dyslexia: four consecutive patients with cortical anomalies. *Ann Neurol* 18: 222–233.

Gambardella A, Palmini A, Andermann F, *et al.* (1996): Usefulness of focal rhythmic discharges on scalp EEG of patients with focal cortical dysplasia and intractable epilepsy. *Electroencephalogr Clin Neurophysiol* 98: 243–249.

Gécz J, Cloosterman D, Partington M (2006): ARX: a gene for all seasons. *Curr Opin Genet Develop* 16: 308–316.

Gleeson JG, Allen KM, Fox JW, Lamperti ED, *et al.* (1998): Doublecortin, a brain-specific gene mutated in human X-linked lissencephaly and double cortex syndrome, encodes a putative signaling protein. *Cell* 92: 63–72.

Gleeson JG, Minnerath S, Kuzniecky RI, *et al.* (2000a): Somatic and germline mosaic mutations in the doublecortin gene are associated with variable phenotypes. *Am J Hum Genet* 67: 574–581.

Gleeson JG, Luo RF, Grant PE, *et al.* (2000b): Genetic and neuroradiological heterogeneity of double cortex syndrome. *Ann Neurol* 47: 265–269.

Golden JA and Harding BN (2004): Pathology and Genetics: Developmental Neuropathology. ISN Neuropath Press.

Granata T, D'Incerti L, Freri E, *et al.* (1999): Schizencephaly: Clinical and genetic findings in a case series. In Spreafico R, Avanzini G, Andermann F (eds). *Abnormal Cortical Development and Epilepsy*. London: John Libbey, pp. 181–189.

Granata T, Freri E, Caccia C, Setola V, Taroni F, Battaglia G (2005): Schizencephaly: clinical spectrum, epilepsy, and pathogenesis. *J Child Neurol* 20: 313–318.

Griffiths PD, Welch RG, Gardner-Medwin D, Gholkar A, McAllister V (1994): The radiological features of hemimegalencephaly including three cases associated with Proteus syndrome. *Neuropediatrics* 25: 140–144.

Guerreiro MM, Andermann E, Guerrini R, *et al.* (2000): Familial perisylvian polymicrogyria: a new familial syndrome of cortical maldevelopment. *Ann Neurol.* 48: 39–48.

Guerrini R, Dobyns B (1998): Bilateral periventricular nodular heterotopia with mental retardation and frontonasal malformation. *Neurology* 51: 499–503.

Guerrini R, Dobyns WB (2014): Malformations of cortical development: clinical features and genetic causes. *Lancet Neurol* 13: 710–726.

Guerrini R and Filippi T (2005): Neuronal migration disorders, genetics, and epileptogenesis. *J Child Neurol* 20: 287–299.

Guerrini R, Parrini E (2010): Neuronal migration disorders. *Neurobiol Dis* 38: 154–166.

Guerrini R, Barba C (2010): Malformations of cortical development and aberrant cortical networks: epileptogenesis and functional organization. *J Clin Neurophysiol* 27: 372–379.

Guerrini R, Dravet C, Raybaud C, *et al.* (1992a). Epilepsy and focal gyral anomalies detected by magnetic resonance imaging: electroclinico-morphological correlations and follow-up. *Dev Med Child Neurol* 34: 706–718.

Guerrini R, Dravet C, Raybaud C, *et al.* (1992b). Neurological findings and seizure outcome in children with bilateral opercular macrogyric-like changes detected by magnetic resonance imaging. *Dev Med Child Neurol* 34: 694–705.

Guerrini R, Dravet C, Bureau M, *et al.* (1996a): Diffuse and localized dysplasias of cerebral cortex: clinical presentation, outcome, and proposal for a morphologic MRI classification based on a study of 90 patients. In: Guerrini R, Andermann F, Canapicchi R, RogerJ, Zifkin BG, Pfanner P (eds). *Dysplasias of Cerebral Cortex and Epilepsy*. Philadelphia-New York: Lippincott-Raven. pp. 255–269.

Guerrini R, Parmeggiani A, Bureau M, *et al.* (1996b): Localized cortical dysplasia: good seizure outcome after sleep-related electrical status epilepticus. In: Guerrini R, Andermann F, Canapicchi R, Roger J, Zifkin B, Pfanner P (eds). *Dysplasias of cerebral cortex and epilepsy*, Philadelphia-New-York: Lippincott-Raven, pp. 329–335.

Guerrini R, Dubeau F, Dulac O, *et al.* (1997): Bilateral parasagittal parieto-occipital polymicrogyria and epilepsy. *Ann Neurol* 41: 65–73.

Guerrini R, Genton P, Bureau M, *et al.* (1998): Multilobar polymicrogyria, intractable drop attack seizures and sleep-related electrical status epilepticus *Neurology* 51: 504–512.

Guerrini R, Barkovich AJ, Sztriha L, Dobyns WB (2000): Bilateral frontal polymicrogyria: a newly recognized brain malformation syndrome. *Neurology* 54: 909–13.

Guerrini R, Moro F, Andermann E, *et al.* (2003): Nonsyndromic mental retardation and cryptogenic epilepsy in women with doublecortin gene mutations. *Ann Neurol* 54: 30–37.

Guerrini R, Mei D, Sisodiya S, *et al.* (2004): Germline and mosaic mutations of FLN1 in men with periventricular heterotopia. *Neurology* 63: 51–56.

Guerrini R, Moro F, Kato M, *et al.* (2007): Expansion of the first PolyA tract of ARX causes infantile spasms and status dystonicus. *Neurology* 69: 427–433.

Guerrini R, Dobyns W, Barkovich A (2008): Abnormal development of the human cerebral cortex: genetics, functional consequences and treatment options. *Trends Neurosci* 31: 154–162.

Guerrini R, Mei D, Cordelli DM, Pucatti D, Franzoni E, Parrini E (2012): Symmetric polymicrogyria and pachygyria associated with TUBB2B gene mutations. *Eur J Hum Genet* 20: 995–998.

Guerrini R, Duchowny M, Jayakar P, *et al.* (2005): Diagnostic methods and treatment options for focal cortical dysplasia. *Epilepsia* 56: 1669–1686.

Guzzetta A, Bonanni P, Biagi L, *et al.* (2007): Reorganisation of the somatosensory system after early brain damage. *Clin Neurophysiol* 118: 1110–1121.

Hakamada S, Watanabe K, Hara K, Miyazaki S (1979): The evolution of electroencephalographic features in lissencephaly syndrome. *Brain Dev* 4: 277–283.

Harding B (1996): Gray matter heterotopia. In: Guerrini R, Andermann F, Canapicchi R, Roger J, Zifkin BG, Pfanner P (eds). *Dysplasias of Cerebral Cortex and Epilepsy*. Philadelphia-New-York: Lippincott-Raven, pp. 81–88.

Harding B, Copp A (1997): Malformations of the nervous system. In: Graham J, Lantos PL (Eds.), *Greenfields Neuropathology*. Edward Arnold, London-Melbourne-Auckland, pp. 521–538.

Heinzen EL, O'Neill AC, Zhu X, *et al.* (2018): *De novo* and inherited private variants in MAP1B in periventricular nodular heterotopia. *PLoS Genet* 14: e1007281.

Hiesberger T, Trommsdorff M, Howell BW, *et al.* (1999): Direct binding of Reelin to VLDL receptor and ApoE receptor 2 induces tyrosine phosphorylation of disabled-1 and modulates tau phosphorylation. *Neuron* 24: 481–489.

Hirotsune S, Fleck MW, Gambello MJ, *et al.* (1998): Graded reduction of Pafah1b1 (Lis1) activity results in neuronal migration defects and early embryonic lethality. *Nat Genet* 19: 333–339.

Hong SE, Shugart YY, Huang DT, *et al.* (2000): Autosomal recessive lissencephaly with cerebellar hypoplasia is associated with human RELN mutations. *Nat Genet* 26: 93–96.

Jaglin XH, Poirier K, Saillour Y, *et al.* (2009): Mutations in the beta-tubulin gene TUBB2B result in asymmetrical polymicrogyria. *Nat Genet* 41: 746–752.

Kato M, Das S, Petras K, *et al.* (2004): Mutations of ARX are associated with striking pleiotropy and consistent genotype-phenotype correlation. *Hum Mutat* 23: 147–159.

Keays DA, Tian G, Poirier K, *et al.* (2007): Mutations in alpha-tubulin cause abnormal neuronal migration in mice and lissencephaly in humans. *Cell* 128: 45–57.

Khalid R, Krishnan P, Andres K, *et al.* (2018): COL4A1 and fetal vascular origins of schizencephaly. *Neurology* 90: 232–234.

Kheradmand Kia S, Verbeek E, Engelen E, *et al.* (2012): RTTN mutations link primary cilia function to organization of the human cerebral cortex. *Am J Hum Genet* 91: 533–540.

Kielar M, Tuy FP, Bizzotto S, *et al.* (2014): Mutations in Eml1 lead to ectopic progenitors and neuronal heterotopia in mouse and human. *Nat Neurosci* 17: 923–933.

Kitamura K, Yanazawa M, Sugiyama N, *et al.* (2002): Mutation of ARX causes abnormal development of forebrain and testes in mice and X-linked lissencephaly with abnormal genitalia in humans. *Nat Genet* 32: 359–369.

Kroner BL, Preiss LR, Ardini MA, Gaillard WD (2008): New incidence, prevalence, and survival of Aicardi syndrome from 408 cases. *J Child Neurol* 23: 531–535.

Kumar RA, Pilz DT, Babatz TD, *et al.* (2010): TUBA1A mutations cause wide spectrum lissencephaly (smooth brain) and suggest that multiple neuronal migration pathways converge on alpha tubulins. *Hum Mol Genet* 19: 2817–2827.

Kuzniecky R, Powers R. (1993): Epilepsia partialis continua due to cortical dysplasia. *J Child Neurol* 8: 386–388.

Kuzniecky R, Berkovic S, Andermann F, Melanson D, Olivier A, Robitaille Y (1988): Focal cortical myoclonus and rolandic cortical dysplasia: clarification by magnetic resonance imaging. *Ann. Neurol* 23: 317–325.

Kuzniecky R, Andermann F, Guerrini R, CBPS Multicenter Collaborative Study (1993): Congenital bilateral perisylvian syndrome: study of 31 patients. *Lancet* 341: 608–612.

Kuzniecky R, Andermann F, Guerrini R, CBPS Multicenter Collaborative Study (1994): The epileptic spectrum in the congenital bilateral perysilvian syndrome. *Neurology* 44: 379–385.

Landy HJ, Curless RG, Ramsay RE, Slater J, Ajmone-Marsan C, Quencer RM (1993): Corpus callosotomy for seizures associated with band heterotopia. *Epilepsia* 34: 79–83.

Lenge M, Barba C, Montanaro D, Aghakhanyan G, Frijia F, Guerrini R (2018): Relationships between morphologic and functional patterns in the polymicrogyric cortex. *Cereb Cortex* 28: 1076–1086.

Lee N, Radtke RA, Gray L, Burger PC, *et al.* (1994): Neuronal migration disorders: positron emission tomography correlations. *Ann Neurol* 35: 290–297.

Lee HK, Kim JS, Hwang YM, *et al.* (1999): Location of the primary motor cortex in schizencephaly. *AJNR Am J Neuroradiol* 20: 163–166.

Lee JH, Huynh M, Silhavy JL, *et al.* (2012): *De novo* somatic mutations in components of the PI3K-AKT3-mTOR pathway cause hemimegalencephaly. *Nat Genet* 44: 941–945.

Leventer RJ, Guerrini R, Dobyns WB (2008): Malformations of cortical development and epilepsy. *Dialogues Clin Neurosci* 10: 47–62.

Leventer RJ, Jansen A, Pilz DT, *et al.* (2010): Clinical and imaging heterogeneity of polymicrogyria: a study of 328 patients. *Brain* 133: 1415–1427.

Lim JS, Kim WI, Kang HC, *et al.* (2015): Brain somatic mutations in MTOR cause focal cortical dysplasia type II leading to intractable epilepsy. *Nat* Med 21: 395–400.

Little AS, Ng YT, Kerrigan JF, Treiman DM, Fram E, Rekate HL (2007): Anterior motor strip displacement in a boy with right frontal gray matter heterotopia undergoing epilepsy surgery. *Epilepsy Behav* 11: 241–246.

Lund C, Striano P, Sorte HS, *et al.* (2016): Exome Sequencing Fails to Identify the Genetic Cause of Aicardi Syndrome. *Mol Syndromol* 7: 234–238.

MacGregor DL, Menezes A, Buncic JR (1993): Aicardi syndrome (AS): – natural history and predictors of severity. *Can J Neurol Sci* 20 (Suppl 2): S36.

Maegaki Y, Yamamoto T, Takeshita K (1995): Plasticity of central motor and sensory pathways in a case of unilateral extensive cortical dysplasia: investigation of magnetic resonance imaging, transcranial magnetic stimulation, and short-latency somatosensory evoked potentials. *Neurology* 45: 2255–2261.

Magen D, Ofir A, Berger L, *et al.* (2015): Autosomal recessive lissencephaly with cerebellar hypoplasia is associated with a loss-of-function mutation in CDK5. *Hum Genet* 134: 305–314.

Mai R, Tassi L, Cossu M, *et al.* (2003): A neuropathological, stereo-EEG, and MRI study of subcortical band heterotopia. *Neurology* 60: 1834–1838.

Maillard LG, Tassi L, Bartolomei F, *et al.* (2017): Stereoelectroencephalography and surgical outcome in polymicrogyria-related epilepsy: A multicentric study. *Ann Neurol* 82: 781–794.

Maloof J, Sledz K, Hogg JP, Bodensteiner JB, Schwartz T, Schochet SS (1994): Unilateral megalencephaly and Tuberous Sclerosis: related disorders? *J Child Neurol* 9: 443–446.

Marín-Padilla M, Parisi JE, Armstrong DL, Sargent SK, Kaplan JA (2002): Shaken infant syndrome: developmental neuropathology, progressive cortical dysplasia, and epilepsy. *Acta Neuropathol* 103: 321–332.

Marusic P, Najm IM, Ying Z, *et al.* (2002): Focal cortical dysplasias in eloquent cortex: functional characteristics and correlation with MRI and histopathologic changes. *Epilepsia* 43: 27–32.

Matsumoto N, Leventer RJ, Kuc JA, *et al.* (2001): Mutation analysis of the DCX gene and genotype/phenotype correlation in subcortical band heterotopia. *Eur J Hum Genet* 9: 5–12.

Mei D, Parrini E, Pasqualetti M, *et al.* (2007): Multiplex ligation-dependent probe amplification detects DCX gene deletions in band heterotopia. *Neurology* 68: 446–450.

Mei D, Lewis R, Parrini E, Lazarou L, Marini C, Pilz D, Guerrini R (2008): High frequency of genomic deletions and duplication in the LIS1 gene in lissencephaly: implications for molecular diagnosis. *J Med Genet* 45: 355–361.

Merello E, Swanson E, De Marco P, *et al.* (2008): No major role for the EMX2 gene in schizencephaly. *Am J Med Genet A* 146A: 1142–1150.

Mirandola L, Mai RF, Francione S, *et al.* (2017): Stereo-EEG: Diagnostic and therapeutic tool for periventricular nodular heterotopia epilepsies. *Epilepsia* 58: 1962–1971.

Mishra-Gorur K, Çağlayan AO, Schaffer AE, *et al.* (2014): Mutations in KATNB1 cause complex cerebral malformations by disrupting asymmetrically dividing neural progenitors. *Neuron* 84: 1226–1239.

Mirzaa GM, Conway RL, Gripp KW, *et al.* (2012): Megalencephaly-capillary malformation (MCAP) and megalencephaly-polydactyly-polymicrogyria-hydrocephalus (MPPH) syndromes: two closely related disorders of brain overgrowth and abnormal brain and body morphogenesis. *Am J Med Genet* A 158A: 269–291.

Mirzaa GM, Conti V, Timms AE, *et al.* (2015): Characterisation of mutations of the phosphoinositide-3-kinase regulatory subunit, PIK3R2, in perisylvian polymicrogyria: a next-generation sequencing study. *Lancet Neurol* 14: 1182–1195.

Morris-Rosendahl DJ, Najm J, Lachmeijer AM, *et al.* (2008): Refining the phenotype of alpha-1a Tubulin (TUBA1A) mutation in patients with classical lissencephaly. *Clin Genet* 74: 425–433.

Muller RA, Behen ME, Muzik O, *et al.* (1998): Task-related activations in heterotopic brain malformations: a PET study. *Neuroreport* 9: 2527–2533.

Muntaner L, Pe'rez-Ferro'n J, Herrera M, Rosell J, Taboada D, Climent S (1997): MRI of a family with focal abnormalities of gyration. *Neuroradiology* 39: 605–608.

Najm IM, Tilelli CQ, Oghlakian R (2007): Pathophysiological mechanisms of focal cortical dysplasia: a critical review of human tissue studies and animal models. *Epilepsia* 48: 21–32.

Nellist M, Brouwer RW, Kockx CE, *et al.* (2015): Targeted Next Generation Sequencing reveals previously unidentified TSC1 and TSC2 mutations. *BMC Med Genet* 16: 10.

Packard AM, Miller VS, Delgado MR (1997): Schizencephaly: Correlations: Septo-optic-dysplasia-schizencephaly: Radiographic and clinical features. *Neurology* 48: 1427–1434.

Paladin F, Chiron C, Dulac O, Plouin P, Ponsot G (1989): Electroencephalographic aspects of hemimegalencephaly. *Dev Med Child Neurol* 31: 377–383.

Palmini A, Andermann F, Olivier A, Tampieri D, Robitaille Y (1991): Focal neuronal migration disorders and intractable partial epilepsy: results of surgical treatment. *Ann Neurol* 30: 750–757.

Palmini A, Gambardella A, Andermann F, *et al.* (1995): Intrinsic epileptogenicity of human dysplastic cortex as suggested by corticography and surgical results. *Ann Neurol* 37: 476–487.

Palmini A, Gambardella A, Andermann F, *et al.* (1996): The human dysplastic cortex is intrinsically epileptogenic. In: Guerrini R, Andermann F, Canapicchi R, Roger J, Zifkin BG, Pfanner P (eds) *Dysplasias of Cerebral Cortex and Epilepsy*. Philadelphia-New York: Lippincott-Raven. pp. 43–52.

Park YD, Hoffman JM, Radtke RA, DeLong GR (1994): Focal cerebral metabolic abnormality in a patient with continuous spike waves during slow-wave sleep. *J Child Neurol* 9: 139–143.

Parrini E, Ramazzotti A, Dobyns WB, *et al.* (2006): Periventricular heterotopia: phenotypic heterogeneity and correlation with Filamin A mutations. *Brain* 129: 1892–1906.

Parrini E, Ferrari AR, Dorn T, Walsh CA, Guerrini R (2009): Bilateral frontoparietal polymicrogyria, Lennox-Gastaut syndrome, and *GPR56* gene mutations. *Epilepsia* 50: 134413–134453.

Parrini E, Rivas IL, Toral JF, Pucatti D, Giglio S, Mei D, Guerrini R (2011): In-frame deletion in FLNA causing familial periventricular heterotopia with skeletal dysplasia in males. *Am J Med Genet A* 155A: 1140–1146.

Parrini E, Conti V, Dobyns WB, Guerrini R (2016): Genetic Basis of Brain Malformations. *Mol Syndromol* 7: 220–233.

Pavone L, Curatolo P, Rizzo R, *et al.* (1991): Epidermal nevus syndrome: A neurologic variant with hemimegalencephaly, giral malformation, mental retardation, seizures, and facial hemihypertrophy. *Neurology* 41 (2 (Pt 1)): 266–271.

Pelayo R, Barasch E, Kang H, Marion R, Moshé LS (1994): Progressively intractable seizures, focal alopecia, and hemimegalencephaly. *Neurology* 44: 969–971.

Peserico A, Battistella P, Bertoli P, Drigo P (1988): Unilateral hypomelanosis of Ito with hemimegalencephaly. *Acta Paediatr Scand* 77: 446–447.

Piao X, Hill RS, Bodell A, *et al.* (2004): G protein-coupled receptordependent development of human frontal cortex. *Science* 303: 2033–2036.

Pilz DT, Kuc J, Matsumoto N, *et al.* (1999): Subcortical band heterotopia in rare affected males can be caused by missense mutations in DCX (XLIS) or LIS1. *Hum Mol Genet* 8: 1757–1760.

Pisano T, Barkovich J, Leventer R, *et al.* (2012): Peritrigonal and temporo-occipital heterotopia with corpus callosum and cerebellar dysgenesis. *Neurology* 79: 1244–1251.

Pizzo F, Roehri N, Catenoix H, *et al.* (2017): Epileptogenic networks in nodular heterotopia: A stereoelectroencephalography study. *Epilepsia* 58: 2112–2123.

Poduri A, Evrony GD, Cai X, *et al.* (2012): Somatic activation of AKT3 causes hemispheric developmental brain malformations. *Neuron* 74: 41–48.

Poirier K, Lebrun N, Broix L, *et al.* (2013): Mutations in TUBG1, DYNC1H1, KIF5C and KIF2A cause malformations of cortical development and microcephaly. *Nat Genet* 45: 639–647.

Preul MC, Leblanc R, Cendes F, *et al.* (1997): Function and organization in dysgenetic cortex. Case report. *J Neurosurg* 87: 113–121.

Pulsifer MB, Brandt J, Salorio CF, Vining EP, Carson BS, Freeman JM (2004): The cognitive outcome of hemispherectomy in 71 children. *Epilepsia* 45: 243–254.

Pupillo GT, Andermann F, Dubeau F (1996): Bilateral sylvian parieto-occipital polymicrogyria. *Neurology* 46 (Suppl 2): A303.

Quirk JA, Kendall B, Kingsley DPE, Boyd SG, Pitt MC (1993): EEG features of cortical dysplasia in children. *Neuropediatrics* 24: 193–199.

Ramantani G, Koessler L, Colnat-Coulbois S, *et al.* (2013): Intracranial evaluation of the epileptogenic zone in regional infrasylvian polymicrogyria. *Epilepsia* 54: 296–304.

Reiner O, Carrozzo R, Shen Y, *et al.* (1993): Isolation of a Miller-Dieker lissencephaly gene containing G protein beta-subunit-like repeats. *Nature* 364: 717–721.

Richardson MP, Koepp MJ, Brooks DJ, *et al.* (1998): Cerebral activation in malformations of cortical development. *Brain* 121 (Pt 7): 1295–1304.

Richman DP, Stewart RM, Caviness VS Jr (1974): Cerebral microgyria in a 27-weeks fetus: an architectonic and topographic analysis. *J Neuropathol Exp Neurol* 33: 374–384.

Rivière JB, van Bon BW, Hoischen A, *et al.* (2012a): *De novo* mutations in the actin genes ACTB and ACTG1 cause Baraitser-Winter syndrome. *Nat Genet* 44 (S1–2): 440–444.

Rivière JB, Mirzaa GM, O'Roak BJ, *et al.* (2012b): *De novo* germline and postzygotic mutations in *AKT3*, *PIK3R2* and *PIK3CA* cause a spectrum of related megalencephaly syndromes. *Nat Genet* 44: 934–940.

Robain O, Gelot A (1996): Neuropathology of Hemimegalencephaly. In: Guerrini R, Andermann F, Canapicchi R, Roger J, Zifkin BG, Pfanner P. eds *Dysplasias of Cerebral cortex and Epilepsy*. Philadelphia-New York: Lippincott-Raven. pp. 89–92.

Robin NH, Taylor CJ, McDonald-McGinn DM, *et al.* (2006): Polymicrogyria and deletion 22q11.2 syndrome: window to the etiology of a common cortical malformation. *Am J Med Genet* A 140: 2416–2425.

Ross ME, Swanson K, Dobyns WB (2001): Lissencephaly with cerebellar hypoplasia (LCH): a heterogeneous group of cortical malformations. *Neuropediatrics* 32: 256–263.

Ruton MC, Expert-Bezançon MC, Bursztyn J, Mselati JC, Robain O (1994): Polymicrogyrie bioperculaire associée a une ophtalmoplégie congénitale par atteinte du noyau du nerf moteur oculaire commun. *Rev Neurol* 150: 363–369.

Sakuta RH, Alkawa H, Takashima S, Yoza A, Ryo S (1989): Epidermal nevus syndrome with hemimegalencephaly. *Brain Dev* 11: 191–194.

Salamon N, Andres M, Chute DJ, *et al.* (2006): Contralateral hemimicrencephaly and clinical-pathological correlations in children with hemimegalencephaly. *Brain* 129: 352–365.

Santos NF, Secolin R, Brandão-Almeida IL, *et al.* (2008): A new candidate locus for bilateral perisylvian polymicrogyria mapped on chromosome Xq27. *Am J Med Genet* 146A: 1151–1157.

Sato Y, Shibasaki J, Aida N, *et al.* (2018): Novel *COL4A1* mutation in a fetus with early prenatal onset of schizencephaly. *Hum Genome Var* 5: 4.

Scherer C, Schuele S, Minotti L, Chabardes S, Hoffmann D, Kahane P (2005): Intrinsic epileptogenicity of an isolated periventricular nodular heterotopia. *Neurology* 65: 495–496.

Sheen VL, Dixon PH, Fox JW, *et al.* (2001): Mutations in the X-linked filamin 1 gene cause periventricular nodular heterotopia in males as well as in females. *Hum Mol Genet* 10: 1775–1783.

Sheen VL, Ganesh VS, Topcu M, *et al.* (2004a): Mutations in ARFGEF2 implicate vesicle trafficking in neural progenitor proliferation and migration in the human cerebral cortex. *Nat Genet* 36: 69–76.

Sheen VL, Basel-Vanagaite L, Goodman JR, *et al.* (2004b): Etiological heterogeneity of familial periventricular heterotopia and hydrocephalus. *Brain Dev* 26: 326–334.

Sicca F, Kelemen A, Genton P, *et al.* (2003): Mosaic mutations of the LIS1 gene cause subcortical band heterotopia. *Neurology* 61: 1042–1046.

Sim JC, Scerri T, Fanjul-Fernández M, *et al.* (2016): Familial cortical dysplasia caused by mutation in the mammalian target of rapamycin regulator NPRL3. *Ann Neurol* 79: 132–137.

Staudt M, Krägeloh-Mann I, Holthausen H, Gerloff C, Grodd W (2004): Searching for motor functions in dysgenic cortex: a clinical transcranial magnetic stimulation and functional magnetic resonance imaging study. *J Neurosurg* 101: 69–77.

Tassi L, Colombo N, Garbelli R, *et al.* (2002): Focal cortical dysplasia: neuropathological subtypes, EEG, neuroimaging and surgical outcome. *Brain* 125: 1719–1732.

Tassi L, Colombo N, Cossu M, *et al.* (2005): Electroclinical, MRI and neuropathological study of 10 patients with nodular heterotopia, with surgical outcomes. *Brain* 128: 321–337.

Taylor DC, Falconer MA, Bruton CJ, Corsellis JAN (1971): Focal dysplasia of the cerebral cortex in epilepsy. *J Neurol Neurosurg Psychiatry* 34: 369–387.

Tinkle BT, Schorry EK, Franz DN, Crone KR, Saal HM (2005): Epidemiology of hemimegalencephaly: a case series and review. *Am J Med Genet A* 139: 204–211.

Uyanik G, Morris-Rosendahl DJ, Stiegler J, *et al.* (2007): Location and type of mutation in the LIS1 gene do not predict phenotypic severity. *Neurology* 69: 442–447.

Verloes A, Di Donato N, Masliah-Planchon J, *et al.* (2015): Baraitser-Winter cerebrofrontofacial syndrome: delineation of the spectrum in 42 cases. *Eur J Hum Genet* 23: 292–301.

Villard L, Nguyen K, Cardoso C, *et al.* (2002): A locus for bilateral perisylvian polymicrogyria maps to Xq28. *Am J Hum Genet* 70: 1003–1008.

Vigevano F, Aicardi J, Lini M, Pasquinelli A (1984): La sindrome del nevo sebaceo lineare: presentazione di una casistica multicentra. *Boll Lega It Epil* 45/46: 59–63.

Wang D, Zeesman S, Tarnopolsky MA, Nowaczyk MJ (2013): Duplication of AKT3 as a cause of macrocephaly in duplication 1q43q44. *Am J Med Genet A* 161: 2016–2019.

Widdess-Walsh P, Jeha L, Nair D, Kotagal P, Bingaman W, Najm I (2007): Subdural electrode analysis in focal cortical dysplasia: predictors of surgical outcome. *Neurology* 69: 660–667.

Wieck G, Leventer RJ, Squier WM, *et al.* (2005): Periventricular nodular heterotopia with overlying polymicrogyria. *Brain* 128: 2811–2821.

Williams D, Elster A (1990): Cranial MR imaging in hypomelanosis of Ito. *J Comput Assist Tomogr* 14: 981–983.

Yakovlev PI, Wadsworth RC (1946): Schizencephalies; a study of the congenital clefts in the cerebral mantle; clefts with hydrocephalus and lips separated. *J Neuropathol Exp Neurol* 5: 169–206.

Ying Z, Gonzalez-Martinez J, Tilelli C, Bingaman W, Najm I (2005): Expression of neural stem cell surface marker CD133 in balloon cells of human focal cortical dysplasia. *Epilepsia* 46: 1716–1723.

Yoneda Y, Haginoya K, Kato M, *et al.* (2013): Phenotypic spectrum of COL4A1 mutations: porencephaly to schizencephaly. *Ann Neurol* 73: 48–57.

Zaremba J, Wislawski J, Bidzinski J, Kanski J, Bogna S (1978): Jadassohn's naevus phakomatosis: a report of two cases. *J Ment Def Res* 22: 91–102.

IMPRIM'VERT®

Achevé d'imprimer en mai 2019 par Corlet Imprimeur - 14110 Condé-en-Normandie
Dépôt légal : mai 2019 - n° d'imprimeur : 201207 - *Imprimé en France*